IMMUNOLOGY
and SEROLOGY
in Laboratory Medicine

evolve

❖ *To access your Student Resources, visit:*

http://evolve.elsevier.com/Turgeon/immunology/

Evolve® Student Resources for ***Turgeon: Immunology and Serology in Laboratory Medicine*** offers the following features:

Student Resources

- **Additional Review Questions**
  A set of more than 330 review questions and answers/explanations provides extra review and practice.

- **Weblinks**
  Links to places of interest on the web specifically for clinical laboratory science students.

- **Content Updates**
  Find out the latest information on relevant issues in the field of immunology.

FOURTH EDITION

IMMUNOLOGY
and SEROLOGY
in Laboratory Medicine

Mary Louise Turgeon, EdD, MT(ASCP), CLS(NCA)

Clinical Professor
Program Director
Department of Medical Laboratory Science
Northeastern University
Boston, Massachusetts
Clinical Adjunct Assistant Professor
School of Medicine
Tufts University
Boston, Massachusetts

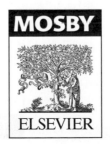

MOSBY

ELSEVIER

MOSBY
ELSEVIER

11830 Westline Industrial Drive
St. Louis, Missouri 63146

IMMUNOLOGY AND SEROLOGY IN LABORATORY
MEDICINE, Fourth Edition

ISBN: 978-0-323-04382-3

Library of Congress Cataloging-in-Publication Data

Turgeon, Mary Louise.
    Immunology and serology in laboratory medicine / Mary Louise Turgeon. — 4th ed.
        p. ; cm.
    Rev. ed. of: Immunology & serology in laboratory medicine / Mary Louise Turgeon.
3rd ed. c2003.
    Includes bibliographical references and index.
    ISBN 978-0-323-04382-3 (hardcover : alk. paper) 1. Immunodiagnosis. 2. Serodiagnosis.
I. Turgeon, Mary Louise. Immunology & serology in laboratory medicine. II. Title.
    [DNLM: 1. Allergy and immunology—Laboratory Manuals. 2. Immunologic Techniques—
Laboratory Manuals. 3. Immunologic Tests—Laboratory Manuals. 4. Serology—Laboratory
Manuals. QW 525 T936i 2009]
    RB46.5.T87 2009
    616.07'56—dc22

                                                                    2008020408

ISBN: 978-0-323-04382-3

Publishing Director: Andrew Allen
Managing Editor: Ellen Wurm-Cutter
Publishing Services Manager: Patricia Tannian
Senior Project Manager: Anne Altepeter
Cover Design Direction: Paula Catalano
Interior Designer: Paula Catalano

Printed in China

Last digit is the print number: 9 8 7 6 5 4 3

To my husband, Dick Mordaunt,

and

Annie

Cheers!

to the adventure of changes in latitudes and attitudes

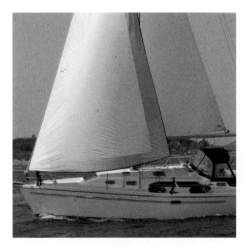

Reviewers

Margaret B. Boone, BS, MT(ASCP)SBB, CLS(NCA)
Program Director, Clinical Laboratory Technician Program
Louisiana Technical College
Lafayette, Louisiana

Jill Dennis, MEd, BSMT (ASCP), CLS(NCA)
Program Director and Assistant Professor
Clinical Laboratory Science Program
Thomas University
Thomasville, Georgia

Patricia Kelly, BSMT, MBA, (AMT), (ASCP)BB
Program Director
Medical Laboratory Technology Program
Mississippi Delta Community College
Moorhead, Mississippi

Preface

The intention of the fourth edition of *Immunology and Serology in Laboratory Medicine* is to continue to fulfill the needs of clinical laboratory technician (CLT) and clinical laboratory science (CLS) students and their instructors for a text that encompasses the most current theory, practice, and clinical applications in the fields of immunology and serology. Practicing medical technologists and practitioners in other allied health disciplines can use this text as a reference.

The purpose of this edition continues to be to describe the basic concepts of immunology, to elucidate the underlying theory of procedures performed in clinical immunology and serology laboratories, to summarize clinical features and present case studies of selected infectious diseases and autoimmune disorders, and to discuss concepts of transplantation and tumor immunology.

ORGANIZATION

The major topical areas are organized into four primary sections. The entire content of the book has been reviewed and updated. New procedures applicable to a student laboratory have been added to relevant chapters. The initial two parts provide foundation knowledge and skills that progress from basic immunologic mechanisms and serologic concepts to the theory of laboratory procedures, including molecular techniques. The latter two parts emphasize medical applications of importance to clinical laboratory science. In addition, the latter two parts contain representative disorders of infectious and immunologic origin, as well as such topics as transplantation and tumor immunology. The sequence of the parts is designed to accommodate the core needs of clinical laboratory students in basic concepts, the underlying theory of procedures, and immunologic manifestations of infectious diseases. Because the needs of some students are more advanced in immunopathology, these topics are presented later in the book to allow students to analyze, evaluate abnormalities, and exercise critical thinking skills based on their knowledge of the preceding parts. Students may study specific components of the book, depending on the length and objectives of the course.

DISTINCTIVE FEATURES AND LEARNING AIDS

This new edition of *Immunology and Serology in Laboratory Medicine* capitalizes on the strengths of previous editions.
- A topical outline is presented at the beginning of each chapter. These outlines should be of value to students in the organization of the material and may be of convenience to instructors in preparing lectures.

- Illustrations, photographs, and summary tables are used to visually clarify various conceptual themes and arrange detailed information.
- Chapter highlights and review questions are provided at the conclusion of each chapter.
- Additional clinical case studies, procedures appropriate for a student laboratory, and more review questions have been added to this edition.

As in the previous editions, representative procedures are organized according to the format suggested by the Clinical Laboratory and Standards Institute (CLSI). This format introduces students to the typical procedural write-up encountered in a working clinical laboratory.

NEW TO THIS EDITION

What's significantly new in the fourth edition? The knowledge base in the field of immunology continues to expand logarithmically. In Part I, information related to inflammation and T lymphocytes has been expanded. Representative procedures have been added.

Part II, The Theory of Immunologic and Serologic Procedures, has been reorganized. New chapters related to quality assessment and point-of-care testing have been added. Representative procedures have been added. Chapters on laboratory safety, basic laboratory techniques, and molecular techniques have been expanded.

In Part III, Chapter 16, A Primer on Vaccines, has been added as the importance of vaccines continues to become evident. Representative case studies have been added to the chapters in this section.

Part IV, Immunologically and Serologically Related Disorders, presents the latest information related to transplantation. In addition, knowledge related to tumor immunology has been revised.

Although the content of immunology continues to expand, *Immunology and Serology in Laboratory Medicine* is written for beginning students in immunology who need an emphasis on the medical aspects of the discipline and the practical aspects of serology. The fourth edition should provide students with a basic foundation in the theory and practice of clinical immunology and practical serology in a one- or two-term course at either CLT or CLS levels of instruction.

ANCILLARIES

For the Instructor

Evolve

The companion Evolve website offers several features to aid instructors:

- **Test Bank:** A test bank of more than 990 multiple-choice questions that feature answers and explanations, cognitive levels, and page number references to the text is provided. A basic medical terminology quiz is also included. The test bank can be used as review in class or for test development. More than 330 of the questions in the instructor test bank are available for student use.
- **PowerPoint Presentations:** One PowerPoint presentation per chapter, this feature can be used "as is" or as a template to prepare lectures.
- **Image Collection:** All of the images from the book are available as .jpg files and can be downloaded into PowerPoint presentations. The figures can be used during lectures to illustrate important concepts.
- **Case Studies:** Case studies are provided for additional opportunity for student application of chapter content in real-life scenarios.
- **Procedures:** This feature presents more hands-on procedures of techniques used in laboratories that are less frequently used.

- Sample syllabi for CLT and CLS one- and two-semester courses are available.
- **Answers to Additional Review Questions:** Students have access to more than 330 questions that test their knowledge on the concepts presented in the book. The questions and answers are available to instructors.

For the Student

Evolve

The student resources on Evolve include:

- **Additional Review Questions:** A set of more than 330 multiple-choice questions provides extra review and practice.
- **Weblinks:** The links lead to web locations of interest specifically for clinical laboratory science students.

Mary L. Turgeon
Boston, Massachusetts

Acknowledgments

My objective in writing *Immunology and Serology in Laboratory Medicine* continues to be to integrate basic science concepts and procedural theory in immunology and serology with relevant medical applications. Because the body of knowledge in immunology continues to expand, writing and revising a book that addresses the holistic needs of those in the clinical sciences continues to be a challenge. In addition, this book continues to provide me with the opportunity to share my experience and insight as a medical educator with others.

I am most appreciative of the efforts extended on my behalf by Loren Wilson, my original acquisitions editor, and Ellen Wurm-Cutter, my developmental editor for my past three books as well as my new managing editor, at Elsevier. I am thrilled that Anne Altepeter has served as the senior project manager for another one of my books. Thank you.

Contents

Part I Basic Immunologic Mechanisms

1 An Overview of Immunology, 1
2 Antigens and Antibodies, 8
3 Cells and Cellular Activities of the Immune System: Granulocytes and Mononuclear Cells, 31
4 Cells and Cellular Activities of the Immune System: Lymphocytes and Plasma Cells, 49
5 Soluble Mediators of the Immune System, 78

Part II The Theory of Immunologic and Serologic Procedures

6 Safety in the Immunology-Serology Laboratory, 103
7 Quality Assurance and Quality Control, 113
8 Basic Serologic Laboratory Techniques, 120
9 Point-of-Care Testing, 131
10 Agglutination Methods, 135
11 Electrophoresis Techniques, 147
12 Labeling Techniques in Immunoassay, 158
13 Automated Procedures, 170
14 Molecular Techniques, 180

Part III Immunologic Manifestations of Infectious Diseases

15 The Immune Response in Infectious Diseases, 189
16 A Primer on Vaccines, 198
17 Streptococcal Infections, 206
18 Syphilis, 215
19 Vector-Borne Diseases, 229
20 Toxoplasmosis, 247
21 Cytomegalovirus, 255
22 Infectious Mononucleosis, 266
23 Viral Hepatitis, 275
24 Rubella Infection, 299
25 Acquired Immunodeficiency Syndrome, 308

Part IV Immunologically and Serologically Related Disorders

26 Hypersensitivity Reactions, 329
27 Immunoproliferative Disorders, 349
28 Autoimmune Disorders, 365
29 Systemic Lupus Erythematosus, 392
30 Rheumatoid Arthritis, 412
31 Solid Organ Transplantation, 425
32 Bone Marrow Transplantation, 448
33 Tumor Immunology, 461

Appendixes

A Answers to Review Questions, 481
B Representative Diagnostic Assays in Medical Laboratory Immunology, 485

Glossary, 493

Index, 513

PART I

Basic Immunologic Mechanisms

1   Overview of Immunology
2   Antigens and Antibodies
3   Cells and Cellular Activities of the Immune
       System: Granulocytes and Mononuclear Cells

4   Cells and Cellular Activities of the Immune
       System: Lymphocytes and Plasma Cells
5   Soluble Mediators of the Immune System

CHAPTER 1

An Overview of Immunology

History of Immunology
What Is Immunology?
Function of Immunology
Body Defenses: Resistance to Microbial Disease
    First Line of Defense
    Natural Immunity
    Adaptive Immunity

Comparison of Innate and Adaptive Immunity
Chapter Highlights
Review Questions
Bibliography

Learning Objectives

At the conclusion of this chapter, the reader should be able to:
* Define the term *immunology*.
* Explain the functions of the immune system.

* Describe the first line of defense, natural immunity, and adaptive immunity as body defense systems against microbial diseases.
* Compare innate and adaptive immunity.

HISTORY OF IMMUNOLOGY

Louis Pasteur is generally considered to be the "Father of Immunology." The science of immunology arose from the knowledge that those who survived one of the common infectious diseases of the past rarely contracted the disease again. As early as 430 BC, Thucydides recorded during the plague in Athens that individuals who had previously contracted the disease recovered, and he recognized their "immune" status.

Beginning about 1000 AD, the Chinese practiced a form of immunization by inhaling dried powders derived from the crusts of smallpox lesions. In the fifteenth century, powdered smallpox "crusts" were inserted with a pin into the skin. When this practice became popular in England, it was discouraged at first, partly because the practice of inoculation occasionally killed or disfigured a patient.

The first step to safer immunization, starting about 1774, was to substitute material derived from the lesion of a cowpox (vaccinia) for inoculation against smallpox. Cowpox is a benign disease caused by infection with a virus closely related to the smallpox (variola) virus. Table 1-1 lists some historic benchmarks in immunology.

WHAT IS IMMUNOLOGY?

Immunology is defined as the study of the molecules, cells, organs, and systems responsible for the recognition and disposal of foreign **(nonself)** material; how body components respond and interact; the desirable and undesirable consequences of immune interactions; and the ways in which the immune system can be advantageously manipulated to protect against or treat disease. Immunologists in the Western Hemisphere generally exclude from the study of immunology the relationship among cells during embryonic development.

The immune system is composed of a large, complex set of widely distributed elements, with the following distinctive characteristics:
* Specificity
* Memory
* Mobility
* Replicability
* Cooperation between different cells or cellular products

Specificity and memory are characteristics of lymphocytes (see Chapter 4). Various specific and nonspecific elements of the immune system demonstrate mobility, including T and

Table 1-1	Significant Milestones in Immunology	
Date	Scientist(s)	Discovery
1798	Jenner	Smallpox vaccination
1862	Haeckel	Phagocytosis
1880-1881	Pasteur	Live, attenuated chicken cholera and anthrax vaccines
1883-1905	Metchnikoff	Cellular theory of immunity through phagocytosis
1885	Pasteur	Therapeutic vaccination
		First report of live "attenuated" vaccine for rabies
1890	Von Behring, Kitasata	Humoral theory of immunity proposed
1891	Koch	Demonstration of cutaneous (delayed-type) hypersensitivity
1900	Ehrlich	Antibody formation theory
1902	Portier, Richet	Immediate-hypersensitivity anaphylaxis
1903	Arthus	Arthus reaction of intermediate hypersensitivity
1938	Marrack	Hypothesis of antigen-antibody binding
1944		Hypothesis of allograft rejection
1949	Salk, Sabin	Development of polio vaccine
1951	Reed	Vaccine against yellow fever
1953		Graft-versus-host reaction
1957	Burnet	Clonal selection theory
1957		Interferon
1958-1962		Human leukocyte antigens (HLAs)
1964-1968		T-cell and B-cell cooperation in immune response
1972		Identification of antibody molecule
1975	Köhler	First monoclonal antibodies
1985-1987		Identification of genes for T-cell receptor
1986		Monoclonal hepatitis B vaccine
1986	Mosmann	Th1 versus Th2 model of T-helper-cell function
1996-1998		Identification of toll-like receptors
2001		FOXP3, the gene directing regulatory-T-cell development
2005	Frazer	Development of human papilloma-virus vaccine

B lymphocytes, **immunoglobulins (antibodies),** complement, and **hematopoietic cells.** For this reason, local sensitization (e.g., insect bite) can result in systemic sensitization. In addition, specific and nonspecific cellular components of the immune system can replicate. Cooperation is required for optimal functioning of the immune system. Cooperative interaction involves specific cellular elements, cell products, and nonlymphoid elements.

FUNCTION OF IMMUNOLOGY

The function of the immune system is to recognize "self" from "nonself" and to defend the body against nonself. Such a system is necessary for survival. The distinction of self from nonself is made by an elaborate, specific recognition system. Specific cellular elements of the immune system include the lymphocytes. The immune system also has nonspecific effector mechanisms that usually amplify the specific functions. Nonspecific components of the immune system include mononuclear phagocytes, polymorphonuclear leukocytes, and soluble factors (e.g., complement).

Nonself substances range from life-threatening infectious microorganisms to a lifesaving organ transplant. The desirable consequences of immunity include natural resistance, recovery, and acquired resistance to infectious diseases. A deficiency or dysfunction of the immune system can cause many disorders. Undesirable consequences of immunity include allergy, rejection of a transplanted organ, or an **autoimmune disorder,** in which the body's own tissues are attacked as if they were foreign. Over the last decade a new concept, the "danger theory," has challenged the classic self-nonself viewpoint; although popular, it has not been widely accepted by immunologists (see Chapter 4).

BODY DEFENSES: RESISTANCE TO MICROBIAL DISEASE

Before a pathogen can invade the human body, it must overcome the resistance provided by the body's immune system, which consists of nonspecific and specific defense mechanisms (Figure 1-1).

First Line of Defense

The first line of defense, or first barrier to infection, is unbroken skin and mucosal membrane surfaces. These surfaces are essential in forming a physical barrier to many microorganisms because this is where foreign materials usually first contact the host. Keratinization of the upper layer of the skin and the constant renewal of the skin's epithelial cells, which repairs breaks in the skin, assist in the protective function of skin and mucosal membranes. In addition, the normal flora (microorganisms normally inhabiting the skin and membranes) deter penetration or facilitate elimination of foreign microorganisms from the body.

Secretions are also an important component in the first line of defense against microbial invasion. Mucus adhering to the membranes of the nose and nasopharynx traps microorganisms, which can be expelled by coughing or sneezing. Sebum (oil) produced by the sebaceous glands of the skin and lactic acid in sweat both possess antimicrobial properties. The production of earwax (cerumen) protects the auditory canals from infectious disease. Secretions produced in the elimination of liquid and solid wastes (e.g., urinary and gastrointestinal processes) are important in physically removing potential pathogens from the body. The acidity and alkalinity of the fluids of the stomach and intestinal tract, as well as the acidity of the vagina, can destroy many potentially infectious microorganisms. Additional protection is provided to the respiratory tract by the constant motion of the cilia of the tubules.

In addition to the physical ability to wash away potential pathogens, tears and saliva also have chemical properties

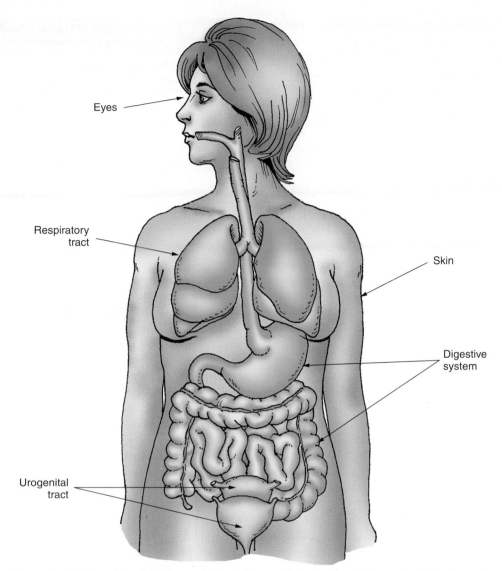

Figure 1-1 **Natural body defenses.** Body fluids, specialized cells, fluids, and resident bacteria (normal biota) allow the respiratory, digestive, urogenital, integumentary, and other systems to defend the body "naturally" against microbial infection.

that defend the body. The enzyme **lysozyme,** which is found in tears and saliva, attacks and destroys the cell wall of susceptible bacteria, particularly certain gram-positive bacteria. Immunoglobulin A (IgA) antibody is another important protective substance in tears and saliva.

The body has a variety of barrier-assisting defenses that protect against disease as the first line of defense. Although varying among individuals, these barriers assist in the general resistance to infectious organisms.

Natural Immunity

Natural (innate or **inborn) resistance** is one of the two ways that the body resists infection after microorganisms have penetrated the first line of resistance. The second form, acquired resistance, which specifically recognizes and selectively eliminates exogenous (or endogenous) agents, is discussed later.

Natural immunity is characterized as a nonspecific mechanism. If a microorganism penetrates the skin or mucosal

membranes, a second line of cellular and humoral defense mechanisms becomes operational (Box 1-1). The elements of natural resistance include phagocytic cells, complement, and the acute inflammatory reaction (see Chapter 3). Despite their relative lack of specificity, these components are essential because they are largely responsible for natural im-

Box 1-1	Components of the Natural Immune System
Cellular	
Mast cells	
Neutrophils	
Macrophages	
Humoral	
Complement	
Lysozyme	
Interferon	

munity to many environmental microorganisms. Phagocytic cells, which engulf invading foreign material, constitute the major cellular component. Complement proteins are the major **humoral** (fluid) component of natural immunity (see Chapter 5). Other substances of the humoral component include lysozymes and interferon, sometimes described as "natural antibiotics." Interferon is a family of proteins produced rapidly by many cells in response to viral infection; it blocks the replication of virus in other cells.

Tissue damage produced by infectious or other agents results in **inflammation,** a series of biochemical and cellular changes that facilitate the **phagocytosis** (engulfment and destruction) of microorganisms or damaged cells. If the degree of inflammation is sufficiently extensive, it is accompanied by an increase in the plasma concentration of acute-phase proteins or reactants, a group of glycoproteins. Acute-phase proteins are sensitive indicators of the presence of inflammatory disease and are especially useful in monitoring such conditions (see Chapter 5).

Adaptive Immunity

If a microorganism overwhelms the body's natural resistance, a third line of defensive resistance exists. Acquired, or adaptive, immunity is a more recently evolved mechanism that allows the body to recognize, remember, and respond to a specific stimulus, an **antigen.** Adaptive immunity can result in elimination of microorganisms and recovery from disease, and the host often acquires a specific immunologic memory. This condition of memory or recall (acquired resistance) allows the host to respond more effectively if reinfection with the same microorganism occurs.

Adaptive immunity, as with natural immunity, is composed of cellular and humoral components (Box 1-2). The major cellular component of acquired immunity is the lymphocyte (see Chapter 4); the major humoral component is the antibody (see Chapter 2). Lymphocytes selectively respond to nonself materials (antigens), which leads to immune memory and a permanently altered pattern of response or adaptation to the environment. Most actions in the two categories of the adaptive response, humoral-mediated immunity and cell-mediated immunity, are exerted by the interaction of antibody with complement and the phagocytic cells (natural immunity) and of T cells with macrophages (Table 1-2).

Box 1-2	Components of the Adaptive Immune System

Cellular
T lymphocytes
B lymphocytes
Plasma cells

Humoral
Antibodies
Cytokines

Table 1-2	Characteristics of Humoral-Mediated and Cell-Mediated Immunity	
	Humoral-Mediated Immunity	Cell-Mediated Immunity
Mechanism	Antibody mediated	Cell mediated
Cell type	B lymphocytes	T lymphocytes
Mode of action	Antibodies in serum	Direct cell-to-cell contact or soluble products secreted by cells
Purpose	Primary defense against bacterial infection	Defense against viral and fungal infections, intracellular organisms, tumor antigens, and graft rejection

Humoral-Mediated Immunity

If specific antibodies have been formed to antigenic stimulation, they are available to protect the body against foreign substances. The recognition of foreign substances and subsequent production of antibodies to these substances define immunity. Antibody-mediated immunity to infection can be acquired if the antibodies are formed by the host or if they are received from another source; these two types of acquired immunity are called active immunity and passive immunity, respectively (Table 1-3).

Active immunity can be acquired by natural exposure in response to an infection or natural series of infections, or through intentional injection of an antigen. The latter, **vaccination,** is an effective method of stimulating antibody production and memory (acquired resistance) without contracting the disease. Suspensions of antigenic materials used for immunization may be of animal or plant origin. These products may consist of living suspensions of weak or attenuated cells or viruses, killed cells or viruses, or extracted bacterial products, such as the altered and no-longer-poisonous toxoids used to immunize against diphtheria and tetanus. The selected agents should stimulate the production of antibodies, without clinical signs and symptoms of disease in an **immunocompetent** host (able to recognize a foreign antigen and build specific antigen-directed antibodies), and result in permanent antigenic memory. Booster vaccinations may be needed in some cases to expand the pool of memory cells. The mechanism of antigen recognition and antibody production is discussed in Chapter 2.

Artificial **passive immunity** is achieved by infusion of serum or plasma containing high concentrations of antibody. This form of passive immunity provides immediate antibody protection against microorganisms (e.g., hepatitis A) by administering preformed antibodies. These antibodies have been produced by another person or animal that has been actively immunized. The recipient will benefit only temporarily from passive immunity, as long as the antibodies persist in the circulation.

In addition, passive immunity can be acquired naturally by the fetus through the transfer of antibodies by the mater-

Table 1-3	Comparison of Types of Acquired Immunity			
	Type	Mode of Acquisition	Antibody Produced by Host	Duration of Immune Response
Active	Natural	Infection	Yes	Long
	Artificial	Vaccination	Yes	Long*
Passive	Natural	Transfer in vivo or colostrum	No	Short
	Artificial	Infusion of serum/plasma	No	Short

*Immunocompetent host.

nal circulation in utero. Maternal antibodies are also transferred to the newborn after parturition in the prelactation fluid, colostrum. For the newborn to have lasting protection, active immunity must occur.

Immediate hypersensitivity is a subset of the body's antibody-mediated mechanisms. This subset consists of the reactions primarily mediated by IgE, a class of immunoglobulins with unique biologic properties. The most dramatic and devastating systemic manifestation of immediate hypersensitivity is **anaphylaxis.** In addition to IgE-dependent hypersensitivity, two other immunoglobulin-dependent (antibody-dependent) mechanisms and a fourth, cell-mediated, delayed-hypersensitivity mechanism exist (Table 1-4; see also Chapter 26).

Cell-Mediated Immunity

Cell-mediated immunity consists of immune activities that differ from antibody-mediated immunity. Lymphocytes are the unique bearers of immunologic specificity, which depends on their antigen receptors. The full development and expression of immune responses, however, require that nonlymphoid cells and molecules primarily act as amplifiers and modifiers.

Cell-mediated immunity is moderated by the link between T lymphocytes and phagocytic cells (i.e., monocytes-macrophages).

A B lymphocyte can probably respond to a native antigenic determinant of the appropriate "fit." A T lymphocyte responds to antigens presented by other cells in the context of **major histocompatibility complex (MHC)** proteins. The T lymphocyte does not directly recognize the antigens of microorganisms or other living cells, such as **allografts** (tissue from a genetically different member of the same species, e.g., a human kidney), but rather recognizes when the antigen is present on the surface of an antigen-presenting cell (APC), the macrophage. APCs were at first thought to be limited to cells of the **mononuclear phagocyte system.** Recently, however, other types of cells (e.g., endothelial, glial) have been shown to possess the ability to "present" antigens.

Lymphocytes are immunologically active through various types of direct cell-to-cell contact and by the production of soluble factors (see Chapter 5). Nonspecific soluble factors are made by or act on various elements of the immune system (see Chapter 5). These molecules are collectively called **cytokines.** Some mediators that act between leukocytes are called **interleukins.**

The term **delayed hypersensitivity** is often used synonymously with the term **cell-mediated immunity.** However, delayed hypersensitivity refers to the slow appearance of a secondary response in the skin, reflected by the subtle difference in the time required for a delayed response to occur (e.g., tuberculin skin test).

Under some conditions, the activities of cell-mediated immunity may not be beneficial. Suppression of the

Table 1-4	Classification of Hypersensitivity Reactions			
	Type I	Type II	Type III	Type IV
	Anaphylactic	**Cytotoxic**	**Immune complex**	**T-cell dependent**
Antibody	IgE	IgG Possibly other	IgG IgM	None
Complement involved	No	Yes	Yes	No
Cells involved	Mast cells Basophils	Red blood cells White blood cells Platelets	Host tissue cells	T cells Macrophages
Examples	Anaphylaxis Hay fever Food allergy	Transfusion reactions Hemolytic disease of newborn Thrombocytopenia	Arthus reaction Serum sickness Pneumonitis	Allergy of infection Contact dermatitis

normal adaptive immune response (**immunosuppression**) by drugs or other means is necessary in conditions such as organ transplantation, hypersensitivity, and autoimmune disorders.

COMPARISON OF INNATE AND ADAPTIVE IMMUNITY

Traditionally, the immune system has been divided into the innate and adaptive components, each with a different function and role. The **innate immune system,** an ancient form of host defense, appeared before the adaptive immune system. Some form of innate immunity probably exists in all multicellular organisms. Innate immune recognition is mediated by germline-encoded receptors, which means the specificity of each receptor is genetically predetermined. Germline-encoded receptors evolved by natural selection to have defined specificities for infectious microorganisms. The problem is that every organism has a limit as to the number of genes it can encode in its **genome.** Consequently, the innate immune response may not be able to recognize every possible antigen, but rather may focus on a few large groups of microorganisms, called **pathogen-associated molecular patterns (PAMPs).** The receptors of the innate immune system that recognize these PAMPs are called **pattern-recognition receptors** (e.g., toll-like receptors).

Mechanisms of innate immunity (e.g., phagocytes) and the alternative complement pathways are activated immediately after infection and quickly begin to control multiplication of infecting microorganisms. By comparison, the **adaptive immune system** is organized around two classes of cells, T and B lymphocytes. When an individual lymphocyte encounters an antigen that binds to its unique antigen receptor site, activation and proliferation of that lymphocyte occur. This is called **clonal selection** and is responsible for the basic properties of the adaptive immune system. Random generation of a highly diverse database of antigen receptors allows the adaptive immune system to recognize virtually any antigen. The downside to this recognition is the inability to distinguish foreign antigens from "self" antigens. Activation of the adaptive immune response can be harmful to the host when the antigens are self or environmental antigens.

CHAPTER HIGHLIGHTS

- Immunology is defined as the study of the molecules, cells, organs, and systems responsible for the recognition and disposal of nonself material; how body components respond and interact; desirable or undesirable consequences of immune interactions; and ways the immune system can be manipulated to protect against or treat disease.
- The function of the immune system is to recognize "self" from "nonself" and to defend the body against nonself.

- The first line of defense against infection is unbroken skin and mucosal membrane surfaces; secretions are also important.
- Natural resistance is one of the two ways that the body resists infection if microorganisms penetrate the first line of resistance.
- Acquired resistance specifically recognizes and selectively eliminates exogenous or endogenous agents. Tissue damage produced by infectious or other agents results in inflammation. If sufficiently extensive, inflammation is accompanied by an increase in the plasma concentration of acute-phase proteins, a group of glycoproteins.
- If a microorganism overwhelms the body's natural resistance, a third line of defensive resistance, acquired (or adaptive) immunity, allows the body to recognize, remember, and respond to a specific stimulus, an antigen. Antibody-mediated immunity to infection can be acquired if the antibodies are formed by the host (active immunity) or received from another source (passive immunity).
- Immediate hypersensitivity is a subset of the body's antibody-mediated effector mechanisms primarily mediated by IgE.
- Cell-mediated immunity differs from antibody-mediated immunity.
- Lymphocytes are immunologically active through direct cell-to-cell contact and production of cytokines for specific immunologic functions, such as recruitment of phagocytic cells to the site of inflammation.
- Often used synonymously with cell-mediated immunity, delayed hypersensitivity refers to the slow appearance of a secondary response in the skin.
- The main difference between the innate and adaptive immune systems is the mechanisms and receptors used for immune recognition.

REVIEW QUESTIONS

Questions 1-5. Match the following terms to their appropriate definitions or descriptions. (Use each answer only once.)

1. _____ Immune system
2. _____ Lymphocytes
3. _____ Cooperative interaction
4. _____ Nonspecific immune elements
5. _____ Autoimmune disorder

   a. T and B types.
   b. Specific cellular elements, cell products, and non-lymphoid elements.
   c. Mononuclear phagocytes.
   d. Condition in which the body's own tissues are attacked as if they were foreign.
   e. Can protect against or can be manipulated to treat disease.

6. The first line of defense in protecting the body from infection includes all the following components *except:*
   a. Unbroken skin.
   b. Normal microbial flora.
   c. Phagocytic leukocytes.
   d. Secretions such as mucus.

7. Natural immunity is characterized as being:
   a. Innate or inborn.
   b. Able specifically to recognize exogenous or endogenous agents.
   c. Able selectively to eliminate exogenous or endogenous agents.
   d. Part of the first line of body defenses against microbial organisms.

Questions 8 and 9. Complete the chart below from the following list of choices:
   a. Lymphocytes
   b. Macrophages
   c. Mucus
   d. Interferons

Components of the Natural Immune System

Cellular	Mast cells
	Neutrophils
	8. _____
Humoral	Complement
	Lysozyme
	9. _____

10. Another term for adaptive immunity is:
    a. Antigenic immunity.
    b. Acquired immunity.
    c. Lymphocyte reactive immunity.
    d. Phagocytosis.

11. Humoral components of the adaptive immune system include:
    a. T lymphocytes.
    b. B lymphocytes.
    c. Antibodies.
    d. Saliva.

Questions 12-23. Complete the table below, choosing from the following answers:

Possible answers for questions 12-15:
   a. Infusion of serum of plasma
   b. Transfer in vivo or by colostrum
   c. Vaccination
   d. Infection

Possible answers for questions 16-19:
   a. Yes
   b. No

Possible answers for questions 20-23:
   a. Short
   b. Long

Comparison of the Types of Adaptive Immunity

Type	Mode of Acquisition	Antibody Produced by Host	Duration of Response
Active natural	12. _____	16. _____	20. _____
Artificial active	13. _____	17. _____	21. _____
Passive natural	14. _____	18. _____	22. _____
Artificial passive	15. _____	19. _____	23. _____

24. Immediate hypersensitivity consists of the reactions primarily mediated by the _____ class of immunoglobulins.
    a. IgM
    b. IgG
    c. IgE
    d. IgA

25. The most immediate and severe manifestation of immediate hypersensitivity reaction is:
    a. Anaphylaxis.
    b. Anaphylactoid.
    c. Itching.
    d. Sneezing.

26. Delayed hypersensitivity is also referred to as:
    a. Humoral immunity.
    b. Cell-mediated immunity.
    c. B-cell hypersensitivity.
    d. Cytotoxic hypersensitivity.

BIBLIOGRAPHY

Barrett JT: *Textbook of immunology,* ed 5, St Louis, 1988, Mosby.
Bergsma J: Illness, the mind, and the body: cancer and immunology: an introduction, *Theor Med* 15(4):337-347, 1994.
Claman HN: The biology of the immune system *JAMA* 268(20):2888-2892, 1992.
Medzhitov R, Janeway C Jr: Innate immunity *N Engl J Med* 343(5):338-344, 2000.

CHAPTER 2

Antigens and Antibodies

Antigen Characteristics
    General Characteristics of Antigens
    Histocompatibility Antigens
    Autoantigens
    Blood Group Antigens
Chemical Nature of Antigens
Physical Nature of Antigens
    Foreignness
    Degradability
    Molecular Weight
    Structural Stability
    Complexity
General Characteristics of Antibodies
Immunoglobulin Classes
    IgM
    IgG
    IgA
    IgD
    IgE
Antibody Structure
    Typical Immunoglobulin Molecule
    Fab, Fc, and Hinge Molecular Components
    Structure of Other Immunoglobulins
Immunoglobulin Variants
    Isotype Determinants
    Allotype Determinants
    Idiotype Determinants

Antibody Synthesis
    Primary Antibody Response
    Secondary (Anamnestic) Response
Functions of Antibodies
Antigen-Antibody Interaction: Specificity
    and Cross-Reactivity
    Antibody Affinity
    Antibody Avidity
    Immune Complexes
Molecular Basis of Antigen-Antibody Reactions
    Types of Bonding
    Goodness of Fit
    Detection of Antigen-Antibody Reactions
    Influence of Antibody Types on Agglutination
Monoclonal Antibodies
    Discovery of the Technique
    Monoclonal Antibody Production
    Uses of Monoclonal Antibodies
ABO Blood Grouping (Forward Antigen Typing)
    Procedure
Serum Protein Electrophoresis Procedure
Chapter Highlights
Review Questions
Bibliography

Learning Objectives

At the conclusion of this chapter, the reader should be able to:
- Define the terms *antigen* and *antibody*.
- Name and describe the characteristics of each of the five immunoglobulin classes.
- Draw and describe a typical immunoglobulin G (IgG) molecular structure.
- Name the four phases of an antibody response.

- Describe the characteristics of a primary and secondary (anamnestic) response.
- Compare the terms antibody *avidity* and antibody *affinity*.
- Describe the method of production of a monoclonal antibody.

ANTIGEN CHARACTERISTICS

General Characteristics of Antigens

An **antigen** is a substance that stimulates antibody formation and has the ability to bind to an antibody. Foreign substances can be **immunogenic** or **antigenic** (capable of provoking an immune response) if their membrane or molecular components contain structures recognized as foreign by the immune system. These structures are called **antigenic determinants,** or epitopes. An **epitope,** as part of an antigen, reacts specifically with an antibody or T-lymphocyte receptor.

Not all surfaces act as antigenic determinants. Only prominent determinants on the surface of a protein are normally recognized by the immune system, and some of these

are much more immunogenic than others. An immune response is directed against specific determinants, and resultant antibodies will bind to them, with much of the remaining molecule being immunogenic.

The cellular membrane of mammalian cells chemically consists of proteins, phospholipids, cholesterol, and traces of polysaccharide. Polysaccharides (carbohydrates) in the form of either glycoproteins or glycolipids can be found attached to the lipid and protein molecules of the membrane. When antigen-bearing cells, such as red blood cells (RBCs), from one person, a donor, are transfused into another person, a recipient, they can be immunogenic. Outer surfaces of bacteria, such as the capsule or the cell wall, as well as the surface structures of other microorganisms, can also be immunogenic.

Cellular antigens of importance to immunologists include histocompatibility antigens, autoantigens, and blood group antigens (see later ABO Blood Grouping procedure). The normal immune system responds to foreignness by producing antibodies. For this reason, microbial antigens are also important to immunologists in the study of the immunologic manifestations of infectious disease.

Histocompatibility Antigens

Nucleated cells such as leukocytes and tissues possess many cell surface protein antigens that readily provoke an immune response if transferred into a genetically different **(allogenic)** individual of the same species. Some of these antigens, which constitute the **major histocompatibility complex (MHC)** (Plate 1), are much more potent than others in provoking an immune response. The MHC is referred to as the **human leukocyte antigen (HLA)** system in humans because its gene products were originally identified on white blood cells (WBCs, leukocytes). These antigens are second only to the ABO antigens in influencing the survival or graft rejection of transplanted organs. HLAs are the subject of numerous scientific investigations because of the strong association between individual HLAs and immunologic disorders (see Chapter 31).

Autoantigens

The evolution of a recognition system that can recognize and destroy "nonself" material must also have safeguards to prevent damage to "self" antigens. The body's immune system usually exercises tolerance to self antigens, but in some situations, antibodies may be produced in response to normal self antigens. This failure to recognize self antigens can result in autoantibodies directed at hormones, such as thyroglobulin (see Chapter 28).

Blood Group Antigens

Blood group substances are widely distributed throughout the tissues, blood cells, and body fluids. When foreign RBC antigens are introduced to a host, a transfusion reaction or hemolytic disease of the newborn can result (see Chapter 26). In addition, certain antigens, especially those of the Rh system, are integral structural components of the erythrocyte (RBC) membrane. If these antigens are missing, the erythrocyte membrane is defective and results in hemolytic anemia. When antigens do not form part of the essential membrane structure (e.g., A, B, and H antigens), the absence of antigen has no effect on membrane integrity.

CHEMICAL NATURE OF ANTIGENS

Antigens, or **immunogens,** are usually large, organic molecules that are either proteins or large polysaccharides and rarely, if ever, lipids. Antigens, especially cell surface or membrane-bound antigens, can be composed of combinations of the biochemical classes (e.g., glycoproteins or glyco-

lipids). For example, histocompatibility HLAs are glycoprotein in nature and are found on the surface membranes of nucleated body cells composed of both solid tissue and most circulating blood cells (e.g., granulocytes, monocytes, lymphocytes, thrombocytes).

Proteins are excellent antigens because of their high molecular weight and structural complexity. Lipids are considered inferior antigens because of their relative simplicity and lack of structural stability. However, when lipids are linked to proteins or polysaccharides, they may function as antigens. Nucleic acids are poor antigens because of relative simplicity, molecular flexibility, and rapid degradation. Anti–nucleic acid antibodies can be produced by artificially stabilizing them and linking them to an immunogenic carrier. Carbohydrates (polysaccharides) by themselves are considered too small to function as antigens. In the case of erythrocyte blood group antigens, protein or lipid carriers may contribute to the necessary size, and the polysaccharides present in the form of side chains confer immunologic specificity.

PHYSICAL NATURE OF ANTIGENS

Important factors in the effective functioning of antigens include foreignness, degradability, molecular weight (MW), structural stability, and complexity.

Foreignness

Foreignness is the degree to which antigenic determinants are recognized as nonself by an individual's immune system. The immunogenicity of a molecule depends to a great extent on its degree of foreignness. For example, if a transplant recipient receives a donor organ with several major HLA differences, the organ is perceived as foreign and is subsequently rejected by the recipient. Normally, an individual's immune system does not respond to self antigens.

Degradability

For an antigen to be recognized as foreign by an individual's immune system, sufficient antigens to stimulate an immune response must be present. Foreign molecules are rapidly destroyed and thus cannot provide adequate antigenic exposure. In the case of vaccination, an adequate dose of vaccine at appropriate intervals must be administered for an immune response to be stimulated.

Molecular Weight

The higher the MW, the better the molecule will function as an antigen. The number of antigenic determinants on a molecule is directly related to its size. For example, proteins are effective antigens because of a large MW.

Although large foreign molecules (MW >10,000 D) are better antigens, **haptens,** which are tiny molecules, can bind to a larger carrier molecule and behave as antigens. If a hapten is chemically linked to a large molecule, a new surface structure is formed on the large molecule, which may function as an antigenic determinant.

Structural Stability

If a molecule is an effective antigen, structural stability is mandatory. If a structure is unstable (e.g., gelatin), the molecule will be a poor antigen. Similarly, totally inert molecules are poor antigens.

Complexity

The more complex an antigen, the greater is its effectiveness. Complex proteins are better antigens than large, repeating polymers such as lipids, carbohydrates, and nucleic acids, which are relatively poor antigens.

GENERAL CHARACTERISTICS OF ANTIBODIES

Antibodies are specific glycoproteins referred to as immunoglobulins. Many antibodies can be isolated in the gamma-globulin fraction of protein by electrophoresis separation (Figure 2-1). The term *immunoglobulin* (Ig) has replaced "gamma globulin" because not all antibodies have gamma electrophoretic mobility. Antibodies can be found in blood plasma and in many body fluids (e.g., tears, saliva, colostrum).

The primary function of an antibody in body defenses is to combine with antigen, which may be enough to neutral-

ize bacterial toxins or some viruses. A secondary interaction of an antibody molecule with another effector agent (e.g., complement) is usually required to dispose of larger antigens (e.g., bacteria).

Determining Ig concentration can be of diagnostic significance in infectious and autoimmune diseases. Test methods to detect the presence and concentration of immunoglobulins are discussed in Chapters 10 through 14 and in chapters relating to specific diseases.

IMMUNOGLOBULIN (Ig) CLASSES

Five distinct classes of immunoglobulin molecules are recognized in most higher mammals: IgM, IgG, IgA, IgD, and IgE. These Ig classes differ from each other in characteristics such as MW and sedimentation coefficients (Table 2-1).

IgM

Immunoglobulin M accounts for about 10% of the Ig pool, and it is largely confined to the intravascular pool because of its large size. This antibody is produced early in an immune response and is largely confined to the blood. IgM is effective in agglutination and cytolytic reactions. In humans, IgM is found in smaller concentrations than either

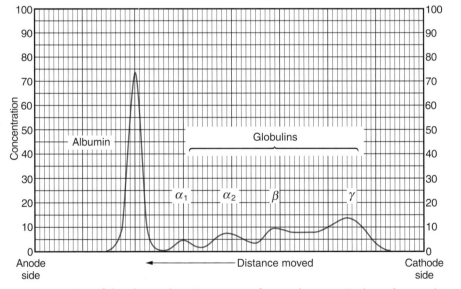

Figure 2-1   Tracing of the electrophoretic pattern of normal serum. *(Redrawn from Kaplan LA, Pesce AJ, Kazmierczak SC, editors:* Clinical chemistry: theory, analysis, correlation, *ed 4, St Louis, 2003, Mosby.)*

Table 2-1	**Characteristics of Immunoglobulin Classes**				
	IgM	**IgG**	**IgA**	**IgE**	**IgD**
Molecular weight (daltons, D)	900,000	160,000	360,000	200,000	160,000
Sedimentation coefficient	19S	7S	11S	8S	7S
Carbohydrate (%)	12	8	7	12	12
Subclasses	—	IgG1-4	α_1, α_2	—	—
Serum concentration, adults (mg/dL)*	50-200	800-1600	150-400	0.002-0.05	1.5-40
Half-life (days)	5	21	6	2	—

*Conversion factors: IgG, 1 mg = 11.5 IU; IgA, 1 mg = 57.7 IU; IgM, 1 mg = 117 IU; IgD, 1 mg = 709 IU.

IgG or IgA. The molecule has five individual heavy chains, with MW of 65,000 daltons (D); the whole molecule has MW of 900,000 D and sedimentation coefficient of 19S.

Normal values of IgM are 60 to 250 mg/dL (70-290 IU/mL) for males and 70 to 280 mg/dL (80-320 IU/mL) for females. Fifty percent of adult levels is present at 4 months of age, and adult levels are reached by 8 to 15 years. Cord blood contains greater than 20 mg/dL. IgM is usually undetectable in cerebrospinal fluid (CSF).

Immunoglobulin M is decreased in *primary* (genetically determined) Ig disorders as well as *secondary* Ig deficiencies (acquired disorders associated with certain diseases). IgM can be increased in the following conditions:

- Infectious diseases, such as subacute bacterial endocarditis, infectious mononucleosis, leprosy, trypanosomiasis, malaria, and actinomycosis.
- Collagen disorders, such as scleroderma.
- Hematologic disorders, such as polyclonal gammopathies, monocytic leukemia, and monoclonal gammopathies (e.g., Waldenström's macroglobulinemia).

IgG

The major immunoglobulin in normal serum is IgG. It diffuses more readily than other immunoglobulins into the extravascular spaces, and it neutralizes toxins or binds to microorganisms in extravascular spaces. IgG can cross the placenta. In addition, when IgG complexes are formed, complement can be activated. IgG accounts for 70% to 75% of the total Ig pool. It is a 7S molecule, with an MW of approximately 150,000 D. One of the subclasses, IgG3, is slightly larger (170,000 D) than the other subclasses.

Normal human adult serum values of IgG are 800 to 1800 mg/dL (90-210 IU/mL). In infants 3 to 4 months old the IgG level is approximately 350 to 400 mg/dL (40-45 IU/mL), gradually increasing to 700 to 800 mg/dL (80-90 IU/mL) by the end of the first year of life (Figure 2-2). The average adult level is achieved before age 16 years. Other body fluids containing IgG include cord blood (800-1800 mg/dL) and CSF (2-4 mg/dL).

Decreased levels of IgG can be manifested in primary (genetic) or secondary (acquired) Ig deficiencies. Significant increases of IgG are seen in the following conditions:

- Infectious diseases, such as hepatitis, rubella, and infectious mononucleosis.
- Collagen disorders, such as rheumatoid arthritis and systemic lupus erythematosus.
- Hematologic disorders, such as polyclonal gammopathies, monoclonal gammopathies, monocytic leukemia, and Hodgkin's disease.

IgA

Immunoglobulin A represents 15% to 20% of the total circulatory Ig pool. It is the predominant immunoglobulin in secretions such as tears, saliva, colostrum, milk, and intestinal fluids. IgA is synthesized largely by plasma cells located on body surfaces. If produced by cells in the intestinal wall, IgA may pass directly into the intestinal lumen or diffuse into the blood circulation. As IgA is transported through intestinal epithelial cells or hepatocytes, it binds to a glycoprotein called the "secretory" component. The secretory piece protects IgA from digestion by gastrointestinal proteolytic enzymes. It forms a complex molecule named *secretory IgA*, which is critical in protecting body surfaces against invading microorganisms because of its presence in seromucous secretions (e.g., tears, saliva, nasal fluids, colostrum).

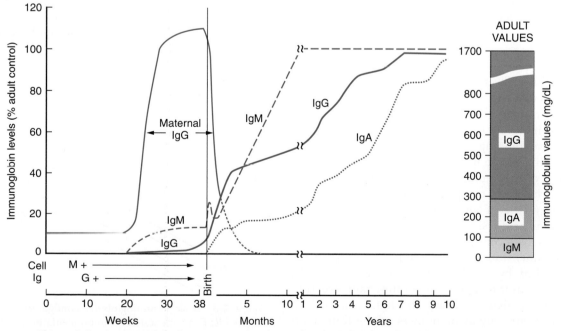

Figure 2-2 Immunoglobulin concentration in newborns, infants, and children. *(Redrawn from Bauer JD: Clinical laboratory methods, ed 9, St Louis, 1982, Mosby.)*

IgA monomer is present in relatively high concentrations in human serum, including a concentration of 90 to 450 mg/dL (55-270 IU/mL) in normal adult humans. Twenty-five percent of the adult IgA level is reached at the end of the first year of life, and 50% at 3½ years. The average adult level is attained by age 16 years. IgA concentration in cord blood is greater than 1 mg/dL, and CSF contains 0.1 to 0.6 mg/dL.

IgA is decreased in primary or secondary Ig deficiencies. Significant increases in serum IgA concentration of are associated with the following:

- Infectious diseases, such as tuberculosis and actinomycosis.
- Collagen disorders, such as rheumatoid arthritis.
- Hematologic disorders, such as polyclonal gammopathies, monocytic leukemia, and monoclonal gammopathy (e.g., IgA myeloma).
- Liver disease, such as Laennec's cirrhosis and chronic active hepatitis.

IgD

Immunoglobulin D is found in very low concentrations in plasma, accounting for less than 1% of the total Ig pool. IgD is extremely susceptible to proteolysis and is primarily a cell membrane Ig found on the surface of B lymphocytes in association with IgM.

IgE

Immunoglobulin E is a trace plasma protein found in the blood plasma of unparasitized individuals (MW, 188,000 D). IgE is crucial because it mediates some types of hypersensitivity (allergic) reactions, allergies, and anaphylaxis and is generally responsible for an individual's immunity to invading parasites. The IgE molecule is unique in that it binds strongly to a receptor on mast cells and basophils and, together with antigen, mediates the release of histamines and heparin from these cells.

ANTIBODY STRUCTURE

Antibodies exhibit diversity among the different classes, which suggests that they perform different functions in addition to their primary function of antigen binding. Essentially, each Ig molecule is bifunctional; one region of the molecule involves binding to antigen, and a different region mediates binding of the immunoglobulin to host tissues, including cells of the immune system and the first component (C1q) of the classic complement system.

The primary core of an antibody consists of the sequence of amino acid residues linked by the peptide bond. All antibodies have a common, basic polypeptide structure with a three-dimensional configuration. The polypeptide chains are linked by covalent and noncovalent bonds, which produce a unit composed of a four-chain structure based on pairs of identical heavy and light chains. IgG, IgD, and IgE occur only as monomers of the four-chain unit; IgA occurs in both monomeric and polymeric forms;

and IgM occurs as a pentamer with 5 four-chain subunits linked together.

Typical Immunoglobulin Molecule

The basic unit of an antibody structure is the homology unit or **domain.** A typical molecule has 12 domains, arranged in two heavy (H) and two light (L) chains, linked through cysteine residues by disulfide bonds so that the domains lie in pairs (Figure 2-3). The antigen-binding portion of the molecule (N-terminal end) shows such heterogeneity that it is known as the variable (V) region; the remainder is composed of relatively constant amino acid sequences, the *constant* (C) region. Short segments of about 10 amino acid residues within the variable regions of antibodies (or T-cell receptor [TCR] proteins) form loop structures called complementary-determining regions (CDRs). Three hypervariable loops, also called CDRs, are present in each antibody H chain and L chain. Most of the variability between different antibodies or TCRs is located within these loops.

The IgG molecule provides a classic model of antibody structure, appearing Y shaped under electron microscopy (Figure 2-4). If the molecule is chemically treated to break interchain disulfide bonds, the molecule separates into four polypeptide chains. Light chains are small chains (25,000 D) common to all Ig classes. The L chains are of two subtypes, kappa (κ) and lambda (λ), which have different amino acid sequences and are antigenically different. In humans, about 65% of Ig molecules have κ chains, whereas 35% have λ chains. The larger H chains (50,000-77,000 D) extend the full length of the molecule.

A general feature of the Ig chains is their amino acid sequence. The first 110 to 120 amino acids of both L and H chains have a variable sequence and form the V region; the remainder of the L chains represents the C region, with a similar amino acid sequence for each type and subtype. The remaining portion of the H chain is also constant for each type and has a hinge region. The class and subclass of an Ig molecule are determined by its H-chain type.

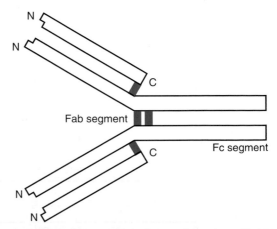

Figure 2-3 Basic immunoglobulin configuration. *(Redrawn from Turgeon ML:* Fundamentals of immunohematology, *ed 2, Baltimore, 1995, Williams & Wilkins.)*

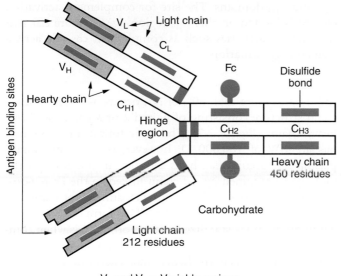

V_L and V_H = Variable regions
C_L and C_H = Constant regions

Figure 2-4   Basic structure of IgG. *(Redrawn from Turgeon MI · Fun-damentals of immunohematology, ed 2, Baltimore, 1995, Williams & Wilkins.)*

Fab, Fc, and Hinge Molecular Components

A typical monomeric IgG molecule consists of three globular regions (two Fab regions and an Fc portion) linked by a flexible hinge region. If the molecule is digested with a proteolytic enzyme such as papain, it splits into three approximately equal-size fragments (Figure 2-5). Two of these fragments retain the ability to bind antigen and are called the antigen-binding fragments (Fab fragments). The third fragment, which is relatively homogeneous and is sometimes crystallizable, is called the Fc portion. If IgG is treated with another proteolytic enzyme, pepsin, the molecule separates somewhat differently. The Fc fragment is split into tiny peptides and thus is completely destroyed. The two Fab fragments remain joined to produce a fragment called F(ab)'2. This fragment possesses two antigen-binding sites. If F(ab)'2 is treated to reduce its disulfide bonds, it breaks into two Fab fragments, each of which has only one antigen-binding site. Further disruption of the interchain disulfide bonds in the Fab fragments shows that each contains a light chain and half of a heavy chain, which is called the Fd fragment.

Electron microscopy studies of IgG reveal that the Fab regions of the molecule are mobile and can swing freely

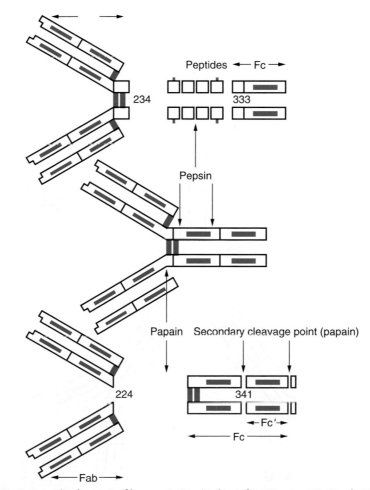

Figure 2-5   Enzymatic cleavage of human IgG1. *(Redrawn from Turgeon ML: Fundamentals of immunohematology, ed 2, 1995, Williams & Wilkins.)*

around the center of the molecule as if it were hinged. This hinge consists of a group of about 15 amino acids located between the C_{H1} and C_{H2} regions. The exact sequence of amino acids in the hinge is variable and unique for each Ig class and subclass. Because amino acids can rotate freely around peptide bonds, the effect of closely spaced proline amino acid residues is production of a "universal joint," around which the Ig chains can swing freely. A remarkable feature of the hinge region is the presence of a large number of hydrophilic and proline residues. The hydrophilic residues tend to open up this region and thus make it accessible to proteolytic cleavage with enzymes such as pepsin and papain. This region also contains all the interchain disulfide bonds except for IgD, which has no interchain links.

Structure of Other Immunoglobulins

IgM

The IgM molecule is structurally composed of five basic subunits. Each subunit consists of two κ or two λ light chains and two mu (μ) heavy chains. The individual monomers of IgM are linked together by disulfide bonds in a circular fashion (Figure 2-6). A small, cysteine-rich polypeptide, the J chain, must be considered an integral part of the molecule. IgM has carbohydrate residues attached to the C_{H3} and C_{H4} domains. The site for complement activation by IgM is located on this C_{H4} region. IgM is more efficient than IgG in activities such as complement cascade activation and agglutination.

IgA

In humans, more than 80% of IgA occurs as a typical four-chain structure consisting of paired κ or λ chains and two heavy chains (Figure 2-7). The basic four-chain monomer has an MW of 160,000 D; however, in most mammals, plasma IgA occurs mainly as a dimer. In dimeric IgA the molecules are joined by a J chain linked to the Fc regions. Secretory IgA exists mainly in the 11S dimeric form and has an MW of 385,000 D (Figure 2-8). This form of IgA is present in fluids and is stabilized against proteolysis when combined with another protein, the secretory component. In humans, variations in the heavy chains account for the subclasses IgA1 and IgA2.

IgD

The IgD molecule has an MW of 184,000 D and consists of two κ or λ light chains and two delta (δ) heavy chains (Figure 2-9). It has no interchain disulfide bonds between its heavy chains and an exposed hinge region.

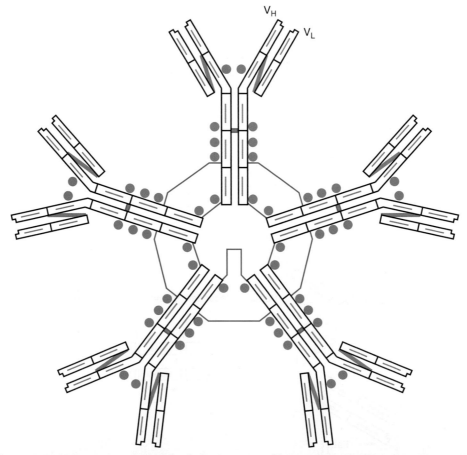

Figure 2-6   Pentameric polypeptide chain structure of human IgM. *(Redrawn From Turgeon ML: Fundamentals of immunohematology, ed 2, Baltimore, 1995, Williams & Wilkins.)*

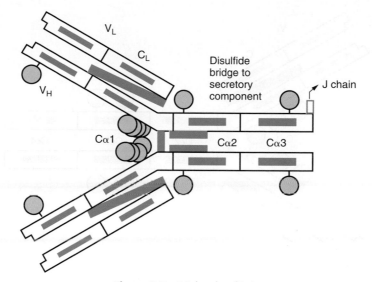

V_L

C_L

V_H

Disulfide bridge to secretory component

J chain

$C\alpha1$

$C\alpha2$

$C\alpha3$

Figure 2-7   Molecule of IgA.

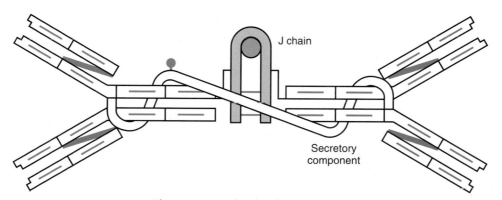

J chain

Secretory component

Figure 2-8   Molecule of secretory IgA.

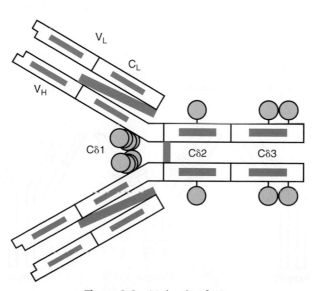

V_L

C_L

V_H

$C\delta1$

$C\delta2$

$C\delta3$

Figure 2-9   Molecule of IgD.

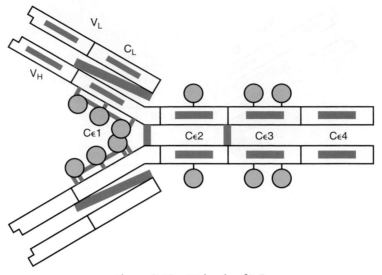

Figure 2-10   Molecule of IgE.

IgE

The IgE molecule is composed of paired κ or λ light chains and two epsilon (ε) heavy chains (Figure 2-10). It is unique in that its Fc region binds strongly to a receptor on mast cells and basophils and, together with antigen, mediates the release of histamines and heparin from these cells.

IMMUNOGLOBULIN VARIANTS

An **antigenic determinant** is the specific chemical determinant group or molecular configuration against which the immune response is directed. Because they are proteins, immunoglobulins themselves can function as effective antigens when used to immunize mammals of a different species. When the resulting antiimmunoglobulins or antiglobulins are analyzed, three principal categories of antigenic determinants can be recognized: isotype, allotype, and idiotype (Figure 2-11 and Table 2-2).

Isotype Determinants

The isotypic class of antigenic determinants is the dominant type found on the immunoglobulins of all animals of a species. The heavy-chain, constant-region structures asso-

ciated with the different classes and subclasses are termed *isotypic variants*. Genes for isotypic variants are present in all healthy members of a species. Determinants in this category include those specific for each Ig class, such as gamma (γ) for IgG, mu (μ) for IgM, and alpha (α) for IgA, as well as the subclass-specific determinants κ and λ.

Allotype Determinants

The second principal group of determinants is found on the immunoglobulins of some, but not all, animals of a species. Antibodies to these allotypes **(alloantibodies)** may be produced by injecting the immunoglobulins of one animal into another member of the same species. The allotypic determinants are genetically determined variations representing the presence of allelic genes at a single locus within a species. Typical allotypes in humans are the Gm specificities on IgG (Gm is a marker on IgG). In humans, five sets of allotypic markers have been found: Gm, Km, Mm, Am, and Hv.

Idiotype Determinants

A result of the unique structures on light and heavy chains, individual determinants characteristic of each antibody are called the **idiotypes.** The idiotypic determinants are located

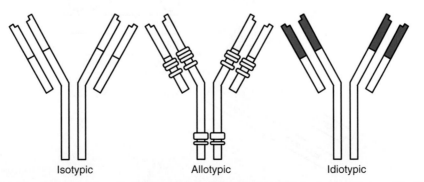

Figure 2-11   Variants of antibodies; antigenic determinants. *(Redrawn from Turgeon ML: Fundamentals of immunohematology, ed 2, Baltimore, 1995, Williams & Wilkins.)*

Table 2-2	**Immunoglobulin Variants**		
Variant	Distribution	Location	Examples
Isotype	All variants in normal persons	C_H C_H C_L	IgM, IgE IgA1, IgA2 Kappa subtype Lambda subtype
Allotype	Genetically controlled alternate forms—not present in all persons	Mainly C_H/C_L Sometimes V_H/V_2	Gm groups in humans
Idiotype	Individually specific to each immunoglobulin molecule	Variable regions	Probably one or more hypervariable regions forming the antigen-combining site

C, Constant region; *H,* heavy chain; *L,* light chain; *V,* variable region; *Gm,* marker on IgG.

in the variable part of the antibody associated with the hypervariable regions that form the antigen-combining site.

ANTIBODY SYNTHESIS

When an antigen is initially encountered, the cells of the immune system recognize the antigen as nonself and either elicit an immune response or become tolerant of it, depending on the circumstances. An immune reaction can take the form of cell-mediated immunity (immunity dependent on T cells and macrophages) or may involve the production of antibodies (B lymphocytes and plasma cells) directed against the antigen.

Production of antibodies is induced when the host's lymphocytes come in contact with a foreign antigenic substance that binds to its receptor. This triggers activation and proliferation, or **clonal selection.** Clonal expansion of lymphocytes in response to infection is necessary for an effective immune response (Figure 2-12). However, it requires 3 to 5 days for a sufficient number of clones to be produced and to differentiate into antibody-producing cells. This allows time for most pathogens to damage host tissues and cells.

Whether a cell-mediated response or an antibody response takes place depends on the way in which the antigen is presented to the lymphocytes; many immune reactions display both types of responses. The antigenicity of a foreign substance is also related to the route of entry. Intravenous and intraperitoneal routes are stronger stimuli than subcutaneous and intramuscular routes.

Subsequent exposure to the same antigen produces a memory response, or **anamnestic response,** and reflects the outcome of the initial challenge. In the case of antibody production, the quantity of IgM/IgG varies.

Primary Antibody Response

Although the duration and levels of antibody (titer) depend on the characteristics of the antigen and the individual, an IgM antibody response proceeds in the following four phases after a foreign antigen challenge (see Figure 2-12):
1. *Lag* phase: no antibody is detectable.
2. *Log* phase: the antibody titer increases logarithmically.

3. *Plateau* phase: the antibody titer stabilizes.
4. *Decline* phase: the antibody is catabolized.

Secondary (Anamnestic) Response

Subsequent exposure to the same antigenic stimulus produces an antibody response that exhibits the same four phases as the primary responses (see Figure 2-12). Repeated exposure to an antigen can occur many years after the initial exposure, but clones of memory cells will be stimulated to proliferate with subsequent production of antibody by the individual. An anamnestic response differs from a primary response as follows:
1. *Time.* A secondary response has a shorter lag phase, a longer plateau, and a more gradual decline.
2. *Type of antibody.* IgM-type antibodies are the principal class formed in the primary response. Although some IgM antibody is formed in a secondary response, the IgG class is the predominant type formed.
3. *Antibody titer.* In a secondary response, antibody levels attain a higher titer. The plateau levels in a secondary response are typically tenfold or greater than the plateau levels in the primary response.

An example of an anamnestic response can be observed in hemolytic disease, when an Rh-negative mother is pregnant with an Rh-positive baby (see Chapter 26). During the mother's first exposure, the Rh-positive RBCs of the fetus leak into the maternal circulation and elicit a primary response. Subsequent pregnancies with Rh-positive fetuses will elicit a secondary (anamnestic) response.

Vaccination is the application of primary and second responses. Humans can become immune to microbial antigens through artificial and natural exposure. A vaccine is designed to provide artificially acquired active immunity to a specific disease (e.g., hepatitis B). Booster vaccine (repeated antigen exposure) allows for an anamnestic response, with an increase in antibody titer and clones of memory cells (see Chapter 16).

FUNCTIONS OF ANTIBODIES

The principal function of an antibody is to bind antigen, but antibodies may also exhibit secondary effector functions and behave as antigens. The significant secondary ef-

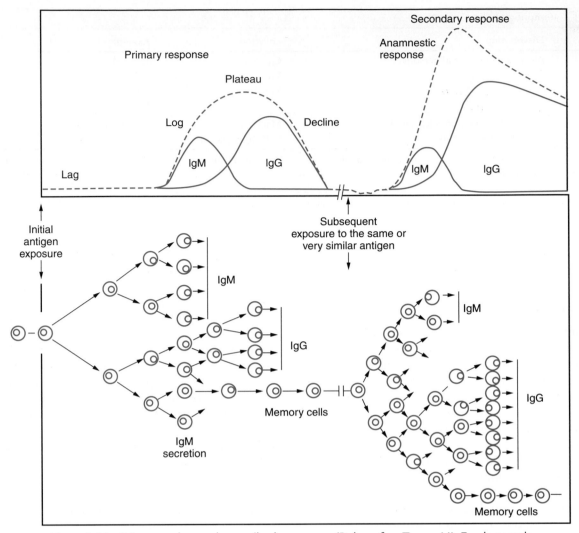

Figure 2-12   Primary and secondary antibody response. *(Redrawn from Turgeon ML:* Fundamentals of immunohematology, *ed 2, Baltimore, 1995, Williams & Wilkins.)*

fector functions of antibodies are complement fixation and placental transfer (Table 2-3). The activation of complement is one of most important effector mechanisms of IgG1 and IgG3 molecules (see Chapter 5). IgG2 seems to be less effective in activating complement; IgG4, IgA, IgD, and IgE are ineffective in terms of complement activation. In humans, most of the IgG subclass molecules are capable of crossing the placental barrier; no consensus exists on whether IgG2 crosses the placenta. Passage of antibodies across the placental barrier is important in the etiology of hemolytic disease of the newborn and in conferring passive immunity to the newborn during the first few months of life.

ANTIGEN-ANTIBODY INTERACTION: SPECIFICITY AND CROSS-REACTIVITY

The ability of a particular antibody to combine with a particular antigen is referred to as its **specificity.** This property resides in the portion of the Fab molecule called the combining site, a cleft formed largely by the hypervariable regions of heavy and light chains. Evidence indicates that an antigen may bind to larger, or even separate, parts of the variable region. The closer the fit between this site and the antigen determinant, the stronger are the noncovalent forces (e.g., hydrophobic or electrostatic bonds) between them, and the higher is the affinity between the antigen and antibody. Binding depends on a close three-dimensional fit, allowing weak intermolecular forces to overcome the normal repulsion between molecules. When more than one combining site interacts with the same antigen, the bond has greatly increased strength.

Antigen-antibody reactions can show a high level of specificity. Specificity exists when the binding sites of antibodies directed against determinants of one antigen are not com-

Table 2-3	Comparison of Properties of Immunoglobulins				
	IgM	IgG	IgA	IgD	IgE
Complement fixation	3+	0-2+	No	No	No
Placental transfer	No	Yes	No	No	No

plementary to determinants of another, dissimilar antigen. When some of the determinants of an antigen are shared by similar antigenic determinants on the surface of apparently unrelated molecules, a proportion of the antibodies directed against one type of antigen will also react with the other type of antigen; this is called **cross-reactivity.** Antibodies directed against a protein in one species may also react in a detectable manner with the homologous protein in another species.

Cross-reactivity occurs between bacteria that possess the same cell wall polysaccharides as mammalian erythrocytes. Intestinal bacteria, as well as other substances found in the environment, possess "A-like" or "B-like" antigens similar to the A and B erythrocyte antigens. If A or B antigens are foreign to an individual, production of anti-A or anti-B occurs, despite lack of previous exposure to these erythrocyte antigens. Cross-reacting antibodies of this type are *heterophile* antibodies.

Antibody Affinity

Affinity is the initial force of attraction that exists between a single Fab site on an antibody molecule and a single epitope or determinant site on the corresponding antigen. The antigen is univalent and is usually a hapten. Several types of noncovalent bonds hold an epitope and binding site close together (see Type of Bonding).

Antibody Avidity

Each four-polypeptide-chain antibody unit has two antigen-binding sites, which allows them to be potentially multivalent in their reaction with an antigen. The functional combining strength of an antibody with its antigen is called **avidity,** in contrast to affinity, the binding strength between an antigenic determinant (epitope) and an antibody-combining site (Figure 2-13). When a multivalent antigen combines with more than one of an antibody's combining sites, the strength of the bonding is significantly increased. For the antigen and antibody to dissociate, all the antigen-antibody bonds must be broken simultaneously.

Decreased avidity can result when an antigen (e.g., hapten) has only one antigenic determinant (monovalent).

Immune Complexes

The noncovalent combination of antigen with its respective, specific antibody is called an **immune complex.** An immune complex may be of the small **(soluble)** or large **(precipitating)** type, depending on the nature and proportion of antigen and antibody. Under conditions of antigen or antibody excess, soluble complexes tend to predominate. If equivalent amounts of antigen and antibody are present, a precipitate may form. However, all antigen-antibody complexes will not precipitate, even at equivalence.

Antibody can react with antigen that is fixed or localized in tissues or that is released or present in the circulation. Once formed in the circulation, the immune complex is usually removed by phagocytic cells through the interaction of the Fc portion of the antibody with complement and cell surface receptors.

Under normal circumstances, this process does not lead to pathologic consequences, and it may be viewed as a major host defense against the invasion of foreign antigens. It is only in unusual circumstances that the immune complex persists as a soluble complex in the circulation, escapes phagocytosis, and is deposited in endothelial or vascular structures (where it causes inflammatory damage, the principal characteristic of immune complex disease), is deposited in organs (e.g., kidney), or inhibits useful immunity (e.g., tumors, parasites). The level of circulating immune complex is determined by the rate of formation, the rate of clearance, and most importantly the nature of the complex

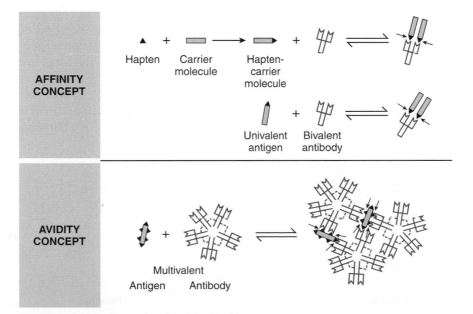

Figure 2-13 Affinity versus avidity. *(From Zane HD:* Immunology: theoretical and practical concepts in laboratory medicine, *Philadelphia, 2001, Saunders.)*

formed. Detection of immune complexes and the identification of the associated antigens are important to the clinical diagnosis of immune complex disorders.

MOLECULAR BASIS OF ANTIGEN-ANTIBODY REACTIONS

The basic Y-shaped Ig molecule is a bifunctional structure. The variable (V) regions are primarily concerned with antigen binding. When an antigenic determinant and its specific antibody combine, they interact through the chemical groups found on the surface of the antigenic determinant and on the surface of the hypervariable regions of the Ig molecule. Although the constant (C) regions do not form the antigen-binding sites, the arrangement of the C regions and hinge region give the molecule segmental flexibility, which allows it to combine with separated antigenic determinants.

Types of Bonding

Bonding of an antigen to an antibody results from the formation of multiple, reversible, intermolecular attractions between an antigen and amino acids of the binding site. These forces require proximity of the interacting groups. The optimum distance separating the interacting groups varies for different types of bond; however, all these bonds act only across a very short distance and weaken rapidly as that distance increases.

The bonding of antigen to antibody is exclusively *noncovalent*. The attractive force of noncovalent bonds is weak compared with covalent bonds, but the formation of multiple noncovalent bonds produces considerable total binding energy. The strength of a single antigen-antibody bond (antibody affinity) is produced by the summation of the attractive and repulsive forces. The four types of noncovalent bonds involved in antigen-antibody reactions are hydrophobic bonds, hydrogen bonds, van der Waals forces, and electrostatic forces.

Hydrophobic Bonds

The major bonds formed between antigens and antibodies are hydrophobic. Many of the nonpolar side chains of proteins are hydrophobic. When antigen and antibody molecules come together, these side chains interact and exclude water molecules from the area of the interaction. The exclusion of water frees some of the constraints imposed by the proteins, which results in a gain in energy and forms an energetically stable complex.

Hydrogen Bonds

Hydrogen bonding results from the formation of hydrogen bridges between appropriate atoms. Major hydrogen bonds in antigen-antibody interactions are O–H–O, N–H–N, and O–H–N.

Van der Waals Forces

Van der Waals forces are nonspecific, attractive forces generated by the interaction between electron clouds and hydrophobic bonds. These bonds result from minor asymmetry in the charge of an atom caused by the position of its electrons. They rely on the association of nonpolar, hydrophobic groups so that contact with water molecules is minimized. Although extremely weak, van der Waals forces may become collectively important in an antigen-antibody reaction.

Electrostatic Forces

Electrostatic forces result from the attraction of oppositely charged amino acids located on the side chains of two amino acid residues. The relative importance of electrostatic bonds is unclear.

Goodness of Fit

The strongest bonding develops when antigens and antibodies are close to each other and when the shapes of the antigenic determinants and the antigen-binding site conform to each other. This complementary matching of determinants and binding sites is referred to as "goodness of fit" (Figure 2-14).

A good fit will create ample opportunities for the simultaneous formation of several noncovalent bonds and few opportunities for disruption of the bond. If a poor fit exists, repulsive forces can overpower any small forces of attraction. Variations from the ideal complementary shape will produce a decrease in the total binding energy because of increased repulsive forces and decreased attractive forces. Goodness of fit is important in determining the binding of an antibody molecule for a particular antigen.

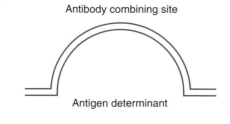

Good fit

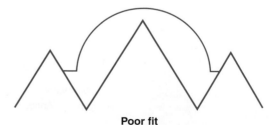

Poor fit

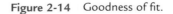

Figure 2-14   Goodness of fit.

Detection of Antigen-Antibody Reactions

In vitro tests detect the combination of antigens and antibodies. **Agglutination** is the process in which particulate antigens (e.g., cells) aggregate to form larger complexes in the presence of a specific antibody. Agglutination tests are widely used in immunology to detect and measure the consequences of antigen-antibody interaction. Other tests include the following:

- *Precipitation reactions* combine soluble antigen with soluble antibody to produce insoluble complexes that are visible.
- *Hemolysis testing* involves the reaction of antigen and antibody with a cellular indicator (e.g., lysed RBCs).
- *Enzyme-linked immunosorbent assay* (ELISA) measures immune complexes formed in an in vitro system.

The principles of immunologic methods are discussed in Part II of this text. Detection and quantitation of immunoglobulins is important in the laboratory investigation of infectious diseases and immunologic disorders (Table 2-4).

Influence of Antibody Types on Agglutination

Immunoglobulins are relatively positively charged, and after sensitization or coating of particles, they reduce the **zeta potential** (electron cloud surrounding an RBC), which is the difference in electrostatic potential between the net charge at the cell membrane and the charge at the surface of shear. Antibodies can bridge charged particles by extending beyond the effective range of the zeta potential, which results in the erythrocytes closely approaching each other, binding, and agglutinating.

Antibodies differ in their ability to agglutinate. IgM-type antibodies, sometimes referred to as "complete antibodies," are more efficient than IgG or IgA antibodies in exhibiting in vitro agglutination when the antigen-bearing erythrocytes are suspended in physiologic (0.85%) sodium chloride (saline). Antibodies that do not exhibit visible agglutination of saline-suspended erythrocytes, even when bound to the cell's surface membrane, are considered to be nonagglutinating antibodies and have been called "incomplete antibodies." Incomplete antibodies may fail to exhibit agglutination because the antigenic determinants are located deep within the surface membrane or may show restricted movement in their hinge region, causing them to be functionally monovalent.

MONOCLONAL ANTIBODIES

Monoclonal antibodies are purified antibodies cloned from a single cell. These antibodies exhibit exceptional purity and specificity and are able to recognize and bind to a specific antigen.

Discovery of the Technique

In 1975, Köhler, Milstein, and Jerne discovered how to fuse lymphocytes to produce a cell line that was both immortal and a producer of specific antibodies. These scientists were awarded the Nobel Prize in Physiology and Medicine in 1984 for developing this **hybridoma** (cell hybrids) from different lines of cultured myeloma cells (plasma cells derived from malignant tumor strains). To induce the cells to fuse, they used Sendai virus, an influenza virus that characteristically causes cell fusion. Initially, the scientists immunized donors with sheep erythrocytes to provide a marker for the normal cells. The hybrids were tested to determine if they still produced antibodies against the sheep erythrocytes. Köhler discovered that some of the hybrids were manufacturing large quantities of specific anti–sheep erythrocyte antibodies.

This technique is referred to as *somatic cell hybridization*. The resulting hybrid cells secrete the antibody that is characteristic of the parent cell (e.g., anti–sheep erythrocyte antibodies). The multiplying hybrid cell culture is a hybridoma. Hybridoma cells can be cloned (the process in which single cells are selected and grown). The immunoglobulins derived from a single clone of cells are termed *monoclonal antibodies* (MAbs).

Monoclonal Antibody Production

Modern methods for producing MAbs are refinements of the Köhler's original technique. Basically, the hybridoma technique enables scientists to inoculate crude antigen mixtures into mice and then select clones producing specific antibodies against a single cell surface antigen (Figure 2-15). The process of producing MAbs takes 3 to 6 months.

Mice are immunized with a specific antigen; several doses are given to ensure a vigorous immune response. After 2 to 4 days, spleen cells are mixed with cultured mouse myeloma cells. Myeloma parent cells that lack the enzyme hypoxanthine phosphoribosyl transferase are selected because these cells cannot use hypoxanthine derived from the culture medium to manufacture purines and pyrimidines and, if unfused, will not survive in the culture medium. In addition, the mouse myeloma cell lines usually do not secrete immunoglobulins, thus simplifying the purification process.

Polyethylene glycol (PEG) rather than Sendai virus is added to the cell mixture to promote cell membrane fusion. Only 1 in 200,000 spleen cells actually forms a viable hybrid with a myeloma cell. Normal spleen cells do not survive in culture. The fused-cell mixture is placed in a medium containing hypoxanthine, aminopterin, and thymidine (HAT medium). Aminopterin is a drug that prevents myeloma cells from making their own purines and

Table 2-4	Role of Specific Immunoglobulins in Diagnostic Tests		
	IgG	IgM	IgA
Agglutination	1+	3+	Negative
Complement fixation	1+	3+	1+
Time of appearance after exposure to antigen (days)	3-7	2.5	3-7
Time to reach peak titer (days)	7-21	5-14	7-21

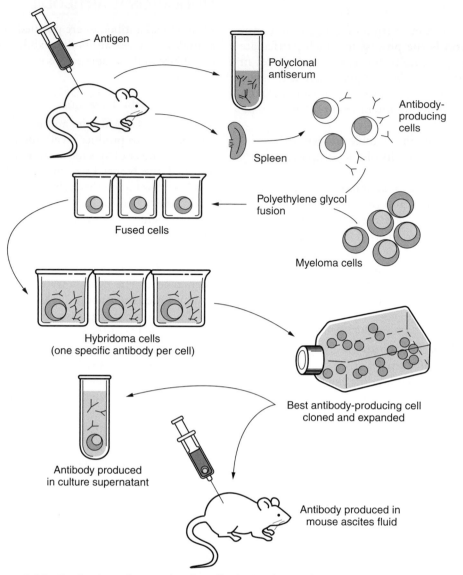

Figure 2-15   Production of monoclonal antibody (MAb). *(Redrawn from Forbes BA, Sahm DF, Weissfeld AS:* Bailey & Scott's diagnostic microbiology, *ed 12, St Louis, 2007, Mosby.)*

pyrimidines; they cannot use hypoxanthine from the medium, so they will die.

Hybrids resulting from the fusion of spleen cells and myeloma cells contain transferase provided by the normal spleen cells. Consequently, the hybridoma cells are able to use the hypoxanthine and thymidine in the culture medium and survive. They divide rapidly in HAT medium, doubling in number every 24 to 48 hours. About 300 to 500 hybrids can be generated from the cells of a single mouse spleen, although not all will be making the desired antibodies. After the hybridomas have been growing for 2 to 4 weeks, the supernatant is tested for specific antibody using methods such as ELISA. Clones that produce the desired antibody are grown in mass culture and recloned to eliminate non–antibody-producing cells.

Antibody-producing clones lose their ability to synthesize or secrete antibody after being cultured for several months. Hybridoma cells usually are frozen and stored in small aliquots. The cells may then be grown in mass culture or injected intraperitoneally into mice. Because hybridomas are tumor cells, they grow rapidly and induce the effusion of large quantities of fluid into the peritoneal cavity. This ascites fluid is rich in MAbs and can be easily harvested.

Uses of Monoclonal Antibodies

The greatest impact of MAbs in immunology has been on the analysis of cell membrane antigens. Because they have a single specificity rather than the range of antibody molecules present in the serum, MAbs have multiple clinical applications that include the following:

- Identifying and quantifying hormones.
- Typing tissue and blood.
- Identifying infectious agents.
- Identifying clusters of differentiation for the classification of leukemias and lymphomas and follow-up therapy.

- Identifying tumor antigens and autoantibodies.
- Delivering immunotherapy.

ABO Blood Grouping (Forward Antigen Typing) Procedure

Principle

The ABO blood groups (A, B, AB, and O) represent the antigens expressed on the erythrocytes (red blood cells, RBCs) of each group.

Reagent typing sera contains specific antibodies to A antigen and B antigen. When unknown patient RBCs are mixed with known antibody A or antibody B, agglutination of the RBCs will occur if a specific antigen-antibody reaction occurs. This is called *direct blood typing*.

Specimen Collection and Preparation

No special preparation of the patient is required before specimen collection. The patient must be positively identified when the specimen is collected, and the specimen must be labeled at the bedside. Specimen labels include the patient's full name, the date, the patient's hospital identification number, and the phlebotomist's initials. Bar coding is now a popular method of identification as well.

Blood should be drawn by aseptic technique. A minimum of 2 mL of anticoagulated blood (lavender-top evacuated tube) is required. Hemolysis or contamination with bacteria renders a specimen unsuitable for testing. If the test cannot be performed immediately, the specimen should be refrigerated (2° to 8° C).

Reagents, Supplies, and Equipment

Reagents

- Commercial blood grouping antisera
- Anti-A and anti-B typing sera (store at 4° C)
- Group A and Group B reagent RBCs (store at 4° C)
- *Note:* Reagents must be used before the expiration date published on the label.

Supplies

- 10 × 75–mm test tubes
- Normal saline (0.9% NaCl)
- Disposable pipettes
- Marking pen

Equipment

- Centrifuge
- Magnifier reading device

Quality Control

- Positive control: known group A reagent RBCs should demonstrate agglutination with anti-A typing serum.
- Positive control: known group B reagent RBCs should demonstrate agglutination with anti-B typing serum.
- Negative control: known group A reagent RBCs should *not* demonstrate agglutination with anti-B typing serum.

- Negative control: known group B reagent RBCs should *not* demonstrate agglutination with anti-A typing serum.

Procedure Steps

1. Check the patient's name and identification number on the blood specimen and requisition.
2. Prepared a 2% to 5% suspension of the patient's RBCs in normal saline.
3. Label two test tubes, one with the letter A and the other with B.
4. To the tube labeled A, add 1 drop of anti-A antiserum.
5. To the tube labeled B, add 1 drop of anti-B antiserum.
6. Using a disposable pipette, add 1 drop of the cell suspension to each of the test tubes.
7. Mix well, and centrifuge the test tubes for 15 seconds at 3400 rpm.
8. Resuspend the cells with gentle agitation, and examine macroscopically for agglutination (see Agglutination Reactions).

Reporting and Interpretation of Results

Agglutination is an indication of an antigen-antibody bonding reaction.

- If anti-A yields agglutination with RBCs, the erythrocytes have the corresponding A antigen or group A.
- If anti-B yields agglutination with RBCs, the erythrocytes have the corresponding B antigen or group B.
- If anti-A yields agglutination with RBCs and anti-B yields agglutination with RBCs, the erythrocytes have both the corresponding A antigen and B antigen on the cellular membrane. This is a *group AB reaction*.
- If anti-A yields no agglutination with RBCs, the erythrocytes do not have the corresponding A antigen or group A. If anti-B yields no agglutination with RBCs, the erythrocytes do not have the corresponding B antigen or group B. This is a *group O reaction*.

Agglutination Reactions

Anti-A	Anti-B	Blood Group
Positive	Negative	A
Negative	Positive	B
Positive	Positive	AB
Negative	Negative	O

Sources of Error

Clinical Sources

Discrepancies in forward typing can result from conditions such as weak antigens, altered expression of antigens caused by disease, chimerism, or excessive blood group substances. Excess of blood group–specific substance caused by disorders (e.g., carcinoma of stomach and pancreas) that neutralize the reagent anti-A and anti-B can produces a false-negative or weak reaction in forward typing. Incorrect typing can result from additional antigens (e.g., acquired A-like and B-like antigens) or antibody-sensitized RBCs (e.g., autoimmune disorders).

If a patient has been recently transfused with non–group-specific blood, mixed-filed agglutination may be observed.

Technical Sources

- Antisera should not be cloudy, and need to be refrigerated unless being used.
- Do not rely on the color of tubes to identify reagent antisera. All tubes must be properly labeled.
- Do not perform tests at temperatures higher than room temperature.
- Observe for agglutination with a well-lit background.
- Record results immediately after observation.

Clinical Applications

Direct blood grouping is the first step in proper blood grouping. *Reverse grouping* involves using known reagent RBCs with blood serum for the detection of A or B antibodies.

Limitations

Reverse cell typing using a patient's serum containing isoantibodies should be performed to verify the results.

References

Turgeon ML: *Fundamentals of immunohematology,* ed 2, Baltimore, 1995, Williams & Wilkins, pp 344-346.

Serum Protein Electrophoresis Procedure

Principle

Serum protein electrophoresis is used to separate and quantitate serum proteins based on electrophoretic mobility on cellulose acetate.

Proteins are large molecules composed of amino acids. Depending on electron distributions resulting from covalent or ionic bonding of structural subgroups, proteins have different electrical charges at a given pH. Based on electrical charge, serum proteins can be fractionated into five classic fractions: albumin, alpha-1 (α_1), alpha-2 (α_2), beta (β), and gamma (γ) proteins. For the following method, the pH is 8.8. After the proteins are separated, the plate is placed in a solution of sulfosalicylic acid and Ponceau S to stain the protein bands. The intensity of the stain for each band is related to protein concentration.

Specimen Collection and Preparation

No special preparation of the patient is required before specimen collection. The patient must be positively identified when the specimen is collected, and the specimen must be labeled at the bedside. Specimen labels include the patient's full name, the date, the patient's hospital identification number, and the phlebotomist's initials. Bar coding is now a popular method of identification as well.

Blood should be drawn by aseptic technique. A minimum of 2 mL of whole blood (red-top evacuated tube) is required. Hemolysis or contamination with bacteria renders a specimen unsuitable for testing. Plasma should be avoided. Cerebrospinal fluid (CSF) may be used if concentrated approximately 100 times; urine may be used if concentrated up to 300 times, depending on original protein concentration.

Storage and Stability

If the test cannot be performed immediately, the specimen should be refrigerated (2° to 6° C) for 48 hours. CSF and urine specimens may be used after proper concentration with a concentrator. Inaccurate results may be obtained if specimens are left uncovered, because of evaporation.

Quality Control

For electrophoresis serum control, Kemtrol Serum Control–Normal or Kemtrol Serum Control–Abnormal may be used to verify all phases of the procedure and should be used on each test run. Refer to the package insert provided with the control for assay values.

Reagents, Supplies, and Equipment*

Chemical Needed (not provided in kit)

- Absolute methanol, reagent grade
- 5% acetic acid (v/v); add 50 mL of glacial acetic acid to 950 mL of deionized water.

Reagents and Supplies

1. Ponceau S stain; aqueous solution of 0.5% (w/v) Ponceau S in 10% (w/v) sulfosalicylic acid.
- **Preparation for use:** One vial of Ponceau S Stain is dissolved in 1 L of deionized water. Mix until thoroughly dissolved.
- **Storage and stability:** The stain may be stored as packaged or in a tightly closed staining dish at 15° to 30° C. The unopened stain is stable until the expiration date on the bottle.
- **Signs of deterioration:** The stain should be a homogeneous mixture free of precipitate. Do not use if excessive evaporation occurs or with large amounts of precipitate.
- **Warning:** Do not ingest.
2. Electra HR Buffer; tris-barbital–sodium barbital buffer.
- **Preparation for use:** Dissolve one package of dry buffer in 750 mL of deionized water. The buffer is ready for use when all material is dissolved and completely mixed.
- **Storage and stability:** The packaged buffer is stable until the expiration date on the package. Diluted buffer is stable for 2 months at 15° to 30° C when stored tightly closed.
- **Signs of deterioration:** Discard packaged buffer if the material shows signs of dampness or discoloration. Discard unused diluted buffer if it becomes turbid.
- **Warning:** Do not ingest; the buffer can be toxic.
3. Clear Aid polyethylene glycol (PEG).
- **Preparation for use:** Mix 30 parts glacial acetic acid with 70 parts absolute methanol and 4 parts Clear Aid. Stir until well mixed.

---

*Helena Laboratories, Beaumont, Texas.

- **Storage and stability:** Prepared Clear Aid should be stored in a tightly closed container at 15° to 30° C to prevent evaporation of the methanol. Clear Aid is stable until the expiration date on the bottle.
- **Signs of deterioration:** Clear Aid should be clear and colorless. It may appear cloudy when cold. Do not use if discolored. Discard the prepared solution if the plates appear cloudy after the clearing procedure.
- **Warning:** Do not ingest; the buffer can be toxic.
4. Titan III cellulose acetate plate.
- **Preparation for use:** The plates are ready for use as packaged.
- **Storage and stability:** The plates should be stored at 15° to 30° C and are stable indefinitely.
5. PermaClear solution; *N*-methylpyrrolidinone and PEG.
- **Preparation for use:** Add 55 mL of PermaClear to 45 mL of deionized water to make a working clearing solution. Mix well.
- **Storage and stability:** PermaClear should be stored at 15° to 30° C. It is stable until the expiration date on the bottle.
- **Signs of deterioration:** Discard solution if the plates turn white or do not clear as expected.
- **Warning:** Do not pipette by mouth; vapor is harmful. Flush affected areas with copious amounts of water if splashed. Seek immediate attention for eyes.

Equipment
- Hardware (available from Helena Laboratories in kit* or by order): Super Z applicator,* Super Z sample well plate (2),* Super Z aligning base,* Super Z-12 applicator,* Super Z-12 sample well plate (2),* Super CPK aligning base,* Zip Zone chamber,* 1000 staining set, 5-μL microdispenser and tubes,* Bufferizer.*
- Consumable (available from Helena Laboratories in kit* or by order): Zip Zone prep,* Titan III cellulose acetate plates,* glue stick,* blotter pads,* Titan plastic envelopes,* Helena marker,* Titan identification labels, Ponceau S stain,* Electra HR Buffer,* Clear Aid,* PermaClear,* electrophoresis serum control, Zip Zone chamber wicks,* Kemtrol Serum Control–Normal,* Kemtrol Serum Control–Abnormal,* Titan identification labels,* IOD, EWS digital power supply.
- Any high-quality scanning densitometer with visible transmittance capability can be used.
- Centrifuge (optional).
- Magnifier reading device (optional).

Quality Control Procedure: Step-by-Step Method
A. Titan III Plate Preparation
1. Properly code the required number of Titan III plates by marking on the glossy, hard side with a Helena marker. The identification mark should be placed in one corner so that it is always aligned with Sample No. 1.

---

*Product is provided in the serum protein kits.

2. Soak the plates for 20 minutes in diluted Electra HR Buffer. The plates should be soaked in the Bufferizer according to the instructions. Alternately, the plates may be wetted by slowly and uniformly lowering a rack of plates into the buffer so that air is not trapped in the plates. The same soaking buffer may be used for soaking up to 12 plates, or for approximately 1 week if stored tightly closed. If used longer, residual solvents from the plate may build up in the buffer, or evaporation may alter buffer concentration.

B. Electrophoresis Chamber Preparation
1. Pour approximately 100 mL of diluted Electra HR Buffer into each of the outer sections of the electrophoresis chamber. Do not use the same buffer in which the plates were soaked for electrophoresis.
2. Wet two disposable wicks in the buffer. Stand them lengthwise (on edge) in the buffer compartments. Fold the top edge of each wick over each support bridge, making sure the bottom edge is in the buffer and touching the bottom of the chamber. Press the top edge down over the bridge until the wick makes contact with the buffer and there are no air bubbles under the wicks.
3. Cover the chamber to saturate the air with buffer. Discard electrophoresis buffer after use.

C. Sample Application
1. Fill each well in the sample plate with 3 μL of sample using the microdispenser. Expel the samples as a bead on the tip of the glass tube; then touch this bead to the well. Cover the samples with a glass slide if they are not used within 2 minutes.
2. Prime the applicator by depressing the tips into the sample wells three or four times. Apply this loading to a piece of blotter paper. Priming the applicator makes the second loading much more uniform. Do not load applicator again at this point, but proceed quickly to the next step.
3. Remove the wetted Titan III plate from the buffer with the fingertips, and blot once firmly. Before placing the plate in the aligning base, place a drop of water or buffer on the center of the aligning base, to prevent the plate from shifting during the sample application. Place the plate in the aligning base, cellulose acetate side up, aligning the bottom edge of the plate with the black line marked "Center Application." The identification mark should be aligned with Sample No. 1.
4. Apply the sample to the plate by gently depressing the applicator tips into the sample well three or four times and promptly transferring the applicator to the aligning base. Press the button down and hold for 5 seconds.

D. Electrophoresis
1. Quickly place the cellulose acetate plate(s) side down, in the electrophoresis chamber. Place a weight (e.g., glass slide, coin) on the plates to ensure contact with the

wicks. Cover the chamber securely, and wait 30 seconds for the plates to equilibrate.

2. Electrophorese the plates for 15 minutes at 180 volts. Power must be applied within 5 minutes after plates have been placed in the chamber.

E. Visualization of the Protein Bands

1. At the end of the electrophoresis time, remove the plate(s) from the chamber. Place the plates in 40 to 50 mL of Ponceau S stain (sufficient volume to cover the plates) for 6 minutes. When staining two or more plates, carry out the protocol vertically in a rack. The stain may be reused until the plate background contains stain precipitate.

2. Destain in three successive 2-minute washes of 5% acetic acid or until the plate background is white. The plates may be dried and stored as a permanent record at this point, if stored in a plastic envelope to protect the surface. If a transparent background is desired (densitometry), proceed to the next step.

If using Clear Aid solution:

3. Dehydrate by rinsing the plate(s) in two absolute-methanol washes, 2 minutes for each wash. Allow the plates to drain for 5 to 10 seconds before placing in the next solution.

4. Place the plates into the clearing solution for 5 to 10 minutes.

5. Drain off excess solution, then place the plates, acetate side up, onto a blotter and into an IOD or other drying oven at 50° to 60° C for 15 minutes or until dry.

If using PermaClear solution:

3. Place the plate(s) into the diluted PermaClear solution for 2 minutes.

4. Drain off excess solution by holding plates vertically for 1 minute. Then place the plate, acetate side up, onto a blotter and into an IOD or other drying oven at 50° to 60° C for 15 minutes or until dry.

F. Evaluation of the Protein Bands

Scan the plates in a densitometer using a 525-nm filter and the narrow slit (size 4).

Stability of End Product

The completed, dried serum protein plate is stable for an indefinite period and may be stored in Titan plastic envelopes.

Calibration

The Optical Density Step Tablet should be used to ensure the linearity of the instrument, and a Neutral Density Densitometer Control should be used to validate the zero adjustment and quantitation by the instrument.

Calculation of the Unknown

The CliniScan-3 and other Helena densitometers with computer accessories will automatically print the relative percent and the absolute values for each band. Alternately, the relative percent of each band can be calculated manually by referring to the operator's manual provided with the densitometer.

The relative percent of each band is calculated by the following formula:

(Number of integration units of the band ÷
Total integration units) × 100 =
Relative percent of total integration units of the band

Relative percent × Total serum =
Absolute value of protein per band

Results

The fastest moving band, and normally the most prominent, is the albumin band found closest to the anodic edge of the plate. The faint band next to this is alpha-1 globulin, followed by alpha-2, beta, and gamma globulins. Prealbumin is seldom visible with this system.

Reference Values

Each laboratory should establish its own range. However, the reference values for serum protein electrophoresis on cellulose acetate stained with Ponceau S were determined from a study of 51 normal subjects. The following values are for illustrative purposes only:

Protein Fraction	Concentration (g/dL)
Albumin	3.63-4.91
Alpha-1	0.11-0.35
Alpha-2	0.65-1.17
Beta	0.74-1.26
Gamma	0.58-1.74

Clinical Interpretation

Electrophoresis is used to identify the presence or absence of aberrant proteins and to identify when different groups of proteins are increased or decreased in serum or urine. It is frequently ordered to detect and identify monoclonal proteins (excessive production of one specific immunoglobulin). Protein and immunofixation electrophoresis are ordered to help detect, diagnose, and monitor the course and treatment of conditions associated with these abnormal proteins (e.g., multiple myeloma).

References

Lab tests at a glance, May 2006, www.labtestsonline.org.

Helena Laboratories, Beaumont, Texas, 2007.

CHAPTER HIGHLIGHTS

- Foreign substances can be immunogenic if their membrane or molecular components contain structures (antigenic determinants or epitopes) that are recognized as foreign by the immune system. The normal immune system responds to foreignness by producing antibodies.

- Cellular antigens of importance to immunologists include MHC groups and HLAs, autoantigens, and blood group antigens. Some of these antigens (e.g., MHC) are much more potent than others in provoking an immune response.

- Antigens are usually large, organic molecules that are either proteins or polysaccharides. Although large foreign molecules are better antigens, haptens (can bind to larger carrier molecules and behave as antigens.
- Antibodies that are specific glycoproteins are known as immunoglobulins. Many antibodies can be isolated in the gamma-globulin fraction of protein by electrophoresis separation. The primary function of an antibody in body defenses is to combine with antigen.
- Five distinct classes of immunoglobulin molecules are recognized: IgM, IgG, IgA, IgD, and IgE. Antibodies exhibit diversity among the different classes, suggesting different functions in addition to their primary function of antigen binding.
- A typical monomeric IgG molecule consists of three globular regions (two Fab regions and Fc portion) linked by a flexible hinge region.
- An antigenic determinant is the specific chemical determinant group or molecular configuration against which the immune response is directed. Because they are proteins, immunoglobulins can function as effective antigens when used to immunize mammals of a different species. When the resulting antiimmunoglobulins or antiglobulins are analyzed, three principal categories of antigenic determinants can be recognized: isotype, allotype, and idiotype.
- Production of antibodies is induced when the host's immune system comes into contact with a foreign antigenic substance and reacts to this antigenic stimulation. When an antigen is initially encountered, the cells of the immune system recognize the antigen as "nonself" and elicit an immune response or become tolerant of it. An immune reaction can be cell-mediated immunity (dependent on T cells and macrophages) or may involve the production of antibodies directed against the antigen.
- After a foreign antigen challenge, an IgM antibody response proceeds in four phases: lag, log, plateau, and decline. Subsequent exposure to the same antigenic stimulus produces an anamnestic (secondary) response, which exhibits the same four phases but differs from a primary response in time, type of antibody produced, and antibody titer.
- Specificity is the ability of a particular antibody to combine with one antigen instead of another.
- Affinity is the bonding strength between an antigenic determinant and antibody-combining site, whereas avidity is the strength with which a multivalent antibody binds a multivalent antigen.
- Agglutination and other tests (precipitation reactions, hemolysis testing, ELISA) are widely used in immunology to detect and measure the consequences of antigen-antibody interaction.
- Monoclonal antibodies (MAbs) are purified antibodies cloned from a single cell. MAbs bound to cell surface antigens now provide a method for classifying and identifying specific cellular membrane characteristics and leukocyte antigens.

REVIEW QUESTIONS

1. A synonym for an antigenic determinant is:
   a. Immunogen.
   b. Epitope.
   c. Binding site.
   d. Polysaccharide.

2. Genetically different individuals are referred to as:
   a. Allogenic.
   b. Heterogenic.
   c. Autogenic.
   d. Isogenic.

3. Antigenic substances can be composed of:
   a. Large polysaccharides.
   b. Proteins.
   c. Glycoproteins.
   d. All the above.

4. Which of the following characteristics of an antigen is the *least* important?
   a. Foreignness.
   b. Degradability.
   c. Molecular weight
   d. Presence of large, repeating polymers.

5. The chemical composition of an antibody is:
   a. Protein.
   b. Lipid.
   c. Carbohydrate.
   d. Glycoprotein.

Questions 6-10. Match the following characteristics with the appropriate antibody class (use an answer only once).

6. _____ IgM

7. _____ IgG

8. _____ IgA

9. _____ IgE

10. _____ IgD

    a. Highest in plasma/serum concentration in normal individuals.
    b. Shortest half-life.
    c. 19S.
    d. Can exist as a dimer.
    e. No known subclasses.

Questions 11-15. Match the following characteristics with the appropriate antibody.

11. _____ IgG

12. _____ IgM

13. _____ IgA

14. _____ IgD

15. _____ IgE
    a. Predominant immunoglobulin in secretions.
    b. Increased in infectious diseases, collagen disorders, and hematologic disorders.
    c. Mediates some types of hypersensitivity reactions.
    d. Primarily a cell membrane immunoglobulin.
    e. Produced early in an immune response.

Questions 16-18. Match each of the following antigenic determinant terms with its appropriate definition.

16. _____ Isotype

17. _____ Allotype

18. _____ Idiotype
    a. Found on the immunoglobulins of some, but not all, animals of a species.
    b. Dominant type found on immunoglobulins of all animals of a species.
    c. Individual determinants characteristic of each antibody.

Questions 19-22. Arrange the sequence of events of a typical antibody response.

19. _____

20. _____

21. _____

22. _____
    a. Plateau
    b. Lag phase
    c. Log phase
    d. Decline

23. Which of the following statements is *false* about an anamnestic response versus a primary response?
    a. Has a shorter lag phase.
    b. Has a longer plateau.
    c. Antibodies decline more gradually.
    d. IgM antibodies predominate.

24. Which type of antibody is capable of placental transfer?
    a. IgM
    b. IgG
    c. IgA
    d. IgD

Questions 25-28. Match the following terms and their respective definitions.

25. _____ Specificity

26. _____ Affinity

27. _____ Avidity

28. _____ Immune complex
    a. Strength of a bond between a single antigenic determinant and an individual combining site.
    b. Noncovalent combination of an antigen with its respective specific antibody.
    c. Ability of an antibody to combine with one antigen instead of another.
    d. Strength with which a multivalent antibody binds to a multivalent antigen.

29. Which of the following type(s) of bonding is (are) involved in antigen-antibody reactions?
    a. Hydrophobic
    b. Hydrogen
    c. Van der Waals
    d. All the above

30. Monovalent antibodies have also been referred to as:
    a. Complete antibodies.
    b. Incomplete antibodies.

31. Which of the following is an accurate statement about monoclonal antibodies (MAbs)?
    a. MAbs are antibodies engineered to bind to a single epitope.
    b. MAbs are purified antibodies cloned from a single cell.
    c. MAbs are used to classify and identify specific cellular membrane characteristics.
    d. All the above are correct.

32. Antigens are characterized by all the following *except* that they:
    a. Are usually large organic molecules.
    b. Are usually lipids.
    c. Can be glycolipids or glycoproteins.
    d. Are also called immunogens.

33. The immunogenicity of an antigen depends greatly on:
    a. Its biochemical composition.
    b. Being structurally unstable.
    c. Its degree of foreignness.
    d. Having a low molecular weight.

34. Antibodies are also referred to as:
    a. Immunoglobulins.
    b. Haptens.
    c. Epitopes.
    d. Gamma globulins.

Questions 35-39. Match the following immunoglobulins with the appropriate description.

35. _____ IgM

36. _____ IgG

37. _____ IgA

38. _____ IgE

39. _____ IgD

  a. Accounts for 10% of Ig pool, largely confined to the intravascular space.
  b. Mediates some types of hypersensitivity.
  c. Found in tears, saliva, colostrum, milk, and intestinal secretions.
  d. Makes up less than 1% of total immunoglobulins.
  e. Diffuses more readily into extravascular spaces, neutralizes toxins, and binds to microorganisms.

Questions 40 and 41. Label the components of the basic immunoglobulin (Ig) configuration in the following figure.

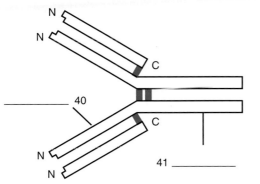

(Redrawn from Turgeon ML: Fundamentals of immunohematology, ed 2, Baltimore, 1995, Williams & Wilkins.)

Possible answers for question 40:
  a. Fc segment
  b. Fab segment
  c. Hinge region
  d. Disulfide bond

Possible answers for question 41:
  a. Fc segment
  b. Fab segment
  c. Hinge region
  d. Disulfide bond

42. Which of the following statements about IgM is *false*?
  a. Composed of five basic subunits.
  b. More efficient in the activation of the complement cascade and agglutination than IgG.
  c. Predominant in an initial antibody response.
  d. Predominant in a secondary (anamnestic) response.

Questions 43-46. Label the four phases of an antibody response on the following figure, choosing from the following answers:
  a. Log
  b. Plateau
  c. Lag
  d. Decline

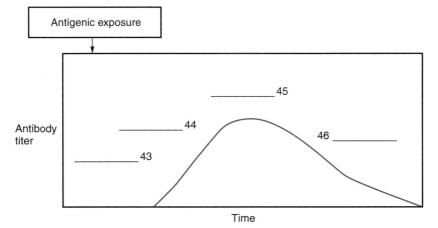

(Redrawn from Turgeon ML: Fundamentals of immunohematology, ed 2, Baltimore, 1995, Williams & Wilkins.)

47. In a secondary (anamnestic) response, all the following characteristics are correct *except:*
    a. IgG is the predominant antibody type.
    b. It has a shorter lag phase.
    c. The antibody titer is lower.
    d. It has a more gradual decline in antibody response.

48. Bonding of antigen to antibody consists of:
    a. Hydrogen bonding.
    b. Van der Waals forces.
    c. Electrostatic forces.
    d. Noncovalent bonding.

49. The strongest bond of antigen and antibody chiefly results from the:
    a. Type of bonding.
    b. Goodness of fit.
    c. Antibody type.
    d. Quantity of antibody.

50. Monoclonal antibodies have all the following characteristics *except:*
    a. Purified antibodies.
    b. Cloned from a single cell.
    c. Engineered to bind to a single specific antigen.
    d. Frequent occurrence in nature.

BIBLIOGRAPHY

Baron EJ, Peterson LR, Finegold SM: *Bailey and Scott's diagnostic microbiology,* ed 9, St Louis, 1994, Mosby.

Barrett JT: *Textbook of immunology,* ed 5, St Louis, 1988, Mosby.

Bellanti JA: *Immunology: basic processes,* Philadelphia, 1979, Saunders.

Medzhitov R, Janeway C: Innate immunity, *N Engl J Med* 343(5):338-344, 2000.

McDougal JS, McDuffie FC: Detection and significance of immune complexes, *Adv Clin Chem* 24:4, 1985.

Ritzmann SE, Daniels JC, editors: *Serum protein abnormalities,* Boston, 1985, Little, Brown.

Ritzmann SE, editor: *Physiology of immunoglobulins,* New York, 1982, Alan R Liss.

Roitt IM: *Essential immunology,* ed 5, Oxford, England, 1984, Blackwell Scientific Publications.

Turgeon ML: *Fundamentals of immunohematology,* ed 2, Baltimore, 1995, Williams & Wilkins.

CHAPTER 3

Cells and Cellular Activities of the Immune System: Granulocytes and Mononuclear Cells

Origin and Development of Blood Cells
Granulocytic Cells
    Neutrophils
    Eosinophils and Basophils
Process of Phagocytosis
    Chemotaxis
    Adherence
    Engulfment
    Digestion
    Subsequent Phagocytic Activity
Monocytes-Macrophages
    Mononuclear Phagocyte System
    Host Defense Functions
Acute Inflammation
Sepsis

Cell Surface Receptors
Disorders of Neutrophils
    Noninfectious Neutrophil-Mediated Inflammatory
        Disease
    Abnormal Neutrophil Function
    Congenital Neutrophil Abnormalities
Monocyte-Macrophage Disorders
    Gaucher's Disease
    Niemann-Pick Disease
Disease States Involving Leukocyte Integrins
Case Studies
Screening Test for Phagocytic Engulfment
Chapter Highlights
Review Questions
Bibliography

Learning Objectives

At the conclusion of this chapter, the reader should be able to:

- Describe the general functions of granulocytes, monocytes-macrophages, and lymphocytes and plasma cells as components of the immune system.
- Explain the process of phagocytosis.
- Discuss the role of monocytes-macrophages in cellular immunity.
- Define and compare acute inflammation and sepsis.

- Briefly describe cell surface receptors.
- Name and compare the signs and symptoms of disorders of neutrophil function.
- Compare the signs and symptoms of two monocyte-macrophage disorders.
- Describe states involving the leukocyte integrins.
- Analyze case studies related to defects of neutrophils.

The entire leukocytic cell system is designed to defend the body against disease. Each cell type has a unique function and behaves both independently and, in many cases, in cooperation with other cell types. Leukocytes can be functionally divided into the general categories of granulocyte, monocyte-macrophage, and lymphocyte–plasma cell. The primary phagocytic cells are the polymorphonuclear neutrophilic (PMN) leukocytes and the mononuclear monocytes-macrophages. The response of the body to pathogens involves "cross-talk" among many immune cells, including macrophages, dendritic cells, and CD4 T cells (Figure 3-1). The lymphocytes participate in body defenses primarily through the recognition of foreign antigen and production of antibody. Plasma cells are antibody-synthesizing cells.

ORIGIN AND DEVELOPMENT OF BLOOD CELLS

Embryonic blood cells, excluding the lymphocyte type of white blood cell (WBC), originate from the mesenchymal tissue that arises from the embryonic germ layer, the meso-derm. The sites of blood cell development, **hematopoiesis,** follow a definite sequence in the embryo and fetus:

1. The first blood cells are primitive red blood cells (erythroblasts; RBCs) formed in the islets of the yolk sac during the first 2 to 8 weeks of life.
2. Gradually the liver and spleen replace the yolk sac as the sites of blood cell development. By the second month of gestation, the liver becomes the major site of hematopoiesis, and granular types of leukocytes have made their initial appearance. The liver and spleen predominate from about 2 to 5 months of fetal life.
3. In the fourth month of gestation, bone marrow begins to produce blood cells. After the fifth fetal month, bone marrow begins to assume its ultimate role as the primary site of hematopoiesis.

The cellular elements of the blood are produced from a common, multipotential, **hematopoietic** (blood-producing) cell, the stem cell. After stem cell differentiation, blast cells arise for each of the major categories of cell types: erythrocytes, megakaryocytes, granulocytes, monocytes-macrophages, lymphocytes, and plasma cells. Subsequent maturation of these

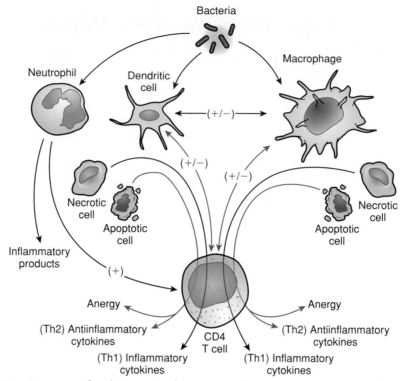

Figure 3-1   Response of pathogens, involving cross-talk among many immune cells, including macrophages, dendritic cells, and CD4 T cells. Macrophages and dendritic cells are activated by the ingestion of bacteria and by stimulation through cytokines (e.g., interferon-γ) secreted by CD4 T cells. Alternatively, CD4 T cells that have an antiinflammatory profile (type 2 helper T cells [Th2]) secrete interleukin-10, which suppresses macrophage activation. CD4 T cells become activated by stimulation through macrophages or dendritic cells. For example, macrophages and dendritic cells secrete interleukin-12, which activates CD4 T cells to secrete inflammatory (type 1 helper T-cell [Th1]) cytokines. Depending on numerous factors (e.g., the type of organism and the site of infection), macrophages and dendritic cells respond by inducing either inflammatory or antiinflammatory cytokines or causing a global reduction in cytokine production (anergy). Macrophages or dendritic cells that have previously ingested necrotic cells induce an inflammatory cytokine profile (Th1). Ingestion of apoptotic cells can induce either an antiinflammatory cytokine profile or anergy. A plus sign indicates upregulation, and a minus sign indicates downregulation; in cases in which both a plus sign and a minus sign appear, either upregulation or downregulation may occur, depending on a variety of factors. *(Modified from Hotchkiss RS, Karl IE: N Engl J Med 348(2):138, 2003.)*

cells will produce the major cellular elements of the circulating blood, the erythrocytes (RBCs), thrombocytes, and specific types of leukocytes (WBCs). In normal peripheral or circulating blood, the following types of leukocytes can be found in order of frequency: neutrophils, lymphocytes, monocytes, eosinophils, and basophils.

GRANULOCYTIC CELLS

Granulocytic leukocytes can be further subdivided on the basis of morphology into neutrophils, eosinophils, and basophils. Each of these begins as a multipotential stem cell in the bone marrow.

Neutrophils

The neutrophilic leukocyte, particularly the polymorphonuclear (PMN) type, provides an effective host defense against bacterial and fungal infections. Although the monocytes-macrophages and other granulocytes are also phagocytic

cells, the neutrophil is the principal leukocyte associated with phagocytosis and a localized inflammatory response. The formation of an inflammatory exudate (pus), which develops rapidly in an inflammatory response, is composed primarily of neutrophils and monocytes.

Mature neutrophils are found in two evenly divided pools, the circulating and marginating pools. The marginating granulocytes adhere to the vascular endothelium. In the peripheral blood, these cells are only in transit to their potential sites of action in the tissues. Movement of granulocytes from the circulating pool to the peripheral tissues occurs by a process called **diapedesis** (movement through the vessel wall). Once in the peripheral tissues, the neutrophils are able to carry out their function of phagocytosis.

The granules of segmented neutrophils contain various antibacterial substances, including lysosomal hydrolases, lysozyme, and peroxidase. Some of these granules are typical lysosomes. During the phagocytic process, however, the powerful antimicrobial enzymes that are released also disrupt the integrity of the cell itself. Neutrophils are also steadily lost to the respiratory, gastrointestinal (GI), and urinary systems, where they participate in generalized phagocytic activities. An alternate route for the removal of neutrophils from the circulation is phagocytosis by cells of the mononuclear phagocyte system.

Eosinophils and Basophils

Although capable of participating in phagocytosis, eosinophils and basophils possess less phagocytic activity. The ineffectiveness of these cells results from both the small number of cells in the circulating blood and the lack of powerful digestive enzymes. Both eosinophils and basophils, however, are functionally important in body defense.

Eosinophils

The eosinophil is considered to be a homeostatic regulator of inflammation. Functionally, this means that the eosinophil attempts to suppress an inflammatory reaction to prevent the excessive spread of the inflammation. The eosinophil may also play a role in the host defense mechanism because of its ability to kill certain parasites.

A functional property related to the membrane receptors of the eosinophil is the cell's ability to interact with the larval stages of some helminth parasites and damage them through oxidative mechanisms. Certain proteins released from eosinophilic granules damage antibody-coated *Schistosoma* parasites and may account for damage to endothelial cells in hypereosinophilic syndromes.

Basophils

Basophils have high concentrations of heparin and histamine in their granules, which play an important role in acute, systemic, hypersensitivity reactions (see Chapter 26). Degranulation occurs when an antigen such as pollen binds to two adjacent immunoglobulin E (IgE) antibody molecules located on the surface of mast cells. The events resulting from the release of the contents of these basophilic granules include increased vascular permeability, smooth muscle spasm, and vasodilation. If severe, this reaction can result in anaphylactic shock.

A newly identified class of compounds, the **leukotrienes,** mediate the inflammatory functions of leukocytes. The observed systemic reactions related to leukotrienes were previously attributed to the slow-reacting substance of anaphylaxis.

PROCESS OF PHAGOCYTOSIS

Phagocytosis can be divided into six stages: chemotaxis, adherence, engulfment, phagosome formation, fusion, and digestion and destruction (Figure 3-2). The physical occurrence of damage to tissues, either by trauma or microbial multiplication, releases substances such as activated complement components and products of infection to initiate phagocytosis.

Chemotaxis

Various phagocytic cells continually circulate throughout the blood, lymph, GI system, and respiratory tract. When trauma occurs, the neutrophils arrive at the site of injury and can be found in the initial exudate in less than 1 hour. Monocytes are slower in moving to the inflammatory site. Macrophages resident in the tissues of the body are already in place to deal with an intruding agent. Additional macrophages from the bone marrow and other tissues can be released in severe infections.

Segmented neutrophils are able to gather quickly at the site of injury because they are actively motile. The marginating pool of neutrophils, adhering to the endothelial lining of nearby blood vessels, migrates through the vessel wall to the interstitial tissues. Mediators produced by microorgan-

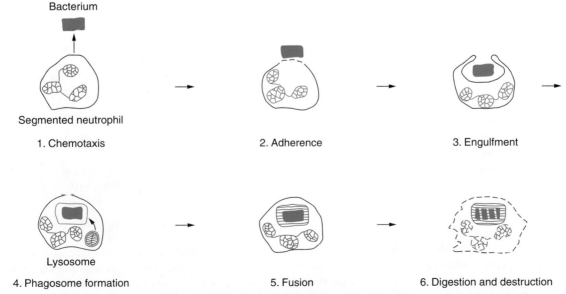

Figure 3-2 Process of phagocytosis. *(Redrawn from Turgeon ML: Clinical hematology: theory and procedures, ed 4, Philadelphia, 2005, Lippincott–Williams & Wilkins.)*

isms and by cells participating in the inflammatory process include **interleukin-1 (IL-1),** which is released by macrophages in response to infection or tissue injury. Another is **histamine,** released by circulating basophils, tissue mast cells, and blood platelets. Mediators cause capillary and venular dilation.

Cells are guided to the site of injury by the chemoattractant substances. This event is termed **chemotaxis.** A "chemotactic response" is defined as a change in the direction of movement of a motile cell in response to a concentration gradient of a specific chemical, chemotaxin. Chemotaxins can induce both a positive movement toward and a negative movement away from a chemotactic response. Antigens function as chemoattractants and when antigenic material is present in the body, phagocytes are attracted to its source by moving up its concentration gradient.

Phagocytes detect antigens using various cell surface receptors. The speed of phagocytosis can be greatly increased by recruiting the following two attachment devices present on the surface of phagocytic cells:

- **Fc receptor:** binds the Fc portion of antibody molecules, chiefly immunoglobulin G (IgG). The IgG attaches to the organism through its Fab site.
- **Complement receptor:** the third component of complement, C3, also binds to organisms and then attaches to the complement receptor.

This coating of the organisms by molecules that speed up phagocytosis is termed **opsonization,** and the Fc portion of antibody and C3 are called **opsonins.** The steps in opsonization are as follows:

1. Antibody attached to the surface of a bacterium minimally binds the Fc phagocyte receptor.
2. Complement C3b is attached to the surface of the bacterium and binds loosely to the phagocyte C3b receptor.
3. Both antibody and C3b are attached to the surface of the bacterium and bound tightly to the phagocyte, allowing greater opportunity for the phagocyte to engulf the bacterium.

Adherence

The "leukocyte adhesion cascade" is a sequence of adhesion and activation events that ends with the cell exerting its effects on the inflamed site (see Acute Inflammation, p. 38). At least five steps appear to be necessary for effective leukocyte recruitment to the site of injury: capture, rolling, slow rolling, firm adhesion, and transmigration.

The process known as capture (tethering) represents the first contact of a leukocyte with the activated endothelium. Capture occurs after margination, which allows phagocytes to move in a position close to the endothelium. P-selectin on endothelial cells is the primary adhesion molecule for capture and the initiation of rolling. In addition, many studies suggest that L-selectin also has an important role in capture. Other cell adhesion molecules (CAMs) have been implicated in capture, although their level of actual involvement varies (e.g., PECAM-1, ICAM-1,

VE-cadherin, LFA-1 [CD11a/CD18], IAP [CD47], VLA-4 [$4\beta_1$-integrin]).

The inflammatory response begins with a release of inflammatory chemicals into the extracellular fluid. Sources of these inflammatory mediators, the most important of which are histamine, prostaglandins, and cytokines, are injured tissue cells, lymphocytes, mast cells, and blood proteins. The presence of these chemicals promotes the reactions to inflammation (redness, heat, swelling, pain).

The transit time through the microcirculation and, more specifically, the contact time during which the leukocyte is close to the endothelium, appears to be a key parameter in determining the success of the recruitment process, as reflected in firm adhesion.

Engulfment

On reaching the site of infection, phagocytes engulf and destroy the foreign matter (Figure 3-3). Eosinophils can also undergo this process, except that they kill parasites. After the phagocytic cells have arrived at the site of injury, the bacteria can be engulfed through active membrane invagination. Pseudopodia are extended around the pathogen, pulled by interactions between the Fc receptors and Fc antibody portions on the opsonized bacterium. Pseudopodia meet and fuse, thereby internalizing the bacterium and enclosing it in a phagocytic vacuole, or **phagosome.**

The principal factor in determining whether phagocytosis can occur is the physical nature of the surface of both the bacteria and the phagocytic cell. The bacteria must be more hydrophobic than the phagocyte. Some bacteria, such as *Diplococcus pneumoniae,* possess a hydrophilic capsule and are not normally phagocytized. Most nonpathogenic bacteria are easily phagocytized because they are very hydrophobic. The presence of certain soluble factors such as complement,

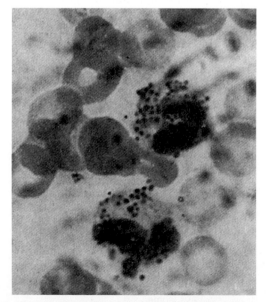

Figure 3-3 Two phagocytic cells have engulfed numerous *Staphylococcus aureus* cells. *(From Barrett JT: Textbook of immunology, ed 5, St Louis, 1988, Mosby.)*

a plasma protein, coupled with antibodies, and chemicals such as acetylcholine enhance the phagocytic process. Enhancement of phagocytosis through opsonization can speed up the ingestion of particles. If the surface tensions are conducive to engulfment, the phagocytic cell membrane invaginates. This invagination leads to the formation of an isolated vacuole (phagosome) within the cell.

Digestion

Digestion follows ingestion of particles, with the required energy primarily provided by anaerobic glycolysis. Granules in the phagocyte cytosol then migrate to and fuse with the phagosome to form the phagolysosome. These granules contain degradatory enzymes of the following three types:

1. *Primary,* or azurophilic, granules containing enzymes (e.g., lysozyme, myeloperoxidase).
2. *Secondary,* or specific, granules containing substances such as lactoferrin.
3. *Tertiary* granules containing substance such as capsases.

Degranulation of the neutrophil releases antibacterial substances (e.g., lactoferrin, lysozyme, defensin) from the granules; released enzymes promote bactericidal activity by increasing membrane permeability. *Elastase,* one of several substances that can damage host tissues, is also released. The myeloperoxidase granules are responsible for the action of the oxygen-dependent, myeloperoxidase-mediated system. Hydrogen peroxide (H_2O_2) and an oxidizable cofactor serve as major factors in the actual killing of bacteria within the vacuole. Other oxygen-independent systems, such as alterations in pH, lysozymes, lactoferrin, and the granular cationic proteins, also participate in the bactericidal process. Monocytes are particularly effective as phagocytic cells because of the large amounts of lipase in their cytoplasm. Lipase is able to attack bacteria with a lipid capsule, such as *Mycobacterium tuberculosis.* Monocytes are further able to bind and destroy cells coated with complement-fixing antibodies because of the presence of membrane receptors for specific components or types of immunoglobulin.

Release of lytic enzymes results in destruction of neutrophils and their subsequent phagocytosis by macrophages. Macrophage digestion proceeds without risk to the cell unless the ingested material is toxic. If the ingested material damages the lysosomal membrane, however, the macrophage will also be destroyed because of the release of lysosomal enzymes.

During phagocytosis, cells demonstrate increased metabolic activity, referred to as "respiratory burst." This results in the production by the phagocyte of large quantities of reactive oxygen species (ROS), which are released into the phagocytic vesicle. This phenomenon is achieved by the activity of the enzyme reduced nicotinamide-adenine dinucleotide phosphate (NADPH) oxidase. Together, the granule-mediated and NADPH oxidase–mediated effects elicit microbicidal results. NADPH oxidase forms the centerpiece of the phagocyte-killing mechanism and is activated in about 2 seconds. The NADPH oxidase generates ROS by generating the superoxide radical (O_2^-); the associated cyanide-insensitive increase in oxygen consumption is the respiratory burst.

The importance of the oxygen-dependent microbicidal mechanism is dramatically illustrated by patients with chronic granulomatous disease (CGD), a severe congenital deficit in bacterial killing that results from the inability to produce superoxide. CGD results from defects in the genes encoding individual components of the enzyme system responsible for oxidant production. Acquisition of oxidase activity occurs in the course of myeloid cell maturation, and the genes for several of its components have been identified. This system also lends itself to analysis of the transcriptional and translational events that occur during cellular differentiation and under the influence of specific cytokines.

Rather than being discarded by exocytosis, some peptides undergo an important separate process at this stage. Instead of being eliminated, they attach to a host molecule called **major histocompatibility complex (MHC)** class II and are expressed on the surface of the cell within a groove on the MHC molecule (antigen presentation).

Subsequent Phagocytic Activity

If invading bacteria are not phagocytized at entry into the body, they may establish themselves in secondary sites such as the lymph nodes or various body organs. These undigested bacteria produce a secondary inflammation, where neutrophils and macrophages again congregate. If bacteria escape from secondary tissue sites, a bacteremia will develop. In patients who are unresponsive to antibiotic intervention, this situation can prove fatal.

MONOCYTES-MACROPHAGES

In the past the mononuclear monocyte-macrophage was known only as a "scavenger cell." Only recently has its role as a complex cell of the immune system in the host defense against infection been recognized.

Mononuclear Phagocyte System

The macrophage and its precursors (Figure 3-4) are widely distributed throughout the body. These cells constitute a physiologic system, the **mononuclear phagocyte system** (previously "reticuloendothelial system"), which includes promonocytes and their precursors in the bone marrow, monocytes in the circulating blood, and macrophages in tissues. This collection of cells is considered to be a "system" because of their common origin, similar morphology, and shared functions, including rapid phagocytosis mediated by receptors for IgG and the major fragment of C3.

Macrophages and monocytes, migrate freely into the tissues from the blood to replenish and reinforce the macrophage population (Figure 3-5). Cells of the macrophage system originate in the bone marrow from the multipotential stem cell. This common, committed progenitor cell can differentiate into either the granulocyte or the monocyte-macrophage pathway, depending on the microenvironment and chemical regulators. Maturation and differentiation of these

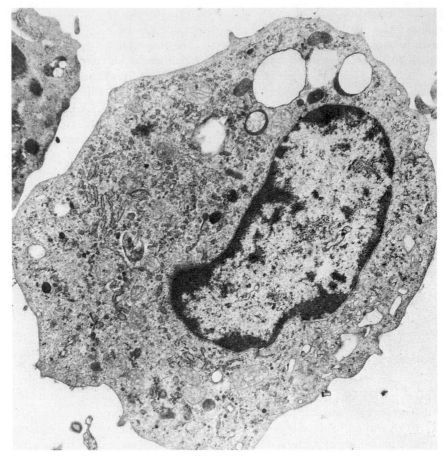

Figure 3-4   Electron micrograph of a macrophage. *(From Barrett JT: Textbook of immunology, ed 5, St Louis, 1988, Mosby.)*

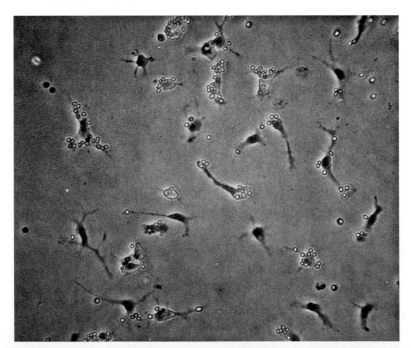

Figure 3-5   Macrophages in culture. Note their elongated form, indicative of their motility. The cellular refractile bodies are erythrocytes that the macrophages are phagocytosing. *(From Barrett JT: Textbook of immunology, ed 5, St Louis, 1988, Mosby.)*

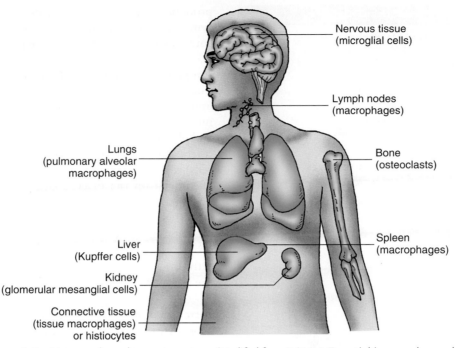

Figure 3-6 Mononuclear phagocyte system. *(Modified from Roitt IM: Essential immunology, ed 5, Oxford, 1984, Blackwell Scientific.)*

cells may occur in various directions. Circulating monocytes may continue to be multipotential and give rise to different types of macrophages.

Macrophages exist as either "fixed" or "wandering" cells. Specialized macrophages such as the pulmonary alveolar macrophages are the "dust phagocytes" of the lung that function as the first line of defense against inhaled foreign particles and bacteria. Fixed macrophages line the endothelium of capillaries and the sinuses of organs such as the bone marrow, spleen, and lymph nodes. Macrophages, along with the network of reticular cells of the spleen, thymus, and other lymphoid tissues, are organized into the mononuclear phagocyte system (Figure 3-6).

Functionally, the most important step in the maturation of macrophages is the cytokine-driven conversion of the normal resting macrophage to the activated macrophage. Macrophages can be activated during infection by the release of macrophage-activating cytokines such as interferon gamma (IFN-γ) and granulocyte colony-stimulating factor (G-CSF), from T lymphocytes specifically sensitized to antigens from the infecting microorganisms. This interaction constitutes the basis of cell-mediated immunity. In addition, macrophages exposed to an endotoxin release a hormone, tumor necrosis factor alpha (TNF-α, cachectin), which can activate macrophages itself under certain in vitro conditions.

The terminal stage of development in the mononuclear phagocyte cell line is the multinucleated giant cell, which characterizes granulomatous inflammatory diseases such as tuberculosis. Both monocytes and macrophages can be shown in the lesions in these diseases before the formation of giant cells, thought to be precursors to the multinucleated cells.

Host Defense Functions

Functionally, monocytes-macrophages have phagocytosis as their major role, but these cells perform at least three distinct but interrelated functions in host defense. The categories of host defense functions of monocytes-macrophages include phagocytosis, antigen presentation and induction of the immune response, and secretion of biologically active molecules.

Phagocytosis

The principal functions of mononuclear phagocytes in body defenses result from the changes that take place in these functions when the macrophage is activated (Box 3-1). Macrophages carry out the fundamental function of ingesting and killing invading microorganisms such as intracellular parasites, *M. tuberculosis,* and some fungi. In addition, macrophages remove and eliminate such extracellular pathogens as pneumococci from the blood circulation. The macrophage also has the capacity to phagocytize particulate and aggregated soluble materials. This process is enhanced by the presence of receptors on the surface of the Fc portion of IgG and C3. The ability to internalize soluble substances supports the increased microbicidal and tumoricidal ability of activated macrophages.

Another important phagocytic function of macrophages is their ability to dispose of damaged or dying cells. Macrophages lining the sinusoids of the spleen are particularly important in ingesting aging erythrocytes. They are also

Increased Activity in Activated Macrophages
Antigen presentation
Chemotaxis
Glucose transport and metabolism
Microbicidal activity
Phagocytosis (variable activity, depending on particle)
Phagocytosis-associated respiratory burst
Pinocytosis
Tumoricidal activity

Increased Constituents in Activated Macrophages
Acid hydrolases
Angiogenesis factor
Arginase
Collagenase
Complement components*
Cytolytic proteinase
Fibronectin
Interleukin-1
Interferon (alpha and beta)
Plasminogen activator
Tumor necrosis factor(cachectin)†

Decreased Constituents in Activated Macrophages
Apolipoprotein E and lipoprotein lipase
Elastase
Prostaglandins, leukotrienes

Constituent Demonstrating No Change in Activated Macrophages
Lysoenzyme

Modified from Johnston RB: *N Engl J Med* 318(12):749, 1988.
*Increased or no change.
†When stimulated.

involved in removing tissue debris, repairing wounds, and removing debris as embryonic tissues replace one another.

Phagocytic activity increases when there is tissue damage and inflammation, which releases substances that attract macrophages. Activated macrophages migrate more vigorously in response to chemotactic factors and should enter sites of inflammation (e.g., locations of infection or cancer) more efficiently than resting macrophages. Migration of monocytes into different body tissues appears to be a random phenomenon in the absence of localized inflammation. An essential factor in the protective function of monocytes is the capacity of the cell to move through the endothelial wall of blood vessels (diapedesis) to the site of microbial invasion in tissues. The attracting forces for monocytes, chemotactic factors, include complement products and chemoattractants derived from neutrophils, lymphocytes, or cancer cells.

The activity of mononuclear phagocytes against cancer cells in humans is less well understood than the phagocytosis of microorganisms. Phagocytes are thought to suppress the growth of spontaneously arising tumors. The ability of these cells to control malignant cells may not involve phagocytosis, but it may be related to secreted cellular products such as lysosomal enzymes, oxygen metabolites (e.g., H_2O_2),

proteinases, and TNF-α, (cachectin). The proteolytic enzymes present on the surface membrane of monocytes could also have a role in tumor rejection.

Antigen Presentation and Induction of Immune Response
The phagocytic property of the macrophage is particularly important in the processing of antigens as part of the immune response. Macrophages are believed to process antigens and physically present this biochemically modified and more reactive form of antigen to lymphocytes (particularly T-helper cells) as an initial step in the immune response. Recognition of antigen on the macrophage surface by T lymphocytes, however, requires an additional match of the surface MHC class II gene product. This gene product is the Ia product in the mouse and D gene region product in humans. With proper recognition, the macrophage secretes a lymphocyte-activating factor (IL-1), lymphocyte proliferation ensues, and the immune response (T-cell/B-cell response) is facilitated.

Secretion of Biologically Active Molecules
Monocytes-macrophages release many factors associated with host defense and inflammation. These cells serve as supportive "accessory" cells to lymphocytes, at least partly by releasing soluble factors. In cellular immunity, monocytes assume a "killer" role in that they are activated by sensitized lymphocytes to phagocytize offending cells or antigen particles. This is important in fields such as tumor immunology.

In addition to their phagocytic properties, monocytes-macrophages are able to synthesize a number of biologically important compounds, including transferrin, complement, interferon, pyrogens, and certain growth factors. Approximately 100 distinct substances have been identified as being secreted by monocytes-macrophages.

Blood monocytes and tissue macrophages are primary sources of the polypeptide hormones called IL-1, which have a particularly potent effect on the inflammatory response. IL-1 also supports B-lymphocyte proliferation and antibody production, as well as T-lymphocyte production of lymphokines. The increased synthesis of IL-1 by activated macrophages could contribute to enhancement of the immune response. Endotoxin also induces the synthesis of IL-1. This effect is achieved at least partly by stimulation of the macrophages to release TNF-α, which then stimulates the production of IL-1 by endothelial cells and macrophages. Activated macrophages release much more TNF-α than do resting macrophages that are exposed to endotoxin. Both TNF-α and IL-1 can induce the fever and synthesis of acute-phase reactants (discussed later) that characterize inflammation.

ACUTE INFLAMMATION

Tissue damage results in **inflammation,** a series of biochemical and cellular changes that facilitate the phagocytosis of invading microorganisms or damaged cells (Figure 3-7). If inflammation is sufficiently extensive, it is accompa-

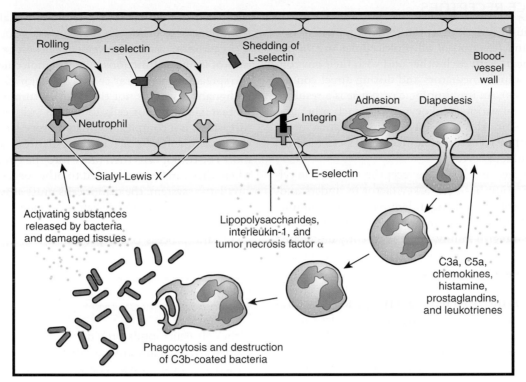

Figure 3-7   Acute inflammatory response. Neutrophils are among the first cells to arrive at the scene of an infection and are important contributors to the acute inflammatory response. As the neutrophil rolls along the blood vessel wall, the L-selectin on its surface binds to carbohydrate structures such as sialyl-Lewis^x on the adhesion molecules on the vascular endothelium, and its progress is eventually halted. As the neutrophil becomes activated, it replaces L-selectin with other cell-surface adhesion molecules, such as integrins. These molecules bind E-selectin, which is present on the blood vessel wall as a result of the influence of inflammatory mediators such as bacterial lipopolysaccharides and the cytokines interleukin-1 and tumor necrosis factor alpha (TNF-α). The activated neutrophil then enters the tissues, where it is attracted to the infection site by a number of chemoattractants. The neutrophil can then phagocytose and destroy the C3b-coated bacteria. *(Modified from Delves PJ, Roitt, IM: N Engl J Med 343(1)37, 2000.)*

nied by an increase in the plasma concentration of acute-phase reactants (see Chapter 5).

Inflammation is characterized by redness, heat, swelling, and pain. The primary objective of inflammation is to localize and eradicate the irritant and repair the surrounding tissue. The inflammatory response involves the following three major stages:
1. Dilation of capillaries to increase blood flow.
2. Microvascular structural changes and escape of plasma proteins from the bloodstream.
3. Leukocyte transmigration through endothelium and accumulation at the site of injury.

Once inflammation is triggered, it must be appropriately resolved, or pathologic tissue damage will occur. In some diseases, however, the body's defense system (immune system) inappropriately triggers an inflammatory response when no foreign substances are present. In these autoimmune disorders the body's normally protective immune system causes damage to its own tissues (see Chapter 28). The body responds as if normal tissues are infected or somehow abnormal.

SEPSIS

If an inflammation overwhelms the whole body, systemic inflammatory response syndrome (SIRS) is diagnosed. When caused by infection, the term *sepsis* is applied. Vasodilation and organ dysfunction are serious problems that may lead to septic shock and death. Inflammatory disorders (e.g., asthma, autoimmune disorders, sepsis) can be major causes of death.

Sepsis is an infection-induced syndrome defined as the presence of two or more of the following features of systemic inflammation:
- Fever or hypothermia
- Leukocytosis or leukopenia
- Tachycardia and tachypnea
- Supranormal minute ventilation

Early biochemical events in sepsis include the key element, cytokines. The most widely investigated cytokines are TNF, IL-1, and interleukin-8 (IL-8), which are generally proinflammatory, and interleukin-6 (IL-6) and interleukin-10 (IL-10), which tend to be antiinflammatory. IL-8 may have an especially important role in promoting tissue inflammation.

CELL SURFACE RECEPTORS

Cellular communication is essential to development, tissue organization, and function of all multicellular organisms. Cells communicate with each other and with their environment through soluble mediators and during direct contact (e.g., phagocytosis). An immunologic response is a result of the interactions of various leukocytes with each other and with other cells in the body. These interactions occur through cell surface receptors that mediate cell-cell binding, or "adhesion," of leukocytes.

Discovery of several cell surface receptors involved in cellular communication has been a key factor in understanding the mechanisms underlying inflammatory and immune phenomena. Three protein families—the immunoglobulin (Ig) family, the integrin family, and the recently designated selectin family—form a network of cellular interactions in the immune system.

Members of the Ig superfamily include antigen-specific receptors, such as the T-cell receptor (TCR) and surface immunoglobulin (sIg), as well as antigen-independent receptors and their counterreceptors, such as CD2 and lymphocyte function–associated antigen-3. Ig superfamily members function in cell activation, differentiation, and cell-cell interaction. In some cases, both an adhesion receptor and the counterreceptor to which it binds are members of the Ig superfamily.

Three selectin family molecules—endothelial cell adhesion molecule-1, leukocyte adhesion molecule (LAM-1, Mel-14), and CD62, also known as platelet activation–dependent granule–external membrane protein and granule membrane protein of 140 kilodaltons (GMP-140)—have been implicated in a number of leukocyte adhesion phenomena, including leukocyte homing to lymphoid tissue. Selectins are expressed on both leukocytes and endothelial cells. Mel-14 functions early in neutrophil-endothelium adhesion.

The integrin family consists of at least 14 alpha/beta heterodimers divided into subfamilies with distinct structural and functional characteristics. The subfamily of leukocyte integrins contains three members: LFA-1, Mac-1, and p150,95. These molecules are glycoproteins composed of noncovalently associated alpha and beta subunits. LFA-1 is expressed on all leukocytes, whereas Mac-1 and p150,95 are found primarily on granulocytes and monocytes.

The integrin family is phylogenetically ancient. Integrin family members engage in interactions with cell surface ligands and extracellular matrix (ECM) components. ECM components, including fibronectin, collagen, and laminin, have been shown to be ligands for members of the beta-1 and beta-3 subfamilies. Members of these subfamilies are of great significance in embryogenesis, growth and repair, and hemostasis. The leukocyte integrins, or beta-2 subfamily, have been shown to be involved in a diverse number of leukocyte adhesion-dependent phenomena, giving them a critical role in inflammatory and immune responses. The term "integrin" was initially used to emphasize that these receptors integrate signals from the extracellular environment with the intracellular cytoskeleton. A signal is transduced from outside to inside the cell.

In addition to the involvement of these receptors in a variety of immune functions, integrin molecules play a role in the spread of malignant cells. The major cause of death in malignant disease is not the primary tumor but rather the **metastasis** of tumor cells to distant sites within the body. Metastasis is a complex, multistep process that begins with the detachment of a few tumor cells from the primary tumor. The tumor cells then move into the circulatory system, where they can be transported to other organs. While in the circulatory system, the tumor cells must survive the natural defense system of the body before attaching to and invading the tissues of another organ. A better understanding of the metastatic process could provide the basis for diagnostic and therapeutic strategies.

DISORDERS OF NEUTROPHILS

Noninfectious Neutrophil-Mediated Inflammatory Disease

Although neutrophils provide the major means of defense against bacterial and fungal infections, they can also be destructive to host tissues. The same oxidative and nonoxidative processes that destroy microorganisms can affect adjacent host tissues. A number of disease states correspond to inappropriate phagocytosis (Box 3-2), as with prolonged activation of NADPH oxidase. This process occurs when the phagocytes attempt to engulf particles that are too large. The phagocyte releases oxygen radicals and granule contents onto the particle, but these escape into the surrounding tissues, generating tissue damage. This is often observed in response to dust inhalation and smoking (e.g., nicotine) and in persistent infections such as cystic fibrosis. In addition, many autoimmune diseases are thought to be caused by inappropriate activation of the process of phagocytosis, whereby the body attacks its own cells and tissues. Examples

Box 3-2	Noninfectious Neutrophil-Mediated Diseases*

Autoimmune arthritides
Autoimmune vasculitis
Dermatophytic disorders
    Autoimmune bullous dermatoses
    Behçet's disease
    Psoriasiform dermatoses
    Pyoderma gangrenosum
    Sweet's syndrome
Glomerulonephritis
Gout
Inflammatory bowel disease
Malignant neoplasms at site of chronic inflammation
Myocardial infarction
Respiratory disorders
    Adult respiratory distress syndrome
    Asthma and allergic asthma
    Emphysema

*Signs, symptoms, and injury may be partly mediated by neutrophils.

include rheumatoid arthritis, multiple sclerosis, and Graves' disease.

Abnormal Neutrophil Function

Patients with quantitative or qualitative defects of neutrophils have a high rate of infection, which illustrates the importance of the neutrophil to body defenses. Individuals with a marked decrease of neutrophils (neutropenia) or severe defects in neutrophil function frequently have recurrent systemic bacterial infections (e.g., pneumonia), disseminated cutaneous pyogenic lesions, and other types of life-threatening bacterial and fungal infections.

Leukocyte mobility may be impaired in some diseases (e.g., rheumatoid arthritis, cirrhosis, CGD). Defective locomotion or leukocyte immobility can also be seen in patients receiving steroids and in those with lazy leukocyte syndrome. A marked defect in the cellular response to chemotaxis, an important step in phagocytosis, can be seen in patients with diabetes mellitus, Chédiak-Higashi anomaly (syndrome), or sepsis, as well as in those with high levels of antibody immunoglobulin E (IgE), as in Job's syndrome.

Congenital Neutrophil Abnormalities

A small number of patients have congenital abnormalities of neutrophil structure and function (Box 3-3).

Chédiak-Higashi Syndrome

The Chédiak-Higashi syndrome represents a qualitative disorder of neutrophils. It is a rare familial disorder inherited as an autosomal recessive trait and expressed as an abnormal granulation of neutrophils. Neutrophils having giant granules display impaired chemotaxis and delayed killing of ingested bacteria.

Chronic Granulomatous Disease

The chronic granulomatous diseases (CGDs) are a genetically heterogeneous group of disorders of oxidative metabolism affecting the cascade of events required for hydrogen peroxide production by phagocytes. Multiple types of inheritance of the disorder have been described, including sex linked (X chromosome linked) in 66%, autosomal recessive in 34%, and autosomal dominant in less than 1% of cases. Patients with the autosomal recessive form may have a less severe clinical course than patients with the X-linked form.

The onset of CGD is during infancy, with one third of patients dying before age 7 years because of infections. It was observed that in the presence of normal or elevated leukocyte counts, the neutrophilic granulocytes in vitro ingested and destroyed only streptococci, not staphylococci. Subsequent testing revealed that the cells from patients with CGD can phagocytize non–H_2O_2-producing bacteria such as *Staphylococcus aureus* and gram-negative rods (e.g., Enterobacteriaceae), but they cannot destroy them. In the X-linked form the defective leukocytes fail to exhibit increased anaerobic metabolism during phagocytosis because of a cytochrome b_{558} deficiency (which expresses itself as a defect in the 91,000-dalton glycoprotein membrane anchor of the cytochrome complex); or these defective leukocytes produce H_2O_2 because of a myeloperoxidase deficiency.

Patients with CGD have infections with catalase-positive bacteria and fungi affecting the skin, lungs, liver, and bones. They also develop granuloma resulting from a lack of resolution of inflammatory foci, even after the infection has been eliminated. This leads to extensive granuloma formation and, in some circumstances, impairment of physiologic processes (e.g., obstruction of esophagus or urinary tract).

Complement Receptor 3 (CR3) Deficiency

The CR3 deficiency is a rare condition inherited as an autosomal recessive trait. A deficiency of CR3 on phagocytic cells presents as a leukocyte adhesion deficiency. Leukocyte adhesion deficiency type 1 (LAD-1) is caused by a deficiency of CD18. LAD-2 is caused by absent sialyl–Lewis X (CD15s).

A CR3 deficiency in neutrophils is associated with marked abnormalities of adherence-related functions, including decreased aggregation of neutrophils to each other after activation, decreased adherence of neutrophils to endothelial cells, poor adherence and phagocytosis of opsonized microorganisms, defective spreading, and decreased diapedesis and chemotaxis. Patients may also lack an intravascular marginating pool of neutrophils. Defects in T lymphocytes are characterized by faulty lymphocyte-mediated cytotoxicity, with poor adherence to target cells. Abnormalities of B lymphocytes have also been observed.

Clinically, a deficiency can manifest as delayed separation of the umbilical cord. Other signs and symptoms include early onset of bacterial infections, including skin infections, mucositis, otitis, gingivitis, and periodontitis. A depressed inflammatory response and neutrophilia can be observed.

Myeloperoxidase Deficiency

A deficiency of myeloperoxidase is inherited as an autosomal recessive trait on chromosome 17. Myeloperoxidase is an iron-containing heme protein responsible for the peroxidase activity characteristic of azurophilic granules; it accounts for the greenish color of pus. Human neutrophils contain many granules of various sizes that are morphologically, biochemically, and functionally distinct. The azurophilic granules normally contain myeloperoxidase. In this disorder, azurophilic granules are present, but myeloperoxidase is decreased or absent. If phagocytes are deficient in myeloperoxidase, the patient's phagocytes manifest a mild

Box 3-3	Congenital Neutrophil Abnormalities

Chédiak-Higashi syndrome (anomaly)
Chronic granulomatous disease (CGD)
Complement receptor 3 (CR3) deficiency
Myeloperoxidase deficiency
Specific granule deficiency

to moderate defect in bacterial killing and a marked defect in fungal killing in vitro.

Persons with a myeloperoxidase deficiency are generally healthy and do not have an increased frequency of infection, probably because of other microbicidal mechanisms compensating for the deficiency. Patients with diabetes and myeloperoxidase deficiency, however, may have deep fungal infections caused by *Candida* species.

Specific Granule Deficiency

Specific granule deficiency is believed to be an autosomal recessive disease. It is caused by a failure to synthesize specific granules and some contents of other granules during differentiation of neutrophils in the bone marrow. Patients with specific granule deficiency have recurrent, severe bacterial infections of the skin and deep tissues, with a depressed inflammatory response.

MONOCYTE-MACROPHAGE DISORDERS

Monocyte-macrophage has been shown to be abnormal in a variety of diseases (Table 3-1). The abnormality is partial, and no related association with increased susceptibility to infection has been established. In cases of severely depressed migration of monocytes, however, it is likely that this dysfunction predisposes a patient to infection because other defects of host defense coexist in these disorders.

The signs and symptoms of abnormalities of monocyte-macrophage function are extremely evident in some conditions. The profound defect of phagocytic killing exhibited by patients with CGD results in the formation of subcutaneous abscesses and abscesses in the liver, lungs, spleen, and lymph nodes. Cancer patients with a defective monocyte cytotoxicity may develop this defect because tumors have the ability to release factors that suppress the generation of toxic oxygen metabolites by macrophages. In newborn infants, depressed chemotaxis, killing, and decreased synthesis of the phagocytosis-promoting factors fibronectin, C3,

and complement factor B have been observed. In addition, the newborn's macrophages may not respond effectively to infection because the lymphocytes have impaired the production of the macrophage activator IFN-γ.

Qualitative disorders of monocytes-macrophages reflect manifest as lipid storage diseases, including a number of rare autosomal recessive disorders. The expression in macrophages of a systemic enzymatic defect permits the accumulation of cell debris normally cleared by macrophages. The macrophages are particularly prone to accumulate undegraded lipid products. Resistance to infection can be impaired, at least partially, because of a defect in macrophage function. Disorders of this type include Gaucher's disease and Niemann-Pick disease.

Gaucher's Disease

An inherited disease caused by a disturbance in cellular lipid metabolism, Gaucher's disease most frequently affects children. Prognosis varies; with mild disease the patient may live a relatively normal life, whereas with severe disease the patient may die prematurely.

The disorder represents a deficiency of β-glucocerebrosidase, the enzyme that normally splits glucose from its parent sphingolipid, glucosylceramide. As the result of this enzyme deficiency, cerebroside accumulates in histiocytes (macrophages). Gaucher's cells are rarely found in the circulating blood; the typical cell is large, with one to three eccentric nuclei and a characteristically wrinkled cytoplasm. These cells are found in the bone marrow, spleen, and other organs of the mononuclear phagocyte system. Production of erythrocytes and leukocytes decreases as these abnormal cells infiltrate the bone marrow.

Niemann-Pick Disease

Niemann-Pick disease is similar to Gaucher's disease, also an inherited abnormality of lipid metabolism. Niemann-Pick disease affects infants and children, with an average life expectancy of 5 years.

This disorder represents a rare autosomal recessive deficiency of the enzyme sphingomyelinase, characterized by massive accumulation of sphingomyelin in the mononuclear phagocytes. The characteristic cell in this disorder, Pick's cell, is similar in appearance to Gaucher's cell, although the cytoplasm of the cell is foamy.

DISEASE STATES INVOLVING LEUKOCYTE INTEGRINS

Leukocyte adhesion deficiency (LAD) ultimately leads to recurrent and often-fatal bacterial and fungal infections. The etiology of this very rare condition (about 300 cases have been diagnosed worldwide) is mutations in the gene or chromosome.

There are several types of LAD based on genotypes and phenotypes. Two genotypes have been identified, LAD-1 and LAD-2. LAD-1 can affect people of all racial groups. LAD-2 has been reported only in people from the Middle East and

Table 3-1	Primary and Secondary Abnormalities of Monocyte-Macrophage Function	
Abnormality	**Condition/Group**
Defect in phagocyte killing	Chronic granulomatous disease, corticosteroid therapy, newborn infants, viral infections
Defective monocyte cytotoxicity	Cancer, Wiskott-Aldrich syndrome
Defective release of macrophage-activating factors	Acquired immunodeficiency syndrome (AIDS), intracellular infections (e.g., lepromatous leprosy, tuberculosis, visceral leishmaniasis)
Depressed migration	AIDS, burns, diabetes, immunosuppressive therapy, newborn infants
Impaired phagocytosis	Congenital deficiency of CD11 to CD18, monocytic leukemia, systemic lupus erythematosus

Brazil. LAD-1 patients have a deficiency of β_2-integrin sub-unit (CD18). The phenotypes are severe, moderate, and novel or variant. LAD-2 is described as the failure to convert guanosine diphosphate (GDP) mannose to fructose.

Patients have a history of delayed separation of the umbilical cord, gingivitis, recurrent and persistent bacterial or fungal skin infections, and impaired wound healing. A lack of pus formation has also been noted. Patients frequently develop severe, life-threatening infections, although their neutrophil counts are usually elevated (25.0×10^9/L). Affected individuals do not have increased susceptibility to viral infections or malignant neoplasms.

Patients with LAD-2 have a characteristic facial appearance, short stature, limb malformations, and severe developmental delay.

Adhesion defects can also be caused by two common drugs, epinephrine and corticosteroids. Both demarginate neutrophils from the peripheral vasculature, although the mechanism is not understood. Epinephrine acts by causing endothelial cells to release cyclic adenosine monophosphate (cAMP), which in turn interrupts adherence.

CASE STUDY

History and Physical Examination

This family had a son who had died at age 2 weeks because of overwhelming bacterial infection. When their newborn daughter began developing recurrent infections, she was immediately taken to a pediatrician.

Laboratory Data

Hemoglobin and hematocrit: within normal range.
Total WBC count: 62.0×10^9/L.
Absolute leukocyte counts: above normal for each leukocyte type.
Leukocyte differential: neutrophils 76%; lymphocytes 22%; eosinophils 2%.
Flow cell cytometry:
  T lymphocytes: normal proportions of CD4+ and CD8+ cells.
  B lymphocytes (CD19+): elevated.
  Natural killer (NK) cells: elevated.
  CD18+ lymphocytes: 5%.
Serum Ig fractions: within reference ranges.

Treatment

The infant was given busulfan cyclophosphamide and antithymocyte serum for 10 days. She received mature-T-lymphocyte–depleted bone marrow transplanted from her mother. This was followed by a short period of immunosuppressive therapy.

She recovered from the procedures and did well clinically.

Questions and Discussion

1. What laboratory test is of the greatest diagnostic value in diagnosing this patient?

Flow cytometry is used to assess the presence of the beta-2 integrins CD11a/CD18 (LFA-1 or α_L/β_2) on leukocytes, CD11b/CD18 (Mac-1 or α_M/β_2) on myeloid cells, and CD11c/CD18 (p150,95 or α_X/β_2) on myeloid cells.

2. What value in the reported flow cytometry results is diagnostic?

The presence of 5% CD18+ lymphocytes suggests defective leukocyte adhesion.

3. Can leukocyte adhesion deficiency be misdiagnosed?

Yes; LAD diseases potentially could be misdiagnosed as "severe infection with appropriate leukocytosis" or a "leukemoid reaction."

Diagnosis

Leukocyte adhesion deficiency (LAD).

CASE STUDY

History and Physical Examination

This 6-year-old white male patient was taken to a pediatrician because of recurring abscesses since age 1 month. The current abscesses were lanced, and he was placed on antibiotic therapy.

The patient had two brothers who had died in infancy of infections. His parents and two sisters are healthy.

Laboratory Data

Hemoglobin and hematocrit: slightly decreased.
Total leukocyte count: elevated.
Differential leukocyte count: increased percentage of segmented neutrophils.
Immunoglobulin profile: polyclonal elevation of all Ig classes.
Nitroblue tetrazolium (NBT) test (automated): reduction of unstimulated and stimulated neutrophils.
Culture of abscess revealed *Staphylococcus aureus*.

Questions and Discussion

1. Does this boy's condition appear to be gender related?

Yes; because his brothers died of infections but his sisters are normal, an X-linked disorder would be suspected.

2. What is the significance of reduced neutrophil activity in the NBT test?

Reduction in NBT activity indicates that this boy's neutrophils could engulf but could not kill *Staphylococcus* because of impaired intracellular killing ability.

3. Why are the bacteria not killed?

The neutrophils fail to kill the bacteria because the cells either fail to consume oxygen or fail to produce hydrogen peroxide during phagocytosis.

Diagnosis

Chronic granulomatous disease (CGD).

Screening Test for Phagocytic Engulfment

Principle

A mixture of bacteria and phagocytes is incubated and ex-amined for the presence of engulfed bacteria. This simple procedure may be useful in supporting the diagnosis of im-paired neutrophilic function in conjunction with clinical signs and symptoms (Figure 3-8).

Specimen Collection and Preparation

No special preparation of the patient is required before specimen collection. The patient must be positively identi-fied when the specimen is collected. The specimen label should be completed at the bedside and should include the patient's full name, date, patient's hospital identification number, and phlebotomist's initials.

Blood should be drawn by an aseptic technique. A mini-mum of 2 mL of heparinized blood (green-top evacuated tube) or 15 to 20 heparinized capillary tubes are required. The specimen should be centrifuged, and the test should be performed promptly.

Reagents, Supplies, and Equipment

- Broth culture of *Bacillus subtilis* or *Staphylococcus* coagu-lase-negative species
- Microscope slides
- Pasteur pipettes and rubber bulb
- 12 × 75–mm test tubes
- Wright's stain

Quality Control

A fresh, heparinized sample of blood from a healthy volun-teer should be tested simultaneously.

Procedure

1. Label two 12 × 75–mm test tubes: "patient" and "control."
2. Add 4 to 8 drops of the buffer coat from either the pa-tient's heparinized blood or the normal control to the respectively labeled test tubes.
3. Add 2 to 3 drops of the bacterial broth culture to each tube.
4. Incubate both tubes at room temperature or 37° C for 30 minutes.
5. Place 1 drop of the incubated specimen on a glass slide, and prepare a smear.
6. Air-dry the slides, and stain with Wright's stain.

Wright's Stain Procedure

a. Cover each smear generously with filtered Wright's stain, and allow the stain to remain on the slide for at least 5 minutes.

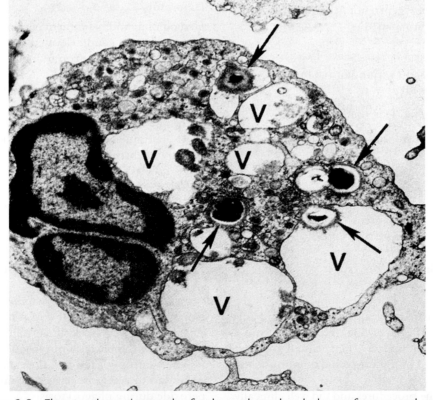

Figure 3-8 Electron photomicrograph of polymorphonuclear leukocyte from normal control patient incubated with staphylococci for 30 minutes. Many bacteria *(arrows)* in various stages of destruction are evident within the cell. Note the cytoplasmic vacuoles *(V)* around and adjacent to degenerating bacteria. *(From Bauer JD: Clinical laboratory methods, ed 9, St Louis, 1982, Mosby.)*

b. Slowly add distilled water or buffer to the stain until the buffer begins to overflow the stain. Watch for the appearance of a metallic luster.

c. Gently blow on the slide to mix the stain and buffer.

d. Allow the buffer to remain on the slide for at least 5 minutes.

e. Gently wash the stain and buffer off the slide with distilled water.

f. Air-dry or carefully blot the slide between two sheets of bibulous (highly absorbent) paper.

7. Place a drop of immersion oil on each smear, and examine microscopically with the oil (×100) immersion objective.

Reporting Results

Positive: demonstration of the engulfment of bacteria.
Negative: no engulfment of bacteria.

Sources of Error

This procedure may produce false-negative results if the blood specimen is not fresh or if a coagulase-positive *Staphylococcus* specimen is used. It is important to distinguish between granules and cocci. In addition, the bacteria must be intracellular and not extracellular for the test to be positive.

Clinical Applications

The failure of phagocytes to engulf bacteria can support the diagnosis of neutrophilic dysfunction; however, these results must be used in conjunction with patient signs and symptoms.

Limitations

This is a simple screening procedure for engulfment. The presence of engulfed bacteria does not demonstrate that the bacteria have been destroyed.

CHAPTER HIGHLIGHTS

- The entire leukocytic cell system is designed to defend the body against disease. Each cell type has a unique function and behaves both independently and, in many cases, in cooperation with other cell types.
- The primary phagocytic cells are the neutrophilic leukocytes and the mononuclear monocytes-macrophages.
- The neutrophilic leukocyte provides an effective host defense against bacterial and fungal infections. Although the monocytes-macrophages and other granulocytes are also phagocytic cells, the neutrophil is the principal leukocyte associated with phagocytosis and a localized inflammatory response.
- Phagocytosis can be divided into movement of cells, engulfment, and digestion.
- Cells communicate with each other and with their environment through soluble mediators and during direct contact (e.g., phagocytosis). These interactions occur through cell surface receptors that mediate cell-cell binding ("adhesion") of leukocytes.
- Three protein families (immunoglobulin, integrin, selectin) are associated in a network of cellular interactions in the immune system.
- Qualitative monocyte-macrophage disorders manifest as lipid storage diseases, including a number of rare autosomal recessive disorders.
- Leukocyte adhesion deficiency ultimately leads to recurrent and often-fatal bacterial and fungal infections.

REVIEW QUESTIONS

1. The major site of hematopoiesis in the second month of gestation is the:
   a. Yolk sac.
   b. Spleen.
   c. Liver.
   d. Bone marrow.

2. The principal type of leukocyte in the process of phagocytosis is the:
   a. Eosinophil.
   b. Basophil.
   c. Monocyte.
   d. Neutrophil.

3. Chronic granulomatous disease represents a defect of:
   a. Oxidative metabolism.
   b. Abnormal granulation of neutrophils.
   c. Diapedesis.
   d. Chemotaxis.

4. A primary function of the eosinophil is:
   a. Phagocytosis.
   b. Suppression of the inflammatory response.
   c. Reacting in acute, systemic hypersensitivity reactions.
   d. Antigen recognition.

5. The cells of the mononuclear phagocyte system include:
   a. Monocytes and promonocytes.
   b. Monocytes and macrophages.
   c. Lymphocytes and monocytes.
   d. Both a and b.

6. The host defense function(s) of monocytes-macrophages include(s):
   a. Antigen presentation.
   b. Phagocytosis.
   c. Secretion of biologically active molecules.
   d. All the above.

7. The surface MHC class II gene product is important in:
    a. Antigen recognition by T lymphocytes.
    b. Antigen recognition by B lymphocytes.
    c. Synthesis of antibody by plasma cells.
    d. Phagocytosis.

Questions 8-12. Match the appropriate monocyte-macrophage abnormality with its respective condition.

8. _____ Defect in phagocytic killing

9. _____ Defective monocyte cytotoxicity

10. _____ Defective release of macrophage-activating factors

11. _____ Depressed migration

12. _____ Impaired phagocytosis

    a. Wiskott-Aldrich syndrome
    b. Burns or diabetes
    c. Systemic lupus erythematosus
    d. Corticosteroid therapy
    e. Intracellular infections

Questions 13-16. Arrange the steps of phagocytosis in the proper sequence.

13. _____

14. _____

15. _____

16. _____

    a. Digestion of bacteria.
    b. Increase in chemoattractants at site of tissue damage.
    c. Ingestion of bacteria.
    d. Movement of phagocytic cells.

Questions 17-20. Match the following cell types to their respective functions. (An answer can be used more than once.)

17. _____ Polymorphonuclear neutrophilic (PMN) leukocytes

18. _____ Lymphocytes

19. _____ Mononuclear monocytes-macrophages

20. _____ Plasma cells

    a. Primary phagocytic cells.
    b. Antibody-synthesizing cells.
    c. Recognition of foreign antigen and production of antibody.

Questions 21-23. Arrange the sites of blood cell development (hematopoiesis) in the embryo and fetus in the correct sequence of development.

21. _____ Site of initial red blood cell production

22. _____ Predominant site from 2 to 5 months of fetal life

23. _____ Ultimate site of primary hematopoiesis

    a. Liver and spleen
    b. Yolk sac
    c. Bone marrow

24. Patients with a marked decrease in neutrophils or severe defects in neutrophil function have:
    a. A high rate of infection.
    b. Recurrent systemic bacterial infections.
    c. Recurrent life-threatening fungal infections
    d. All the above.

Questions 25-28. Match each disorder/deficiency to its characteristics.

25. _____ Chronic granulomatosus disease

26. _____ Lazy leukocyte syndrome

27. _____ Chédiak-Higashi anomaly

28. _____ Myeloperoxidase deficiency

    a. Marked defect in cellular response to chemotaxis.
    b. Failure to exhibit increased anaerobic metabolism during phagocytosis.
    c. Mild to marked defect in bactericidal ability of neutrophils.
    d. Defective leukocyte locomotion.

29. Which statement about eosinophils is false?
    a. Are homeostatic regulators of inflammation.
    b. Attempt to suppress an inflammatory reaction.
    c. Are able to kill most parasites.
    d. Interact with the larval stages of some helminth parasites.

30. Which statement about basophils is false?
    a. Have a high concentration of heparin in the granules.
    b. Have a high concentration of histamine in the granules
    c. React with two adjacent IgA molecules on mast cells.
    d. Are associated with anaphylactic shock.

31. The cells that constitute the physiologic, mononuclear phagocyte system do *not* include:
    a. Promonocytes and their precursors.
    b. Monocytes in circulating blood.
    c. Macrophages in tissues.
    d. Polymorphonuclear neutrophils.

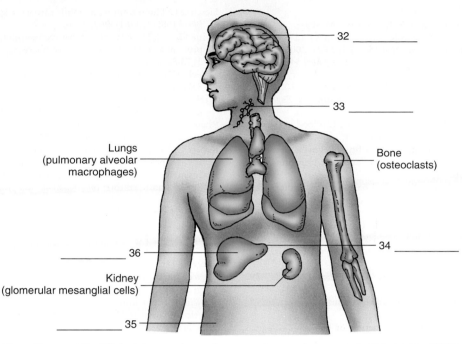

(From Turgeon ML: Clinical hematology: theory and procedures, ed 4, Philadelphia, 2005, Lippincott Williams & Wilkins)

Questions 32-36. Identify the types of mononuclear phagocytic cells found in the various locations shown in the illustration. Choose from the following answers:

    a. Kupffer cells
    b. Macrophages
    c. Microglial cells
    d. Histiocytes

Questions 37-40. Name the steps in the process of phagocytosis shown in the illustration. Choose from the following answers:

    a. Engulfment
    b. Chemotaxis
    c. Phagosome formation
    d. Adherence

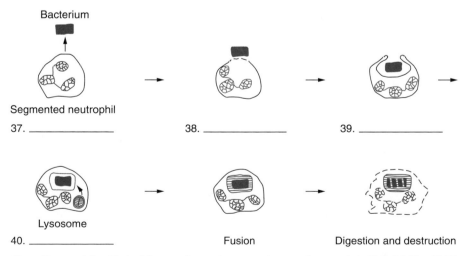

(From Turgeon ML: Clinical hematology: theory and procedures, ed 4, Philadelphia, 2005, Lippincott Williams & Wilkins)

BIBLIOGRAPHY

Barrett J: *Textbook of immunology,* ed 5, St Louis, 1988, Mosby.

Charo IF, Ransohoff RM: The many roles of chemokines and chemokine receptors in inflammation, *N Engl J Med* 354(6):610-621, 2006.

Delves PJ, Roitt IM: The immune system. Part I, *N Engl J Med* 343(1):37-49, 2000.

Etzion A: Integrins: the molecular glue of life, *Hosp Pract* 35(3):102, 2000.

Frenette PS: Locking a leukocyte integrin with statins, *N Engl J Med* 345(19):1419-1421, 2001.

Frenette PS, Wagner DD: Adhesion molecules. Part II. Blood vessels and blood cells, *N Engl J Med* 335(1):43-45, 1996.

Green CE et al: Dynamic shifts in LFA-1 affinity regulate neutrophil rolling, arrest, and transmigration on inflamed endothelium, *Blood* 107(5):2101-2110, 2006.

Grosser T, Fries S, Fitzgerald GA: Biological basis for the cardiovascular consequences of COX-2 inhibition: therapeutic challenges and opportunities, *J Clin Invest* 116:4-15, 2006.

Hansson G: Inflammation, atherosclerosis, and coronary artery disease, *N Engl J Med* 352(16):1685-1695, 2005.

Hotchkiss RS, Karl IE: The pathophysiology and treatment of sepsis, *N Engl J Med* 348(2):138-150, 2003.

Johnston RB: Monocytes and macrophages, *N Engl J Med* 318(12):747-752, 1988.

Katz P: Clinical and laboratory evaluation of the immune system, *Med Clin North Am* 69(3):453-459, 1985.

Larson RS, Springer TA: Structure and function of leukocyte integrins, *Immunol Rev* 114:181-217, 1990.

Lieschke G: Fluorescent neutrophils throw the spotlight on inflammation, *Blood* 108(13):3961-3962, 2006.

Ledue TB et al: The relationship between serum levels of lipoprotein (a) and proteins associated with the acute-phase response, *Clin Chim Acta* 223(1-2):73-82, 1993.

Malech HL, Malech JI: Neutrophils in human diseases, *N Engl J Med* 317(11):687-692, 1987.

Myeloperoxidase: a novel addition to multimarker testing in acute coronary syndromes, *MEDCO Forum* 13(32):1-2, 2006.

Rhen T, Cidlowski JA: Antiinflammatory action of glucocorticoids: new mechanisms for old drugs, *N Engl J Med* 353(16):1711-1722, 2005.

Robert C, Kupper TS: Inflammatory skin diseases, T cells, and immune surveillance, *N Engl J Med* 340(24):1817-1828, 1999.

Rotrosen D: The respiratory burst oxidase. In Gallin JI, Goldstein IM, Snyderman R, editors: *Inflammation: basic principles and clinical correlates,* ed 2, New York, 1992, Raven.

Serhan CN, Chiang N: Putting the brakes on neutrophils, *Blood* 107(5):1742-1743, 2006.

Sysmex: XE-IG Master, the first to know about inflammation, September 2003.

Turgeon ML: *Fundamentals of immunohematology,* ed 2, Baltimore, 1995, Williams & Wilkins.

Turgeon ML: *Clinical hematology,* ed 4, Philadelphia, 2005, Lippincott Williams & Wilkins.

Wheeler AP, Bernard GR: Treating patients with severe sepsis, *N Engl J Med* 340(3):207-214, 1999.

CHAPTER 4

Cells and Cellular Activities of the Immune System: Lymphocytes and Plasma Cells

Lymphocytes and Plasma Cells
    Sites of Lymphocyte Development
    Circulation of Lymphocytes
Lymphoid and Nonlymphoid Surface Membrane Markers
T Lymphocytes
    T-Lymphocyte Subsets
    Antigen Processing and Antigen Presentation to T Cells
    Antigen Recognition by T Cells
    T-Independent Antigen Triggering
Natural Killer and K-Type Lymphocytes
    Natural Killer Cells
    K-Type Lymphocytes
B Lymphocytes
    Cell Surface Markers
    B-Cell Activation
Other Types of Lymphocytes

Plasma Cell Biology
Alterations in Lymphocyte Subsets
    Changes with Aging
Evaluation of Suspected Defects
    Cell-Mediated Immune System
    Humoral System
    Lymphocyte Testing
Immunologic Disorders
    Primary Immunodeficiency Disorders
    Secondary Immunodeficiency Disorders
    Immune-Mediated Disease
Case Study
Classic Enumeration of T Lymphocytes
Chapter Highlights
Review Questions
Bibliography

Learning Objectives

At the conclusion of this chapter, the reader should be able to:
- Name and describe the function of primary and secondary lymphoid tissue.
- Explain the function of T lymphocytes in immunity.
- Explain the function of B lymphocytes in immunity.
- Describe the evaluation of suspected lymphocytic or plasma cell defects.

- Name and compare disorders of immunologic (lymphocytic or plasma cell) origin.
- Compare the categories of immunodeficiency disorders.
- Analyze representative case studies.

LYMPHOCYTES AND PLASMA CELLS

Lymphocytes represent the only immunologically specific cellular components of the immune system (Figure 4-1). The adaptive component of innate immunity is organized around two classes of specialized cells, **T lymphocytes** and **B lymphocytes.** Any immune response involves the interaction of many different cell types, and cell-mediated and antibody-mediated responses cannot be separated. T cells play an important role in the regulation of virtually all immune responses by providing help for antibody production by B lymphocytes (B cells) and by providing growth factors for B cells, T cells, and several other cell types. The cytotoxic subset of lymphocytes performs important effector functions; it is one of the cell types responsible for destroying virally infected cells, tumor cells, and allogeneic transplant cells.

In addition to the activities of the granulocytes and monocytes-macrophages, the lymphocytes and plasma cells are the cornerstone of the immune system. Lymphocytes recognize foreign antigens, directly destroy some cells, and produce antibodies as plasma cells.

Sites of Lymphocyte Development

In mammalian immunologic development, the precursors of lymphocytes arise from **progenitor cells** of the yolk sac and liver (Figure 4-2). Later in fetal development and throughout the life cycle, the bone marrow becomes the sole provider of undifferentiated progenitor cells, which can further develop into **lymphoblasts.** Continued cellular development and proliferation of lymphoid precursors occur as the cells travel to the primary and secondary lymphoid tissues.

Primary Lymphoid Tissue

In mammals, both the bone marrow (and/or fetal liver) and thymus are classified as primary or "central" lymphoid organs (Figure 4-3).

Thymus. Early in embryonic development, the stroma and nonlymphoid epithelium of the thymus are derived from the third and fourth pharyngeal pouches. This structure, located in the mediastinum, exercises control over the entire immune system. It is believed that the development of diversity occurs mainly in the thymus and bone marrow, al-

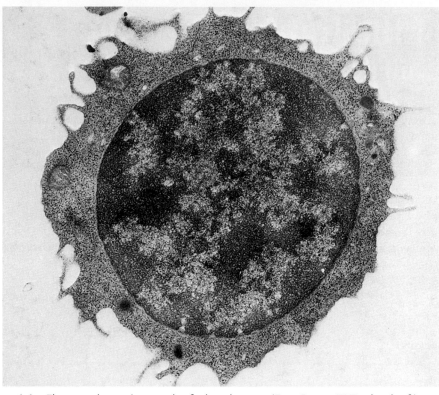

Figure 4-1   Electron photomicrograph of a lymphocyte. *(From Barrett JT:* Textbook of immunology, *ed 5, St Louis, 1988, Mosby.)*

though clonal expansion can occur anywhere in the peripheral lymphoid tissue.

Progenitor cells that migrate to the thymus proliferate and differentiate under the influence of the humoral factor thymosin. These lymphocyte precursors with acquired surface membrane antigens are referred to as thymocytes. The reticular structure of the thymus allows a significant number of lymphocytes to pass through it to become fully **immunocompetent** (able to function in the immune response), thymus-derived T cells. The thymus also regulates immune function by secretion of multiple soluble hormones.

Many cells die in the thymus and apparently are phagocytsized, a mechanism to eliminate lymphocyte clones reactive against self. Viable cells migrate to the secondary tissues. The absence or abnormal development of the thymus results in a T-lymphocyte deficiency. Involution of the thymus is the first age-related change occurring in the immune system of humans. The thymus gradually loses up to 95% of its mass during the first 50 years of life (Figure 4-4). The

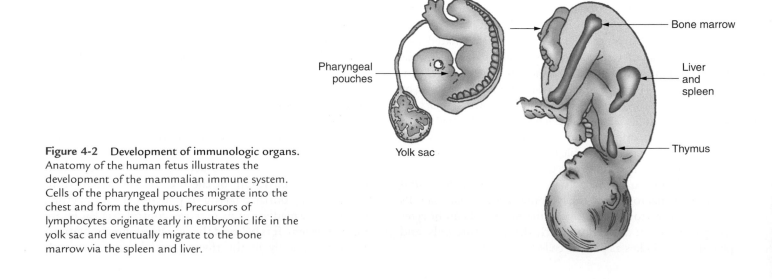

Figure 4-2   **Development of immunologic organs.** Anatomy of the human fetus illustrates the development of the mammalian immune system. Cells of the pharyngeal pouches migrate into the chest and form the thymus. Precursors of lymphocytes originate early in embryonic life in the yolk sac and eventually migrate to the bone marrow via the spleen and liver.

Pharyngeal pouches

Yolk sac

Bone marrow

Liver and spleen

Thymus

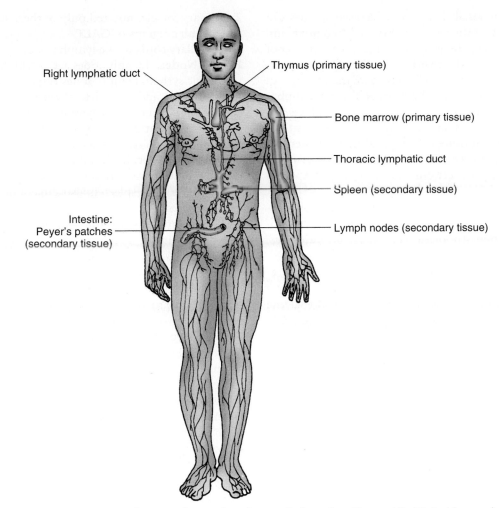

Figure 4-3   Human primary and secondary tissues. *(Redrawn from Turgeon ML: Clinical hematology: theory and procedures, ed 4, Philadelphia, 2005, Lippincott Williams & Wilkins.)*

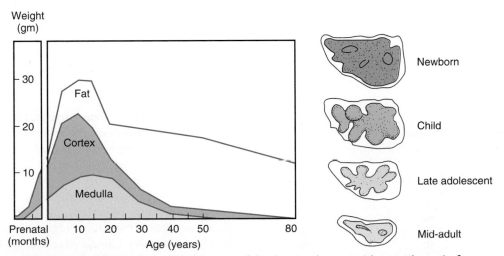

Figure 4-4   Thymic development. Histology of the thymus changes with age. The main feature of these changes is a loss of cellularity with increasing age.

accompanying functional changes of decreased synthesis of thymic hormones and the loss of ability to differentiate immature lymphocytes are reflected in an increased number of immature lymphocytes both within the thymus and as circulating peripheral blood T cells. Most of the changes in immune function, such as dysfunction of T and B lymphocytes, elevated levels of circulating immune complexes, increases in autoantibodies, and monoclonal gammopathies are correlated to involution of the thymus (see Chapter 27). Immune senescence may account for the increased susceptibility of older adults to infections, autoimmune disease, and neoplasms.

Bone Marrow. The bone marrow is the source of progenitor cells. These cells can differentiate into lymphocytes and other hematopoietic cells (e.g., granulocytes, erythrocytes, and megakaryocyte populations). In mammals the bone marrow also supports eventual differentiation of mature T and B lymphocytes, probably from a common lymphoid cell progenitor. It is believed that the bone marrow and **gut-associated lymphoid tissue (GALT)** may also play a role in the differentiation of progenitor cells into B lymphocytes.

Secondary Lymphoid Tissues

The secondary lymphoid tissues include lymph nodes, spleen, GALT, thoracic duct, bronchus-associated lymphoid tissue (BALT), skin-associated lymphoid tissue, and blood. Mature lymphocytes and accessory cells (e.g., antigen-presenting cells) are found throughout the body, although the relative percentages of T and B cells vary in different locations (Table 4-1).

Proliferation of the T and B lymphocytes in the secondary or peripheral lymphoid tissues (Figure 4-5) is primarily dependent on antigenic stimulation.

The T lymphocytes or T cells populate the following:
1. Perifollicular and paracortical regions of the lymph nodes
2. Medullary cords of the lymph nodes
3. Periarteriolar regions of the spleen
4. Thoracic duct of the circulatory system
   The B lymphocytes or B cells multiply and populate:
1. Follicular and medullary (germinal centers) of the lymph nodes

2. Primary follicles and red pulp of the spleen
3. Follicular regions of GALT
4. Medullary cords of the lymph nodes

Lymph Nodes. Lymph nodes act as lymphoid filters in the lymphatic system. Lymph nodes respond to antigens introduced distally and routed to them by afferent lymphatics (Figure 4-6). Generalized lymph node reactivity can occur after systemic antigen challenge (e.g., serum sickness).

Spleen. The spleen acts as a lymphatic filter within the blood vascular tree. It is an important site of antibody production in response to intravenous particulate antigens (e.g., bacteria). The spleen is also a major organ for the clearance particles.

Gut-Associated Lymphoid Tissue. GALT includes lymphoid tissue in the intestines (Peyer's patches) and the liver. GALT features immunoglobulin A (IgA) production and involves a unique pattern of lymphocyte recirculation. Pre-B cells develop in Peyer's patches and, after meeting antigen from the gut, many enter the general circulation and then return back to the gut. GALT is also important for the development of tolerance to ingested antigens.

Thoracic Duct. Thoracic duct lymph is a rich source of mature T cells. Chronic thoracic duct drainage can cause T-cell depletion and has been used as a method of immunosuppression.

Bronchus-Associated Lymphoid Tissue. BALT includes lymphoid tissue in the lower respiratory tract and in the hilar lymph nodes. It is mainly associated with IgA production to inhaled antigens.

Skin-Associated Lymphoid Tissue. Antigens introduced through the skin are presented by epidermal Langerhans cells, which are bone marrow–derived accessory cells. These epidermal cells then interact with lymphocytes in the skin and in draining lymph nodes.

Blood. The blood is an important lymphoid organ and immunologic effector tissue. Circulating blood has enough mature T cells to produce a graft-versus-host reaction. In addition, blood transfusions have been responsible for inducing acquired immunologic tolerance in kidney allograft patients.

Blood is the most frequently sampled lymphoid organ. It is assumed that what is found in blood samples represents what is present in other lymphoid tissues. Although this may be a true representation, it is not always accurate.

Circulation of Lymphocytes

The mature T lymphocyte survives for several months or years, whereas the average life span of the B lymphocytes is only a few days. Lymphocytes move freely between the blood and lymphoid tissues. This activity, referred to as **lymphocyte recirculation,** enables lymphocytes to come in contact with processed foreign antigens and to disseminate antigen-sensitized memory cells throughout the lymphoid system. Clonal expansion may occur regionally, as in lymph nodes draining a contact allergic reaction, and then the whole body becomes susceptible to rechallenge because T cells recirculate (but generally are excluded from returning to the

Table 4-1	Approximate Percentage of Lymphocytes in Lymphoid Organs	
Lymphoid Organ	T Lymphocytes (%)	B Lymphocytes (%)
Thymus	100	0
Blood	80	20
Lymph nodes	60	40
Spleen	45	55
Bone marrow	10	90

Modified from Claman HN: *JAMA* 268(20):2792, 1992.

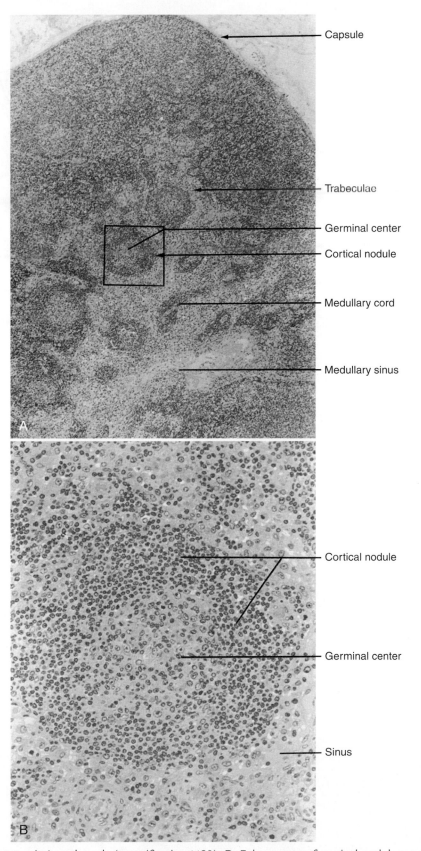

Figure 4-5   A, Lymph node (magnification ×90). **B,** Enlargement of cortical nodule seen in *A* (×450). *(From Anthony CP, Thibodeau GA: Textbook of anatomy and physiology, ed 12, St Louis, 1987, Mosby.)*

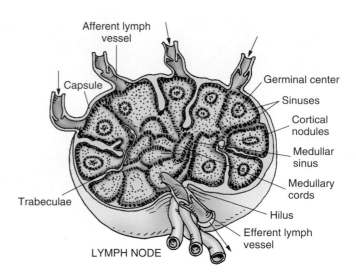

Figure 4-6 **Structure of a lymph node.** Several valved afferent lymphatics bring lymph to the node. An efferent lymphatic leaves the node at the hilus. Note that the artery and vein enter and leave at the hilus. *(Redrawn from Anthony CP, Thibodeau GA: Textbook of anatomy and physiology, ed 12, St Louis, 1987, Mosby.)*

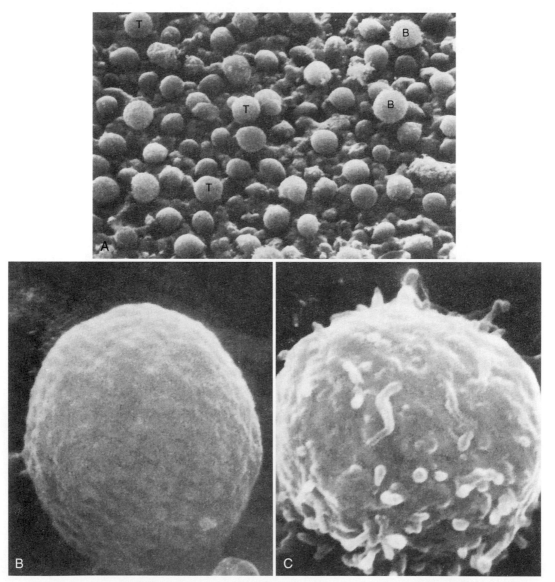

Figure 4-7 Scanning electron photomicrographs of lymphocyte cell surface membranes: **A,** T and B lymphocytes; **B,** T lymphocyte; **C,** B lymphocyte. *(From Polliack A et al:* J Exp Med *138:607, 1973.)*

thymus). Research has shown that a pool of T-cell clonal elements is developed by a combination of positive selection of those clones able to recognize and react to foreign antigens, and negative selection (purging) of those clones able to interact with self-antigens in a damaging way.

Recirculation of lymphocytes back to the blood is through the major lymphatic ducts. Lymphocytes enter the lymph node from the blood circulation via arterioles and capillaries to reach the specialized postcapillary venules. From the venule the lymphocytes enter the node and will either remain in the node or pass through the node and return to the circulating blood. Lymphatic fluid, lymphocytes, and antigens from certain body sites enter the lymph node through the **afferent lymphatic duct** and exit the lymph node through the **efferent lymphatic duct** (see Figure 4-6).

LYMPHOID AND NONLYMPHOID SURFACE MEMBRANE MARKERS

Before 1979, human lymphocytes could be classified as T or B cells. Observation of these cells on electron microscopy revealed that T lymphocytes have a relatively smooth surface compared with the rough pattern of the B lymphocytes (Figure 4-7).

The introduction of **monoclonal antibody (MAb)** testing led to the present identification of surface membrane markers on lymphocytes and other cells. In practical terms, surface markers are used to identify and enumerate various lymphocyte subsets, establish lymphocyte maturity, classify leukemias, and monitor patients on immunosuppressive therapy.

Cell surface molecules recognized by MAbs are called antigens (because antibodies can be produced against them) or markers (because they identify and discriminate between, or "mark," different cell populations). Originally, surface markers were named according to the antibodies that reacted with them, but a uniform nomenclature system has now been adopted. In this system a surface marker that identifies a particular lineage or differentiation stage with a defined structure, and that can be identified with a group or cluster of MAbs, is called a member of a **cluster of differentiation** (CD). Markers can be categorized as follows:

1. Some markers are specific for cells of a particular lineage or maturational pathway.
2. Some markers vary in expression, depending on the state of activation or differentiation of the same cells. For example, when CD antigen identification is used to classify lymphocyte subsets, most helper T lymphocytes are CD3+, CD4+, and CD8−; most cytotoxic T lymphocytes are CD3+, CD4−, and CD8+. In addition to using CD classification for the identification and separation of lymphocytes, CD antigens are involved in various lymphocyte functions, most often the following:
   - Promotion of cell-to-cell interactions and adhesion.
   - Transduction of signals that lead to lymphocyte activation.

T LYMPHOCYTES

Most total circulating lymphocytes are T cells derived from bone marrow progenitor cells that mature in the thymus gland (Table 4-2). These cells are responsible for cellular immune responses and are involved in the regulation of antibody reactions in conjunction with B lymphocytes.

During cellular development, T-lymphocyte function–associated antigens vary in expression (Figure 4-8). Some antigens appear early in cellular development and remain on mature T cells. Others appear at an early or intermediate stage of cellular maturation and are lost before maturity. When mature T cells leave the thymus, their T-cell receptors (TCRs) are either CD4+ or CD8+, and the cells gain functional maturity with their entry into the peripheral blood circulation.

T cells develop into a variety of clones. Each lymphocyte displays a single type of structurally unique receptor. The repertoire of antigen receptors in the entire population of lymphocytes is extremely large and diverse. This increases the probability that an individual lymphocyte will encoun-

Table 4-2	Lymphocyte Characteristics		
Type	Function(s)	Phenotypic Marker	Peripheral Blood (% of Total)
Helper T (Th) cells	Stimulate B-cell growth and differentiation *(humoral immunity)* Macrophage activation by secreted cytokines *(cell-mediated immunity)*	CD3+, CD4+, CD8−	50-60
Cytotoxic T (Tc) cells	Lysis of virus-infected cells, tumor cells, and allografts *(cell-mediated immunity)* Macrophage activation by secreted cytokines *(cell-mediated immunity)*	CD3+, CD4−, CD8+	20-25
Natural killer (NK) cells	Lysis of virus-infected cells, *(antibody-dependent cellular cytotoxicity)*	Fc receptor for IgG or cells CD16	~10
B cells	Antibody production *(humoral immunity)*	Fc receptors, MHC class II, CD19, CD21	10-15

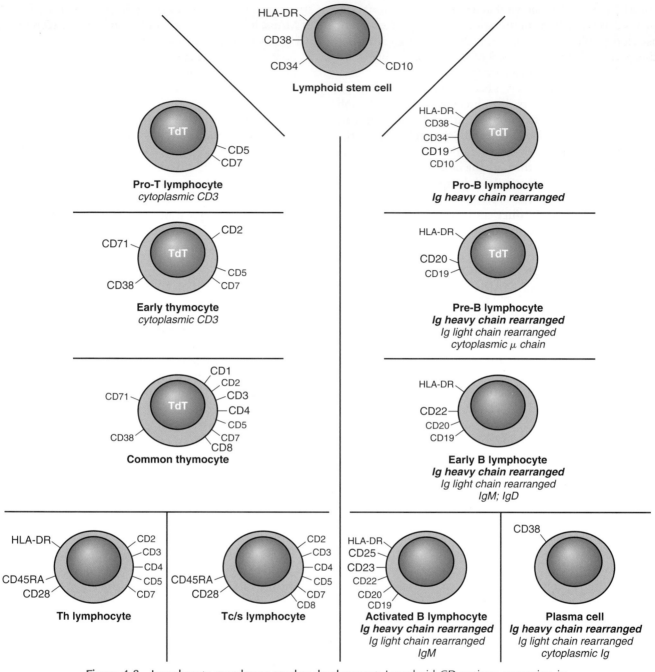

Figure 4-8   Lymphocyte membrane marker development. Lymphoid CD antigen expression in T lymphocytes. *TdT,* Terminal deoxynucleotidyl transferase.

ter an antigen that binds to its receptor, thereby triggering activation and proliferation of the cell. This process, **clonal selection,** accounts for most of the basic properties of the adaptive immune system.

Antigen receptors for common environmental pathogens need to be reinvented by every generation of cells. Because the binding sites of antigen receptors arise from random genetic mechanisms, the receptor repertoire contains binding sites that can react not only with infectious microorgan-

isms, but also with innocuous environmental antigens and "self" antigens.

T-Lymphocyte Subsets

The CD4+ subset was initially described as representing the "helper-inducer" T cell; the CD8+ subset was initially described as representing the "suppressor-cytotoxic" T cells. The complexity of the T cells has increased, with recent reports describing subpopulations of the cells. T cells can be subdivided into several populations using various operational and phenotypic parameters.

Helper T Lymphocytes

Helper T lymphocytes, or T-helper (Th) cells, can be assigned to one of several subsets, including the following:

- Helper T type 1 **(Th1)** cells are responsible for cell-mediated effector mechanisms.
- Helper T type 2 **(Th2)** cells play a greater role in the regulation of antibody production.
- Regulatory T **(Treg)** cells are an immunoregulatory type of Th cells.

These divisions are not absolute, with considerable overlap or redundancy in function among the different subsets. This classification is based on the in vitro blends of cytokines they produce. Th1 and Th2 cells can promote development of cytotoxic cells and are believed to develop from Th0 cells. Th1 cells interact most effectively with mononuclear phagocytes; Th2 release cytokines that are required for B-cell differentiation (Figure 4-9).

Characterized by high interferon-gamma (IFN-γ) production, Th1 responses promote elimination of intracellular pathogens (Figure 4-10, *A*). Characterized by interleukin-4 (IL-4) and IL-5, Th2 responses promote a different type of effector response that involves immunoglobulin E (IgE) production and eosinophils capable of elimination of larger extracellular pathogens, such as helminths (Figure 4-10, *B*). In situations of repeated pathogen exposure or persistent infections, the polarization of T-cell responses serves to focus the antigen-specific response on a specific effector pathway.

The following factors can influence the terminal differentiation of lymphocytes:

- Type of antigen-presenting cell (APC).
- Affinity of the specific antigenic peptide.
- Types of co-stimulatory (costimulatory) molecules expressed by APCs.
- Cytokines acting on T cell during primary activation through TCR.

A hierarchy is apparent among these factors and is determined by how they influence T-cell differentiation. Certain cytokines acting directly on T cells during primary activation appear the most proximal or direct mediators of CD4+ T-cell differentiation. The presence of interleukin-12 (IL-12) during primary T-cell activation leads to strong development of Th1 responses, and IL-4 promotes Th2 development. Activation through the TCR is a requirement for initiating terminal differentiation, but the signals from the TCR appear to be "phenotype neutral."

Certain T cells carry out delayed-hypersensitivity reactions. These T cells react with antigen major histocompatibility complex (MHC) class II on APCs and create their effects mainly through cytokine production. These cells generally are of the CD4+ phenotype.

T cells can also be differentiated into two populations depending on whether they use an alpha-beta (TCR2) or a gamma-delta (TCR1) antigen receptor. The TCR consists of

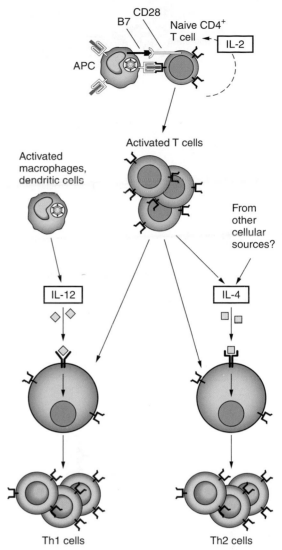

Figure 4-9 Differentiation of naive CD4+ helper T (Th) cells into Th1 and Th2 effector cells. After their activation by antigen and costimulators, naive helper T cells may differentiate into Th1 and Th2 cells under the influence of cytokines. Interleukin-12 *(IL-12)* produced by microbe-activated macrophages and dendritic cells stimulates differentiation of CD4+ T cells into Th1 effectors. In the absence of IL-12, the T cells themselves (and perhaps other cells) produce interleukin-4 *(IL-4)*, which stimulates their differentiation into Th2 effectors. *APC,* Antigen-presenting cell. *(Redrawn from Abbas AK, Lichtman AH:* Basic immunology: functions and disorders of the immune system, *ed 3, Philadelphia, 2008, Saunders.)*

a heterodimer and a number of associated polypeptides that form the CD3 complex. The dimer recognizes processed antigen associated with an MHC molecule. The CD3 complex is required for receptor expression and is involved in signal transduction. TCR1 cells constitute less than 5% of total lymphocytes but appear in greater proportions in some sites (e.g., skin, vagina). TCR1 cells appear to recognize different antigens than TCR2 cells, including carbohydrate and intact protein antigens. In addition, some TCR1 cells do not

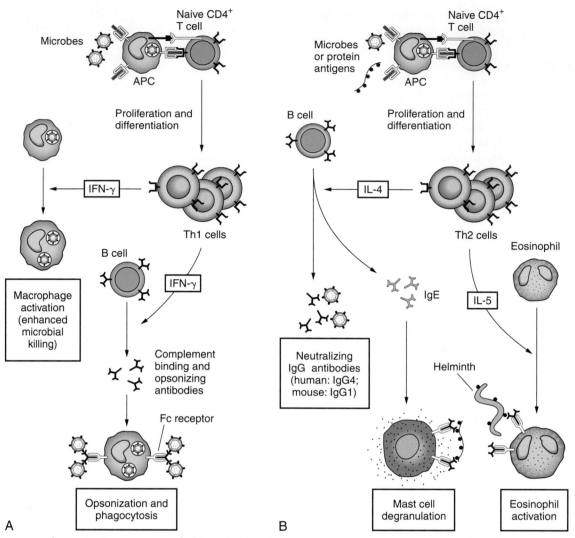

Figure 4-10   Functions of Th1 and Th2 subsets of CD4+ helper T lymphocytes. **A,** Th1 cells produce the cytokine interferon-gamma (*IFN-γ*), which activates phagocytes to kill ingested microbes and stimulates the production of antibodies that promote the ingestion of microbes by the phagocytes. **B,** Th2 cells specific for microbial or nonmicrobial protein antigens produce the cytokines interleukin-4 *(IL-4)*, which stimulates the production of IgE antibody, and IL-5, which activates eosinophils. IgE participates in the activation of mast cells by protein antigens and coats helminths for destruction by eosinophils. Th2 cells also stimulate the production of other antibodies (IgG4 in humans) that neutralize microbes and toxins but do not bind to Fc receptors or activate complement efficiently. *(Redrawn from Abbas AK, Lichtman AH: Basic immunology: functions and disorders of the immune system, ed 3, Philadelphia, 2008, Saunders.)*

require antigen to be processed or to be presented by MHC molecules.

T-Regulatory Lymphocytes.   Treg cells are immunoregulatory Th cells that control autoimmunity in the peripheral blood through "dominant tolerance." Types of Treg cells include the following:

- Natural CD4+ Treg cells
- Th3 cells
- Tr1 cells
- CD8+ Treg cells

Natural Treg cells, characterized by constitutive expression of CD25, are developed primarily in the thymus from positively selected thymocytes with a relatively high avidity for "self" antigens. Natural Treg cells represent approximately 5% to 10% of the total CD4+ T-cell population. The signal to develop into Treg cells is thought to come from interactions between the TCR and the MHC class II–"self" peptide complex expressed on the thymic stroma. In humans, natural Treg cells express CD4 and CD25.

Other types of Treg cells that can develop in the periphery are Tr1 and Th3. *Tr1* cells are CD4+ and are functionally induced by interleukin-10 (IL-10). These Treg cells in turn secrete IL-10 and regulate the immune system. *Th3* progenitor cells are also CD4+. In vitro, CD4+ cells have been shown to secrete transforming growth factor beta (TGF-β). *CD8+* Treg cells are less well characterized and reportedly capable of suppressing CD4+ cells in vitro.

Cytotoxic T Lymphocytes

Cytotoxic T lymphocytes, or T-cytotoxic (Tc) cells, are effector cells found in the peripheral blood that are capable of directly destroying virally infected target cells. Most Tc cells are CD8+ and recognize antigen on the target cell surface associated with MHC class I molecules (HLA-A, HLA-B, HLA-C) or MHC class I alone. This process is demonstrated by the immune response to virus-infected cells or tumor cells (Figure 4-11). In addition to destruction of virally infected, MHC class I–bearing targets, Tc cells are major effectors in allograft organ rejection. Tc cells express either CD4 or CD8, depending on the MHC antigen restriction that governs their antigen recognition (i.e., class I or class II antigens) (Figure 4-12).

Suppressor T lymphocytes, or T-suppressor (Ts) cells, are functionally defined T cells that downregulate the actions of other T and B cells. Ts cells have no unique markers. Although antigen-specific suppression was described in 1970, and many investigators believe that Ts cells are critical in various phases of immunoregulation, peripheral tolerance, and autoimmunity, their mode of action is unclear. Many Ts cells are CD8+ and may operate through secretion of free TCRs.

Antigen Processing and Antigen Presentation to T Cells

Antigen-presenting cells (APCs) are a group of functionally defined cells capable of taking up antigens and presenting them to lymphocytes in a form that they can recognize. APCs take up antigens (e.g., dendritic cells, macrophages, B cells, even tissue cells) in various ways. Some antigens are collected in the periphery and transported to the secondary lymphoid tissues; other APCs normally reside in lymphoid tissues and intercept antigen as it arrives. B cells recognize antigen in a native form.

There are two major pathways of antigen processing for the APC and target cell: endogenous and exogenous.

The *endogenous pathway* processes proteins that have been internalized, processed into fragments, and reexpressed at the cell surface membrane in association with MHC molecules. In this pathway, proteins in the cytoplasm are cleaved into peptide fragments about 20 amino acids in length. These fragments are then transported into the lumen of the endoplasmic reticulum by the transporter associated with the antigen-processing complex, where the fragments encounter newly formed, heavy-chain molecules of MHC class I and their associated beta$_2$-microglobulin (β$_2$m) light chains. The heavy chain, light chain, and peptide form a *trimeric* complex, which is then transported to and expressed on the cell surface. T cells that express the CD8+ cell surface marker recognize antigens that are presented by MHC class I molecules. CD8+ functions as a co-receptor (coreceptor) in this process, binding to an invariant region of the MHC class I molecule.

In the *exogenous pathway,* soluble proteins are taken up from the extracellular environment, generally by specialized or "professional" APCs. The antigens are then processed in a series of intracellular acidic vesicles called *endosomes*. During this process, the endosomes intersect with vesicles that are transporting MHC class II molecules to the cell surface. CD4+ T cells recognize antigens that are presented by MHC class II molecules. As with CD8, the CD4 molecule functions as a coreceptor, increasing the strength of the interaction between the T cell and the APC.

For both systems of antigen presentation, recognition of the antigen by the T cells is described as being "MHC restricted"; that is, the T cells recognize only antigen presented by "self" MHC molecules.

Antigen Recognition by T Cells

T cells are "clonally restricted" so that each T cell expresses a receptor that is able to interact with a given peptide. Each lymphocyte makes only one type of antigen receptor and can recognize only a very limited number of antigens. Because receptors differ on each clone of cells, the entire lymphocyte population has an enormous number of different, specific antigen receptors.

The TCR of most T lymphocytes is composed of an alpha and beta polypeptide chain, with constant regions located close to the cell surface and the part that binds to the antigenic peptide of appropriate fit located away from the cell surface. The difference in the structure of the distal regions of the alpha and beta chains allows the development of different clones of T cells. The TCR reacts with antigen in the context of MHC class I or II molecules on an APC (Figure 4-13).

T cells recognize protein antigens in the form of peptide fragments presented at the cell surface by MHC I or MHC II molecules. When the antigen-specific TCR on the T-cell surface (specifically the zeta-beta chains) of the CD3 complex interacts with the appropriate peptide-MHC complex, it triggers phosphorylation of the intracellular domains of the CD3 zeta chains. Subsequently, the zeta-associated protein 70 (ZAP-70) binds to the phosphorylated zeta chains and is activated.

Simultaneous coligation of the cell marker CD4 (or CD8) with the MHC class II (or I) molecule results in the phosphorylation of particular kinases. These events stimulate the activation of at least three intracellular signaling cascades. T-cell activation also requires a second costimulatory signal (e.g., interaction between marker CD28 on T cell and marker CD80 on APC). This interaction also triggers several intracellular signaling pathways. Activation of T cells can lead to the following:

- Cell division
- Cytokine secretion by T cell
- Expression by T cell of antigens associated with activated state

Activated T cells frequently express "activation antigens" (Table 4-3). Expression of CD69 occurs within 12 hours of

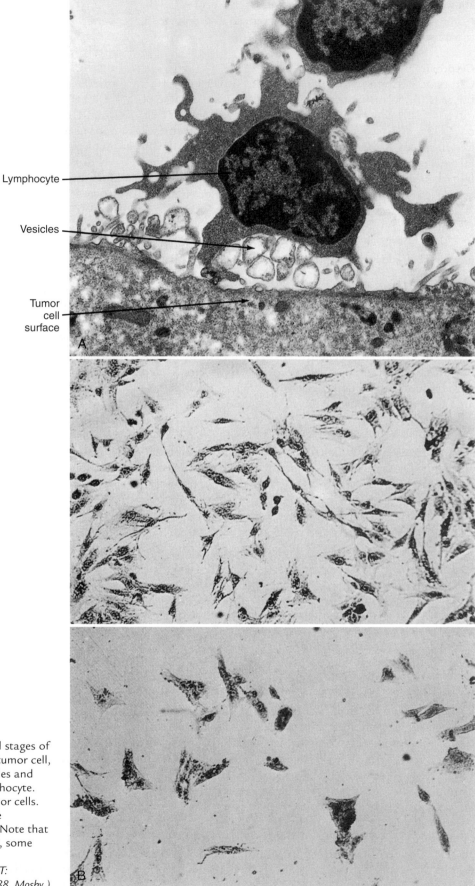

Lymphocyte

Vesicles

Tumor
cell
surface

A

B

Figure 4-11   A, Transmission electron photomicrograph demonstrating the initial stages of the attack of a cytotoxic lymphocyte on a tumor cell, only a portion of which is seen. Note vesicles and blebs of cytoplasm being shed by the lymphocyte. **B,** Effects of cytotoxic lymphocytes on tumor cells. *1,* Tumor cells before contact with immune lymphocytes. *2,* Tumor cells after contact. Note that many cells have detached from the surface, some cells are swollen, and few cells exhibit the morphology of normal cells. *(From Barrett JT: Textbook of immunology, ed 5, St Louis, 1988, Mosby.)*

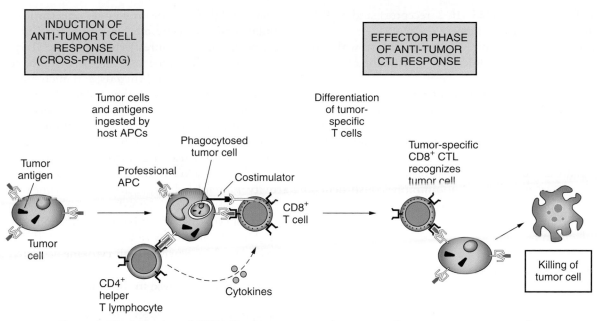

Figure 4-12   Induction of CD8+ T-cell responses against tumors. Responses to tumors may be induced by *cross-priming* (or cross-presentation), in which the tumor cells and tumor antigens are taken up by specialized ("professional") antigen-presenting cells *(APCs)*, processed, and presented to T cells. In some cases, B7 costimulators expressed by the APCs provide the second signals for the differentiation of the CD8+ T cells. APCs may also stimulate CD4+ helper T cells, which provide the second signals for cytotoxic T lymphocyte *(CTL)* development. Differentiated CTLs kill tumor cells without a requirement for costimulation or T-cell help. *(From Abbas AK, Lichtman AH:* Basic immunology: functions and disorders of the immune system, *ed 3, Philadelphia, 2008, Saunders.)*

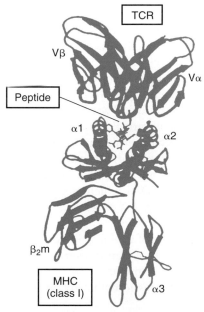

Figure 4-13   Recognition of peptide-MHC by TCR. This ribbon diagram is drawn from the crystal structure of the extracellular portion of a peptide–major histocompatibility complex *(MHC)* bound to a T-cell antigen receptor *(TCR)* that is specific for the peptide displayed by the MHC molecule. The peptide can be seen attached to the cleft at the top of the MHC molecule, and one residue of the peptide contacts the variable *(V)* region of a TCR. *(Redrawn from Bjorkman PJ:* MHC restriction in three dimensions: a view of T cell receptor/ligand interactions, *Cell 89:167-170, 1997. © Cell Press; with permission.)*

Table 4-3	T-Cell Activation Profile
Components	**Reference Range (% positive)**
CD2	75-92
CD3	63-84
CD69+ and CD3+	0-2
CD25+ and CD2+	0-5
CD71+ and CD2+	0-8
HLA-DR+ (class II HLA) and CD3+	1-9
TCR alpha-beta	59-84
TCR gamma-delta	0-10

Data from Associated Regional and University Pathologists (ARUP): *Interpretive data guide,* ed 2, Salt Lake City, Utah, 1999, ARUP, p 473.
CD, Cluster of differentiation; *HLA,* human leukocyte antigen; *TCR,* T-cell receptor.

activation, followed by CD25 (IL-2 receptor) and CD71 (transferrin receptor) in 1 to 3 days.

Alternatively, in the case of Tc cells, interaction with antigen through the specific TCR leads to destruction of target cells.

If a cell does not receive a full set of signals, it will not divide, and it may even become anergic. Peripheral T cells generally exist in a resting state (G0 or G1). T-cell activation is a complex reaction involving transmembrane signaling and intracellular enzyme activation steps. It is through soluble cytokines that the T-cell regulation influences the action of other T cells, accessory cells, and nonimmune constituents. When activated by the proper signals, T cells may carry out one or more of the following functions:

1. Proliferation
2. Differentiation
3. Production of cytokines
4. Development of effector function

T-Independent Antigen Triggering

Some antigens, particularly polysaccharide polymers (e.g., dextran), can trigger B cells without help from T cells. These *T-independent antigens* generally are not strong, provoke mainly IgM responses, and induce minimal immunologic memory.

NATURAL KILLER AND K-TYPE LYMPHOCYTES

A subpopulation of circulating lymphocytes (~10%), the natural killer (NK) and K-type lymphocytes lack conventional antigen receptors of T or B cells. These cells are classified as "effector" lymphocytes that produce mediators (e.g., interferon, IL-2).

Although these cells were previously classified as "null cells," MAbs demonstrate that NK and K-type cells express a variety of surface membrane markers (Table 4-4). Most of these cells lack CD3 but express CD2, CD16, CD56, CD57, and occasionally CD8.

Natural Killer Cells

A total of 70% to 80% of NK cells have the appearance of large granular lymphocytes (LGLs). Up to about 75% of LGLs function as NK cells, and LGLs appear to account fully for the NK activity in mixed-cell populations.

Table 4-4	Natural Killer (NK) Cell Profile
Components	**Reference Interval (% positive)**
CD2	75-92
CD3	63-84
CD5	61-88
CD7	73-94
CD8	14-39
CD16	1-12
CD56	7-27
CD57	1-26

Data from ARUP: *Interpretive data guide*, ed 2, Salt Lake City, Utah, 1999, ARUP, p 473.

Natural killer cells destroy target cells through an extracellular, nonphagocytic mechanism referred to as a "cytotoxic reaction, MHC-unrestricted cytolysis." Target cells include tumor cells, some cells of the embryo, cells of the normal bone marrow and thymus, and microbial agents. Increasing evidence suggests that a considerable number of NK cells may be present in other tissues, particularly in the lungs and liver, where they may play important roles in inflammatory reactions and in host defense, including defense against certain viruses (e.g., cytomegalovirus, hepatitis). NK cells will actively kill virally infected target cells, and if this activity is completed before the virus has time to replicate, a viral infection may be stopped.

Several cytokines affect NK cell activation and proliferation. NK cells are highly responsive to IL-2, IL-7, and IL-12. These cytokines generate high cytokine-activated killer activity in these cells. In addition, NK cells synthesize a number of cytokines involved in the modulation of hematopoiesis and immune responses and in the regulation of their own activities.

Target cell recognition and the molecular identification and analysis of the involved NK cell receptors are undergoing intensive research. These molecules are mainly classified under the family of **cell adhesion molecules (CAMs).** The main class of effector CAMs shown to mediate NK cell functions is the leukocyte integrins, more specifically, the beta-2 class of integrins.

Several NK cell surface molecules involved in target cell recognition and binding have been identified. NK cells recognize targets using several cell surface molecular receptors (e.g., CD2, CD69, NKR-P1) and a high density of the Fc receptor CD16 of IgG (FC-R III). They also receive inhibitory signals from MHC class I on potential target cells, transduced by a "killer inhibitory receptor" on the NK cell. CD56 may mediate interactions between effector and target cells. NK cells are able to bind and lyse antibody-coated nucleated cells through a membrane Fc receptor that can recognize a part of the heavy chain of immunoglobulins. This enables NK cells to mediate *antibody-dependent, cell-mediated cytotoxic* (ADCC) activities. Some, if not all, of the activation of NK cells is mediated by CD16, which exerts a regulatory role in their cytolytic function. NK cells respond to cross-linking of CD16 and CD69 as follows:

- Increasing the rate of proliferation of NK cells.
- Elevating the levels of tumor necrosis factor production within 4 hours of stimulation.
- Increasing the expression of CD69 on the cell surface of NK cells.
- Increasing the cytotoxicity activity against a normally resistant cell line (P815).

K-Type Lymphocytes

K-type killer cells are mononuclear cells that can kill target cells sensitized with antibody, which they engage through their Fc receptors. Most K-type cells are non-T, non-B lymphocytes, but macrophages and eosinophils can also have K-cell activity.

K-type cells exhibit a different cytotoxic mechanism than NK cells. The target cell must be coated with low concentrations of IgG antibody, referred to as an *ADCC reaction.* An ADCC reaction may be exhibited by both K cells and phagocytic and nonphagocytic myelogenous-type leukocytes. K cells are capable of lysing tumor cells. Although morphologically similar to a small lymphocyte, the precise lineage of the K cell is uncertain.

B LYMPHOCYTES

B cells represent a small proportion of the circulating peripheral blood lymphocytes. B1 and B2 cells are B-cell subsets. B1 cells are distinguished by the CD5 marker, appear to form a self-renewing set, respond to a number of common microbial antigens, and occasionally generate autoantibodies. B2 cells account for the majority of the B lymphocytes in adults. This subset generates a greater diversity of antigen receptors and responds effectively to T-dependent antigen.

B cells are derived from progenitor cells through an antigen-independent maturation process occurring in the bone marrow and GALT. Participation of B cells in the humoral immune response is accomplished by reacting to antigenic stimuli through division and differentiation into plasma cells. Plasma cells or antibody-forming cells are terminally differentiated B cells. These cells are entirely devoted to antibody production, a primary host defense against microorganisms.

The specific antibodies produced are able to bind to infected cells and free organisms bearing the antigen, then inactivate those cells or organisms and destroy them. The condition of hyperacute rejection of transplanted organs is also mediated by B cells. In addition, antigenic stimulation prompts B cells to multiply.

Cell Surface Markers

Primitive B-cell precursors have delta chains in their cytoplasm and no immunoglobulin (Ig) on their surface. More differentiated (but still immature) B cells have intact cytoplasmic IgM and surface IgM. Mature B cells lose their cytoplasmic IgM and add surface IgD to the surface IgM. These changes appear to occur in the absence of antigen and depend on cytokines. In humans there is evidence of four types of B-cell markers, described next.
1. The best studied B-cell surface marker is the Ig receptor. This receptor is actually an antibody molecule with antigenic specificity. According to the clonal selection theory, B cells exist in the body with Ig receptors specific for antigen before exposure to the antigenic substances. When specific antigen exposure does occur, the antigen will select the B cell having an Ig receptor with the best fit. After binding and cooperative interaction with T cells, B cells undergo transformation into plasma cells. The secreted antibody in turn has the same specificity as the Ig receptor on the B cell. Virtually all the antibody produced by plasma cells is secreted (plasma cells have few Ig receptors), but 90% of the antibody produced by B cells is expressed as

surface Ig receptors. Some antigens (e.g., lipopolysaccharides from some gram-negative organisms) can bind to the Ig receptor and also stimulate an antibody response independent of T-cell cooperation (T-independent antigens). This type of response is generally of low intensity and is class-restricted to the production of IgM antibody.

B cells have **surface immunoglobulin (sIg)** (except for very immature lymphocytes and mature plasma cells) that are normally polyclonal (i.e., kappa and lambda light chains are present on cytoplasmic membrane of B cells). Mu and delta heavy chains are usually found with either kappa or lambda chains on any one cell surface. Gamma and alpha chains are rarely found on the surface of properly prepared, normal lymphocytes.
2. An Fc receptor that specifically binds the Fc portion of IgG antibody may function to aid B cells in binding to antigen already bound to antibody.
3. Receptors that bind fragments of the cleaved complement component C3 have been reported on the surface of approximately 75% of B cells. This receptor binds C3b, iC3b (inactivated C3b), and C3d, but the function of these receptors is not completely understood.
4. B-cell surface antigens coded by the MHC class II genes are a fourth type of B-cell marker in humans.

B-Cell Activation

B cells can be stimulated in their resting state to enlarge, develop synthetic machinery, divide, mature, and secrete antibody. The proper signals for this sequence depend on the type of triggers, which can be specific or nonspecific and polyclonal. Specific activation involves the antigen that is complementary to the particular Ig on the surface. Nonspecific activation occurs with B-cell mitogens.

Efficient antibody production to complex protein antigens requires T-cell help, which in turn develops from APC presentation of antigen to the T cell. Activated T cells secrete a variety of cytokines that, together with the specific antigen, trigger the B cell to develop into an antibody-secreting cell. This process also involves "class switching."

In the immune response to a foreign protein, the first antibodies to appear are of the IgM class (or **isotype**). As the response proceeds, other isotypes (IgG, IgA, and IgE) emerge from Ig class switching. The isotype switch has considerable clinical importance because each of the four major isotypes has specialized biologic properties. IgG is the principal class of antibody in interstitial fluids, and IgA is the protective antibody of mucosal surfaces. Isotype switching requires collaboration between antibody-synthesizing B cells and helper CD4+ T cells. The B cell uses IgM molecules on its surface to capture the antigen and present the antigen to the T cell. Contact between the collaborating lymphocytes is enhanced by complementary pairs of CAMs. Some CAMs (e.g., CD4, MHC class II antigens) are constitutively expressed on the surface of T and B cells, whereas others are induced. For example, contact between B and T cells induces the T cell to express a ligand for the B-cell surface molecule CD40. In turn, CD40 interacts with the newly expressed

CD40 ligand on the T cell, which leads to the expression of another B-cell surface molecule, B7. The latter's partner on the surface of the T lymphocyte is CD28. These cooperative and synergistic interactions between the T cell and B cell induce the secretion of cytokines such as IL-2 and IL-4.

Isotype switching requires two signals. The first is delivered by an interleukin and the second by the binding of CD40 to its ligand on the T cell. In the process of switching from IgM synthesis to IgE synthesis, IL-4 makes the IgE gene in the B cell accessible to the switch machinery initiated when CD40 binds to its ligand. In this process the gene that encodes the variable region (part of antibody molecule that contains antigen-binding site) moves from its position near the gene that encodes for IgM to a position near the gene that encodes for IgE.

OTHER TYPES OF LYMPHOCYTES

"Virgin" or "naive" lymphocytes are cells that have not encountered their specific antigen. These cells do express high-molecular-weight variants of leukocyte common antigen.

Memory cells are populations of long-lived T or B cells that have been stimulated by antigen. These cells can make a quick response to a previously encountered antigen. Memory B cells carry surface IgG as their antigen receptor; memory T cells express the CD45RO variant of the leukocyte common antigen and increased levels of CAMs (e.g., LFA-3, VLA-4).

PLASMA CELL BIOLOGY

The function of **plasma cells** is the synthesis and excretion of immunoglobulins. Plasma cells are not normally found in the circulating blood but are found in the bone marrow in concentrations that do not normally exceed 2%. Plasma cells arise as the end stage of B-cell differentiation into a large, activated plasma cell.

The pathway from the B lymphocyte to the antibody-synthesizing plasma cell forms when the B cell is antigenically stimulated and undergoes transformation because of the stimulation of various interleukins. The immune antibody response begins when individual B lymphocytes encounter an antigen that binds to their specific Ig surface receptors. After receiving an appropriate "second signal" provided by interaction with helper T cells, these antigen-binding B cells undergo transformation and proliferation to generate a clone of mature plasma cells that secrete a specific type of antibody.

An increase in plasma cells can be seen in a variety of nonmalignant disorders, such as viral disease (e.g., rubella, infectious mononucleosis), allergic conditions, chronic infections, and collagen diseases. In plasma cell dyscrasias the plasma cells can be greatly increased or can completely infiltrate the bone marrow (e.g., multiple myeloma, Waldenström's macroglobulinemia).

Antibody molecules secreted by plasma cells consist of four chains (two light chains and two heavy chains, based on molecular weight) and can be enzymatically cleaved into Fab ("antigen-binding") and Fc ("crystallizable") fragments. The Fab portion binds antigen and contains the light chains and their antigenic markers (kappa, lambda), as well as heavy chains.

The Fc fragment contains the markers that distinguish the different classes of antibody and sites that will bind and activate complement and bind to Fc receptors on cells. The amino acid sequence for most of the antibody protein is constant, except for the antigen-binding portion of the molecule that has a hypervariable region and accounts for the various antigenic specificities that the antibody is programmed to recognize.

ALTERATIONS IN LYMPHOCYTE SUBSETS

The normal functioning of helper cells and suppressor cells in the immune response can be reversed under certain conditions. For example, the target cell for human T-cell leukemia or immunodeficiency virus (HIV) is phenotypically a helper cell but functionally a suppressor cell. Functionally, the helper-inducer subset of cells signal B cells to generate antibodies, control production and switching of types of antibodies formed, and activate suppressor cells. The suppressor-cytotoxic lymphocytes control and inhibit antibody production either by suppressing helper cells or by turning off B-cell differentiation. The normal ratio of helper cells and suppressor cells (~2:1) can be reversed under certain conditions.

Changes with Aging

Except for inconsistent values seen in extremely elderly persons, the total number of T cells in the peripheral blood is relatively stable throughout adult life. However, there is a change in the distribution of T-cell subpopulations. A decrease in the number of suppressor cells and an increase in the helper cell population are demonstrated in older adults.

The effect of aging on the immune response is highly variable, but the ability to respond immunologically to disease is age related. Faulty immunologic reactions, such as aberrant functioning of immunoregulatory cells, effector T cells, and antibody-producing B cells, may contribute to poor immunity in older adults. Functional deficits of T lymphocytes have been identified with aging, causing impairment of cell-mediated immunity. In addition, skin testing reveals decreases in the intensity of delayed hypersensitivity in older adults. The proliferative response of T lymphocytes to mitogens or antigens such as *Mycobacterium tuberculosis* or varicella-zoster virus is impaired.

A decrease in Th cells is the primary cause of impaired humoral response in older adults. Although the total number of B cells and total Ig concentration remain unchanged, the serum concentration of IgM is decreased, and IgA and IgG concentrations are increased.

EVALUATION OF SUSPECTED DEFECTS

Although more than 50 genetically determined immunodeficiency syndromes have been reported since 1952, defects in immunity were considered rare until acquired immunodefi-

Table 4-5	Initial Evaluation of Suspected Immunodeficiency
Suspected Deficiency	**Appropriate Laboratory Procedures**
All suspected immunodeficiencies	Complete blood count with platelet evaluation Erythrocyte sedimentation rate
Antibody deficiency	Screen for anti-A and anti-B isoagglutinins Screen for antibodies to diphtheria or tetanus toxoids
T-cell deficiency	Absolute lymphocyte count Intradermal skin test to *Candida albicans* 1:1000 or 1:100
Phagocytic cell deficiency	Absolute neutrophil count Nitroblue tetrazolium test

ciency syndrome (AIDS) emerged more than 25 years ago. This growing list of primary and secondary diseases now encompasses all major components of the immune system, including lymphocytes, phagocytic cells, and complement proteins (Table 4-5). Clinical and laboratory tests for the evaluation of patients with suspected disorders must be informative, reliable, and cost-effective.

A complete blood cell (CBC) count and erythrocyte sedimentation rate (ESR) are among the most cost-effective screening tests. If the ESR is normal, chronic bacterial infection is unlikely. If the absolute neutrophil count is normal, congenital and acquired neutropenias and severe chemotactic defects are eliminated. If the absolute lymphocyte count is normal, the patient is not likely to have a severe T-cell defect. The absolute lymphocyte count is the number of lymphocytes in the total white blood cell (WBC) population (Box 4-1).

Cell-Mediated Immune System

Deficiencies of cell-mediated immunity (discussed in detail later) are often suspected in individuals with recurrent viral, fungal, parasitic, and protozoal infections. Patients with AIDS exhibit some of the most severe manifestations of cell-mediated immunity (see Chapter 25).

One avenue of testing involves delayed-hypersensitivity skin testing to determine the integrity of the patient's cell-mediated immune response. More than 90% of normal adults will react to one of the following antigens within 48 hours after antigen exposure: *Candida albicans,* trichophyton, tetanus toxoid, mumps, and streptokinase-streptodor-

Box 4-1	Determination of Absolute Lymphocyte Count

Absolute number of lymphocytes =
   Total leukocyte count × Percentage (%) of lymphocytes
Total leukocyte count = 25×10^9/L
Relative percentage (%) of lymphocytes = 76%
Absolute number = 19×10^9/L

nase. Reactivity to histoplasmin or purified protein derivative (PPD) is positive in patients with active infection or previous exposure to histoplasmosis or tuberculosis, respectively; therefore these tests are not useful in the assessment of anergy.

The number of T lymphocytes, the primary effector cells in cell-mediated reactions, can be determined by several techniques. The "gold standard" was the E technique (erythrocyte rosette formation) but the development of MAbs has replaced this technique. Mabs are a quick and specific method for determining the number of T lymphocytes. These immunofluorescent techniques use fluorescent microscopy or the fluorescence-activated cell sorter (FACS). Additional testing can include functional testing or measurement of biologic response modifiers such as IL-2 (T-cell growth factor).

Humoral System

The humoral system can be screened for abnormalities by quantitating the concentrations of IgM, IgG, and IgA. An initial simple screening can be determined by the presence and titer of antibodies to type A and B red blood cell (RBC) antigens.

Lymphocyte Testing

In functional testing, phenotypes are enumerated in proportional relationship to one another. Functional assays evaluate the response of lymphocytes to nonspecific mitogens. In the case of T lymphocytes, mitogens (e.g., pokeweed) or specific antigens (e.g., PPD) are used. Functional testing of B lymphocytes is confined to determining the response to pure B-cell mitogen such as *Staphylococcus aureus*–Cowan strain and antibody production. These substances initiate deoxyribonucleic acid (DNA) synthesis and mitosis or production of antibodies, to determine which cells are functioning abnormally. A patient may have a normal proportion of phenotypically defined suppressor cells, but functional tests might show that those cells are impaired.

Several tests were used before the introduction of highly specific fluorescent MAb testing to distinguish T and B cells. T lymphocytes were defined by their ability to form rosettes with sheep erythrocytes (Figure 4-14); they were further subclassified by their ability to form rosettes with Ig or bovine erythrocytes coated with **complement** (a soluble blood protein consisting of nine components, C1-C9, which if activated can lead to rupture of the cellular membrane). This test demonstrated that the surface membrane of T cells had receptors for attachment to normal sheep erythrocytes. B cells had membrane-bound antibody and receptors, including the complement (C3) receptor. The presence of the C3 receptor could be demonstrated by the ability of B cells to bind erythrocytes with complement to form the erythrocyte-antibody-complement rosettes. B lymphocytes were indisputably characterized by their surface membrane Ig markers. Using these techniques, a population of non-B, non-T cells could also be shown.

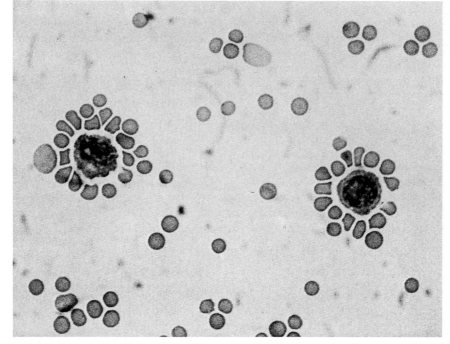

Figure 4-14 Rosettes in Giemsa-stained, cytocentrifuged preparation from normal adult peripheral blood sample. *(From Bauer JD:* Clinical laboratory methods, *ed 9, St Louis, 1982, Mosby.)*

IMMUNOLOGIC DISORDERS

A breakdown in any part of the immune mechanism can lead to disease. Disorders with an immunologic origin can involve progenitor cells, phagocytosis (see Chapter 3), T cells, B cells, or complement (see Chapter 5).

Immunologic disorders can be divided into primary processes (dysfunction in the immune organ itself) and acquired, or secondary, processes (disease or therapy causing an immune defect). A third category, diseases mediated through immune mechanisms, can also be included. Because of its complexity and contemporary importance, AIDS is discussed separately in Chapter 25. Other immunoproliferative and autoimmune disorders are presented in Chapters 27 to 30.

Immunodeficiency disorders may be caused by defects in the quality (defects) or quantity (deficiencies) of lymphocytes and may be congenital or acquired. These conditions may be combined disorders or may involve either T cells or B cells (Table 4-6).

Table 4-6	Examples of T-Cell and B-Cell Disorders	
T-Cell Disorder	**B-Cell Disorder**
Congenital	
Thymic hypoplasia (DiGeorge's syndrome)	Bruton's agammaglobulinemia
Acquired	
Acquired immunodeficiency syndrome	Autoimmune disorders
Hodgkin's disease	Multiple myeloma
Chronic lymphocytic leukemia	
Systemic lupus erythematosus	

Primary Immunodeficiency Disorders

Classic primary immunodeficiency disorders (PIDs) are usually monogenic (mendelian) disorders affecting host defenses (Box 4-2). More than 200 clinical phenotypes of PID have been described, about 100 of which now have a well-defined molecular genetic basis. Diseases associated with a primary defect in the immune response comprise about 40% T-cell disorders, 50% B-cell disorders, 6% phagocytic abnormalities, and 4% complement alterations (Figure 4-15). The most common T-cell deficiency states are those associated with a concurrent B-cell abnormality. Primary immunodeficiency disorders are predominantly seen (75%) in children under age 5 years.

T-Cell and Combined Immunodeficiency Disorders
DiGeorge's Syndrome

Etiology. This T-cell defect is a congenital anomaly that represents faulty embryogenesis of the endodermal derivation of third and fourth pharyngeal pouches, which results in aplasia of the parathyroid and thymus glands. At autopsy, parathyroid and a vestigial thymus may be found in ectopic locations. The newborn may exhibit various facial and vascular anomalies, collectively referred to as pharyngeal pouch syndrome. In addition to the established embryonic cause of DiGeorge's syndrome, a question of a nutrient (zinc) deficiency in utero has been suggested as a cause of this process.

Signs and Symptoms. DiGeorge's syndrome is present at birth. Initial manifestations can include hypocalcemic tetany, unusual facies, and congenital heart defects. An increased susceptibility to viral, fungal, and disseminated bacterial infections (e.g., acid-fast bacilli, *Listeria monocytogenes, Pneumocystis jiroveci/carinii*) result from the defect of T cells

Box 4-2	Primary Immunodeficiency Diseases

T Cells

Combined immunodeficiency
    Thymic alymphoplasia
    Swiss type
    Adenosine deaminase deficiency
    Nezelof syndrome
DiGeorge's syndrome (thymic hypoplasia)
Wiskott-Aldrich syndrome
Chronic mucocutaneous candidiasis
Immunodeficiency associated with nucleoside phosphorylase
    deficiency
Short-limbed dwarfism
Ataxia-telangiectasia
Thymoma
Leukocyte adhesion deficiency (LAD)

B Cells

Selected IgA deficiency associated with:
    Normal state
    Allergy
    Autoimmune disease
    Central nervous system disease
    Gastrointestinal disorders
    Malignancy
    Pulmonary infections
X-linked infantile agammaglobulinemia
X-linked immunodeficiency with hyper-IgM
Common variable hypogammaglobulinemia
Selective IgM deficiency
IgG subclass deficiency

Modified from Graziano FM, Bell CL: *Med Clin North Am* 69(3):445, 1985.

normally controlled by cell-mediated immunity. Infants usually die of sepsis during the first year of life.

Immunologic Manifestations. Peripheral lymphoid tissue appears to be normal except for depletion of T cells in the thymus-dependent zones, such as subcortical region of the lymph nodes and perifollicular and periarteriolar lymphoid sheaths of the spleen. Lymph node paracortical areas and thymus-dependent regions of the spleen show variable degrees of depletion.

In the circulating blood, lymphopenia is generally present, although in some cases the concentration of lymphocytes is normal. However, an abnormally high CD4+/CD8+ ratio is present because of a decrease in CD8+ cells. Most patients with DiGeorge's syndrome have a decreased percentage of cells expressing the CD3+ (mature T cell) antigen. Because patients do demonstrate lymphocytes capable of differentiating to the more mature surface markers such as CD4+, a small rudimentary thymus is believed to be present in these patients. Lymphocytic responsiveness to antigenic and mitogenic stimulation can be absent, reduced, or normal depending on the degree of thymic deficiency. Cell-mediated immune reactions such as delayed hypersensitivity and skin allograft rejections, however, are absent or feeble.

Serum Ig concentrations are near normal. IgA may be diminished and IgE elevated. Antibody response to primary antigenic stimulation may be unimpaired.

Nezelof Syndrome (Cellular Immunodeficiency with Immunoglobulins)

Etiology. An autosomal recessive pattern of inheritance is often seen. The defect appears to exist on chromosome 14q13.1.

Signs and Symptoms. Nezelof syndrome is the PID most likely to be confused with AIDS in the pediatric age group. Infants have failure to thrive, recurrent or chronic pulmonary infections, oral or cutaneous candidiasis, chronic diarrhea, recurrent skin infections, gram-negative sepsis, urinary tract infections, and severe varicella.

Immunologic Manifestations. Nezelof syndrome is characterized by lymphopenia, neutropenia, and eosinophilia. In addition, diminished lymphoid tissue and abnormal thymus architecture are observed. Peripheral lymphoid tissues are hypoplastic and demonstrate paracortical lymphocyte depletion. Lymphocyte responses to mitogens, antigens, and allogeneic cells are profoundly depressed but not totally absent. Serum levels of most of the five Ig classes are normal or increased. Antibody-forming capacity has been reported as normal in one third of cases.

Severe Combined Immunodeficiency

Etiology. Severe combined immunodeficiency (SCID) is caused by inappropriate development of progenitor cells into lymphocyte precursors. This hereditary and invariably fatal disorder in infants results from the lack of both T and B cells and the consequent inability to synthesize antibody.

Recently, mutations in the IL-2 receptor complex, a hematopoietic growth factor, have been shown to cause X-linked SCID in humans. Two modes of inheritance are known: autosomal recessive and X-linked recessive. X-linked recessive SCID is thought to be the most common form of SCID in the United States, which accounts for the 3:1 male/female ratio with the disorder.

Half the patients with autosomal SCID have a concomitant deficiency of adenosine deaminase (ADA), an aminohy-

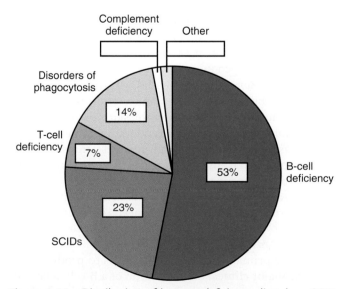

Figure 4-15 Distribution of immunodeficiency disorders. *SCIDs,* Severe combined immunodeficiencies.

drolase that converts adenosine to inosine. Analysis by complementary (copy) DNA (cDNA) probe has revealed that the deficiency results from a hereditable point mutation in the ADA gene. Another variant with a severe deficiency in T-cell immunity but normal B-cell concentrations is associated with purine nucleotide phosphorylase deficiency.

There are two main forms of defective expression of MHC antigens. In a less common cause of SCID, "bare lymphocyte syndrome," an MHC class I antigen deficiency, is present. In another form of defective expression, MHC class I antigen deficiency plus the absence of class II antigens is present. Patient lymphocytes cannot be typed by standard serologic cytotoxicity tests.

Signs and Symptoms.   No important differences in signs and symptoms exist between the two major genetic types of SCID. Initial manifestations of SCID are repeated debilitating infections beginning within the first 6 months of life. These are dominated by bacterial, viral, and fungal infections of the respiratory and intestinal systems and skin. Infants with SCID usually die within 3 years of birth from lung abscesses, *Pneumocystis* pneumonitis, or a common viral disorder such as chickenpox or measles.

Immunologic Manifestations.   The thymus and other lymphoid organs are severely hypoplastic. The bone marrow is devoid of lymphoblasts, lymphocytes, and plasma cells. Lymphocytes are also absent from lymphoid tissues such as the spleen, tonsils, appendix, and intestinal tract. Variable hypogammaglobulinemia with decreased serum IgM and IgA levels and poor to absent antibody production are representative characteristics. Moderate lymphocytopenia is detectable early in infancy. T-cell functions are decreased. The circulating blood contains no CD4+, CD8+, or CD3+ cells. The percentage of B cells is usually normal.

Patients with the X-linked form of SCID usually appear similar to those with the autosomal recessive form, except they tend to have an increased percentage of B cells. However, the defect affects B-lineage cells as well as T-lineage cells.

Chronic Mucocutaneous Candidiasis

Etiology.   Chronic mucocutaneous candidiasis (CMC) results from a primary defect in cell-mediated immunity. T cells specifically fail to recognize only the *Candida* antigen.

Signs and Symptoms.   Patients with CMC usually survive to adulthood. The characteristic manifestation is *Candida* infection of mucous membranes, scalp, skin, and nails. Endocrine abnormalities, often polyendocrinopathies, are frequently associated with fungal manifestations. Sudden death from adrenal insufficiency has been reported in patients with CMC.

Immunologic Manifestations.   Patients demonstrate normal skin reactions to testing with all antigens except *Candida*.

B-Cell and Antibody Deficiency Disorders

Because the primary function of B cells is to produce antibody, the major clinical manifestation of a B-cell deficiency is an increased susceptibility to severe bacterial infections.

Selective IgA deficiency is the most common B-cell disorder, affecting 1 in 400 to 800 persons. Because IgA is the primary immunoglobulin in secretions, a deficiency contributes to pulmonary infections, gastrointestinal (GI) disorders, and allergic respiratory disorders. Most cases (50% of reported cases are associated with Ig deficiencies) are autoimmune in nature, including rheumatoid arthritis (RA), systemic lupus erythematosus (SLE), thyroiditis, and pernicious anemia.

Bruton's X-Linked Agammaglobulinemia

Etiology.   This is a classic example of an X-linked agammaglobulinemia, in which a disease-causing variant in the gene coding for Bruton's tyrosine kinase (BTK) leads to arrest of B-cell development at the pre B-cell stage.

Signs and Symptoms.   X-linked agammaglobulinemia occurs primarily in young boys, but scattered cases have been identified in girls. Manifestations begin in the first or second year of life. Hypersusceptibility to infection does not develop until 9 to 12 months after birth because of passive protection by residual maternal immunoglobulin. Thereafter, patients repeatedly acquire infections with high-grade extracellular pyogenic organisms such as streptococci. This disorder is characterized by sinopulmonary and central nervous system (CNS) infectious episodes and severe septicemia, but patients are not abnormally susceptible to common viral infection (excluding fulminant hepatitis) or to enterococci or most gram-negative organisms. Chronic fungal infections are not usually present.

An autoimmune phenomenon, especially a juvenile RA type of disease, has also been associated with X-linked agammaglobulinemia. In addition, patients are highly vulnerable to a malignant form of dermatomyositis that eventually involves destructive T-cell infiltration surrounding the small vessels of the CNS. In addition to infections and connective tissue disorders, agammaglobulinemic patients also have hemolytic anemia, drug eruptions, atopic eczema, allergic rhinitis, and asthma.

Immunologic Manifestations.   The diagnosis of X-linked agammaglobulinemia is suspected if serum concentrations of IgG, IgA, and IgM are notably below the appropriate level for the patient's age. Tests for natural antibodies to blood group substances and for antibodies to antigens given during standard courses of immunization (e.g., diphtheria) are useful in distinguishing this disorder from transient hypogammaglobulinemia of infancy (see later discussion).

B cells are virtually absent from bone marrow and lymphoid tissues. A deficiency or absence of peripheral B lymphocytes is usually noted in this disorder. If present, B cells are unresponsive to T cells and incapable of antibody synthesis or secretion. Surface immunoglobulins are absent. However, patients do have normal numbers of CD3+ and CD8+ cells, and many have normal CD4+ cells. Male children possess normal T-cell function; therefore, homograft rejection mechanisms are intact, and delayed-hypersensitivity reaction for both tuberculin and skin contact types can be elicited.

Common Variable Immunodeficiency

Etiology. Common variable immunodeficiency (CVID) is a form of primary acquired agammaglobulinemia, occurring equally in males and females. The etiology of CVID seems to be heterogeneous, with abnormalities of B-cell maturation, antibody production, antibody secretion, or T-cell regulation. Family clusters have been reported in which first-degree relatives of patients with selective IgA deficiency have a high incidence of abnormal Ig concentration, autoantibodies, autoimmune disease, and malignant neoplasms. Recent findings of rare alleles or deletions of MHC class III genes in patients with IgA deficiency of CVID suggest that the susceptibility gene(s) is (are) on chromosome 6.

Signs and Symptoms. CVID usually manifests in the second or third decade of life. The signs and symptoms include frequent sinopulmonary infections, diarrhea, endocrine and autoimmune disorders, and malabsorption (e.g., vitamin B_{12}). Intestinal giardiasis is also prevalent.

Immunologic Manifestations. Both the concentration and near absence of serum and secretory IgA are thought to represent the most common and well-defined PID. The pattern of inheritance suggests that an autosomal function of antibodies is usually compromised. The number of B cells is typically normal or mildly depressed. Despite a normal number of circulating Ig-bearing B lymphocytes and the presence of lymphoid cortical follicles, blood lymphocytes do not differentiate into Ig-producing cells. In most patients the defect appears to be intrinsic to the B cell. The primary defect in Ig synthesis may be caused by the absence or dysfunction of CD4+ cells or by increased CD8+ supressor cell activity. Therefore, both cellular immunity and Ig production are impaired by the interaction between helper and suppressor T-cell subsets. Lymph nodes lack plasma cells, but they may show striking follicular hyperplasia.

The total IgG level may be normal, but a subclass (usually IgG2 or IgG3) is deficient. Both IgA and IgM may be detectable, but IgM levels may be elevated.

In addition, some patients may have thymoma and refractory anemia.

Immunoglobulin Subclass Deficiencies

Some patients have deficiencies of one or more subclasses of IgG despite normal total IgG serum concentrations. Most of those with absent or very low concentrations of IgG2 have been patients with selective IgA deficiency.

Selective IgA Deficiency

Etiology. An isolated absence mode is often seen in pedigrees containing individuals with CVID. IgA deficiency has been noted to evolve into CVID, and rare alleles and deletions of MHC class III genes in both conditions suggest a common basis.

Signs and Symptoms. IgA deficiency is typically associated with poor health. Infections occur predominantly in the respiratory, GI, and urogenital tracts. There is no clear evidence that patients have any increased susceptibility to viral agents.

IgA deficiency has been noted in patients treated with phenytoin, sulfasalazine, penicillamine, and gold, suggesting that environmental factors may lead to expression of the defect.

Immunologic Manifestations. As many as 44% of patients with selective IgA deficiency demonstrate antibodies to IgA. Severe or fatal anaphylactic reactions after intravenous (IV) administration of blood products containing IgA and anti-IgA antibodies (particularly IgE anti-IgA antibodies) have occurred.

Immunodeficiency with Elevated IgM (Hyper-M)

Etiology. A sex-linked mode of inheritance has been noted in some pedigrees. The abnormal gene in the X-linked type has been localized to Xq24-Xq27. However, more than one genetic cause is suspected.

Signs and Symptoms. Patients with hyper-IgM defect become symptomatic during the first or second year of life, with recurrent pyogenic infections, including otitis media, sinusitis, pneumonia, and tonsillitis. Hemolytic anemia and thrombocytopenia have been observed. Transient, persistent, or cyclic neutropenia is a common feature.

Immunologic Manifestations. This disorder is characterized by extremely low concentrations of IgG and IgA and, most frequently, greatly elevated concentrations of polyclonal IgM. Normal or slightly reduced numbers of IgM and IgD B lymphocytes have been observed.

Transient Hypogammaglobulinemia of Infancy

Unlike patients with Bruton's X-linked agammaglobulinemia or CVID, patients with transient hypogammaglobulinemia of infancy can synthesize antibodies to A and B erythrocyte antigens, if they lack the antigen(s), and to diphtheria and tetanus toxoids. Antibody production usually occurs by 6 to 11 months of age. This antibody production occurs before Ig levels become normal.

X-Linked Lymphoproliferative Disease (Duncan's Disease)

Etiology. Duncan's disease is caused by a recessive trait. The defective gene has been localized to the Xq26-Xq27 region.

Signs and Symptoms. The disease is characterized by an inadequate immune reaction to infection with Epstein-Barr virus (EBV). Infected patients are apparently healthy until they experience infectious mononucleosis (see Chapter 22). Two thirds of more than 100 patients studied died of overwhelming EBV-induced B-cell proliferation during mononucleosis. A majority of patients surviving the primary infection developed hypogammaglobulinemia and/or B-cell lymphomas.

Immunologic Manifestations. A marked impairment in production of antibodies to the EBV nucleus has been noted in affected patients. In contrast, titers of antibodies to the viral capsid antigen range from zero to extremely elevated.

Antibody-dependent, cell-mediated cytotoxicity against EBV-infected cells has been low in many patients. NK cell function is also depressed. There is also a deficiency in long-lived T-cell immunity to EBV.

Partial Combined Immunodeficiency Disorders
Wiskott-Aldrich Syndrome (Immunodeficiency with Thrombocytopenia and Eczema)

Etiology. The primary defect in this uncommon X-linked recessive pediatric disease is caused by a specific inability to respond to polysaccharide antigens (e.g., pneumococci). An immunodeficiency and poor humoral immune response to bacterial polysaccharide antigen result.

Signs and Symptoms. Wiskott-Aldrich syndrome is characterized by the triad of thrombocytopenic purpura, increased susceptibility to infection, and eczema (atopic dermatitis). Affected boys rarely survive beyond 10 years of age. Thrombocytopenia and bleeding are common. Platelets are small, with an intrinsic defect. Patients usually die from sepsis, hemorrhage, or malignancy.

Immunologic Manifestations. Progressive deterioration of the thymus leads to a defect in cellular immunity and the attrition of T-cell populations from the lymph nodes and spleen. Decreased numbers of T cells and alteration in the normal T4/T8 ratio of lymphocytes are manifested. Serum levels of IgM are low, but IgG concentrations are usually normal. IgA levels are normal or elevated, and IgE levels are usually elevated.

Hereditary Ataxia-Telangiectasia

Etiology. This autosomal recessive disorder apparently results from the coexistence of a T-cell deficiency with a defect in DNA repair, which leads to extreme nonrandom chromosomal instability. The sites of chromosomal breakage involve chromosomes 7 and 14 in more than 50% of patients.

Signs and Symptoms. Ataxia-telangiectasia is characterized by ataxia and choreoathetosis in infancy. Multiple telangiectases appear on exposed oculocutaneous surfaces during childhood. A high incidence of malignancy (e.g., lymphoma) is also seen. Children with this disorder eventually die of respiratory insufficiency and sepsis.

Immunologic Manifestations. The thymus is hypoplastic or dysplastic, and the thymus-dependent zones of the lymph nodes are void of cells. About 80% of patients lack serum and secretory IgA, and some develop IgG antibodies to injections of IgA. The signs and symptoms of the disease appear to result from a concomitant T-cell deficiency, a deficiency of DNA repair, and disordered IgG synthesis.

Hyperimmunoglobulinemia E Syndrome

Etiology. This disorder has a presumed autosomal dominant pattern of inheritance.

Signs and Symptoms. Hyperimmunoglobulinemia E syndrome is a relatively rare PID characterized by recurrent severe staphylococcal abscesses. Patients have histories from infancy of staphylococcal abscesses involving the skin, lungs, joints, and other sites; persistent pneumatoceles develop as a result of the recurrent pneumonias. Pruritic dermatitis also occurs.

Immunologic Manifestations. Patients have elevated levels of serum IgE and IgD; usually, normal concentrations of IgG, IgA, and IgM are present. Poor antibody and cell-mediated responses to neoantigens are demonstrated. In addition, a decreased percentage of T cells with the memory receptor (CD45RO) has been noted.

T-Cell Activation Defects

Some patients with defective activation of T cells have experienced the following:
- Defective surface expression of the CD3-TCR complex caused by mutation in the gene encoding the CD3 gamma subunit.
- Defective signal transduction from the TCR to intracellular metabolic pathways.
- Pretranslational defect in IL-2 or other cytokine production.

These conditions are characterized by the presence of T cells that appear phenotypically normal but fail to proliferate or produce cytokines in response to stimulation with mitogens, antigens, or other signals delivered to the T-cell antigen receptor. Patient problems are similar to those of other T-cell–deficient individuals, and some patients with severe T-cell activation defects may clinically resemble patients with SCID.

Other Primary Immunodeficiencies

In addition to hereditary or congenital disorders of lymphocytes, several PIDs involve the complement system and phagocytic cells.

Complement Deficiency. Deficiencies in all of the components of the complement system have been described (see Chapter 5). These deficiencies are genetic in origin. Unusual susceptibility to infection is characteristic of some of these components, particularly deficiencies involving C3, C5, C6, and C7 (Table 4-7).

A functional deficiency of the polymorphonuclear neutrophilic (PMN) leukocytes is chronic granulomatous disease (CGD; see Chapter 3). This fatal syndrome usually begins with the onset of symptoms during the first year of life.

Table 4-7	Complement Deficiencies
Deficient Component	**Common Types of Infections**
C1 (r/q)	Gram positive, mainly respiratory
C2	Gram positive, recurrent respiratory; meningitis, sepsis, tuberculosis
C3	Gram positive, recurrent
C4	Gram positive; sepsis, meningitis
C5	Meningitis *(Neisseria meningitidis)*, disseminated gonococcal infection
C6	Meningitis *(N. meningitidis)*, disseminated gonococcal infection
C7	Meningitis *(N. meningitidis)*
C8	Meningitis *(N. meningitidis)*, disseminated gonococcal infection
C9	Meningitis *(N. meningitidis)*

Box 4-3	Secondary Immunodeficiencies

Hematologic Lymphoproliferative Disorders
Hodgkin's disease and lymphoma
Leukemia, myeloma, macroglobulinemia
Agranulocytosis and aplastic anemia
Sickle cell disease

Other Systemic Processes and Metabolic Disorders
Nephrotic syndrome
Protein-losing enteropathy
Diabetes mellitus
Malnutrition
Hepatic disease
Uremia
Aging

Viral Infection
Acquired immunodeficiency syndrome (AIDS)

Surgical Procedures and Trauma
Splenectomy
Burns

Immunosuppressive Agents
Antimetabolites
Corticosteroids
Radiation

Modified from Graziano FM, Bell CL: *Med Clin North Am* 69(3):445, 1985.

Secondary Immunodeficiency Disorders

A secondary immunodeficiency can result from a disease process that causes a defect in normal immune function, which leads to a temporary or permanent impairment of one or multiple components of immunity in the host (Box 4-3). Patients with secondary immunodeficiencies, which are much more common than primary deficiencies, have an increased susceptibility to infections, as seen in the PIDs.

Immunosuppressive agents and burns are major causes of secondary immunodeficiencies. Immunosuppressive agents have been demonstrated to affect, in varying degrees, every component of the immune response. In burn patients, *septicemia* is a common complication in those who survive the initial period of hemodynamic shock. The mechanism that seems most critical in thermal injury is disruption of the skin; however, interference with phagocytosis and deficiencies of serum Ig and complement levels have also been observed.

Immune-Mediated Disease

The immune system is normally efficient in eliminating foreign antigens. The nature of the antigen or the genetic makeup of the host, however, can cause alterations of the immune response that can be injurious and can lead to immune-mediated disease (Table 4-8). In these disorders the immune response is normal, but the reactivity is heightened, prolonged, or inappropriate.

A major concern is allergic reactions, characterized by an immediate response on exposure to an offending antigen and the release of mediators (e.g., histamine, leukotrienes, prostaglandins) capable of initiating signs and symptoms

Table 4-8	Immune-Mediated Disease	
Type	**Cause/Disease**
Allergic hypersensitivity	Foods, drugs, aeroallergens (dust, pollens, molds)
Contact hypersensitivity	Poison ivy, nickel, cosmetics
Transfusion Reactions	
Autoimmune disease	Systemic lupus erythematosus, rheumatoid arthritis, vasculitis syndromes, hemolytic anemia, idiopathic thrombocytopenia, pernicious anemia, Goodpasture's syndrome, myasthenia gravis, Graves' disease

(see Chapter 26). Although allergic reactions are associated with IgE, not all allergic reactions are IgE mediated. Complement activation by immune complexes or through the alternative complement pathway has been shown to release complement C3a and C5a anaphylatoxins, which are capable of producing similar reactions.

Autoimmune disease is thought to be caused by antibody or T-cell sensitization with autologous "self" antigens (see Chapter 28). Postulated mechanisms of this process include the following:

- *Altered antigen or neoantigen.* Such antigens may be created by chemical, physical, or biologic processes. Hemolytic anemia caused by a drug interaction is an example of this process occurring in RBCs.
- *Shared or cross-reactive antigens.* Evidence suggests that poststreptococcal disease occurs through this mechanism.

CASE STUDY

History and Physical Examination

A 38-year-old Caucasian woman presented to the emergency department of her local hospital with increasing difficulty in breathing. She also reported that she has experienced chronic diarrhea for the past 18 months.

Her physical examination revealed a cachectic woman with bilateral rales and splenomegaly. After a chest x-ray film confirmed the presence of pneumonia and bronchiectasis, the patient was admitted to the hospital.

The patient's condition worsened. Her respiratory insufficiency increased, and she developed renal failure and disseminated intravascular coagulation (DIC). She was subsequently transferred to a tertiary care medical center.

Medical History

The patient had a childhood history of multiple episodes of bronchitis and middle ear infections **(otitis media).** In her late 20s she developed sinusitis, frequent diarrhea, and a chronic productive cough. She had two bouts of pneumonia, one of which required hospitalization. One year before

Assay	Patient's Results	Reference Range
Complete Blood Count		
Hemoglobin	9.8 g/dL	11.5-13.5 g/dL
Hematocrit	24%	34%-42%
Total leukocyte count	9.0×10^9/L	$4.5\text{-}9.0 \times 10^9$/L
PMNs	87%	40%-60%
Lymphocytes	13%	20%-40%
Absolute lymphocytes	1.17×10^9/L	$>1.1 \times 10^9$/L
Other		
Stool culture	Normal biota (flora)	Normal biota (flora)
Ova and parasite examination	*Giardia lamblia*	Negative for all ova and parasites
Serum total protein	5.5 g/dL	
Serum electrophoresis	Hypogammaglobulinemia	
Immunoelectrophoresis		
IgM	0.7 g/L	0.6-2.5 g/L
IgG	2.2 g/L	6.8-15.5 g/L
IgA	Undetectable	0.7-3.0 g/L
Follow-Up		
CD4+	20%	35%-55%
CD8+	26%	18%-32%
Absolute CD4 count	0.26×10^9/L	$>0.43 \times 10^9$/L

the current episode, the patient developed extreme difficulty in breathing when exercising. During the past year she lost almost 30 pounds and became so weak that she could no longer lead a normal life.

Family History

She had no family history of frequent infections, immuno-deficiency, or autoimmune disorders.

Laboratory Data

On admission to the tertiary medical center, a blood count, serum protein, serum protein electrophoresis, immuno-globulin electrophoresis, stool culture, and ova and parasite examination were administered (see the chart above).

The patient was found to be anergic. Tetanus, rubella, and diphtheria titers were nonprotective despite previous immunizations.

The patient was diagnosed with common variable immu-nodeficiency (CVID). She was treated with IV immunoglob-ulin monthly. She also received metronidazole for *Giardia lamblia* intestinal infection. After 1 year of Ig therapy, the patient gained weight and returned to a normal lifestyle.

Questions and Discussion

1. Does the patient's medical history suggest an immuno-deficiency?

A history of repeated infections in childhood is sugges-tive of an immunologic defect.

2. Which laboratory findings are significant?

Hypogammaglobulinemia is a hallmark of CVID. The laboratory finding of a decreased number of CD4+ lympho-cytes and decreased Ig levels is important. *G. lamblia* is often detected in CVID patients.

3. How often is CVID diagnosed in adults?

CVID usually manifests in the second or third decade of life.

Diagnosis

Common variable immunodeficiency (CVID).

Classic Enumeration of T Lymphocytes

Principle

This classic procedure is a centrifugation technique for separating lymphocytes from other formed elements in blood. T lymphocytes from erythrocytes and granulocytes are measured in whole blood using a density gradient of fi-coll (synthetic sucrose polymer) material. Mononuclear cells form a layer at the top of the gradient; erythrocytes and granulocytes settle to the bottom of a conical-shaped centrifuge tube.

Note: Modern laboratories identify and enumerate lym-phocyte subsets through the use of flow cytometry. Flow cy-tometry allows for the use of monoclonal antibodies (MAbs) to react with cell surface membrane antigens.

Reagents

- Heparin: 1000 U/mL
- Ficoll-Hypaque solution (diatrizoate sodium/meglumine)
- Phosphate buffer solution (PBS)
- RPMI-1640 supplemented with 10 mM glutamine and 15% fetal bovine serum (FBS).
- AET (0.14 M). Dissolve 1.967 g AET in 35 mL di-H_2O. Adjust to pH 8.0 with 1.0 N NaOH. Bring volume to

50 mL with di-H$_2$O. Store at 2° to 8° C. Check pH every 2 weeks.

Procedure

AET-Treated SRBC

1. Wash sheep red blood cells (SRBCs) four times with PBS.
2. Add 4 volumes AET to 1 volume packed SRBCs in a 15 m conical tube (1 mL AET + 0.25 mL packed SRBCs).
3. Mix well. Incubate in a 37° C water bath for 30 minutes. Shake vigorously.
4. Wash three times with PBS.
5. Store in PBS at 2° to 8° C for up to 3 days.

SRBC-Absorbed FBS

1. Mix 10 volumes FBS with 1 volume packed SRBCs.
2. Incubate at 37° C for 30 minutes.
3. Incubate at 2° to 8° C for 30 minutes.
4. Centrifuge at 400 g for 10 minutes.
5. Collect the FBS; filter-sterilize. Store aliquots at −20° C.

Preparation of Peripheral Blood Lymphocytes (PBLs)

1. Draw peripheral blood into syringe containing 10 U/mL heparin.
2. Dilute the blood 1:1 with PBS.
3. Layer 30 mL diluted blood onto 20 mL Ficoll-Hypaque solution.
4. Centrifuge at 1550 rpm for 30 minutes, room temperature.
5. Aspirate, and discard the supernatant.
6. Carefully collect the interface of PBLs and transfer into a clean tube.
7. Fill the tube with PBS. Centrifuge at 1550 rpm for 10 minutes.
8. Wash the pellet twice with PBS.
9. Count the cells, and resuspend to 10^7 cells/mL in PBS.

Separation of T Cells

1. Mix 1 mL AET-treated SRBCs with 10 mL FBS.
2. Mix an equal volume of PBLs with a 1% (v/v) mixture of AET-SRBC-FBS in a 50-mL tube.
3. Incubate in a 37° C water bath for 10 minutes.
4. Centrifuge at 200 g for 10 minutes. Ensure that the cells have pelleted; if not, recentrifuge for 5 minutes.
5. Place the tube upright on ice for 60 minutes.
6. Layer supernatant over 15 mL Ficoll-Hypaque, leaving 7.5 mL fluid above the pellet.
7. Resuspend the pellet by rotating the tube along the long axis.
8. Stand upright for 1 minute. Remove the top 5 mL, and layer on Ficoll-Hypaque.
9. Rotate as above, and transfer to gradient tube.
10. Wash the tube with 5 mL PBS, and add to gradient.
11. Centrifuge at 300 g for 40 minutes, room temperature.
12. Collect the B cells at the interface. Wash three times with PBS.
13. Suspend the SRBC–T-cell pellet. Centrifuge at 300 g for 10 minutes.
14. Aspirate all the supernatant. Break up the cell pellet by gently shaking.
15. Add 9 mL distilled H$_2$O, and shake for 4 seconds.
16. Add 1 mL 10× PBS with shaking.
17. Immediately fill the tube with 1× PBS.
18. Centrifuge at 300 g for 10 minutes, and wash twice with PBS.

CHAPTER HIGHLIGHTS

- Lymphocytes represent the cellular components of the specific system of body defense. These cells function cooperatively in cell-mediated or humoral immunity.
- The primary lymphoid organs in mammals are the bone marrow (and/or fetal liver) and thymus.
- The secondary lymphoid tissues include the lymph nodes, spleen, and Peyer's patches in the intestine. Proliferation of the T and B lymphocytes in the secondary or peripheral lymphoid tissues is primarily dependent on antigenic stimulation.
- Several major categories of lymphocytes are recognized by the presence of cell surface membrane markers. These categories are T and B cells and natural killer (NK) and K-type lymphocytes.
- The function of plasma cells is the synthesis and excretion of immunoglobulins.
- Monoclonal antibody (MAb) testing led to the present identification of surface membrane markers. Relating MAbs to cell surface antigens now provides a method for classifying and identifying specific cellular membrane characteristics. The "gold standard" has previously been the E rosette technique. The current method of testing uses flow cytometery with immunofluorescence.
- Immunologic disorders can be divided into primary, secondary (acquired), and those mediated through immune mechanisms. Diseases associated with a primary immunodeficiency comprise 40% T-cell disorders, 50% B-cell disorders, 6% phagocytic abnormalities, and 4% complement alterations. The most common T-cell deficiency states are those associated with a concurrent B-cell abnormality.

REVIEW QUESTIONS

1. A function of the cell-mediated immune response *not* associated with humoral immunity is:
   a. Defense against viral and bacterial infection.
   b. Initiation of rejection of foreign tissues and tumors.
   c. Defense against fungal and bacterial infection.
   d. Antibody production.

2. The primary or central lymphoid organs in humans are the:
    a. Bursa of Fabricius and thymus.
    b. Lymph nodes and thymus.
    c. Bone marrow and thymus.
    d. Lymph nodes and spleen.

3. All the following are a function of T cells *except:*
    a. Mediation of delayed-hypersensitivity reactions.
    b. Mediation of cytolytic reactions.
    c. Regulation of the immune response.
    d. Synthesis of antibody.

Questions 4-7. Match the type of lymphocyte with its function (use an answer only once).

4. _____ T cells

5. _____ B cells

6. _____ K-type lymphocytes

7. _____ Natural killer (NK) cells

    a. Antibody-dependent, cell-mediated cytotoxicity (ADCC) reaction
    b. Cellular immune response
    c. Cytotoxic reaction
    d. Humoral response
    e. Phagocytosis

Questions 8-10. Match the surface membrane marker with the appropriate normal T-cell type.

8. _____ CD4

9. _____ CD8

10. _____ CD3

    a. All or most T lymphocytes
    b. Helper-inducer T cells
    c. Suppressor-cytotoxic T cells

Questions 11-14. Match the types of cell with an appropriate condition or disease.

11. _____ Decreased helper cells

12. _____ Increased helper cells

13. _____ Decreased suppressor cells

14. _____ Increased suppressor cells

    a. Kawasaki's disease
    b. Infectious mononucleosis
    c. Acquired immunodeficiency syndrome (AIDS)
    d. Acute graft-versus-host disease

15. All the following are B-cell surface membrane markers *except:*
    a. sIg.
    b. F_C receptor.
    c. C3 receptor.
    d. CD4.

Questions 16-21. Match the following congenital or acquired disorders with the major type of lymphocyte affected.

16. _____ Thymic hypoplasia

17. _____ AIDS

18. _____ Chronic lymphocytic leukemia

19. _____ Systemic lupus erythematosus

20. _____ Multiple myeloma

21. _____ Bruton's agammaglobulinemia

    a. Congenital T-cell disorder
    b. Congenital B-cell disorder
    c. Acquired T-cell disorder
    d. Acquired B-cell disorder

22. Most diseases associated with a primary defect are _____ disorders.
    a. T-cell
    b. B-cell
    c. Complement
    d. Phagocytic

23. Severe combined immunodeficiency is caused by:
    a. T-cell depletion.
    b. B-cell depletion.
    c. Inappropriate development of stem cells.
    d. Phagocytic dysfunction.

24. DiGeorge's syndrome is caused by:
    a. Faulty embryogenesis.
    b. Deficiency of calcium in utero.
    c. Inappropriate stem cell development.
    d. Autosomal recessive disorder.

25. The major clinical manifestation of a B-cell deficiency is:
    a. Impaired phagocytosis.
    b. Diminished complement levels.
    c. Increased susceptibility to bacterial infections.
    d. Increased susceptibility to parasitic infections.

26. Bruton's agammaglobulinemia is a(n):
    a. Acquired disorder.
    b. Autosomal genetic disorder.
    c. Sex-linked genetic disorder.
    d. Disorder occurring primarily in young females.

27. Which of the following disorders does *not* result in a secondary immunodeficiency?
    a. Sickle cell disease
    b. Uremia
    c. AIDS
    d. Poison ivy hypersensitivity

28. The primary lymphoid tissues in mammals are:
    a. Thymus and bursa of Fabricius.
    b. Thymus and bone marrow.
    c. Thymus and fetal liver.
    d. Both b and c.

29. In mammalian immunologic development, the precursors of lymphocytes arise from progenitor cells of the:
    a. Yolk sac.
    b. Bone marrow.
    c. Liver.
    d. Both a and c.

30. The thymus is embryologically derived from the:
    a. Yolk sac.
    b. Pharyngeal pouches.
    c. Lymphoblasts.
    d. Bone marrow.

31. Identify the sites of secondary tissue on the body diagram.
    a. A, B, and C
    b. B, C, and D
    c. B, D, and E
    d. C, D, and E

32. The process of aging causes the thymus to:
    a. Decrease in size.
    b. Not change over time.
    c. Lose cellularity.
    d. Both a and c.

33. T lymphocytes can also be referred to as:
    a. Mast cells.
    b. Memory cells.
    c. Phagocytic cells.
    d. Short-lived cells.

34. Which of the following characteristics of T lymphocytes is false?
    a. Can form a suppressor/cytotoxic subset.
    b. Can be helpers/inducers.
    c. Can be CD4+ or CD8+.
    d. Can synthesize and secrete immunoglobulin.

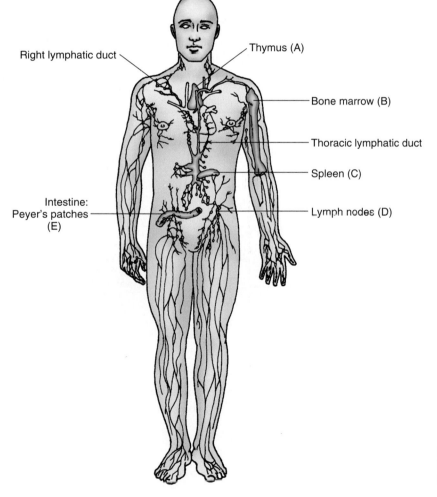

Right lymphatic duct

Thymus (A)

Bone marrow (B)

Thoracic lymphatic duct

Spleen (C)

Intestine: Peyer's patches (E)

Lymph nodes (D)

See question 31. *(Redrawn from Turgeon ML: Clinical hematology: theory and procedures, ed 4, Philadelphia, 2005, Lippincott Williams & Wilkins.)*

Questions 35 and 36. Match each type of lymphocyte to the appropriate function.

35. _____ T lymphocytes

36. _____ B lymphocytes

    a. Cellular immune response
    b. Humoral antibody response

Questions 37-39. Match each to the appropriate function.

37. _____ Cytotoxic or effector T cells

38. _____ Helper or regulator T cells

39. _____ Suppressor T cells

    a. Secrete a variety of cytokines.
    b. Recognize antigens associated with MHC class I.
    c. Inhibit response of helper T cells.

40. Natural killer cells:
    a. Produce interferon.
    b. Produce IL-2.
    c. Were previously called "null cells."
    d. All the above.

41. K-type cells:
    a. Synthesize antibody.
    b. Secrete antibody.
    c. Destroy by cytotoxic reaction.
    d. Phagocytize target cells.

Questions 42-45. Complete the chart, choosing from the following answers for appropriate procedures:
    a. Screening for anti-A and anti-B isoagglutinins
    b. Erythrocyte sedimentation rate
    c. Absolute neutrophil count
    d. Absolute lymphocyte count

Initial Evaluation of Suspected Immunodeficiency

Suspected Immunodeficiency	Appropriate Laboratory Procedures
All suspected deficiencies	42. _____ Complete blood count with platelet evaluation
Antibody deficiency	43. _____ Screening for antibodies to diphtheria or tetanus toxoids
T-cell deficiency	44. _____ Intradermal skin test
Phagocytic cell deficiency	45. _____

46. Calculate the absolute lymphocyte count, when the following conditions exist:

$$\text{Total leukocyte count} = 20 \times 10^9/\text{L}$$
$$\text{Relative \% of lymphocytes} = 50\%$$

    a. $5 \times 10^9/\text{L}$
    b. $10 \times 10^9/\text{L}$
    c. $15 \times 10^9/\text{L}$
    d. $20 \times 10^9/\text{L}$

Questions 47-49. Select an appropriate B-cell disorder for each category (may use an answer more than once):
    a. Chronic lymphocytic leukemia
    b. Bruton's agammaglobulinemia
    c. Autoimmune disorder

T-Cell Disorder	B-Cell Disorder
Congenital	
DiGeorge's syndrome	47. _____
Acquired	
AIDS	48. _____
Hodgkin's disease	
Systemic lupus erythematosus	49. _____

Questions 50-53. Identify the distribution of immunodeficiencies shown in the illustration.

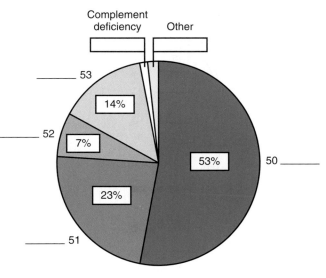

    a. T-cell disorder
    b. B-cell disorder
    c. Severe combined immunodeficiencies (SCIDs)
    d. Disorders of phagocytosis

BIBLIOGRAPHY

Alberts B et al: *Molecular biology of the cell,* ed 2, New York, 1989, Garland Publications.

Antibody deficiency: a review of literature, Denville, NJ, 2004, Biotest.

Arnaiz-Villena A et al: Primary immunodeficiency caused by mutation in the gene encoding the CD-3-(gamma) subunit of the T lymphocyte receptor, *N Engl J Med* 327(8):327-529, 1992.

Buckley RH: Immunodeficiency diseases, *JAMA* 268(20):268-2797, 1992.

Busby J, Caranasos GJ: Immune function, autoimmunity, and selective immunoprophylaxis, *Med Clin North Am* 69(3):69-465, 1985.

Claman HN: The biology of the immune response, *JAMA* 268(20):2790-2796, 1992.

Cooper MD, Lawton AR: The development of the immune system, *Sci Am* 1974, pp 59-70.

D'Andrea AD: Cytokine receptors in congenital hematopoietic disease, *N Engl J Med* 330(12):330-839, 1994.

Denny T et al: Lymphocyte subsets in healthy children during the first 5 years of life, *JAMA* 267(11):267-1484, 1992.

Geha RS, Rosen FS: The genetic basis of immunoglobulin-class switching, *N Engl J Med* 330(14):330-1008, 1994.

Graziano FM, Bell CL: The normal immune response and what can go wrong. In Corman LC, Katz P, editors: *Medical Clinics of North America: Symposium on Clinical Immunology I,* Philadelphia, 1985, Saunders.

Heinzel FP: Infections in patients with humoral immunodeficiency, *Hosp Pract* 1989, pp 97-123.

Jiang H, Chess L: Regulation of immune response by T cells, *N Engl J Med* 354(11):354-1166, 2006.

Medzhitov R, Janeway C Jr: Innate immunity, *N Engl J Med* 343(5):343-338, 2000.

National Primary Immunodeficiency Resource Center: Primary immunodeficiency syndromes—leukocyte adhesion deficiency, 2004, http://npi.jmfworld.org.

Nightengale SL: New therapy for severe combined immunodeficiency disease, *JAMA* 263(22):2995, 1990.

Schejbel L, Garred P: Primary immunodeficiency: complex genetics disorders? *Clin Chem* 53(2):159, 2007.

Sneller MC: New insights into common variable immunodeficiency, *Ann Intern Med* 118(9):118-720, 1993.

Turgeon ML: *Clinical hematology,* ed 4, Philadelphia, 2004, Lippincott Williams & Wilkins.

Turgeon ML: *Fundamentals of immunohematology,* ed 2, Baltimore, 1995, Williams & Wilkins.

Yocum MW, Kelso JM: Common variable immunodeficiency: the disorder and treatment, *Mayo Clin Proc* 66:6-83, 1991.

CHAPTER 5

Soluble Mediators of the Immune System

The Complement System
  Activation of Complement
  Enzyme Activation
  Complement Receptors
  Effects of Complement Activation
Classic Pathway
  Recognition
  Amplification of Proteolytic Complement Cascade
  Membrane Attack Complex
Alternate Pathway
Mannose-Binding Lectin Pathway
Biologic Functions of Complement Proteins
  Alterations in Complement Levels
Diagnostic Evaluation
  Assessment of Complement
  Select Complement Deficiencies
Other Soluble Mediators of Immune Response
  Cytokines
  Interleukins

Interferons
Tumor Necrosis Factor
Hematopoietic Stimulators
  Stem Cell Factor (*c-kit* Ligand)
  Colony-Stimulating Factors
  Transforming Growth Factors
  Chemokines
  Assessment of Cytokines
Acute-Phase Proteins
  Overview
  Synthesis and Catabolism
  C-Reactive Protein
  Case Study
  Other Acute-Phase Reactants
  Assessment Methods
C-Reactive Protein Rapid Latex Agglutination Test
Chapter Highlights
Review Questions
Bibliography

Learning Objectives

At the conclusion of this chapter, the reader should be able to:

- Name and compare the three complement activation pathways.
- Describe the mechanisms and consequences of complement activation.
- Explain the biologic functions of the complement system.
- Name and describe alterations in complement levels.

- Briefly describe the assessment of complement levels.
- Compare other types of nonspecific mediators of the immune system, including cytokines, interleukins, tumor necrosis factor, hematopoietic growth factors, and chemokines.
- Discuss the clinical applications of C-reactive protein.
- Compare acute-phase reactant methods.
- Analyze an acute-phase protein case study.

The immune system is composed of the phylogenetically oldest, highly diversified **innate immune system** and the **adaptive immune system.** Some components of the innate or **natural immune system** (e.g., phagocytosis) are discussed in previous chapters. This chapter discusses the other components of the innate immune system: the complement system and other circulating effector proteins of innate immunity, including cytokines and acute-phase reactants.

Regulatory mechanisms of complement are finely balanced. The activation of complement is focused on the surface of invading microorganisms, with limited complement deposited on normal cells and tissues. If the mechanisms that regulate this delicate balance malfunction, the complement system may cause injury to cells, tissues, and organs, such as destruction of the kidneys in systemic lupus erythematosus or hemolytic anemias.

THE COMPLEMENT SYSTEM

Complement is a heat-labile series of 18 plasma proteins, many of which are enzymes or proteinases. Collectively, these proteins are a major fraction of the beta-1 and beta-2 globulins.

The complement system proteins are named with a capital C followed by a number. A small letter after the number indicates that the protein is a smaller protein resulting from the cleavage of a larger precursor by a protease. Several complement proteins are cleaved during activation of the complement system; the fragments are designated with lowercase suffixes, such as C3a and C3b. Usually, the larger fragment is designated "b" and the smaller fragment, "a." The exception is the designation of the C2 fragments; the larger fragment is designated C2a and the smaller fragment, C2b.

Proteins of the alternative activation pathway are called factors and are symbolized by letters such as B. Control proteins include the inhibitor of C1 (C1 INH), factor I, and factor H.

The complement system displays three overarching physiologic activities (Table 5-1). These are initiated in various ways through the following three pathways (Table 5-2):

1. Classic pathway
2. Alternate pathway
3. Mannose-binding lectin pathway

The three pathways converge at the point of cleavage of C3 to C3b, the central event of the common final pathway, which in turn leads to the activation of the lytic complement sequence, C5 through C9, and cell destruction (Figure 5-1).

Activation of Complement

Normally, complement components are present in the circulation in an inactive form. In addition, the control proteins C1 INH, factor I, factor H, and C4-binding protein (C4-bp) are normally present to inhibit uncontrolled complement activation. Under normal physiologic conditions, activation of one pathway probably also leads to activation of another pathway, as follows:

- The **classic pathway** is initiated by the bonding of the C1 complex, consisting of C1q, C1r, and C1s, to antibodies bound to an antigen on the surface of a bacterial cell.
- The **alternate pathway** is initiated by contact with a foreign surface such as the polysaccharide coating of a microorganism and the covalent binding of a small amount of C3b to hydroxyl groups on cell surface carbohydrates and proteins. The pathway is activated by low-grade cleavage of C3 in plasma.

Table 5-1	Three Main Physiologic Activities of the Complement System
Activity	**Responsible Complement Protein**
Host Defense Against Infection	
Opsonization	Covalently bonded fragments of C3 and C4
Chemotaxis and leukocyte activation	C5a, C3a, and C4a; anaphylatoxin leukocyte receptors
Lysis of bacterial and mammalian cells	C5-C9 membrane attack complex
Interface between Innate and Adaptive Immunity	
Augmentation of antibody	C3b and C4b bound to immune complexes and to antigen
Responses	C3 receptors on B cells and antigen-presenting cells
Enhancement of immunologic memory	C3b and C4b bound to immune complexes and to antigen; C3 receptors on follicular dendritic cells
Disposal of Waste	
Clearance of immune complexes from tissues	C1q; covalently bonded fragments of C3 and C4
Clearance of apoptotic cells	

Modified from Walport MJ: *N Engl J Med* 344(14):1058, 2001.

Table 5-2	Initiators of Three Complement Activation Pathways
Pathway	**Initiators**
Classic	Immune complexes
	Apoptotic cells
	Certain viruses and gram-negative bacteria
	C-reactive protein bound to ligand
Alternate	Various bacteria, fungi, viruses, or tumor cells
Mannose-binding lectin	Microbes with terminal mannose groups

Modified from Walport MJ: *N Engl J Med* 344(14):1058, 2001.

- The **mannose-binding lectin pathway** is initiated by binding of the complex of mannose-binding lectin and associated serine proteases (MASP1 and MASP2) to arrays of mannose groups on the surface of a bacterial cell.

Enzyme Activation

After complement is initially activated, each enzyme precursor is activated by the previous complement component or complex, which is a highly specialized proteinase. This converts the enzyme precursor to its catalytically active form by limited proteolysis.

The pathways leading to the cleavage of C3 are triggered enzyme cascades. During this activation process, a small peptide fragment is cleaved, a membrane-binding site is exposed, and the major fragment binds. As a consequence, the next active enzyme of the sequence is formed. Because each enzyme can activate many enzyme precursors, each step is amplified until the C3 stage; therefore the whole system forms an amplifying cascade.

Complement Receptors

Various cell types express surface membrane glycoproteins that react with one or more of the fragments of C3 produced during complement activation and degradation. The functions of these receptors depend on the type of cell and often are incompletely understood. Complement receptor 1 (CR1) is important in enhancing phagocytosis, and CR3 is also important in such host defense mechanisms.

Effects of Complement Activation

The activation of complement and the products formed during the **complement cascade** have a variety of physiologic and cellular consequences. Physiologic consequences include blood vessel dilation and increased vascular permeability. The cellular consequences include the following:

- Cell activation, such as production of inflammatory mediators.
- **Cytolysis** or **hemolysis,** if the cells are erythrocytes. The most important biologic role of complement in blood group serology is the production of cell membrane lysis of antibody-coated targets.
- **Opsonization,** which renders cells vulnerable to phagocytosis.

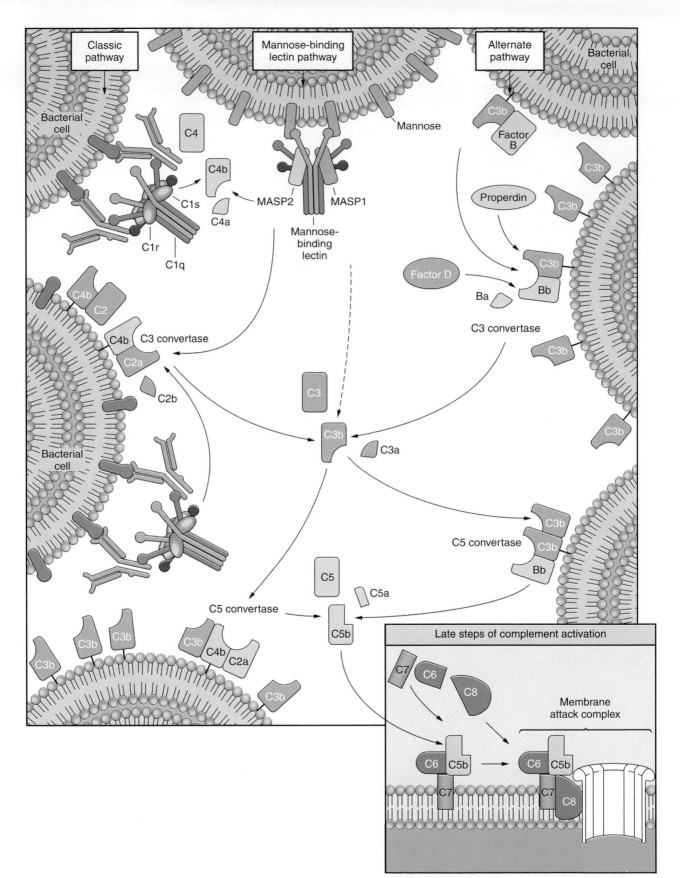

Figure 5-1 Three activation pathways of complement: classic, mannose-binding lectin, and alternate. The three pathways converge at the point of cleavage of C3. The classic pathway is initiated by the binding of the C1 complex (which consists of C1q, two molecules of C1r, and two molecules of C1s) to antibodies bound to an antigen on the surface of a bacterial cell. The mannose-binding lectin pathway is initiated by binding of the complex of mannose-binding lectin and the associated serine proteases 1 and 2 (MASP1 and MASP2) to arrays of mannose groups on the surface of a bacterial cell. The alternate pathway is initiated by the covalent binding of a small amount of C3b to hydroxyl groups on cell surface carbohydrates and proteins and is activated by low-grade cleavage of C3 in plasma. *(Redrawn from Walport MJ:* N Engl J Med *344(14):1058, 2001.)*

In addition to the function of complement as a major effector of antigen-antibody interaction, physiologic concentrations of complement have been found to induce profound alteration in the molecular weight, composition, and solubility of immune complexes. The activation of complement may also play a role in mediating hypersensitivity reactions. This process may occur either from direct alternative pathway activation by immunoglobulin E (IgE)–antigen complexes or through a sequence initiated by the activated Hageman coagulation factor that causes the generation of plasmin, which subsequently activates the classic pathway. In either case, activation of complement components from C3 onward leads to the generation of the anaphylatoxins in an immediate-hypersensitivity reaction.

CLASSIC PATHWAY

The classic complement pathway is one of the major effector mechanisms of antibody-mediated immunity. The principal components of the classic pathway are C1 through C9. The sequence of component activation—C1, 4, 2, 3, 5, 6, 7, 8, and 9—does not follow the expected numeric order.

C3 is present in the plasma in the largest quantities; fixation of C3 is the major quantitative reaction of the complement cascade. Although the principal source of synthesis of complement in vivo is debatable, the majority of the plasma complement components are made in hepatic parenchymal cells, except for **C1** (a calcium-dependent complex of the three glycoproteins C1q, C1r, and C1s), which is primarily synthesized in the epithelium of the gastrointestinal and urogenital tracts.

The classic pathway is composed of three major stages:
1. recognition,
2. amplification of proteolytic complement cascade, and
3. membrane attack complex (MAC).

Recognition

The recognition unit of the complement system is the C1 complex: C1q, C1r, and C1s, an interlocking enzyme system. In the classic pathway the first step is initiation of the pathway triggered by recognition by complement factor C1 of antigen-antibody complexes on the cell surface. When C1 complex interacts with aggregates of immunoglobulin G (IgG) with antigen on a cell's surface, two C1-associated proteases, C1r and C1s, are activated. A single IgM molecule is potentially able to fix C1, but at least two IgG molecules are required for this purpose. The amount of C1 fixed is directly proportional to the concentration of IgM antibodies, although this is not true of IgG molecules. C1s is weakly proteolytic for free intact C2, but it is highly active against C2 that has complexed with C4b molecules in the presence of magnesium (Mg^{++}) ions. This reaction will occur only if the C4bC2 complex forms close to the C1s.

The resultant C2a fragment joins with C4b to form the new *C4bC2a* enzyme, or classic pathway *C3 convertase*. The catalytic site of the C4bC2a complex is probably in the C2a peptide. A smaller C2b fragment from the C2 component is lost to the surrounding environment.

Amplification of Proteolytic Complement Cascade

Once C1s is activated, the proteolytic complement cascade is amplified on the cell membrane through sequential cleavage of complement factors and recruitment of new factors, until a cell surface complex containing C5b, C6, C7, and C8 is formed.

The complement cascade reaches its full amplitude at the C3 stage, which represents the heart of the system. The C4bC2a complex, the classic pathway C3 convertase, activates C3 molecules by splitting the peptide, *C3 anaphylatoxin,* from the N-terminal end of the peptide of C3. This exposes a reactive binding site on the larger fragment, *C3b*. Consequently, clusters of C3b molecules are activated and bound near the C4bC2a complex. Each catalytic site can bind several hundred C3b molecules, even though the reaction is very efficient because C3 is present in high concentration. Only one C3b molecule combines with C4bC2a to form the final proteolytic complex of the complement cascade.

Membrane Attack Complex

The membrane attack complex (MAC) is a unique system that builds up a lipophilic complex in cell membranes from several plasma proteins.

To initiate C5b fixation and the MAC, C3b splits C5a from the alpha chain of C5. No further proteinases are generated in the classic complement sequence. Other bound C3b molecules not involved in the C4b2a3b complex form an opsonic macromolecular coat on the erythrocyte or other target, which renders it susceptible to immune adherence by C3b receptors on phagocytic cells.

When fully assembled in the correct proportions, C7, C6, C5b, and C8 form the MAC (see Figure 5-1, *inset*). The C5bC6 complex is hydrophilic, but with the addition of C7, it has additional detergent and phospholipid-binding properties as well. The presence of both hydrophobic and hydrophilic groups within the same complex may account for its tendency to polymerize and form small protein *micelles* (a packet of chain molecules in parallel arrangement). It can attach to any lipid bilayer within its effective diffusion radius, which produces the phenomenon of reactive lysis on innocent "bystander" cells. Once membrane bound, C5bC6C7 is relatively stable and can interact with C8 and C9.

The C5bC6C7C8 complex polymerizes C9 to form a tubule (pore), which spans the membrane of the cell being attacked, allowing ions to flow freely between the cellular interior and exterior. By complexing with C9, the osmotic cytolytic reaction is accelerated. This tubule is a hollow cylinder with one end inserted into the lipid bilayer and the other projecting from the membrane. A structure of this form can be assumed to disturb the lipid bilayer sufficiently to allow the free exchange of ions as well as water molecules across the membrane. Ions flow out, but large molecules stay in, causing water to flood into the cell. The consequence in a living cell is that the influx of sodium (Na^+) ions and H_2O leads to disruption of osmotic balance, which produces cell lysis.

ALTERNATE PATHWAY

The alternate pathway shows points of similarity with the classic sequence. Both pathways generate a C3 convertase that activates C3 to provide the pivotal event in the final common pathway of both systems. However, in contrast to the classic pathway, which is initiated by the formation of antigen-antibody reactions, the alternate complement pathway is predominantly a non–antibody-initiated pathway.

Microbial and mammalian cell surfaces can activate the alternate pathway in the absence of specific antigen-antibody complexes. Factors capable of activating the alternate pathway include inulin, **zymosan** (polysaccharide complex from surface of yeast cells), bacterial polysaccharides and endotoxins, and the aggregated IgG2, IgA, and IgE. In paroxysmal nocturnal hemoglobinuria (PNH), the patient's erythrocytes act as an activator and result in excessive lysis of these erythrocytes. This nonspecific activation is a major physiologic advantage because host protection can be generated before the induction of a humoral immune response.

A key feature of the alternate pathway is that the first three proteins of the classic activation pathway—C1, C4, and C2—do not participate in the cascade sequence. The C3a component is considered to be the counterpart of C2a in the classic pathway. C2 of the classic pathway structurally resembles factor B of the alternate pathway. The omission of C1, C4, and C2 is possible because activators of the alternate pathway catalyze the conversion of another series of normal serum proteins, which leads to the activation of C3. It was previously believed that **properdin,** a normal protein of human serum, was the first protein to function in the alternate pathway; thus the pathway was originally named after this protein.

The uptake of factor B onto C3b occurs when C3b is bound to an activator surface. However, C3b in the fluid phase or attached to a nonactivator surface will preferentially bind to factor H and so prevent *C3b,B* formation. C3b and factor B combine to form C3b,B, which is converted into an active C3 convertase, C3b,Bb. This results from the loss of a small fragment, *Ba* (glycine-rich α_2-globulin believed to be physiologically inert), through the action of the enzyme, factor D. The C3b,Bb complex is able to convert more C3 to C3b, which binds more factor B; and so the feedback cycle continues.

The major controlling event of the alternate pathway is **factor H,** which prevents the association between C3b and factor B. Factor H blocks the formation of C3b,Bb, the catalytically active C3 convertase of the feedback loop. Factor H (formerly "beta$_1$H") competes with factor B for its combining site on C3b, eventually leading to C3 inactivation. Factors B and H apparently occupy a common site on C3b. The factor that is preferentially bound to C3b depends on the nature of the surface to which C3b is attached. Polysaccharides are called "activator surfaces" and favor the uptake of factor B on the chain of C3b, with the corresponding displacement of factor H. In this situation, binding of factor H is inhibited, and consequently factor B will replace H at the common binding site. When factor H is excluded, C3b is thought to be formed continuously in small amounts. An-

other controlling point in the amplification loop depends on the stability of the C3b,Bb convertase. Ordinarily C3b,Bb decays because of the loss of Bb, with a half-life of approximately 5 minutes. However, if properdin (P) binds to C3b,Bb, forming C3b,BbP, the half-life is extended to 30 minutes.

The association of numerous C3b units, factor Bb, and properdin on the surface of an aggregate of protein or the surface of a microorganism has potent activity as a *C5 convertase*. With the cleavage of C5, the remainder of the complement cascade continues as in the classic pathway.

MANNOSE-BINDING LECTIN PATHWAY

Mannose-binding lectin is a member of a family of calcium-dependent lectins, the collectins (collagenous lectins), and is homologous in structure to C1q. Mannose-binding lectin, a pattern-recognition molecule of the innate immune system, binds to arrays of terminal mannose groups on a variety of bacteria.

A deficiency of mannose-binding lectin is caused by one of three point mutations in its gene, each of which reduces levels of the lectin. After the discovery that the binding of mannose-binding lectin to mannose residues can initiate complement activation, the mannose-binding lectin–associated serine protease (MASP) enzymes were discovered. MASP activates complement by interacting with two serine proteases called MASP1 and MASP2. These components make up the mannose-binding lectin pathway.

BIOLOGIC FUNCTIONS OF COMPLEMENT PROTEINS

The biologic functions of the complement system fall into the following two general categories:
1. Cell lysis by the membrane attack complex (MAC).
2. Biologic effects of proteolytic fragments of complement.

The first category is the situation in which the MAC leads to osmotic lysis of a cell.

The second category encompasses multiple other effects of complement in immunity and inflammation that are mediated by the proteolytic fragments generated during complement activation. These fragments may remain bound to the same cell surfaces where complement has been activated or may be released into the blood or extracellular fluid. In either situation, active fragments mediate their effects by binding to specific receptors expressed on various types of cells, including phagocytic leukocytes and the endothelium. (See Table 5-3.)

In contrast, the absence of an integral component of the classic, alternative, or terminal lytic pathways can lead to decreased complement activation and a lack of complement-mediated biologic functions.

Alterations in Complement Levels

The complement system can cause significant tissue damage in response to abnormal stimuli. Biologic effects of complement activation can occur as a reaction to persistent

Table 5-3	Selected Complement Components and Functions
Complement Component(s)	**Function**
C5-C9	Lysis of cells
C3B, IC3B	Opsonization in phagocytosis
C5A>C3A>>C4A	Anaphylatoxins/inflammation (vascular responses)
C5A	Polymorphonuclear leukocyte activation
Classic complement pathway, C3B, ?iC3b, C3dg	Immune complex removal B-lymphocyte activation

infection or an autoantibody response to "self" antigens. In these infectious or autoimmune conditions, the inflammatory or lytic effects of complement may contribute significantly to the pathology of the disease.

Complement activation is also associated with intravascular **thrombosis,** which leads to ischemic injury to tissues. Complement levels may be abnormal in certain disease states (e.g., rheumatoid arthritis, systemic lupus erythematosus [SLE]) and in some genetic disorders.

Table 5-4	Complement Deficiency in Humans
Deficiency	**Associated Disease**
C1q	SLE-like syndrome; decreased secondary to agammaglobulinemia
C1r	SLE-like syndrome; dermatomyositis, vasculitis, recurrent infections and chronic glomerulonephritis, necrotizing skin lesions, arthritis
C1s	SLE, SLE-like syndrome
C1 INH	Hereditary angioedema, lupus nephritis
C2	Recurrent pyogenic infections, SLE, SLE-like syndrome, discoid lupus, membranoproliferative glomerulonephritis, dermatomyositis, synovitis, purpura, Henoch-Schönlein purpura, hypertension, Hodgkin's disease, chronic lymphocytic leukemia, dermatitis herpetiformis, polymyositis
C3	Recurrent pyogenic infections, SLE-like syndrome, arthralgias, skin rash
C3 inactivator	Recurrent pyogenic infections, urticaria
C4	SLE-like syndrome, SLE, dermatomyositis-like syndrome, vasculitis
C5	*Neisseria* infections, SLE
C5 dysfunction	Leiner's disease, gram-negative skin and bowel infection
C6	*Neisseria* infections, SLE, Raynaud's phenomenon, scleroderma-like syndrome, vasculitis
C7	*Neisseria* infections, SLE, Raynaud's phenomenon, scleroderma-like syndrome, vasculitis
C8	*Neisseria* infections, xeroderma pigmentosa, SLE-like syndrome

Modified from Cassidy JT, Petty RE: Immunodeficiency and arthritis. In Cassidy JT, editor: *Textbook of pediatric rheumatology,* New York, 1982, John Wiley & Sons; Wedgewood RJ, Rosen FS, Paul HW: *Birth Defects* 19:345, 1983; and Pahwa R et al: *Springer Semin Immunopathol* 1:355, 1978.
SLE, Systemic lupus erythematosus.

Elevated Complement Levels

Complement can be elevated in many inflammatory conditions. Increased complement levels are often associated with inflammatory conditions, trauma, or acute illness such as myocardial infarction because separate complement components (e.g., C3) are acute-phase proteins. However, these elevations are common and nonspecific. Therefore, increased levels are of limited clinical significance.

Decreased Complement Levels

Low levels of complement suggest one of the following biologic effects:

- Complement has been excessively activated recently.
- Complement is currently being consumed.
- A single complement component is absent because of a genetic defect.

Specific component deficiencies are associated with a variety of disorders (Table 5-4). Deficiencies of complement account for a small percentage of primary immunodeficiencies (<2%), but depression of complement levels frequently coexists with SLE and other disorders associated with an immunopathologic process (Box 5-1).

Deficiencies in any of the protein components of complement are usually caused by a genetic defect that leads to abnormal patterns of complement activation. If regulatory components are absent, excess activation may occur at the wrong time or at the wrong site. The potential consequences of increased activation are excess inflammation and cell lysis and consumption of complement components.

Hypocomplementemia can result from the complexing of IgG or IgM antibodies capable of activating complement. Depressed values of complement are associated with diseases that give rise to circulating immune complexes. Because of the rapid normal turnover of the complement

Box 5-1	Diseases Associated with Hypocomplementemia

Rheumatic Diseases with Immune Complexes
Systemic lupus erythematosus
Rheumatoid arthritis (with extraarticular disease)
Systemic vasculitis
Essential mixed cryoglobulinemia

Glomerulonephritis
Poststreptococcal type
Membranoproliferative type

Infectious Diseases
Subacute bacterial endocarditis
Infected atrioventricular shunts
Pneumococcal sepsis
Gram-negative sepsis
Viremias (e.g., hepatitis B surface antigenemia, measles)
Parasitic infections (e.g., malaria)

Deficiency of Control Proteins
C1 inhibitor deficiency: hereditary angioedema
Factor I deficiency
Factor H deficiency

proteins—within 1 or 2 days of the cessation of complement activation by immune complexes—complement levels return to normal rapidly.

The following three types of complement deficiency can cause increased susceptibility to pyogenic infections:
1. Deficiency of the opsonic activities of complement.
2. Any deficiency that compromises the lytic activity of complement.
3. Deficient function of the mannose-binding lectin pathway.

Increased susceptibility to pyogenic bacteria (e.g., *Haemophilus influenzae, Streptococcus pneumoniae*) occurs in patients with defects of antibody production, complement proteins of the classic pathway, or phagocyte function. The sole clinical association between inherited deficiency of MAC components and infection is with neisserial infection, particularly *Neisseria meningitidis*. Low levels of mannose-binding lectin in young children with recurrent infections suggest that the mannose-binding lectin pathway is important during the interval between the loss of passively acquired maternal antibody and the acquisition of a mature immunologic repertoire of antigen exposure.

DIAGNOSTIC EVALUATION

During immune complex reactions, certain complement proteins become physically bound to the tissue in which the immunologic reaction is occurring. These proteins can be demonstrated in tissue by appropriate immunopathologic stains. The most frequent evaluation of complement is by serum/plasma assay (Table 5-5). Complement components (e.g., C3 and C4) can be assessed by nephelometry. These assays are useful in diagnosis and monitoring of patients.

Assessment of Complement

The procedures discussed next can be used in diagnostic immunology.

C1 Esterase Inhibitor (C1 Inhibitor)

C1 measures the activity and concentration of C1 inhibitor in serum. A deficiency of this protein is characteristic of hereditary angioedema (HAE; see later discussion). Some patients demonstrate catalytically inactive protein.

C1r, C1s, C2, C3, C4, C5, C6, C7, C8

Homozygous deficiencies predispose a patient to autoimmune disease (especially SLE) and to arthritis, chronic glomerulonephritis, infections, and vasculitis.

C1q

The complement component C1q is evaluated in serum. Decreased levels can be demonstrated in patients with hypocomplementemic urticarial vasculitis, severe combined immunodeficiency (SCID), or X-linked hypogammaglobulinemia.

C1q Binding

This procedure measures the binding of immune complexes containing IgG1, IgG2, or IgG3 and IgM to the complement component C1q. High values of C1q binding are associated with the presence of circulating immune complexes of the type that interacts with the classic pathway of complement activation. This test can be useful as a prognostic tool at diagnosis and during remission of acute myelogenous leukemia.

C2

The most common complement deficiency is of C2. It is an autosomal recessive disorder; the C2 gene is on chromosome 6 in the major histocompatibility complex (MHC). The incidence is 1:28,000 to 1:40,000; the carrier state is 1.2% in the general population.

Half of patients with homozygous C2 deficiency have no symptoms; those with symptoms have infections with *S. pneumoniae, N. meningitidis,* and *H. influenzae.* Fifty percent of symptomatic patients exhibit a lupus-like disorder with photosensitivity and rash.

C3

Also an acute-phase protein, elevated C3 can indicate an acute inflammatory disease. Although C3 lies at the junction of the two pathways, it is much more severely depressed when activation occurs via the alternative pathway. Extremely decreased levels are seen in patients with poststreptococcal glomerulonephritis and in those with inherited (C3) complement deficiency. This component is also decreased in cases of severe liver disease and in SLE patients with renal disease.

C3b Inhibitor (C3b Inactivator)

The C3b component of complement causes low complement C3 levels, the absence of C3PA in serum, and high C3b levels. A deficiency of C3b inhibitor is associated with an increased predisposition to infection.

C3PA (C3 Proactivator, Properdin Factor B)

The factor B component is consumed by activation of the alternative complement pathway. Assessment of C3PA indicates whether a decreased level of C3 results from the classic or alternate pathways of complement activation. Decreased

Table 5-5	Interpretation of Complement Activation by Individual Components				
Complement Determination	**Classic Pathway**	**Alternate Pathway**	**Improper Specimen***	**Inflammation**
C3	Decreased	Decreased	Normal	Increased
C4	Decreased	Normal	Decreased	Increased

*Results if specimen is improperly stored or too old.

levels of C3 and C4 demonstrate activation of the classic pathway. Decreased levels of C3 and C3PA with a normal level of C4 indicate complement activation via the alternative pathway (see Table 5-5).

Activation of the classic pathway (and sometimes with accompanying alternative pathway activation) is associated with disorders such as immune complex diseases, various forms of vasculitis, and acute glomerulonephritis. Activation of the alternative pathway is associated with many disorders, including chronic hypocomplementemic glomerulonephritis, disseminated intravascular coagulation (DIC), septicemia, subacute bacterial endocarditis, PNH, and sickle cell anemia.

In SLE, both the classic and the alternative pathway are activated.

C4

The C4 level often provides the most sensitive indicator of disease activity. C4 is also an acute-phase reactant. Elevated C4 levels can indicate an acute inflammatory reaction or a malignant condition. Measurement of C4 may demonstrate inflammation or infection long before it is clinically evident by standard assessment methods (e.g., total white blood count [WBC] and leukocyte differential, febrile response, or elevated erythrocyte sedimentation rate [ESR]).

C4 is destroyed only when the classic pathway is activated. A decreased C4 level with elevated anti-n-DNA and antinuclear antibody (ANA) titers confirm the diagnosis of SLE in a patient. In these cases of SLE, the periodic assessment of C4 can be useful in monitoring the progress of the disorder. Patients with extremely low C4 in the presence of normal levels of the C3 component may be demonstrating the effects of a genetic deficiency of either C1 inhibitor or C4. Reduction of C3 and C4 components implies that activation of the classic pathway has been initiated.

C4 Allotypes

The antigenically distinct forms of C4A and C4B are located on chromosome 6 in the MHC. C4 allotypes in conjunction with specific human leukocyte antigens (HLAs) are markers for disease susceptibility.

C5

A genetic deficiency of the C5 component is associated with increased susceptibility to bacterial infection and is expressed as an autoimmune disorder (e.g., SLE). Patients with dysfunction of C5 (Leiner's disease) are predisposed to infections of the skin and bowel, characterized by eczema. Their C5 level is normal, but the C5 component fails to promote phagocytosis.

C6

A decreased quantity of C6 predisposes an individual to significant *Neisseria* (bacterial) infections.

C7

A decreased level of C7 is associated with Raynaud's phenomenon, sclerodactyly, telangiectasia, and severe bacterial infections caused by *Neisseria* species.

C8

A decreased quantity of C8 is associated with SLE. A C8 deficiency makes patients highly susceptible to *Neisseria* infections.

Select Complement Deficiencies

Properdin Deficiency

Properdin acts to stabilize the alternative pathway C3 convertase (C3bBb). A deficiency leads to bacterial infections, often meningococcemia. This disorder is an X-linked recessive trait.

Hereditary Angioedema

This disorder is a deficiency in a complement protein. Infections are not usually a significant problem. HAE is autosomal dominant, unlike other complement deficiencies. Two types exist: type 1 (low antigen level and low functional protein) and type 2 (normal antigen level with low function).

Familial Mediterranean Fever

This defect in protease in peritoneal and synovial fluid is transmitted as an autosomal recessive trait on chromosome 16. Patients with the defect experience recurrent episodes of fever and inflammation in the joints and the pleural and peritoneal fluid.

OTHER SOLUBLE MEDIATORS OF IMMUNE RESPONSE

Cytokines

Migratory inhibitory factor (MIF) was the first cytokine activity to be described. MIF performs a T-cell–derived activity that immobilizes macrophage migration, which may cause retention and accumulation of phagocytes at sites of inflammation.

Research continues, and the list of individual cytokines steadily increases. Cytokines are synthesized and secreted by the cells associated with innate and adaptive immunity in response to microbial and other antigen exposure. (See Tables 5-6 and 5-7.)

The generic term **cytokines** has become the preferred name for this class of mediators. Because many cytokines are made by leukocytes and act on other leukocytes, they are

Table 5-6	Examples of Cytokines of Innate and Adaptive Immunity	
Innate Immunity	**Adaptive Immunity**
Chemokines	Interferon-gamma (IFN-γ)
Interferons type 1 (IFN-α, IFN-β)	Interleukin-2 (IL-2)
Interleukin-1 (IL-1)	Interleukin-4 (IL-4)
Interleukin-6 (IL-6)	Interleukin-5 (IL-5)
Interleukin-10 (IL-10)	Interleukin-13 (IL-13)
Interleukin-12 (IL-12)	Lymphotoxin (Lt)
Interleukin-15 (IL-15)	Transforming growth factor beta
Interleukin-18 (IL-18)	(TGF-β)
Tumor necrosis factor (TNF)	

Table 5-7	Comparative Features of Innate and Adaptive Immunity	
	Innate Immunity	**Adaptive Immunity**
Examples	TNF-α, IFN-β, IL-1, IL-12	IFN-γ, IL-2, IL-4, IL-5
Major cell source	Macrophages, NK cells	T lymphocytes
Major physiologic function	Mediators of innate immunity and inflammation (local and systemic)	Regulation of lymphocyte growth and differentiation Activation of effector cells (macrophages, eosinophils, mast cells)
Stimuli	LPS (endotoxin), bacterial peptidoglycans, viral RNA, T-cell–derived cytokines (e.g., IFN-β)	Protein antigens
Quantity produced	Possibly high, detectable in serum	Usually low, usually undetectable in serum
Effects on body	Local and systemic	Usually local
Roles in disease	Systemic diseases	Local tissue injury
Inhibitors	Corticosteroids	Cyclosporine, FK-506

Modified from Abbas AK, Lichtman AH, Pober JS: *Cellular and molecular immunology*, ed 4, Philadelphia, 2000, Saunders.
TNF, Tumor necrosis factor; *IFN,* interferon; *IL,* interleukin; *LPS,* lipopolysaccharides.

also referred to by the imperfect but descriptive term, **interleukins** (ILs). As cytokines are discovered and characterized, they are assigned a number using a standard nomenclature (e.g., IL-1).

Cytokines are polypeptide products of activated cells that control a variety of cellular responses and thereby regulate the immune response. Many cytokines are released in response to specific antigens; however, cytokines are nonspecific in that their chemical structure is not determined by the stimulating antigen. Most cytokines have multiple activities and act on numerous cell types. Hematopoietic and lymphoid cell compartments are regulated by a complex network of interacting cytokines. The **colony-stimulating factors** (CSFs) and the ILs have been shown to play important roles in normal proliferation, differentiation, and activation of several hematopoietic and lymphoid lineages. (See Table 5-8 and 5-9.)

Cytokines have a variety of roles in host defense. In innate immunity, cytokines mediate early inflammatory reactions to microbial organisms and stimulate adaptive immune responses. In contrast, in adaptive immunity, cytokines stimulate proliferation and differentiation of antigen-stimulated lymphocytes and activate specialized effector cells (e.g., macrophages).

Cytokines are very potent even in minute concentrations. Their action is usually limited to affecting cells in the local area of their production, but they can have systemic effects as well.

As a group, cytokines differ molecularly but share the following activities:

- Secrete cytokines in rapid bursts, synthesized in response to cellular activation.
- Bind to specific membrane receptors on target cells.
- Regulate receptor expression in T and B cells, which drives positive amplification or negative feedback.
- Act on different cell types.
- Excite the same functional effects with multiple cytokines (redundancy).
- Act close to the site of synthesis either on the same cell or on a nearby cell.
- Influence the synthesis and actions of other cytokines.

Cytokines act on other cells by bonding to cytokine receptors on the surface of cells. Individual cytokines have characteristic functions and differ in how they transduce signals as a result of binding. All cytokine receptors consist of one or more transmembrane proteins whose extracellular portions are responsible for cytokine binding and whose cytoplasmic portions are responsible for initiating the intracellular signaling pathways. These six pathways are as follows:

1. Janus kinase (JAK/STAT) pathway
2. Tumor necrosis factor (TNF) receptor signaling by TRAFs (tumor necrosis receptor–associated factor)
3. TNF receptor signaling by death domains
4. Toll receptor signaling
5. Receptor-associated tyrosine kinases
6. G-protein signaling

Interleukins

Many different individual and superfamilies of ILs have been identified. A characteristic of ILs is that secreted peptides and proteins mediate local interactions between leukocytes but do not bind antigen. ILs include molecules that are made by and that act on lymphocytes.

Interleukins have widely overlapping functions. These molecules modulate inflammation and immunity by regulating growth, mobility, and differentiation of lymphoid cells. Each of the ILs has been shown to be a distinct molecule by gene cloning and sequencing. In addition, each IL functions through a separate receptor system.

Interferons

The interferons (IFNs) are a group of cytokines discovered in virally infected cultured cells. This interference with viral replication in the cells by another virus led to the name "interferons."

The IFNs are one of the body's natural defensive responses to foreign components (e.g., microbes, tumors, antigens). IFNs are among the most broadly active physiologic regulators, enhancing the expression of specific genes, inhibiting cell proliferation, and augmenting immune effec-

Table 5-8	Origin and Immunoregulatory Activity of Cytokines	
Cytokines	**Origin**	**Prominent Biologic Activities**
Interleukins (ILs)		
IL-1 superfamily	Both IL-1α and IL-1β are produced by monocytes-macrophages and dendritic cells.	Original members: IL-1α, IL-1β, and IL-1 receptor antagonist (IL-1RA). IL-1α and IL-1β are proinflammatory cytokines involved in immune defense against infection. IL-1RA is a molecule that competes for receptor binding with IL-1α and IL-1β, blocking their role in immune activation. Principal function of IL-1: mediator of host inflammatory response to infections and other inflammatory stimuli. These cytokines increase the expression of adhesion factors on endothelial cells to enable transmigration of leukocytes to sites of infection and reset the hypothalamic thermoregulatory center, leading to increased body temperature (fever), which helps immune system fight infection. IL-1 also important in regulation of hematopoiesis.
IL-2 (formerly "T-cell growth factor")	T cells	Has high capacity to induce activation of almost all clones of cytotoxic cells. Increases cytotoxic functions of T-killer and NK cells; promotes production of perforins and IFN-γ by these cells. Activates monocytes-macrophages to synthesize and secrete TNF-α, IL-1β, IL-6, IL-8, G-CSF, and GM-CSF.
IL-3 (formerly "multicolony colony-stimulating factor")	Activated T cells	Promotes expansion of early blood cells (hematopoiesis) that differentiate into all known mature cell types. Supports growth and differentiation of T cells from bone marrow through immune response.
IL-4	T cells, mast cells	Induces differentiation of naive helper T cells (Th0 cells) to Th2 cells. On activation by IL-4, Th2 cells subsequently produce additional IL-4. Cell that initially produces IL-4 and induces Th0 differentiation has not been identified. Early activation of resting B cells: upregulates MHC class II production (induces HLA-DR molecules on B cells, macrophages) and governs B-cell isotype switching to IgG1 and IgE. Key regulator in humoral and adaptive immunity.
IL-5	T-helper type 2 (Th2) cells and mast cells	Principal function: activate eosinophils and serve as link between T-cell activation and eosinophilic inflammation. Stimulates growth and differentiation of eosinophils and activates mature eosinophils (IL-5 expressed on eosinophils). Growth and differentiation–inducing factor for activated T and B cells; induces class-specific B-cell differentiation (IgA production).
IL-6	Macrophages, T cells, osteoblasts	Functions in both innate immunity and adaptive immunity; in latter, stimulates growth of B cells that have differentiated into antibody producers. IL-1, TNF, and IL-6 appear to be major factors that induce the acute-phase response.
IL-7	Stromal cells of red bone marrow and thymus	Stimulates proliferation of lymphoid progenitors; important for proliferation during certain stages of B-cell maturation and in T-cell and NK survival, development, and homeostasis.
IL-8	Macrophages and certain types of epithelial cells (e.g., endothelium)	Potent stimulator of neutrophils in chemotaxis. Activates "respiratory burst" and release of both specific and azurophilic granular contents.
IL-9	T cells (specifically by CD4+ helper cells)	Promotes proliferation of T cells, thymocytes, and mast cells. Supports proliferation of some T-cell lines and of bone marrow–derived mast cell progenitors; supports growth of erythroid blast-forming units.

Select data from http://www.copewithcytokines.de/cope.cgi; http://en.wikipedia.org/wiki/Interleukins; http://www.gene.ucl.ac.uk/nomeclature/genefamily/il.php, 2007.

IFN, Interferon; *TNF,* tumor necrosis factor; *G-CSF,* granulocyte colony-stimulating factor; *GM,* granulocyte-macrophage; *MHC,* major histocompatibility complex; *NK,* natural killer; *APCs,* antigen-presenting cells.

Continued

Table 5-8	Origin and Immunoregulatory Activity of Cytokines—cont'd	
Cytokines	**Origin**	**Prominent Biologic Activities**
Interleukins—cont'd		
IL-10	Monocytes, Th2 cells, B cells	Inhibits activated macrophages; displays potent abilities to suppress antigen presentation capacity of APCs. Released by cytotoxic T (Tc) cells to inhibit the actions of NK cells during immune response to viral infection. IL-10 is stimulatory toward certain T cells, mast cells, and B cells.
IL-11	Bone marrow stroma	Acts in a manner similar to IL-6 on hematopoietic progenitor cells. IL-11 has been shown to synergize with IL-3 to stimulate production of megakaryocyte and myeloid progenitors and to increase number of Ig-secreting B lymphocytes in vivo and in vitro.
IL-12 (NK stimulatory factor)	B cells, macrophages	Although it shares functional properties of enhancing cytotoxic function of NK cells and activated T cells with IL-2, IL-12 appears to act through a distinct mechanism independent of IL-2. Biologic actions of IL-12 include stimulating production of IFN-γ by NK and T cells, stimulating differentiation of naive T cells into Th1 cells, and enhancing cytolytic functions of activated NK cells and CD8+ Tc cells. Growth factor for activated NK/LAK cells.
IL-13	T cells	Possesses many biologic effects similar to IL-4 but appears to have less effect on T or B cells than IL-4. Major action of IL-13 on macrophages is to inhibit their activation and to antagonize IFN-γ. Important mediator of allergic inflammation and disease. Functions of IL-13 overlap considerably with those of IL-4, especially changes induced on hematopoietic cells, but these effects are probably less important given the more potent role of IL-4. IL-13 acts more prominently as a molecular bridge linking allergic inflammatory cells to nonimmune cells, altering physiologic function. It is associated primarily with induction of airway disease and also has antiinflammatory properties.
IL-14 (high-molecular-weight B-cell growth factor, HMW-BCGF)	T cells and malignant B cells	Acts as BCGF in proliferation of both normal and cancerous B cells. Hyperproduction of IL-14 enables progression of B-cell non-Hodgkin's lymphoma (NHL-B); conversely, its antibodies slow down growth of NHL-B.
IL-15	T cells	Biologically similar to IL-2; acts as synergist, particularly in LAK cell induction process; increases antitumoral activities of T-killer and NK cells, and can be chemoattractant for T lymphocytes; endogenous IL-15 is key condition for IFN-γ synthesis. IL-15 produced in response to viral infection and other signals that trigger innate immunity; homologous to IL-2. Function of IL-15 is to promote proliferation of NK cells. Maintenance of memory cells does not appear to require persistence of the original antigen; instead, survival signals for memory lymphocytes are provided by cytokines such as IL-15.
IL-16	Monocytes, CD8+ lymphocytes, B lymphocytes	Acts as a T-cell chemoattractant; increases mobility of CD8+ and CD4+ T cells, and with IL-2, promotes their activation. IL-16 is found in B lymphocytes. Recruits and activates many other cells expressing CD4 molecule, including monocytes, eosinophils, and dendritic cells.
IL-17	CD4+ lymphocytes	Induces granulopoiesis through G-CSF; can reinforce antibody-dependent tumor cell destruction; participates in regulation of many cytokines (IL-1, IL-4, IL-6, IL-10, IL-12, IFN-γ). Histamine and serotonin increase production of IL-17. IL-17 mimics many proinflammatory actions of TNF-α and TNF-β.
IL-18	Macrophages	Acts as synergist with IL-12 in some effects, especially induction of IFN-γ production and inhibition of angiogenesis; high IFN-γ production under integrated effect of IL-18 and IL-12 suppresses tumor growth. IL-18 stimulates production of IFN-γ by NK cells and T cells, synergistic with IL-12.

Table 5-8	Origin and Immunoregulatory Activity of Cytokines—cont'd	
Cytokines	**Origin**	**Prominent Biologic Activities**
Interleukins—cont'd		
IL-19	Monocytes	Lipopolysaccharides (LPS) and GM-CSF stimulate synthesis of IL-19, which is then upregulated in monocytes. Biologic function similar to that of IL-10; regulates functions of macrophages and suppresses activities of Th1 and Th2.
IL-20	Activated keratinocytes, monocytes	Biologic activities similar to those of IL-10, and can stimulate tumor growth. Regulates proliferation and differentiation of keratocytes during inflammation, particularly inflammation associated with the skin. Causes expansion of multipotential hematopoietic progenitor cells.
IL-21	Various lymphocytes	Regulates hematopoiesis and immune response and influences development of lymphocytes; similar to IL-2 and IL-15 in antitumor defense system; promotes high production of T lymphocytes, fast growth and maturation of NK cells, and fast growth of B lymphocytes. Has potent regulatory effects on immune cells, interacting with cell surface IL-21 receptor, expressed in bone marrow cells and various lymphocytes.
IL-22	Activated T cells	Similar to IL-10, but does not prohibit production of proinflammatory cytokines through monocytes in response to LPS; somewhat similar to IFN-α, -β, and -γ.
IL 23	—	Newly discovered cytokine that shares some in vivo functions with IL-12. IL-23 is important part of inflammatory response against infection; as proinflammatory cytokine, it enhances T-cell priming and stimulates production of proinflammatory molecules (IL-1, IL-6, TNF-α, NOS-2, chemokines), resulting in inflammation.
IL-24	Activated monocytes-macrophages, Th2 cells	Appears to participate in cell survival and proliferation by inducing rapid activation of particular transcription factors called STAT-1 and STAT-3; predominantly released by and acts on nonhematopoietic (skin, lung, reproductive) tissues. Performs important roles in wound healing and cancer, cell death occurs in cancer cells/cell lines after exposure to IL-24.
IL-25	Th2 cells, mast cells	Biologically characterized as a member of IL-17 cytokine family. Supports proliferation of cells in lymphoid lineage. Induces production of other cytokines (IL-4, IL-5, IL-13) in multiple tissues, which stimulate the expansion of eosinophils. Important molecule in controlling immunity of the gut; implicated in chronic inflammation associated with gastrointestinal tract; identified in chromosomal region associated with autoimmune diseases such as inflammatory bowel disease (IBD), although no direct evidence suggests that IL-25 plays a role in IBD.
IL-26	Expressed in certain herpes-virus-transformed T cells, but not in primary stimulated T cells.	Induces rapid phosphorylation of transcription factors STAT-1 and STAT-3, which enhance IL-10 and IL-8 secretion and expression of CD54 molecule on surface of epithelial cells.
IL-27	—	Has important function in regulating activity of B and T lymphocytes; belongs to the IL-12 family.
IL-28	—	Plays role in immune defense against viruses.
IL-29	—	Plays important role in host defenses against microbes; its gene is highly upregulated in cells infected with virus.
IL-30 (also IL27p28)	New name of p28, a subunit of IL27	Interleukin 30 (IL-30), a member of the long-chain 4-helix bundle cytokine family, and EBI3 form the IL-27 heterdimer, which is expressed by antigen-presenting cells. IL-27 triggers expansion of antigen-specific naive CD4-positive T cells and promotes polarization toward a Th1 phenotype with expression of gamma-interferon. IL-27 acts in synergy with IL-12 and binds to WSX1.
IL-31	Produced preferentially by Th2 cells. Receptor subunits expressed in activated monocytes and unstimulated epithelial cells.	Believed to play role in skin inflammation.

Continued

Table 5-8	Origin and Immunoregulatory Activity of Cytokines—cont'd	
Cytokines	Origin	Prominent Biologic Activities
Interleukins—cont'd		
IL-32	Monocytes-macrophages	Can induce cells of immune system (e.g., monocytes-macrophages) to secrete TNF-α in addition to chemokines such as IL-8.
		Induces expression of TNF-α, and IL-8 in THP-1 monocytic cells. Expression of IL-32 is induced in human peripheral lymphocyte cells after mitogen stimulation, in human epithelial cells by IFN-γ, and in NK cells after exposure to IL-12/IL-18 combination.
		Involved in activation induced cell death. Expression of IL-32 is upregulated in T-killer and NK-cells after cell activation, and IL-32β is predominant isoform in activated T cells. IL-32 is expressed specifically in T cells undergoing cell death; enforced expression of IL-32 induces apoptosis; downregulation rescues the cells from apoptosis.
IL-33	T-helper cells	Induces type 2 cytokine production from Th cells.
		Mediates biologic effects by interacting with orphan IL-1 receptor, activating intracellular molecules in certain signaling pathways that drive production of type 2 cytokines (e.g., IL-4, IL-5, IL-13) from polarized Th2 cells.
		Constitutive expression of IL-33 is found in smooth muscle cells and bronchial epithelial cells. Expression in primary lung or dermal fibroblasts and keratinocytes is inducible by treatment with TNF-α and IL-1β; these two cytokines only induce low-level expression in dendritic cells and macrophages.
Interferons (IFNs)		
IFN-α	Leukocytes	Antiviral, increased MHC class I expression.
IFN-β	Fibroblasts, epithelial cells	Antiviral, increased MHC class I expression.
IFN-γ	T cells, NK cells	Major macrophage activator; induces MHC class II molecules on many cells and can synergize with TNF; augments NK cell activity; antagonist to IL-4.

Table 5-9	Immunoregulatory Activity of Other Cytokines	
Factor	Target Cells	Prominent Biologic Activities
Tumor Necrosis Factor (TNF)		
TNF-α (cachectin)	Macrophages, NK cells	Local inflammation, endothelial activation
TNF-β (lymphotoxin)	T cells, B cells	Killing, endothelial activation
Tumor necrosis family	T cells, mast cells	
CD40 ligand		B-cell activation, class switching
TNF Family		
CD27 ligand	T cells	Stimulates T-cell proliferation
CD30 ligand	T cells	Stimulates T- and B-cell proliferation
Chemokines		
Membrane cofactor protein (MCP-1)	Macrophages, others	Chemotactic for monocytes

Modified from Claman HN: *JAMA* 268(20):2791, 1992; Janeway C, Travers P, *Immunobiology*, ed 3, New York, 1997, Garland; and Abbas AK, Lichtman AH, Pober JS: *Cellular and molecular immunology*, ed 4, Philadelphia, 2000, Saunders.

tor cells. IFNs have been demonstrated to act as antiviral agents, immunomodulators, and antineoplastic agents.

Type I IFNs mediate the early innate immune response to viral infections. They consist of two distinct groups of proteins, IFN-α and IFN-β, that are structurally quite different, but that bind to the same cell surface receptor and induce similar biologic responses.

Interferon-gamma is the principal macrophage-activating cytokine and serves a critical function in innate immunity and in specific cell-mediated immunity. It stimulates expression of MHC class I and class II molecules and co-stimulates antigen-presenting cells (APCs), promotes the differentiation of naive CD4+ T cells to the helper T cell type 1 (Th1) subset and inhibits the proliferation of Th2 cells. In addition, IFN-γ acts on B cells to promote switching to certain IgG subclasses, activates neutrophils, and stimulates the cytolytic activity of natural killer (NK) cells. It is also antagonistic to IL-4. INF-γ is of most immunologic interest because of its diverse effects on the immune response. Its ability to augment the activity of many cytokines has resulted in clinical trials in a number of different diseases.

Tumor Necrosis Factor

Tumor necrosis factor is the principal mediator of the acute inflammatory response to gram-negative bacteria and other infectious microbes. TNF is responsible for many of the systemic complication of severe infections. The TNF receptor family either stimulates gene transcription or induces apoptosis in a variety of cells. The gene-encoding TNF-α is located in the HLA region between the HLA-DR and HLA-B loci.

TNF-α and TNF-β share similar activities. The principal physiologic functions of TNF are (1) to stimulate the recruitment of neutrophils and monocytes to sites of infection and (2) to activate these cells to eradicate microbes.

In low concentrations, TNF acts on leukocytes and endothelium to induce acute inflammation. At moderate concentrations, TNF mediates the systemic effects of inflammation. In severe infections, TNF is produced in large amounts and causes clinical and pathologic abnormalities (e.g., septic shock). When TNFs gain access to the circulation during infection, they mediate a series of reactions that induce shock and can result in death. The syndrome, *septic shock,* is a complication of severe gram-negative bacterial sepsis.

HEMATOPOIETIC STIMULATORS

Stem Cell Factor (*c-kit* Ligand)

Stem cell factor is a cytokine that interacts with a tyrosine kinase membrane receptor, the protein product of the cellular oncogene *c-kit*. The cytokine that interacts with this receptor is called *c-kit* ligand, or stem cell factor, because it acts on immature stem cells.

Stem cell factor is needed to make bone marrow stem cells responsive to other CSFs, but it does not cause colony formation itself. Stem cell factor may also play a role in sustaining the viability and proliferative capacity of immature T cells in the thymus and mast cells in mucosal tissues.

Colony-Stimulating Factors

A variety of CSFs, such as granulocyte (G-CSF) and granulocyte-macrophage (GM-CSF), are also made by T cells. These pathways provide a link between the lymphoid and hematopoietic systems. For example, G-CSF and GM-CSF regulate the production of granulocytes and monocytes, thus enabling the T-cell system to promote the inflammatory response.

The biologic activity of CSF is measured by its ability to stimulate hematopoietic progenitor cells to form colonies in semisolid medium. These proteins are necessary for the survival, proliferation, and differentiation of precursor cells of the immune system.

The CSFs are potentially important in the treatment of human disease. GM-CSF is being used in a number of clinical trials to increase circulating leukocytes in patients with AIDS, other immunocompromised patients (e.g., recovering from chemotherapy), and bone marrow transplant recipients.

Transforming Growth Factors

As with the IFNs, transforming growth factors (TGFs) were identified as products of virally transformed cells. These factors were found to induce phenotypic transformation in nonneoplastic cells and subsequently were named "transforming growth factors." TGF-β is a group of five cytokines released by many cell types, including macrophages and platelets. TGF-β is known to be a potent inhibitor of IL-1–induced T-cell proliferation.

The principal action of TGF-β in the immune system is to inhibit the proliferation and activation of lymphocytes and other leukocytes. It inhibits the proliferation and differentiation of T cells and the activation of macrophages.

Chemokines

Chemokines are a large family of structurally homologous cytokines that stimulate transendothelial leukocyte movement from the blood to tissue site of infection and regulate the migration of polymorphonuclear leukocytes (PMNs) and mononuclear leukocytes within tissues (see Chapter 3). The largest family consists of *CC* chemokines that attract mononuclear cells to sites of chronic inflammation, such as monocyte chemoattractant protein 1 (MCP-1). A second family of chemokines consists of *CXC* chemokines, of which interleukin-8 (CXCL8) is the prototype. CXCL8 attracts PMNs to sites of acute inflammation, activates monocytes, and may direct the recruitment of these cells to vascular lesions. The third family, *CX3*, forms a cell-adhesion receptor capable of arresting cells under physiologic flow conditions. TNF-α–converting enzyme can cleave CX3CL1 from the cell membrane.

Other functions of various chemokines include the following:

- Increasing the affinity of leukocyte integrins for their ligands on endothelium (e.g., ICAM-1, ICAM-2, VCAM-1).
- Regulating the traffic of lymphocytes and other leukocytes through peripheral lymphoid tissues.
- Maintaining normal migration of immune cells into lymphoid organs, or other specialized cells to particular sites.

Assessment of Cytokines

Defects in cytokine production can lead to autoimmunity (Table 5-10). Traditional methods for assessment of cytokines include the following:

- Bioassays
- Enzyme-linked immunosorbent assay (ELISA)
- Intracellular staining
- Ribonuclease protection assay
- Polymerase chain reaction (PCR)
  New methods of measurement include the following:
- Multiplexed assay using the FlowMetrix: quantify multiple cytokines simultaneously.
- Intracellular staining using flow cytometry.
- Cord blood mononuclear cells stimulated by allergens (celELISA).
- Real-time PCR for lymph nodes or spleen
- Eli spot assays
- Enhanced immunoassays for cytokines
- Biotrak assay: high-sensitivity ELISA

Table 5-10	Defects in Cytokine Production that Can Lead to Autoimmunity	
Cytokine or Protein	**Defect**	**Disorder**
IL-1 receptor antagonist	Underexpression	Arthritis
IL-2	Overexpression	IBD
IL-7		
IL-10		
IL-2 receptor	Overexpression	IBD
IL-10 receptor	Overexpression	IBD
IL-3	Overexpression	Demyelinating syndrome
TNF-α	Overexpression	IBD, arthritis, vasculitis
	Underexpression	SLE
IFN-γ	Overexpression in skin	SLE
TGF-β	Underexpression	Systemic wasting syndrome, IBD
TGF-β receptor in T cells	Underexpression	SLE

Modified from Davidson A, Diamond B: *N Engl J Med* 345(5):345, 2001.
IL, Interleukin; *IBD,* inflammatory bowel disease; *TNF,* tumor necrosis factor; *SLE,* systemic lupus erythematosus; *IFN,* interferon; *TGF,* transforming growth factor.

ACUTE-PHASE PROTEINS

The acute-phase response is an innate body defense. This response is a nonspecific indicator of an inflammatory process.

Overview

A group of glycoproteins associated with the acute-phase response are collectively called **acute-phase proteins** or **acute-phase reactants.** The various acute-phase proteins rise at different rates and in varying levels in response to tissue injury (e.g., inflammation, infection, malignant neoplasia, various diseases or disorders, trauma, surgical procedures, drug response). The increased synthesis of these proteins takes place shortly after a trauma and is initiated and sustained by proinflammatory cytokines.

The main biologic sign of inflammation is an increase in the erythrocyte sedimentation rate (ESR). In addition to the ESR, measurement of the plasma concentration of acute-

Box 5-2	Major Applications of Acute-Phase Protein Measurements

Monitoring the progress of diagnosed disease activity.
Assessing response to therapy in inflammatory diseases (e.g., rheumatoid arthritis, juvenile chronic arthritis, ankylosing spondylitis, Reiter's syndrome, psoriatic arthropathy, vasculitis, rheumatic fever).
Detection of complications of a known disease (e.g., immune complex deposition, postsurgical infection).

phase reactants is usually a good indicator of local inflammatory activity and tissue damage. More than 20 acute-phase proteins have a definable role in inflammation (Box 5-2). These reactants constitute the majority of the serum glycoproteins (Table 5-11).

Acute-phase reactants include **C-reactive protein** (CRP), inflammatory mediators (e.g., complement components C3 and C4), fibrinogen, transport proteins such as haptoglobin, inhibitors (e.g., α_1-antitrypsin), and α_1-acid glycoprotein. Profiles of inflammatory changes yield detailed information but rarely provide major evidence for diagnosis or treatment.

Produced by the liver under the control of IL-6, CRP is a parameter of inflammatory activity. Serum concentrations can increase 1000-fold with an acute inflammatory reaction. Persistent increases in CRP can also occur in chronic inflammatory disorders (e.g., autoimmune disease, malignancy).

C-reactive protein is prominent among the acute-phase proteins because its changes show great sensitivity. Changes in CRP are independent of those of ESR and parallel the inflammatory process. CRP is a direct and quantitative measure of the acute-phase reaction and, as a result of its fast kinetics, provides adequate information of the actual clinical situation (see upcoming discussion). In contrast, ESR is an indirect measure of the acute-phase reaction. It reacts much slower to changes of inflammatory activity and is influenced by other factors. ESR can be falsely normal in conditions such as polyglobulinemia, cryoglobulinemia, and hemoglobinopathy. ESR may also be spuriously high in the absence of inflammation in patients with anemia or hypergammaglobulinemia.

Table 5-11	Examples of Clinically Useful Acute-Phase Proteins		
Protein	**Normal Concentration (g/L)**	**Concentration in Acute Inflammation (g/L)**	**Response Time (hr)**
C-reactive protein	0.0008-0.004	0.4	6-10
Alpha$_1$-antichymotrypsin	0.3-0.6	3.0	10
Alpha$_1$-antitrypsin	2.0-4.0	7.0	24
Orosomucoid	0.5-1.4	3.0	24
Haptoglobin	1.0-3.0	6.0	24
Fibrinogen	2.0-4.5	10.0	24
C3	0.55-1.2	3.0	48-72
C4	0.2-0.5	1.0	48-72
Ceruloplasmin	0.15-0.6	2.0	48-72

Synthesis and Catabolism

All the acute-phase proteins are synthesized rapidly in response to tissue injury. The elevation is twofold to fivefold in certain disease states. In addition, strenuous exercise triggers an inflammatory response similar to that in sepsis. Indices of the inflammatory response, especially to exercise, include leukocytosis, release of inflammatory mediators and acute-phase reactants, tissue damage, priming of various white blood cell lines, production of free radicals, activation of complement, coagulation, and fibrinolytic cascades.

Acute-phase proteins have different kinetics and various degrees of increase. Some, the "negative" acute-phase proteins, actually decrease, possibly resulting from a loss of protein from the vascular space. In addition, acute-phase proteins can be modified by causes other than inflammation (e.g., low fibrinogen in DIC, very low haptoglobin in hemolysis, elevated α_1-acid glycoprotein [orosomucoid] in renal insufficiency, elevated transferrin in iron deficiency). In addition, liver insufficiency or leakage through the kidney or gut lesions can lower these reactants.

The rate of change and peak concentration of separate acute-phase reactants vary with the component and the clinical situation. In acute inflammation, CRP and α_1-antichymotrypsin levels become elevated within the first 12 hours. The complement components, C3 and C4, and ceruloplasmin do not rise for several days.

Acute-phase proteins do not always change in parallel. This mismatch in acute-phase protein levels is most often the result of increased catabolism and elimination from the circulation of certain proteins. Differences may also be caused by discrepancies in rates of synthesis. Most acute-phase proteins have half-lives of 2 to 4 days, but CRP has a half-life of 5 to 7 hours. For this reason, CRP falls much more rapidly than the other acute-phase proteins when the patient recovers.

C-Reactive Protein

Traditionally, CRP has been used clinically for monitoring infection, autoimmune disorders, and more recently, healing after a myocardial infarction (MI). Levels of CRP parallel the course of the inflammatory response and return to lower, undetectable levels as the inflammation subsides. CRP demonstrates a large incremental change, with as much as a 100-fold increase in concentration in acute inflammation, and is the fastest responding and most sensitive indicator of acute inflammation. CRP increases faster than ESR in responding to inflammation, whereas the leukocyte count may remain within normal limits despite infection. An elevated CRP can signal infection many hours before it can be confirmed by culture results; therefore treatment can be prompt. Because of these characteristics, CRP is the method of choice for screening for inflammatory and malignant organic diseases and monitoring therapy in inflammatory diseases.

Elevations of CRP occur in about 70 disease states, including septicemia and meningitis in neonates, infections in immunosuppressed patients, burns complicated by infection, serious postoperative infections, MI, malignant tumors, and rheumatic disease. Measurement of CRP may add to the diagnostic procedure in select cases (e.g., differentiation between bacterial and a viral infection). An extremely elevated CRP suggests a possible bacterial infection (see later procedure description). In general, CRP is advocated as an indicator of bacterial infection in at-risk patients in whom the clinical assessment of infection is difficult to make, but a lack of specificity rules out CRP as a definitive diagnostic tool.

Levels of CRP rise after tissue injury or surgery. In uncomplicated cases, CRP level peaks about 2 days after surgery and gradually returns to normal levels within 7 to 10 days. If the CRP level is persistently elevated or returns to an increased level, it may indicate underlying sepsis preceding clinical signs and symptoms and should alert the clinician to postoperative complications.

In clinical practice, CRP is particularly useful when serial measurements are performed. The course of the CRP level may be useful for monitoring the effect of treatment and for early detection of postoperative complications or intercurrent infections. In rheumatoid arthritis (RA), CRP reflects both short-term and long-term disease activity. Monitoring of CRP levels allows for early prediction of response to a particular drug, often months before clinical and radiologic confirmation is possible. In disorders such as RA, CRP can be used to assess the effect of antiinflammatory drugs (e.g., aspirin) and the nature of their action. Aspirin-like drugs do not suppress acute-phase proteins in inflammation, allowing optimal therapy in the shortest time and minimizing ongoing inflammation and joint damage. Assessment of CRP is also valuable in monitoring therapy and disease activity in other arthritides. Rheumatic fever and Crohn's disease can also be monitored by CRP. In addition, CRP assessment has been found to enhance the value of traditional enzyme measurements in MI.

In a number of chronic inflammatory diseases, however, CRP is an unreliable indicator. CRP values may be normal when other acute-phase proteins are altered in disorders such as SLE, dermatomyositis, and ulcerative colitis. SLE shows little or no CRP response despite apparently active inflammation.

Both CRP and low-density lipoprotein (LDL) cholesterol are known to be elevated in persons at risk for cardiovascular disease. CRP level may be a stronger predictor of cardiovascular events than the LDL cholesterol, an established benchmark of cardiovascular risk.

CASE STUDY

Signs and Symptoms

A 39-year-old woman was admitted for a cholecystectomy. She had a history of chronic cholecystitis; recent x-ray studies revealed stones in the gallbladder and a large stone in the biliary duct (Figure 5-2). During surgery a large stone was removed from the duct, and a cholangiogram showed no further obstructions of the hepatic or common bile ducts.

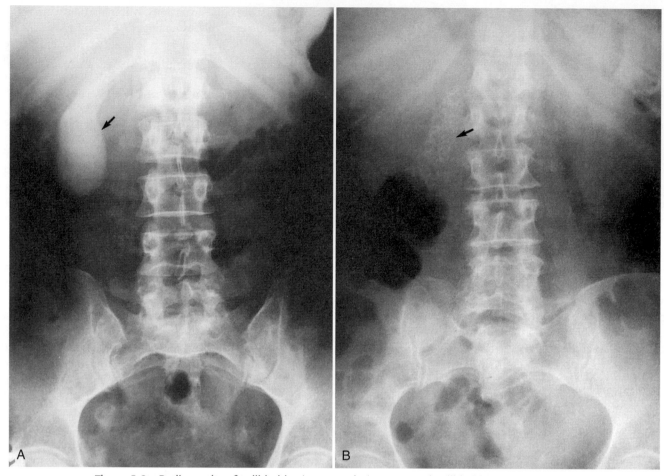

Figure 5-2   Radiographs of gallbladder (contrast dye). **A,** Normal gallbladder *(arrow)*. **B,** Gallbladder filled with stones *(arrow)*.

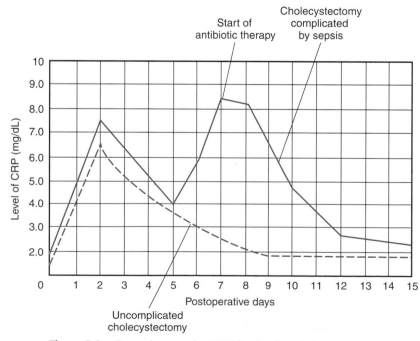

Figure 5-3   C-reactive protein *(CRP)* levels after cholecystectomy.

The patient became febrile 1 day after surgery. A 48-hour postoperative complete blood count (CBC) and CRP were ordered (Figure 5-3). On the seventh postoperative day, she had abdominal pain and began vomiting. A CBC, ESR, CRP, and blood culture were ordered at that time. The patient was started on a broad-spectrum antibiotic and discharged on the thirteenth hospital day.

Laboratory Data

At 48 hours after surgery, the CBC was within normal limits and the CRP was 11 g/L. A repeat CRP on the sixth day after surgery was 7 g/L.

Results after the episode of abdominal pain showed a normal CBC and ESR and a CRP value of 15 g/L. The blood culture was positive for *Pseudomonas* species.

Questions and Discussion

1. Which test was the most rapid and sensitive indicator of infection?

The CRP was the most sensitive indicator of infection and was consistent with the patient's febrile state. Neither the WBC count nor the ESR was elevated.

2. Is the CRP diagnostic?

No; CRP level is suggestive of inflammation or infection, but it is not diagnostic. The growth of *Pseudomonas* in the blood culture was diagnostic of sepsis.

3. Why was the CRP elevated immediately after surgery?

The CRP was elevated after surgery because any tissue trauma will cause an elevation. The levels of acute-phase proteins such as CRP should decline within a few days after surgery.

Diagnosis

Postoperative infection.

Other Acute-Phase Reactants

Alpha$_1$-antitrypsin is an acute-phase protein that increases in acute inflammatory reactions. Generalized vasculitis, such as occurs in immune complex disease, may result in inappropriately low levels of α_1-antitrypsin, probably resulting from increased elimination of complexes with leukocyte lysosomal enzymes.

Defects in the complement components C3a and C5a and the opsonin C3b result in serious infections. In addition, immune complex disease and gram-negative bacteremia result in low levels of complement components, particularly C3 and C4, because the components are consumed during complement activation. Acute inflammation leads to normal or slightly elevated levels. If both disorders are present, complement consumption may be masked, making it deceptive to use complement measurement as the only index of immune complex deposition in disease. The detection of complement breakdown products is more useful than the measurement of total complement component concentrations. It is more desirable to measure C3 break-

down products than total C3 in conditions such as peritonitis or pancreatitis.

Lymphomas may result in a marked increase in C1 esterase inhibitor, with little other change.

Ceruloplasmin, often measured as serum copper, is used to monitor Hodgkin's disease; increases are considered specific indicators of relapse. Although not definitely established, ceruloplasmin monitoring may provide similar information in non-Hodgkin's lymphoma.

Assessment Methods

Inflammation almost always follows acute tissue damage. Diagnostic categories of acute inflammation can include bacterial causes and nonbacterial causes such as trauma, chronic inflammation, or viral disease. Many laboratory tests have been advocated for early diagnosis of acute inflammation: total WBC count (including the absolute count and the percentage of band and segmented neutrophils, as determined by 100-cell differential count on peripheral blood smear), acute-phase proteins, and the ESR.

The ESR ("sedrate") is a nonspecific indicator of disease, with increased sedimentation of erythrocytes seen in acute and chronic inflammation and malignancies. Although nonspecific, ESR is one of the most frequently performed laboratory tests.

In addition to these hematologic tests, several tests are of direct value in immunologic testing. These procedures include a simple phagocytic cell function test and the determination of CRP.

C-Reactive Protein Rapid Latex Agglutination Test

Principle

The CRP agglutination test (CRP Wampole Laboratories, Cranbury, NJ) is based on the reaction between patient serum containing CRP as the antigen and the corresponding antihuman (CRP) antibody coated to the treated surface of latex particles. The coated particles enhance the detection of an agglutination reaction when antigen is present in the serum being tested. The clinical applications of CRP evaluation include detecting inflammatory diseases, particularly infections. It is also a useful indicator in screening for organic disease, both inflammatory and malignant disease, and in monitoring therapy in inflammatory diseases. Because CRP is more rapidly synthesized than other acute-phase proteins, assays of CRP are the measurement of choice in suspected inflammatory conditions.

Specimen Collection and Preparation

No special preparation of the patient is required before specimen collection. The patient must be positively identified when the specimen is collected, and the specimen should be labeled at the bedside. Specimen labels include the patient's full name, the date, the patient's hospital identification number, and the phlebotomist's initials.

Blood should be drawn by an aseptic technique. A minimum of 2 mL of clotted blood (red-top evacuated tube) is required. The specimen should be centrifuged promptly and an aliquot of serum removed. Lipemia, hemolysis, or contamination with bacteria renders a specimen unsuitable for testing. Although icteric and turbid specimens have given valid results, fresh non–heat-inactivated serum is recommended for the test.

If the test cannot be performed immediately, the specimen should be refrigerated (2° to 8° C) for no longer than 24 hours. If additional delay occurs, the serum should be frozen at −20° C or below. Frozen serum should be thawed rapidly at 37° C. Repeat freezing and thawing must be avoided. If the specimen is turbid on thawing, it should be centrifuged to clear it before use.

Preliminary Specimen Preparation

Serum must be at room temperature. Prepare a 1:5 dilution of patient serum by pipetting 0.1 mL of serum into a test tube and adding 0.4 mL of the commercially prepared glycine-saline buffer diluent. Mix the contents thoroughly.

Reagents, Supplies, and Equipment

Materials provided in IMMUNEX kit: latex reagent, concentrated diluent 20×, positive control, negative control, glass slide.

Materials required but not provided in kit: stirrers, conventional test tubes, distilled water, serologic pipettes.

Reagents

- IMMUNEX CRP Latex Reagent (latex particles sensitized with antihuman CRP [sheep]); contains buffer and preservative, sodium azide 0.1%.

  Note: Store at 2° to 8° C. Do not freeze CRP latex reagent. Shake gently and thoroughly before use.
- Concentrated diluent (glycine-saline buffer in kit); contains preservative sodium azide 2%.

  Prepare a 1:20 dilution of the concentrated diluent by mixing the contents of the concentrated diluent vial with 190 mL of distilled water.

  Note: Store the prepared diluent at 2° to 8° C. Properly stored reagent is stable until expiration date indicated on the label. Reagent that does not produce appropriate quality control results should be discarded after verification by repeat testing. Discard if contaminated (i.e., evidence of cloudiness or particulate material in solution).

Supplies and Equipment

- Capillary pipettes
- Applicator sticks
- Glass slide (in kit) (Clean only with distilled water; *do not use detergent.*)
- Stopwatch or timer
- 12 × 75–mm test tubes
- Serologic pipettes (1 mL graduated) and safety pipetter
- Calibrated pipetter (optional)

Quality Control

Positive Control Serum (Human)

Provided in kit.

Contains buffer, stabilizer, and preservative, sodium azide 0.1%.

Store at 2° to 8° C.

Note: Failure to observe a positive reaction with this serum indicates deterioration of the latex reagent and/or positive control.

Negative Control Serum (Human)

Provided in kit.

Contains buffer, stabilizer, and preservative, sodium azide 0.1%.

Store at 2° to 8° C.

Note: A smooth or slightly granular reaction must be observed with the negative control. If agglutination is exhibited with this control, the test should be repeated. If repeat testing produces the same results, the reagents should be replaced.

A positive and a negative control must be tested with each unknown patient specimen.

CAUTION: Because the control sera are derived from human sources, they should be handled at Biosafety Level 2 in the same manner as clinical serum specimens (see Chapter 6).

Procedure

Note: All reagents and specimens must be at room temperature before testing.

Reagent Check Test

1. Place 1 drop of the Positive Control on a section of the slide and 1 drop of the Negative Control on another section.
2. Test each control according to Procedure Steps, beginning with step 4.
3. Observe results immediately at 2 minutes.
4. The Positive Control must show agglutination, whereas the Negative Control should appear uniformly turbid.

Procedural Steps

1. Specimens should be tested undiluted and diluted 1:10 with the prepared diluent.
2. Place 1 drop (~50 μL) of undiluted specimen into one of the rings on the slide and 1 drop (~50 μL) of the diluted 1:10 specimen into another ring.
3. Place 1 drop each of Positive Control and Negative Control into two more rings on the slide.
4. Resuspend the CRP latex reagent by gently mixing until the suspension is homogeneous. Using the dropper provided, add 1 drop of the CRP latex reagent to each serum specimen and to each control.
5. Using separate applicator sticks, mix each specimen and each control thoroughly. The contents of the mixtures should be spread evenly over the entire area of their respective divisions on the slide.

6. Tilt the slide back and forth, slowly and evenly, 8 to 10 times per minute, for 2 minutes. Place the slide on a flat surface and observe immediately for macroscopic agglutination using a direct light source.

WARNING: The latex reagent, controls, and buffer contain sodium azide as a preservative. Sodium azide may react with lead and copper plumbing to form highly explosive metal azides. On disposal, flush with a large volume of water to prevent azide buildup.

Reporting Results

In patients who are free of inflammation and tissue necrosis, CRP is absent from the serum or present in concentrations below 0.5 mg/dL. Reference range mean values are 0.01 mg/dL in newborns and less than 0.05 mg/dL in adult men and nonpregnant women.

Positive Reaction

Agglutination of the latex suspension is a positive result. A positive reaction is reported when either the undiluted specimen or the 1:5 diluted specimen demonstrates agglutination or when both exhibit agglutination.

Negative Reaction

The absence of visible agglutination and the presence of opaque fluid constitute a negative reaction. A negative reaction is reported only when both the undiluted specimen and the 1:5 diluted specimen exhibit no visible agglutination.

Procedural Notes

Specimen collection and handling are important to the quality of the test. Strict adherence must be paid to technique, with a special emphasis on drop size, complete mixing, reaction time, and temperature of reagents.

The strength of a positive reaction may be graded as follows:

1+ Very small clumping with an opaque fluid background.
2+ Small clumping with a slightly opaque fluid background.
3+ Moderate clumping with a fairly clear fluid background.
4+ Large clumping with a clear fluid background.

Sources of Error

False-positive results may be observed if serum specimens are lipemic, hemolyzed, or heavily contaminated with bacteria. If the reaction time is longer than 2 minutes, a false-positive result may also be produced from a drying effect.

False-negative results may be observed in undiluted serum specimens because of high levels of CRP (antigen excess). A 1:5 dilution of serum is also tested for this reason.

Limitations

Because the latex slide agglutination test is a qualitative and semiquantitative procedure, other methods such as nephelometry should be used for quantitative determination of CRP level when indicated. The strength of the agglutination reaction is not always indicative of the CRP concentration. Weak reactions may be produced in samples with elevated or low CRP values. Results may vary depending on the patient's condition.

This 2-minute slide latex agglutination test has a detection level of 1 mg CRP/dL; therefore, patients with CRP values less than 1 mg/dL may go undetected. The sensitivity of the procedure has been assessed at 93%.

Clinical Applications

With the onset of a substantial inflammatory event (e.g., infection, MI, surgery), the CRP level usually increases significantly (>tenfold) above the reference range values for healthy individuals. The test is clinically useful in early detection of inflammatory diseases (particularly infections), as an indicator in screening for organic diseases, and in monitoring patient progress.

Reference

Package insert, June 2006, IMMUNEX CRP, Inverness Medical Professional Diagnostics, Princeton, N.J.

CHAPTER HIGHLIGHTS

- The complement system is a heat-labile series of 18 plasma proteins, many of which are enzymes or proteinases. Normally, complement components are present in the circulation in an inactive form.
- Complement is composed of three interrelated enzyme cascades: the classic, the alternate, and the mannose-binding lectin pathways.
- Complement levels may be abnormal in certain disease states. Increased complement levels are often associated with inflammatory conditions, trauma, and acute illness. Separate complement components (e.g., C3) are acute-phase proteins.
- The biologic functions of the complement system fall into two general categories: cell lysis by the membrane attack complex or biologic effects of proteolytic fragments of complement.
- Cytokines are a family of proteins that are synthesized and secreted by the cells associated with innate and adaptive immunity in response to microbial and other antigen exposure.
- Cytokines also participate in host defense. In innate immunity, cytokines mediate early inflammatory reactions to microbial organisms and stimulate adaptive immune responses. In contrast, in adaptive immunity, cytokines stimulate proliferation and differentiation of antigen-stimulated lymphocytes and activate specialized effector cells (e.g., macrophages).
- The interferons are a group of cytokines discovered in virally infected cultured cells. IFNs are one of the body's natural defensive responses to foreign components (e.g., microbes, tumors, and antigens).

- Tumor necrosis factor is the principal mediator of the acute inflammatory response to gram-negative bacteria and other infectious microbes. TNF is responsible for many of the systemic complications of severe infections.
- Hematopoietic stimulators include stem cell factor, a cytokine that acts on immature stem cells.
- Chemokines are a large family of structurally homologous cytokines that stimulate transendothelial leukocyte movement from the blood to tissue site of infection and regulate the migration of polymorphonuclear leukocytes and mononuclear leukocytes within tissues. Chemokines appear to control the phased arrival of different cell populations at sites of inflammation.
- The acute-phase response is an innate body defense. This response is a nonspecific indicator of an inflammatory process.
- C-reactive protein is used clinically for monitoring infection, autoimmune disorders, and more recently, healing after a myocardial infarction. CRP levels parallel the course of the inflammatory response and return to lower, undetectable levels as the inflammation subsides.

REVIEW QUESTIONS

1. The complement system is:
   a. A heat-labile series of plasma proteins.
   b. Composed of many proteinases.
   c. Composed of three interrelated pathways.
   d. All the above.

2. All the following are complement-controlling proteins *except:*
   a. C1 (INH).
   b. Factor I.
   c. Factor H.
   d. C3.

3. Various cell types express surface membrane glycoproteins that react with one or more of the fragments of _____ produced during complement activation and degradation.
   a. C1
   b. C3
   c. C5
   d. C8

4. All the following result from complement activation *except:*
   a. Decreased cell susceptibility to phagocytosis.
   b. Blood vessel dilation and increased vascular permeability.
   c. Production of inflammatory mediators.
   d. Cytolysis or hemolysis.

Questions 5-8. Complete the following activation sequence of the classic complement pathway:
   C1-C_(5)-C_ _(6)-_ _-C3-_C(7) _-C6-C7- C_(8) _ _-C9
   a. 2
   b. 4
   c. 5
   d. 8

9. Which complement component is present in the greatest quantity in plasma?
   a. 2
   b. 3
   c. 4
   d. 8

Questions 10-12. Arrange the three stages of the classic complement pathway in their correct sequence.

10. _____

11. _____

12. _____
   a. Enzymatic activation
   b. Membrane attack
   c. Recognition

13. Fixation of the C1 complement component is related to each of the following factors *except:*
   a. Molecular weight of the antibody.
   b. The presence of IgM antibody.
   c. The presence of most IgG subclasses.
   d. Spatial constraints.

14. At which stage does the complement system reach its full amplitude?
   a. C1q, C1r, C1s complex
   b. C2
   c. C3
   d. C4

15. Which of the following is *not* a component of the membrane attack complex?
   a. C3b
   b. C6
   c. C7
   d. C8

16. The final steps (C8 and C9) in complement activation lead to:
   a. Cell lysis.
   b. Phagocytosis.
   c. Immune opsonin adherence.
   d. Virus neutralization.

Questions 17-20. Select the appropriate pathway response.

17. _____ Activated by antigen-antibody complexes

18. _____ Generates a C3 convertase

19. _____ Activated by microbial and mammalian cell surfaces

20. _____ Terminates in a membrane attack complex

    a.   Classic pathway
    b.   Alternate pathway
    c.   Both a and b

21. The alternate complement pathway is/can be:
    a.   Initiated by the formation of antigen-antibody reactions.
    b.   Predominantly a non–antibody-initiated pathway.
    c.   Activated by factors such as endotoxins.
    d.   Both b and c.

22. Which of the following conditions can be associated with hypercomplementemia?
    a.   Myocardial infarction
    b.   Systemic lupus erythematosus
    c.   Glomerulonephritis
    d.   Subacute bacterial endocarditis

Questions 23-26. Match the following complement deficiency states in humans with their respective deficient components. (Use an answer only once.)

23. _____ C2

24. _____ C5

25. _____ C6

26. _____ C7

    a.   *Neisseria* infections
    b.   Leiner's disease
    c.   Raynaud's phenomenon
    d.   Recurrent pyogenic infections

27. A (The) nonspecific component(s) of the immune system is (are)
    a.   Complement.
    b.   T cells.
    c.   Both a and b.

Questions 28-31. Match the following.

28. _____ Interleukin-1 (IL-1)

29. _____ Interleukin-2 (IL-2)

30. _____ Interleukin-3 (IL-3)

31. _____ Interleukin-5 (IL-5)

    a.   T-cell growth factor
    b.   Lymphocyte-activating factor
    c.   B cell growth factor 2
    d.   Multicolony colony-stimulating factor

Questions 32-35. Match the following.

32. _____ Interleukin-6 (IL-6)

33. _____ Interleukin-7 (IL-7)

34. _____ Interleukin-8 (IL-8)

35. _____ Interleukin-12 (IL-12)

    a.   NK cell stimulatory factor
    b.   Monocyte-derived neutrophil chemotactic factor
    c.   Interferon beta-2
    d.   Lymphopoietin-1

Questions 36-39. Match the following.

36. _____ Interleukin-1 (IL-1)

37. _____ Interleukin-2 (IL-2)

38. _____ Interleukin-3 (IL-3)

39. _____ Interleukin-4 (IL-4)

    a.   Enhances cytolytic activity of lymphokine-activated killer cells (LAK).
    b.   Potent mediator in acute-phase response.
    c.   Stimulates hematopoietic cells.
    d.   Enhances production of IgG and inhibits production of IgE by activated B cells.

Questions 40-43. Match the following.

40. _____ Interleukin-5 (IL-5)

41. _____ Interleukin-6 (IL-6)

42. _____ Interleukin-7 (IL-7)

43. _____ Interleukin-8 (IL-8)

    a.   Induction of secretion of Ig.
    b.   Inflammatory cytokine.
    c.   Stimulates early B-cell progenitor cells.
    d.   Shares many activities with IL-4.

Questions 44-47. Match the following.

44. _____ Interleukin-9 (IL-9)

45. _____ Interleukin-10 (IL-10)

46. _____ Interleukin-11 (IL-11)

47. _____ Interleukin-12 (IL-12)

    a.   Inhibits cytokine synthesis.
    b.   Increases the number of IgG-secreting B lymphocytes.
    c.   Stimulates proliferation of T cells and mast cells.
    d.   Enhances the activity of cytotoxic effector T cells.

Questions 48-51. Match the following.

48. _____ Interleukin-13 (IL-13)

49. _____ Interleukin-14 (IL-14)

50. _____ Interleukin-15 (IL-15)

51. _____ Interleukin-16 (IL-16}

  a. Inhibits activation of macrophages.
  b. Promotes proliferation of NK cells.
  c. Acts as a T-cell chemoattractant.
  d. Acts as a B-cell growth factor.

Questions 52-55. Match the following.

52. _____ Interleukin-17 (IL-17)

53. _____ Interleukin-18 (IL-18)

54. _____ Interleukin-19 (IL-19)

55. _____ Interleukin-20 (IL-20)

  a. Acts as a synergist with IL-12.
  b. Suppresses activities of Th1 and Th2.
  c. Associated with skin inflammations.
  d. Induces granulopoiesis.

Questions 56-59. Match the following:

56. _____ Interleukin-21 (IL-21)

57. _____ Interleukin-22 (IL_22)

58. _____ Interleukin-23 (IL-23)

59. _____ Interleukin-25 (IL-25)

  a. Promotes increased production of T cells.
  b. Somewhat similar to IFN-α, IFN-β, and IFN-γ.
  c. Also called SF20.
  d. Shares some in vivo functions with IL-12.

Questions 60-63. Indicate true statements with the letter "A," and false statements with the letter "B."

60. _____ Cytokines secreted by lymphocytes are also called lymphokines.

61. _____ Cytokines are polypeptide products of activated cells.

62. _____ Cytokines are released only in response to specific antigens.

63. _____ Most cytokines have multiple activities and act on numerous cell types.

Questions 64-67. Match each term to its appropriate description. (Use each answer only once.)

64. _____ Interleukins

65. _____ Interferons

66. _____ Tumor necrosis factor

67. _____ Colony-stimulating factors

  a. Unable to stimulate T-cell proliferation.
  b. Act(s) between leukocytes.
  c. Discovered in virally infected cells.
  d. Provide(s) a link between the lymphoid hematopoietic system.

68. Transforming growth factors:
  a. Are products of virally transformed cells.
  b. Can be a potent inhibitor of IL-1–induced T-cell proliferation in their beta form.
  c. Are important in inflammation, tumor defense, and cell growth.
  d. All the above.

69. Which activity is associated with interferon?
  a. Enhances phagocytosis.
  b. Retards expression of specific genes.
  c. Promotes complement-mediated cytolysis.
  d. Interferes with viral replication.

70. Tumor necrosis factor (TNF) differs from IL-1 in that TNF is *not* able to:
  a. Mediate an acute inflammatory reaction.
  b. Increase the expression of IL-2 receptors.
  c. Enhance the proliferation and differentiation of B lymphocytes.
  d. Stimulate T-cell proliferation.

Questions 71-73. Match the following.

71. _____ Tumor necrosis factor

72. _____ Colony-stimulating factors

73. _____ Transforming growth factors

  a. Stimulates hematopoietic growth factor.
  b. Encoding gene located in HLA region between HLA-DR and HLA-B loci.
  c. Induce phenotypic transformation in nonneoplastic cells.

BIBLIOGRAPHY

Charo IF, Ransohoff RM: The many roles of chemokines and chemokine receptors in inflammation, *N Engl J Med* 354(6):610-621, 2006.

D'Andrea AD: Cytokine receptors in congenital hematopoietic disease, *N Engl J Med* 330(12):839-846, 1994.

Donahue RE, Yang Y-C, Clark SC: Human P40 T-cell growth factor (interleukin-9) supports erythroid colony formation, *Blood* 75(12):2271-2275, 1990.

Fort MM et al: IL-25 induces IL-4, IL-5, and IL-13 and Th2-associated pathologies in vivo, *Immunology* 5/6:985-995, 2001.

Frank MM: Complement in the pathophysiology of human disease, *N Engl J Med* 316:1525, 1987.

Frucht DM: IL-23: a cytokine that acts on memory T cells, *Sci STKE 2002* 114:PE1, 2002.

Gabay C, Kushner I: Acute-phase proteins and other systemic responses to inflammation, *N Engl J Med* 340(6):448-454, 1999.

Hansson GK: Inflammation, atherosclerosis, and coronary artery disease, *N Engl J Med* 352(16):1685-1695, 2005.

Human Gene Nomenclature Committee (HUGO), 2007, www.gene.ucl.ac.uk.

Hurst SD et al: New IL-17 family members promote Th1 or Th2 responses in the lung: in vivo function of the novel cytokine IL-25, *J Immunol* 169(1):443-453, 2002.

Ibelgaufts H: COPE cytokines & cells online pathfinder encyclopedia, version 19.4, 2007, www.copewithcytokines.de.

Kelleher K et al: Human interleukin-9, *Blood* 77(7):1436-1441, 1991.

Knutsen AP, Fischer TJ: Immunodeficiency diseases. In Lawlor GJ, Fischer TJ, editors: *Manual of allergy and immunology,* ed 2, Boston, 1988, Little, Brown.

Larchmann PJ, Rosen FS: Genetic defects of complement in man, *Springer Semin Immunopathol* 1:339-353, 1978.

Larson RS, Springer TA: Structure and function of leukocyte integrins, *Immunol Rev* 18:181-217, 1990.

Liblau RS, Fugger L: Tumor necrosis factor-alpha and disease progression in multiple sclerosis, *N Engl J Med* 326(4):272, 1992.

MacKay IR, Rosen RS: Allergy and allergic diseases, *N Engl J Med* 344:109-113, 2001.

Marsik C et al: The C-reactive protein +1444C/T alteration modulates the inflammation and coagulation response in human endotoxemia, *Clin Chem* 52(10):1952-1957, 2006.

Medzhitov R, Janeway C Jr: Innate immunity, *N Engl J Med* 343:338-344, 2000.

Muller-Eberhardt HJ: Complement abnormalities in human disease, *Hosp Pract* 13(12):65-76, 1978.

Parham C et al: A receptor for the heterodimeric cytokine IL-23 is composed of IL-23Rβ1 and a novel cytokine receptor subunit, IL-23R, *J Immunol* 168(11):5699-5708, 2002.

Pedrazzi AH: Acute phase proteins: clinical and laboratory diagnosis: a review, *Ann Pharm Fr* 56(3):108-114, 1998.

Peter JB: *The use and interpretation of tests in medical laboratory immunology,* ed 8, Los Angeles, 1991-92, Specialty Laboratories.

Rhen T, Cidlowski JA: Antiinflammatory action of glucocorticoids: new mechanisms for old drugs, *N Engl J Med* 353(16):1711-1723, 2005.

Ridker et al: Comparison of C-reactive protein and low-density lipoprotein cholesterol levels in the prediction of first cardiovascular events, *N Engl J Med* 347:1557-1565, 2002.

Roberts WL et al: Evaluation of four automated high-sensitivity C-reactive protein methods: implications for clinical and epidemiological applications, *Clin Chem* 46(4):461-468, 2000.

Ruddy S: Complement. In Rose NR, Friedman H, Fahey JL, editors: *Manual of clinical laboratory immunology,* ed 3, Washington, DC, 1986, American Society of Microbiology.

Soiffer R et al: Interleukin-12 augments cytolytic activity of peripheral blood lymphocytes from patients with hematologic and solid malignancies, *Blood* 82(9):2790-2796, 1993.

Taga K, Mostowski H, Tosato G: Human interleukin-10 can directly inhibit T cell growth, *Blood* 81(11):2964-2971, 1993.

Tagaya Y: Time to restore individual rights for IL-2 and IL-15? *Blood* 108(2):409, 2006.

Tizmann SE, Daniels JC, editors: *Serum protein abnormalities,* Boston, 1975, Little, Brown.

Tulin EE et al: SF20/IL-25, a novel bone marrow stroma-derived growth factor that binds to mouse thymic shared antigen-1 and supports lymphoid cell proliferation, *J Immunol* 167(11):6338-6347, 2001.

Turgeon ML: *Fundamentals of immunohematology,* ed 3, Baltimore, 1999, Williams & Wilkins.

Van Leeuwen MA, van Rijswijk MH: Acute phase proteins in the monitoring of inflammatory disorders, *Baillieres Clin Rheumatol* 8(3):531-552, 1994.

Waldmann TA: The multichain interleukin-2 receptor, *JAMA* 263(2):272-274, 1990.

Walport MJ: Complement, *N Engl J Med* 344:1058-1065, 1140-1144, 2001.

Wheeler AP, Bernard GR: Treating patients with severe sepsis, *N Engl J Med* 340:208, 1999.

PART II

The Theory of Immunologic and Serologic Procedures

6 Safety in the Immunology-Serology Laboratory
7 Quality Assurance and Quality Control
8 Basic Serologic Laboratory Techniques
9 Point-of-Care Testing
10 Agglutination Methods

11 Electrophoresis Techniques
12 Labeling Techniques in Immunoassay
13 Automated Procedures
14 Molecular Techniques

CHAPTER 6

Safety in the Immunology-Serology Laboratory

Safety Regulations and Practices
Prevention of Transmission of Infectious Diseases
Safe Work Practices for Infection Control
Protective Techniques for Infection Control
  Selection and Use of Gloves
  Facial Barrier Protection and Occlusive Bandages
  Laboratory Coats or Gowns as Barrier Protection
Handwashing
Specimen-Processing Protection
Additional Laboratory Hazards
Decontamination of Work Surfaces,
  Equipment, and Spills

Disposal of Infectious Laboratory Waste
  Containers for Waste
  Final Decontamination of Waste Materials
Disease Prevention
  Immunization
  Screening Tests
  Postexposure Prophylaxis
Basic First-Aid Procedures
Chapter Highlights
Review Questions
Bibliography

Learning Objectives

At the conclusion of this chapter, the reader should be able to:

- Discuss the occupational transmission of hepatitis B virus (HBV) and human immunodeficiency virus (HIV).
- Describe the practice of Standard Blood and Body Fluid Precautions.
- Explain the proper handling of hazardous material and waste management, including infectious waste, chemicals, and radioactive waste.
- Describe the basic aspects of infection control policies, including the use of personal protective equipment or devices (gowns, gloves, goggles) and the purpose of Standard Precautions.

- Compare preexposure and postexposure prophylactic measures for handling potential occupational transmission of certain pathogens (HBV, HCV, HIV).
- Demonstrate the proper decontamination of a work area at the start and completion of work and after a hazardous spill.
- Explain the process of properly segregating and disposing of various types of waste products generated in the clinical laboratory.

In the immunology-serology laboratory, precautions must be taken to prevent accidental exposure to infectious diseases and other laboratory hazards. Clinical laboratory personnel are routinely exposed to potential hazards in their day-to-day activities. The importance of safety and correct first-aid procedures cannot be overemphasized. Many accidents do not just happen; they are caused by carelessness or lack of proper communication. For this reason, the practice of safety should be uppermost in the mind of any worker in a clinical laboratory.

SAFETY REGULATIONS AND PRACTICES

Safety standards for clinical laboratories are initiated, governed, and reviewed by several agencies or committees. These include the U.S. Department of Labor's Occupational Safety and Health Administration (OSHA); the Clinical and Laboratory Standards Institute (CLSI), a nonprofit educational organization providing a forum for development, promotion, and use of national and international standards; the Centers for Disease Control and Prevention (CDC), part of the U.S. Department of Health and Human Services' Public Health Service; the College of American Pathologists (CAP); and The Joint Commission (TJC), formerly Joint Commission on Accreditation of Healthcare Organizations (JCAHO).

All laboratories need programs to minimize risks to the health and safety of employees, volunteers, and patients. Suitable physical arrangements, an acceptable work environment, and appropriate equipment need to be available to maintain safe operations. Adherence to general safety practices will reduce the risk of inadvertent contamination with blood or body fluids, as follows:

1. Staff must wear laboratory coats and must be additionally protected from contamination by infectious agents.
2. Food and drinks should not be consumed in work areas or stored in the same area as specimens. Containers, refrigerators, or freezers used for specimens should be marked as containing a biohazard.
3. Specimens needing centrifugation are capped and placed into a centrifuge with a sealed dome.
4. A gauze square is used when opening rubber-stoppered test tubes to minimize aerosol production (introduction of substances into the air).
5. Autodilutors or safety bulbs are used for pipetting. Pipetting of any clinical material by mouth is strictly forbidden.

Each laboratory must have an up-to-date safety manual. This manual should contain a comprehensive listing of approved policies, acceptable practices, and precautions, including Standard Blood and Body Fluid Precautions. Specific standards that conform to current state and federal requirements (e.g., OSHA regulations) must be included in the manual. Other sources of mandatory and voluntary standards include TJC, CAP, CLSI, and CDC.

PREVENTION OF TRANSMISSION OF INFECTIOUS DISEASES

According to the CDC concept of **Standard Precautions,** all human blood and other body fluids are treated as potentially infectious for human immunodeficiency virus (HIV), hepatitis B virus (HBV), and other blood-borne microorganisms that can cause disease in humans. Compliance with the OSHA Bloodborne Pathogens Standard and the Occupational Exposure Standard is required to provide a safe work environment. OSHA mandates that the employer do the following:

- Educate and train all health care workers in Standard Precautions and in preventing blood-borne infections.
- Provide proper equipment and supplies (e.g., gloves).
- Monitor compliance with the protective biosafety policies.

Blood is the most important source of HIV, HBV, and other blood-borne pathogens in the occupational setting. HBV can be present in extraordinarily high concentrations in blood, but HIV is usually found in lower concentrations. HBV may be stable in dried blood and blood products at 25° C for up to 7 days. HIV retains infectivity for more than 3 days in dried specimens at room temperature and for more than 1 week in an aqueous environment at room temperature.

Both HBV and HIV may be *indirectly* transmitted. Viral transmission can result from contact with inanimate objects, such as work surfaces or equipment contaminated with infected blood or certain body fluids. If the virus is transferred to the skin or mucous membranes by hand contact between a contaminated surface and nonintact skin or mucous membranes, it can produce viral exposure.

Medical personnel must remember that HBV and HIV are different diseases caused by unrelated viruses. The most feared hazard of all, the transmission of HIV through occupational exposure, is among the least likely to occur. The modes of transmission for HBV and HIV are similar, but the potential for transmission in the occupational setting is greater for HBV than HIV.

The transmission of hepatitis B can also be fatal, and it is more probable than transmission of HIV. OSHA estimates that occupational exposures account for 5900 to 7400 cases of HBV infection annually. Although the number of cases has sharply declined since hepatitis B vaccine became available in 1982, approximately 800 health care workers become infected with HBV each year after occupational exposure.

The likelihood of infection after exposure to blood infected with HBV or HIV depends on the following factors:

- Concentration of HBV or HIV; viral concentration is higher for HBV than HIV.
- Duration of the contact.
- Presence or skin lesions or abrasions on the hands or exposed skin of the health care worker.
- Immune status of the health care worker for HBV.

Both HBV and HIV may be *directly* transmitted by various portals of entry. In the occupational setting, however, the following situations may lead to infection:

- Percutaneous (parenteral) inoculation of blood, plasma, serum, or certain other body fluids from accidental needlesticks.
- Contamination of the skin with blood or certain body fluids without overt puncture, caused by scratches, abrasions, burns, weeping, or exudative skin lesions.
- Exposure of mucous membranes (oral, nasal, or conjunctival) to blood or certain body fluids, as the direct result of pipetting by mouth, splashes, or spattering.
- Centrifuge accidents or the improper removal of rubber stoppers from test tubes, producing droplets. If these aerosol products are infectious and come in direct contact with mucous membranes or nonintact skin, direct transmission of virus can result.

Most exposures do not result in infection. The risk varies not only with the type of exposure but also with the amount of infected blood in the exposure, the length of contact with the infectious material, and the amount of virus in the patient's blood or body fluid/tissue at exposure. Studies report that the average risk of HIV transmission is approximately 0.3% after percutaneous exposure to HIV-infected blood and 0.09% after mucous membrane exposure.

SAFE WORK PRACTICES FOR INFECTION CONTROL

Use of CDC Standard Precautions is an approach to infection control that prevents occupational exposures to blood-borne pathogens. It eliminates the need for separate isolation procedures for patients known or suspected to be infectious. The application of Standard Precautions also eliminates the need for warning labels on specimens.

OSHA requires laboratories to have a personal protective equipment (PPE) program. The components of this regulation include the following:

- A workplace hazard assessment, with a written hazard certification.
- Proper equipment selection.
- Employee information and training, with written competency certification.
- Regular reassessment of work hazards.

Laboratory personnel should not rely solely on PPE to protect themselves against hazards. They should also apply PPE standards when using various forms of safety protection.

A clear policy on institutionally required Standard Precautions is needed. For usual laboratory activities, PPE consists of gloves and a laboratory coat or gown; other equipment such as masks would normally not be needed. Standard Precautions are intended to supplement rather than replace handwashing recommendations for routine infection control. The risk of nosocomial transmission of HBV, HIV, and other blood-borne pathogens can be minimized if laboratory personnel are aware of and adhere to essential safety guidelines.

PROTECTIVE TECHNIQUES FOR INFECTION CONTROL

Selection and Use of Gloves

Gloves for medical use are either sterile surgical or nonsterile examination gloves made of vinyl or latex. There are no reported differences in barrier effectiveness between intact latex and intact vinyl gloves. Tactile differences have been observed between the two types of gloves, with latex gloves providing more tactile sensitivity; however, either type is usually satisfactory for phlebotomy and as a protective barrier during technical procedures. Latex-free gloves should be available for personnel with sensitivity to usual glove material. Rubber household gloves may be used for cleaning procedures.

General guidelines related to the selection and general use of gloves include the following:

1. Use sterile gloves for procedures involving contact with normally sterile areas of the body or during procedures where sterility has been established and must be maintained. Use nonsterile examination gloves for procedures that do not require the use of sterile gloves.
2. Wear gloves when processing blood specimens, reagents, or blood products, including reagent red blood cells. Gloves should be changed frequently and immediately if they become visibly contaminated with blood or certain body fluids or if physical damage occurs.
3. Do not wash or disinfect latex or vinyl gloves for reuse. Washing with detergents may cause increased penetration of liquids through undetected holes in the gloves. Rubber gloves may be decontaminated and reused, but disinfectants may cause deterioration. Rubber gloves should be discarded if they have punctures, tears, or evidence of deterioration or if they peel, crack, or become discolored.
4. Using items potentially contaminated with human blood or certain body fluids (e.g., specimen containers, laboratory instruments, countertops).

Care must be taken to avoid indirect contamination of work surfaces or objects in the work area. Gloves should be properly removed or covered with an uncontaminated glove or paper towel before answering the telephone, handling laboratory equipment, or touching doorknobs.

As a result of the 1988 CDC modifications, some institutions have relaxed recommendations for using gloves for phlebotomy procedures by skilled phlebotomists in settings where the prevalence of blood-borne pathogens is known to be very low. Institutions or organizations that choose to modify the policy of requiring gloves for all phlebotomies must periodically reevaluate their policy and must provide gloves to all personnel who want to use gloves for phlebotomy.

The guidelines for the use of gloves during phlebotomy procedures include the following:

1. Gloves must be used by phlebotomists who have cuts, scratches, or other breaks in their skin. The presence of skin lesions will increase the likelihood of infection subsequent to skin exposure.
2. Gloves should be worn when the phlebotomist judges that hand contamination may occur (e.g., when performing phlebotomy on an uncooperative patient).
3. Gloves must be worn when performing fingersticks and heelsticks on infants and children.
4. Gloves must be worn when receiving phlebotomy training.
5. Gloves should be changed between each patient contact.

Facial Barrier Protection and Occlusive Bandages

Facial barrier protection should be used if there is a potential for splashing or spraying of blood or certain body fluids. Masks and facial protection should be worn if mucous membrane contact with blood or body fluids is anticipated. All disruptions of exposed skin, including defects on the arms, face, and neck, should be covered with a water-impermeable occlusive bandage.

Laboratory Coats or Gowns as Barrier Protection

A color-coded, two–laboratory coat or equivalent system should be used whenever laboratory personnel are working with potentially infectious specimens. The garment worn in the laboratory must be changed or covered with an uncontaminated coat when leaving the immediate work area. Garments should be changed immediately if grossly contaminated with blood or body fluids to prevent seepage through to street clothes or skin. Contaminated coats or gowns should be placed in an appropriately designated biohazard bag for laundering. Disposable plastic aprons are recommended if blood or certain body fluids may be splashed. Aprons should be discarded into a biohazard container.

The introduction of water-retardant gowns has been the greatest change in many PPE practices.

HANDWASHING

Frequent handwashing is an important safety precaution. It should be performed after contact with patients and laboratory specimens (Box 6-1). Gloves should be used as an adjunct to, not a substitute for, handwashing.

Table 6-1	Preparation of Diluted Household Bleach		
Volume Bleach	Volume H$_2$O	Ratio	Sodium Hypochlorite
1 mL	9 mL	1:10	0.5%

The efficacy of handwashing in reducing transmission of microbial organisms has been demonstrated. At the very minimum, hands should be washed with soap and water (if visibly soiled) or with soap and water or by hand antisepsis with an alcohol-based handrub (if not visibly soiled) in the following situations:

1. After completing laboratory work and before leaving the laboratory.
2. After removing gloves. The Association for Professionals in Infection Control and Epidemiology reports that extreme variability exists in the quality of gloves, with leakage in 4% to 63% of vinyl gloves and 3% to 52% of latex gloves.
3. Before eating, drinking, applying makeup, and changing contact lenses, and before and after using the bathroom.
4. Before all activities that involve hand contact with mucous membranes or breaks in the skin.
5. Immediately after accidental skin contact with blood, body fluids, or tissues.
   a. If the contact occurs through breaks in gloves, the gloves should be removed immediately and the hands thoroughly washed.
   b. If accidental contamination occurs to an exposed area of the skin or because of a break in gloves, wash first with a liquid soap, rinse well with water, and then apply a 1:10 dilution of bleach (Table 6-1) or 50% isopropyl or ethyl alcohol. The bleach or alcohol is left on skin for at least 1 minute before final washing with liquid soap and water.

Two important points in the practice of hand hygiene technique follow* (see Box 6-1):

- When decontaminating hands with a waterless antiseptic agent (e.g., alcohol-based handrub), apply product to the palm of one hand and rub hands together, covering all surfaces of hands and fingers, until hands are dry. Follow the manufacturer's recommendations on the volume of product to use. If an adequate volume of an alcohol-based handrub is used, it should take 15 to 25 seconds for hands to dry.
- When washing with a non-antimicrobial or antimicrobial soap, wet hands first with warm water, apply 3 to 5 mL of detergent to hands, and rub hands together vigorously for *at least* 15 seconds, covering all surfaces of the hands and fingers. Rinse hands with warm water, and dry thoroughly with a disposable towel. Use the towel to turn off the faucet.

Box 6-1	Guidelines for Handwashing and Hand Antisepsis in Health Care Settings

- Wash hands with a non-antimicrobial soap and water, or an antimicrobial soap and water when hands are visibly dirty or contaminated with proteinaceous material.
- If hands are not visibly soiled, use an alcohol-based waterless antiseptic agent for routinely decontaminating hands in all other clinical situations.
- Waterless antiseptic agents are highly preferable, but hand antisepsis using an antimicrobial soap may be considered in settings where time constraints are not an issue and easy access to hand hygiene facilities can be ensured, or in rare instances when a caregiver is intolerant of the waterless antiseptic product used in the institution.
- Decontaminate hands after contact with a patient's intact skin.
- Decontaminate hands after contact with body fluids or excretions, mucous membranes, nonintact skin, or wound dressings, as long as hands are not visibly soiled.
- Decontaminate hands if moving from a contaminated body site to a clean body site during patient care.
- Decontaminate hands after contact with inanimate objects in the immediate vicinity of the patient.
- Decontaminate hands before caring for patients with severe neutropenia or other forms of severe immune suppression.
- Decontaminate hands after removing gloves.

From US Department of Health and Human Services, Centers for Disease Control and Prevention: *Fed Register* 66(218):56680, 2001; *MMWR* 51(RR16): 1-44, 2002.

*US Department of Health and Human Services, Centers for Disease Control and Prevention (CDC): Guideline for hand hygiene in health-care settings, *MMWR* 51(RR16):1-44, 2002.

SPECIMEN-PROCESSING PROTECTION

Specimens should be transported to the laboratory in plastic, leakproof bags. Protective gloves should always be worn for handling any type of biologic specimen.

Substances can become airborne when the stopper (cap) is popped off a blood-collecting container, a serum sample is poured from one tube to another, or a serum tube is centrifuged. When the cap is being removed from a specimen tube or a blood collection tube, the top should be covered with a disposable gauze pad or a special protective pad. Gauze pads with an impermeable plastic coating on one side can reduce contamination of gloves. The tube should be held away from the body and the cap gently twisted to remove it. Snapping off the cap or top can cause some of the contents to aerosolize. When not in place on the tube, the cap should still be kept in the gauze and not placed directly on the work surface or countertop.

Specially constructed plastic splash shields are used in many laboratories for the processing of blood specimens. The tube caps are removed behind or under the shield, which acts as a barrier between the worker and the specimen tube. This is designed to prevent aerosols from entering the nose, eyes, or mouth. Laboratory safety boxes are commercially available and can be used for unstoppering tubes or doing other procedures that might cause spattering. Splash shields and safety boxes should be periodically decontaminated.

When specimens are being centrifuged, the tube caps should always be kept on the tubes. Centrifuge covers must be used and left on until the centrifuge stops. The centrifuge should be allowed to stop by itself and should not be manually stopped by the worker.

Another step to lessen the hazard from aerosols is to exercise caution in handling pipettes and other equipment used to transfer human specimens, especially pathogenic materials. These materials should be discarded properly and carefully.

ADDITIONAL LABORATORY HAZARDS

It cannot be overemphasized that clinical laboratories present many potential hazards simply because of the nature of the work done. Besides biologic hazards, other hazards in the clinical laboratory include open flames, electrical equipment, glassware, chemicals of varying reactivity, flammable solvents, and toxic fumes.

In addition to the safety practices common to all laboratory situations, certain procedures are mandatory in a medical laboratory. Proper procedures for the handling and disposal of toxic, radioactive, and potentially carcinogenic materials must be included in the safety manual. Information regarding the hazards of particular substances must be included as a safety practice and to comply with the legal right of workers to know about the hazards associated with these substances. Some chemicals (e.g., benzidine) previously used in the laboratory are now known to be carcinogenic and have been replaced with safer chemicals.

DECONTAMINATION OF WORK SURFACES, EQUIPMENT, AND SPILLS

Sodium hypochlorite solutions are inexpensive and effective broad-spectrum germicidical solutions. Generic sources of sodium hypochlorite include household chlorine bleach. Concentrations of 1:10 to 1:100 free chlorine are effective depending on the amount of organic material present on the surface to be cleaned and disinfected. Many chlorine bleaches (available at grocery stores) are not registered by the U.S. Environmental Protection Agency (EPA) for use as surface disinfectants and are unacceptable surface disinfectants. The EPA encourages the use of registered products because the agency reviews them for safety and performance when the products are used according to label instructions. When unregistered products are used for surface disinfection, users do so at their own risk. EPA-registered chemical germicides may be more compatible with certain materials that could be corroded by repeated exposure to sodium hypochlorite, especially the 1:10 dilution.

While wearing gloves, all work surfaces should be cleaned and sanitized at the beginning and end of the shift with a 1:10 dilution of household bleach. Instruments such as scissors or centrifuge carriages should be sanitized daily with a diluted solution of bleach. It is equally important to clean and disinfect work areas frequently during the workday, and before and after each shift.. Studies have demonstrated that HIV is inactivated rapidly after being exposed to common chemical germicides at concentrations much lower than used in practice. Diluted household bleach prepared daily inactivates HBV in 10 minutes and HIV in 2 minutes. Disposable materials contaminated with blood must be placed in containers marked "Biohazard" and properly discarded.

Hepatitis C virus (HCV), HBV, and HIV have never been documented as being transmitted from a housekeeping surface (e.g., countertops). However, an area contaminated by blood or body fluids needs to be treated as potentially hazardous and requires prompt removal and surface disinfection.

Strategies differ for decontaminating spills of blood and other body fluids, based on the setting. The cleanup procedure depends on the porosity of the surface and volume of the spill. The following protocol is recommended for managing spills in a clinical laboratory:

1. Wear gloves and a laboratory coat.
2. Absorb the blood with disposable towels. Bleach solutions are less effective in the presence of high concentrations of protein. Remove as much liquid blood or serum as possible before decontamination.
3. Using a diluted bleach (1:10) solution, clean the spill site of all visible blood.

4. Wipe down the spill site with paper towels soaked with diluted bleach.
5. Place all disposable materials used for decontamination into a biohazard container.

Decontaminate nondisposable equipment by soaking overnight in a dilute (1:10) bleach solution and rinsing with methyl alcohol and water before reuse. Disposable glassware or supplies that have come in contact with blood should be autoclaved or incinerated. Staff should receive training in environmental surface, infection control strategies and procedures as part of an overall infection control and safety program.

DISPOSAL OF INFECTIOUS LABORATORY WASTE

The control of infectious, chemical, and radioactive waste is regulated by a variety of government agencies, including OSHA and the U.S. Food and Drug Administration (FDA). Legislation and regulations that affect laboratories include the Resource Recovery and Conservation Act, the Toxic Substances Control Act, clean air and water laws, "right to know" laws, and HAZCOM (chemical hazard communication). Laboratories should implement applicable federal, state, and local laws that pertain to hazardous material and waste management by establishing safety policies. Laboratories with multiple agencies should follow the guidelines of the most stringent agency. Safety policies should be reviewed and signed annually or whenever a change is instituted. Employers are responsible for ensuring that personnel follow the safety policies.

OSHA has defined **infectious waste** as blood and blood products, contaminated "sharps," pathologic wastes, and microbiologic wastes. Infectious waste is packaged for disposal in color-coded containers and labeled as such with the standard symbol for biohazards (Figure 6-1).

Infectious waste (e.g., contaminated gauze squares and test tubes) must be discarded into proper biohazard containers with the following characteristics:
1. Conspicuously marked "Biohazard" with the universal biohazard symbol.
2. Universal color: orange, orange and black, or red.
3. Rigid, leakproof, and puncture resistant. (Cardboard boxes lined with leakproof plastic bags are available.)
4. Used for blood and other potentially infectious body fluids, as well as disposable materials contaminated with blood or fluid.

Containers for Waste

Containers must be easily accessible to personnel needing them and must be located in the laboratory areas where they are typically used. They should be constructed in such a manner that their contents will not spill out if the container is tipped over accidentally.

Biohazard Containers

Body fluid specimens, including blood, must be placed in well-constructed biohazard containers with secure lids to prevent leakage during transport and for future disposal. Contaminated specimens and other materials used in laboratory tests should be decontaminated before reprocessing for disposal, or should be placed in special impervious bags for disposal, in accordance with established waste removal policies. If outside contamination of the bag is likely, a second bag should be used.

Hazardous specimens and potentially hazardous substances should be tagged and identified as such. The tag should read "Biohazard," or the biologic hazard symbol should be used. All persons working in the laboratory area must be informed about the meaning of the tags and precautions to take for each.

Contaminated equipment must be placed in a designated area for storage, washing, decontamination, or disposal. With the increased use of disposable PPE (e.g., gloves), the volume of waste for disposal will increase.

Biohazard Bags

Although rigid, impermeable containers are used for disposal of sharps and broken glassware, plastic bags are appropriate for disposal of most infectious waste materials. Plastic bags with the biohazard symbol and lettering prominently visible can be used in secondary metal or plastic containers. These containers can be decontaminated or disposed of regularly, or immediately when visibly contaminated. These biohazard bags should be used for all blood, body fluids, tissues, and other disposable materials contaminated with infectious agents and should be handled with gloves.

If the primary infectious waste containers are red plastic bags, they should be kept in secondary metal or plastic cans.

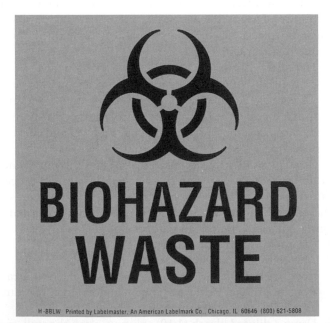

Figure 6-1   Biohazard symbol. *(From Rodak BF, Fritsma GA, Doig K: Hematology: clinical principles and applications, ed 3, St Louis, 2007, Saunders.)*

Extreme care should be taken not to contaminate the exterior of these bags. If they do become contaminated on the outside, the entire bag must be placed into another red plastic bag. Secondary plastic or metal cans should be decontaminated regularly, and immediately after any grossly visible contamination, with an agent such as a 1:10 solution of household bleach.

Final Decontamination of Waste Materials

Terminal disposal of infectious waste should be by incineration; an alternate method is terminal sterilization by autoclaving. If incineration is not done in the health care facility or by an outside contractor, all contaminated disposables should be autoclaved before leaving the facility for disposal with routine waste. Disposal of medical waste should be done by licensed organizations to ensure that no environmental contamination or aesthetic problem occurs. The U.S. Congress has passed various acts and regulations regarding the proper handling of medical waste to assist the EPA to carry out this process in the most prudent manner.

DISEASE PREVENTION

Immunization

A well-planned and implemented immunization program is an important component of a health care organization's infection prevention and control program. When planning these programs, valuable resources are available from the Advisory Committee on Immunization Practices (ACIP) and the Hospital Infection Control Practices Advisory Committee (HICPAC). The characteristics of the health care workers employed and the individuals served should be considered, as well as the requirements of regulatory agencies and local, state, and federal regulations.

In their recommendations for immunization of health care workers, ACIP and HICPAC identify the health care workers whose maintenance of immune status is especially important, which includes laboratory staff. Other individuals are recognized as being at risk for exposure to and possible transmission of diseases that can be prevented by immunizations. The ACIP/HICPAC recommendations are divided into the following three categories:

1. Immunizing agents strongly recommended for health care workers.
2. Other immunologic agents that are or may be indicated for health care workers.
3. Other vaccine-preventable diseases.

All health care organizations should include the strongly recommended immunizations. To determine whether to include other immunologic agents, the incidence of the vaccine-preventable diseases within the community served needs to be reviewed. Also, comparing the demographics of the workforce pool with the disease pattern within the community will determine which of these immunologic agents are indicated for the specific organization's program. Other vaccines may not be routinely administered but may be considered after an injury or exposure incident or for immunocompromised or older health care workers.

The ACIP/HICPAC recommendations determine which vaccines to include based on documented nosocomial transmission and significant risk for acquiring or transmitting the following vaccine-preventable diseases:

- Hepatitis B
- Influenza
- Measles
- Mumps
- Rubella
- Varicella

Optional immunizations include hepatitis A, diphtheria, pneumococcal disease, and tetanus. Because health care workers are not at greater risk for acquiring these diseases than the general population, they should seek recommendations for these immunizations from their primary care provider.

Screening Tests

Purified Protein Derivative (PPD, Mantoux) Tuberculin Skin Test

If recently exposed to an individual with active tuberculosis (TB) infection, a health care worker may not yet have a positive TB skin test reaction. The worker may need a second skin test 10 to 12 weeks after the last exposure to the infected person. It can take several weeks after infection for the immune system to react to the TB skin test. If the reaction to the second test is negative, the worker probably does not have latent TB infection. Strongly positive "reactors," with skin test diameters greater than 15 mm and symptoms suggestive of TB, should be evaluated clinically and microbiologically. Two sputum specimens, collected on successive days, should be investigated for TB by microscopy and culture.

QuantiFERON-TB Gold

QuantiFERON-TB Gold (QFT) is a blood test used to detect infection with TB bacteria. The QFT measures the response to TB proteins when they are mixed with a small amount of blood. Currently, few health departments offer the QFT. If your health department does offer the QFT, only one visit is required, at which time your blood is drawn for the test.

Rubella

All phlebotomists and laboratory staff need to demonstrate immunity to rubella. If antibodies are not demonstrable, vaccination is necessary.

Hepatitis B Surface Antigen

All phlebotomists and laboratory staff need to demonstrate immunity to hepatitis B. If a positive test is not demonstrable, vaccination is necessary.

Postexposure Prophylaxis

Although the most important strategy for reducing the risk of occupational HIV transmission is to prevent occupational exposures, plans for postexposure management of health care personnel should be in place. The CDC has issued guidelines for the management of health care personnel exposure to HIV and recommendations for postexposure prophylaxis (PEP).*

These guidelines outline considerations in determining whether health care personnel should receive PEP and in choosing the type of PEP regimen. For most HIV exposures that warrant PEP, a basic 4-week, two-drug regimen is recommended. For HIV exposures that pose an increased risk of transmission, a three-drug regimen may be recommended.

Special circumstances are also discussed in the guidelines, including delayed exposure report, unknown source person, pregnancy in an exposed woman, resistance of the source virus to antiviral agents, and toxicity of PEP regimens. Occupational exposures should be considered urgent medical concerns.

Hepatitis B Virus Exposure

After skin or mucosal exposure to blood, the ACIP recommends **immunoprophylaxis,** depending on several factors. If an individual has not been vaccinated, hepatitis B immune globulin (HBIG) is usually given, within 24 hours if practical, and concurrently with hepatitis B vaccine postexposure injuries. Recommendations for HBV postexposure management include initiation of the hepatitis B vaccine series to any susceptible, unvaccinated person who sustains an occupational blood or body fluid exposure. PEP with HBIG and hepatitis B vaccine series should be considered for occupational exposures after evaluation of the hepatitis B surface antigen (HBsAg) status of the source and the vaccination and vaccine-response status of the exposed person. The specific protocol for these measures is determined by the institution's infection control division. Postvaccination testing for the development of antibody to HBsAg (anti-HBsAg) for persons at occupational risk who may have had needlestick exposures necessitating PEP should be done to ensure that the vaccination has been successful.

Hepatitis C Virus Exposure

Immune globulin and antiviral agents (e.g., interferon with or without ribavirin) are not recommended for PEP of hepatitis C. For HCV postexposure management, the HCV status of the source and the exposed person should be determined, and for health care personnel exposed to an HCV-positive source, follow-up HCV testing should be performed to determine if infection develops. After exposure to blood of a patient infected or suspected of being infected with HCV, immune globulin should be given as soon as possible. No vaccine is currently available.

In addition, special circumstances (see previous PEP section) should be addressed during consultation with local experts or the National Clinicians' Post-Exposure Prophylaxis Hotline ([PEPline] 1-888-448-4911).

---

*Updated US Public Health Service guidelines for the management of occupational exposures to HBV, HCV, and HIV and recommendations for postexposure prophylaxis, *MMWR* 50(RR-11), 2001.

Human Immunodeficiency Virus

Transmission of HIV is believed to result from intimate contact with blood and body fluids from an infected person. Casual contact with infected persons has not been documented as a mode of transmission. If there has been occupational exposure to a potentially HIV-infected specimen or patient, the antibody status of the patient or specimen source should be determined, if it is not already known. If the source is a patient, voluntary consent should be obtained, if possible, for testing for HIV antibodies as soon as possible. High-risk exposure prophylaxis includes the use of a combination of antiretroviral agents to prevent seroconversion.

The CDC bases PEP guidelines on the determined risks of transmission, stratified as highest risk, increased risk, and no risk. "Highest risk" exists when there has been occupational exposure both to a large volume of blood (as with deep percutaneous injury or a cut with large-diameter hollow needle previously used in source patient's vein or artery) and to blood containing a high titer of HIV (known as a high viral load), to fluids containing visible blood, or to specific other potentially infectious fluids or tissue, including semen, vaginal secretions, and cerebrospinal, peritoneal, pleural, pericardial, and amniotic fluids.

If a known or suspected parenteral exposure takes place, a technician or technologist may request follow-up monitoring for HBV or HIV antibodies. This monitoring and follow-up counseling must be provided free of charge. If voluntary informed consent is obtained, the source of the potentially infectious material and the technician/technologist should be tested immediately. The laboratory technologist should also be tested at intervals after exposure. An injury report must be filed after parenteral exposure.

An **enzyme immunoassay (EIA)** screening test is used to detect antibodies to HIV. Before any HIV result is considered positive, the result is confirmed by **Western blot (WB)** analysis. A negative antibody test for HIV does not confirm the absence of virus. There is a "window period" after HIV infection during which detectable antibody is not present. In these patients, detection of antigen is important; a polymerase chain reaction (PCR) assay for HIV DNA can be used for this purpose, and a p24 antigen test is used for screening blood donors for HIV antigen.

If the source patient is seronegative, the exposed worker should be screened for antibody again at 3 and 6 months. If the source patient is at high risk for HIV infection, more extensive follow-up of both the worker and the source patient may be needed.

If the source patient or specimen is HIV positive (HIV antibodies, WB, HIV antigen, or HIV DNA by PCR), the blood of the exposed worker should be tested for HIV antibodies within 48 hours, if possible. Exposed workers who are initially seronegative for the HIV antibody should be tested again 6 weeks after exposure. If this test is negative, the worker should be tested again at 12 weeks and 6 months after exposure. Most reported seroconversions have occurred between 6 and 12 weeks after exposure. PEP should be started immediately and according to policies set by the institution's infection control program. A policy of "hit hard, hit early" should generally be in place.

During the early follow-up after exposure, especially the first 6 to 12 weeks, the worker should follow the recommendations of the CDC regarding the transmission of acquired immunodeficiency syndrome (AIDS), as follows:

1. Refrain from donating blood or plasma.
2. Inform potential sex partners of the exposure.
3. Avoid pregnancy.
4. Inform health care providers of their potential exposure, so they can take necessary precautions.
5. Do not share razors, toothbrushes, or other items that could become contaminated with blood.
6. Clean and disinfect surfaces on which blood or body fluids have spilled.

The exposed worker should be advised of and alerted to the risks of infection and evaluated medically for any history, signs, or symptoms consistent with HIV infection. Serologic testing for HIV antibodies should be made available to all health care workers who are concerned that they may have been infected with HIV.

Occupational exposures should be considered urgent medical concerns to ensure timely postexposure management and administration of HBIG, hepatitis B vaccine, and HIV PEP.

BASIC FIRST-AID PROCEDURES

Because there are so many potential hazards in a clinical laboratory, knowledge of **basic first aid** should be an integral part of any educational program. A key rule in dealing with laboratory emergencies is to *keep calm,* which may not always be easy but is important to the victim's well-being. Keep crowds of people away, and give the victim plenty of fresh air. Because injuries can be extreme and immediate care is critical, application of the proper first-aid procedures must be thoroughly understood by every person in the medical laboratory.

In serious laboratory accidents, medical assistance should be summoned while first aid is being administered. For general accidents, competent medical help should be sought as soon as possible after the first-aid treatment has been completed. In cases of chemical burns, especially involving the eyes, rapid treatment is essential.

Remember that first aid is useful not only in your working environment, but also at home and in your community. It deserves your earnest attention and study.

CHAPTER HIGHLIGHTS

- Clinical laboratories have instituted Standard Blood and Body Fluid Precautions, or Standard Precautions, to prevent parenteral, mucous membrane, and nonintact skin exposures of health care workers to bloodborne pathogens such as HIV and HBV.

- Although HIV has been isolated from blood, semen, vaginal secretions, saliva, tears, breast milk, cerebrospinal fluid, amniotic fluid, and urine, only blood, semen, vaginal secretions, and possibly breast milk have been implicated in transmission of HIV to date.

- Medical personnel should be aware that HBV and HIV are different diseases caused by unrelated viruses. The most feared hazard of all, the transmission of HIV through occupational exposure, is among the least likely to occur if proper safety practices are followed.

- The control of infectious, chemical, and radioactive waste is regulated by a variety of government agencies (e.g., OSHA, FDA).

REVIEW QUESTIONS

1. Which of the following is *primarily* responsible for safeguards and regulations to ensure a safe and healthful workplace?
   a. Occupational Safety and Health Administration (OSHA)
   b. Clinical Laboratory Improvement Amendments of 1988 (CLIA '88)
   c. Centers for Disease Control and Prevention (CDC)
   d. All the above

2. The simplest and most important step in the proper handling of any hazardous substance is:
   a. Wearing disposable gloves.
   b. Wearing safety glasses.
   c. Properly labeling containers.
   d. Using a biosafety hood.

3. The term *Standard Precautions* refers to:
   a. Treating all specimens as if they are infectious.
   b. Assuming that every direct contact with a body fluid is infectious.
   c. Treating only blood or blood-tinged specimens as infectious.
   d. Both a and b.

4. The CDC Bloodborne Pathogen Standard and the OSHA Occupational Exposure Standard mandate:
   a. Education and training of all health care workers in standard precautions.
   b. Proper handling of chemicals.
   c. Calibration of equipment.
   d. Fire extinguisher maintenance.

5. The single most common source of human immunodeficiency virus in the occupational setting is:
   a. Saliva.
   b. Urine.
   c. Blood.
   d. Cerebrospinal fluid.

Questions 6-9. Indicate true statements with the letter "A," and false statements with the letter "B."

6. _____ Sterile gloves need to be worn for all laboratory procedures.

7. _____ Hands should be washed after removing gloves.

8. _____ Hands should be washed before leaving the laboratory.

9. _____ Hands should be washed before and after using the bathroom.

10. Gloves for medical use may be:
    a. Sterile or nonsterile.
    b. Latex or vinyl.
    c. Used only once.
    d. All the above.

Questions 11 and 12:

Diluted bleach for disinfecting work surfaces, equipment, and spills should be prepared daily by preparing a (11) _____ dilution of household bleach. This dilution requires (12) _____ mL of bleach diluted to 100 mL with H_2O.

11. a. 1:5
    b. 1:10
    c. 1:20
    d. 1:100

12. a. 1
    b. 10
    c. 25
    d. 50

13. Infectious waste must be discarded into containers with all the following characteristics *except:*
    a. Marked "Biohazard."
    b. Has standard biohazard symbol.
    c. Orange, orange and black, or red.
    d. Made of sturdy cardboard for landfill disposal.

14. Clinical laboratory personnel need to have demonstrable immunity to:
    a. Rubella.
    b. Polio.
    c. Hepatitis B.
    d. Both a and c.

BIBLIOGRAPHY

Miller LE: Recommended concentrations of bleach, *Lab Med* 21(2):116, 1990.

National Committee for Clinical Laboratory Standards: *Clinical laboratory waste management: approved guideline,* Villanova, Pa, 1993, NCCLS Document GP5-A.

Sebazcp S: Considerations for immunization programs, 2005. www.infectioncontroltoday.com/articles/0a1feat4.html.

Turgeon ML: *Linné & Ringsrud's clinical laboratory science,* ed 5, St Louis, 2007, Mosby.

US Department of Health and Human Services, Centers for Disease Control and Prevention (CDC): *Guidelines for environmental infection control in health-care facilities,* Atlanta, 2003, CDC.

CDC: Surveillance of healthcare personnel with HIV/AIDS, as of December 2002, www.cdc.gov/ncidod/hip/Blood/hivpersonnel.htm, 2005.

CDC: *Guidelines for environmental infection control in health-care facilities,* Atlanta, 2003.

CDC: Update: provisional public health service recommendations for chemoprophylaxis after occupational exposure to HIV, *MMWR* 45:468-472, 1996.

CDC, Hospital Infection Control Practices Advisory Committee (HICPAC): *Guidelines for isolation precautions in hospitals,* Atlanta, 1996.

US Department of Health and Human Services: Protection against viral hepatitis: recommendations of the Immunization Practices Advisory Committee, *MMWR* 39:1-23, 1990.

US Department of Labor, Occupational Safety and Health Administration (OSHA): Occupational exposure to bloodborne pathogens: final rule, *Fed Register* 29 CFR 1910.1030(235), 64003-64182, 1991.

OSHA: Occupational exposure to hazardous chemicals in laboratories: final rule, *Fed Register* 29 CFR 1910.1450, 55(21), 3327-3335, 1990.

CHAPTER 7

Quality Assurance and Quality Control

Clinical Laboratory Regulatory and Accrediting
  Organizations
Nonanalytical Factors Related to Testing Accuracy
  Qualified Personnel
  Established Laboratory Policies
  Laboratory Procedure Manual
  Test Requisitioning
  Patient Identification, Specimen Procurement,
    and Labeling
  Preventive Maintenance of Equipment
  Appropriate Testing Methods
  Inaccurate Results
Errors Related to Phase of Testing
Quality Descriptors
  Terms
  Coefficient of Variation

Sensitivity and Specificity
Predictive Values
Monitoring Quality
  Proficiency Testing
  Control Specimens
Reference Range Statistics
Testing Outcomes
Validating New Procedures
Chapter Highlights
Review Questions
Bibliography

Learning Objectives

At the conclusion of this chapter, the reader should be able to:

- Identify the regulatory and accrediting organizations that influence quality assessment in clinical laboratories.
- Describe the eight nonanalytical factors related to testing accuracy.
- Identify and give examples of the three categories of errors related to phase of testing.
- Define the terms *accuracy, precision, reproducibility,* and *reliability.*
- Describe the use of the coefficient of variation, and give the formula.
- Define true positive, true negative, false positive, and false negative.

- Provide the equations for calculating percent sensitivity and percent specificity.
- Define positive predictive value and negative predictive value.
- Describe the process of proficiency testing.
- Explain the use of control specimens.
- Cite seven causes for a control value being out of the acceptable range or out of control.
- Define the terms *mean, median, mode, standard deviation,* and *reference range.*
- Discuss issues related to testing outcomes.
- Describe how a new procedure is validated.

The introduction of routine **quality assurance (QA)** programs and **quality control (QC)** in the clinical laboratory was a major advance in improving the accuracy and reliability of testing. This process assures the clinician ordering the test that the testing method has been done in the best possible way to provide the most useful information in diagnosing or managing a patient. QA indicators and QC are tools to ensure that reported laboratory results are of the highest quality.

CLINICAL LABORATORY REGULATORY AND ACCREDITING ORGANIZATIONS

The U.S. Congress enacted the Clinical Laboratory Improvement Amendments of 1988 (CLIA '88) in response to the concerns about laboratory testing errors. The final CLIA rule, Laboratory Requirements Relating to Quality Systems

and Certain Personnel Qualification, was published in the *Federal Register* in January 2003. Enactment of CLIA established a minimum threshold for all aspects of clinical laboratory testing.

Voluntary standards have been set by The Joint Commission (TJC), the Commission on Office Laboratory Accreditation (COLA), and the College of American Pathologists (CAP).

NONANALYTICAL FACTORS RELATED TO TESTING ACCURACY

Qualified Personnel

The competence of personnel is an important determinant of the quality of the laboratory result. Only properly certified personnel can perform *nonwaived assays* (see Chapter 9 for levels of laboratory testing).

Procedure name
Name of the test method
Principle and purpose of the test
Specimen collection and storage
Quality control
Reagents, supplies, and equipment
Procedural protocol
Expected or normal (reference) values
Procedural notes:
    Sources of error
    Limitations
    Clinical applications

Modified from Clinical and Laboratory Standards Institute: *Clinical laboratory technical procedure manual: approved guideline,* ed 4, Wayne, Pa, 2002, CLSI Document GP2-A4.

Established Laboratory Policies

Laboratory policies should be included in a laboratory reference manual that is available to all hospital personnel. Each laboratory must have an up-to-date safety manual. This manual contains a comprehensive listing of approved policies, acceptable practices, and precautions, including Standard Blood and Body Fluid Precautions. Specific regulations that conform to current state and general requirement, such as Occupational Safety and Health Administration (OSHA) regulations, must be included in the manual.

Laboratory Procedure Manual

A complete laboratory procedure manual for all analytical procedures performed within the laboratory must be provided. The manual must be reviewed regularly, in some cases annually, by the supervisory staff and updated, as needed.

A complete laboratory procedure manual for all procedures performed within the laboratory must be provided. The Clinical and Laboratory Standards Institute (CLSI), formerly the National Committee for Clinical Laboratory Standards (NCCLS), recommends that these manuals follow a specific pattern for how procedures are organized (Box 7-1).

Test Requisitioning

A laboratory test request must include the (1) patient identification data, (2) time and date of specimen collection, (3) source of the specimen, and (4) analyses to be performed. The information on the accompanying specimen container must match exactly the patient identification on the test request.

Patient Identification, Specimen Procurement, and Labeling

Patients must be carefully identified. For outpatients, identification may be validated with two forms of identification. Using established specimen-processing information, the clinical specimens must be properly labeled or identified once obtained from the patient. An important rule is that the analytical result can only be as good as the specimen. Specimens must be efficiently transported to the laboratory.

For elimination of the most frequent source of pretesting error, a patient must be positively identified when a blood specimen is obtained. This specimen must be properly collected and labeled. In general, hemolyzed specimens should not be used for serologic testing.

Preventive Maintenance of Equipment

Microscopes, centrifuges, and other pieces of equipment need to be cleaned and checked for accuracy. A preventive maintenance schedule should be followed for all automated equipment. Failure to monitor equipment regularly can produce inaccurate test results and lead to expensive repairs.

Appropriate Testing Methods

Each laboratory must have an assessment routine for all procedures, performed on a daily, weekly, or monthly basis, to detect problems. When such problems are indicated, they must be corrected as soon as possible.

Another part of a quality control program concerns the way new procedures are validated before they are included among the methods routinely used by the laboratory. Each laboratory must determine the **reproducibility** (or **confidence limits**) for each procedure used and establish acceptable limits of variation for control specimens.

Inaccurate Results

Inaccuracies in testing can be systematic or sporadic. **Systematic** errors can be eliminated by a program that monitors equipment, reagents, and other supplies. Sporadic or isolated errors in technique can produce false-positive and false-negative results, depending on the technique used for testing (Box 7-2).

An important aspect of quality is documentation of results. CLIA regulations mandate that any problem or situa-

False-Positive Errors
Overcentrifugation of serum cell mixture
Dirty glassware
Hemolyzed patient serum
Inadequate dispersal of centrifuged serum cell mixture
Extended incubation

False-Negative Errors
Omitting patient serum from test mixture
Omitting reagent from test mixture
Undercentrifugation of serum cell mixture
Vigorous shaking of centrifuged serum cell mixture

False-Positive or False-Negative Errors
Incorrect labeling of test tubes
Addition of wrong reagent to test tube
Erroneously reading or interpreting results
Inaccurately recording results
Expired or improperly stored reagents

Incorrect test request
Specimen obtained from wrong patient
Specimen procured at wrong time
Specimen collected in wrong tube or container
Blood specimens collected in wrong order
Incorrect labeling of specimen
Improper processing of specimen

Recording results inaccurately
Verbally reporting results for wrong patient

tion that might affect the outcome of a test result be recorded and reported. These incidents can involve specimens that are improperly collected, labeled, or transported to the laboratory or problems concerning prolonged turnaround times for test results. There must be a reasonable attempt to correct the problems or situation, and all steps in this process must be documented.

ERRORS RELATED TO PHASE OF TESTING

The Institute for Quality Laboratory Medicine has developed measures to evaluate quality in the laboratory based on the phases of testing: preanalytical, analytical, and postanalytical.

Errors occurring during the analytical phase of testing within clinical laboratories are now relatively rare. Currently, most laboratory errors are related to the preanalytical and postanalytical phases of testing. To guarantee the highest-quality laboratory results and to comply with CLIA regulations, various preanalytical factors need to be considered (Boxes 7-3 and 7-4).

QUALITY DESCRIPTORS

Quality control activities include monitoring the performance of laboratory instruments, reagents, other testing products, and equipment. A written record of QC activities for each procedure or function should include details of deviation from the usual results, problems, or failures in functioning or in the analytical procedure and any corrective action taken in response to these problems. All solutions and kits used in testing must be carefully checked before actual use in testing patient samples.

Definitions

Quality control consists of procedures used to detect errors that result from test system failure, adverse environmental conditions, and differences between technologists, as well as the monitoring of the accuracy and precision of test performance over time. Accrediting agencies require monitoring and documentation of quality assessment records. Docu-

mentation of QC includes preventive maintenance records, temperature charts, and QC charts for specific assays.

Quality control monitors the accuracy and *reproducibility* of results through the use of control specimens. The diagnostic usefulness of a test and its procedure is assessed by using statistical evaluations, such as descriptions of the accuracy and **reliability** of the test and its methodology.

The terms accuracy and precision are often used to describe quality. **Accuracy** describes how close a test result is to the true value. **Precision** describes how close the test results are to one another when repeated analyses of the same specimen are performed. It is possible to achieve great precision, with all laboratory personnel who perform the same procedure arriving at the same answer, but without accuracy if the answer does not represent the actual value being tested. Accuracy can be improved by the following:

- Use of properly standardized procedures.
- Statistically valid comparisons of new methods with established reference methods.
- Use of samples of known values (controls).
- Participation in proficiency testing programs.

The precision of a test, its **reproducibility,** may be expressed as the **standard deviation (SD)** or the derived **coefficient of variation (CV).** A procedure may be extremely accurate, yet so difficult to perform that individual laboratory personnel are unable to arrive at values that are close enough to be clinically meaningful.

Precision can be ensured by the proper inclusion of standards, reference samples, or control solutions; statistically valid, replicate determinations of a single sample; or duplicate determinations of sufficient numbers of unknown samples. Day-to-day and between-run precision is measured by inclusion of blind samples and control specimens.

Coefficient of Variation

The CV can be used to compare the standard deviations of two samples. Standard deviations cannot be compared directly without considering the mean. The CV can be used to compare 1 day's work with that of a similar day or to compare test results from one laboratory with the same type of test results from another laboratory. The coefficient of variation in percent is equal to the standard deviation divided by the mean, as follows:

$$CV(\%) = \frac{SD}{Mean} \times 100$$

Sensitivity and Specificity

Laboratory results should provide medically useful information, including the *specificity* and *sensitivity* of the tests being ordered and reported. Both specificity and sensitivity are desirable characteristics for a test, but in different clinical situations, one is generally preferred over the other.

Assessing the sensitivity and specificity of a test requires four entities: tests positive, tests negative, disease present (positive), and disease absent (negative). True positives are those subjects who have a positive test result and who also have the disease in question. True negatives represent those who have a negative test result and who do not have the disease. False positives are those who have a positive test result but do not have the disease. False negatives are those subjects who have a negative test result but do have the disease.

Sensitivity

The **sensitivity** of a test is defined as the proportion of subjects with the specific disease or condition who have a positive test result (i.e., assay correctly predicts with a positive result):

$$\text{Sensitivity (\%)} = \frac{\text{True positives}}{\text{True positives} + \text{False negatives}} \times 100$$

Practically, sensitivity represents how much of a given substance is measured; the more sensitive the test, the smaller the amount of assayed substance that is measured.

Specificity

The **specificity** of a test is defined as the proportion of subjects without the specific disease or condition who have a negative test result (i.e., assay correctly excludes with a negative result):

$$\text{Specificity (\%)} = \frac{\text{True negatives}}{\text{False positive} + \text{True negatives}} \times 100$$

Practically, specificity represents what is being measured. A highly specific test measures only the assay substance in question; it does not measure interfering or similar substances.

Predictive Values

To assess the **predictive value (PV)** for a test, the sensitivity, specificity, and prevalence of the disease in the population being studied must be known. The prevalence of a disease is the proportion of a population who have the disease. The incidence is the number of subjects found to have the disease within a defined period, such as 1 year, in a population of 100,000.

A positive predictive value for a test indicates the number of patients with an abnormal test result who have the disease, compared with all patients with an abnormal result:

$$\text{Positive PV} = \frac{\text{Number of patients with disease and with abnormal test results}}{\text{Total number of patients with abnormal test results}}$$

$$\text{Positive PV} = \frac{\text{True positives}}{\text{True positives} + \text{False positives}}$$

A *negative predictive value* for a test indicates the number of patients with a normal test result who do not have the disease, compared with all patients with a normal (negative) result:

$$\text{Negative PV} = \frac{\text{True negatives}}{\text{True Negatives} + \text{False Negatives}}$$

MONITORING QUALITY

Proficiency Testing

Proficiency testing (PT) is incorporated into the CLIA requirements. In addition to the use of internal QC programs, each laboratory should participate in an external PT program as a means of verification of laboratory accuracy. Periodically, a laboratory tests a specimen that has been provided by a government agency, professional society, or commercial company. Identical samples are sent to a group of laboratories participating in the PT program, Each laboratory analyzes the specimen, reports the results to the agency, and is evaluated and graded on those results compared with results from other laboratories. In this way, quality control between laboratories is monitored.

Control Specimens

A QC program for the laboratory makes use of a **control specimen,** a specimen with a known value that is similar in composition to the patient's blood.

A control specimen must be carried through the entire test procedure and treated in exactly the same way as any unknown specimen; it must be affected by all the variables that affect the unknown specimen. Control specimens are used because repeated determinations on the same or different portions (or *aliquots*) of the same sample will not give identical values. Many factors can produce variations in laboratory analyses. With a properly designed control system, it is possible to monitor testing variables.

If the control value in a determination is out of the acceptable range (out of control), one or more of the following factors may be responsible:
1. Deterioration of reagents or standards.
2. Faulty instrument or equipment.
3. Dirty glassware.
4. Lack of attention to timing or incubation temperature.
5. Use of a method not suited to the needs and facilities of the laboratory.
6. Use of poor technique by the technologist doing the test.
7. Statistics: a certain percentage of all determinations will be statistically out of control.

REFERENCE RANGE STATISTICS

In analytical immunology and serology testing using methods such as enzyme immunoassay, quantitative reference range statistics can be used. Statistically, the **reference range** for a particular measurement in most cases is related to a normal, bell-shaped curve (Figure 7-1). This **gaussian curve** has been shown to be correct for virtually all types of biologic, chemical, and physical measurements. A statistically valid series of individuals who are thought to represent a normal, healthy group are measured, and the average value is calculated. This mathematical average is defined as the "mean" ($\overline{X}$, called the "X-bar"). The distribution of all values around the average for the particular

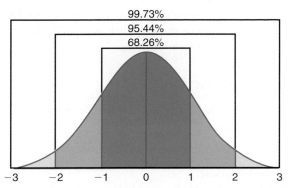

Figure 7-1 Normal distribution curve. *(From Turgeon ML:* Linné and Ringsrud's clinical laboratory science: the basics and routine techniques, *ed 5, St Louis, 2007, Mosby.)*

group measured is described statistically by the standard deviation (SD).

Mean Mathematical average calculated by dividing the sum of all individual values by the number of values.

Median Middle value in a body of data; if all the variables are arranged in order of increasing magnitude, the median is the variable that falls halfway between the highest and lowest variables.

Mode Value that occurs most frequently in a mass of data.

Use of the mean, median, and mode is explained in the following example:

A series of results reported for a laboratory test
on seven different specimens = 7, 2, 3, 6, 5, 4, and 2

The *mean* is the mathematical average and is calculated by taking the sum of the values (29) and dividing by the number of values (7) in the list. The mean is 4.1 (rounded off to 4).

The *median* equals the middle value. To find the median, the list of numbers must first be ranked according to magnitude: 2, 2, 3, 4, 5, 6, 7. There are seven values in the list, and the median is the middle value, 4.

The *mode* is the value most frequently occurring value, or 2 in this example.

The **standard deviation (SD)** is the square root of the variance of the values in any one observation or in a series of test results. In a normal population, 68% of the values will be clustered above and below the average and defined statistically as falling within the "first standard deviation" (±1 SD) (see Figure 8-1). The second standard deviation (±2 SD) represents 95% of the values falling equally above and below the average, and 99.7% is included within the third standard deviation (±3 SD). (Again, variations occur equally above and below the average value [or mean] for any measurement.) Thus, in determining reference values for a particular measurement, a statistically valid series of people are chosen and assumed to represent a healthy population. These people are then tested, and the results are averaged.

The reference range is the range of values that includes 95% of the test results for a healthy reference population. The term replaces "normal values" or "normal range." The limits (or range) of normal are defined in terms of the standard deviation from the average value. Thus, "normal" or "reference" values are stated as a range of values, in terms of SD units.

TESTING OUTCOMES

Before physicians can determine whether a patient has a disease, they must know what is acceptable for a representative population of similar patients (e.g., same age, same gender, same ethnicity), as well as the analytical method used for an assay. Further, an individual may show daily, circadian, physiologic variations.

Biometrics, the science of statistics applied to biologic observations, is a rapidly expanding field that attempts to describe these variations. The selection of a group on whom to base "reference groups" is another problem confronting the individual laboratory. To develop reference values ("normal values"), the proper statistical tools of sampling, selection of the comparison group, and analysis of data must be used by the manufacturer of testing kits or individual laboratories.

Although generally accepted values are published, reference values will vary, especially between laboratories and between geographic locations. Each laboratory must give the physician information concerning the range of reference values for that particular laboratory.

VALIDATING NEW PROCEDURES

The QC program also determines how new procedures are validated before being included as one the methods routinely used by the laboratory. Each laboratory must determine the reproducibility (or confidence limits) for each procedure used and establish acceptable limits of variation for control specimens. The QC program includes calculation of the mean (or average value) and standard deviation and the preparation of control charts for each procedure.

CHAPTER HIGHLIGHTS

- Quality assurance indicators and quality control (QC) are tools to ensure that reported laboratory results are of the highest quality.
- The Clinical Laboratory Improvement Amendments of 1988 (CLIA '88) established a minimum threshold for all aspects of clinical laboratory testing.
- Voluntary QC standards have been set by TJC, COLA, and CAP.
- Nonanalytical factors related to testing accuracy include qualified personnel; established policies; procedure manual; test requisitioning; patient identification, speci-

men procurement, and labeling; preventive maintenance of equipment; appropriate testing methods; and inaccurate results.

- The Institute for Quality Laboratory Medicine has developed measures to evaluate quality in the laboratory based on the phase of testing: preanalytical, analytical, and postanalytical.

- Quality control monitors the accuracy and reproducibility of results through control specimens. *Accuracy* describes how close a test result is to the true value. **Precision** describes how close the test results are to one another when repeated analyses of the same specimen are performed. It is possible to have great precision, but without accuracy if the answer does not represent the actual value tested.

- The precision of a test, its reproducibility, may be expressed as standard deviations (SD) or the derived coefficient of variation (CV), used to compare SDs of two samples. A procedure may be extremely accurate but so difficult that values are not clinically meaningful.

- Assessing sensitivity and specificity of a test involves tests positive, tests negative, disease present (positive), and disease absent (negative). **Sensitivity** is the proportion of subjects with a specific disease or condition who have a positive test result. **Specificity** is the proportion of subjects without the specific disease or condition who have a negative test result.

- Assessing the predictive value (PV) requires knowledge of the sensitivity, specificity, and disease prevalence. **Prevalence** is the proportion of a population who have the disease. **Incidence** is the number of subjects who have the disease within a defined period per 100,000 population.

- Proficiency testing (PT) is incorporated into the CLIA requirements. In addition to internal QC programs, each laboratory should participate in an external PT program to verify laboratory accuracy.

- A control specimen has a known value and is similar in composition to the patient's blood. A control value out of the acceptable range (out of control) may result from deterioration of reagents, faulty equipment, dirty glassware, lack of attention to timing or temperature, use of inappropriate methods, poor technique, and statistical percentage out of control.

- Reference range for a particular measurement is usually a normal bell-shaped curve.

- Mean is the mathematical average of the values. Median is the middle value. Mode is the most frequently occurring value. Standard deviation (SD) is the square root of the variance of the values.

- Reference range is the range of values that includes 95% of the test results for a healthy reference population; formerly "normal values" or "normal range."

- Biometrics attempts to describe statistical variations in biologic observation.

- Each laboratory must determine the reproducibility for each new procedure and establish acceptable limits of variation for control specimens.

REVIEW QUESTIONS

Questions 1 to 3. Match the factors *(a-c)* with the three phases of testing.

1. _____ Preanalytical

2. _____ Analytical

3. _____ Postanalytical

   a. Accuracy in testing.
   b. Patient identification.
   c. Critical value reporting.

Questions 4 to 6. Match the errors with the phase of testing. (An answer may be used more than once.)

4. _____ Blood from the wrong patient.

5. _____ Specimen collected in wrong tube.

6. _____ Quality control outside of acceptable limits.

   a. Preanalytical
   b. Analytical
   c. Postanalytical

Questions 7 to 9. Match the terms with the definitions.

7. _____ Accuracy

8. _____ Control

9. _____ Precision

   a. How close results are to one another when repeatedly analyzed.
   b. Describes how close a test result is to the true value.
   c. Specimen is similar to patient's blood; known concentration of constituent.
   d. Comparison of an instrument measure or reading to a known physical constant.

Questions 10 and 11. Match the terms with the definitions.

10. _____ Sensitivity

11. _____ Specificity

   a. Subjects with specific disease or condition produce a positive result.
   b. Subjects without a specific disease or condition produce a negative result.

Questions 12-16. Indicate the type of error for the following causes of technical errors.

12. _____ Omitting patient serum or reagent from the test mixture.

13. _____ Dirty glassware.

14. _____ Addition of the wrong reagent.

15. _____ Inaccurately recording results.

16. _____ Hemolyzed patient serum.

 a. False-positive error
 b. False-negative error
 c. False-positive or false-negative error

Questions 17-20. Insert the missing elements in the list below, choosing from the following answers:

 a. Quality control
 b. Sources of error
 c. Principle and purpose of the test
 d. Procedural protocol

A written procedural protocol should contain this information in the following order:
 Procedure name
 Name of test method

17. _____
 Specimen collection and storage

18. _____
 Reagents, supplies, and equipment

19. _____
 Expected or normal (reference) values
 Procedural notes

20. _____
 Limitations

BIBLIOGRAPHY

Astion ML, Shojania KG, Hamill TR, et al: Classifying laboratory incident reports to identify problems that jeopardize safety, *Am J Clin Pathol* 120:18-26, 2003.

Burtis CA, Ashwood ER, Bruns DB, editors: *Tietz fundamentals of clinical chemistry,* ed 6, St Louis, 2008, Saunders.

Campbell JB, Campbell JM: *Laboratory mathematics: medical and biological applications,* ed 5, St Louis, 1997, Mosby.

Clinical and Laboratory Standards Institute: *Training and competence assessment: approved guideline,* ed 2, Wayne, Pa, 2004, CLSI Document GP21-A2.

Clinical and Laboratory Standards Institute: *Clinical laboratory technical procedure manual: approved guideline,* ed 4, Wayne, Pa, 2002, CLSI Document GP2-A4.

Lasky FD: Technology variations: strategies for assuring quality results. In Quality control for the future, *Lab Med* 36(10):617-620, 2005.

National Committee for Clinical Laboratory Standards: *Continuous quality improvement: essential management approaches and their use in proficiency testing: approved guideline,* ed 2, Wayne, Pa, 2004, NCCLS Document GP22-A2.

Institute for Medicine (IOM): To err is human, 2005. www.iom.edu.

Turgeon ML: *Linné and Ringsrud's clinical laboratory science: the basics and routine techniques,* ed 5, St Louis, 2007, Mosby.

US Department of Health and Human Services, Centers for Medicare and Medicaid Services, Centers for Disease Control and Prevention: Clinical Laboratory Improvement Amendments (CLIA): equivalent quality control procedures, Brochure #4, 2004.

US Department of Health and Human Services, Centers for Medicare and Medicaid Services: Laboratory requirements relating to quality systems and certain personnel qualifications: amendments, final rule, *Fed Register* 42 CFR 405, 16:3640-3714, 2003.

US Department of Health and Human Services, Health Care Financing Administration: Clinical Laboratory Improvement Amendments of 1988. Medicare, Medicaid, and CLIA Programs. Laboratory requirements relating to quality systems and certain personnel qualifications: final rule, *Fed Register* 42 CFR 493, 2003.

Yost J, Mattingly P: CLIA and equivalent quality control: options for the future. In Quality control for the future, *Lab Med* 36(10):614-616, 2005.

CHAPTER 8

Basic Serologic Laboratory Techniques

Procedures Manual
Blood Specimen Preparation
Types of Specimens Tested
Inactivation of Complement
Pipettes
    Graduated Pipettes
    Serologic Pipettes
    Inspection and Use
Pipetting Techniques
    Manual Pipettes
    Automatic Pipettes

Dilutions
    Diluting Specimens
    Dilution Factor
    Single Dilutions
    Serial Dilutions
Serial Dilutions Exercise
Antibody Testing
    Antibody Titer
Chapter Highlights
Review Questions
Bibliography

Learning Objectives

At the conclusion of this chapter, the reader should be able to:

- Identify and explain the parts of a procedure.
- Describe the preparation of blood specimens for testing.
- Provide examples of the types of specimens that can be tested using immunologic procedures.
- Describe how complement is inactivated in a serum sample.
- Describe the differences between the two types of pipettes typically used in the immunology-serology laboratory.

- Describe and demonstrate pipetting techniques using manual and automatic pipettes.
- Define *dilution*.
- Calculate the concentration of a substance using the dilution factor.
- Calculate the concentration of a single dilution.
- Explain the preparation of a serial dilution.
- Compare the characteristics of the acute and chronic phases of illness.
- Define *antibody titer*.

Serologic testing has long been an important part of diagnostic tests in the clinical laboratory for viral and bacterial diseases. Immunologic testing is done in many areas of the clinical laboratory—microbiology, chemistry, toxicology, immunology, hematology, surgical pathology, cytopathology, immunohematology (blood banking)—and a great variety of specimens are tested. Rapid testing is typically used in the laboratory as well in home-testing kits.

The advent of **monoclonal antibody (MAb)** technology has led to the development of highly specific and sensitive immunoassays. Common serologic and immunologic tests include pregnancy tests for **human gonadotropin hormone (hCG)** and tests for infectious mononucleosis and syphilis.

PROCEDURES MANUAL

The procedures manual must be a complete document of current techniques and approved policies that is available at all times in the immediate bench area of laboratory personnel. It is extremely important that all personnel periodically review this manual. The manual should comply with the Clinical and Laboratory Standards Institute (CLSI, formerly NCCLS) format for a procedures manual (see Box 7-1). The procedural format found in this text generally follows these guidelines.

Alternate techniques can be included with each procedure if more than one technique is acceptable. New pages must be dated and initialed when inserted, and removed pages must be retained for 5 years with the date of removal and the reason for removal indicated. It may be legally necessary to identify the procedure followed for a particular reason.

Procedures used in immunology apply many techniques common to other scientific disciplines such as chemistry. In the field of immunology, many different serologic techniques are used to detect the interaction of antigens with antibodies. These methods are suitable for the detection and quantitation of antibodies to infectious agents, as well as microbial and nonmicrobial antigens (see Part III chapters).

BLOOD SPECIMEN PREPARATION

After blood has been obtained from a patient, it should be allowed to clot, and the serum should be promptly removed for testing. Clotting and clot retraction should take place at room temperature or in the refrigerator, depending on the protocol for the specific procedure. Complete clot retraction normally takes about 1 hour. After clot retraction, the clot should be loosened from the sides of the test tube with an applicator stick and centrifuged for 10 minutes at a moderate speed.

After centrifugation, serum can be transferred to a labeled tube with a Pasteur pipette and rubber bulb. If the serum is contaminated with erythrocytes, it should be recentrifuged. The serum-containing tube should be sealed.

Excessive heat and bacterial contamination are avoided. Heat coagulates the proteins, and bacterial growth alters protein molecules. If the test cannot be performed immediately, the serum should be refrigerated. In most cases, if the testing cannot be done within 72 hours, a serum specimen must be frozen at −20° C. Standard Precautions must be followed when blood specimens are handled.

For some testing, the serum complement must first be inactivated (see following discussion). If the protein complement is not inactivated, it will promote lysis of the red blood cells and other types of cells and can produce invalid results. Complement is also known to interfere with certain tests for syphilis.

TYPES OF SPECIMENS TESTED

The majority of immunology tests are done on serum, although body fluids may also be tested. *Lipemia, hemolysis,* or any bacterial contamination can make the specimen unacceptable. *Icteric* or turbid serum may give valid results for some tests but may interfere with others. Blood specimens should be collected before a meal to avoid the presence of *chyle,* an emulsion of fat globules that often appears in serum after eating, during digestion. Contamination with alkali or acid must be avoided because these substances have a denaturing effect on serum proteins and make the specimens useless for serologic testing.

Other specimens include urine for pregnancy tests and tests for urinary tract infection. It is important that the urine specimen be collected after thorough cleaning of the external genitalia to prevent contamination of microbiologic assays. Urine for the hCG assay (pregnancy test) must be collected at a suitable time interval after fertilization, to allow the concentration of the hCG hormone to rise to a significant detectable level.

Any specimen must be collected into a suitable container to prevent in vitro changes that could affect the assay results. Proper handling and storage of the specimen until testing are essential. Immunologic assays are also done on cerebrospinal fluid (CSF), other body fluids, and swabs of various body exudates and discharges. The established protocol for each specific assay must be followed in terms of specimen collection requirements and conditions for the assay itself.

INACTIVATION OF COMPLEMENT

Some procedures require the use of inactivated serum. *Inactivation* is the process that destroys complement activity. Complement is known to interfere with the reactions of certain syphilis tests and complement components (e.g., C1q). It can agglutinate latex particles and cause a false-positive reaction in latex passive agglutination assays. Complement may also cause lysis of the indicator cells in hemagglutination assays.

Complement in body fluids can be inactivated by heating to 56° C for 30 minutes. When more than 4 hours has elapsed since inactivation, a specimen can be reinactivated by heating it to 56° C for 10 minutes.

PIPETTES

Pipettes are used in the immunology-serology laboratory for the quantitative transfer of reagents and the preparations of serial dilution of specimens such as serum (Figure 8-1). Although semiautomated micropipettes have replaced traditional glass pipettes in the laboratory, traditional methods may still be needed at times.

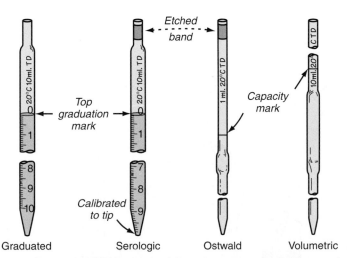

Figure 8-1 **Types of manual pipettes.** *TD,* To deliver. *(From Turgeon ML:* Linné & Ringsrud's clinical laboratory science: the basics and routine techniques, *ed 5, St Louis, 2007, Mosby.)*

Graduated Pipettes

A way to deliver a particular amount of liquid is to deliver the amount of liquid contained between two calibration marks on a cylindrical tube, or pipette. Such a pipette is called a graduated pipette, or measuring pipette. It has several graduation, or calibration, marks. Graduated pipettes are used when great accuracy is not required, although these pipettes should not be used with any less care than volumetric pipettes. Graduated pipettes are used primarily for measuring reagents, but they are not calibrated with sufficient tolerance for measuring standard or control solutions, unknown specimens, or filtrates.

A graduated pipette is a straight piece of glass tubing with a tapered end and graduation marks on the stem separating it into parts. Depending on the size used, graduated pipettes can be used to measure parts of a milliliter or many milliliters. These pipettes come in various sizes, or capacities, including 0.1, 0.2, 1.0, 2.0, 5.0, 10, and 25 mL. If 4 mL of deionized water is to be measured into a test tube, a 5-mL graduated pipette would be the best choice.

Because graduated pipettes require draining between two marks, they introduce one more source of error, compared with the volumetric pipettes, which have only one calibration mark. This makes measurements with the graduated pipette less precise. Because of this relatively poor precision, the graduated pipette is used when speed is more important than precision (e.g., measurement of reagents) and is generally not considered accurate enough for measuring samples and standard solutions.

Serologic Pipettes

Another pipette used in the laboratory, the serologic pipette, looks similar to the graduated pipette. However, the orifice, or tip opening, is larger in the serologic pipette than in other pipettes. The rate of fall of liquid is much too fast for great accuracy or precision.

The serologic pipette is recognized by a frosted ring at the noncalibrated end, with calibrations extending to the tip. The letters TD (to deliver) appear on the pipette, and for quick recognition, each size of pipette has an imprinted, color-coded band that indicates the volume. The serologic pipette is usually allowed to empty by gravity. Depending on the calibration, the remaining drop needs to be expelled to deliver the full volume.

Each serologic pipette is marked with identifying numerals (e.g., 10 mL in $1/10$). The first of these numbers represents the total capacity of the pipette. The second number represents the smallest gradation into which the pipette is divided. In the example cited, therefore, the total pipette volume is 10 mL. Markings then divide it into 1-mL sections, and each mL is further divided into tenths. Sizes of serologic pipettes most frequently used are 10 mL in $1/10$, 5 mL in $1/10$, 2 mL in $1/10$, 2 mL in $1/100$, 1 mL in $1/10$, and 1 mL in $1/100$. For greatest accuracy, the smallest pipette that will hold the desired volume should be used.

Inspection and Use

Before use, glass pipettes should be inspected for broken or chipped ends or contamination. A safety bulb must be used to aspirate liquid into the pipette, as well as to dispense it.
- Aspirate liquid to about 1 inch (2.5 cm) above the top (zero) line of the pipette.
- Raise the pipette vertically to avoid the introduction of air bubbles, and wipe off the exterior surface with a clean gauze or tissue square.
- Working at eye level, slowly lower the liquid so that the meniscus is at zero.

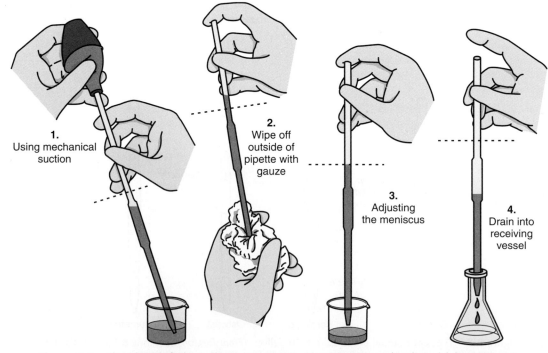

1. Using mechanical suction

2. Wipe off outside of pipette with gauze

3. Adjusting the meniscus

4. Drain into receiving vessel

Figure 8-2   Pipetting technique. *(From Turgeon ML:* Linné & Ringsrud's clinical laboratory science: the basics and routine techniques, *ed 5, St Louis, 2007, Mosby.)*

- Aspirate the contents of the pipette into the appropriate test tube or vessel.
- Wear gloves during pipetting procedures in compliance with Standard Precautions.

PIPETTING TECHNIQUES

Manual Pipettes

It is important to develop through practice a good technique for handling pipettes (Figure 8-2). With few exceptions, the same general steps apply to pipetting with all manual pipettes (Box 8-1).

Laboratory accidents frequently result from improper pipetting techniques. The greatest potential hazard is when mouth pipetting is done instead of mechanical suction. *Mouth pipetting is never acceptable in the clinical laboratory.*

After the pipette has been filled above the top graduation mark, removed from the vessel, and held in a vertical position, the meniscus must be adjusted. The **meniscus** is the curvature in the top surface of a liquid (Figure 8-3). The pipette should be held in such a way that the calibration mark is at eye level. All readings must be made with the eye at the level of the meniscus. The delivery tip is touched to the inside wall of the original vessel, not the liquid, and the meniscus of the liquid in the pipette is eased, or adjusted, down to the calibration mark.

Before the measured liquid in the pipette is allowed to drain into the receiving vessel, any liquid adhering to the

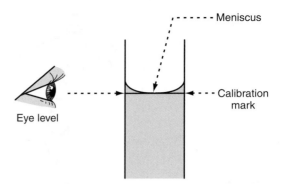

Figure 8-3 Reading the meniscus. *(From Turgeon ML:* Linné & Ringsrud's clinical laboratory science: the basics and routine techniques, *ed 5, St Louis, 2007, Mosby.)*

outside of the pipette must be wiped off with a clean piece of gauze or tissue. If this is not done, any drops present on the outside of the pipette might drain into the receiving vessel along with the measured volume. This would make the volume greater than that specified, and an error would result.

Automatic Pipettes

Automatic pipettes allow fast, repetitive measurement and delivery of solutions of equal volumes. The sampling type measures the substance in question. The sampling-diluting type measures the substance and then adds the desired diluent. The sampling type of automatic pipette is mechanically operated and uses a piston-operated plunger. These are adjustable so that varying amounts of reagent or sample can be delivered with the same device. Disposable and exchangeable tips are available for these pipettes. Automatic pipettes and micropipettors must be calibrated before use.

Micropipettors

Automatic micropipetting devices allow rapid, repetitive measurements and delivery of predetermined volumes of reagents or specimens. The most common type of micropipette used in many laboratories is one that is automatic or semiautomatic, called a micropipettor. These are piston-operated devices that allow repeated, accurate, reproducible delivery of specimens, reagents, and other liquids requiring measurement in small amounts. Many micropipettors are continuously adjustable so that variable volumes of liquids can be dispensed with the same device. Delivery volume is selected by adjusting the settings. Different types or models are available, which allow volume delivery ranging from, for example, 0.5 to 5000 μL. The calibration of these micropipettes should be checked periodically.

The piston, usually in the form of a thumb plunger, is depressed to a stop position on the pipetting device. The tip is placed in the liquid to be measured, and then slowly the plunger is allowed to rise back to the original position (Figure 8-4). This will fill the tip with the desired volume of liquid. The tips are usually drawn along the inside wall of the vessel from which the measured volume is drawn, so that any adhering liquid is removed from the end of the tip. These pipette tips are not usually wiped, as done with the manual pipettes, because the plastic surface is considered

---

Box 8-1	Pipetting with Manual Pipettes

1. Check the pipette to ascertain its correct size, being careful also to check for broken delivery or suction tips.
2. Wearing protective gloves, hold the pipette lightly between the thumb and the last three fingers, leaving the index finger free.
3. Place the tip of the pipette well below the surface of the liquid to be pipetted.
4. Using mechanical suction or an aspirator bulb, carefully draw the liquid up into the pipette until the level of liquid is well above the calibration mark.
5. Quickly cover the suction opening at the top of the pipette with the index finger.
6. Wipe the outside of the pipette dry with a piece of gauze or tissue to remove excess fluid.
7. Hold the pipette in a vertical position with the delivery tip against the inside of the original vessel. Carefully allow the liquid in the pipette to drain by gravity until the bottom of the meniscus is exactly at the calibration mark. To do this, do not entirely remove the index finger from the suction-hole end of the pipette; rather, by rolling the finger slightly over the opening, allow slow drainage to take place.
8. While still holding the pipette in a vertical position, touch the tip of the pipette to the inside wall of the receiving vessel. Remove the index finger from the top of the pipette to permit free drainage. Remember to keep the pipette in a vertical position for correct drainage. In TD (to deliver) pipettes, a small amount of fluid will remain in the delivery tip.
9. To be certain that the drainage is as complete as possible, touch the delivery tip of the pipette to another area on the inside wall of the receiving vessel.

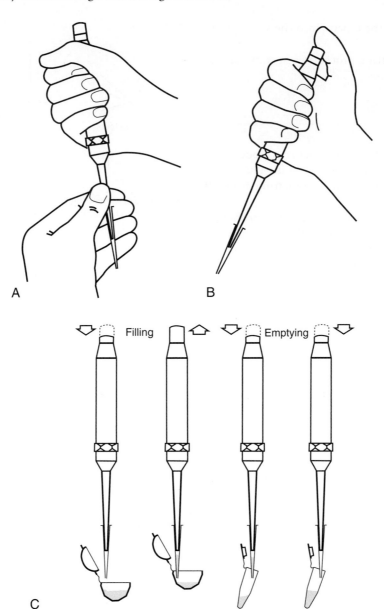

Figure 8-4 **Steps in using piston-type automatic micropipette. A,** Attaching proper tip size for range of pipette volume, and twisting tip as it is pushed onto pipette to give an airtight, continuous seal. **B,** Holding pipette before use. **C,** Follow instructions for filling and emptying pipette tip. *(From Kaplan LA, Pesce A:* Clinical chemistry: theory, analysis, and correlation, *ed 4, St Louis, 2003, Mosby.)*

nonwettable. The tip of the pipette device is then placed against the inside wall of the receiving vessel, and the plunger is depressed. When the manufacturer's directions for the device being used are followed, sample delivery volume is judged to be extremely accurate.

The pipette tips are usually made of disposable plastic, so no cleaning is necessary. Various types of tips are available. Some pipetting devices automatically eject the tip after use. These will also allow the user to insert a new tip as well as remove the used tip without touching it, minimizing infectious biohazard exposures.

The problems encountered with automatic pipetting depend largely on the nature of the solution to be pipetted. Some reagents cause more bubbles than others, and some

are more viscous. Bubbles and viscous solutions can cause problems with measurement and delivery of samples and solutions.

Micropipettors contain or deliver 1 to 500 μL of solution. It is important to follow the individual manufacturer's instructions for the device being used; each may be slightly different. In general, the following steps apply for use of a micropipettor:

1. Attach the proper tip to the pipettor, and set the delivery volume.
2. Depress the piston to a stop position on the pipettor.
3. Place the tip into the solution, and allow the piston to rise back slowly to its original position (this fills the pipettor tip with the desired volume of solution).

4. Some tips are wiped with a dry gauze at this step, and some are not. Follow the manufacturer's directions.
5. Place the tip on the wall of the receiving vessel and depress the piston, first to a stop position where the liquid is allowed to drain, and then to a second stop position where the full dispensing of the liquid takes place.
6. Dispose of the tip in the waste disposal receptacle. Some pipettors automatically eject the used tips, minimizing biohazard exposure.

Automatic Dispensers or Syringes

Many types of automatic dispensers or syringes are used in the laboratory for repetitive adding of multiple doses of the same reagent or diluent. These devices are used for measuring serial amounts of relatively small volumes of the same liquid. The volume to be dispensed is determined by the pipettor setting. Dispensers are available with a variety of volume settings. Some are available as syringes and others as bottle-top devices. Most of these dispensers can be cleaned by autoclaving.

Diluter-Dispensers

In automated instruments, diluter-dispensers are used to prepare a number of different samples for analysis. These devices pipette a selected aliquot of sample and diluent into the instrument or receiving vessel. These devices are primarily of the dual-piston type, with one used for the sample and the other for the diluent or reagent.

DILUTIONS

It is often necessary to make dilutions of specimens being analyzed or to make weaker solutions from stronger solutions in various laboratory procedures. Clinicians must be able to work with various dilution problems and dilution factors. They often need determine the concentration of antibody in each solution, the actual amount of material in each solution, and the total volume of each solution. All dilutions are a form of ratio. **Dilution** is an indication of relative concentration.

Diluting Specimens

In most laboratory determinations, a small sample is taken for analysis, and the final result is expressed as concentration per some convenient standard volume. In a certain procedure, 0.5 mL of blood is diluted to a total of 10 mL with various reagents, and 1 mL of this dilution is then analyzed for a particular chemical constituent. The final result is to be expressed in terms of the concentration of that substance per 100 mL of blood.

Dilution Factor

A dilution factor is used to correct for having used a diluted sample in a determination rather than the undiluted sample. The result (answer) using the dilution must be multiplied by the reciprocal of the dilution made. For example, a dilution factor by which all determination answers are

multiplied to give the concentration per 100 mL of sample (blood) may be calculated as follows.

First, determine the volume of blood that is actually analyzed in the procedure. By use of a simple proportion, it is evident that 0.5 mL of blood diluted to 10 mL is equivalent to 1 mL of blood diluted to 20 mL:

$$\frac{0.5\ mL\ blood}{10\ mL\ solution} = \frac{1\ mL\ blood}{x\ mL\ solution}$$

$$x = \frac{1\ mL\ blood \times 10\ mL}{0.5\ mL} = 20\ mL$$

The concentration of specimen (blood) in each milliliter of solution may be determined, by the use of another simple proportion, to be 0.05 mL of blood per milliliter of solution:

$$\frac{1\ mL\ blood}{20\ mL\ solution} = \frac{x\ mL\ blood}{1\ mL\ solution}$$

$$x = \frac{1\ mL \times 1\ mL}{20\ mL} = 0.05\ mL$$

Because 1 mL of the 1:20 dilution of blood is analyzed in the remaining steps of the procedure, 0.05 mL of blood is actually analyzed (1 mL of the dilution used × 0.05 mL/mL = 0.05 mL of blood analyzed).

To relate the concentration of the substance measured in the procedure to the concentration in 100 mL of blood (the units in which the result is to be expressed), another proportion may be used:

$$\frac{\begin{array}{c}100\ mL\\ (volume\ of\ blood\ desired)\\ \hline 0.05\ mL\\ (volume\ of\ blood\ used)\end{array}} = \frac{Concentration\ desired}{\begin{array}{c}Concentration\ used\\ or\ determined\end{array}}$$

$$Concentration\ desired = \frac{100\ mL \times Concentration\ determined}{0.05\ mL}$$

$$Concentration\ desired = 2000 \times Value\ determined$$

The concentration of the substance being measured in the volume of blood actually tested (0.05 mL) must be multiplied by 2000 in order to report the concentration per 100 mL of blood.

The preceding material may be summarized by the following statement and equations. In reporting results obtained from laboratory determinations, one must first determine the amount of specimen actually analyzed in the procedure and then calculate the factor that will express the concentration in the desired terms of measurement. Thus, in the previous example, the following equations may be used:

$$\frac{\begin{array}{c}0.5\ mL\\ (volume\ of\ blood\ used)\\ \hline 10\ mL\\ (volume\ of\ total\ dilution)\end{array}} = \frac{\begin{array}{c}x\ mL\\ (volume\ of\ blood\ analyzed)\\ \hline 1\ mL\\ (volume\ of\ dilution\ used)\end{array}}$$

$$x = 0.05\ mL\ (volume\ of\ blood\ actually\ analyzed)$$

$$\frac{100 \text{ mL (volume of blood required for expression of result)}}{0.05 \text{ mL (volume of blood actually analyzed)}} = 2000 \text{ (dilution factor)}$$

Single Dilutions

When the concentration of a particular substance in a specimen is too great to be accurately determined, or when there is less specimen available for analysis than the procedure requires, it may be necessary to dilute the original specimen, or further dilute the initial dilution (or filtrate). Such *single dilutions* are usually expressed as a ratio, such as 1:2, 1:5, or 1:10, or as a fraction, ½, ⅕, or ¹⁄₁₀. These ratios or fractions refer to 1 unit of the original specimen diluted to a final volume of 2, 5, or 10 units, respectively. A dilution therefore refers to the volume or number of parts of the substance to be diluted in the total volume, or parts, of the final solution. A dilution is an expression of concentration, not volume; it indicates the relative amount of substance in solution. Dilutions can be made singly or in series.

To calculate the concentration of a single dilution, multiply the original concentration by the dilution expressed as a fraction.

Calculation of Concentration of a Single Dilution

A specimen contains 500 mg of substance per deciliter of blood. A 1:5 dilution of this specimen is prepared by volumetrically measuring 1 mL of the specimen and adding 4 mL of diluent. The concentration of substance in the dilution is:

$$500 \text{ mg/dL} \times ⅕ \times 100 \text{ mg/dL}$$

Note that the concentration of the final solution (or dilution) is expressed in the same units as that of the original solution.

To obtain a dilution factor that can be applied to the determination answer and express it as a concentration per standard volume, proceed as follows. Rather than multiply by the dilution expressed as a fraction, multiply the determination value by the reciprocal of the dilution fraction. In the case of a 1:5 dilution, the dilution factor applied to values obtained in the procedure would be 5, because the original specimen was five times more concentrated than the diluted specimen tested in the procedure.

Use of Dilution Factors

A 1:5 dilution of a specimen is prepared, and an **aliquot** (one of a number of equal parts) of the dilution is analyzed for a particular substance. The concentration of the substance in the aliquot is multiplied by 5 to determine its concentration in the original specimen. If the concentration of the dilution is 100 mg/dL, the concentration of the original specimen is:

$$100 \text{ mg/dL} \times 5 \text{ (dilution factor)} = 500 \text{ mg/dL in blood}$$

Serial Dilutions

Dilutions can also be made in series, in which the original solution is further diluted. A general rule for calculating the concentrations of solutions obtained by dilution in series is to multiply the original concentration by the first dilution (expressed as a fraction), this by the second dilution, and so on, until the desired concentration is known.

Several laboratory procedures, especially serologic methods, make use of a dilution series in which all dilutions, including or following the first one, are the same. Such dilutions are referred to as **serial dilutions** (Table 8-1). A complete dilution series usually contains five or ten tubes, although any single dilution may be made directly from an undiluted specimen or substance. In calculating the dilution or concentration of a substance or serum in each tube of the dilution series, the rules previously discussed apply.

A five-tube twofold dilution may be prepared as follows (Figure 8-5): A serum specimen is diluted 1:2 with buffer. A series of five tubes are prepared, in which each succeeding tube is rediluted 1:2. This is accomplished by placing 1 mL of diluent into each of four tubes (tubes 2 to 5). Tube 1 contains 1 mL of undiluted serum. Tube 2 contains 1 mL of undiluted serum plus 1 mL of diluent, resulting in a 1:2 dilution of serum. A 1-mL portion of the 1:2 dilution of serum is placed in tube 3, resulting in a 1:4 dilution of serum (½ × ½ × ¼). A 1-mL portion of the 1:4 dilution from tube 3 is placed in tube 4, resulting in a 1:8 dilution (¼ × ½ × ⅛). Finally, 1 mL of the 1:8 dilution from tube 4 is added to tube 5, resulting in a 1:16 dilution (⅛ × ½ × ¹⁄₁₆). One milliliter of the final dilution is discarded so that the volumes in all the tubes are equal.

Note that each tube is diluted twice as much as the previous tube, and that the final volume in each tube is the same. The undiluted serum may also be given a dilution value, 1:1.

The concentration of serum in terms of milliliters in each tube is calculated by multiplying the previous concentration (mL) by the succeeding dilution. In this example, tube 1 contains 1 mL of serum, tube 2 contains 1 mL × ½ × 0.5 mL of serum, and tubes 3 to 5 contain 0.25, 0.125, and 0.06 mL of serum, respectively.

Table 8-1	Example of Preparation of a Serial Dilution									
Tube	1	2	3	4	5	6	7	8	9	10
Saline (mL)	1	1	1	1	1	1	1	1	1	1
Patient serum or preceding dilution (mL)	1	1 of 1:2	1 of 1:4	1 of 1:8	1 of 1:16	1 of 1:32	1 of 1:64	1 of 1:128	1 of 1:256	1 of 1:512
Final dilution	1:2	1:4	1:8	1:16	1:32	1:64	1:128	1:256	1:512	1:1024

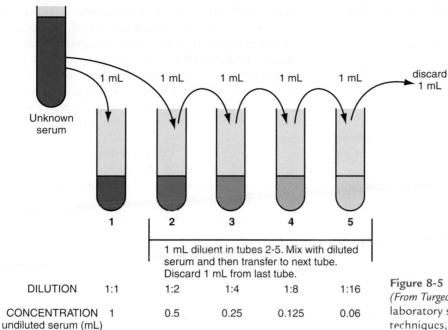

DILUTION	1:1	1:2	1:4	1:8	1:16
CONCENTRATION undiluted serum (mL)	1	0.5	0.25	0.125	0.06

Figure 8-5   Five-tube twofold dilution. *(From Turgeon ML:* Linné & Ringsrud's clinical laboratory science: the basics and routine techniques, *ed 5, St Louis, 2007, Mosby.)*

Other serial dilutions might be fivefold or tenfold; that is, each succeeding tube is diluted five or ten times. A fivefold series would begin with 1 mL of serum in 4 mL of diluent and a total volume of 5 mL in each tube. A tenfold series would begin with 1 mL of serum in 9 mL of diluent and a total volume of 10 mL in each tube. Other systems might begin with a 1:2 dilution and then dilute five succeeding tubes 1:10. The dilutions in such a series would be 1:2, 1:20 ($\frac{1}{2} \times \frac{1}{10} \times \frac{1}{20}$), 1:200 ($\frac{1}{20} \times \frac{1}{10} \times \frac{1}{200}$), 1:2000, 1:20,000, and 1:200,000.

Serial Dilutions Exercise

Principle

Serial dilutions are a method for determining the concentration of a substance (e.g., antibody). The greatest dilution of the sample that yields a positive result is the *end point.* This end point dilution can be expressed as a fraction. The reciprocal of that fraction is called the *titer* of the antibody.

A series of dilutions of a sample is necessary for determining an antibody titer. In serial dilution, each dilution is prepared from the previous dilution. Dilutions can be in large test tubes, macrotitration, or in a miniaturized version, microtitration.

Microtitration is valuable for any procedure in which dilutions are made and red blood cells (RBCs) are used as indicator cells (e.g., hemagglutination). Colorimetric reactions can be performed (e.g., enzyme immunoassay) and quantitated spectrophotometrically with specialized instruments for microtiter plates.

Sample

Anti-A antisera (this reagent contains either human serum or MAb and a blue dye, pontamine sky-blue)

Reagents, Supplies, and Equipment

- Type A RBCs (commercially available or prepared as 4% solution)
- 0.9% (isotonic) saline
- Serologic pipettes, 1 mL
- Aspirator bulb for pipettes
- Test tubes, 12 × 75 mm
- Parafilm or stoppers
- Centrifuge

Procedure

1. Prepared a 1:10 dilution of anti-A antisera by adding 1 mL of anti-A to 9 mL of saline.
2. If commercially prepared cells are not used, prepare a 4% solution of RBCs.
   a. Centrifuge a specimen of blood freshly collected in EDTA at 1500 rpm for 10 minutes.
   b. Remove the plasma, and replace with isotonic saline.
   c. Transfer the solution to a conical centrifuge tube with graduated marks.
   d. Centrifuge again for 10 minutes.
   e. Remove the saline layer, and replace an equivalent amount of isotonic saline.
   f. Repeat this process until the saline on top (supernatant) is clear.
   g. Prepare a 4% solution by suspending 4 mL of packed RBCs in 96 mL of isotonic saline.
   Approximately 4 mL of the final suspension is necessary for this practice exercise.
3. Label eight 12 × 75–mm test tubes as: (1) 10, (2) 20, (3) 40, (4) 80, (5) 160, (6) 320, (7) 640, and (8) 1280. The numbers 10 to 1280 represent the dilution in each tube.

4. Using a 1-mL serologic pipette, add 0.25 mL of isotonic saline to tubes 2 through 8.
5. Add 0.25 mL of anti-A antiserum to tubes and 1 and 2, using a clean serologic pipette.
6. Mix tube 2 by gently drawing the fluid up and down 10 times.
7. Transfer 0.25mL from tube 2 to tube 3, and mix with a pipette.
8. Repeat step 7, transferring and mixing up to tube 8. Discard the last 0.25 mL of the dilution from tube 8.
9. Using a 1-mL serologic pipette, add 0.25 mL of the 4% type A RBCs to each tube. Mix gently by covering each tube and inverting it several times.
10. Centrifuge for 1 minute at 1500 rpm.
11. Observe for agglutination (clumping of RBCs) by gently shaking the red cell button off the bottom of the tube.
12. Observe. With a positive reaction, RBCs remain agglutinated. The size of the clumps decreases, but any visible clumping is a positive reaction. A negative reaction (end point) is no agglutination of RBCs.
13. Record the results. The titer is the last tube in which visible agglutination can be observed. The titer is the reciprocal of the highest dilution. If tube 6 with a 1:320 dilution is the last positive tube, the end point dilution as a fraction is 1:320 and the titer, 320.

Interpretation of Results

In clinical immunology the titer of an antibody in an individual's serum can have clinical significance depending on the antibody in question. Antibody titers are sometimes used to evaluate a person's immune status. Titers may be obtained over time, as with acute and convalescent specimens for infectious diseases or monitoring of a mother's titer for blood group antibodies during pregnancy.

ANTIBODY TESTING

In obtaining specimens for serologic testing, it is important to consider the phase of the disease and the condition of the patient at the time of specimen collection. This is especially important in assays for diagnosis of infectious diseases. If serum is being tested for antibody levels with a specific infectious organism, generally the blood should be drawn during the **acute phase** of the illness—when the disease is first discovered or suspected—and another sample drawn during the **convalescent phase,** usually about 2 weeks later. Accordingly, these samples are called "acute" and "convalescent" serum. A difference in the amount of antibody present, or the antibody titer, may be noted when the two different samples are tested concurrently. Some infections, such as legionnaires' disease or hepatitis, may not manifest a rise in titer until months after the acute infection.

Antibody Titer

A central concept of serologic testing is the manifestation of a rise in *titer,* or concentration, of an antibody. The antibody **titer** is defined as the reciprocal of the highest dilution of the patient's serum in which the antibody is still detectable. That is, the titer is read at the highest dilution of serum that gives a positive reaction with the antigen. If a serum sample has been diluted 1:64 and reacts positively with the antigen suspension used in the testing process, and if the next highest dilution of 1:128 does not give a positive reaction, the titer is read as 64. A "high titer" indicates that there is a relatively high concentration of the antibody present in the serum.

Determination of the concentration of antibody (titer) for a specific antigen involves the following two steps:
1. Preparing a serial dilution of the antibody-containing solution (e.g., serum).
2. Adding an equal volume of antigen suspension to each dilution.

A high titer indicates that a considerable amount of antibody is present in the serum. For most pathogenic infections, an increase in the patient's titer of two doubling dilutions, or from a positive result of 1:8 to a positive result of 1:32 over several weeks, is an indication of a current infection. This is known as a "fourfold rise" in the antibody titer.

CHAPTER HIGHLIGHTS

- Traditional serologic tests have been done for viral and bacterial diseases. Other common tests include pregnancy tests for human gonadotropin hormone (hCG) and immunologic tests for infectious mononucleosis and syphilis.
- The procedures manual describes current techniques (in CLSI format) and approved policies and is always available to laboratory personnel.
- After a blood sample has clotted, serum should be promptly removed for testing or frozen at −20° C. Standard Precautions must be followed when blood specimens are handled.
- Lipemia, hemolysis, and bacterial contamination can make the specimen unacceptable. Icteric or turbid serum may give valid results or may interfere. Blood specimens should be collected before a meal to avoid chyle. Contamination with alkali or acid must be avoided.
- Some procedures require inactivated serum. Complement can be inactivated by heating to 56° C for 30 minutes, or after 4 hours, reinactivated by heating for 10 minutes.
- A graduated pipette delivers the liquid between two calibration marks. A serologic pipette resembles the graduated pipette, but has a frosted ring and enlarged tip opening.
- Automatic pipettes allow fast, repetitive measurement and delivery of solutions of equal volumes.
- All dilutions are a ratio. Dilution is an indication of relative concentration.
- A dilution factor is used to correct for having used a diluted sample in a determination rather than the undi-

luted sample. The result (answer) using the dilution must be multiplied by the reciprocal of the dilution made.

- When concentration is too great or less specimen is available for analysis, the original specimen may be diluted, or the initial dilution (or filtrate) further diluted. These single dilutions are usually expressed as a ratio (1:2, 1:5, 1:10) or as a fraction (½, ⅕, ¹⁄₁₀).
- A dilution is the volume or number of parts of the substance to be diluted in the total volume, or parts, of the final solution. A dilution is an expression of concentration, the relative amount of substance in solution. Dilutions can be made singly or in series.
- In a dilution series, all dilutions, including or following the first one, are the same, called serial dilutions.
- A complete dilution series usually contains five or ten tubes, although any single dilution may be made directly from an undiluted specimen or substance.
- When testing antibody levels for a specific infectious organism, blood should be drawn during both the acute phase and the convalescent phase.
- A difference in the amount of antibody present, or the antibody titer, may be noted when two different samples are tested concurrently. A rise in titer is central to serologic testing.
- The antibody *titer* is defined as the reciprocal of the highest dilution of the patient's serum in which the antibody is still detectable.

REVIEW QUESTIONS

1. A written procedural protocol should contain the following information in this order: _____, _____, _____, _____ (choose from *a-d*).
   a. Specimen collection and storage
   b. Reference values
   c. Reagents, supplies, and equipment
   d. Procedural method

   a. A, B, C, D
   b. B, C, A, D
   c. A, C, D, B
   d. None of the above

2. Factors that can denature, coagulate, or alter protein molecules include:
   a. Heat.
   b. Strong acid solution.
   c. Strong alkali solution.
   d. All the above.

3. If testing cannot be done within _____ hours of collection, a serum specimen should be frozen at −20° C.
   a. 24
   b. 48
   c. 72
   d. 96

4. Complement can be inactivated in human serum by heating to _____° C.
   a. 25
   b. 37
   c. 45
   d. 56

5. A specimen should be reinactivated when more than _____ hour(s) has/have elapsed since inactivation.
   a. 1
   b. 2
   c. 4
   d. 8

6. A graduated pipette can be used when:
   a. Extreme accuracy is not needed.
   b. Very precise accuracy is needed.
   c. Precision is more important than speed.
   d. Speed is more important than precision.

7. A meniscus is the:
   a. Curvature in the top surface of a liquid.
   b. Zero mark on a pipette.
   c. Last marking on a serologic pipette.
   d. Flat line of liquid in a pipette.

8. Automatic pipettes have the advantage of:
   a. Being fast.
   b. Allowing repetitive measurement of solutions.
   c. Delivering equal volumes of solutions.
   d. All the above.

9. A dilution is a(n):
   a. Ratio of volume or number of parts of the substance to be diluted in the total volume, or parts, of the final solution.
   b. Indication of relative concentration.
   c. Frequently used measure in serologic testing.
   d. All the above.

10. If a serial dilution is prepared in 1:2 dilutions, the final dilution in tube 6 is:
    a. 1:25
    b. 1:32
    c. 1:64
    d. 1:256

Questions 11 and 12. To dilute a serum specimen 1:10,

11. _____ part of serum is needed.
    a. 1
    b. 1
    c. 0.5
    d. 0.2

and

12. _____ parts of distilled water to reach the total volume is needed.
    a. 10
    b. 9
    c. 4.5
    d. 0.1

13. Serum for detection of antibodies should be drawn during the:
    a. Acute phase of illness only.
    b. Acute and convalescent phases of illness.
    c. Convalescent phase of illness only.
    d. Acute and convalescent phases, as well as 6 months after an illness.

14. A central concept of serologic testing is:
    a. Antigen-antibody interaction.
    b. Determination of antibody composition.
    c. Quantitation of antigen titer.
    d. Manifestation of a rise in antibody titer.

BIBLIOGRAPHY

Campbell JM, Campbell JB: *Laboratory mathematics: medical and biological applications,* ed 5, St Louis, 1997, Mosby.

Bishop ML, Fody EP, Schoeff L: *Clinical chemistry: principles, procedures, correlations,* ed 5, Philadelphia, 2005, Lippincott–Williams & Wilkins.

Burtis CA, Ashwood ER, Bruns DB, editors: *Tietz fundamentals of clinical chemistry,* ed 6, St Louis, 2008, Saunders.

Kaplan LA, Pesce AJ, Kazmiercazk SC: *Clinical chemistry: theory, analysis, correlation,* ed 4, St Louis, 2003, Mosby.

Turgeon M.L.: *Linné & Ringsrud's clinical laboratory science: the basics and routine techniques,* ed 5, St Louis, 2007, Mosby.

CHAPTER 9

Point-of-Care Testing

Testing Categories
Quality Control Standards
Non–Instrument-Based Testing
Card Pregnancy Test

Chapter Highlights
Review Questions
Bibliography

Point-of-care testing (POCT) is defined as laboratory assays performed near the patient. Development of new POCT assays is increasing at a rapid rate. POCT testing can include home test kits and handheld monitors. The major advantage is the speed of obtaining the results. The major drawback is cost, particularly if a large volume of testing is done. Other areas of concern include maintenance of quality control (QC) and quality assurance (QA).

TESTING CATEGORIES

Diagnostic testing that is not performed within a traditional laboratory is called "waived testing" by The Joint Commission (TJC, formerly JCAHO). The Clinical Laboratory Improvement Acts of 1988 (CLIA '88) subjects all clinical laboratory testing to federal regulation and inspection. According to CLIA '88, test procedures are grouped into one of four following categories:
1. Waived tests. Simple procedures with little chance of negative outcomes if performed inaccurately.
2. Moderately complex tests. More complex than waived tests but usually automated (e.g., enzyme immunoassays).
3. Highly complex tests. Usually nonautomated or complicated tests requiring considerable judgment (e.g., serum protein electrophoresis).
4. Provider-performed microscopy tests. Slide examinations of freshly collected body fluids.

Test complexity is determined by criteria that assess knowledge, training, reagent and material preparation, operational technique, QC/QA characteristics, maintenance and troubleshooting, and interpretation and judgment. Any over-the-counter test approved by the U.S. Food and Drug Administration (FDA) is automatically placed into the "waived" category. POCT falls within the "waived" or "moderately complex" category.

QUALITY CONTROL STANDARDS

All laboratory testing must meet the same quality standards regardless of where it is performed. State and city governments may enact mandatory regulations, including qualifications of personnel performing the test, which may be more (but not less) stringent than federal regulations. Voluntary participation in QA programs is also available.

The Centers for Disease Control and Prevention (www.cdc.gov) invites providers to participate in a new performance evaluation program (HIV Rapid Testing MPEP) that offers external evaluation of rapid tests for human immunodeficiency virus (e.g., OraQuick Rapid HIV-1 Antibody Test) and other licensed tests (e.g., MedMira Reveal Rapid HIV-1 Test).

Ultimate responsibility and control of POCT reside within the CLIA-certified laboratory and require a minimum of one laboratory staff member to be responsible for each POCT program.

Written policies and procedures must be available to all laboratory personnel for patient preparation, specimen collection and preservation, instrument calibration, policies for QC and remedial actions, equipment performance evaluations, procedures for test performance, result report, and recording. The greatest source of error is preanalytical error, such as patient identification and specimen collection.

NON–INSTRUMENT-BASED TESTING

In immunology and serology testing, most POCT testing is done by manual rapid test methods, such as pregnancy testing. More rapid tests are being developed for the identification of infectious organisms, such as group A streptococci and HIV, in emergency rooms, in hospital settings, and even at home.

Card Pregnancy Test*

Principle

The OSOM Card Pregnancy Test (Genzyme Diagnostics; Figure 9-1) is a solid phase, sandwich-format immunochromatographic assay for the qualitative detection of human chorionic gonadotropin (hCG).

Urine is added to the sample well, and the sample migrates through reaction pads, where hCG, if present in the sample, binds to a monoclonal anti-hCG dye conjugate. The sample then migrates across a membrane toward the "results window," where the labeled hCG complex is captured at a test line region containing immobilized rabbit anti-hCG. Excess conjugate will flow past the test line region and

---

*Modified from product directional insert for Genzyme Diagnostics OSOM Card Pregnancy Test.

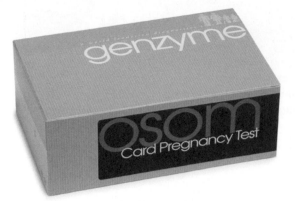

Figure 9-1   Pregnancy test kit, an example of POCT. *(From Turgeon ML:* Linné & Ringsrud's clinical laboratory science, *ed 5, St Louis, 2007, Mosby.)*

will be captured at a control line region containing an immobilized antibody directed against the anti-hCG dye conjugate (with or without hCG complexed to it).

The appearance of two black bands in the results window, one at "T: Test" and the other at "C: Control," indicates the presence of hCG in the sample. If a detectable level of hCG is not present, only the control band will appear in the results window.

Specimen

No filtration or centrifugation of urine specimens is required for testing with the OSOM Card Pregnancy Test. Urine specimens may be collected in any clean, dry, plastic or glass container. For early determination of pregnancy, the first morning specimen of urine is recommended because it usually contains the highest concentration of hCG.

Urine specimens may be stored at room temperature (15°-30° C) for up to 8 hours, or refrigerated (2°-8° C) for up to 72 hours. If specimen has been stored refrigerated, allow it to warm to room temperature before use.

Reagents, Supplies, and Equipment

Kit Contents
- OSOM Card Pregnancy Test devices are individually pouched, each containing a disposable pipette.
1. Store at room temperature, 15° to 30° C (59°-86° F), out of direct sunlight.
2. Do not remove the test device from the pouch until needed. Test devices are stable in the unopened foil pouches until the expiration date printed on the kit or foil pouch.
3. *Note:* The lot numbers may be different on the foil pouch and the kit.
4. Dispose of all used test devices, pipettes, and specimens in suitable biohazard waste containers.
5. Several tests can be run at the same time. Use a new pipette with each test to avoid contamination errors.
6. *Do not freeze.*

Materials Required But Not Provided
- Clock or timer
- Sample collection cups or tubes
- Positive and negative controls

Quality Control and Quality Assurance

Quality control requirements should be established in accordance with local, state, and federal regulations or accreditation requirements.

Internal Quality Control

Several controls are incorporated into each OSOM Card Pregnancy Test for routine QC checks. It is recommended that these procedural controls be documented for each sample as part of daily quality control.

The same labeled conjugate antibody results in the appearance of both the test and the control bands. The appearance of the control band in the results window is an internal positive procedural control that validates the following:
- Test system. Ensures that the detection component of both the test line and the control line is intact, that adequate volume was added, and that adequate capillary migration of the sample has occurred; also verifies proper assembly of the test device.
- Indicates that an adequate volume of fluid was added to the sample well for capillary migration to occur. If the control band does not appear at the read time, the test is invalid. Appearance of the control band should be documented as part of the daily quality control.
- The clearing of the background in the results area may be documented as a "negative" procedural control. It also serves as an additional capillary flow control. At the read time, the background should appear white to light gray and should not interfere with the reading of the test. The test is invalid if the background fails to clear and obscures the formation of a distinct control band.
- If the control band fails to appear with a repeat assay, do not report patient results. If the control band does not appear when running the test, the test cassette or kit may have been stored or handled improperly, or the foil pouch may not have been intact.

External Quality Control

The manufacturer recommends that external hCG controls be run with each new lot and with each new untrained operator. A commercial control, OSOM hCG Urine Control, is designed for this purpose.

Procedure

1. Patient specimens and control material must be brought to room temperature (15°-30° C; 59°-86° F) before testing.
2. Remove the test device and pipette from the pouch. Place the device on a flat surface.

3. Squeeze the bulb of the pipette, and insert the barrel into the patient sample. Release the bulb, and draw up enough sample to fill the barrel to the line indicated on the pipette. *Do not overfill.*
4. Expel the entire contents of the barrel (135 μL) into the sample well of the test device. No drop counting is required.
5. Discard the pipette in a suitable biohazard waste container.
6. Read the results at 3 minutes. Results are invalid after the stated read time. The use of a timer is recommended.

Reporting Results

Positive
Two separate black or gray bands, one at "T: Test" and the other at "C: Control," are visible in the results window, indicating that the specimen contains detectable levels of hCG. Although the intensity of the test band may vary with different specimens, the appearance of two distinct bands should be interpreted as a "positive" result.

Negative
If no band appears at "T" and a black or gray band is visible at the "C" position, the test can be considered "negative," indicating that a detectable level of hCG is not present.

Invalid
If no band appears at "C" or incomplete or beaded bands appear at either the "T" or the "C" position, the test is invalid. The test should be repeated using another OSOM Card Pregnancy Test device.

Note: The test is valid if the control line appears by the stated read time, regardless of whether the sample has migrated all the way to the end of the sample window.

Clinical Applications
Human CG is not normally detected in the urine specimens of healthy men and nonpregnant women.

In normal pregnancy, 20 mIU/mL hCG is reported to be present in urine 2 to 3 days before the first missed menstrual period. The levels of hCG continue to increase up to 200,000 mIU/mL at the end of the first trimester.

Limitations
• This assay is capable of detecting only whole-molecule (intact) hCG. It cannot detect the presence of free hCG subunits. Therefore, this test should only be used for the qualitative detection of hCG in urine for the early determination of pregnancy.
• For diagnostic purposes, hCG test results should always be used with other methods and in the context of the patient's clinical information (e.g., medical history, symptoms, results of other tests, clinical impression). Ectopic pregnancy cannot be distinguished from normal pregnancy by hCG measurements alone.

• If the hCG level is inconsistent with or unsupported by clinical evidence, results should also be confirmed by an alternative hCG method. Test results should be confirmed using a quantitative hCG assay before any critical medical procedure.
• Interfering substances may falsely depress or falsely elevate results. These interfering substances may cause false results over the entire range of the assay, not only at low levels, and may indicate the presence of hCG when there is none. As with any immunochemical reaction, unknown interferences from medications or endogenous substances may affect results.
• Infrequently, hCG levels may appear consistently elevated and could be caused by, but are not limited to, the following:

   Trophoblastic or nontrophoblastic neoplasms. These abnormal physiologic states may falsely elevate hCG levels and should not be diagnosed with this test.
   Human CG–like substances.

• Because of the high degree of sensitivity of the assay, specimens tested as "positive" during the initial days after conception may later be "negative" because of natural termination of the pregnancy.
• Overall, natural termination occurs in 22% of clinically unrecognized pregnancies and 31% of other pregnancies. In the presence of weakly positive results, it is good laboratory practice to sample and test again after 48 hours.
• If the test band appears very faint, it is recommended that a new sample be collected 48 hours later and tested using another OSOM Card Pregnancy Test device.
• Dilute urine specimens may not have representative levels of hCG.
• Detection of very low levels of hCG does not rule out pregnancy; low levels of hCG can occur in apparently healthy, nonpregnant subjects. Additionally, postmenopausal specimens may elicit weak positive results because of low hCG levels unrelated to pregnancy. In a normal pregnancy, hCG values double approximately every 48 hours. Patients with very low levels of hCG should be sampled and tested again after 48 hours, or tested with an alternative method.
• Some antipsychotic drugs are known to cause false-positive results in pregnancy tests.

Cross-Reactivity
The addition of luteinizing hormone (300 mIU/mL of LH), follicle-stimulating hormone (1000 mIU/mL of FSH), or thyroid-stimulating hormone (1000 μIU/mL of TSH) to negative urine serum specimens gives negative results in the OSOM Card Pregnancy Test.

The following substances were added to urine specimens containing 0 or 20 mIU/mL hCG. The substances at the concentrations listed below were not found to affect the performance of the test.

Interfering Substance	Concentration
Acetaminophen	20 mg/dL
Acetoacetic acid	2000 mg/dL
Acetylsalicylic acid	20 mg/dL
Amitriptyline	100 mg/dL
Amphetamines	10 µg/mL
Ascorbic acid	20 mg/dL
Atropine	20 mg/dL
Benzoylecgonine	10 mg/dL
Bilirubin	2 mg/dL
Caffeine	20 mg/dL
Cannabinol	10 mg/dL
Chlorpromazine	5 mg/dL
Codeine	10 mg/dL
Desipramine	20 mg/dL
Diazepam	2 mg/dL
Ephedrine	20 mg/dL
Estradiol	25 ng/mL
Estriol	1 mg/dL
Ethanol	200 mg/dL
Gentisic acid	20 mg/dL
Glucose	2000 mg/dL
Hemoglobin	250 mg/dL
Human albumin	2000 mg/dL
β-Hydroxybutyrate	2000 mg/dL
Ibuprofen	40 mg/dL
Imipramine	100 mg/dL
Lithium	3.5 mg/dL
Methadone	10 mg/dL
Mezoridazine	1 mg/dL
Morphine	6 µg/mL
Nortriptyline	100 mg/dL
Phenobarbital	15 mg/dL
Phenylpropanolamine	20 mg/dL
Pregnanediol	1500 µg/dL
Progesterone	40 ng/mL
Proteins	2000 mg/dL
Salicylic acid	20 mg/dL
Tetracycline	20 mg/dL
Thioridazine	2 mg/dL

Reference

OSOM Card Pregnancy Test, Genzyme Diagnostics, December 2007.

CHAPTER HIGHLIGHTS

- Point-of-care testing (POCT) involves laboratory assays performed near the patient and includes home test kits and handheld monitors.
- The major advantage of POCT is speed; the major drawback is cost.
- Testing can be divided into waived, moderately complex, highly complex, and provider-performed microscopy tests. POCT is in either the waived or the moderately complex category.

- State and city governments may enact mandatory POCT regulations that are more stringent than federal regulations.
- Written POCT policies and procedures must be available to all laboratory personnel.
- The greatest source of POCT error is preanalytical errors.
- Most POCT is done by manual rapid tests (e.g., pregnancy testing).

REVIEW QUESTIONS

1. A major advantage of POCT is:
   a. Faster turnaround time.
   b. Lower cost.
   c. Better quality than traditional testing.
   d. Both a and c.

2. POCT assays are usually in the _____ CLIA category.
   a. waived
   b. provider-performed microscopy
   c. moderately complex
   d. highly complex

3. Over-the-counter test kits are in the _____ CLIA category.
   a. waived
   b. provider-performed microscopy
   c. moderately complex
   d. highly complex

Questions 4-7. Indicate whether each characteristic is true with the letter "A" or false with the letter "B."

Important characteristics to consider when selecting a POCT kit are:

4. _____ Rapid turnaround time.

5. _____ Easy-to-perform protocol.

6. _____ Storage of temperature reagents.

7. _____ Length of time until expiration.

BIBLIOGRAPHY

Burtis CA, Ashwood ER, Bruns DB, editors: *Tietz fundamentals of clinical chemistry,* ed 6, St Louis, 2008, Saunders.

Kaplan LA, Pesce AJ, Kazmiercazk SC: *Clinical chemistry: theory, analysis, and correlation,* ed 4, St Louis, 2003, Mosby.

Joint Commission on Accreditation of Healthcare Organizations: *2005-2006, Comprehensive accreditation manual for laboratory and point-of-care testing,* Oak Brook Terrace, 2005, Department of Communications Laboratory Accreditation Program, JCAHO.

National Committee for Clinical Laboratory Standards: *Physician's office laboratory guidelines: tentative guidelines,* ed 3, Villanova, Pa, 1995, NCCLS Document POL ½-T3 and POL 3-R.

Turgeon ML: *Linné & Ringsrud's clinical laboratory science,* ed 5, St Louis, 2007, Mosby.

CHAPTER 10

Agglutination Methods

Principles of Agglutination
Latex Agglutination
Pregnancy Testing
    Human Chorionic Gonadotropin
    Agglutination Inhibition
Pregnancy Testing Protocols
Flocculation Tests
Direct Bacterial Agglutination
Hemagglutination
    Mechanisms of Agglutination
    Methods of Enhancing Agglutination

Graded Agglutination Reactions
    Microplate Agglutination Reactions
ABO Blood Grouping (Reverse Serum Grouping)
Chapter Highlights
Review Questions
Bibliography

Learning Objectives

At the conclusion of this chapter, the reader should be able to:

- Describe the principles of agglutination.
- Identify and compare the characteristics of agglutination methods.
- Explain methods for enhancing agglutination.
- Describe the characteristics of graded agglutination reactions.

- Explain agglutination reactions of the ABO blood group procedure.
- Discuss the principles of pregnancy testing, including sources of error.

PRINCIPLES OF AGGLUTINATION

Precipitation and agglutination are the visible expression of the aggregation of antigens and antibodies through the formation of a framework in which antigen particles or molecules alternate with antibody molecules (Figure 10-1). **Precipitation** is the term for the aggregation of soluble test antigens. **Agglutination** describes the aggregation of particulate test antigens.

Agglutination of particles to which soluble antigen has been absorbed produces a serum method of demonstrating precipitins. Examples of artificial carriers include latex particles and colloidal charcoal. Cells unrelated to the antigen, such as erythrocytes coated with antigen in a constant amount, can be used as biologic carriers. Whole bacterial cells can contain an antigen that will bind with antibodies produced in response to that antigen when it was introduced into the host.

The quality of test results depends on the following factors:

- Time of incubation with the antibody source (i.e., patient serum).
- Amount and avidity of an antigen conjugated to the carrier.
- Conditions of the test environment (e.g., pH, protein concentration).

Agglutination tests are easy to perform and in some cases are the most sensitive tests currently available. These tests have a wide range of applications in the clinical diagnosis of noninfectious immune disorders and infectious disease.

LATEX AGGLUTINATION

In latex agglutination procedures (Box 10-1), antibody molecules can be bound to the surface of latex beads. Many antibody molecules can be bound to each latex particle, increasing the potential number of exposed antigen-binding sites. If an antigen is present in a test specimen such as the C-reactive protein, the antigen will bind to the combining sites of the antibody exposed on the surface of the latex beads, forming visible cross-linked aggregates of latex beads and antigen (Figure 10-2). In some systems (e.g., pregnancy testing, rubella antibody testing), latex particles can be coated with antigen. In the presence of serum antibodies, these particles agglutinate into large, visible clumps.

Procedures based on latex agglutination must be performed under standardized conditions. The amount of antigen-antibody binding is influenced by factors such as pH, osmolarity, and ionic concentration of the solution. A variety of conditions can produce false-positive or false-negative reactions in agglutination testing (see Table 10-3).

Coagglutination and **liposome-enhanced** testing are variations of latex agglutination (Figure 10-3). Coagglutination uses antibodies bound to a particle to enhance the visibility of agglutination. It is a highly specific method but

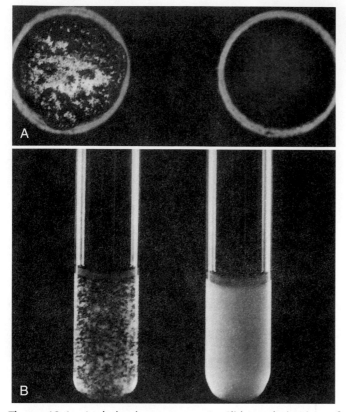

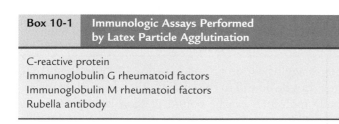

Figure 10-1 Agglutination patterns. **A,** Slide agglutination of bacteria with known antisera or known bacteria. *Left,* Positive reaction; *right,* negative reaction. **B,** Tube agglutination. *Left,* Positive reaction; *right,* negative reaction. *(From Barrett JT: Textbook of immunology, ed 5, St Louis, 1988, Mosby.)*

Box 10-1	Immunologic Assays Performed by Latex Particle Agglutination

C-reactive protein
Immunoglobulin G rheumatoid factors
Immunoglobulin M rheumatoid factors
Rubella antibody

may not be as sensitive as latex agglutination for detecting small quantities of antigen.

PREGNANCY TESTING

The principle of antigen and antibody interaction has been applied to pregnancy testing since the first agglutination tests were developed in the 1960s. These assays replaced animal testing.

Human Chorionic Gonadotropin

Pregnancy tests are designed to detect minute amounts of **human chorionic gonadotropin (hCG),** a glycoprotein hormone secreted by the trophoblast of the developing embryo that rapidly increases in the urine or serum during early stages of pregnancy.

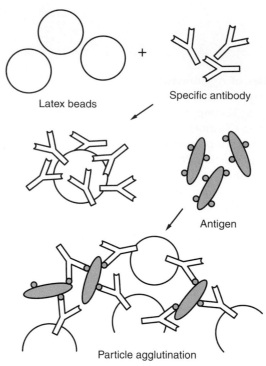

Figure 10-2 Alignment of antibody molecules bound to surface of a latex particle and latex agglutination reaction. *(Redrawn from Forbes BA, Sahm DF, Weissfeld AS: Bailey and Scott's diagnostic microbiology, ed 12, St Louis, 2007, Mosby.)*

This glycoprotein hormone consists of two noncovalently linked subunits, alpha (α) and beta (β). The α unit is identical to that found in luteinizing hormone (LH), follicle-stimulating hormone (FSH), and thyroid-stimulating hormone (TSH). The β subunit has a unique carboxy-terminal region. Using antibodies made against the β subunit will cut down on cross-reactivity with the other three hormones. Accordingly, many pregnancy test kits contain monoclonal antibody (MAb) directed against the β subunit to increase the specificity of the reaction.

For the first 6 to 8 weeks after conception, hCG helps to maintain the corpus luteum and stimulate the production of progesterone. As a general rule, the level of hCG should double every 2 to 3 days. Pregnant women usually attain serum concentrations of 10 to 50 mIU of hCG in the week after conception. If a test is negative at this stage, the test should be repeated within a week. Peak levels are reached approximately 2 to 3 months after the last menstrual period (LMP).

Agglutination Inhibition

The determination of in vitro agglutination inhibition depends on incubation of the patient's specimen with anti-hCG, followed by the addition of latex particles coated with hCG. If hCG is present, it neutralizes the antibody; thus no agglutination of latex particles is seen. If no hCG is present, agglutination occurs between the anti-hCG and hCG-coated latex particles.

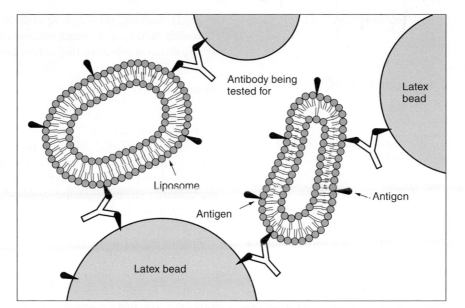

Figure 10-3   Diagram of liposome-enhanced latex agglutination reactions. *(Redrawn from Neo-Planotest Ducoclox Slide Test, Organon Teknika Corp., Durham, NC.)*

Pregnancy Testing Protocols

Principle

Rapid direct monoclonal latex slide agglutination test for detection of hCG is based on the principle of agglutination between latex particles coated with anti-hCG antibodies and hCG, if present, in the test specimen.

Specimen

The first morning urine specimen is required because it contains the highest concentration of hormone. It should have a specific gravity of at least 1.018. Collect the urine specimen in a clean glass or plastic container. It may be refrigerated for up to 2 days or frozen at −20° C for at least 1 year.

Thaw frozen samples by placing the frozen specimen in a water bath at 37 ° C and then mixing thoroughly before use. If turbidity or precipitation is present after thawing, filtering or centrifuging is recommended. Specimens containing blood, large amounts of protein, or excessive bacterial contamination should not be used. *Do not refreeze.*

Materials

- hCG-coated latex particles (yellow label)
- Positive and negative controls
- Stirrers, disposable pipettes, black glass slides, filter paper, centrifuge

Sample Procedure

1. Ensure that all reagents are at room temperature.
2. On clean slide, label positive control, negative control, and patient sample.
3. Using the disposable pipette provided, place 1 drop of patient urine in the central circle on the glass slide.

Place 1 drop of negative control and 1 drop of positive control into the circles on either side of the patient sample, using a new disposable pipette for each.
4. Add 1 drop of well-shaken latex antigen reagent to each circle.
5. Mix well, using a new stirrer for each circle. Spread the mixture over the entire circle.
6. Rock the slide gently back and forth for 2 minutes.
7. Observe immediately for agglutination.

Technical Sources of Error

Reagents should never be expired; latex reagent must be well shaken, and agglutination should be read within 3 minutes to avoid erroneous results caused by evaporation.

Results

Agglutination within 2 minutes represents a positive reaction.
No agglutination represents a negative reaction.

False-Positive Results

If a patient has been given an hCG injection (e.g., Pregnyl) to trigger ovulation or to lengthen the luteal phase of the menstrual cycle, trace amounts can remain in the patient's system for as long as 10 days after the last injection. This will produce a false-positive result. Two consecutive quantitative hCG blood assays can circumvent this problem. If the hCG level increases by the second test, the patient is probably pregnant.

Chorioepithelioma, hydatidiform mole, or excessive ingestion of aspirin may give false-positive results.

In men, a test identical to that used for pregnancy may be performed to detect the presence of a testicular tumor. If MAb against the β subunit is not used, other hormones with the same α unit may cross-react and cause a false-positive reaction.

False-Negative Results

Testing before reaching detectable levels of hCG will yield false-negative results.

Reference

Direct Monoclonal Latex Pregnancy test kit. Plasmatec package insert, January 2000, www.plasmatek.uk.com.

Alternate Procedural Protocols

Latex agglutination slide tests have been replaced in many circumstances (e.g., home testing; see Chapter 9) by one-step chromatographic color-label immunoassays for the qualitative detection of hCG in urine (e.g., ClearView HCG II and ClearView HCG Easy, Wampole Laboratories, Princeton, NJ).

Another variation is one-step chromatographic color-label immunoassay for use with urine or serum (e.g., Wampole PreVue HCG Stick or Cassette, Status HCG).

FLOCCULATION TESTS

Flocculation tests for antibody detection are based on the interaction of soluble antigen with antibody, which results in the formation of a precipitate of fine particles. These particles are macroscopically or microscopically visible only because the precipitated product is forced to remain in a confined space.

Flocculation testing can be used in syphilis serologic testing (see Chapter 18). These tests are the classic *Venereal Disease Research Laboratories* (VDRL) and the **rapid plasma reagin** (RPR) tests. In the VDRL test an antibody-like protein, reagin, binds to the test antigen, cardiolipid-lecithin–coated cholesterol particles, and produces the particles that flocculate (see EVOLVE website for traditional VDRL procedures). In the RPR test the antigen, cardiolipid-lecithin–coated cholesterol with choline chloride, also contains charcoal particles that allow for macroscopically visible flocculation.

DIRECT BACTERIAL AGGLUTINATION

Direct agglutination of whole pathogens can be used to detect antibodies directed against the pathogens. The most basic tests measure the antibody produced by the host to antigen determinants on the surface of a bacterial agent in response to infection with that bacterium. In a thick suspension of the bacteria, the binding of specific antibodies to surface antigens of the bacteria causes the bacteria to clump together in visible aggregates. This type of agglutination is called bacterial agglutination.

The formation of aggregates in solution is influenced by electrostatic and other forces; therefore certain conditions are usually necessary for satisfactory results. The use of sterile physiologic saline with free positive ions in the agglutination procedure enhances the aggregation of bacteria because most bacterial surfaces exhibit a negative charge that causes them to repel each other. Because it allows more time for antigen-

antibody reaction, tube testing is considered more sensitive than slide testing. The small volume of liquid used in slide testing requires rapid reading before the liquid evaporates.

HEMAGGLUTINATION

The hemagglutination method of testing detects antibodies to erythrocyte antigens. The antibody-containing specimen can be serially diluted and a suspension of red blood cells (RBCs) added to the dilutions. If a sufficient concentration of antibody is present, the erythrocytes are cross-linked and agglutinated. If nonreacting antibody or an insufficient quantity of antibody is present, the erythrocytes will fail to agglutinate.

By binding different antigens to the RBC surface in indirect hemagglutination or passive hemagglutination (PHA), the hemagglutination technique can be extended to detect antibodies to antigens other than those present on the cells (Box 10-2; see also Pregnancy Testing Protocols). Chemicals such as chromic chloride, tannic acid, and glutaraldehyde can be used to cross-link antigens to the cells.

Some antibodies (e.g., IgG) do not directly agglutinate erythrocytes. This incomplete or blocking type of antibody may be detected by using an enhancement medium such as **antihuman globulin (AHG)** reagent. If AHG reagent is added, this second antibody binds to the antibody present on the erythrocytes (see procedure in Chapter 26).

Mechanisms of Agglutination

Agglutination is the clumping of particles that have antigens on their surface, such as erythrocytes, by antibody molecules that form bridges between the antigenic determinants. This is the end point for most tests involving erythrocyte antigens. Agglutination is influenced by a number of factors and is believed to occur in two stages: sensitization and lattice formation.

Sensitization

The first phase of agglutination, sensitization, represents the physical attachment of antibody molecules to antigens on the erythrocyte membrane. The combination of antigen and antibody is a reversible chemical reaction. Altering the physical conditions can result in the release of antibody from the antigen-binding site. When physical conditions are purposely manipulated to break the antigen-antibody complex, with subsequent release of the antibody into the surrounding medium, the procedure is referred to as an **elution.**

The amount of antibody that will react is affected by the equilibrium constant, or affinity constant, of the antibody. In

Box 10-2	Immunologic Assays Performed by Indirect Hemagglutination

Antinuclear ribonucleoprotein
Anti-Sm
Antithyroglobulin and antithyroid microsome
Rubella antibodies
Sheep cell agglutination titer

most cases the higher the equilibrium constant, the higher is the rate of association and the slower the rate of dissociation of antibody molecules. The degree of association between antigen and antibody is affected by a variety of factors and can be altered in some cases in vitro by altering some of the factors that influence antigen-antibody association, include:

- Particle charge
- Electrolyte concentration and viscosity
- Antibody type
- Antigen-antibody ratio
- Antigenic determinants
- Physical conditions: pH, temperature, duration of incubation

Particle Charge. Inert particles such as latex, RBCs, and bacteria have a net negative surface charge called the **zeta potential** (Figure 10-4). The concentration of salt in the reaction medium has an effect on antibody uptake by the membrane-bound erythrocyte antigens. Sodium (Na^+) and chloride (Cl^-) ions in a solution have a shielding effect. These ions cluster around and partially neutralize the opposite charges on antigen and antibody molecules, which hinders antibody-antigen association. By reducing the ionic strength of a reaction medium (e.g., using low-ionic-strength saline [LIS]), antibody uptake is enhanced. Charges can be overcome by centrifugation, addition of charged molecules (e.g., albumin, LIS), or enzyme pretreatment to permit the cross-linking that results in agglutination (Table 10-1).

Antibody Type. Immunoglobulin M (IgM) antibodies are more efficient at agglutination because their large size and multivalency permit more effective bridging of the space between cells caused by zeta potential. Immunoglobulin G (IgG) antibodies are too small to overcome electrostatic

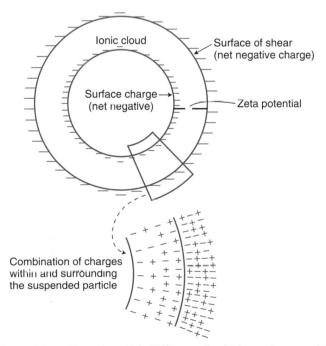

Figure 10-4 **Zeta potential.** Difference in electrostatic potential between net charge at cell membrane and charge at surface of shear. *(From Turgeon ML: Fundamentals of immunohematology, ed 2, Baltimore, 1995, Williams & Wilkins.)*

Table 10-1	Techniques to Reduce Zeta Potential
Technique	**Action**
Enzyme pretreatment of red blood cells	Removes negatively charged sialic acid residues from cell surface membrane.
Addition of colloids (e.g., albumin)	Increases electrical conductivity of environment.
Centrifugation	Mechanical process to force red blood cells closer together.

Modified from Lehman CA: *Saunders manual of clinical laboratory science*, Philadelphia, 1998, Saunders, p 391.

forces between cells. Use of AHG forms cross-links between antibody molecules that have bound to the surface of RBCs. This promotes formation of agglutination and allows visual observation of an antigen-antibody reaction.

Antigen-Antibody Ratio. Under conditions of antibody excess, there is a surplus of molecular antigen-combining sites not bound to antigenic determinants.

Precipitation reactions depend on a **zone of equivalence,** the zone in which optimum precipitation occurs because the number of multivalent sites of antigens and antibodies are approximately equal. For a precipitation reaction to be detectable, the reaction must occur in the zone of equivalence. In this zone, each antibody or antigen binds to more than one antigen or antibody, respectively, forming a stable lattice or network (see later discussion). This "lattice hypothesis" is based on the assumptions that each antibody molecule must have at least two binding sites and that an antigen must be multivalent.

On either side of the zone of equivalence, precipitation is prevented because of an excess of either antigen or antibody. If excessive antibody concentration is present, the phenomenon known as the **prozone phenomenon** occurs and can result in a false-negative reaction. In this case, antigen combines with only one or two antibody molecules, and no cross-linkages are formed. This phenomenon can be overcome by serially diluting the antibody-containing serum until optimum amounts of antigen and antibody are present in the test system.

If an excess of antigen occurs, the **postzone phenomenon** occurs, in which small aggregates (clumps) are surrounded by excess antigen, and no lattice formation is established. Excess antigen can block the presence of a small amount of antibody. To correct postzone phenomenon, a repeat blood specimen should be collected a week or more later. If an active antibody reaction is occuring in vivo, the titer of antibody will increase and should be detectable. Repeated negative results generally suggest that the patient has the specific antibody being tested for by the procedure.

Antigenic Determinants. The placement and number of antigenic determinants both affect agglutination. For example, the A blood group antigen has more than 1.5 million sites/RBC, whereas the Kell blood group antigen has about 3500 to 6000 sites/RBC. If the number of antigenic sites is small or if the antigenic sites are buried deep in the cell membranes, antibodies will be unable physically to contact antigenic sites.

Steric hindrance is an important physiochemical effect that influences antibody uptake by cell surface antigens. If dissimilar antibodies with approximately the same binding constant are directed against antigenic determinants located close to each other, the antibodies will compete for space in reaching their specific receptor sites. The effect of this competition can be mutual blocking, or steric hindrance, and neither antibody type will be bound to its respective antigenic determinant. Steric hindrance can occur whenever a conformational change in the relationship of an antigenic receptor site to the outside surface occurs. In addition to antibody competition, competition with bound complement, other protein molecules, or the action of agents that interfere with the structural integrity of the cell surface can produce steric hindrance.

pH. The pH of the medium used for testing should be near physiologic conditions, or optimum pH of 6.5 to 7.5. At a neutral pH, high electrolyte concentrations act to neutralize net negative charge of particles.

Temperature and Length of Incubation. The optimum temperature needed to reach equilibrium in an antibody-antigen reaction differs for different antibodies. IgM antibodies are cold reacting (thermal range, 4°-22° C), and IgG antibodies are warm reacting, with an optimum temperature of reaction at 37° C.

The duration of incubation required to achieve maximum results depends on the rate of association and dissociation of each specific antibody. In laboratory testing, incubation times range from 15 to 60 minutes. The optimum time of incubation varies, depending on the class of immunoglobulin and how tightly an antibody attaches to its specific antigen.

Lattice Formation

Lattice formation, or the establishment of cross-links between sensitized particles (e.g., erythrocytes) and antibodies resulting in aggregation, is a much slower process than the sensitization phase. The formation of chemical bonds and resultant lattice formation depend on the ability of a cell with attached antibody on its surface to come close enough to another cell to permit the antibody molecules to bridge the gap and combine with the antigen receptor site on the second cell. As antigens and antibodies combine, a multimolecular lattice increases in size until it precipitates out of solution as a solid particle. Cross-linking is influenced by factors such as the zeta potential.

Methods of Enhancing Agglutination

Techniques used to enhance agglutination include the following:
- Centrifugation
- Treatment with proteolytic enzymes
- Use of colloids
- Antihuman globulin (AHG) testing

Treatment with proteolytic enzymes and use of colloids or AHG techniques could be applied in the immunology laboratory.

Centrifugation attempts to overcome the problem of distance by subjecting sensitized cells to a high gravitational force that counteracts the repulsive effect and physically forces the cells together.

Enzyme treatment alters the zeta potential or dielectric constant to enhance the chances of demonstrable agglutination. Mild proteolytic enzyme treatment can strip off some of the negative charges on the cell membrane by removing surface sialic acid residues (cleaving sialoglycoproteins from the cell surface), which reduces the surface charge of cells, lowers the zeta potential, and permits cells to come closer together for chemical linking by specific antibody molecules.

Some IgG antibodies will agglutinate if the zeta potential is carefully adjusted by the addition of colloids and salts.

In some cases, antigens may be so deeply embedded in the membrane surface that the previous techniques will not bring the antigens and antibodies close enough to cross-link. The AHG test is frequently incorporated into the protocol of many laboratory techniques to facilitate agglutination. The direct AHG test can be used to detect disorders such as hemolytic disease of the newborn, transfusion reactions, and differentiation of immunoglobulin from complement coating of erythrocytes.

Graded Agglutination Reactions

Observation of agglutination is initially made by gently shaking the test tube containing the serum and cells and viewing the lower portion, the button, with a magnifying glass as it is dispersed. Because agglutination is a reversible reaction, the test tube must be treated delicately, and hard shaking must be avoided; however, all the cells in the button must be resuspended before an accurate observation can be determined. Attention should also be given to whether discoloration of the fluid above the cells, the *supernatant*, is present. Rupture or hemolysis of erythrocytes is as important a finding as agglutination.

The strength of agglutination (Table 10-2 and Figure 10-5), called **grading,** uses a scale of 0 or "negative" (no agglutination) to 41 (all erythrocytes clumped). Table 10-3 describes false-positive and false-negative reactions. **Pseudoagglutination,** or false appearance of clumping, may rarely

Table 10-2	Grading Agglutination Reactions
Grade	**Description**
Negative	No aggregates.
Mixed field	A few isolated aggregates; mostly free-floating cells; supernatant appears red.
Weak (+/−)	Tiny aggregates barely visible macroscopically; many free erythrocytes; turbid and reddish supernatant.
1+	A few small aggregates just visible macroscopically; many free erythrocytes; turbid and reddish supernatant.
2+	Medium-sized aggregates; some free erythrocytes; clear supernatant.
3+	Several large aggregates; some free erythrocytes; clear supernatant.
4+	All erythrocytes are combined into one solid aggregate; clear supernatant.

READING AGGLUTINATION

GRADE	DESCRIPTION		APPEARANCE	
	Cells	Supernate	Macroscopic*	Microscopic†
0	No agglutinates	Dark, turbid, homogeneous	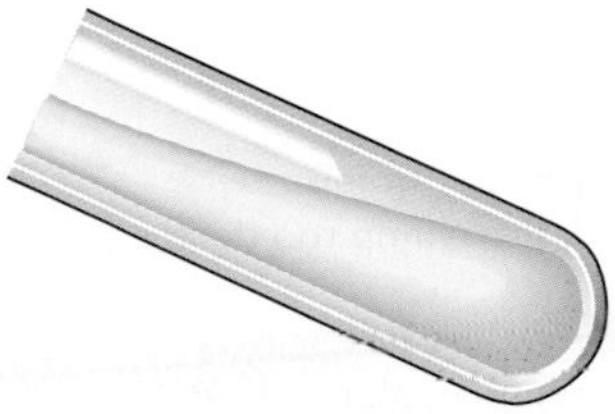	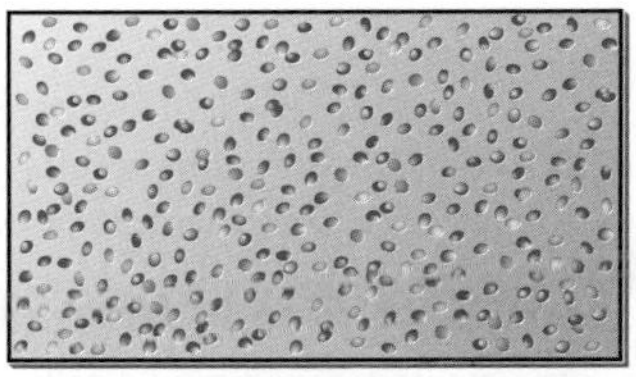
w+	Many tiny agglutinates Many free cells May not be visible without microscope	Dark, turbid	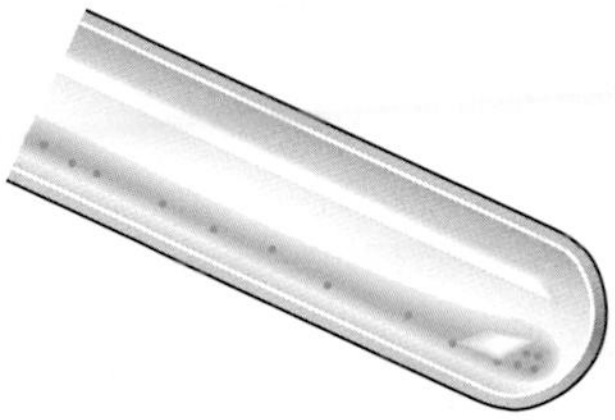	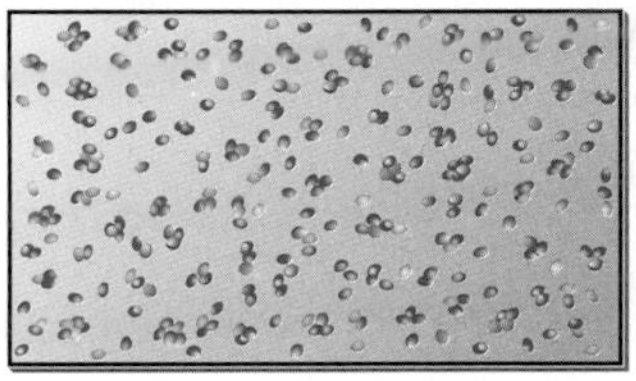
1+	Many small agglutinates Many free cells	Turbid	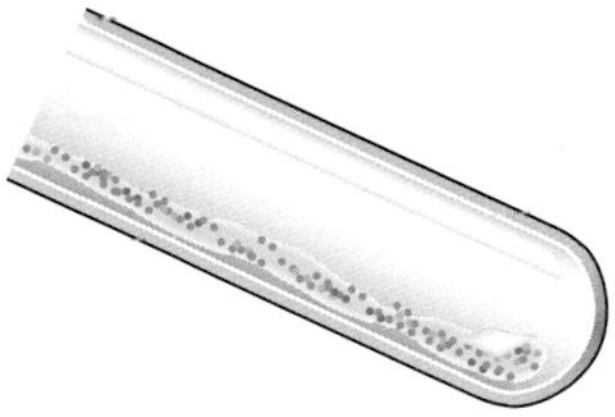	
2+	Many medium-sized agglutinates Moderate number of free cells	Clear	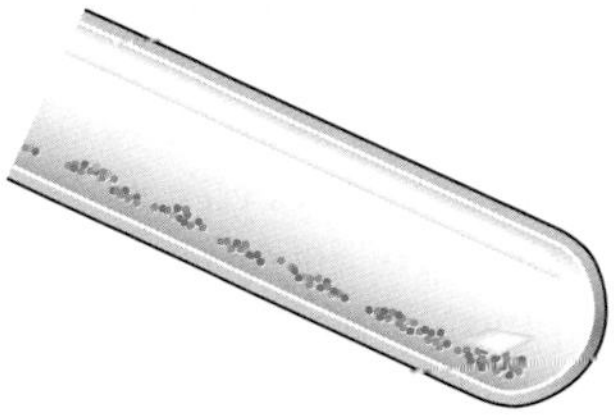	
3+	Several large agglutinates Few free cells	Clear	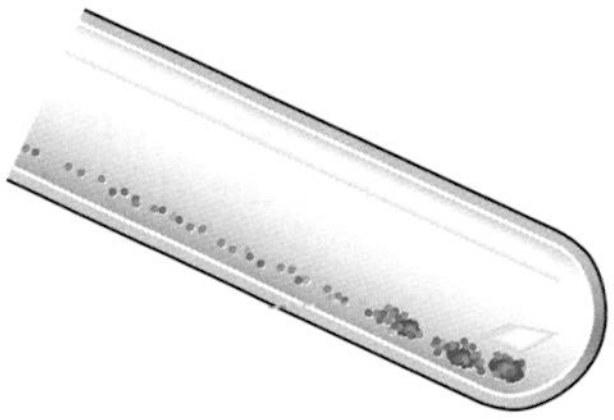	
4+	One large, solid agglutinate No free cells	Clear	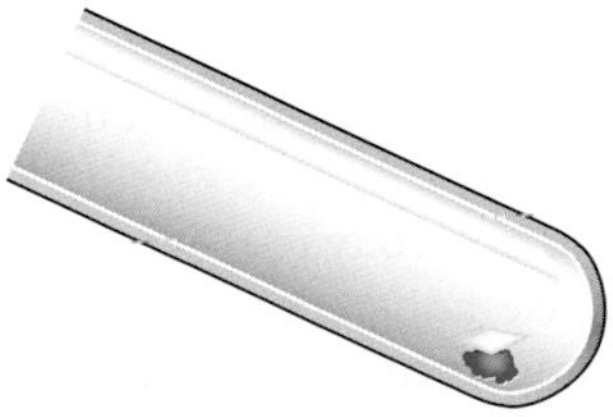	

*For any one grade, readings can be on a scale from weak+ to strong+ (e.g., grade 2 can be scored as 2+w, 2+, or 2+s, depending on the number and size of agglutinates).
†Microscopic readings are generally performed to differentiate pseudoagglutination (rouleaux) from true agglutination, to detect mixed-field reactions, and to confirm a negative reaction.

Figure 10-5   Reading red blood cell agglutination reactions. *(From Lehman CA:* Saunders Manual of Clinical Laboratory Science, *Philadelphia, 1998, Saunders, pp 394-395.)*

Table 10-3	Causes of False-Positive and False-Negative Agglutination Testing Reactions	
Cause	**Correction**
False-Positive Reactions	
Contaminated equipment or reagents may cause particles to clump.	Store equipment and reagent in clean, dust-free environment, and handle with care. Use negative quality control (QC) steps.
Autoagglutination.	Use a control with saline and no antibody as a negative control. If positive, patient's result is invalid.
Delay in reading slide reactions results in drying out of mixture.	Follow procedural directions and read reactions exactly as specified.
Overcentrifugation causes the cells or particles to clump too tightly.	Calibrate centrifuge to proper speed and time.
False-Negative Reactions	
Inadequate washing of red blood cells in antihuman globulin (AHG) testing* may result in unbound immunoglobulins neutralizing the reagent.	Wash cells according to directions. Use positive and negative QC steps.
Failure to add AHG reagent.	Use positive QC steps.
Contaminated or expired reagents.	Use positive and negative QC steps.
Improper incubation.	Follow procedural protocol exactly. Use positive and negative QC steps.
Delay in reading slide reactions.	Follow procedural protocol exactly. Use positive and negative control steps.
Undercentrifugation.	Calibrate centrifuge to proper speed and time.
Prozone phenomenon.	Dilute patient serum containing antibody, and repeat the procedure.

*See Chapter 26.

occur because of the presence of rouleaux formation. *Rouleaux formation* can be encountered in patients with high or abnormal types of globulins in their blood, such as in multiple myeloma, or after receiving dextran as a plasma expander. On microscopic examination the erythrocytes appear as rolls resembling stacks of coins. To disperse the pseudoagglutination, a few drops of physiologic NaCl (saline) can be added to the reaction tube, remixed, and reexamined. This procedure, *saline replacement,* should be performed carefully after pseudoagglutination is suspected. It should never be done before the initial testing protocol is followed; a false-negative result may occur from the dilutional effect of the saline.

Microplate Agglutination Reactions

Serologic testing has usually been performed by slide or test tube techniques, but the increased emphasis on cost containment has stimulated interest in microtechniques as an alternative to conventional methods.

Micromethods for RBC antigen and antibody testing are either hemagglutination or solid-phase adherence assays. These methods are also considered simpler to perform. Use of microplates allows for the performance of a large number of tests on a single plate, which eliminates time-consuming steps such as labeling test tubes.

A microplate is a compact plate of rigid or flexible plastic with multiple wells. The wells may be U shaped or have a flat-bottom configuration. The U-shaped well has been used most often in immunohematology. The volume capacity of each well is approximately 0.2 mL, which pre-

vents spilling during mixing. Samples and reagents are dispensed with small-bore Pasteur pipettes. These pipettes are recommended because they deliver 0.025 mL, which prevents splashing. After the specimens and reagents are added to the wells, they are mixed by gentle agitation of the plates. The microplate is then centrifuged for an immediate reading.

Countertop or floor-model centrifuges are suitable if they are equipped with special rotors that can accommodate microplate centrifuge carriers and are capable of speeds of 400 to 2000 rpm. Smaller plates can be centrifuged in serologic centrifuges with an appropriate adapter.

After centrifugation, the cell buttons are resuspended by gently tapping the microplate or by using a flat-topped mechanical shaker. A shaker provides a more consistent and standard resuspension of the cells than manual tapping. After the cells are resuspended, the wells are examined with an optical aid or over a well-lit surface. A positive reaction will settle in a diffuse, uneven button; negative reactions are manifested by a smooth, compact button. Detection of weakly positive reactions is enhanced by allowing the RBCs to settle.

ABO Blood Grouping (Reverse Grouping)

Principle

The reverse (serum) typing procedure to confirm ABO blood grouping is based on the presence or absence of the antibodies, anti-A and anti-B, in serum. If these antibodies are present in serum, agglutination should be demonstrated when the serum is combined with reagent erythrocytes expressing either A or B antigens.

Reverse typing is a cross-check for forward typing (see Chapter 2 procedure). Because of the lack of synthesized immunoglobulins in newborn and very young infants, this procedure is not performed on specimens from these patients.

Specimen

No special preparation of the patient is required before specimen collection. The patient must be positively identified when the specimen is collected. The specimen must be labeled at the bedside, and the label must include the patient's first and last name, the date when the specimen is collected, and the patient's hospital identification number. The time of collection and the phlebotomist's initials should be written on the required form.

Blood should be drawn by aseptic technique and the specimen tested as soon as possible. Approximately 5 to 7 mL of blood should be collected in a red-top (no anticoagulant) or lavender-top (EDTA) evacuated tube.

Hemolysis is undesirable. If a delay in testing is necessary, the blood should be refrigerated.

Reagents, Supplies, and Equipment

- Reagent erythrocytes: A1 and B (A2 optional)
- Disposable test tubes, 10 × 75 mm
- Disposable pipettes, 4⅝-inch plastic or Pasteur
- High-intensity lamp or optical magnifying lens
- Centrifuge

Quality Control

Reagent erythrocytes should be tested daily with known antisera.

Procedure

1. Label two 10X 75 mm test tubes one with the letter A, the other with the letter B. <u>A</u> and <u>B</u>. Label each with the last three digits of the laboratory number. *Note:* The letters <u>A</u> and <u>B</u> should be underlined to denote <u>reverse</u> grouping.
2. To each test tube, add 2 drops of the serum or plasma to be tested, using a disposable pipette.
3. To the tube labeled <u>A</u>, add 1 drop of the thoroughly mixed A_1 reagent erythrocytes.
4. To the tube labeled <u>B</u>, add 1 drop of the thoroughly mixed B reagent erythrocytes.
5. Mix well and centrifuge both test tubes for 15 seconds at 3400 rpm.
6. Resuspend the cells by gentle agitation, and examine macroscopically for agglutination; record results.

Reporting Results

Agglutination indicates that an antibody specific for either the A antigen or the B antigen is present in the serum or plasma being tested. Grade all positive reactions.

Reactions of Patient Serum and Reagent Erythrocytes			
A1 Cells	B Cells	Antibody	Blood Group
+	+	Anti-A and anti-B	O
0	+	Anti-B	A
+	0	Anti-A	B
0	0	Neither	AB

Procedure Notes

A hemolyzed specimen is unsuitable for this test. As in the forward typing, testing must be conducted at room temperature or colder. If the expected results of both forward and reverse typing are not demonstrated, either a variation in the patient or a technical error may exist.

Biologic Sources of Error

If a patient has been recently transfused with non–group-specific blood, *mixed-field agglutination* may be observed. If large quantities of non–group-specific blood have been transfused, determination of the correct ABO grouping may be impossible.

Discrepancies in forward typing can result from conditions such as weak antigens, altered expression of antigens caused by disease, chimerism, or excessive blood group substances. Excess amounts of blood group–specific soluble substances present in the plasma in certain disorders (e.g., carcinoma of stomach or pancreas) neutralize the reagent anti-A or anti-B, leaving no unbound antibody to react with the patient's erythrocytes. This excess of blood group–specific substance produces a false-negative or weak reaction in the forward grouping. If the patient's erythrocytes are washed with saline, the substance should be removed, and a correct grouping can be observed.

Incorrect typing can also result from additional antigens, caused by the following:

- Polyagglutinable RBCs
- Acquired B-like antigen; acquired A-like antigen
- Complexes attached to RBCs
- Agents causing nonspecific erythrocyte agglutination
- Antibody-sensitized RBCs: effect of colloids and anti-antibodies (e.g., hemolytic disease of newborn, incompatible transfusion, autoimmune process)

Discrepancies in serum (reverse) grouping can result from additional or missing antibodies, caused by the following:

- Passively acquired isoagglutinins
- Alloantibodies
- Rouleaux formation
- Auto-anti-I; iso-anti-I
- Anti-A1 in A*x*, A2, and A2B blood
- Anti-H in A1B, A1, B, and Bombay blood
- Anti-IA and IA

Causes of weak or missing antibodies include the following:

- Deteriorated reagent erythrocytes
- Hypogammaglobulinemic or elderly patients
- Newborn infants

- Chimerism
- Rare variants of A or B

Technical Sources of Error

Each manufacturer provides, with each package of antiserum, detailed instructions for the use of anti-A and anti-B. Because the details vary, it is important to follow the directions for the specific antiserum in use.

Procedures that apply to *all* tests for ABO grouping include the following:

1. Do not rely on the color of dyes to identify reagent antisera. All tubes must be properly labeled.
2. Do not perform tests at temperatures higher than room temperature (20°-24° C).
3. Perform observations of agglutination with a well-lit background, not a warm viewbox.
4. Record results immediately after observation.
5. Remember that contaminated blood specimens, reagents, or supplies may interfere with the test results.

Limitations

Antisera prepared from human sources are capable of detecting A1 and A2 groups. Except in the case of newborn and very young infants, a reverse cell typing should also be performed to verify the results of forward typing.

CHAPTER HIGHLIGHTS

- Agglutination of particles to which soluble antigen has been adsorbed produces a serum method of demonstrating precipitins. Examples of artificial carriers include latex particles and colloidal charcoal. Cells unrelated to the antigen, such as erythrocytes coated with antigen in a constant amount, can be used as biologic carriers.
- In latex agglutination procedures, antibody molecules can be bound to the surface of latex beads. If an antigen is present in a test specimen, the antigen will bind to the combining sites of the antibody exposed on the surface of the latex beads, forming visible cross-linked aggregates of latex beads and antigen.
- Flocculation tests for antibody detection are based on the interaction of soluble antigen with antibody, which results in the formation of a precipitate of fine particles.
- Direct bacterial agglutination can be used to detect antibodies directed against pathogens.

REVIEW QUESTIONS

1. The quality of test results in an agglutination reaction depends on all the following *except:*
   a. Duration of incubation.
   b. Amount of antigen conjugated to the carrier.
   c. Avidity of antigen conjugated to the carrier.
   d. Whether the carrier is artificial or biologic.

2. Flocculation procedures differ from latex agglutination procedures because:
   a. Antigen is bound to a carrier.
   b. Antibody is bound to a carrier.
   c. Soluble antigen reacts with antibody.
   d. Flocculation procedures are only qualitative.

3. In the hemagglutination technique, antihuman globulin is used as an enhancement medium to detect _____ antibodies.
   a. IgM
   b. IgG
   c. IgD
   d. IgE

4. The prozone phenomenon can result in a (an):
   a. False-positive reaction.
   b. False-negative reaction.
   c. Enhanced agglutination.
   d. Diminished antigen response.

5. The effect of competing antibodies seeking to attach to antigen sites is called:
   a. Prozone phenomenon.
   b. Ionic strength.
   c. Steric hindrance.
   d. Sensitization.

6. All the following are methods that can be used to enhance agglutination of IgG antibodies *except:*
   a. Centrifugation.
   b. Treatment with proteolytic enzymes.
   c. Acidifying the mixture.
   d. Using colloids.

Questions 7-10. Match the following grades of agglutination with the appropriate description.

7. _____ Mixed field

8. _____ 1+

9. _____ 2+

10. _____ 4+

   a. All the erythrocytes are combined into one solid aggregate; clear supernatant.
   b. Few isolated aggregates; supernatant appears red.
   c. Medium-sized aggregates; clear supernatant.
   d. A few small aggregates; turbid and reddish supernatant.
   e. Several large aggregates; clear supernatant.

11. A classic technique for the detection of viral antibodies is:
   a. Passive hemagglutination.
   b. Indirect hemagglutination.
   c. Hemagglutination inhibition.
   d. Latex particle agglutination.

Questions 12-16. Match each term to its definition.

12. _____ Precipitation

13. _____ Agglutination

14. _____ Coagglutination

15. _____ Flocculation

16. _____ Hemagglutination

    a. Aggregation of particulate test antigens.
    b. Aggregation of soluble test antigens.
    c. Uses antibodies bound to a particle to enhance visibility of agglutination.
    d. Agglutination of erythrocytes in tests for antibody detection.
    e. Based on the interaction of soluble antigen with antibody, resulting in formation of a precipitate of fine particles.

17. Artificial or biologic carriers that can be used in an agglutination reaction include:
    a. Latex particles.
    b. Colloidal charcoal.
    c. Erythrocytes coated with antigen in a constant amount.
    d. All the above.

Questions 18 and 19. Identify the components (*a* and *b*) of a latex agglutination reaction in the figure.

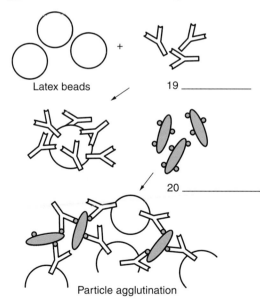

(*Redrawn from Forbes BA, Sahm DF, Weissfeld AS:* Bailey and Scott's diagnostic microbiology, *ed 12, St Louis, 2007, Mosby.*)

    a. Antigen
    b. Specific antibody

20. Sensitization:
    a. Is the first phase of agglutination.
    b. Represents the physical attachment of antibody molecules to antigens on the RBC membrane.
    c. Is an irreversible reaction.
    d. Both a and b.

21. Agglutination can be used to enhance reactions by all the following means *except:*
    a. Decreasing ionic strength of the reaction.
    b. Centrifugation.
    c. Increasing pH of the reaction.
    d. Using colloids and antihuman globulin.

Questions 22-24. Match each grade of agglutination with its respective description.

22. _____ Negative

23. _____ Weak (1+ or 2+)

24. _____ 3+

    a. Tiny aggregates that are barely visible macroscopically.
    b. Several large aggregates.
    c. All erythrocytes combined into one solid aggregate.
    d. No aggregates.

25. All the following statements are correct regarding human pregnancy testing *except:*
    a. Tests detect human chorionic gonadotropin (hCG).
    b. The hCG is secreted by the trophoblast of the developing embryo.
    c. Presence of hCG rapidly increases in urine or serum.
    d. Presence of hCG in maternal urine or serum persists throughout pregnancy.

26. All the following statements are correct regarding hCG *except:*
    a. Helps to maintain the corpus luteum.
    b. Stimulates production of progesterone.
    c. Detectable within 102 hours after the last expected menstrual period.
    d. Reaches peak levels at 2 to 3 months after the last menstrual period.

27. The most common laboratory method for detecting hCG is:
    a. Latex agglutination.
    b. Enzyme-linked immunosorbent assay.
    c. Immunofluorescence.
    d. Antibody titration.

28. In the latex agglutination method for the detection of hCG, no agglutination indicates:
    a. Absence of hCG.
    b. Presence of hCG.
    c. Absence of hCG, a positive test.
    d. Presence of hCG, a negative test.

29. A urine specimen for pregnancy testing _____ be frozen.
    a. may
    b. may not

30. A false-positive reaction in a latex agglutination test for hCG can be caused by all the following *except:*
    a. Chorioepithelioma.
    b. Hydatidiform mole.
    c. Taking oral contraceptives.
    d. Excessive ingestion of aspirin.

BIBLIOGRAPHY

Aloisi RM: *Principles of immunology and immuno-diagnostics,* Philadelphia, 1988, Lea & Febiger.

Baines W, Noble P: Sensitivity limits of latex agglutination tests, *Am Clin Lab* 12(3):14-18, 1993.

Forbes BA, Sahm DF, Weissfeld AS: *Bailey and Scott's diagnostic microbiology,* ed 12, St Louis, 2007, Mosby.

Henry JB, editor: *Clinical diagnosis and management,* ed 18, Philadelphia, 1991, Saunders.

Kaplan LA, Pesce AJ, Kazmierczak SC: *Clinical chemistry,* ed 4, St Louis, 2003, Mosby, p 234.

Lehman CA: *Saunders manual of clinical laboratory science,* Philadelphia, Saunders, p 391.

Turgeon ML: *Fundamentals of immunohematology,* ed 2, Baltimore, 1995, Williams & Wilkins.

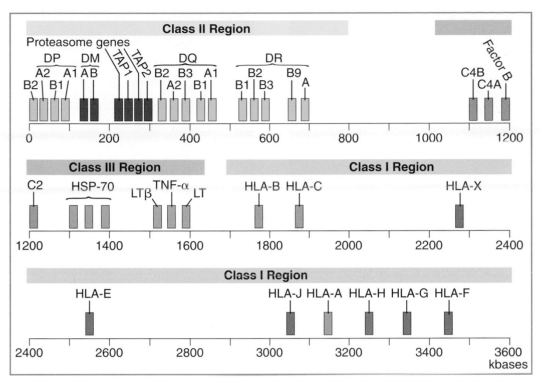

Plate 1 Human major histocompatibility complex. *(From Abbas AK et al: Cellular and molecular immunology, ed 6, Philadelphia, 2007, Saunders.)*

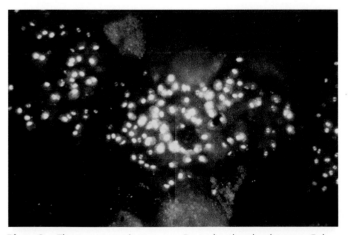

Plate 2 Fluorescent microscopy. Bronchoalveolar lavage. Calcufluor white stain. Fluorescent cysts with coccoid bodies. Impression: Pneumocystosis. *(From Mahon CR et al: Textbook of diagnostic microbiology, ed 3, St Louis, 2007, Saunders.)*

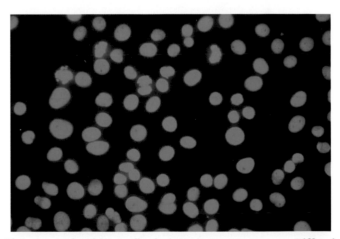

Plate 3 Antinuclear Antibody (ANA). *Homogeneous* or *Diffused:* A solid staining of the nucleus with or without apparent masking of the nucleoli. **Nuclear antigens present:** dsDNA, nDNA, DNP histone. **Disease association:** High titers are suggestive of systemic lupus erythematosus (SLE); lower titers are suggestive of SLE or other connective tissue diseases. *(Courtesy INOVA Diagnostics, Inc, San Diego, Calif.)*

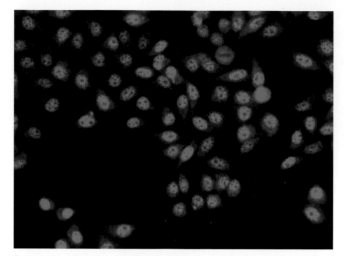

Plate 4   Antinuclear Antibody (ANA). *Homogenous:* The chromosome region of mitotic cells demonstrates the same smooth, homogeneous staining pattern. *(Courtesy INOVA Diagnostics, Inc, San Diego, Calif.)*

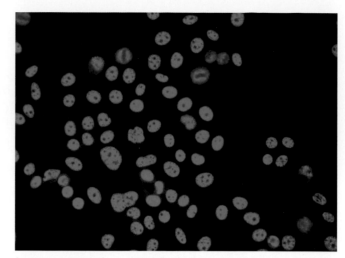

Plate 5   Antinuclear Antibody (ANA). *Speckled:* A fine or grainy-appearing staining of the nucleus, generally without fluorescent staining of the nucleoli. **Nuclear antigens present:** Sm, RNP, Scl-70, SS-A, SS-B, and other antigen/antibody systems not yet characterized. **Disease association:** High titers suggestive of systemic lupus erythematosus (Sm antibody), mixed connective tissue disease (RNP antibody), scleroderma (Scl-70 antibody), or Sjogren's syndrome-sicca complex (SS-B antibody); lower titers may be suggestive of other connective tissue diseases. *(Courtesy INOVA Diagnostics, Inc, San Diego, Calif.)*

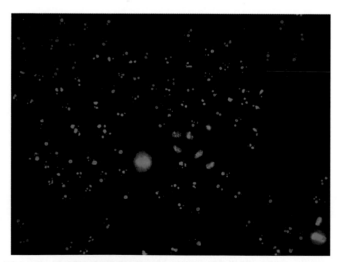

Plate 6   Antinuclear Antibody (ANA). *Nucleolar:* Large, coarse, speckled staining within the nucleus, generally less than 6 in number per cell, with or without occasional fine speckles. **Nuclear antigens present:** 4-6S RNA and other unknown nuclear antigens. **Disease association:** High titers are prevalent in scleroderma and Sjogren's syndrome. *(Courtesy INOVA Diagnostics, Inc, San Diego, Calif.)*

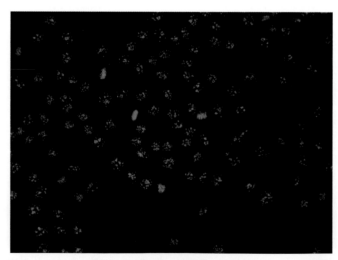

Plate 7   Antinuclear Antibody (ANA). *Centromere:* A discrete, speckled staining pattern. The nuclear speckles are very discrete and usually in some multiple of 46 (23-46 speckles per nucleus). **Nuclear antigens present:** Chromosomal centromere (kinetochore). **Disease association:** Highly suggestive of CREST syndrome, a variant of progressive systemic sclerosis (PSS). *(Courtesy INOVA Diagnostics, Inc, San Diego, Calif.)*

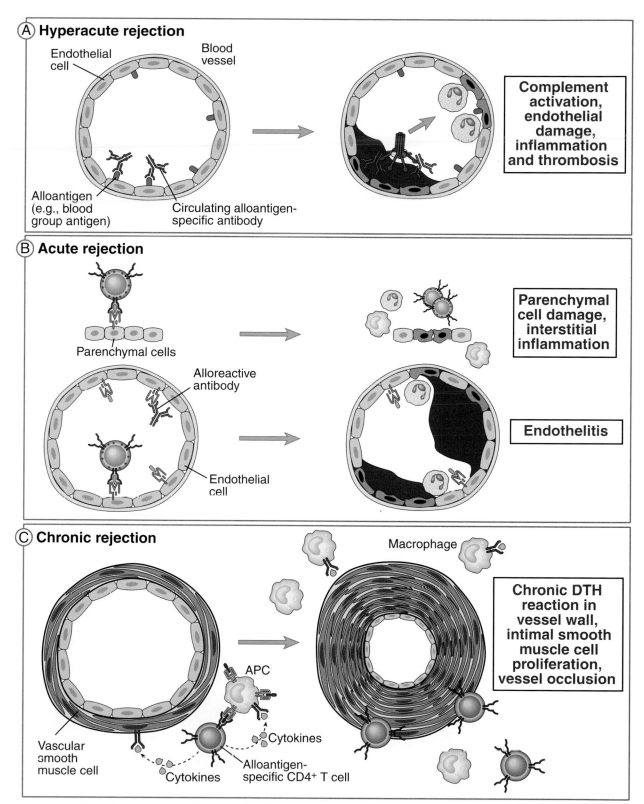

Plate 8 Immune mechanism of graft rejection. *(From Abbas AK et al: Cellular and molecular immunology, ed 6, Philadelphia, 2007, Saunders.)*

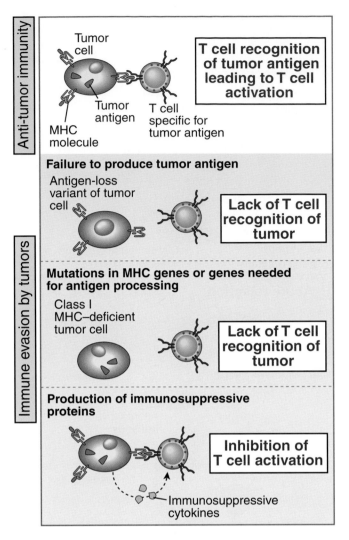

Anti-tumor immunity

Tumor cell

T cell recognition of tumor antigen leading to T cell activation

Tumor antigen

MHC molecule

T cell specific for tumor antigen

Failure to produce tumor antigen

Antigen-loss variant of tumor cell

Lack of T cell recognition of tumor

Mutations in MHC genes or genes needed for antigen processing

Class I MHC–deficient tumor cell

Lack of T cell recognition of tumor

Production of immunosuppressive proteins

Inhibition of T cell activation

Immunosuppressive cytokines

Immune evasion by tumors

Plate 9 Mechanisms by which tumors escape immune defenses. *(From Abbas AK et al: Cellular and molecular immunology, ed 6, Philadelphia, 2007, Saunders.)*

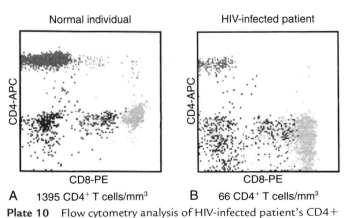

Normal individual

HIV-infected patient

CD4-APC

CD8-PE

CD4-APC

CD8-PE

A   1395 CD4$^+$ T cells/mm^3

B   66 CD4$^+$ T cells/mm^3

Plate 10 Flow cytometry analysis of HIV-infected patient's CD4+ and CD8+ cells. Shown are two-color plots of a control blood sample **(A)** and that of the patient **(B).** The CD4+ T cells are shown in orange *(upper left quadrant),* and the CD8+ T cells are shown in green *(lower right quadrant.)* *(From Abbas AK, Lichtman AH: Basic immunology: functions and disorders of the immune system, ed 3, Philadelphia, 2008, Saunders.)*

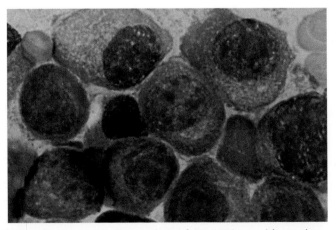

Plate 11 Bone marrow aspirate from patient with myeloma. *(From Nairn R, Helbert M: Immunology for medical students, ed 2, St Louis, 2007, Mosby.)*

CHAPTER 11

Electrophoresis Techniques

Electrophoresis
Immunoelectrophoresis
   Principle
   Normal Appearance of Precipitin Bands
   Clinical Applications
   Source of Error
   Abnormal Appearance of Precipitin Bands
   Polyvalent and Monovalent Antisera

Immunofixation Electrophoresis
   Clinical Applications
Immunofixation Electrophoresis Procedure
Comparison of Techniques
Capillary Electrophoresis
Chapter Highlights
Review Questions
Bibliography

Learning Objectives

At the conclusion of this chapter, the reader should be able to:

- Define *electrophoresis.*
- Describe the electrophoresis technique.
- Identify the fractions into which serum proteins can be divided by electrophoresis.
- Describe the characteristics of immunoelectrophoresis.
- Explain the features of immunofixation electrophoresis.
- Discuss the clinical applications of immunoelectrophoresis.
- Compare immunoelectrophoresis and immunofixation electrophoresis.
- Compare capillary electrophoresis and microchip capillary electrophoresis.
- Describe two electrophoresis separation methods.

ELECTROPHORESIS

Electrophoresis is the migration of charged solutes or particles in an electrical field. Using this principle, charged molecules can be made to move, and different molecules can be separated if they have different velocities in an electrical field.

The electrical field is applied to a solution with oppositely charged electrodes. Charged particles in this solution begin to migrate. Positively charged particles **(cations)** move to the negatively charged (−) electrode; negatively charged particles **(anions)** migrate to the positively charged (+) electrode (Figure 11-1).

Serum proteins are often separated by electrophoresis. **Serum electrophoresis** results in the separation of proteins into five fractions using cellulose acetate as a support medium (Figure 11-2). This separation is based on the rate of migration of these individual components in an electrical field.

Electrophoresis is a versatile analytical technique. Immunoglobulins are separated by electrophoresis using agarose as a support medium. The immunologic applications of electrophoresis include identification of monoclonal proteins in serum or urine, immunoelectrophoresis, and various blotting techniques (see Chapter 14).

IMMUNOELECTROPHORESIS

Immunoelectrophoresis (IEP) involves the electrophoresis of serum or urine followed by immunodiffusion. The size and position of precipitin bands provide the same type of information regarding equivalence or antibody excess as the double-immunodiffusion method. Proteins are differentiated not only by their electrophoretic mobility, but also by their diffusion coefficient and antibody specificity.

Although double immunodiffusion produces a separate precipitation band for each antigen-antibody system in a mixture, it is often difficult to determine all the components in a complex mixture. IEP separates the antigen mixture by electrophoresis before performing immunodiffusion.

Principle

Immunoelectrophoresis is a combination of the techniques of electrophoresis and double immunodiffusion (Figure 11-3). In the first phase, *electrophoresis,* serum is placed in an appropriate medium (e.g., cellulose acetate or agarose), then electrophoresed to separate its constituents according to electrophoretic mobilities: albumin, α_1-, α_2-, β-, and γ-globulin fractions.

After electrophoresis, in the second phase, *immunodiffusion,* the fractions are allowed to act as antigens and to interact with their corresponding antibodies. Antiserum (polyvalent or monovalent) is deposited in a trough cut into the gel to one side and parallel to the line of separated proteins. Incubation allows double immunodiffusion of the antigens and antibodies. Each antiserum diffuses outward, perpendicular to the trough, and each serum protein diffuses outward from its point of electrophoresis. When a favorable antigen/antibody ratio exists **(equivalence),** the antigen-antibody complex becomes visible as precipitin lines or bands. Diffusion is halted by rinsing the plate in 0.85% saline. Unbound protein is washed from the agarose with sa-

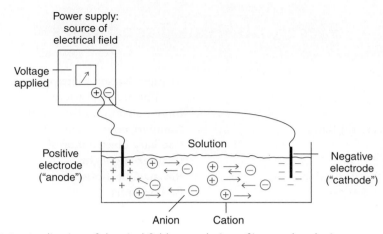

Figure 11-1   Application of electrical field to a solution of ions makes the ions move. *(From Kaplan LA, Pesce AJ, Kazmierczak SC:* Clinical chemistry, *ed 4, St Louis, 2003, Mosby.)*

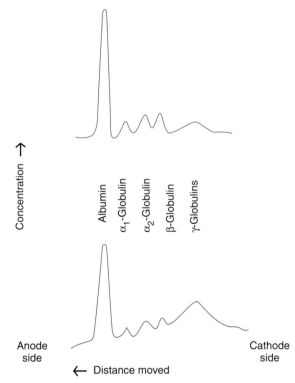

Figure 11-2   Example of the effect of disease (hepatic cirrhosis) on serum protein electrophoresis pattern. *Upper profile,* Distribution characteristic of healthy people. *(From Kaplan LA, Pesce AJ, Kazmierczak SC:* Clinical chemistry, *ed 4, St Louis, 2003, Mosby.)*

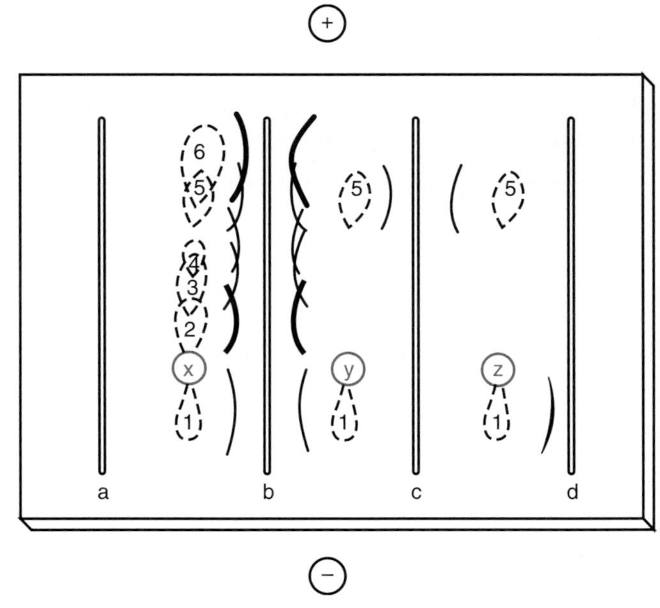

Figure 11-3   Configuration for immunoelectrophoresis. Sample wells are punched in the agar/agarose, sample is applied, and electrophoresis is carried out to separate the proteins in the sample. Antiserum is loaded into the troughs and the gel incubated in a moist chamber at 4° C for 24 to 72 hours. Track *x* represents the shape of the protein zones after electrophoresis; tracks *y* and *z* show the reaction of proteins 5 and 1 with their specific antisera in troughs *c* and *d.* Antiserum against proteins 1 through 6 is present in trough *b. (From Burtis CA, Ashwood ER, Bruns DB:* Tietz fundamentals of clinical chemistry, *ed 6, St Louis, 2008, Saunders.)*

line, and the antigen-antibody precipitin "arcs" are stained with a protein-sensitive stain.

Each line represents one specific protein. Proteins are thus differentiated by their diffusion coefficient and antibody specificity as well as electrophoretic mobility. Antibody diffuses as a uniform band parallel to the antibody trough. If the proteins are homogeneous, the antigen diffuses in a circle, and the antigen-antibody precipitation line resembles a segment or "arc" of a circle. If the antigen is heterogeneous, the antigen-antibody line assumes an elliptical shape.

One arc of precipitation forms for each constituent in the antigen mixture. This technique can be used to resolve the protein of normal serum into 25 to 40 distinct precipitation bands. The exact number depends on the strength and specificity of the antiserum used.

Normal Appearance of Precipitin Bands

Immunoprecipitation bands should be of normal curvature, symmetry, length, position, intensity, and distance from the antigen well and antibody trough (Figure 11-4). In

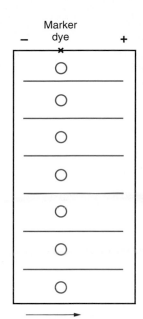

Marker
dye
−   +

Normal control serum

Anti-IgG antiserum (γ specific)

No. 1 patient's serum (1:10 dilution)

Anti-IgA antiserum (α specific)

Normal control serum

Anti-IgM antiserum (μ specific)

No. 1 patient's serum

Polyvalent antiserum

Normal control serum

Anti-λ antiserum

No. 1 patient's serum

Anti-κ antiserum

Normal control serum

Electrophoresis direction

Figure 11-4 Suggested sequence of antigen-antiserum combinations used in immunoelectrophoresis. *(Redrawn from Bauer JD: Clinical laboratory methods, ed 9, St Louis, 1982, Mosby.)*

normal serum, immunoglobulin G (IgG), IgA, and IgM are present in sufficient concentrations of 10 mg/mL, 2 mg/mL, and 1 mg/mL, respectively, to produce precipitin lines. The normal concentrations of IgD and IgE are too low to be detected by IEP.

A normal IgG precipitin band is elongated, elliptical, slightly curved, and clearly visible in undiluted serum and 1:10 diluted serum. An IgG band is located cathodic to the antigen well in the alpha (α) area of the *electrophoretogram*. If monospecific serum is used, it is fused with a thin precipitin line positioned midway between the antigen well and antibody trough and extending into the beta (β) area. The IgM and IgA bands are visible in undiluted serum but disappear at a 1:10 dilution of serum. The IgA band is a flattened, thin arc, slightly cathodic to the well in the α-β position. The IgM line is a barely visible, thin line, slightly cathodic to the antigen well.

Clinical Applications

Immunoelectrophoresis is most often used to determine qualitatively the elevation or deficiency of specific classes of immunoglobulins. Also, IEP is a reliable and accurate method for detecting both structural abnormalities and concentration changes in proteins. It is possible to identify the absence of a normal serum protein (e.g., congenital deficiency of complement component) or alterations in serum proteins. This method can be used to screen for circulating immune complexes, characterize cryoglobulinemia and pyroglobulinemia, and recognize and characterize antibody syndromes and the various dysgammaglobulinemias.

The most common application of IEP is in the diagnosis of a **monoclonal gammopathy,** a condition in which a single

clone of plasma cells produces elevated levels of a single class and type of immunoglobulin. The elevated immunoglobulin is referred to as a **monoclonal protein, M protein,** or **paraprotein.** Monoclonal gammopathies may indicate a malignancy such as multiple myeloma or macroglobulinemia. Antikappa (anti-κ) and antilambda (anti-λ) antisera are necessary for complete typing of the immunoglobulin in the evaluation of the ratio and for the diagnosis of M proteins. The class (heavy [H] chain) and type (light [L] chain) must be established because a patient's prognosis, and treatment may differ depending on the immunoglobulin identified.

Differentiation must also be made between monoclonal and polyclonal gammopathies. A **polyclonal gammopathy** is a secondary condition caused by disorders such as liver disease, collagen disorders, rheumatoid arthritis, and chronic infection. It is characterized by elevation of two or more (often all) immunoglobulins by several clones of plasma cells. Polyclonal increases of proteins are usually twice the normal levels.

The most important application of IEP of urine is the demonstration of **Bence Jones (BJ) protein.** IEP detects very low concentrations of BJ protein (~1-2 mg/dL). If BJ protein is present in a urine specimen, precipitin lines will form with either κ or λ anti-L chain antisera because BJ protein is composed of homogeneous L chains of a single antigen type, either κ or λ. Normal L chains are heterogeneous and include equal concentrations of κ and λ.

Source of Error

Prozone phenomenon is an incomplete precipitin reaction caused by antigen excess (antigen/antibody ratio too high). "Prozoning" should be suspected if a precipitin arc appears to "run" into a trough, if an L chain appears fuzzy when an H chain is increased, or if an arc appears to be incomplete.

Abnormal Appearance of Precipitin Bands

The size and position of precipitin bands provide the same type of information regarding equivalence or antigen-antibody excess as double-immunodiffusion systems. The position and shape of precipitin bands in the IEP assay of serum are relatively stable and reproducible; virtually any deviation is abnormal (Figure 11-5). These abnormalities can be detected by evaluating the following features of the precipitin bands:

- Position of the band in relationship to electrophoretically identified protein fractions.
- Position of the band between the antigen well and the antibody trough.
- Distortion of the curvature or arc formation.
- Thickening (density) and elongation of a band.
- Shortening (inhibition), thinning, or doubling of a band.

Position of Band

The precipitin band may be displaced compared with its normal position in the control serum because molecular charges in the abnormal protein may affect its speed of mi-

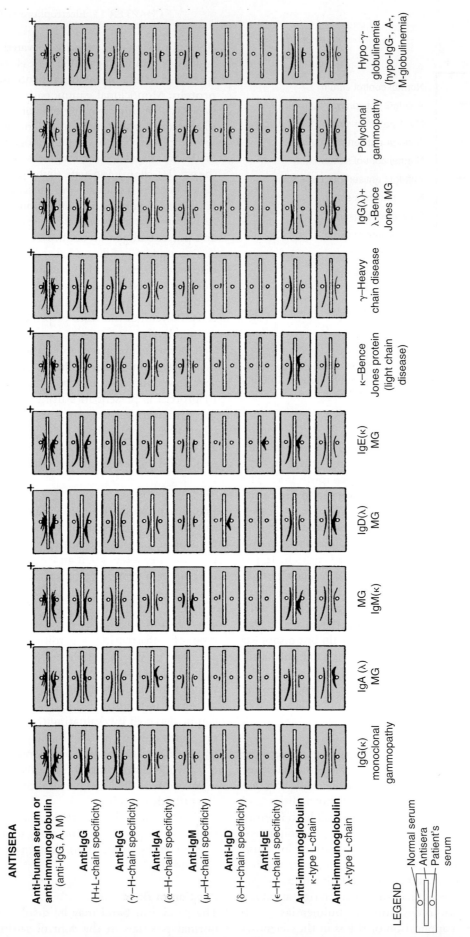

Figure 11-5 Example of immunoglobulin (Ig) profile on immunoelectrophoresis showing abnormal Ig pattern. *(Redrawn from Ritzman SE, Daniels JC:* Laboratory notes—serum proteins, *No. 3, Somerville, NJ, 1973, Behring Diagnostics/Hoechst Pharmaceuticals.)*

gration in the electrophoresis phase of IEP. A precipitin band may form a line of fusion or partial fusion with another protein, indicating the presence of proteins immunologically similar but electrophoretically distinct.

A distinct abnormality in the position of the band is seen in cases of monoclonal IgA gammopathy. The monoclonal IgA band is closer to the antibody trough than normal IgA.

Distortion of Curvature or Arc
An abnormal curvature of the precipitin band can be observed with M proteins because of an antigen excess.

The monoclonal IgG band shows an arc of a circle rather than the elongated, elliptical shape of a normal band. This distortion of IgG reflects the homogeneous nature and limited electrophoretic mobility of the abnormal protein.

Normal IgM and IgD bands are hardly visible, but the monoclonal IgM or IgD bands are skewed arcs of a circle.

Thickening and Elongation
Thickening and elongation can be seen in the presence of M proteins because excess antigen diffuses a greater distance.

Monoclonal IgM, IgG, IgD, and IgA all demonstrate denser-than-normal bands. In addition, monoclonal IgG touches the antisera trough.

Shortening, Thinning, or Doubling
A band may be shortened and incomplete because of inhibition of a segment, resulting from the antibody's reacting with only a portion of the abnormal protein.

Monoclonal IgE elevation leads to a short, thick arc in the antigen well area, extending to the anodal side.

Polyvalent and Monovalent Antisera
Polyvalent antiserum confirms the presence or absence of major protein fractions. *Monospecific antisera* for specific individual immunoglobulins identify only the corresponding proteins. If the nonspecific antisera have combining sites for H and L chains, the combining sites will react with L chains of other immunoglobulins or with the free L chains of BJ protein. H-chain–specific sera do not cross-react with other proteins.

IMMUNOFIXATION ELECTROPHORESIS

Immunofixation electrophoresis (IFE), or simply **immunofixation,** has replaced IEP in the evaluation of monoclonal gammopathies because of its rapidity and ease of interpretation. IFE is a two-stage procedure: (1) agarose gel protein electrophoresis and (2) immunoprecipitation. The test specimen may be serum, urine, cerebrospinal fluid (CSF), or other body fluids. The primary use of IFE in clinical laboratories is for the characterization of monoclonal immunoglobulins.

Clinical Applications
Although IFE was first described in 1964, it was introduced as a procedure for the study of immunoglobulins in 1976. IEP and IFE are complementary techniques best used in the workup of a patient with a suspected monoclonal gammopathy. The laboratory protocol for ruling out monoclonal gammopathy should include high-resolution electrophoresis, IEP of both serum and urine, and a quantitative immunoglobulin assay. These procedures are usually sufficient to detect and characterize monoclonal proteins with a serum concentration of 1 g or more.

The following three variables of protein can be determined using IFE:
1. Antigenic specificity
2. Electrophoretic mobility
3. Quantity or ratio of test and control proteins

Immunofixation Electrophoresis Procedure

Principle
Titan Gel ImmunofiFix is intended for the identification of monoclonal gammopathies in serum, urine, or CSF using high-resolution protein electrophoresis and immunofixation.

In the first step of the IFE procedure, a single specimen is applied to six different positions on an agarose plate, and the proteins are separated according to their net charge by electrophoresis. In the second phase, monospecific antisera are applied to five of the electrophoresis patterns: IgG, IgA, IgM, and κ and λ antisera. A protein fixative solution is applied to the sixth pattern to produce a complete protein reference pattern. The plate is incubated for 10 minutes.

If complementary antigen is present in the proper proportions in the test sample, antigen-antibody complexes form and precipitate. The formation of a stable antigen-antibody precipitate fixes the protein in the gel. After fixation, the gel is washed in deproteination solution (e.g., dilute NaCl), and nonprecipitated proteins are washed out of the agarose, leaving only the antigen-antibody complex. The protein reference pattern and the antigen-antibody precipitation bands are stained with a protein-sensitive stain.

Specimen Collection and Preparation
Fresh human serum, CSF, or urine is the specimens of choice. No special preparation of the patient is required before specimen collection. The patient must be positively identified when the specimen is collected, and the specimen should be labeled at the bedside. Specimen labels should include the patient's full name, the date, the patient's hospital identification number, and the phlebotomist's initials.

Blood should be drawn by aseptic technique. A minimum of 2 mL of clotted blood (red-top evacuated tube) is required. The specimen should be centrifuged promptly and an aliquot of serum removed. Hemolysis or contamination with bacteria renders a specimen unsuitable for testing.

Serum Preparation
1. Dilute serum 1:2 for the serum protein electrophoresis (SPE) reference pattern.
2. Dilute serum 1:10 for the immunofixation electrophoresis (IFE) pattern.

3. When typing mini–monoclonal specimens, if the sample IgG level exceeds 1500 mg/dL, the sample should be diluted 1:20 for the IgG slot only.
4. When typing IgM or λ proteins in specimens containing mini–monoclonal bands, a sample dilution of 1:5 is recommended for the IgM and λ patterns.

Urine Preparation
Detection of BJ proteins (free κ and λ L chains): if necessary, concentrate urine sample to 100 mg/dL of total protein.

Cerebrospinal Fluid Preparation
Concentrate CSF to an IgG level of 100 to 200 mg/dL for typing oligoclonal bands in CSF. Use concentrated specimen for all patterns.

Specimen Storage and Stability
If storage is necessary, serum, CSF, or urine samples may be stored covered at 2° to 6° C for up to 72 hours.

Reagents, Supplies, and Equipment
Reagents and supplies for gel electrophoresis are commercially available from Helena Laboratories, Beaumont, Texas.
- Titan Gel IFE gel
- Titan Gel IFE buffer
- Acid blue stain
- Tital Gel IFE protein fixative
- Antisera to human IgG, IgA, IgM, and κ and λ L chains

The Titan Gel ImmunoFix kit contains gels, buffer, stain, and fixative. In addition, the kit contains:
- Titan Gel IFE sample templates
- Titan Gel IFE antisera templates
- Titan Gel IFE antisera to human IgG, IgA, IgM, and λ and κ L chains; Titan Gel blotters A, C, D, and X

Other materials provided by Helena Laboratories, but not contained in the kit, include:
- ImmunoFix Controls
- Titan Gel IgD and IgE
- Microdispenser and tubes
- Electrophoresis chamber; incubator, oven, dryer (IOD)
- Digital power supply
- Titan Plus power supply
- Titan Gel isoenzyme incubation chamber
- 1000 Staining Set and Titan Rack
- Bufferizer bottoms with lids
- Titan carrying rack

Other Needed Supplies
- Glacial acetic acid
- Destaining solution: 5% acetic acid
- Saline (0.85%)
- Laboratory rotator

CAUTION: Because the control sera are derived from human sources, they should be handled in the same manner as clinical serum specimens (Standard Precautions; see Chapter 6).

WARNING: Sodium azide is used as a preservative.

Quality Control
The ImmunoFix Controls are recommended for use as qualitative controls for verification of the appropriate reactivity of the antisera. The control set contains three monoclonal proteins: IgG κ, IgA λ, and IgM.

Procedure
Part I: Protein Electrophoresis
A. Patient sample preparation.
  Dilute the patient serum samples with 0.85% saline as follows:
  - 1:2 for SPE pattern.
  - 1:10 for identification of all immunoglobulins (IgG, IgA, IgM, κ, λ).
  Note: If necessary, concentrate urine or CSF according to instructions (see Specimen Collection and Preparation).
B. Preparation of electrophoresis chamber.
  1. Dissolve one package of Titan Gel IFE buffer in 1500 mL deionized or distilled water. Mix well for complete dissolution of the buffer.
  2. Pour 40 mL of buffer into each of the inner sections of the Titan Gel chamber. Total buffer volume = 80 mL.
  3. Cover the chamber until ready to use to prevent evaporation.
C. Sample application.
  1. Remove the Titan Gel IFE gel from the protective packing, and discard the paper overlay.
  2. Gently blot the surface of the gel with the Titan Gel blotter C.
  3. Place the sample template on the gel so that the small hole, in the corner of the template, is positioned at the lower left, and the application slits align with the arrows on the gel edges. Proper placement of the template is with the slightly rough side of the slits away from the gel, ensuring uniform absorption of the sample. Apply slight fingertip pressure to the template, making sure there are no air bubbles between it and the gel.
  Note: When wearing protective gloves to perform step 3, place a blotter A over the template, and then apply fingertip pressure. The powder from the gloves can produce artifacts on the gel.
  4. Apply 3.0 μL of the appropriate serum sample dilution or concentrated urine or CSF to the template slits. When using a concentrated sample, apply the concentrate to every position across the gel.
  5. Wait 5 minutes after the last sample has been applied to allow the samples to diffuse into the agarose.
  6. After allowing the samples to absorb into the agarose, gently blot the template with Titan Gel blotter A to remove unabsorbed sample. Then carefully remove the template.
D. Electrophoresis of sample gel.
  1. Place the Titan Gel IFE gel in the inner sections of the electrophoresis chamber (agarose side up) with

the edges of the gel in the buffer. The application point should be on the cathodic (−) side. Two gels may be run per Titan Gel chamber. A maximum of four gels can be run on a Titan Plus power supply.

2. Place the cover on the Titan Gel chamber.
3. Electrophorese the gel at 120 volts for 20 minutes.

Note: An alternate procedure for electrophoresis is described in the package insert.

Part II: Immunofixation

1. Remove the electrophoresed gel from the chamber.
2. Place the gel in the Titan Gel isoenzyme incubator chamber, which has been lined with a damp blotter or filter paper, or return the gel to the protective plastic package. Be sure that the gel is laying flat against the wet blotter. If the gel maintains a bowed shape after removal from the electrophoresis chamber, moisten the blotter in the incubator chamber sufficiently to hold it flat.
3. Apply the IFE controls.
   a. Because the control wells are very small and may be filled with buffer after electrophoresis, blot them carefully with a blotter A to ensure that the wells will hold all control that is applied.
   b. Align the antisera template on the gel so that the slits in the template are aligned over the antisera application areas on the gel. Make sure that the template makes good contact with the agarose, using gentle fingertip pressure along the edges and over the channel dividers.
   c. Apply 2 μL of the controls to the appropriate wells.
   • IgG κ control is applied to both the "G" and "κ" wells.
   • IgA λ control is applied to the "A" and "λ" wells.
   • IgM control is applied to the "M" well only.
   d. Close the incubator chamber, and allow the controls to absorb into the agarose for 2½ minutes.
   e. Open the incubator chamber, and blot the wells with a blotter A to ensure that the excess unabsorbed control material does not float out of the well during antisera application, resulting in a poorly defined control ring.
4. Apply Titan Gel antisera and protein fixative. The antisera and fixative are packaged in dropper vials and can be applied directly to the gel from the vial. No pipetting is required. The IFE protein fixative is applied to the serum protein (SP) position of the gel to develop a complete protein pattern. To apply, squeeze the vial until a drop of antisera or fixative is hanging on the tip of the vial and touching the agarose. Maintain fingertip pressure on the vial, but do not continue to squeeze more antisera from the vial. Pull this drop down the ImmunoFix channel. The antisera (or fixative) will be quickly and evenly applied in this manner.
5. Incubate the gel for 10 minutes at room temperature (15°-30° C) in the closed incubator chamber.
6. Wash and press the gels to clear unprecipitated protein. Note that blotter X is used in the first pressing step and blotter D in the second pressing step. Blotter C is used in both pressing steps and is placed directly on the agarose.
   a. Remove the gel from the incubator chamber and rinse it in 0.85% saline, before removing the antisera template, by quickly dipping the gel in a small container of saline. The antisera template will wash off in the process. This washes excess antisera from the surface and thoroughly wets the surface of the gel.
   b. Remove the antisera template (usually washes off in the saline).
   c. Place one blotter C, wetted in saline, on the surface of the gel, followed by one blotter X.
   d. Place the gel with blotters on the top in the ImmunoSuperPress, tighten it, and press the gels for 5 minutes. Approximately 12 to 15 gels with blotters can be stacked in the press.
   e. Remove the gels from the press, discard the blotters, and place the gels in 0.85% saline for 4 minutes. A single gel can be washed by laying it in a shallow dish and covering it with 50 mL of saline. Up to 12 gels can be placed in the Titan carrying rack and washed in one dish. Place the gels in the wash dish so that they are in a horizontal position (rack must be rotated so that gels change from vertical to horizontal positioning). The Helena Bufferizer Bottom is an appropriately sized wash container to hold the gels in a horizontal position.
   f. Remove the gel(s) from the saline wash. Place one blotter C, wetted in saline, followed by one blotter D on each gel. Place the gels with blotters in the SuperPress for 1 minute.
   g. Remove the gels from the press, and discard the blotters. Dry the gel in a drying oven at 56° to 60° C for 1 minute or until the agarose is completely dry.
7. Stain the gel for 4 minutes in acid blue stain. Again, a single gel can be placed in a shallow staining dish, or 12 gels can be stained together in a 1000 Staining Dish and Titan Rack or Helena Bufferizer Bottom.
8. Place the gels in two washes of destain solution for 2 minutes each, or until the background is clear.
9. Place the gels in IOD at 56° to 60° C until the destain has evaporated and gels are completely dry (~2-4 minutes).
10. Observe the control wells for the presence of precipitin rings indicating appropriate reactivity in the antisera, and interpret results.

Note: The completed, stained, and dried immunofixation gel is stable for an indefinite period of time.

Reporting Results

The majority of monoclonal proteins migrate in the cathodic region of the protein pattern. Because of an abnormality, however, they may migrate anywhere within the globulin region on protein electrophoresis. The monoclonal protein band on the immunofixation pattern will occupy the same migration position and shape as the monoclonal band on the reference protein electrophoresis pattern. The abnormal protein is identified by the corresponding antiserum used.

Procedure Notes

Further testing is required if specimens contain a band on SPE suggestive of a monoclonal protein, but do not react with IgG, IgA, or IgM antisera.

Sources of Error

- Evaporation of uncovered specimens may cause inaccurate results.

- Plasma should not be used because the fibrinogen may adhere to the gel matrix and result in a band in all patterns across the gel.

Clinical Applications

See earlier text section.

Limitations

- Antigen excess will occur if there is not slight antibody excess or antigen-antibody equivalency at the site of precipitation. Antigen excess in IFE is usually caused by a very high level of the immunoglobulin in the patient sample. Dissolution of immunoprecipitation is mani-

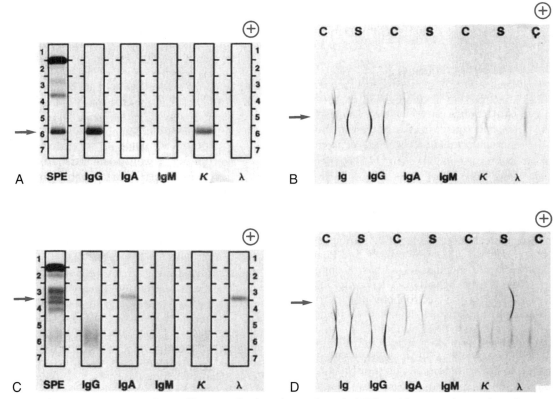

Figure 11-6 Comparison of immunofixation electrophoresis (IFE) and immunoelectrophoresis (IEP) for two patients with monoclonal gammopathies. **A,** Patient specimen with an IgG (κ) monoclonal protein, as identified by IFE. Note the position of monoclonal protein *(arrow)*. After electrophoresis, each track except serum protein electrophoresis *(SPE)* is reacted with its respective antiserum; then all tracks are stained to visualize the respective protein bands. Immunoglobulins G, A, and M *(IgG, IgA, IgM)*; kappa (κ); and lambda (λ) indicate antiserum used on each track. **B,** Same specimen as in *A*, with proteins identified by IEP. Note the position of monoclonal protein *(arrow)*. Normal control *(C)* and patient sera *(S)* are alternated. After electrophoresis, antiserum is added to each trough, as indicated by the labels *Ig, IgG, IgA, IgM, κ,* and λ. The antisera react with separated proteins in the specimens to form precipitates in the shape of arcs. The IgG and κ arcs are shorter and thicker than those in the normal control, showing the presence of the IgG (κ) monoclonal protein. The concentrations of IgA, IgM, and λ-light chains also are reduced. **C,** Patient specimen with an IgA (λ) monoclonal protein identified by the IFE procedure, as described in *A*. **D,** Same specimen as in *C*, with proteins identified by IEP, as described in *B*. The abnormal IgA and λ-arcs for the patient specimen indicate an elevated concentration of a monoclonal IgA (λ) protein. All separations were performed with the Beckman paragon system. *(From Burtis CA, Ashwood ER, Bruns DB: Tietz fundamentals of clinical chemistry, ed 6, St Louis, 2008, Saunders.)*

fested by a loss of protein at the point of highest antigen concentration, resulting in staining in the margins and leaving the central area with little demonstrable protein stain. If this occurs, it may be necessary to adjust the protein content of the sample by preparing a greater dilution than originally used.

Electrophoresing excessive amounts of antigen decreases resolution and requires higher concentrations of antibody. For optimum separation and sufficient intensity for visual detection, care must be taken in adjusting antibody content, sample concentration, time and voltage. The Titan Gel ImmunoFix method has been optimally developed to minimize the antigen excess phenomenon.

- Monoclonal proteins may occasionally adhere to the gel matrix, especially IgM. These bands will appear in all five antisera reaction areas of the gel. However, where the band reacts with the specific antisera for its H chain and L chain, there will be a marked increase in size and staining activity, allowing the band to be identified.
- The level of monoclonal protein in urine may not correlate well with the total protein quantitation.

Reference

Helena Laboratories catalog number 3046.

COMPARISON OF TECHNIQUES

Immunoelectrophoresis (IEP) is technically simpler and less subject to antigen excess phenomenon than immunofixation electrophoresis (IFE). If high concentrations of monoclonal protein with IFE give no visible reactions, IEP is considered to be a better technique for typing large monoclonal gammopathies.

Immunofixation electrophoresis can be optimized to give both greater sensitivity and resolution than IEP. IFE should be reserved for anomalous proteins, which are difficult to characterize by IEP. These include small bands, such as those exhibited in the early stages of monoclonal gammopathies or L-chain disease, and any multiple, closely spaced bands. IFE is easier to interpret than IEP because interpretation is based on examination of a precipitate pattern directly analogous to routine electrophoresis; IFE does not depend

on detecting slight deviations in the shape of a precipitin arc (Figure 11-6 and Table 11-1).

CAPILLARY ELECTROPHORESIS

In capillary electrophoresis (CE) the classic separation techniques of *zone electrophoresis, isotachophoresis, isoelectric focusing,* and *gel electrophoresis* are performed in a small-bore (10- to 100-μm), fused-silica capillary tubes 20 to 200 cm in length (Box 11-1). The CE method is efficient, sensitive, and rapid. High electrical field strengths are used to separate molecules based on differences in charge, size, and hydrophobicity. Sample introduction is accomplished by immersing the end of the capillary into a sample vial and applying pressure, vacuum, or voltage.

Microchip CE was developed in the early 1990s. The advantages of microchip CE include high speed, reduced reagent consumption, integration analysis, and miniaturization. The applications of microchip CE are diverse and include immune disorders.

Conventional CE revolutionized DNA analysis and was vital to the Human Genome Project. Microchip CE is still in the early stages of development, but it has demonstrated distinct advantages compared with traditional CE (Table 11-2).

Box 11-1	Separation Techniques Used in Capillary Electrophoresis (CE)

Capillary Zone Electrophoresis (CZE)
CZE is the most widely used type of CE because of its simplicity and versatility. As long as a molecule is charged, it can be separated by CZE. Also, CZE is simple to perform because the capillary is only filled with buffer. Separation occurs as solutes migrate at different velocities through the capillary. Another advantage of CZE is that it separates anions and cations in the same run, which is not done in other CE methods. However, CZE cannot separate neutral molecules.

Isotachophoresis (ITP)
ITP is a focusing technique based on the migration of the sample components between leading and terminating electrolytes. Solutes with mobilities intermediate to those of the leading and terminating electrolytes stack into sharp, focused zones. Although used as a mode of separation, transient ITP has been used primarily as a sample concentration technique.

Capillary Isoelectric Focusing (CIEF)
CIEF is a separation method that allows amphoteric molecules, such as proteins, to be separated by electrophoresis in a pH gradient generated between the cathode and anode. A solute will migrate to a point where its net charge is zero. At the solute's *isoelectric point* (pI), migration stops, and the sample is focused into a tight zone. In CIEF, once a solute has focused at its pI, the zone is mobilized past the detector by either pressure or chemical means. CIEF is often employed in protein characterization as a mechanism to determine a protein's pI.

Modified from www.chemsoc.org and www.beckmancoulter.com, November 2007.

Table 11-1	Comparison of Immunoelectrophoresis (IEP) and Immunofixation Electrophoresis (IFE)	
Characteristic	**IEP**	**IFE**
Ease of use	Easy	More complex
Sensitivity	Less sensitive	More sensitive
Monoclonal gammopathies	Better for typing large monoclonal gammopathies	Used for difficult-to-characterize anomalous proteins
Interpretation	Challenging	Easier

Table 11-2	Comparison of Traditional Capillary Electrophoresis (CE) and Microchip CE	
Characteristic	**Conventional CE**	**Microchip CE**
Separation channels	Mainly silica: single capillary or capillary array	Glass or polymer
Separation media	Buffers, gels, sieving polymers, microparticles	Buffers, sieving polymers, microparticles
Speed of analysis	Fast (typically minutes)	Very fast (typically seconds)
Integration	Difficult-to-connect capillaries	Easy-to-integrate multiple functions (e.g., PCR-CE)
Potential for growth	Relatively mature	Emerging technology with potential for new designs and applications

Modified from Li SFY, Kricka LJ: *Clin Chem* 52(1):42, 2006.
PCR, Polymerase chain reaction.

CHAPTER HIGHLIGHTS

- Serum electrophoresis results in the separation of proteins into five fractions on cellulose acetate based on the rate of migration of these individual components in an electrical field.
- Immunoelectrophoresis (IEP) involves the electrophoresis of serum or urine followed by immunodiffusion. Proteins are differentiated by electrophoretic mobility as well as by their diffusion coefficient and antibody specificity.
- Immunofixation electrophoresis (IFE) has two stages: agarose gel protein electrophoresis and immunoprecipitation.
- Capillary electrophoresis (CE) and microchip CE are important techniques in the study of various immunoglobulins.

REVIEW QUESTIONS

1. Protein can be separated into _____ fractions by use of serum electrophoresis.
   a. three
   b. four
   c. five
   d. six

2. Which of the following is the *most* common application of immunoelectrophoresis (IEP)?
   a. Identification of the absence of a normal serum protein.
   b. Structural abnormalities of proteins.
   c. Screening for circulating immune complexes.
   d. Diagnosis of monoclonal gammopathies.

3. Abnormalities of precipitin bands in an IEP assay can be evaluated by all the following features *except:*
   a. Position of the band between antigen well and antibody trough.
   b. Position of the band in relationship to electrophoretically identified protein fractions.
   c. General location of the band.
   d. Distortion of the arc formation.

4. Immunofixation electrophoresis (IFE) is best used in the:
   a. Workup of a polyclonal gammopathy.
   b. Workup of a monoclonal gammopathy.
   c. Screening for circulating immune complexes.
   d. Identification of hypercomplementemia.

Questions 5-9. Indicate true statements with the letter "A," and false statements with the letter "B."

5. _____ IEP is technically simpler and less subject to antigen excess phenomenon than IFE.

6. _____ IFE is considered to be a better technique than IEP for typing large monoclonal gammopathies.

7. _____ IFE can be optimized to give greater sensitivity and resolution than IEP.

8. _____ IFE should be reserved for anomalous proteins that are difficult to characterize by IEP.

9. _____ IEP is easier to interpret than IFE.

10. Immunoelectrophoresis (IEP) involves:
    a. Separation of proteins based on the rate of migration of individual components in an electrical field.
    b. Electrophoresis of serum or urine.
    c. Double immunodiffusion following electrophoresis.
    d. All the above.

11. In IEP, proteins are differentiated by:
    a. Electrophoresis.
    b. Diffusion coefficient.
    c. Antibody specificity.
    d. All the above.

12. IEP can divide the proteins of normal serum into _____ distinct precipitation bands.
    a. 5 to 10
    b. 15 to 20
    c. 25 to 40
    d. 45 to 100

13. IEP is useful for clinically detecting:
    a. Structural abnormalities.
    b. Concentration changes in proteins.
    c. Congenital deficiency of some complement components.
    d. All the above.

14. The most common application of IEP of serum is:
    a. Diagnosis of monoclonal gammopathy.
    b. Diagnosis of polyclonal gammopathy.
    c. Diagnosis of autoimmune hemolysis.
    d. Demonstration of Bence Jones (BJ) protein.

15. Immunofixation electrophoresis (IFE) can test:
    a. Serum and urine.
    b. Cerebrospinal fluid.
    c. Whole blood.
    d. Both a and b.

16. The primary use of IFE is:
    a. Characterization of monoclonal immunoglobulins.
    b. Characterization of polyclonal immunoglobulins.
    c. Identification of monoclonal immunoglobulins.
    d. Identification of polyclonal immunoglobulins.

RESOURCES
http://tinyurl.com

BIBLIOGRAPHY
Burtis CA, Ashwood ER, Bruns DB: *Tietz fundamentals of clinical chemistry,* ed 6, St Louis, 2008, Saunders.
Helena Laboratories: Protein electrophoresis and IFE and immunofixation for identification of monoclonal gammopathies, Educational Slide Series, www.helena.com, November 2007.
Kaplan LA, Pesce AJ, Kazmierczak SC: *Clinical chemistry,* ed 4, St Louis, 2003, Mosby.
Killingsworth LM, Warren BM: *Immunofixation for the identification of monoclonal gammopathies,* Beaumont, Texas, 1986, Helena Laboratories.
Li SFY, Kricka LJ: Clinical analysis by microchip capillary electrophoresis, *Clin Chem* 52(1):42, 2006.
Ritzmann EE: Immunoglobulin abnormalities. In Ritzman S, editor: *Serum protein abnormalities: diagnostic and clinical aspects,* Boston, 1976, Little, Brown.
Sun T: Immunofixation electrophoresis procedures. In *Protein abnormalities.* Vol 1. *Physiology of immunoglobulins: diagnostic and clinical aspects,* New York, 1982, Alan R Liss.

CHAPTER 12

Labeling Techniques in Immunoassay

Immunoassay Formats
Types of Labels
Enzyme Immunoassay
    Antigen Detection
    Antibody Detection
Autoimmune Enzyme Immunoassay ANA Screening Test
Chemiluminescence
    Specific Clinical Applications
Immunofluorescence
    Direct Immunofluorescent Assay
    Inhibition Immunofluorescent Assay
    Indirect Immunofluorescent Assay
Direct Fluorescent Antibody Test for *Neisseria gonorrhoeae*

Emerging Labeling Technologies
    Quantum Dots
    SQUID Technology
    Luminescent Oxygen-Channeling Immunoassay
    Signal Amplification Technology
    Magnetic Labeling Technology
    Time-Resolved Fluoroimmunoassay
    Fluorescence Polarization Immunoassay
    Fluorescence in Situ Hybridization
Chapter Highlights
Review Questions
Bibliography

Learning Objectives

At the conclusion of this chapter, the reader should be able to:

- Compare heterogeneous and homogeneous immunoassays.
- Name at least three types of labels that can be used in immunoassay.
- Describe chemiluminescence.
- Describe and compare chemiluminescence, enzyme immunoassay (EIA), and immunofluorescence techniques.

- Briefly compare direct immunofluorescent, inhibition immunofluorescent, and indirect immunofluorescent assays.
- Describe the advantages, disadvantages, and application of Q dots, SQUID technology, luminescent oxygen-channeling immunoassay, fluorescent in situ hybridization, signal amplification technology, and magnetic labeling technology.

IMMUNOASSAY FORMATS

Immunoassays can be divided into heterogeneous and homogeneous immunoassays.

Heterogeneous immunoassays involve a solid phase (microwell, bead) and require washing steps to remove unbound antigens or antibodies. Heterogeneous immunoassays can have a competitive or a noncompetitive format.

Homogeneous immunoassays consists of only a liquid phase and do not require washing steps. Homogeneous immunoassays are faster and easier to automate than heterogeneous immunoassays. In addition, homogeneous immunoassays have competitive formats.

TYPES OF LABELS

The principles and applications of enzyme immunoassays, chemiluminescence, and fluorescent substances as labels are presented in this chapter (Table 12-1).

The original technique of using antigen-coated cells or particles in agglutination techniques may be considered the earliest method for labeling components in immunoassays. Ideal characteristics of a *label* include the quality of being measurable by several methods, including visual inspection. The properties of a label used in an immunoassay

determine the ways in which detection is possible. For example, coated latex particles can be detected by various methods: visual inspection, light scattering (nephelometry), and particle counting. The conversion of a colorless substrate into a colored product in enzyme immunoassay allows for two methods of detection, colorimetry and visual inspection.

Yalow and Berson developed the **radioimmunoassay (RIA)** method in 1959, using a radioactive label that could identify an immunocomponent at very low concentrations. In the 1960s, researchers began to search for a substitute for the successful RIA method because of the inherent drawbacks of using radioactive isotopes as labels (e.g., radioactive waste, short shelf life). Currently, chemiluminescent reactions have replaced most RIAs in the clinical laboratory. Relatively simple and cost-effective, chemiluminescence technology has sensitivity at least as good as RIA.

ENZYME IMMUNOASSAY

There are two general approaches to diagnosing diseases or conditions by immunoassay: testing for specific antigens or testing for antigen-specific antibodies. **Enzyme-linked immunosorbent assay (ELISA),** also known as **enzyme**

Table 12-1 Examples of Immunoassay Types

Type	Antibody	Comments
Enzyme immunoassay (EIA; enzyme-linked immunosorbent assay, ELISA)	Enzyme-labeled antibody (e.g., horseradish peroxidase)	Competitive ELISA Noncompetitive (e.g., direct ELISA, indirect ELISA)
Chemiluminescence	Chemiluminescent molecule–labeled antibody (e.g., isoluminol or acridinium ester labels)	Competitive or sandwich immunoassay
Electrochemiluminescence	Electrochemiluminescent molecule–labeled antibody (e.g., ruthenium label)	—
Fluoroimmunoassay	Fluorescent molecule–labeled antigen (e.g., europium or fluorescein label)	Heterogeneous (e.g., time-resolved immunofluoroassay) Homogeneous (e.g., fluorescence polarization immunoassay)

immunoassay (EIA), is designed to detect antigens or antibodies by producing an enzyme-triggered color change.

The EIA method uses a nonisotopic label that offers the advantage of safety. EIA is usually an objective measurement that provides numerical results. Some EIA procedures provide diagnostic information and measure immune status (e.g., detect either total antibody IgM or IgG).

The EIA method uses the catalytic properties of enzymes to detect and quantitate immunologic reactions. An enzyme-labeled antibody or enzyme-labeled antigen conjugate is used in immunologic assays (Box 12-1). The enzyme with its substrate detects the presence and quantity of antigen or antibody in a patient specimen. In some tissues an enzyme-labeled antibody can identify antigenic locations.

Various enzymes are used in enzyme immunoassay (Table 12-2). Common enzyme labels are horseradish peroxidase, alkaline phosphatase, glucose-6-phosphate dehydrogenase,

Table 12-2 Enzymes Used in Enzyme Immunoassay

Enzyme	Source
Acetylcholinesterase	*Electrophorous electicus*
Alkaline phosphatase	*Escherichia coli*
β-Galactosidase	*Escherichia coli*
Glucose oxidase	*Aspergillus niger*
Glucose-6-phosphate dehydrogenase (G6PD)	*Leuconostoc mesenteroides*
Lysozyme	Egg white
Malate dehydrogenase	Pig heart
Peroxidase	Horseradish

and beta-galactosidase. To be used in EIA, an enzyme must fulfill the following criteria:
- High degree of stability
- Extreme specificity
- Absence from the antigen or antibody
- No alteration by inhibitor within the system

In a representative EIA test, a plastic bead or plastic plate is coated with antigen (e.g., virus) (Figure 12-1). The antigen reacts with antibody in the patient serum. The bead or plate is then incubated with an enzyme-labeled antibody conjugate. If antibody is present, the conjugate reacts with the antigen-antibody complex on the bead or plate. The enzyme activity is measured spectrophotometrically after the addition of the specific chromogenic substrate. For example, peroxidase cleaves its substrate, o-dianisidine, causing a color change. In some cases the test can be read subjectively.

The results of a typical test are calculated by comparing the spectrophotometric reading of patient serum to that of a control or reference serum. The advantage of an objective enzyme test is that results are not dependent on a technician's interpretations. In general, the EIA procedure is faster and requires less laboratory work than comparable methods (see Autoimmune Enzyme Immunoassay ANA Screening Test).

Antigen Detection

The EIAs for antigen detection (e.g., hepatitis B surface antigen [HBsAg]) have four steps. Antigen-specific antibody is attached a solid-phase surface (e.g., plastic beads). Patient

Box 12-1 Examples of Enzyme Immunoassays

Borrelia burgdorferi (IgG and IgM)
Cytomegalovirus (IgG and IgM)
Cytomegalovirus (Ag)
Hepatitis A virus (total Ab)
Hepatitis B virus (HBV)
  Anti-HBs
  Anti-HBc
  Anti-HBe
  Anti-HBc (IgM)
  HBs Ag
  HBe Ag
Hepatitis delta virus (total Ab)
HIV Ab
HIV Ag
HTLV I Ab
HTLV-II Ab
Human B-lymphotropic virus Ab
Rubella virus (IgG and IgM)
Toxoplasma gondii (IgG and IgM)

Ig, Immunoglobulin; *Ab*, antibody; *Ag*, antigen; *HIV*, human immunodeficiency virus; *HTLV*, human T-lymphotropic (leukemia/lymphoma) virus.

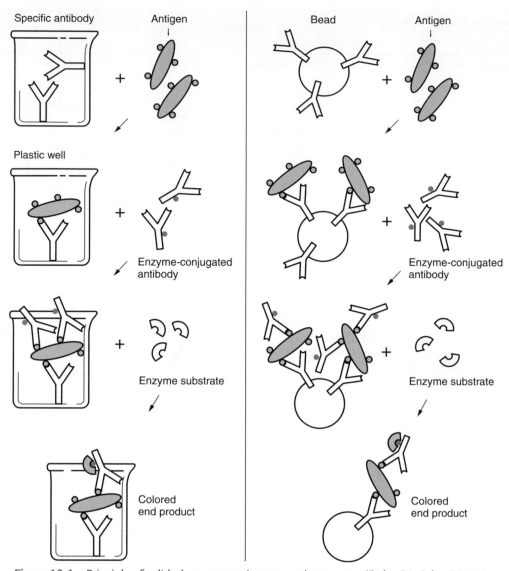

Figure 12-1 Principle of solid-phase enzyme immunosorbent assay. *(Forbes BA, Sahm DF, Weissfeld AS:* Bailey and Scott's diagnostic microbiology, *ed 12, St Louis, 2007, Mosby.)*

serum that may contain the antigen is added. Next, an enzyme-labeled antibody specific to the antigen **(conjugate)** is added. Finally, chromogenic substrate is added, which changes color in the presence of the enzyme. The amount of color that develops is proportional to the amount of antigen in the patient specimen.

Antibody Detection

There are three types of EIAs for antibody detection: noncompetitive, competitive, and capture.

Noncompetitive EIA takes place when a specific antigen is attached to a solid-phase surface, such as a plastic bead or microtiter well. Patient serum that could contain antibody (e.g., CMV IgG, HIV antibody) is added to the solid-phase surface, followed by an enzyme-labeled antibody specific to the test antibody. The added chromogenic substrate changes color if the enzyme is present. The amount of color that de-

velops is proportional to the amount of antibody in the patient serum.

Competitive EIA involves using a solid-phase surface to which specific antigen is attached. Patient serum potentially containing antibody (e.g., hepatitis B core antibody) and an enzyme-labeled antibody specific to the test antibody (conjugate) are mixed. Chromogenic substrate is then added, which changes color in the presence of the enzyme. The amount of color that develops is inversely proportional to the amount of antibody in the patient serum.

Capture EIA is designed to detect a specific type of antibody, such as immunoglobulin M (IgM) or IgG, cytomegalovirus (CMV) IgM, rubella IgM, or *Toxoplasma* IgM. Antibody specific for IgM or IgG is attached to a solid-phase surface (plastic bead, microtiter well). The patient specimen potentially containing IgM or IgG is added. Specific antigen is then added. Finally, chromogenic substrate is added, which in the presence of the enzyme, changes color. The amount of color that develops is proportional to the amount of antigen-specific IgM or IgG in the patient serum.

Autoimmune Enzyme Immunoassay ANA Screening Test*

Principle

Purified antigens (dsDNA, histones, SS-A/Ro, SS-B/La, Sm, Smrnp, Scl-70, Jo-1, centromere and other antigens extracted from Hep-2 nucleus) are bound to microwells. Antibodies to these antigens, if present in diluted serum, bind in the microwells (*ANA*, antinuclear antibody). Washing of the microwells removes unbound serum antibodies. Horseradish peroxidase–conjugated antihuman IgG immunologically binds to the bound patient antibodies, forming a "conjugate-antibody-antigen" sandwich. Washing of the microwells removes unbound conjugate. An enzyme substrate in the presence of bound conjugate hydrolyzes to form a blue color. The addition of an acid stops the reaction, forming a yellow end product. The intensity of the color is measured photometrically at 450 nm.

Specimen Collection and Preparation

No special preparation of the patient is required before specimen collection. The patient must be positively identified when the specimen is collected, and the specimen is labeled at the bedside. Specimen labels must include the patient's full name, the date the specimen is collected, the patient's hospital identification number, and the phlebotomist's initials.

Blood should be drawn by aseptic technique. A minimum of 2 mL of clotted blood (red-top evacuated tube) is required. The specimen should be centrifuged promptly and the serum removed.

Store the serum at 2° to 8° C. Freeze serum at −20° C if not tested within 24 hours.

The Clinical and Laboratory Standards Institute (CLSI) advises that the specimen should *not* be frozen in a frost-free freezer because the freeze-thaw cycle may be detrimental to serum proteins.

Serum should not be heat inactivated because this may cause false-positive results.

Reagents, Supplies and Equipment

• EIA ANA Screening Test Kit (Bio-Rad, Hercules, Calif).
Note: All kit components should be stored at 2° to 8° C and can be used until the expiration date printed on the labels.

Reagents

• ANA Screening Test microplate: nuclear antigen–coated wells, sealed in resealable foil pouch with desiccant.
   Store at 2° to 8° C. Do not open pouch until it reaches room temperature.

After removing the required number of wells, return the unused wells immediately to the resealable pouch with dessicant.
• Wash concentrate (16.7×)

Wash Solution Preparation
1. Empty contents of wash concentrate bottle, including any crystals, into a 1-L bottle.
2. If any crystals remain in the bottle, remove by adding some deionized water to the bottle; mix, and pour all contents into the 1-L bottle.
3. Add deionized water to the 1-L bottle to bring the final volume of the solution to 1 L.
4. Insert a magnetic stir bar into the 1-L bottle, and place on a stir plate. Stir the diluted wash solution for a few minutes until all crystals are dissolved. If no stir plate is available, cover the top of the wash solution container, and gently invert back and forth until the crystals are dissolved. Avoid excessive bubbles.
Note: Diluted wash solution is stable for 14 days when stored at 2° to 8° C.
• Sample diluent (ready to use)
   Allow to reach room temperature before use.
• Conjugate
• ANA Screening Test positive control
• Negative control
• Substrate
• Stop solution

Additional Required Items
• EIA frame
• EIA reader (set to 450nm)
• Micropipettors (10 and 100 μL)
• 8-channel repeating pipettor (for washing)
• Deionized water
• Pipettes (1 and 10 mL)
• Graduated cylinder (for wash solution)
• Test tubes (4 and 15 mL)
• Countdown timer

Recommended Items
• Automatic washer
• 100-μL 8-channel micropipettor (for reagent delivery)
• 1-mL minitubes (for sample dilutions)

Quality Control

An ANA positive control, ANA cutoff control, and sample diluent blank must be included with each test run.
• The values for each control must be within the specified range printed on the quality control card included with each kit lot number.
• The results must be as expected for the patient results to be valid.
• The sample diluent optical density (OD) must be ≤ 0.200 or less when zeroed against air.

*Modified from Bio-Rad Autoimmune EIA ANA Screening Test.

If any of these criteria is not met, the results are invalid, and the test should be repeated.

Procedure

1. Collect all reagents, samples, and dilutions necessary before starting the assay.
2. Assign and record wells for controls and samples.
3. Prepared 1:40 working solutions.
   a. Dilute 10 μL of patient serum in 0.4 mL of sample diluent.
   b. Dilute 10 μL of ANA positive control in 0.4 mL of sample diluent.
   c. Dilute 10 μL of ANA cutoff control in 0.4 mL of sample diluent.
   d. Dilute 10 μL of negative control in 0.4 mL of sample diluent.

Note: Discard working solutions after use.

4. Apply diluted samples and controls to wells.
   a. *Controls:* Apply 10 μL of diluted controls (1:40 in sample diluent) to assigned wells.
   b. Add 100 μL of sample diluent as a blank control.
   c. *Patient samples:* Apply 10 μL of diluted patient serum (1:40 in sample diluent) to assigned wells.
5. Incubate wells. Shake plate gently, then incubate for 30 minutes at room temperature (18°-27° C). Do not incubate for more than 40 minutes.
6. Discard incubated samples. After 30 minutes of incubation, discard samples by inverting plate and rapidly flicking the liquid away from the plate.
7. Wash wells. Gently fill five times with approximately 200 μL of wash solution, and discard. Remove all liquid before proceeding.
8. Apply conjugate. Add 100 μL of conjugate to all wells. Discard excess transferred conjugate after use.
9. Incubate wells. Shake plate gently, then incubate for 30 minutes at room temperature (18°-27° C). Do not incubate for more than 40 minutes.
10. Discard incubated conjugate. After 30 minutes of incubation, discard conjugate by inverting plate and rapidly flicking the liquid away from the plate.
11. Wash wells. Gently fill five times with approximately 200 μL of wash solution, and discard. Remove all liquid before proceeding.
12. Develop color. Add 100 μL of substrate to each well. Discard excess transferred substrate after use.
13. Incubate. Shake or tap plate gently to disperse color. Incubate for 30 minutes at room temperature (18°-27°C).
14. Stop color development. After 30 minutes of color development, add 100 μL of stop solution to each well to stop the color development.
15. Read results. Read wells within 30 minutes with an EIA reader set to 450 nm. Zero the reader on the sample diluent blanking control well, then read the color of the control and patient wells.
   a. The ANA positive control well should show yellow color.
   b. The ANA cutoff control well should show yellow color.
   c. The negative control well should show moderate color.
   d. The sample diluent blanking control well should show little or no color.

Reporting Results

Negative: <20 EU (index <0.8)
Borderline positive: 20-25 EU (index 0.8-1.0)
Positive: >25 (index >1.0)

Note: Enzyme units (EUs) are semiquantitative index variables defined by Bio-Rad Laboratories.

Procedure Notes

1. All kit components must be at room temperature.
2. Do not use cutoff or controls from different kit lots. Do not use expired reagents.
3. Avoid contamination of reagents, pipettes, and wells. Keep bottle capped when not in use. Do not reuse wells or pipettes.
4. All wells should be handled in the same sequence and the same manner throughout the test. The test should be performed without interruption.
5. Gently and completely swirl each bottle of liquid reagent and sample before use.
6. Make reliable 1:40 dilutions.
7. Always run an ANA positive control, an ANA cutoff control, and a negative control. Always blank against sample diluent.
8. Do not allow controls, samples, or conjugate to incubate in the strip wells for more than 40 minutes.
9. Thoroughly wash the microtiter wells after each incubation. Remove all liquid before proceeding to the next step. Fill wells, then invert and rapidly flick away the liquid. After complete washing, blot the plate on a paper towel.
10. Transfer to a graduated test tube 1 mL of conjugate for each strip to be run. Discard excess transferred conjugate.
11. Transfer to a graduated test tube 1 mL of substrate for each strip to be run. Discard excess transferred substrate.

Precautions and Warnings

1. Avoid contact with skin and eyes with acidic stop solution. Clean up spills immediately.
2. Although this product uses human serum screened for infectious diseases in cutoff and controls, Standard Precautions must be used.
3. All safety practices described in Chapter 6 need to be followed.
4. Do not use kit beyond its expiration date. The date is printed on kit boxes.
5. Adhere to the protocol specified in the product instruction manual to ensure proper performance of the product.

6. Never mix the contents from different bottles of the same reagent.
7. Use kit components at room temperature.
8. Do not interchange reagents between kit lots.

Clinical Applications

Antinuclear antibodies (ANAs) directed against a variety of macromolecules occur in extraordinarily high frequency in systemic rheumatic disease. Many rheumatic diseases are characterized by the presence of one or more ANAs. The identification of the specific antibody is useful in the detection and diagnosis of the disease.

Reference

Bio-Rad Autoimmune EIA ANA Screening Test, November 2003.

CHEMILUMINESCENCE

Chemiluminescence refers to light emission produced during a chemical reaction and is used extensively in automated immunoassay (see Chapter 13). This methodology has excellent sensitivity and dynamic range. It does not require sample radiation, and nonselective excitation and source instability are eliminated. Most chemiluminescent reagents and conjugates are stable and relatively nontoxic.

In immunoassays, chemiluminescent labels can be attached to an antigen or an antibody. Acridinium esters are highly specific activity labels that can be used to label both antibodies and haptens. Chemiluminescent labels are being used to detect proteins, viruses, oligonucleotides, and genomic nucleic acid sequences in immunoassay. Two formats are used: competitive and sandwich immunoassays.

In a **competitive immunoassay** a fixed amount of labeled antigen competes with unlabeled antigen from a patient specimen for a limited number of antibody-binding sites (Figure 12-2). The amount of light emitted is inversely proportional to the amount of analyte (antigen) measured.

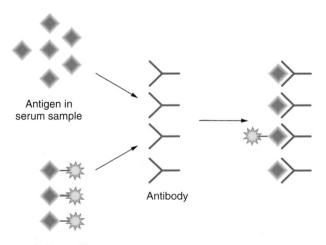

Antigen in serum sample

Antibody

Antigen with chemiluminescent label

Figure 12-2 Format for competitive immunoassays. *(Redrawn from Jandreski MA: Lab Med 29[9]:557, 1998.)*

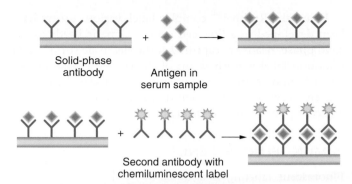

Solid-phase antibody

Antigen in serum sample

Second antibody with chemiluminescent label

Figure 12-3 Format for sandwich immunoassays. *(Redrawn from Jandreski MA: Lab Med 29[9]:557, 1998.)*

In a **sandwich immunoassay** the sample antigen binds to an antibody fixed onto a solid phase; a second antibody, labeled with a chemiluminescent label, binds to the antigen-antibody complex on the solid phase (Figure 12-3). In the sandwich assay the emitted light is directly proportional to the analyte concentration. The detection device for analyses is a simple photomultiplier tube used to detect the emitted light.

Chemiluminescent labels can be divided into five major groups: (1) luminol (2) acridinium esters, (3) peroxyoxalates, (4) dioxetanes, and (5) tris(2,2′bipyridyl)-ruthenium (II).

The direct labels include luminol, acridinium ester, and electrogenerated luminescent chelate from ruthenium and tripropylamine (TPA) complex $[Ru(bpy)^{3+}]$. These labels are attached directly to antigens, antibodies, or deoxyribonucleic acid (DNA) probes, depending on the assay format.

Oxidation of isoluminol by hydrogen peroxide (H_2O_2) in the presence of a catalyst (e.g., microperoxidase) produces a relatively long-lived emission at 425 nm. Oxidation of acridinium ester by alkaline H_2O_2 in the presence of detergent produces a rapid flash of light lasting from 1 to 5 seconds at 429 nm. Peak intensity can be used for the measurement. An alternate method is to use an integrator to measure the entire light output for greater sensitivity.

Enzymes are typically used for indirect labels. *Indirect* labels are attached to antibodies, antigens, and DNA probes, depending on the assay format. Enzyme labels often used in indirect procedures include the following:
- Alkaline phosphatase (ALP)
- Horseradish peroxidase (HRP)
- Beta-galactosidase (β-galactosidase)

An interesting label is native or recombinant *apoaequorin* (from the bioluminescent jellyfish, *Aequoria*). It is activated by reaction with coelenterazine. Light emission at 469 nm is triggered by reaction with calcium chloride.

Specific Clinical Applications

One of many clinical applications of chemiluminescence is a third-generation serum IgE (sIgE) method (ImmunoLite 2000, Diagnostic Products) that is a solid-phase (bead), two-step chemiluminescent EIA. Allergens are covalently lined to a soluble polymer–ligand matrix, allowing immunochemical reactions to occur in liquid phases for random-access automation.

Using the Ru(bpy)$^{3+}$ complex label, various assays have been developed in a flow cell using magnetic beads as the solid phase. Beads are captured at the electrode surface, and unbound label is washed out of the cell by a wash buffer. Label bound to the bead undergoes an electrochemiluminescent reaction, and the emitted light is measured by an adjacent photomultiplier tube.

IMMUNOFLUORESCENCE

Fluorescent labeling is another method used to demonstrate the complexing of antigens and antibodies (Figure 12-4). Fluorescent molecules are used as substitutes for radioisotope or enzyme labels. The fluorescent antibody technique consists of labeling antibody with fluorescein isothiocyanate (FITC), a fluorescent compound with an affinity for proteins, to form a complex (conjugate). This conjugate is able to react with antibody-specific antigen.

Fluorescent techniques are extremely specific and sensitive. Antibodies may be conjugated to other markers in addition to fluorescent dyes; the use of these markers is called colorimetric immunologic probe detection. The use of enzyme-substrate marker systems has been expanded. HRP, ALP, and avidin-biotin conjugated enzyme labels have all been used as visual tags for the presence of antibody. These reagents have the advantage of requiring only a standard light microscope.

Fluorescent conjugates are used in the following popular basic methods:

- Direct immunofluorescent assay
- Inhibition immunofluorescent assay
- Indirect immunofluorescent assay

Direct Immunofluorescent Assay

In the **direct fluorescent antibody (DFA)** technique a conjugated antibody is used to detect antigen-antibody reactions at a microscopic level (Figure 12-5). DFA can be applied to tissue sections or in smears for microorganisms (Plate 2).

Fluorescein-conjugated antibodies bound to the fluorochrome FITC are used to visualize many bacteria in direct specimens (see Direct Fluorescent Antibody Test for *Neisseria gonorrhoeae*). HRP conjugated to antibody, the immunoperoxidase stain, can be used to detect cytomegalovirus (CMV), other viruses, or nucleic acids in cells. In biotin-avidin, enzyme-conjugated methods, single-stranded nucleic

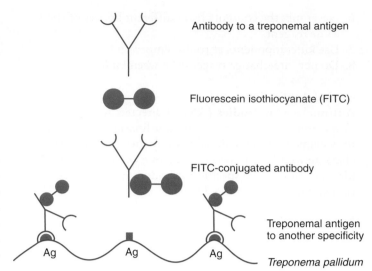

Figure 12-5 Direct fluorescent antibody (DFA) technique. After the labeling of a specific antibody with FITC, it can be reacted with its antigen and identified microscopically.

acid probes, antimicrobial antibodies, or antibiotin antibodies can be bound to the small molecule *biotin*. These molecules have a strong affinity for the protein *avidin*, which has four binding sites. Biotin bound to avidin or antibody can be complexed to fluorescent dyes or to color-producing enzymes to form specific detector systems. This system can be applied to the detection of nucleic acids in organisms such as CMV, hepatitis B virus (HBV), Epstein-Barr virus (EBV), and *Chlamydia*.

The chemical manipulation in labeling antibodies with fluorescent dyes to permit detection by direct microscopic examination does not seriously impair antibody activity (i.e., ability of fluorescent antibody conjugate to react specifically with its homologous antigen). Monoclonal antibodies (MAbs) have also been successfully conjugated to fluorescein for the detection of chlamydiae, rabies virus, and other pathogens in directly stained specimens.

When absorbing light of one wavelength, a fluorescent substance emits light of another (longer) wavelength. In **fluorescent antibody (FA)** microscopy, the incident or exciting light is often blue-green to ultraviolet. The light is provided by a high-pressure mercury arc lamp with a primary (e.g., blue-violet) filter between the lamp and the object that passes only fluorescein-exciting wavelengths. The color of the emitted light depends on the nature of the substance. Fluorescein gives off yellow-green light, and the rhodamines fluoresce in the red portion of the spectrum. The color observed in the fluorescent microscope depends on the secondary or barrier filter used in the eyepiece. A yellow filter absorbs the green fluorescence of fluorescein and transmits only yellow. Fluorescein fluoresces an intense apple-green color when excited.

Inhibition Immunofluorescent Assay

The inhibition immunofluorescent assay is a blocking test in which an antigen is first exposed to unlabeled antibody, then to labeled antibody, and is finally washed and examined. If the unlabeled and labeled antibodies are both ho-

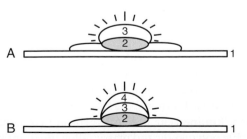

Figure 12-4 Principles of direct and indirect fluorescent techniques. **A,** Direct fluorescence. **B,** Indirect fluorescence. *1,* Microscopic slide; *2,* cell (cytoplasm and nucleus); *3,* antiserum (conjugate in *A,* unconjugate in *B*); *4,* conjugated antiglobulin serum.

mologous to the antigen, there should be no fluorescence. This result confirms the specificity of the FA technique. Antibody in an unknown serum can also be detected and identified by the inhibition test.

Indirect Immunofluorescent Assay

The basis for **indirect fluorescent assay (IFA)** is that antibodies (immunoglobulins) not only react with homologous antigens, but also can act as antigens and react with anti-immunoglobulins (Box 12-2).

The serologic method most widely used for the detection of diverse antibodies is the indirect immunofluorescent assay (IFA). Immunofluorescence is used extensively in the detection of autoantibodies and antibodies to tissue and cellular antigens. For example, antinuclear antibodies (ANAs)—a heterogeneous group of circulating immunoglobulins that react with the whole nucleus or nuclear components (e.g., nuclear proteins, DNA, histones) in host tissues—are frequently assayed by indirect fluorescence. By using tissue sections that contain a large number of antigens, it is possible to identify antibodies to several different antigens in a single test. The antigens are differentiated according to their different staining patterns.

Immunofluorescence can also be used to identify specific antigens on live cells in suspension (i.e., flow cytometry). When a live, stained-cell suspension is put through a fluorescence-activated cell sorter (FACS), which measures its fluorescent intensity, the cells are separated according to their particular fluorescent brightness. This technique permits the isolation of different cell populations with differ-

ent surface antigens (e.g., CD4+ and CD8+ lymphocytes) (see Chapter 4).

In the IFA the antigen source (e.g., whole *Toxoplasma* microorganism, virus in infected tissue culture cells) to the specific antibody being tested is affixed to the surface of a microscope slide. The patient's serum is diluted and placed on the slide to cover the antigen source. If antibody is present in the serum, it will bind to its specific antigen. Unbound antibody is then removed by washing the slide. In the second phase, antihuman globulin (AHG, directed specifically against IgM or IgG) conjugated to a fluorescent substance that will fluoresce when exposed to ultraviolet light is placed on the slide. This conjugated marker for human antibody will bind to the antibody already bound to the antigen on the slide and will serve as a marker for the antibody when viewed under a fluorescent microscope.

A major problem in interpreting IFA results is background staining. For most IFAs, laboratories must choose a screening dilution because undiluted specimens will show background staining resulting from nonspecific binding or clinically insignificant levels of circulating autoantibodies. The screening dilution plays a critical role: the more dilute the specimen becomes, the less sensitive but more specific the procedure.

An example of a changing clinical situation is that many laboratories have replaced indirect immunofluorescence, once the standard for ANA testing, with the enzyme immunoassay. Less labor and technical experience are cited as reasons for switching away from indirect immunofluorescence. However, the trade-off may not be valuable if patients have antibody titers of less than 1:160.

Box 12-2	Examples of Immunologic Assays Performed by Indirect Fluorescent Antibody (IFA) Technique

Antiadrenal antibodies
Antibody (HR-ANA)
Anticentriole antibodies
Anticentromere antibodies
Anti–glomerular basement membrane antibodies
Anti–islet cell antibodies
Anti–liver-kidney microsomal (LKM) antibodies
Antimitochondrial
Antimyelin
Antimyocardial
Antinuclear antibody
Anti–parietal cell
Antiplatelet
Antireticulin
Antiribosome
Antiskin (dermal-epidermal)
Antiskin (interepithelial)
Anti–smooth muscle
Antistriational
Cytomegalovirus (IgM antibody)
Histone-reactive antinuclear antibody (HR-ANA)
Human immunodeficiency virus (total and IgM antibody)
Immunoglobulin M (IgM) antibodies (antigen specific)
Lymphocyte typing
Rubella virus antibody
Toxoplasma gondii antibody

Direct Fluorescent Antibody Test for *Neisseria gonorrhoeae*

Principle

Immunofluorescence is a reliable, simple, rapid test used extensively in the clinical laboratory. The demonstration of microbial antigens is one of the many applications of the direct immunofluorescence procedure; the microbes are incubated with fluorescent-labeled antibodies. Under appropriate conditions, the labeled antibodies bind to specific antigens. Any unbound antibodies are washed off, and the bound antibodies are visualized with a fluorescence microscope.

Neisseria gonorrhoeae is a gram-negative diplococcus that causes urogenital infections. The Syva Microtrak *N. gonorrhoeae* culture confirmation test is a direct fluorescent antibody (FA) assay that uses fluorescein-labeled MAbs that react specifically with *N. gonorrhoeae*. The test is performed on primary culture isolates and requires only a small inoculum. Culture isolates presumptively identified as *N. gonorrhoeae* are transferred to a slide well and stained with fluorescein-labeled anti–*N. gonorrhoeae* reagent antibody (anti-GC/FITC). The antibodies bind specifically to gonococcal antigen. Unbound antibodies are then removed by a rinse step. Under a fluorescence microscope, cultures positive for *N. gonorrhoeae* show apple-green fluorescent staining of the kidney-shaped diplococci.

Procedure

1. You have been given a prepared slide. To prepare this slide, a small inoculum of the presumptive *Neisseria* (gram-negative diplococcus) was emulsified in distilled water, allowed to air-dry, and heat-fixed.
2. Place 30 μL of anti-GC/FITC in each slide well, making sure the entire area of each well is covered.
   Note: If necessary, spread the anti-GC/FITC over the well with the picture tip, taking care not to disturb the fixed specimen.
3. Incubate the slides for 15 minutes at 37° C in a moist chamber. Do not allow the anti-GC/FITC to dry on the slide.
4. Promptly remove the slide from incubation at 15 minutes.
5. Remove the excess anti-GC/FITC without disturbing the smear.
6. Rinse the slide for 5 to 10 seconds with a gentle stream of distilled water from a wash bottle. Hold the slide at a 45-degree angle, and aim the stream of water at the slide surface above the well. Direct a gentle but continuous stream of water back and forth so that the water flows down over the well.
7. Gently shake off the excess water, and thoroughly air-dry the smear.
8. Add a drop of mounting fluid to the slide well. Place a coverslip on the drop, and remove all air bubbles.
9. Immediately after staining, read the slide using a fluorescence microscope (oil-immersion objective ×100). Scan the entire well for fluorescent apple-green–stained kidney-shaped diplococci.

Reporting Results

Positive and negative controls are available to check before reading patient slides.

Positive Results

Positive diagnosis is made when intact, typical diplococci displaying medium to bright fluorescent staining are identified in a fixed, stained smear. Use the appearance of control slides to aid in evaluating patient specimens.

Final report: *Neisseria gonorrhoeae* present.

Negative Results

Negative results are reported when fixed, stained slides are free of characteristic fluorescent staining. The outline of bacterial cells or other cellular material should be visible but will appear nonfluorescent. If no cellular material is visible on the slide, prepare a new smear from the same colonies.

Final report: negative for *Neisseria gonorrhoeae*.

Procedure Notes

Sources of Error

- Thick bacterial smears will not stain adequately. Clumps of bacteria may trap stain and cause misinterpretation. Always prepare a very thin bacterial smear.
- Ensure that smears are completely air-dried before heat fixing. Failure to do so will cause poor fluorescent staining or distortion of cellular morphology.
- Do not overheat specimens during fixation. Overheating will denature the protein, distort morphology, reduce fluorescence intensity, and produce uninterpretable results.

Limitations

Only gram-negative, oxidase-positive diplococci should be tested. If colonies selected for testing show the presence of gram-positive cocci mixed with gram-negative diplococci, obtain a culture that contains only gram-negative diplococci.

Clinical Applications

The direct FA test for *N. gonorrhoeae* is of confirmatory diagnostic value in cases of gonococcal infections. This test allows quick, reliable confirmation of presumptive *N. gonorrhoeae* isolates, eliminating the need for 72-hour carbohydrate utilization testing.

EMERGING LABELING TECHNOLOGIES

Quantum Dots (Q dots)

An advanced labeling technique, quantum dots are semiconductor nanocrystals that are used as fluorescent labeling reagents for biologic imaging. A valuable property of Q dots is that different sizes of crystals produce different signals with a single laser excitation. This seemingly simple physical property implies that different-size Q dots could be directed against different analyte targets, and the Q dots would fluoresce with different colors in a size-dependent manner. This allows for the detection of multiple analytes with a single assay. Q dots are the next step in the evolution of luminescence-based assays.

SQUID Technology

A novel method of target labeling is to tag antibodies with superparamagnetic particles, allow the tagged antibodies to bind with the target antigen, and use a **superconducting quantum interference device (SQUID)** to detect the tagged antigen-antibody complex. The amplitude of the signal is proportional to the number of bound particles and correspondingly to the amount of target. A current application of this technology is its use in the detection of *Listeria monocytogenes*.

Luminescent Oxygen-Channeling Immunoassay

This novel detection technology is based on two different 200-nm latex particles: a sensitizer particle that absorbs energy at 680 nm with generation of singlet oxygen (donor bead) and a chemiluminescer molecule that shifts the emission wavelength to 570 nm (receptor bead). When these particles are in proximity during excitation, singlet oxygen moves from the donor bead to the receptor bead, where it triggers the generation of a luminescent signal. **Luminescent oxygen-channeling immunoassay (LOCI)** technol-

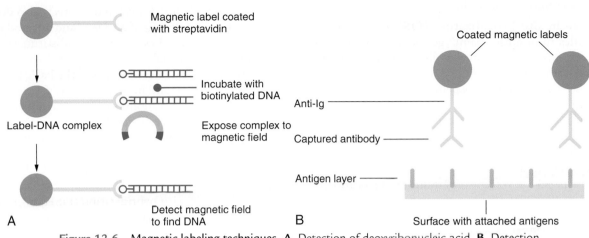

Figure 12-6   Magnetic labeling techniques. **A,** Detection of deoxyribonucleic acid. **B,** Detection of antibodies. *(Redrawn from Adelman L: Adv Med Lab Admin 11[6]:131, 1999. This article has been reprinted with permission from ADVANCE Newsmagazines.)*

ogy is broadly applicable to any molecule that can be determined in a binding assay. The production of end-point ribonucleic acid (RNA) determination by LOCI has been investigated.

Signal Amplification Technology

Tyramide signal amplification (TSA) can be used in a variety of both fluorescent and colorimetric detection applications. TSA protocols are simple and require few changes to standard operating procedures. TSA provides a messenger RNA (mRNA) in situ hybridization protocol that is effective in detecting B-cell clonality in plastic-embedded tissue specimens. Immunoglobulin light-chain mRNA molecules can be detected directly in paraffin-embedded tissue using fluorescein-labeled oligonucleotide probes. TSA amplification enables B cells to be detected in tissue sections without additional processing steps and specially prepared sections. Similar in situ hybridization technology can also be used for the detection of cytokines, such as interferon gamma (IFN-γ) and interleukin-4 (IL-4).

Magnetic Labeling Technology

Magnetic labeling technology is an application of the high-resolution magnetic recording technology developed for the computer disk drive industry. Increased density of microscopic, magnetically labeled biologic samples (e.g., nucleic acid on a biochip) translates directly into reduced sample-processing times. Magnetic labeling can be applied to automated DNA sequences, DNA probe technology, and gel electrophoresis (Figure 12-6).

Compared with other nonradioactive labeling systems, magnetic labels are inherently safe, instrumentation is less expensive, signals are virtually permanent, and spatial resolution is increased.

In a magnetic label–based gel electrophoresis application sphere, DNA is analyzed. DNA is separated into bands using electrophoresis, and magnetic labels are bound to the DNA in each band. By applying and then removing a magnetic field, the magnetic domains in each label are oriented in the same direction, resulting in a net magnetic field near the bands in the direction of the applied field (Figure 12-7).

Time-Resolved Fluoroimmunoassay

"Time-resolved" assay means that fluorescence is measured after a certain period to exclude background-interference fluorescence. This form of immunoassay is heterogeneous with a direct format (sandwich assay), similar to direct ELISA. Time-resolved fluoroimmunoassay uses europium-labeled antibodies. If excited at 340 nm, europium fluoresces at 620 nm. The fluorescence is measured and is directly proportional to the concentration of substance.

Fluorescence Polarization Immunoassay

In this homogeneous competitive fluoroimmunoassay, the polarization of the fluorescence from a fluorescein-antigen conjugate is determined by its rate of rotation during the lifetime of the excited state in solution. Binding to a large antibody molecule slows down the rate of rotation and increases the degree of polarization, and the fluorescence emitted is polarized.

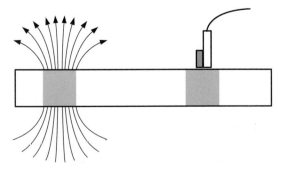

Figure 12-7   Cross-sectional schematic of small region of sequencing gel or nylon membrane with magnetic labels bound to DNA, separated into two bands. *Left,* Arrows on band represent the magnetic field resulting from the magnetized labels. *Right,* Band has a sensor near the surface. *(Redrawn from Adelman L: Adv Med Lab Admin 11[6]:131, 1999. This article has been reprinted with permission from ADVANCE Newsmagazines.)*

Fluorescence in Situ Hybridization

Fluorescence in situ hybridization (FISH) uses fluorescent molecules to brightly "paint" genes or chromosomes. The rapid expansion in the availability of polyclonal and monoclonal antibodies has fostered a dramatic increase in light microscopic immunohistochemistry (IHC) and in situ hybridization.

The FISH molecular cytogenetic technique uses recombinant DNA technology. Probes are short sequences of single-stranded DNA that are complementary to the DNA sequences to be examined. Probes hybridize, or "bind," to the cDNA, and labeled fluorescent tags indicate the location of the sequences. Probes can be locus-specific, centromeric repeat probes or whole-chromosome probes.

In metaphase FISH, a specific nucleic acid sequence (probe) is bound to the homologous segment on a metaphase chromosome affixed to a glass slide. Uniquely, the existence of a region-specific DNA sequence in a nondividing cell can be detected using interphase FISH.

Clinical applications of FISH in the detection of inherited and acquired chromosomal abnormalities include hematopathology and oncology. Many genetic syndromes have been recognized by geneticists, but laboratory tests often are unavailable for confirmation. DiGeorge syndrome is an example of a chromosomal deletion leading to the loss of several genes.

A simple, sensitive method for in situ amplified chemiluminescent detection of sequence-specific DNA and IgG immunoassay has been developed. This immunoassay uses highly active gold nanoparticles as the label and can be confirmed by clinical testing. This method has many desirable features, including rapid detection, selectivity, and minimal instrumentation. The protocol has potentially broad applications for clinical immunoassays and DNA hybridization analysis.

CHAPTER HIGHLIGHTS

- Heterogeneous immunoassays have a solid phase (microwell, bead) and require washing steps to remove unbound antigens or antibodies. Faster and easier to automate, homogeneous immunoassays have only a liquid phase and do not require washing steps.
- The ideal label should be measurable by several methods, including visual inspection.
- Enzyme immunoassay (EIA) uses a nonisotopic label and is safer than but shares the specificity, sensitivity, and rapidity of radioimmunoassay (RIA).
- In EIA antibody detection, the antigen in question is firmly fixed to a solid matrix (microplate well, outside of bead), called solid-phase immunosorbent assay.
- Chemiluminescence is the technology of choice of most immunodiagnostics manufacturers. In competitive and sandwich immunoassays, chemiluminescent labels can be attached to an antigen or an antibody.
- Fluorescent labeling (direct and indirect) also demonstrates the complexing of antigens and antibodies. Fluorescent antibodies are used as substitutes for radioisotope or enzyme labels.
- Fluorescent conjugates are used in the basic methods of direct, inhibition, and indirect immunofluorescent assay. In direct immunofluorescence a conjugated antibody is used to detect antigen-antibody reactions. In the indirect method, antibodies react with homologous antigens but also can act as antigens.
- Emerging labeling technologies include Q dots, SQUID, LOCI, signal amplification, and magnetic labeling.
- Fluorescence in situ hybridization (FISH) is often applied in immunology, hematopathology, and oncology.

REVIEW QUESTIONS

1. Chemiluminescence:
   a. Has excellent sensitivity and dynamic range.
   b. Does not require sample radiation.
   c. Uses unstable chemiluminescent reagents and conjugates.
   d. Both a and b.

Questions 2 and 3. Match the descriptions (*a* and *b*) to the assays.

2. _____ Competitive immunoassay

3. _____ Sandwich immunoassay

   a. Fixed amount of labeled antigen competes with unlabeled antigen from patient specimen for limited number of antibody-binding sites.
   b. Sample antigen binds to antibody fixed onto solid phase; second, chemiluminescent-labeled antibody binds to antigen-antibody complex.

4. Enzyme labels often used in indirect procedures are:
   a. Alkaline phosphatase.
   b. Horseradish peroxidase.
   c. Beta-galactosidase.
   d. All the above.

Questions 5 and 6. Match the following.

5. _____ Enzyme immunoassay (EIA)

6. _____ Immunofluorescent technique

   a. Uses a nonisotopic label.
   b. Uses antibody labeled with fluorescein isothiocyanate (FITC).
   c. Uses colloidal particle consisting of a metal or insoluble metal compound.

Questions 7-9. Match the assays and definitions.

7. _____ Direct immunofluorescent assay

8. _____ Inhibition immunofluorescent assay

9. _____ Indirect immunofluorescent assay

   a. Based on antibodies acting as antigens and reacting with antiimmunoglobulins.

   b. Uses conjugated antibody to detect antigen/antibody reactions.

   c. Antigen first exposed to unlabeled antibody, then labeled antibody.

10. For an enzyme to be used in an EIA, it must meet all the following criteria *except:*

   a. High amount of stability.

   b. Extreme specificity.

   c. Presence in antigen or antibody.

   d. No alteration by inhibitor with the system.

Questions 11 and 12. Fill in the blanks below, choosing from the answers for each.

A fluorescent substance is one that, while (11) _____ light of one wavelength, (12) _____ light of another (longer) wavelength.

11.		12.	
a.	emitting	a.	emits
b.	absorbing	b.	absorbs
c.	generating bright	c.	reduces
d.	generating dull	d.	increases

Questions 13-16. Match the following.

13. _____ Quantum dots (Q dots)

14. _____ SQUID technology

15. _____ Luminescent oxygen-channeling immunoassay (LOCI)

16. _____ Fluorescent in situ hybridization (FISH)

   a. Semiconductor nanocrystals.

   b. Method of tagging antibodies with superparamagnetic particles.

   c. Technology based on two different 200-nm latex particles.

   d. Molecular cytogenetic technique.

BIBLIOGRAPHY

Adelman L: Laboratory technology: magnetic labeling technology, *Adv Med Lab Admin* 11(6):131, 1999.

Forbes BA, Sahm DF, Weissfeld AS: *Bailey and Scott's diagnostic microbiology,* ed 12, St Louis, 2007, Mosby.

Hyde A: Enzyme-linked immunosorbent assay (ELISA): an overview, *Adv Med Lab Professionals,* October 9, 2006, pp 13-16.

Jandreski MA: Chemiluminescence technology in immunoassays, *Lab Med* 29(9):555-560, 1998.

Mark HFL: Fluorescent in situ hybridization as an adjunct to conventional cytogenetics, *Ann Clin Lab Sci* 24(2):153-163, 1994.

McDowell J: Beyond ANA testing, *Clin Lab News,* October 2005.

Sainato D: The coming revolution in assay technologies, *Clin Lab News* 20:26-27, 2000.

Van Den Berg F. Applications of a signal amplification technique for light microscopy, *Clin Lab News* 15:8-9, 1996.

Wang Z et al: In situ amplified chemiluminescent detection of DNA and immunoassay of IgG using special-shaped gold nanoparticles as label, *Clin Chem* 52(10):1958-1962, 2006.

CHAPTER 13

Automated Procedures

Characteristics of Automated Testing
Nephelometry
    Principle
    Physical Basis
    Optical System
    Measuring Methods
    Advantages and Disadvantages
    Clinical Application: Cryoglobulins
Flow-Cell Cytometry
    Fundamentals of Laser Technology
    Principles of Cell Cytometry

Cell Sorting
Eight-Color Immunofluorescence
Clinical Applications
Trends in Immunoassay Automation
    Fluorescent Polarization Immunoassay
Chapter Highlights
Review Questions
Bibliography

Learning Objectives

At the conclusion of this chapter, the reader should be able to:

- Identify and give examples of the three phases in automated testing.
- Describe the principle, advantages, and disadvantages of nephelometry.
- Discuss the analysis and clinical implications of cryoglobulins.

- Explain the principle of flow cell cytometry, and cite clinical applications.
- Discuss current trends in immunoassay.
- List at least three potential benefits of automated immunoassay.

CHARACTERISTICS OF AUTOMATED TESTING

Laboratory automation can be separated into preanalytical, analytical, and postanalytical phases. Accuracy in each of the phases is critical to quality results. The preanalytical phase includes specimen labeling (bar coding preferred), accessioning, and tracking, along with proper test ordering.

The analytical phase involves the following areas:

- Automated results entry
- Quality control
- Validation of results
- Networking to laboratory information systems

Automated analyzers link each specimen to its specific test request. Any results generated must be "verified" (approved or reviewed) by the laboratorian before the data are released to the patient report. Useful data for this verification process include "flags" signifying results outside the reference range, critical or "panic" values (possibly life threatening), values out of the technical range for the analyzer, and failures in other checks and balances built into the system.

The postanalytical phase includes adding to patient cumulative reports, workload recording, and networks to other systems. Quality assurance (QA) procedures, including the use of quality control (QC) solutions, are part of the analytical functions of the analyzer and its interfaced computer. CLIA '88 regulations require the documentation of all QC data associated with any test results reported (see Chapter 7).

NEPHELOMETRY

Nephelometry has become increasingly more popular in diagnostic laboratories and depends on the light-scattering properties of antigen-antibody complexes (Figure 13-1).

The quantity of cloudiness or "turbidity" in a solution can be measured photometrically. When specific antigen-coated latex particles acting as reaction intensifiers are agglutinated by their corresponding antibody, the increased light scatter of a solution can be measured by nephelometry as the macromolecular complexes form. The use of polyethylene glycol (PEG) enhances and stabilizes the precipitates, thus increasing the speed and sensitivity of the technique by controlling the particle size for optimal light-angle deflection. The kinetics of this change can be determined when the photometric results are analyzed by computer.

In immunology, nephelometry is used to measure complement components, immune complexes, and the presence of a variety of antibodies (Box 13-1).

Principle

Formation of a macromolecular complex is a fundamental prerequisite for nephelometric protein quantitation. The procedure is based on the reaction between the protein being assayed and a specific antiserum. Protein in a patient specimen reacts with specific nephelometric antiserum to human proteins and forms insoluble complexes. When light is passed through such a suspension, the resulting complexes of insoluble precipitants scatter incident light in so-

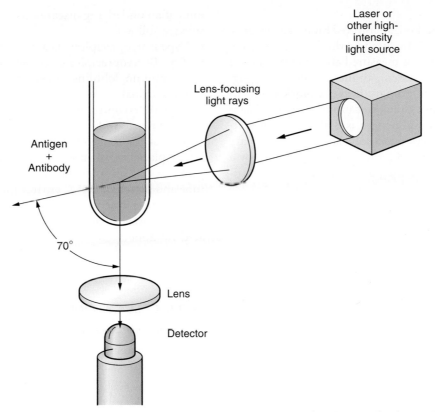

Figure 13-1 Principle of nephelometry for the measurement of antigen-antibody reactions. Light rays are collected in a focusing lens and can ultimately be related to the antigen or antibody concentration in a sample.

Box 13-1	Examples of Immunologic Assays Performed by Nephelometry

Acid α_1-glycoprotein
Albumin
α_1-Antitrypsin
α_2-Macroglobulin
C1 esterase inhibitor (C1 inhibitor)
C3
C3b inhibitor (C3b inactivator)
C3PA (C3 proactivator, properdin factor B)
C4
C6
C7
C8
Ceruloplasmin
Complement components (C1r, C1s, C2, C3, C4, C5, C6, C7, C8)
C-reactive protein (CRP)
Cryofibrinogen
Cryoglobulins
Haptoglobin
Hemopexin
Immunoglobulins
Properdin factor B
Transferrin

lutions. The scattered light can be detected with a photodiode. The amount of scattered light is proportional to the number of insoluble complexes and can be quantitated by comparing the unknown patient values with standards of known protein concentration.

The relationship between the quantity of antigen and the measuring signal at a constant antibody concentration is expressed by the Heidelberger curve. If antibodies are present to excess, a proportional relationship exits between the antigen and the resulting signal. If the antigen overwhelms the quantity of antibody, the measured signal drops.

By optimizing the reaction conditions, the typical antigen-antibody reactions as characterized by the Heidelberger curve are effectively shifted in the direction of high concentration. This ensures that these high concentrations will be measured on the ascending portion of the curve. At concentrations higher than the reference curve, the instrument will transmit an out-of-range warning.

Physical Basis

Nephelometry is based on the principle that light is scattered by a homogeneous particulate solution at a variety of angles. Three types of scatter can occur: (1) scatter around the particles, (2) forward scatter caused by out-of-phase backscatter, and (3) forward scatter exceeding backscatter.

Optical System

In the nephelometric method, an infrared high-performance light-emitting diode (LED) is used as the light source. Because an entire solid angle is measured after convergence of this light through a lens system, an intense measuring signal is available when the primary beam is blocked off. In connection with the lens system, this produces a light beam of high colinearity. The wavelength is 840 nm. Light scattered in the forward direction in a solid angle to the primary beam ranges between 13 and 24 feet and is measured by a silicon photodiode with an integrated amplifier. The electrical signals generated are digitized, compared with reference curves, and converted to protein concentrations.

Measuring Methods

A fixed-time method is used routinely for precipitation reactions. Ten seconds after all reaction components have been mixed, a *cuvette* reading (initial blank measurement) is taken. Six minutes later a second measurement is taken, and after subtraction of the original 1-second blanking value, a final answer is calculated against the multiple-point or single-point calibration in the computerized program memory for the assay.

Advantages and Disadvantages

Nephelometry represents an automated system that is rapid, reproducible, relatively simple to operate, and common in higher-volume laboratories. It has many applications in the immunology laboratory. Currently, instruments using a rate method and fixed-time approach are commercially available with tests for immunoglobulin G (IgG), IgA, IgM, C3, C4, properdin, C-reactive protein (CRP), rheumatoid factor, ceruloplasmin, α_1-antitrypsin, apolipoproteins, and haptoglobins.

The disadvantages of nephelometry include high initial equipment cost and interfering substances such as microbial contamination, which may cause protein denaturation and erroneous test results. Intrinsic specimen turbidity or lipemia may exceed the preset limits. In these cases a clearing agent may be needed before an accurate assay can be performed. In addition, low-molecular-weight immunoglobulins, monoclonal immunoglobulins, and antibovidae antibodies also may produce spurious results in nephelometry.

Clinical Application: Cryoglobulins

Cryoglobulin analysis is frequently requested when patient symptoms such as pain, cyanosis, Raynaud's phenomenon, and skin ulceration on exposure to cold temperatures are present. **Cryoglobulins** are proteins that precipitate or gel when cooled to 0° C and dissolve when heated. In most cases, monoclonal cryoglobulins are IgM or IgG. Occasionally, the macroglobulin is both cryoprecipitable and capable of cold-induced anti-i–mediated agglutination of red blood cells.

Cryoglobulins with a detected monoclonal protein component normally prompt a clinical investigation to determine if an underlying disease exists. Cryoglobulins are classified as follows:

- Type I: cryoprecipitate is a monoclonal IgG, IgA, or IgM.
- Type II: cryoprecipitate is mixed, containing two classes of immunoglobulins, at least one of which is monoclonal.
- Type III: cryoprecipitate is mixed, and no monoclonal protein is found.

To test for the presence of cryoglobulins, blood is collected, placed in warm water, and centrifuged at room temperature. The serum is then put into a graduated centrifuge tube and placed in a 4° C environment for 7 days. If a gel or precipitate is observed, the tube is centrifuged, and the precipitate is washed at 4° C, redissolved at 37° C, and evaluated by double diffusion and immunoelectrophoresis for the content of the cryoglobulin. Newer methods use nephelometry with cold treatment for analysis.

FLOW-CELL CYTOMETRY

Fundamentals of Laser Technology

In 1917, Einstein speculated that under certain conditions, atoms or molecules could absorb light or other radiation and then be stimulated to shed this gained energy. Lasers have now been developed with numerous medical and industrial applications.

The **electromagnetic spectrum** ranges from long radio waves to short, powerful gamma rays (Figure 13-2). Within this spectrum is a narrow band of visible or "white" light, composed of red, orange, yellow, green, blue, and violet light. **Laser** (**l**ight **a**mplification by **s**timulated **e**mission of **r**adiation) light ranges from the ultraviolet (UV) and infrared (IR) spectrum through all the colors of the rainbow. In contrast to other diffuse forms of radiation, laser light is concentrated. It is almost exclusively of one wavelength or color, and its parallel waves travel in one direction. Through the use of fluorescent dyes, laser light can occur in numerous wavelengths. The types of lasers include glass-filled tubes of helium and neon (most common), yttrium-aluminum-garnet (YAG; an imitation diamond), argon, and krypton.

Lasers sort the energy in atoms and molecules, concentrate it, and release it in powerful waves. In most lasers, a medium of gas, liquid, or crystal is energized by high-intensity light, an electrical discharge, or even nuclear radiation. When an atom extends beyond the orbits of its electrons or when a molecule vibrates or changes its shape, it instantly snaps back, shedding energy in the form of a photon. The **photon** is the basic unit of all radiation. When a photon reaches an atom of the medium, the energy exchange stimulates the emission of another photon in the same wavelength and direction. This process continues until a cascade of growing energy sweeps through the medium.

Photons travel the length of the laser and bounce off mirrors. First a few and eventually countless photons synchronize themselves until an avalanche of light streaks between the mirrors. In some gas lasers, transparent disks referred to

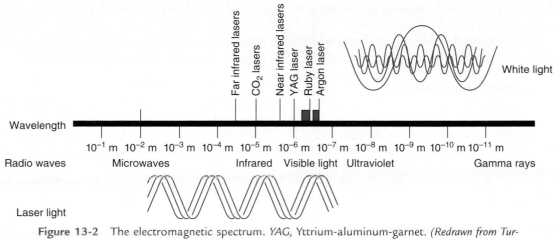

Figure 13-2 The electromagnetic spectrum. *YAG, Yttrium-aluminum-garnet. (Redrawn from Turgeon ML: Clinical hematology: theory and procedures, ed 4, Philadelphia, 2003, Lippincott–Williams & Wilkins.)*

as "Brewster windows" are slanted at a precise angle, which polarizes the laser's light. The photons, which are reflected back and forth, finally gain so much energy that they exit as a powerful beam. The power of lasers to pass on energy and information is rated in watts.

Principles of Cell Cytometry

Flow-cell cytometry combines fluid dynamics, optics, laser science, high-speed computers, and fluorochrome-conjugated monoclonal antibodies (MAbs) that rapidly classify groups of cells within heterogeneous mixtures. The principle of flow cytometry is based on cells being stained in suspension with an appropriate **fluorochrome**—an immunologic reagent, a dye that stains a specific component, or some other marker with specific reactivity. Fluorescent dyes used in flow cytometry must bind or react specifically with the cellular component of interest (e.g., reticulocytes, peroxidase enzyme, DNA content). Fluorescent dyes include acridine orange and thioflavin T.

Pygon is preferred for fluorescein isothiocyanate (FITC) labeling. Krypton is often used as a second laser in dual-analysis systems and serves as a better light source for compounds labeled by tetramethyl- and tetramethylcyclopropyl-rhodamine isothiocyanate.

A suspension of stained cells is pressurized using gas and transported through plastic tubing to a flow chamber within the instrument (Figure 13-3). In the flow chamber the specimen is injected through a needle into a stream of physiologic saline called the *sheath*. The sheath and specimen both exit the flow chamber through a 75-μm orifice. This laminar flow design confines the cells to the center of the saline sheath, with the cells moving in single file.

The stained cells then pass through the laser beam. The laser activates the dye, and the cell fluoresces. Although the fluorescence is emitted throughout a 360-degree circle, it is usually collected by optical sensors located 90 degrees relative to the laser beam. The fluorescence information is then

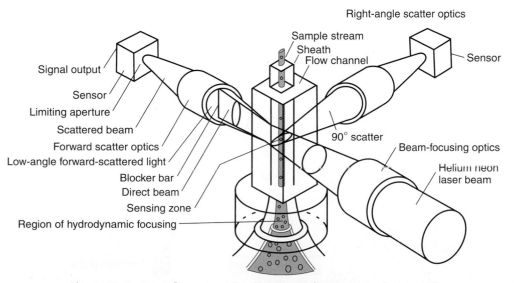

Figure 13-3 Laser flow cytometry. *(Courtesy Ortho Diagnostics, Raritan, NJ.)*

transmitted to a computer, which controls all decisions regarding data collection, analysis, and cell sorting.

Flow cytometry performs fluorescence analysis on single cells. The major applications of this technology follow:

- Identification of cells
- Cell sorting before further analysis

Cell Sorting

In flow cytometry, cells can be sorted from the main cellular population into subpopulations for further analysis (Figure 13-4). Any fresh specimen that can be placed into a single-cell suspension is a valid candidate for **immunophenotyping** (e.g., T cells, B cells, CD34+ stem cells, detection of minimal residual disease in leukemia). Sorting is accomplished using stored computer information.

When the laser strikes a stained cell, the dye creates distinctive colored light that the cytometer recognizes. This fluorescent intensity is recorded and analyzed by the computer, and cells are sorted according to a preprogrammed selection. If the particular cell in the laser beam is of interest, the computer waits the appropriate time for the cell to reach the droplet break-off point within the charging collar. At that point the computer signals the charging collar to administer an electrostatically positive or negative charge to the stream containing the target cell. A droplet containing this cell is then removed from the main stream before the charge has time to redistribute.

This action produces the cell of interest within a liquid drop that has on its surface an electrostatic charge (only the droplet is charged). The droplet falls between a set of deflection plates, which creates an electrical field. The charged droplets are deflected to the left or right, depending on their polarity, and collected for further analysis.

Eight-Color Immunofluorescence

Current fluorescent methods (e.g., BD FACSCanto II flow cytometer) can perform up to eight-color analysis. The BD LSRII flow cytometer, with up to four lasers, can measure up to 16 colors. It can use four MAbs, each directly conjugated to a distinct fluorochrome, per tube of patient cell suspension. The four most common fluorochromes are FITC, phycoerythrin (PE), peridinin chlorophyll protein (PerCP), and allophycocyanin (APC). The first three fluorochromes are excited by the 488-nm line of an argon laser; the fourth fluorochrome is excited by the 633-nm line of a helium-neon or diode laser.

Eight-color immunofluorescence offers the advantages of greater sensitivity and specificity, with increased ability to identify and subclassify individual cells. Improvements in methods and probes may lead to **fluorescence in situ hybridization (FISH)** in suspension as a routine protocol (see Chapter 12) and enable flow cytometry to operate on a molecular level simultaneously to identify chromosomal abnormalities.

A system that uses a flow cytometer, specific data analysis software, and fluorescent latex particles, the Luminex 100 Total System, has been developed by Luminex Technology (Austin, Texas). This system combines advances in

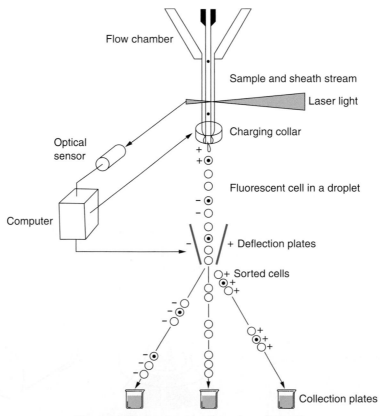

Figure 13-4   Laser and cell-sorting schematic.

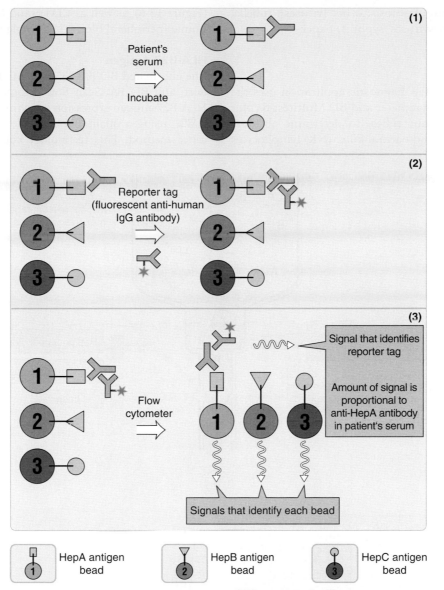

Figure 13-5 Fluorescent microsphere–based immunoassay for antibodies to hepatitis virus (Luminex xMAP technology). This approach is especially valuable when multiple tests must be done. It utilizes aspects of both enzyme-linked immunosorbent assay (ELISA) and flow cytometry. A small amount of sample is known. Polystyrene microspheres are internally color-coded with two fluorescent dyes that can be detected after laser illumination. *(From Nairn R, Helbert M: Immunology for medical students, ed 2, St Louis, 2007, Mosby.)*

computing and optics with a new concept in color coding to create a simple, cost-efficient analysis system (Figure 13-5). Latex beads are coupled to various amounts of two different fluorescent dyes, which are analyzed by the flow cytometer and software to allow the distinct separation of up to 64 slightly different, colored bead sets. The color-coded microspheres identify each unique reaction. Hundreds of microsphere sets can be identified at once in a single sample. Optical technology recognizes each microsphere and provides a precise, quantitative measure simply and in real time.

Currently, up to 64 microsphere sets are recognized. The current FlowMetrix system is compatible with the BD (Franklin Lakes, NJ) FACS Vantage SE System and the BD FACSCalibur, the most widely used flow cytometers for cellular analysis. Because the Luminex technology requires fewer steps to assess multiple parameters, with a high level of sensitivity and accuracy, it is significantly more cost-effective than current methods of analysis. Some immunologic applications already demonstrated with FlowMetrix are human immunodeficiency virus (HIV) and hepatitis B seroconversion; multicytokine measurement; multiplexed allergy testing; DNA-based tissue typing; herpes simplex viral load; IgG, IgA, and IgM assay; IgG subclassification; autoimmunity pane; epitope mapping; human chorionic gonadotropin (hCG) and alpha-fetoprotein; HIV viral load;

and the TORCHS (toxoplasmosis, other [viruses], rubella, cytomegalovirus, herpesviruses, syphilis) panel.

Clinical Applications

Lymphocyte Subsets

A six-color flow cytometry diagnostic application uses the BD FACSCanto II flow cytometer and BD Multitest 6-color TBNK with BD Trucount tubes, to determine absolute counts of mature T, B, and natural killer (NK) lymphocytes

(Figure 13-6), as well as CD4+ and CD8+ T-cell subsets in human peripheral blood, in a single tube.

HLA-B27 Antigen

The automated BD FACSCanto, BD FACSCalibur, BD FAC-Sort, and BD FACScan flow cytometers can rapidly detect HLA-B27 antigen expression in erythrocyte–lysed whole blood (LWB) using a qualitative two-color direct immunofluorescence method. This technology compares the intensity of

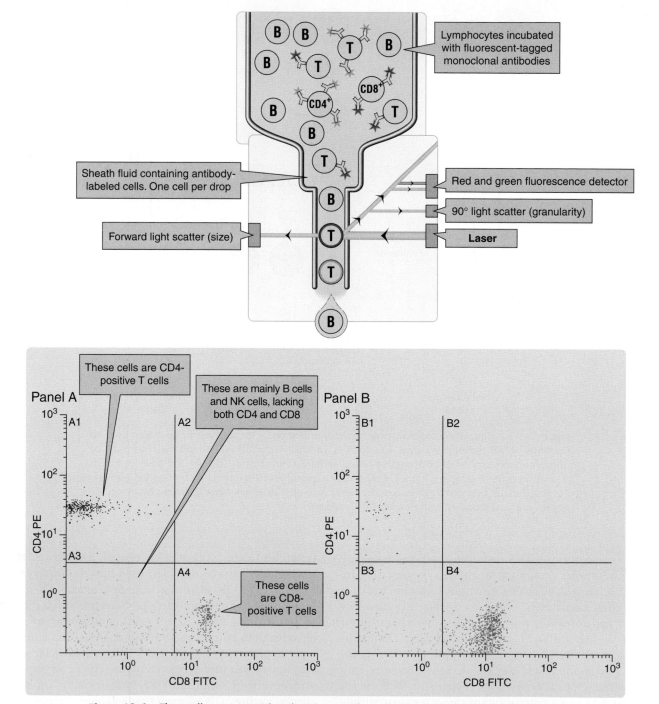

Figure 13-6 **Flow-cell cytometry "dot plots."** In *Panel A,* cells stained with the red CD4 antibody account for 59% of all lymphocytes; this is a normal sample. In *Panel B,* there is a reduction in the number of red-staining CD4+ T cells; this sample is from a patient with HIV infection. *PE,* Phycoerythrin (emits red light); *FITC,* fluorescein isothiocyanate (emits green light). *(From Nairn R, Helbert M: Immunology for medical students, ed 2, St Louis, 2007, Mosby.)*

Table 13-1	Examples of Automated Immunoassays	
Manufacturer	**Instrument**	**Assay Type**
Abbott Diagnostics	AxSym	FPIA/MEIA
Bayer, Inc.	Immuno-1	Latex EIA, ELISA
Beckman Coulter, Inc.	Access	Chemiluminscence
Dade Behring, Inc.	Opus Plus	Fluorescent ELISA
Ortho Diagnostics	Vitros	Chemiluminescence
Tosoh Medics, Inc.	AIA-1200, NexiA	Kinetic fluorescence

Data from *CAP Today* 21(6):24-72, 2007.

FPIA, Fluorescent polarization immunoassay; *MEIA,* microparticle enzyme immunoassay; *EIA,* enzyme immunoassay; *ELISA,* enzyme-linked immunosorbent assay.

T lymphocytes stained with anti–HLA-B27 FITC to a predetermined decision marker during analysis. When anti–HLA-B27 FITC/CD3 PE MAb reagent is added to human whole blood, the fluorochrome-labeled antibodies bind specifically to leukocyte surface antigens. The stained samples are treated with BD FACS lysing solution to lyse erythrocytes, then are washed and fixed before flow cytometric analysis.

This application of flow cytometry is clinically relevant to the evaluation of seronegative spondyloarthropathies.

TRENDS IN IMMUNOASSAY AUTOMATION

Technical advances in methodologies, robotics, and computerization have led to expanded immunoassay automation (Tables 13-1 and 13-2). Newer systems are using chemilumi-

Table 13-2	Examples of Automated Immunoassay Analyzers	
Manufacturer	**Instrument**	**Launch Date/Country**
Abbott Diagnostics	Architect	2000-1999/US
	AxSym/AxSymPlus	1993/worldwide, 1994/US
Awareness Technology, Inc.	ChemWell	1998/US
Beckman Coulter, Inc.	UniCel Dxl 800	2003/US
	UniCel 600Access	2007/US
	Access/Access 2	2001/US
The Binding Site, Inc.	DSX Automated System	2000/Guernsey, UK
BioMérieux Inc.	Vidas and MiniVidas	1989/US
Bio-Rad	BioPlex 2200	2006/Australia
	PR3100TSC	2006/Austria
	Evolis	2001/Germany
Dade Behring, Inc.	Dimension Vista	2006/US
	1500 Opus Plus	1992/US
	Stratus CS Stat	1998
	Fluorometric Analyzer	1997
	Dimension Xpand Plus System with Heterogeneous Module (HM)	2004/US
Diamedix Corp.	Mago Plus Automated EIA Analyzer	1997/Italy
DiaSorin Inc.	ETI-Lab	1996/Italy
Grifols-Quest, Inc.	Triturus	1999/Spain
Hycor Biomedical, Inc.	Hy-Tec 288	1998/US
		1999/Netherlands
	Hy-Tec 480	1994/Switzerland
Inverness Medical	AIMS	2007/Switerland
Olympus America, Inc.	AU400e	2002/Japan
	AU3000i	2007/Japan, Ireland
Ortho Diagnostics	VITROS Eci	1997/US
	VITROS EciQ	2004/US
	Immunodiagnostic System	1997/US
Phadia	ImmunoCAP 250	2004/Japan, Sweden
	ImmunoCAP 100	2003/Japan, Sweden
Roche Diagnostics	Elecsys 2010	1996/Japan, Germany
	Cobas	2006/Japan
Siemens Medical Solutions Diagnostics	ADVIA Centaur	1998/US
	ADVIA Centaur CP	2005/US
	ImmunoLite	1993/US
Tosoh Medics, Inc.	AIA-360	2004/Japan
	AIA-600 II	2000/Japan

Modified from *CAP Today* 21(6):25-71, 2001.

Box 13-2	Potential Benefits of Immunoassay Automation

- Ability to provide better service with less staff.
- Savings on controls, duplicates, dilutions, and repeats.
- Elimination of radioactive labels and associated regulations.
- Better shelf life of reagents, with less disposal of outdated supplies.
- Better sample identification with bar-code labels and primary tube sampling.
- Automation of sample delivery possible.

Modified from Blick K: *J Clin Ligand Assay* 22:6-12, 1999.

nescent labels and substrates rather than the fluorescent labels and detection systems, such as enzyme immunoassays (see Chapter 12). Immunoassay systems have the potential to improve turnaround time with enhanced cost-effectiveness (Box 13-2).

Fluorescent Polarization Immunoassay

The fluorescent polarization immunoassay, the IMx System manufactured by Abbott Laboratories, is an automated analyzer designed to perform microparticle enzyme immunoassay, fluorescence polarization immunoassay, and ion capture technologies. This unique combination allows both high- and low-molecular-weight analytes to be measured. This expands the range of available assays to include tests for endocrine function, fertility, cancer, hepatitis, transplantation, rubella, and congenital disease.

CHAPTER HIGHLIGHTS

- When specific antigen-coated latex particles acting as reaction intensifiers are agglutinated by their corresponding antibody, the increased light scatter of a solution can be measured by nephelometry as the macromolecular complexes form.
- Nephelometry is a rapid and highly reproducible automated method.
- Cryoglobulins are proteins that precipitate or gel when cooled to 0° C and dissolve when heated. In most cases, monoclonal cryoglobulins are IgM or IgG.
- Flow cytometry is based on cells being stained in suspension with an appropriate fluorochrome (immunologic reagent, dye that stains specific component, other marker with specified reactivity).
- Laser light is the most common light source used in flow cytometers.
- Color immunofluorescence uses monoclonal antibodies, each directly conjugated to a distinct fluorochrome, per tube of patient cell suspension. Eight-color immunofluorescence offers the advantages of greater sensitivity and specificity.
- Newer systems in immunoassay automation use chemiluminescent labels and substrates rather than fluorescent labels and detection systems.

REVIEW QUESTIONS

1. Nephelometry measures the light scatter of:
   a. Ions.
   b. Macromolecules.
   c. Antibodies.
   d. Soluble antigens.

2. Nephelometry can be used to assay all the following *except:*
   a. IgM.
   b. IgG.
   c. IgD.
   d. IgA.

3. Cryoglobulins are proteins that precipitate or gel when cooled to:
   a. $-18°$ C.
   b. $0°$ C.
   c. $4°$ C.
   d. $18°$ C.

Questions 4-6. Match the following types of cryoglobulin with their respective descriptions.

4. _____ Type I

5. _____ Type II

6. _____ Type III

   a. Contains two classes of immunoglobulins, at least one of which is monoclonal.
   b. Mixed, no monoclonal protein found.
   c. Monoclonal IgG, IgA, or IgM.

7. Cryoglobulin analysis can be useful in the diagnosis of:
   a. Hypothermia.
   b. Raynaud's phenomenon.
   c. Hepatitis C.
   d. Rheumatoid arthritis.

8. "Laser" is an acronym for:
   a. Light amplification by stimulated emission of radiation.
   b. Light augmentation by stimulated emitted radiation.
   c. Light amplified by stimulated energy radiation.
   d. Large angle stimulation by emitted radiation.

9. All the following are descriptive characteristics of laser light *except:*
   a. Intensity.
   b. Stability.
   c. Polychromaticity.
   d. Monochromaticity.

10. A photon is a:
    a. Basic unit of light.
    b. Basic unit of all radiation.
    c. Component of an atom.
    d. Component of laser light.

11. The major applications of flow-cell technology is:
    a. Identification of cells.
    b. Cell sorting before further analysis.
    c. Diagnosis of autoimmune disease.
    d. Both a and b.

12. Four-color immunofluorescence typically uses:
    a. Fluorescein isothiocyanate (FITC).
    b. Phycoerythrin (PE).
    c. Peridinin chlorophyll protein (PerCP).
    d. All the above.

BIBLIOGRAPHY

Bakke AC: The principles of flow cytometry, *Lab Med* 32:207-211, 2001.

Behring nephelometer system folder, Branchburg, NJ, 1987, Behring Diagnostics.

Blick KE: Current trends in automation of immunoassays, *J Clin Ligand Assay* 22:6-12, 1999.

Hoffman EG: Laboratory evaluation of monoclonal gammopathies, *Can J Med Technol* 49(2):99-115, 1987.

Kaplan LA, Pesce AJ, Kazmierczak SC: *Clinical chemistry: theory, analysis, correlation,* ed 4, St Louis, 2003, Mosby.

Kelliher AS et al: Multiparameter flow cytometry in the clinical lab: present capacities and future projections, *Adv Med Lab Prof* 2001, pp 9-13.

Lovett EJ et al: Application of flow cytometry to diagnostic pathology, *Lab Invest* 50(2):115-140, 1984.

Smalley D, Aller RD: Picturing tomorrow's system, *Cap Today* 15:53-84, 2001.

Turgeon ML: *Clinical hematology: theory and procedures,* ed 3, Philadelphia, 1999, Lippincott-Williams & Wilkins.

CHAPTER 14

Molecular Techniques

Amplification Techniques in Molecular Biology
    Polymerase Chain Reaction
    Modifications in PCR Technique
    Other Amplification Techniques
Analysis of Amplification Products
    Conventional Analysis
    Other Techniques

DNA Sequencing
Branched DNA
Hybridization Techniques
Microarrays
Chapter Highlights
Review Questions
Bibliography

Learning Objectives

At the conclusion of this chapter, the reader should be able to:
- Describe the polymerase chain reaction (PCR) amplification technique.
- Compare various PCR modifications.
- Identify and briefly describe other amplification techniques.
- Describe the "gold standard" of genetic analysis.
- Compare DNA sequencing and branched-DNA protocols.
- Identify and compare three hybridization techniques.
- Explain how microarrays are applied to immunologic testing.
- Discuss the general concept of nucleic acid blotting.
- Compare the characteristics and clinical applications of Southern, Northern, and Western blotting techniques.

Molecular genetic testing is a fast-growing diagnostic discipline in the clinical laboratory. Since the complete human genome (sequence) became available in 2003, molecular genetic testing has been expanded extensively. The clinician needs to remember, however, that even with highly standardized molecular methods, these tests are as susceptible to laboratory errors as any other laboratory procedure.

AMPLIFICATION TECHNIQUES IN MOLECULAR BIOLOGY

Polymerase Chain Reaction

Polymerase chain reaction (PCR) is an in vitro method that amplifies low levels of specific deoxyribonucleic acid (DNA) sequences in a sample to higher quantities suitable for further analysis (Figure 14-1, *A*). To use this technology, the target sequence to be amplified must be known. Typically, a target sequence ranges from 100 to 1000 base pairs (bp) in length. Two short DNA "primers," typically 16 to 20 bp, are used. The **oligonucleotides** (small portions of a single DNA strand) act as a template for the new DNA. These primer sequences are complementary to the 3' ends of the sequence to be amplified.

This enzymatic process is carried out in cycles. Each repeated cycle consists of the following:
- *DNA denaturation.* Separation of the double DNA strands into two single strands through the use of heat.
- *Primer annealing.* Recombination of the oligonucleotide primers with the single-stranded original DNA.
- *Extension of primed DNA sequence.* The enzyme *DNA polymerase* synthesizes new complementary strands by the extension of primers.

Each cycle theoretically doubles the amount of specific DNA sequence present and results in an exponential accumulation of the DNA fragment being amplified **(amplicons).** In general, this process is repeated approximately 30 times. At the end of 30 cycles, the reaction mixture should contain about 2^{30} molecules of the desired product.

After cycling is completed, the amplification products can be examined in various ways. Typically, the contents of the reaction vessel are subjected to *gel electrophoresis*. This allows visualization of the amplified gene segments (e.g., PCR products, bands) and a determination of their specificity. Additional product analysis by probe hybridization or direct DNA sequencing is often performed to verify further the authenticity of the amplicon.

Three important applications of PCR are as follows:
1. Amplification of DNA
2. Identification of a target sequence
3. Synthesis of a labeled antisense probe

The PCR analysis can lead to (1) detection of gene mutations that signify the early development of cancer, (2) identification of viral DNA associated with specific cancers (e.g., human papillomavirus [HPV], a causative agent in cervical cancer), and (3) detection of genetic mutations associated with various diseases, such as coronary artery disease associated with mutations of the gene that encodes for the low-density lipoprotein receptor (LDLR).

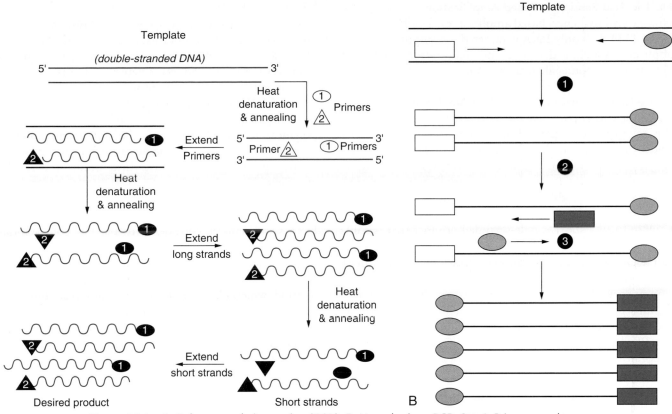

Figure 14-1   A, Polymerase chain reaction (PCR). **B,** Nested primer PCR. *Step 1: Primers anneal to and amplify a broad region of DNA around the gene of interest. Step 2:* Nested primers anneal to the specific gene to be amplified. *Step 3:* Amplification of the desired gene by nested primers. *(Redrawn and modified from Warden BA, Thompson E:* Lab Med *25[7]:453, 1994.)*

The PCR technique has undergone adaptations (Figure 14-1, *B*). One adaptation uses *nested primers* in a two-step amplification process: (1) a broad region of the DNA surrounding the sequence of interest is amplified, followed by (2) another round of amplification to amplify the specific gene sequence to be studied. Another PCR modification successfully differentiates alleles of the same gene.

Modifications In PCR Technique

Reverse-Transcriptase Polymerase Chain Reaction
If the nucleic acid of interest is ribonucleic acid (RNA) rather than DNA, the PCR procedures can be modified to include the conversion of RNA to DNA using **reverse transcriptase (RT)** in the initial steps. RT-PCR is useful in the identification of RNA viral agents, such as human immunodeficiency virus (HIV) and hepatitis C virus (HCV).

Multiplex Polymerase Chain Reaction
Multiplex PCR uses numerous primers within a single reaction tube to amplify nucleic acid fragments from different targets. Specific nucleic acid amplification should occur if the appropriate target DNA is present in the sample tests. Detection may be accomplished by traditional Southern transfer and subsequent nucleic acid probe, by enzyme immunoassay (EIA) methods, or by gene-chip analysis. This technology is limited by (1) the number of primers that can be included in a single reaction, (2) primer-primer interference, and (3) nonspecific nucleic acid amplification.

Real-Time Polymerase Chain Reaction
Real-time PCR uses fluorescence-resonance energy transfer to quantitate specific DNA sequences of interest and identify point mutations. Real-time PCR is particularly appealing because the procedure is less susceptible to amplicon contamination and is more accurate in quantifying the initial copy number.

Other Amplification Techniques

Strand Displacement Amplification
Strand displacement amplification (SDA) is a fully automated method that amplifies target nucleic acid without the use of a thermocycler. A double-strand DNA fragment is created and becomes the target for exponential amplification.

Transcription Mediate Amplification
Transcription mediate amplification (TMA) is another isothermal assay that targets either DNA or RNA, but generates RNA as its amplified product. TMA is used to detect microorganisms (e.g., *Mycobacterium tuberculosis*).

Nucleic Acid Sequence–Based Amplification

Nucleic acid sequence–based amplification (NASBA) is similar to TMA, but only RNA is targeted for amplification. Its applications include detection and quantitation of HIV and detection of cytomegalovirus (CMV).

Ligase Chain Reaction Nucleic Acid Amplification

Oligonucleotide pairs hybridize to target sequences within the gene or the cryptic plasmid. The bound oligonucleotides are separated by a small gap at the target site. The enzyme DNA polymerase uses nucleotides in the ligase chain reaction (LCR) nucleic acid amplification reaction mixture to fill in this gap, creating a ligatable junction. Once the gap is filled, DNA ligase joins the oligonucleotide pairs to form a short, single-stranded product that is complementary to the original target sequence. This product can itself serve as a target for hybridization and ligation of a second pair of oligonucleotides present in the LCR reaction mixture.

Subsequent rounds of denaturation and ligation lead to the geometric accumulation of amplification product. The amplified products are detected in an LCx analyzer (Abbott Laboratories, Abbott Park, Ill) by microparticle EIA.

ANALYSIS OF AMPLIFICATION PRODUCTS

Many of the revolutionary changes that have occurred in research in the biologic sciences, particularly the Human Genome Project, can be directly attributed to the ability to manipulate DNA in defined ways. Molecular genetic testing focuses on examination of nucleic acids (DNA or RNA) by special techniques to determine if a specific nucleotide base sequence is present.

Although nucleic acid testing is in its infancy, its applications have expanded, despite higher costs associated with testing, in various areas of the clinical laboratory. Applications include genetic testing, hematopathology diagnosis and monitoring, and identification of infectious agents. Molecular testing has the following advantages:
- Faster turnaround time
- Smaller required sample volumes
- Increased specificity and sensitivity

Conventional Analysis

Detection of DNA products that result from PCR can be conventionally analyzed using agarose gel electrophoresis after ethidium bromide staining. This technique is simply an extra step after a PCR assay has been run. DNA and other biomolecules can be separated based on charge, size, and shape. DNA has a net negative charge and will migrate toward the anode (positive pole). PCR products are loaded into an agarose gel and electrophoresed. Ethidium bromide is a dye that intercalates into nucleic acids and will fluoresce with an orange color under ultraviolet (UV) irradiation. An image analyzer uses UV light to capture computer images of the PCR products.

Other Techniques

Other techniques are used to enhance both the sensitivity and specificity of amplification techniques. Probe-based DNA detection systems have the advantage of providing sequence specificity and lower detection limits. Other techniques include hybridization protection assay, DNA EIA, automated DNA sequencing technology, single-strand conformational polymorphisms, and restriction fragment length polymorphism (RFLP) analysis. The selection of one technique over another is often based on such factors as sensitivity and specificity profiles, cost, turnaround time, and local experience.

DNA Sequencing

DNA sequencing is considered to be the "gold standard" method by which other molecular methods are compared. DNA sequencing displays the exact nucleotide or base sequence of a fragment of DNA that is targeted. The Sanger method, which uses a series of enzymatic reactions to produce segments of DNA complementary to the DNA being sequenced, is the most frequently used method for DNA sequencing. Automated sequencing techniques use primers with four different fluorescent labels.

1. The first step to sequence a target is usually to amplify it, by cloning or in vitro amplification, usually PCR. Once the amplified DNA is purified from the clinical specimen (the target DNA), it is heat-denatured to separate the double-stranded DNA (dsDNA) into single strands (ssDNA).
2. The second step involves adding primers to the ssDNA; *primers* are short synthetic segments of single-stranded DNA that contain a nucleotide sequence complementary to a short strand of target DNA. The patient's DNA serves as a "template" to copy. DNA polymerase catalyzes the addition of the appropriate nucleotides to the preexisting primer. DNA synthesis is terminated when the deoxynucleotide is embodied into a growing DNA chain.

Branched DNA

Branched DNA (b-DNA) represents an alternative quantitative test that uses signal amplification instead of target amplification. Target DNA or RNA is hybridized at different sites by two types of probes. Branched DNA assays are being used to measure the viral load of hepatitis B virus (HBV), HCV, HIV-1, CMV, and microbial organisms (e.g., *Trypanosoma brucei*).

Versant HIV-1 RNA 3.0 assay (b-DNA), manufactured by Bayer Diagnostics (Bayer Group, Germany), uses branched DNA technology and is the only viral load assay specifically designed to target multiple sequences of the HIV-1 genome with more than 80 nucleic acid probes.

Hybridization Techniques

There are many forms of probe hybridization assays involving the complementary pairing of a probe with a DNA or RNA strand derived from the patient specimen. The common feature of probe hybridization assays is the use of a labeled nucleic acid probe to examine a specimen for a specific, homologous DNA or RNA sequence. The clinical probes are most often labeled with nonradioisotopic molecules such as digoxigenin, alkaline phosphatase, biotin, or a fluorescent compound. The detection systems are conjugate dependent and include chemiluminescent, fluorescent, and calorimetric methodologies.

Liquid-Phase Hybridization

In the liquid-phase hybridization (LPH) assay, both the target nucleic acid and the labeled probe interact in solution. Specific homologous hybrids are subsequently separated from the remaining nucleic acid component, and the hybrids are identified by an appropriate detection system.

Dot Blot and Reverse Dot Blot

These hybridization methods are used in the clinical laboratory for the detection of disorders in which the DNA sequence of the mutated region has been identified (e.g., sickle cell anemia, cystic fibrosis). These techniques are capable of distinguishing homozygous or heterozygous states for a mutation.

Dot Blot. The dot blot hybridization method detects single-base mutations using allele-specific oligonucleotides (ASOs). Unlike other assays, the dot blot does not require enzyme digestion or electrophoretic separation of DNA fragments. The procedure uses labeled oligonucleotide probes of about 15 to 19 bp. DNA is amplified in the region of a known mutation, denatured, and applied to separate areas of a membrane or filter. A probe designed to detect a normal DNA sequence is added to one area; a second probe for the detection of a sequence with the single-base mutation is applied to a second area. Ideally, only the labeled probe whose base sequences perfectly match those of the patient will hybridize.

Reverse Dot Blot. In this variation of the dot blot procedure, the ASO probes are bound to a filter, and denatured DNA from the patient is added to the immobilized ASO. Hybridization occurs only if the patient's DNA contains base sequences that are 100% complementary to those of the probe. A common variation of the reverse dot blot procedure is to bind oligonucleotide probes of a slightly longer length than usual to a 96-well microtiter plate. Biotin is used to label copies of the target sequence. The labeled copies are hybridized in the wells to the bound probes and detected using avidin conjugated to horseradish peroxidase. Subsequent addition of substrate produces a colored reaction that can be read photometrically.

Blotting Protocols

The Southern blot and Northern blot are used to detect DNA and RNA, respectively. These procedures share the following steps:

1. Electrophoretic separation of the patient's nucleic acid.
2. Transfer of nucleic acid fragments to a solid support (e.g., nitrocellulose).
3. Hybridization with a labeled probe of known nucleic acid sequence.
4. Autoradiographic or colorimetric detection of the bands created by the probe–nuclei acid hybrid.

Southern Blot. Specimen DNA is denatured and treated with restriction enzymes to create DNA fragments, and then the ssDNA fragments are separated by electrophoresis. The electrophoretically separated fragments are then blotted to a nitrocellulose membrane, retaining their electrophoretic position and hybridized with radiolabeled single-stranded DNA fragments with sequences complementary to those being sought. The resulting dsDNA bearing the radiolabel is then, if present, detected by radiography.

The Southern blot procedure has clinical diagnostic applications for disorders associated with significant changes in DNA, a deletion or insertion of at least 50 to 100 bp (e.g., fragile X syndrome), and for determination of clonality in lymphomas of T- or B-cell origin. If a single-base mutation changes an enzyme restriction site on the DNA, resulting in an altered band or fragment size, the Southern blot procedure can detect these changes in DNA sequences, referred to as **restriction fragment length polymorphisms (RFLPs).** Single-base mutations that can be determined by Southern blot include sickle cell anemia and hemophilia A.

Northern Blot. Messenger RNA (mRNA) from the specimen is separated by electrophoresis and blotted to a specially modified paper support to result in covalent fixing of the mRNA in the electrophoretic positions. Radiolabeled, single-stranded DNA fragments complementary to the specific mRNA being sought are then hybridized to the bound mRNA. If the specific mRNA is present, the radioactivity is detected by autoradiography.

The derivation of this technique from the Southern blot used for DNA detection has led to the common usage of the term *Northern blot* for the detection of specific mRNA. The Northern blot is not routinely used in clinical molecular diagnostics.

Western Blot. Compared with the Southern blot, which separates and identifies RNA fragments and proteins, and the Northern blot, which concentrates on isolating mRNA, the Western blot is a technique in which proteins are separated electrophoretically, transferred to membranes, and identified through the use of labeled antibodies specific for the protein of interest (Figure 14-2).

The Western blot detects antibodies to specific epitopes of antigen subspecies. Electrophoresis of antigenic material results in separation of the antigen components by molecular weight (MW). Blotting the separated antigen to nitrocellulose, retaining the electrophoretic position, and causing it to react with patient specimen will result in the binding of specific antibodies, if present, to each antigenic "band." Electrophoresis of known MW standards allows for the determination of the MW of each antigenic band to which antibodies may be produced. These antibodies are then detected using EIA reactions that characterize antibody specificity.

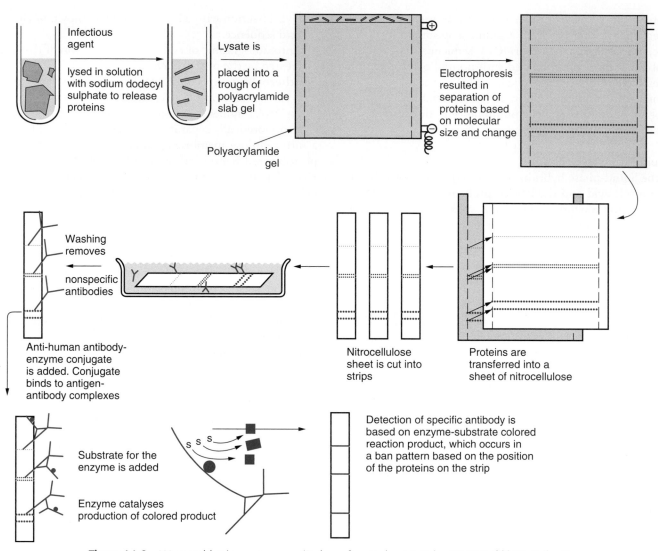

Infectious agent lysed in solution with sodium dodecyl sulphate to release proteins

Lysate is placed into a trough of polyacrylamide slab gel

Polyacrylamide gel

Electrophoresis resulted in separation of proteins based on molecular size and change

Washing removes nonspecific antibodies

Anti-human antibody-enzyme conjugate is added. Conjugate binds to antigen-antibody complexes

Nitrocellulose sheet is cut into strips

Proteins are transferred into a sheet of nitrocellulose

Substrate for the enzyme is added

Enzyme catalyses production of colored product

Detection of specific antibody is based on enzyme-substrate colored reaction product, which occurs in a ban pattern based on the position of the proteins on the strip

Figure 14-2   Western blot immunoassay. *(Redrawn from Forbes BA, Sahm DF, Weissfeld AS:* Bailey & Scott's diagnostic microbiology, *ed 12, St Louis, 2007, Mosby.)*

Western blot is often used to confirm the specificity of antibodies detected by enzyme-linked immunosorbent assay (ELISA) screening procedures.

Microarrays

Microarray (DNA chip) technology has helped to accelerate genetic analysis just as microprocessors accelerated computation (Figure 14-3).

Microarrays are basically the product of bonding or direct synthesis of numerous specific DNA probes on a stationary, often-silicon–based support. The chip may be tailored to particular disease processes. It is easily performed and readily automated. Microarrays are miniature gene fragments attached to glass chips. These chips are used to examine gene activity of thousands or tens of thousands of gene fragments and to identify genetic mutations, using a hybridization reaction between the sequences on the microarray and a fluorescent sample. After hybridization, the chips

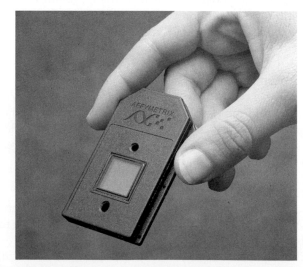

Figure 14-3   Affymetrix GeneChip probe array. *(Courtesy Affymetrix, Santa Clara, Calif.)*

are scanned with high-speed fluorescent detectors, and the intensity of each spot is quantitated (Figure 14-4).

The identity and amount of each sequence are revealed by the location and intensity of fluorescence displayed by each spot. Computers are used to analyze the data (Figure 14-5).

The applications of microarrays in clinical medicine include analysis of gene expression in malignancies (e.g., mutations in BRCA-1, mutations of the tumor-suppressor gene p53, genetic disease testing, viral resistance mutation detection).

The Human Genome GeneChip set (HG-U133 Set; Affymetrix, Santa Clara, Calif), consisting of two GeneChip arrays, contains almost 45,000 probe sets representing more than 39,000 transcripts derived from approximately 33,000 well-substantiated human genes. The sequence clusters were created from the UniGene database, then refined by analysis and comparison with a number of other publicly available databases, including the Washington University EST trace repository and the University of California, Santa Cruz, Golden Path human genome database.

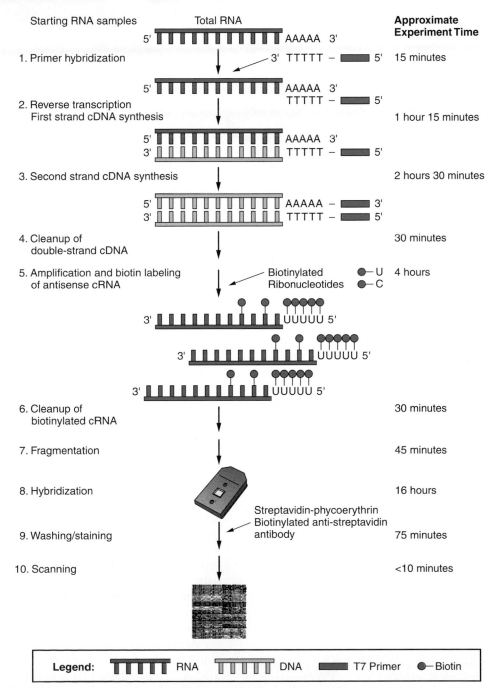

Figure 14-4 Overview of eukaryotic target labeling for GeneChip expression arrays. *(Courtesy Affymetrix, Santa Clara, Calif.)*

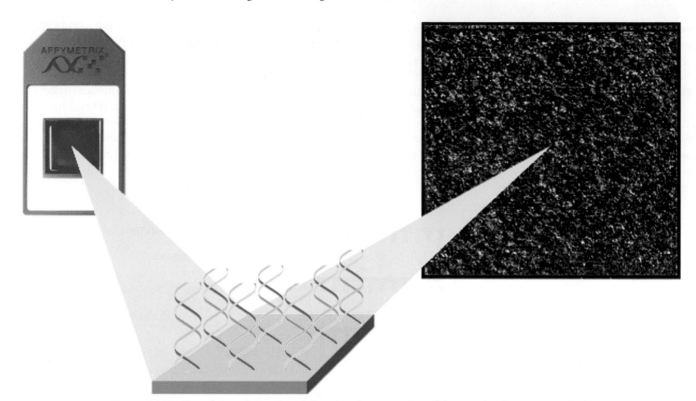

Figure 14-5 Data from an experiment showing the expression of thousands of genes on a single GeneChip probe array. *(Courtesy Affymetrix, Santa Clara, Calif.)*

The HG-U133A array includes representation of the Ref-Seq database sequences and probe sets related to sequences previously represented on the Human Genome U95Av2 array. The HG-U133B array contains primarily probe sets representing EST clusters. The applications of this array include definition of tissue and cell type–specific gene expression and investigation of cellular and tissue responses to the environment (e.g., heat shock; interactions with other cells; exposure to chemical compounds, growth factors, or other signaling molecules). In addition, this array helps to elucidate human cell differentiation by (1) determining which transcripts are increased or decreased during distinct stages in cellular differentiation and (2) detecting what genes are uniquely expressed during different stages of tumorigenesis.

Another genomic microarray, GenoSensor (Vysis, Downer's Grove, Ill), enables researchers to screen for abnormal gene amplifications and deletions with the sensitivity to detect single gene-copy change in a variety of specimens. The GenoSensor system simultaneously screens for gene-copy number changes in 287 targets spotted in triplicate. This permits the screening of proto-oncogenes, tumor suppressor genes, microdeletion syndrome, gene regions, and subtelomeric regions.

CHAPTER HIGHLIGHTS

- Polymerase chain reaction (PCR) is an in vitro method that amplifies low levels of specific DNA sequences in a sample to higher quantities suitable for further analysis.

- PCR, an enzymatic process, is carried out in cycles. Each repeated cycle consists of DNA denaturation, primer annealing, and extension of the primed DNA sequence. Each cycle theoretically doubles the amount of specific DNA sequence present and results in an exponential accumulation of the DNA fragment being amplified (amplicons).

- PCR analysis can lead to detection of gene mutations, identification of viral DNA associated with specific cancers, and detection of genetic mutations.

- Adaptations of the PCR technique include nested primers. Modifications include RT-PCR, multiplex PCR, and real-time PCR.

- Conventional analysis is the use of agarose gel electrophoresis after ethidium bromide staining.

- Probe-based DNA detection systems provide sequence specificity and lower detection limits.

- Selection of technique is based on sensitivity and specificity profiles, cost, turnaround time, and local experience.

- Probe hybridization assays involve the complementary pairing of a probe with DNA or RNA from the patient specimen and include liquid-phase assay, dot blot, and reverse dot blot.

- Southern blot can determine single-base mutations (sickle cell anemia, hemophilia A).

- Northern blot can be used for the detection of specific mRNA. The Northern blot is not routinely used in clinical molecular diagnostics.

- In Western blot, proteins are separated electrophoretically, transferred to membranes, and identified through labeled antibodies. It is used to detect antibodies to specific epitopes of antigen subspecies and confirm the specificity of antibodies detected by ELISA screening.

- Microarrays (DNA chips) are the product of bonding or synthesis of specific DNA probes on a stationary support. These chips are used to examine gene activity and identify genetic mutations in malignancies, genetic disease testing, and detection of virally resistant mutations.

REVIEW QUESTIONS

1. In comparison to serologic assays, nucleic acid testing offers all the following benefits *except:*
   a. Reduced cost.
   b. Enhanced specificity.
   c. Increased sensitivity.
   d. All the above.

2. Polymerase chain reaction (PCR) testing is useful in:
   a. Forensic testing.
   b. Genetic testing.
   c. Disease diagnosis.
   d. All the above.

3. The traditional PCR technique:
   a. Extends the length of the genomic DNA.
   b. Alters the original DNA nucleotide sequence.
   c. Copies the target region of DNA.
   d. Amplifies the target region of RNA.

4. For the PCR reaction to occur, the clinician must provide which of the following?
   a. Oligonucleotide primers.
   b. Individual deoxynucleotides.
   c. Thermostable DNA polymerase.
   d. All the above.

5. The enzyme *reverse transcriptase* converts:
   a. mRNA to cDNA.
   b. tRNA to DNTP.
   c. dsDNA to ssDNA.
   d. Mitochondrial to nuclear DNA.

6. DNA polymerase catalyzes:
   a. Primer annealing.
   b. Primer extension.
   c. Hybridization of DNA.
   d. Hybridization of RNA.

7. The figure below depicts:
   a. Polymerase chain reaction (PCR).
   b. Nested primer PCR.
   c. Western blot analysis.
   d. Southern blot analysis.

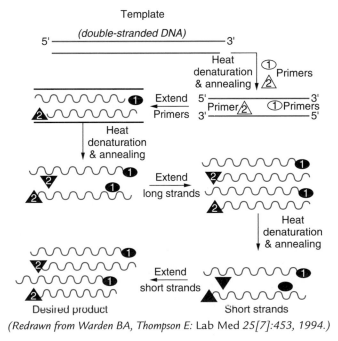

(Redrawn from Warden BA, Thompson E: Lab Med *25[7]:453, 1994.)*

Questions 8-10. Match the method with the appropriate description.

8. _____ Southern blot immunoassay

9. _____ Northern blot immunoassay

10. _____ Western blot immunoassay

   a. Messenger RNA is studied.
   b. Called immunoblot, it is used to detect antibodies to subspecies of antigens.
   c. Single-stranded DNA is studied.

11. Which of the following techniques uses signal amplification?
   a. b-DNA
   b. TMA
   c. NASBA
   d. RT-PCR

12. Which of the following nucleic acid amplification techniques does *not* require the use of a thermocycler?
   a. PCR
   b. SDA
   c. NASBA
   d. TMA

BIBLIOGRAPHY

Bakker E: Is the DNA sequence the gold standard in genetic testing? Quality of molecular genetic tests assessed, *Clin Chem* 52(4):557-558, 2006.

Branca M: One genome—two chips, *Bio-IT World* 1(1):12, 2002.

Capetandes A: Polymerase chain reaction: the making of something big, *Med Lab Observer* 31:26, 1999.

Doty A: Monitoring the quality of nucleic acid testing for infectious disease, *Adv Med Lab Prof* 13(10):12-16, 2001.

Forbes BA, Sahm DF, Weissfeld AS: *Bailey and Scott's diagnostic microbiology,* ed 12, St Louis, 2007, Mosby.

Kazmi S, Krull IS: Proteonomics and the current state of protein separations, *PharmaGenomics* 1(1):14-29, 2001.

Miyake K: Olympus develops DNA computer, *Bio-IT World* 1(1):2, 2002.

Nadder TS: The new millennium laboratory: molecular diagnostics goes clinical, *Clin Lab Sci* 14:252, 2001.

Rohlfs EM, Silverman LM: Molecular diagnosis of inherited disease, *Med Lab Observer* 28:44-52, 1996.

Schena M: *Microarray biochip technology,* Natick, Mass, 2000, Eaton Publishing.

Tang Y, Procop GW, Persing DH: Molecular diagnostics of infectious diseases, *Clin Chem* 43:2021-2038, 1997.

Turgeon ML: *Clinical hematology: theory and procedures,* ed 3, Philadelphia, 1999, Lippincott-Williams & Wilkins.

Uphoff TS: Basic concepts and innovations in molecular diagnosis, *Adv Med Lab Prof* 14(18):13, 2002.

Warden BA, Thompson E: Apolipoprotein E and the development of atherosclerosis, *Lab Med* 25(7):449-455, 1994.

Weiss RL: *Interpretive data guide,* Salt Lake City, 1999, ARUP Laboratories.

Weiss RL, editor: *ARUP's guide to molecular diagnostics clinical laboratory testing,* ed 2, Salt Lake City, 2001, ARUP Laboratories.

Wisecarver J: Amplification of DNA sequences, *Lab Med* 28:191-196, 1997.

PART III

Immunologic Manifestations of Infectious Diseases

15 The Immune Response in Infectious Diseases
16 A Primer on Vaccines
17 Streptococcal Infections
18 Syphilis
19 Vector-Borne Disease
20 Toxoplasmosis
21 Cytomegalovirus
22 Infectious Mononucleosis
23 Viral Hepatitis
24 Rubella Infection
25 Acquired Immunodeficiency Virus (AIDS)

CHAPTER 15

The Immune Response in Infectious Diseases

Characteristics of Infectious Diseases
Development of Infectious Diseases
Bacterial Diseases
Parasitic Diseases
Fungal Diseases
　Histoplasmosis
　Aspergillosis
　Coccidioidomycosis
　North American Blastomycosis
　Sporotrichosis
　Cryptococcosis

Viral, Rickettsial, and Mycoplasmal Diseases
　Herpesviruses
　Herpes Simplex Virus
　Varicella-Zoster Virus
　Human Herpesvirus-6
Laboratory Detection of Immunologic Responses
　Antibody Significance
　TORCH Testing
Chapter Highlights
Review Questions
Bibliography

Learning Objectives

At the conclusion of this chapter, the reader should be able to:
- Describe important characteristics in the acquisition and development of infectious diseases.
- Compare how the body develops immunity to bacterial, parasitic, fungal, and viral, rickettsial, and mycoplasmal diseases.

- Briefly describe the laboratory detection of immunologic responses.

CHARACTERISTICS OF INFECTIOUS DISEASES

The acquisition of an infectious disease (e.g., viral, bacterial, parasitic, fungal) is influenced by factors related to both the microorganism and the host. The following factors can influence exposure to and development of an infectious disease:
- The immune status of an individual. (Immunocompromised individuals have a much higher rate of microbial disease.)
- Overall incidence of an organism in the population.
- Pathogenicity or virulence of the agent.
- Presence of a sufficiently large dose of the agent or organism to produce an infection.
- Appropriate portal of entry.

In many cases the successful dissemination of a microorganism results from spread of the microorganism over long distances by insect vectors or rapidly from country to country by global travelers. Also, some microorganisms are able to multiply in an intracellular habitat, such as in macrophages, and others can display antigen variation, which makes normal immune mechanism control difficult.

Host factors, such as the general health and age of an individual, influence the likelihood of developing an infectious disease and are important determinants of its severity. The very young and the older populations develop infectious diseases more frequently than individuals in other age groups. In addition, a history of previous exposure to a disease or harboring of an organism such as a virus in a dormant condition is also a determining factor in disease development.

DEVELOPMENT OF INFECTIOUS DISEASES

For an infectious disease to develop in a host, the organism must penetrate the skin or mucous membrane barrier (first line of defense) and survive other natural and adaptive body defense mechanisms (see Chapter 1). These mechanisms include phagocytosis, antibody and cell-mediated immunity or complement activation, and associated interacting effector mechanisms. Phagocytosis and complement activation may be initiated within minutes of invasion by a microorganism; however, unless primed by previous contact with the same or similar antigen, antibody and cell-mediated responses do not become activated for several days. Complement and antibodies are the most active constituents against microorganisms free in the blood or tissues, whereas cell-mediated responses are most active against microorganisms that are associated with cells.

The most effective mechanism of body defense in a healthy host depends on factors such as an appropriate portal of entry and the characteristics of each microorganism. The routes of infection or portals of entry can include transmission through oral routes (e.g., food-borne or water-borne contamination), maternal-fetal transmission, insect vectors, sexual transmission, parenteral routes (e.g., injection or transfusion of infected blood), and respiratory transmission. Development of an infectious disease occurs only if a microorganism can evade, overcome, or inhibit normal body defense mechanisms.

BACTERIAL DISEASES

The presence of key substances (e.g., *lysozyme*) and the process of phagocytosis represent major immunologic defense mechanisms against bacteria. A microorganism, however, is able to survive phagocytosis if it possesses a capsule that impedes attachment or a cell wall that interferes with digestion and release of exotoxins, which damage phagocytic and other cells. Most capsules and toxins are strongly antigenic, but antibodies can overcome many of their effects; this is the basis of most antibacterial vaccines.

Examples of representative bacterial diseases of importance in the study of immunology and serology are presented in Chapters 17 and 18.

PARASITIC DISEASES

Parasites are relatively large, may have resistant body walls, and may avoid being phagocytized because of their ability to migrate away from an inflamed area. These differences set parasitic infections apart from bacterial and viral infections, to which some forms of natural and adaptive immunity afford protection. (Toxoplasmosis, a representative disease, is discussed in Chapter 20.)

Immune responses ("effectors") to parasitic infections include immunoglobulins, complement, antibody-dependent cell-mediated cytotoxicity, and cellular defenses such as eosinophils and T cells. Some cestodes, especially in their larval stages, may be eradicated by complement-fixing immunoglobulin G (IgG) antibodies. In addition, some antibodies may cross-react with other parasitic antigens. Increased levels of IgE may be noted in many helminth infections. Activation of both the classic and the alternate complement pathways may occur in some cases of schistosomiasis, and the alternate pathway of complement activation may kill larvae in the absence of antibody (see Chapter 5).

Phagocytosis may have some direct activity against parasitic organisms, but the most effective protection in some parasitic infections is provided by antibody-dependent, cell-mediated cytotoxicity. Macrophages, neutrophils, and eosinophils may demonstrate direct toxicity or phagocytosis toward parasites. The actual attachment of the cytotoxic cells is most frequently mediated by IgG, although IgE may be effective. The role of eosinophils is complex. They may phagocytize immune complexes and act as effector cells in mediating local (type I) reactions, primarily in tissue-stage parasites. T cells are frequently involved in body defenses against parasites. Sequestration of microorganisms is a classic T-cell-dependent hypersensitivity response. In addition, helper T cells may sensitize B cells to specific parasitic antigens.

Other, nonspecific factors (e.g., nonstimulated monocytes) are a major protective mechanism against parasites such as *Giardia* species. Natural killer (NK) cells also have a direct activity against cancer cells and some parasites. Delayed hypersensitivity may be helpful in preventing some parasitic infections but may cause disease in other cases. Deposition of antigen-antibody complexes, demonstrated by Raji cell assays, is responsible for severe pathologic lesions in some parasitic infections. In addition, high levels of circulating IgE may cause hypersensitivity reactions in helminth and cestode infections. Anaphylaxis is a clear risk in echinococcal infections, especially with spontaneous or surgical rupture of a hydatid cyst.

FUNGAL DISEASES

Fungal, or *mycotic*, infections are normally superficial, but a few fungi can cause serious systemic disease, usually entering through the respiratory tract in the form of spores. Disease manifestation depends on the degree and type of immune response elicited by the host. Fungi are common and harmless inhabitants of skin and mucous membranes under normal conditions (e.g., *Candida albicans*). In immunocompromised hosts, however, *Candida* species and other fungi become opportunistic agents that take advantage of the host's weakened resistance. Manifestations of fungal disease may range from unnoticed respiratory episodes to rapid, fatal dissemination of a violent hypersensitivity reaction.

Survival mechanisms of fungi that successfully invade the body are similar to bacterial characteristics and include (1) presence of an antiphagocytic capsule, (2) resistance to digestion within macrophages, and (3) destruction of phagocytes (e.g., neutrophils). Some types of yeast activate complement through the alternative pathway, but it is unknown if this activation has any effect on the microorganism's survival.

Fungal infections are increasing worldwide for a variety of reasons, including the use of immunosuppressive drugs and the development of diseases that result in an immunocompromised host (e.g., AIDS). Serologic tests often play an important role in the diagnosis of these fungal infections (Table 15-1).

Several species of fungi are associated with respiratory disease in humans. These diseases are acquired by inhaling spores from exogenous reservoirs, including dust, bird droppings, and the soil.

Histoplasmosis

Histoplasma capsulatum can be found in soil contaminated with chicken, bird, or bat excreta. Inhalation of spore-laden dust is the source of histoplasmosis.

Histoplasmosis can be difficult to diagnose and can range from asymptomatic to chronic pulmonary disease. In addition, a disseminated form manifesting hepatosplenomegaly with diffuse lymphadenopathy is usually present in varying degrees of severity because of the propensity of the fungus to invade the cells of the mononuclear phagocyte system. Disseminated disease is characterized by fever, anemia, leukopenia, weight loss, and lassitude.

Definitive diagnosis requires isolation in culture and microscopic identification of the fungus, as well as serologic evidence. If an immunodiffusion technique is used, H and M bands appearing together indicate active infection. If only an M band is present, it indicates early infection, chronic infection, or a recent reactive skin test. An H band appears later than the M band and disappears earlier. Disappearance of an H band suggests regression of the infection.

Delayed-hypersensitivity skin testing is confirmed by a rise in complement-fixing antibodies to *Histoplasma* antigens. Titers of 8 and 16 (dilution 1:8, 1:16) are highly suggestive of infection. A titer of 32 or greater usually indicates active infection. A rising titer indicates progressive infection; a decreasing titer suggests regression. Some disseminated infections are nonreactive in **complement fixation (CF)** tests. In addition, recent skin tests in individuals with prior exposure to *H. capsulatum* will produce a rise in the CF titer in 17% to 20% of patients. Cross-reactions in the CF test occur in patients with aspergillosis, blastomycosis, or coccidioidomycosis, but the titers are usually lower. Several follow-up serum samples should be tested at 2- to 3-week intervals.

Aspergillosis

Another opportunistic mycotic infection occurring in humans is aspergillosis, which can be allergic, invasive, or disseminating, depending on pathologic findings in the host. Aspergillosis is usually secondary to another disease. Allergic bronchopulmonary aspergillosis is characterized by allergic reactions to the toxins and endotoxins of the *Aspergillus* species.

Species identification of aspergillosis can be made microscopically. Serologically, skin reactions and immunodiffusion are useful tools for identification, especially if the culture is negative.

Immunodiffusion antibody test with reference antisera and known antigen is a frequently used test for the identification of *Aspergillus* species in almost all clinical types of aspergillosis. Precipitin formation by immunodiffusion is useful in identifying patients with pulmonary eosinophilia, severe allergic aspergillosis, and aspergillomas. The presence of one or more precipitin bands suggests active infection. The precipitin bands correlate with CF titers. In this test the greater the number of bands, the higher is the titer. In general, immunodiffusion measures IgG, and a positive result may suggest past infection. The test is positive in about 90% of sera from patients with aspergilloma and 50% to 70% of patients with allergic bronchopulmonary aspergillosis. A negative test does not exclude aspergillosis.

In addition, the enzyme immunoassay (EIA) can be used to detect IgE and IgG antibodies. ImmunoCAP is a newer method used to detect *Aspergillus niger* IgE in serum.

Enzyme immunoassay is used to detect *Aspergillus* galactomannan antigen in serum. Negative results do not exclude the diagnosis of invasive aspergillosis. A single positive test result should be confirmed by testing a separate serum specimen. Many agents (e.g., antibiotics, food) can cross-react with the assay. The false-positive rate is higher in children than in adults. If invasive aspergillosis is suspected in high-risk patients, serial sampling is recommended.

Hypersensitivity testing is characterized by both immediate and delayed-type hypersensitivity reactions, as a result of the presence of *Aspergillus*-specific immunoglobulin. IgE

Table 15-1	Testing Methods for Fungal Disease
Disease	**Procedure**
Aspergillosis	ImmunoCAP system (solid-phase two-site fluorescent EIA with covalently immobilized antigens)
	IgG to *Aspergillus fumigatus* (≤110 mg/L): 85% of farmers and some persons with no evidence of disease
Histoplasmosis	Complement fixation, immunodiffusion, PCR (sputum, blood, tissue)
	Fungus media, nucleic acid probe
Coccidioidomycosis	Complement fixation using coccidioidin (blood, CSF)
Blastomycosis	Complement fixation (<50% positive in proven cases), immunodiffusion
Sporotrichosis	Latex particle agglutination, EIA, IgG, IgM, IgA (CSF)
Cryptococcosis	Latex agglutination (serum, CSF)

EIA, Enzyme immunoassay; *PCR,* polymerase chain reaction; *CSF,* cerebrospinal fluid.

titers are greatly increased in allergic bronchopulmonary aspergillosis.

Coccidioidomycosis

Coccidioidomycosis is also known as *desert fever, San Joaquin fever,* or *valley fever.* The disease may assume several forms, including primary pulmonary, primary cutaneous, and disseminated. The disease is contracted from inhalation of soil or dust containing the arthrospores of *Coccidioides immitis.*

Hypersensitivity testing using intradermal injections is useful in screening for *C. immitis.* It is usually the first immunologic test to be positive in both asymptomatic and symptomatic cases. Skin testing does not differentiate between recent and past exposures to *C. immitis.* A positive skin test should be followed by other serodiagnostic tests. A negative test in a previously positive person can indicate a disseminated infection and a state of anergy.

The **fluorescent antibody (FA)** test can be applied directly to clinical specimens. This procedure is invaluable for making a rapid and specific identification of fungal structures. In addition to culturing the organism, serologic tests used to confirm the diagnosis of coccidioidomycosis include the tube precipitin test, immunodiffusion, CF, and latex agglutination. The CF test is the most widely used quantitative serodiagnostic test to identify infection with *C. immitis.* It is very effective in detecting disseminated disease. The tube precipitin test is positive in more than 90% of primary symptomatic cases.

Immunodiffusion is equivalent to CF; it can be used as a screening test, but the results should be confirmed by CF. Latex agglutination is not usually a recommended method because it lacks specificity. This creates many false-positive results.

Two antigens have been developed for the serologic identification of circulating antibodies to *C. immitis.* IgM appears 1 to 3 weeks after infection in 90% of symptomatic patients. IgG develops 3 to 6 months after onset of symptoms. Titers of 1:2 to 1:4 are presumptive evidence of an early infection and should be repeated in 3 to 4 weeks. Titers of 1:8 to 1:16 are evidence of active infection, particularly when accompanied by a positive immunodiffusion test. Titers greater than 1:16 occur in 90% to 95% of patients with disseminated coccidioidomycosis.

North American Blastomycosis

Blastomycosis is a chronic fungal disease usually secondary to pulmonary involvement. *Blastomyces dermatitidis* causes tumors in the skin or lesions in the lungs, bones, subcutaneous tissues, liver, spleen, and kidneys.

Serologic diagnosis is problematic because of high cross-reactivity with antigenic components of the organism. Although both immunodiffusion and CF are used, immunodiffusion is considered the better method. CF titers of 8 and 16 are highly suggestive of active infection, and titers of 32 or greater are diagnostic. A decreasing titer indicates regression; however, most patients with blastomycosis have negative CF tests.

Sporotrichosis

This chronic, progressive, subcutaneous lymphatic mycosis is caused by *Sporothrix schenckii.* The disease takes three forms: lymphatic (which is the most common), disseminated, and respiratory. It is characterized by a sporotrichotic chancre at the site of inoculation, followed by the development and formation of subcutaneous nodules along the lymphatics draining the primary lesions. Infection is associated with injuries caused by thorns or splinters. Handlers of peat moss are particularly susceptible to the disease, especially when working in rose gardens.

Laboratory methods of identification include cultures, serologic techniques, and FA-staining technique. Two of the most sensitive tests are yeast cell and latex agglutination. Titers of 80 or greater usually indicate active infection.

Skin testing is also available. Patients with cutaneous infection usually demonstrate negative tests; patients with extracutaneous infections have positive tests.

Cryptococcosis

Cryptococcus neoformans is the etiologic agent of this disease. Infected pigeons are the chief vector. Cryptococcosis is acquired by inhaling yeast. It may initially be asymptomatic or may develop as a symptomatic pulmonary infection. Any organ or tissue of the body may be infected, but localization outside the lungs or brain is relatively uncommon. The disease can be serious in immunocompromised or debilitated patients.

Antigen tests take less time to perform and are more specific than antibody detection. Latex agglutination antigen tests can be performed on serum or cerebrospinal fluid (CSF). Titers of 1:2 suggest infection, although such findings have been found in individuals with no evidence of cryptococcosis. Titers of 1:4 or greater are evidence of an active infection. Higher titers also indicate more severe infections. Positive titers are found in CSF in 95% of cases with involvement of the central nervous system.

The indirect FA test detects antibodies to *C. neoformans.* It is most valuable when antigen tests are negative and can even be combined with an antigen test to determine a patient's prognosis. A positive test suggests a present or recent infection.

Complement fixation is the most specific antibody detection test, but it is very insensitive. Tube agglutination, using serum or CSF that demonstrates a titer of 1:2 or greater, suggests a current or recent infection with *C. neoformans.*

As cryptococcosis progresses, antigens begin to appear, along with a decrease in antibody production. After treatment, a decrease in antigen titer and reappearance of antibodies indicate a good prognosis.

VIRAL, RICKETTSIAL, AND MYCOPLASMAL DISEASES

The characteristic process associated with viral infections is cellular replication, which may or may not lead to cell death. **Interferon** plays a major role in body defenses against viral infections. Antibodies are valuable in preventing entry and blood-borne spread of some viruses, but the ability of other viruses to spread from cell to cell places the burden of adaptive immunity on the T-cell system, which specializes in recognizing altered "self" histocompatibility antigens (histocompatibility leukocyte antigen, HLA). Macrophages may also play a role in immunity. Some of the most virulent viruses to humans are **zoonoses** (e.g., rabies). Other viruses, however, can persist for years without symptoms, then can be reactivated to cause serious disease, possibly including tumors.

New viruses can cause "old" diseases, and "old" viruses can cause new diseases (see Chapters 21 to 25 for representative examples of immunologically important viral diseases). The mutation rates of viruses, especially the ribonucleic acid (RNA) viruses such as human immunodeficiency virus (HIV), are extraordinarily high. Consequently, RNA viruses evolve much more rapidly under selective conditions than their hosts, and contemporary RNA viruses may have descended from a common ancestor only relatively recently. The survival of influenza A and B viruses as new viruses seems to depend on a continual evolution of mutants able to escape patient immunity as a result of preceding viruses. The most frequent cause of "new" viral infections is old viruses that are not natural infections of humans, but rather are accidentally transmitted from other species as zoonoses.

Organisms intermediate between viruses and bacteria are obligatory intracellular organisms with cell walls (e.g., Rickettsiae) and without cell walls but capable of extracellular replication (e.g., *Mycoplasma*). Immunologically, the former are closer to viruses, the latter to bacteria.

Herpesviruses

Two members of the human herpesviruses, **cytomegalovirus (CMV)** and **Epstein-Barr virus (EBV),** are described in detail in Chapters 21 and 22. The following sections briefly describe other members of the human herpesvirus family, including herpes simplex, varicella-zoster, and human herpesvirus-6.

All the human herpesviruses are large, enveloped DNA viruses that replicate within the cell's nucleus. The virus gains an envelope when the virus buds through the nuclear membrane, which has been altered to contain specific viral proteins.

The herpesviruses produce a number of clinical diseases, although they share the basic characteristic of being cell associated, which may partly account for their ability to produce subclinical infections that can be reactivated under appropriate stimuli.

Herpes Simplex Virus

Herpes simplex virus (HSV) can be cultured from the oropharynx in about 1% of healthy adults and from the genital tract of slightly less than 1% of asymptomatic adult women who are not pregnant. HSV is widespread. Humans are the only natural hosts or known reservoir of infection. The incubation period is 2 to 12 days. Incidence of seropositivity

rises to almost 100% in some populations by age 45 years. Antibody prevalence in adults varies greatly with socioeconomic class; 30% to 50% of upper-socioeconomic-class adults have detectable antibody to HSV, compared with 80% to 100% of adults in lower socioeconomic groups.

The most frequent manifestation of HSV infection is the common cold sore or fever blister. HSV has been shown to be related to a wide variety of clinical syndromes, as well as to subclinical infection, occurring with either primary or recurrent disease. Recurrent HSV disease usually results from reactivation of latent virus resting in paraspinal or cranial nerve ganglia that innervate the site of primary infection. Distant sites may be involved. Activated virus presumably travels down the axon to the skin (or other site) and induces disease. In some cases, exogenous reinfection can occur. Recurrence with cell-to-cell spread of virus occurs in the presence of serum-neutralizing antibodies.

Two cross-reacting antigen types of HSV have been identified, type 1 (HSV-1) and type 2 (HSV-2). HSV-1 is generally found in and around the oral cavity and in skin lesions that occur above the waist. HSV-2 is isolated primarily to the genital tract and skin lesions below the waist.

Congenital and Neonatal Infection

Malnutrition, severe illness, many acute childhood illnesses, and prematurity predispose infants and young children to disseminated primary infection. Neonatal HSV infections may be acquired in the antenatal or perinatal period. Active lesions in the mother's genital tract at birth present the greatest risk of infection to the newborn. The spectrum of disease occurring in an infected newborn varies from subclinical to severe. In cases of overwhelming generalized infection, the infant may develop encephalitis and respiratory failure, or hepatic failure with increasing jaundice and adrenal insufficiency may occur. Infants who survive severe infection are frequently left with some neurologic damage and may have recurrent vesicular skin lesions for many years.

Laboratory Diagnosis

Methods for laboratory diagnosis of HSV include isolation of the virus and the direct detection of antigen in tissues or cytologic preparation through the use of immunofluorescence or immunoenzyme methods. In addition, detection of the virus in body fluids (using monoclonal antibodies) can be performed with immunoassays or immunoblot techniques. Serologic diagnosis of primary infections can be demonstrated when a fourfold or greater rise in titer occurs. Titers may rise significantly in early recurrent infection but usually become stable at moderately high levels after multiple recurrences.

Varicella-Zoster Virus

Varicella-zoster virus (VZV) is the cause of two different types of clinical diseases resulting from the same virus infection. Primary infection with the virus results in the clinical manifestations of chickenpox. After a primary infection, the virus enters a latent phase, presumably within nuclei in the dorsal root ganglia. Reactivation of the virus results in the characteristic clinical manifestation of (zoster), shingles.

Epidemiology and Etiology

Humans are the only natural hosts of VZV. **Varicella** primarily affects children age 2 to 5 years. The virus is endemic and highly contagious. Periodic epidemics do occur. The presumed route of transmission is through the respiratory tract.

Zoster is less communicable than varicella. This sporadic disease occurs most frequently in middle-age persons. Antibodies to varicella do not protect against reactivation or clinical zoster. The reactivation of VZV is associated with a depressed immune response. Patients with AIDS, older adults, and immunocompromised persons are at high risk of developing disease. In addition, manipulation of the spinal cord, local radiation therapy, and therapy that suppresses cellular immunity have been associated with triggering the onset of zoster.

Varicella has an incubation period of 14 to 17 days. There may be a 1- to 3-day prodromal period of fever, headache, and malaise. This precedes the eruption of the characteristic red macular rash, which progresses to papules, vesicles, and pustules that crust over and shed without scarring. Successive crops of lesions continue to appear for 2 to 6 days; therefore multiple lesions in various stages of development are present at any one time.

The name of the virus reflects two associated diseases: varicella *(chickenpox)* and zoster *(shingles)*. Primary infection with the virus results in the clinical manifestation of chickenpox. After this, the virus enters a latent phase, presumably within nuclei of neurons in dorsal root ganglia or cranial nerve sensory ganglia. The reactivity of the virus results in the clinical manifestations characteristic of zoster.

Signs and Symptoms

Complications of VZV include pneumonitis, encephalitic conditions, nephritis, hepatitis, myocarditis, arthritis, and Reye's syndrome. Susceptible individuals who are immunosuppressed have a greater risk of complications after VZV exposure. Another complication can include febrile purpura, which can occur a few days after the onset of the rash and is seen in both children and adults. This complication is characterized by thrombocytopenia and hemorrhage into the vesicles. Postinfection purpura, which begins 1 to 2 weeks after the appearance of the rash, is characterized by thrombocytopenia with gastrointestinal, genitourinary, cutaneous, and mucous membrane hemorrhage. More severe hemorrhagic complications include malignant varicella with purpura and purpura fulminans.

Zoster Infection. Zoster infection is characterized by vesicular eruptions, typically confined to one or two adjacent dermatomes. The viral replication follows the nerve fiber. Neuralgia accompanies the skin eruptions and can last for months after the skin heals. Persistent neuralgia can be severe and can last months or longer.

Neonatal Varicella Infection. Neonatal varicella may be acquired in utero or in the perinatal period and can result in congenital abnormalities. The infant is at greatest risk if the mother's illness occurs 4 days or less before delivery.

Laboratory Diagnosis

Laboratory diagnosis of VZV is similar to HSV methods. Serologic methods include *indirect* immunofluorescence, which detects antibodies to specific membrane antigens, and EIA.

Rapid preliminary diagnosis can also be made by *direct* immunofluorescence to detect viral antigens in vesicular lesions. A smear of cells taken from lesions enables direct examination. A presumptive diagnosis can be made by examining scrapings from the base of a vesicular lesion and histologically observing multinucleated giant cells containing intranuclear inclusion bodies, or by observing virus particles on electron microscopy. The best way to confirm VZV infection is to recover the virus in human diploid fibroblast cell cultures.

Antibodies to varicella are detectable within several days of the onset of rash and peak at 2 to 3 weeks. Antibodies to zoster increase more rapidly and are detectable at the onset of clinical symptoms. Because of the rapid turnaround time and correlation with clinical symptoms, serologic methods are preferable to viral isolation methods. In addition, enzyme-linked immunosorbent assay (ELISA) methods are valuable for assessing the immune status of adults.

Human Herpesvirus-6

A "new" virus classified as a herpesvirus because of its shape, size, and in vitro behavior has been recently identified. Genomic analysis shows the virus to be molecularly unrelated to other human herpesviruses. Initially the virus was called B-lymphotropic virus, but subsequent studies indicated that T cells are the primary target of infection. This viral agent is currently classified as **human herpesvirus-6 (HHV-6).**

Patients with serologic evidence of acute HHV-6 infection are reported to experience mild, nonspecific symptoms and cervical lymphadenopathy. The same agent has been implicated as the cause of roseola infantum (exanthema subitum). Up to 75% of infants develop antibody to HHV-6 by age 10 to 11 months, which suggests a high rate of seropositivity in the general population.

Laboratory methods include direct examination by immunofluorescence or immunoperoxidase staining of cells taken from lesions. In addition, polymerase chain reaction (PCR), DNA probes, and serologic methods (e.g., ELISA, radioimmunoassay, indirect immunofluorescence, latex agglutination) can be used.

Culture methods include the cocultivation of the patient's peripheral blood cells with cord blood mononuclear cells and examination of these cultures after 5 to 10 days by electron microscopy. Anticomplement immunofluorescence of infected cell culture has also been used for antibody detection and titration.

LABORATORY DETECTION OF IMMUNOLOGIC RESPONSES

Because immunoglobulin M (IgM) is usually produced in significant quantities during the first exposure of a patient to an infectious agent, the detection of specific IgM can be of diagnostic significance (see Chapter 2). This immunologic characteristic is particularly important in diseases that do not manifest decisive clinical signs and symptoms (e.g., toxoplasmosis) or under those conditions in which a rapid therapeutic decision may be required (e.g., rubella).

Antibody Significance

In many diseases, infected individuals show a spectrum of responses. Some patients may develop and manifest antibodies from a subclinical infection or after colonization of an agent, without actually developing disease. In these patients the presence of antibody in a single serum specimen or a comparative titer of antibody in paired specimens may merely indicate past contact with the agent; the presence of antibodies cannot be used for accurate diagnosis of a recent disease. In comparison, some patients may respond to an antigenic stimulus by producing antibodies that can cross-react with other antigens. These antibodies are nonspecific and may lead to misinterpretation of serologic tests.

Serologic diagnosis of recent infection using acute and convalescent specimens is the method of choice. Except for the detection of IgM or in diseases with no chance of developing an immune response (e.g., rabies virus, botulism toxin), testing a single specimen is usually not recommended. In a number of circumstances, when only one specimen is tested to determine immune status, antibody to past infection or to immunization can be determined.

The testing protocols described in this chapter for the immunologic detection of representative infectious diseases are examples of the types of procedures typically encountered in the immunology-serology laboratory.

TORCH Testing

Procedures that specifically evaluate the presence of IgM or IgG are frequently used to detect CMV, herpesviruses (types 1 and 2), *Toxoplasma gondii,* and rubella. The names of the tests have been grouped under the acronym **TORCH:** *Toxoplasma,* other (viruses), rubella, CMV, herpes (Tables 15-2 and 15-3).

A spectrum of congenital defects called "TORCH syndrome" occurs with maternal exposure to rubella (also to *T. gondii,* CMV, and HSV) Congenital defects may be asymptomatic. A TORCH panel is ordered if a pregnant woman is suspected of having any of the TORCH infections. Rubella infection during the first 16 weeks of pregnancy presents major risks for the unborn baby. If a pregnant woman has a rash and other symptoms of rubella, laboratory tests are required to make the diagnosis. Women infected with *Toxoplasma* or CMV may have flulike symptoms that are not easily differentiated from other illnesses. Antibody testing will help diagnose an infection that may be harmful to the fetus.

Table 15-2	TORCH Antibodies, Immunoglobulin M
Infectious Agent	**Interpretation of Assay**
CMV	Positive: IgM antibody to CMV detected; may indicate current or recent infection; 1.10 IV or greater = positive.
HSV-1, HSV-2	Positive (>1.10 IV): IgM antibody to HSV detected (ELISA); may indicate a current or recent infection.
Rubella	Positive: 1.10 IV or greater; IgM antibody to rubella detected; may indicate current or recent infection or immunization.
Toxoplasma gondii	Positive: 1.10 IV or greater; significant level of antibody detected; may indicate current or recent infection.

Modified from Associated Regional and University Pathologists: ARUP test reference guide, 2008. www.arup-lab.com.
TORCH, Toxoplasma, other (viruses), rubella, CMV, herpes; *CMV,* cytomegalovirus; *HSV,* herpes simplex virus; *ELISA,* enzyme-linked immunosorbent assay.

Table 15-3	TORCH Antibodies, Immunoglobulin G
Infectious Agent	**Interpretation of Assay**
CMV antibody	Positive: 1.10 or greater; IgG antibody to CMV detected; may indicate current or previous CMV infection.
HSV-1, HSV-2	Positive: 1.10 or greater; IgG antibody to HSV detected (ELISA); may indicate current or previous HSV infection.
Rubella	Positive: 10 IU/mL or greater; IgG antibody to rubella detected; may indicate current or previous exposure/immunization to rubella.
Toxoplasma gondii	≥6 IU/mL: negative 9 IU/mL or greater = positive. Results may indicate current or past infection.

Modified from Associated Regional and University Pathologists: ARUP test reference guide, 2008. www.arup-lab.com.

In addition, a TORCH panel may be ordered on the newborn if the infant shows any signs suggestive of these infections, such as exceptionally small size relative to gestational age, deafness, mental impairment, seizures, heart defects, cataracts, enlarged liver or spleen, low platelet level, and jaundice.

Toxoplasmosis

Toxoplasmosis infection during pregnancy can cause congenital infection and manifestations, such as mental retardation and blindness. Hydrocephalus, intracranial calcification, and retinochoroiditis are the most common manifestations of tissue damage from congenital toxoplasmosis.

Neonatal screening program based on detecting IgM antibodies against *T. gondii* alone would identify 70% to 80% of congenital toxoplasmosis cases. The prevalence of congenital toxoplasmosis is 1 per 10,000 live births in the United States, where 85% of women of childbearing age are susceptible to acute infection with *T. gondii.*

Cytomegalovirus

Cytomegalovirus is the most common congenital virus infection in the world. Both primary and recurrent infection can result in fetal infection. The birth prevalence of congenital CMV infection varies from 0.3% to 2.4%, and at least 90% of congenitally infected infants have no clinical signs. CMV causes illnesses ranging from no clinical signs to prematurity, encephalitis, deafness, hematologic disorders, and death.

Congenital CMV infection is described in 30,000 to 40,000 newborns each year in the United States; approximately 9000 of these children have permanent neurologic sequelae. The death rate from symptomatic congenital CMV infection is approximately 30%.

Rubella

Rubella virus infection during early pregnancy can lead to severe birth defects known as *congenital rubella syndrome.* Sequelae of rubella virus infection include three distinct neurologic syndromes, as follows:
• Postinfectious encephalitis after acute infection.
• Neurologic manifestations after congenital infection.
• Rare neurodegenerative disorder, *progressive rubella panencephalitis,* that can follow either congenital or postnatal infection.

CHAPTER HIGHLIGHTS

• For an infectious disease to be acquired by a host, the microorganism must penetrate the skin or mucous membrane barrier and survive other natural and adaptive body defense mechanisms.
• Phagocytosis and complement activation may be initiated within minutes of the invasion of a microorganism; however, unless primed by previous contact with the same or similar antigen, antibody and cell-mediated responses do not become activated for several days.
• The mechanism of body defense most effective in a healthy host depends on the microorganism. Defenses such as phagocytosis are highly effective in bacterial immunity; T cells are frequently involved in body defenses against parasites.
• Sequestration of microorganisms is a classic T-cell-dependent hypersensitivity response.
• IgM is usually produced in significant quantities after the first exposure to an infectious agent. This is important in diseases that do not manifest decisive clinical signs and symptoms or under conditions requiring a rapid therapeutic decision.
• TORCH procedures evaluate the presence of IgM to detect *Toxoplasma,* other viruses, rubella, CMV, and herpes.

• In most cases, serologic diagnosis of recent infection using acute and convalescent specimens is the method of choice. The testing of a single specimen is not recommended.

REVIEW QUESTIONS

1. Factors that influence the development of an infectious disease include all the following *except* the:
   a. Immune status of the individual.
   b. Incidence of an organism in the population.
   c. Pathogenicity of the agent.
   d. Sole presence of the agent or microorganism.

Questions 2-5. Match the appropriate immunologic defense mechanism *(a-d)* with the class of microorganism.

2. _____ Bacteria

3. _____ Yeast

4. _____ Viruses

5. _____ Parasites

   a. Interferon.
   b. Lysozymes and phagocytosis.
   c. Immunoglobulins, complement, antibody-dependent cell-mediated cytotoxicity, and cellular defenses.
   d. Possibly the activation of complement.

6. The detection of _____ can be of diagnostic significance during the first exposure of a patient to an infectious agent.
   a. IgM
   b. IgG
   c. IgA
   d. IgD

7. Serologic procedures for the diagnosis of recent infection should include:
   a. Only an acute specimen.
   b. Only a convalescent specimen.
   c. Acute and convalescent specimens.
   d. Acute, convalescent, and 6-month postinfection specimens.

8. An important factor affecting microbial disease development is the:
   a. Ability of some microorganisms to multiply in an intracellular habitat.
   b. Display of antigen variation.
   c. Presence of a related microorganism.
   d. Both a and b.

9. For an infectious disease to develop in a host, the organism must initially:
   a. Survive phagocytosis.
   b. Be in the log phase of multiplication.
   c. Penetrate the skin or mucous membrane barrier.
   d. Be present in the host for 7 to 10 days.

Questions 10-12. Match each type of infectious disease to the appropriate description.

10. _____ Bacterial disease

11. _____ Viral disease

12. _____ Parasitic disease

    a. Affected by such immune responses as immunoglobulin; complement; and antibody-dependent cell-mediated cytotoxicity.

    b. Inhibited by antibiotics, lysozymes, and phagocytosis.

    c. Stimulates production of, and is in turn inhibited by, interferon.

13. The first type of antibody that may be apparent in the immune response to an infectious disease is:
    a. IgM.
    b. IgG.
    c. IgD.
    d. IgA.

14. A distinguishing characteristic of the herpesviruses is that:
    a. They are cell-associated viruses.
    b. They are enveloped RNA.
    c. Humans are the only known reservoir of infection.
    d. Both a and c.

15. Up to _____ of infants develop antibody to HHV-6 by 10 to 11 months of age.
    a. 25%
    b. 50%
    c. 75%
    d. 95%

16. Varicella-zoster virus causes:
    a. Chickenpox.
    b. Shingles.
    c. Measles.
    d. Both a and b.

17. Varicella-zoster virus can be reactivated in:
    a. AIDS patients.
    b. Elderly persons.
    c. Immunocompromised persons.
    d. All the above.

18. Rapid preliminary diagnosis of varicella-zoster can be made in the laboratory by:
    a. Direct immunofluorescence.
    b. Viral isolation.
    c. ELISA method.
    d. Complement fixation.

19. Histoplasmosis is caused by a:
    a. Bacterium.
    b. Parasite.
    c. Fungus.
    d. Virus.

20. Aspergillosis is:
    a. An opportunistic organism.
    b. Caused by a parasite.
    c. A cause of skin infections.
    d. A relatively mild disease.

21. The first test to be positive in coccidioidomycosis is:
    a. Fluorescent antibody.
    b. Hypersensitivity testing.
    c. Complement fixation.
    d. Culture of the organism.

Questions 22-24. Match the following.

22. _____ Blastomycosis

23. _____ Sporotrichosis

24. _____ Cryptococcosis

    a. Subcutaneous lymphatic mycosis.
    b. Vector in infected pigeons.
    c. Chronic fungal disease.

BIBLIOGRAPHY

Associated Regional and University Pathologists (ARUP) Laboratories: *Aspergillus* testing, 2007. www.aruplab.com.

Davidson RA: Immunology of parasitic infections, *Med Clin North Am* 69(4):751-757, 1985.

Forbes BA, Sahm DF, Weissfeld AS: *Bailey and Scott's diagnostic microbiology,* ed 12, St Louis, 2007, Mosby.

Kilbourne ED: New viral diseases, *JAMA* 264(1):68-70, 1990.

Neto EC, Rubin R, Schulte J, Giugliani R: Newborn screening for congenital infectious diseases, *Emerg Infect Dis,* June 2004 (serial on Internet). http://www.cdc.gov.

Pastuszak AL et al: Outcome after maternal varicella infection in the first 20 weeks of pregnancy, *N Engl J Med* 330(13):901-906, 1994.

Playfair JHL: *Immunology at a glance,* Oxford, 1979, Blackwell Scientific Publications.

Turgeon ML: Bloodborne infectious diseases. In Turgeon ML, editor: *Fundamentals of immunohematology,* ed 2, Baltimore, 1996, Williams & Wilkins.

CHAPTER 16

A Primer on Vaccines

Vaccine Approval
Vaccines in Biodefense
History and Use of Vaccines
Concerns about Vaccines
Characteristics of a Vaccine
Host Response to Vaccination
Representative Vaccines
   HIV/AIDS
   Anthrax
   Cytomegalovirus

Hay Fever
Human Papillomavirus
Influenza
Leukemia
Polio
Smallpox
Chapter Highlights
Review Questions
Bibliography

Learning Objectives

At the conclusion of the chapter, the reader should be able to:

- Identify the federal agency that regulates vaccine products.
- Describe vaccine policy and the role of vaccines in public safety.
- Briefly describe the history and use of several specific vaccines.
- Explain some new targets and technologies for vaccines.
- Identify at least three essential characteristic of a vaccine.

- Based on immunologic principles, describe host response to vaccination.
- Analyze the problems associated with AIDS vaccine development and use.
- Describe the development and application of human papillomavirus vaccine.
- Compare and contrast the applications of at least four vaccines.

Of all the public health measures against infections, vaccination is the most cost-effective strategy. We become immune to microbial antigens through artificial and natural means. Vaccines give us artificially acquired, active immunity to a specific disease.

VACCINE APPROVAL

The **Center for Biologics Evaluation and Research (CBER)** regulates vaccine products. Many of these are childhood vaccines that have contributed to a significant reduction of vaccine-preventable diseases. According to the U.S. Centers for Disease Control and Prevention (CDC), vaccines have reduced preventable infectious diseases to an all-time low, and few people now experience the devastating effects of measles, pertussis, and other illnesses.

Vaccine development is an important focus of research related to acquired immunodeficiency syndrome (AIDS), malaria, and other devastating diseases.

VACCINES IN BIODEFENSE

In regard to bioterrorism, the goal of the U.S. Food and Drug Administration (FDA) is to foster the development of vaccines. Many products (e.g., FDA-regulated vaccines) could be affected by bioterrorism. Pathogens or pathogen products adapted for biologic warfare include the following:

- Smallpox (variola)
- Anthrax *(Bacillus anthracis)*
- Plague *(Yersinia pestis)*
- Tularemia *(Francisella tularensis)*
- Brucellosis *(Brucella abortus, B. melitensis, B. suis, B. canis)*
- Q fever *(Coxiella burnetii)*
- Botulinum toxin (produced by *Clostridium botulinum*)
- Staphylococcal enterotoxin B

HISTORY AND USE OF VACCINES

Edward Jenner, an English physician, discovered one of the fundamentals principles of immunization more than 200 years ago. His observations and experiments with smallpox vaccine paved the way for the development of rabies vaccine by Louis Pasteur and many other vaccines (e.g., diphtheria, typhoid fever).

The concept of **vaccination,** or deliberately introducing a potentially harmful microbe into a patient, initially met with suspicion and outrage. Current vaccines are considered safer and more protective than early products. Children now receive vaccines to numerous diseases (e.g., German measles [rubella]) once common in childhood. Adults require updates of certain vaccinations (e.g., tetanus).

More recently, a vaccine was approved in 2006 for adults over age 60 to reduce the risk of shingles (reactivation of varicella virus) in those who had chickenpox in childhood. International travelers frequently require vaccination to endemic diseases in a particular country (e.g., hepatitis A). Health care professionals are now protected against hepatitis B through the use of vaccines. Also, each year, many adults prepare for winter and the "flu season" by receiving flu vaccine.

The use of vaccines has spread to pets and livestock as well (e.g., rabies, Lyme disease, feline leukemia).

CONCERNS ABOUT VACCINES

Vaccination requirements, even well-accepted laws on "classic" childhood diseases (e.g., polio, measles, pertussis), have been resisted in recent years based on philosophic, political, scientific, and ideologic issues. In the past 20 years, the number of recommended pediatric vaccines has increased dramatically despite unproven theories alleging connections between vaccines and illnesses, including autism, diabetes, and multiple sclerosis. An estimated 1% to 3% of U.S. children are excused by their parents from vaccine requirements, with rates as high as 15% to 20% in a few communities.

A vaccine for hepatitis E virus (HEV) vaccine has raised ethical concerns in Nepal. Testing the recombinant protein (rHEV) vaccine in a civilian population led to concerns that residents might not have access to the vaccines after the clinical trials concluded. Hepatitis E is common (endemic) in Nepal.

CHARACTERISTICS OF A VACCINE

The purpose of a vaccine is to stimulate active immunity and to create an immune memory so that exposure to the active disease microorganism will stimulate an already-primed immune system to fight the disease. Most vaccines can be divided into the following two types:

- Live, attenuated vaccines
- Nonreplicating vaccines

Traditionally prepared vaccines are preparations of inactivated ("killed") or live, attenuated ("weakened") bacteria or viruses; parts of the microorganisms; or toxoids (inactivated toxins) from the disease-causing agent. Newer synthetic vaccines use subunit vaccines, conjugate vaccines, and naked DNA vaccines. Critical to the protective effect of *subunit vaccines* (vaccines consisting of components of the pathogens) are additives called *adjuvants,* which amplify the immune response. Currently, an aluminum salt−based substance called "alum" and an oil-based substance called "MF59" are two adjuvants licensed for clinical use.

No vaccine is totally effective or 100% safe. To be FDA approved (Table 16-1), a vaccine must meet specific requirements, as follows:

1. Produce protective immunity with only minimal side effects.

2. Be immunogenic enough to produce a strong and measurable immune response.
3. Be stable during its shelf life, with potency remaining at a proper level.

Inactivated vaccines are stored in a powdered form and are reconstituted before administration. Live, attenuated vaccines require refrigeration.

Recently recommended vaccines include a new measles-mumps-rubella-varicella vaccine for 1-year-old children and a tetanus-diphtheria-pertussis vaccine for people age 11 to 65 years.

HOST RESPONSE TO VACCINATION

Classic preventive vaccines are designed to mimic the effects of natural exposure to microbes. The earliest host response to vaccination is called the **innate immune response.** This response is an evolutionarily ancient system of host defense that occurs within minutes or hours after vaccination. The dendritic cell is critical to this response. **Dendritic cells** can sense components of bacteria, viruses, parasites, and fungi through **pathogen-recognition receptors.** One class of these receptors is the **toll-like receptor (TLR);** at least 10 have been described. As a group, TLRs can sense a wide variety of microbial stimuli (e.g., lipopolysaccharides, viral/bacterial DNA).

The intracelluar TLR signaling within dendritic cells is mediated by at least four adapter proteins. Once dendritic cells decode and integrate the signals generated by sensing microbial molecules with TLRs, the cells convey this information to naive antigen-specific T cells, which launch an immune response.

Over time, vaccine-induced immunity wanes; this may result in increased susceptibility later in life (e.g., varicella [shingles]). A second dose of vaccine could improve protection from both primary vaccine failure and waning vaccine-induced immunity.

REPRESENTATIVE VACCINES

Many different vaccines are currently available. Some emphasize public health safety (e.g., anthrax), and others prevent the return of epidemic disease.

HIV/AIDS

Vaccines such as the one to provide a immunity to human immunodeficiency virus (HIV) continue to be a problem because of the enormous genetic diversity and other unique features of the HIV-B viral envelope protein. An estimated 14,000 new HIV infections occur daily worldwide.

Preventive vaccines are given to HIV-negative individuals to prevent HIV infection. Therapeutic vaccines are administered to HIV-positive patients to improve their immune system. Currently, no HIV/AIDS vaccines are approved for use, although many are in clinical trials.

The status of HIV vaccines to date follows:

1. There are no proven effective therapeutic or preventive HIV vaccines.

Table 16-1	Status of Licensure and Recommendations for New Vaccines*				
Vaccine	Manufacturer	BLA Submitted to FDA	BLA Age Indications†	FDA Licensure	Status of AAP/CDC Recommendations‡
MCV4 (Menactra)	Sanofi Pasteur	December 2003	11-55 years	Licensed 14 Jan 05	AAP: aappolicy.aappublications.org/cgi/content/full/pediatrics;116/2/496 CDC: cdc.gov/mmwr/preview/mmwrhtml/rr5407a1.htm
		Supplement to original BLA: March 2005	2-10 years	Licensed 18 Oct 07	ACIP: cdc.gov/mmwr/preview/mmwrhtm/mm5648a4.htm
Varicella virus second dose (Varivax)	Merck	Supplement to original BLA: second dose	Children 12 months to 12 years (3-month minimum interval)	Licensed 5 Apr 05	AAP: aappolicy.aappublications.org/cgi/content/full/pediatrics;120/1/221 CDC: cdc.gov/mmwr/preview/mmwrhtml/rr5604a1.htm
Tdap (Boostrix)	GlaxoSmithKline (GSK)	July 2004	10-18 years	Licensed 3 May 05	AAP: aappolicy.aappublications.org/cgi/content/full/pediatrics;117/3/965 CDC: cdc.gov/mmwr/preview/mmwrhtml/rr5503a1.htm
Tdap (Adacel)	Sanofi Pasteur	August 2004	11-64 years	Licensed 10 Jun 05	AAP: aappolicy.aappublications.org/cgi/content/full/pediatrics;117/3/965 CDC Adolescent: cdc.gov/mmwr/preview/mmwrhtml/rr5503a1.htm CDC Adult: cdc.gov/mmwr/preview/mmwrhtml/rr5517a1.htm ACIP in Pregnancy: cdc.gov/nip/recs/provisional_recs/tdap-preg.pdf
MMRV (ProQuad)	Merck	August 2004	Same as for MMR dose 1 or dose 2; 12 months to 12 years	Licensed 6 Sep 05	CDC: cdc.gov/mmwr/preview/mmwrhtml/mm5447a4.htm
Hepatitis A (VAQTA)	Merck	Supplement to original BLA	≥12 months	Licensed 15 Aug 05	AAP: aappolicy.aappublications.org/cgi/content/full/pediatrics;120/1/189 CDC: cdc.gov/mmwr/preview/mmwrhtml/rr5507a1.htm
Hepatitis A (Havrix)	GlaxoSmithKline (GSK)	Supplement to original BLA	≥12 months	Licensed 18 Oct 05	AAP: aappolicy.aappublications.org/cgi/content/full/pediatrics;120/1/189 CDC: cdc.gov/mmwr/preview/mmwrhtml/rr5507a1.htm
Hepatitis A and hepatitis B (Twinrix)	GlaxoSmithKline (GSK)	May 2006	≥18 years	Licensed 28 Mar 07	CDC: Pending notice in MMWR
Rotavirus (RotateQ)	Merck	April 2005	2, 4, and 6 months	Licensed 3 Feb 06	CDC: cdc.gov/mmwr/preview/mmwrhtml/rr5512a1.htm AAP: aappolicy.aappublications.org/cgi/content/full/pediatrics;119/1/171
Rotavirus (Rotarix)	GlaxoSmithKline (GSK)	June 2007	2 and 4 months	To be reviewed	Pending FDA licensure
Herpes zoster vaccine (ZostaVax)	Merck	April 2005	≥60 years	Licensed 25 May 06	ACIP Recommendation: cdc.gov/nip/recs/provisional_recs/zoster-11-20-06.pdf

From American Academy of Pediatrics: *Red Book* online, 2003; updated 12/11/07; http://aapredbook.aappublications.org/news/vaccstatus.shtml.
*Information from vaccine manufacturers, ACIP meetings, and AAP.
†Age licensure can change following FDA review; not final until package insert approved.
‡ACIP recommendations do not become official until approved by the CDC Director and Department of HHS and publication in *Morbidity and Mortality Weekly Report.*

Table 16-1	Status of Licensure and Recommendations for New Vaccines—cont'd				
Vaccine	Manufacturer	BLA Submitted to FDA	BLA Age Indications†	FDA Licensure	Status of AAP/CDC Recommendations‡
HPV (Gardasil)	Merck	December 2005	9-26 years (3 doses)	Licensed 8 Jun 06	ACIP: cdc.gov/mmwr/preview/mmwrhtml/ rr56e312a1.htm AAP: aapredbook.org/news/hpv-provisional.pdf
HPV (Cervarix)	GlaxoSmithKline (GSK)	March 2007	Data not available	To be reviewed	Pending FDA licensure
Hib/DTaP/IPV (Pentacel)	Sanofi Pasteur	July 2005	2, 4, 6, and 15 to 18 months	To be reviewed	Pending FDA licensure
DTaP/IPV (Kinrix)	GlaxoSmithKline (GSK)	June 2007	4-6 years	To be reviewed	Pending FDA licensure
Influenza (Fluarix)	GlaxoSmithKline (GSK)	May 2005	≥18 years	Licensed 31 Aug 05	CDC: cdc.gov/flu/about/qa/vaxprioritygroups. htm
Influenza (FluLaval)	GlaxoSmithKline (GSK)	March 2006	≥18 years	Licensed 5 Oct 06	CDC: cdc.gov/flu/about/qa/vaxprioritygroups. htm
CAIV-T (FluMist)	MedImmune	July 2006	24 months to 59 months	Licensed 19 Sept 07	Pending AAP and ACIP recommendations
Influenza (Afluria)	CSL Biotherapies	March 2007	≥18 years	Licensed 28 Sept 07	CDC: cdc.gov/flu/about/qa/vaxprioritygroups. htm

BLA, Biologics license application; *FDA,* US Food and Drug Administration; *AAP,* American Academy of Pediatrics; *ACIP,* Advisory Committee on Immunization Practices; *MCV4,* meningococcal conjugate vaccine; *MMRV,* measles, mumps, rubella, varicella; *Tdap,* tetanus toxoid, reduced diphtheria toxoid, and acellular pertussis vaccine, adsorbed; *HPV,* human papillomavirus vaccine; *Hib, Haemophilus influenzae* b, *DTaP,* diphtheria, tetanus, pertussis; *IPV,* inactivated poliovirus vaccine; *CAIV-T,* cold-adapted influenza vaccine, trivalent.

2. There is a lack of knowledge related to the ability of a vaccine to induce HIV-specific immune responses that are effective in preventing or treating HIV infection.
3. Therapeutic HIV vaccine research is still in early stages.

Vaccine Development

The goal in producing HIV vaccines is to destroy HIV or keep the virus in check so that it causes no further damage. An ideal vaccine would stop progressive immunodeficiency and restore the immune system to a healthy state.

The requirements for a preventive HIV vaccine are to generate both humoral and cellular immunity against HIV in the host before exposure to the virus. After initial exposure to HIV, the generation of cellular immune responses against HIV may take time to develop, which makes neutralizing antibodies against free virus important to reduce the initial spread of the virus in the body.

In the United States, research is based on the use of subunit proteins found in the envelope of HIV. Vaccine research scientists are trying to develop the following three types of HIV vaccines:

1. Preventive or prophylactic vaccines to protect individuals from HIV infection.
2. Therapeutic vaccines to prevent HIV infected patients from progressing to AIDS.

3. Perinatal vaccines for administration to HIV-infected pregnant women to prevent transmission of HIV to the fetus.

Scientists hope that therapeutic and perinatal administration of vaccine will reach a high level of success. Challenges associated with HIV vaccine development include the following:

- A high rate of viral mutation and recombination.
- No clearly defined, natural immunity to HIV.
- HIV infects cells that are critical to the immune body defenses, and HIV is transmitted as a free virus and within infected cells.

Vaccine Problems

Problems associated with HIV vaccine development are plagued by the lack of scientific understanding of HIV infection and the complex biology of HIV disease/AIDS. Once inside a host cell, HIV is capable of integrating itself into the genetic material of infected cells. For a vaccine to be effective, it needs to produce a constant state of immune protection, not only to block viral entry to most cells, but also to continue to block newly produced viruses over the infected person's lifetime.

Researchers have identified the following specific problem areas:

- A lack of knowledge related to the critical components in the body's immune response to HIV infection.

- The high risk of using the entire weakened or inactive HIV in a vaccine.
- The extensive rate of viral mutation as HIV replicates. Strains worldwide vary by as much as 35% in terms of the proteins that make up the outer coat of the virus. Even an infected person can experience a change in viral protein by as much as 10% over years. This genetic diversity may require an effective vaccine to be based on multiple viral strains.
- The protective effect of a vaccine may last only a short time, and frequent mandatory booster vaccinations would be impractical and expensive.
- Vaccinated persons could become more susceptible to HIV infection because of vaccine-induced enhancement of infection.
- No vaccine clinical trial to date has demonstrated stimulation of the cellular components of the immune system in the way needed to destroy HIV.
- Animal models have severe limitations, including the possibility of integration of DNA into the human genome from monkeys.
- No research studies have successfully demonstrated which immune responses correlate with protection from HIV infection.

Vaccine research scientists in 2000 lowered their expectations and settled for a vaccine that would not completely prevent HIV infection. It is estimated that a vaccine with only 30% effectiveness against HIV (vs. usual 85%-95% effectiveness of other infectious disease vaccines) can begin to eradicate the virus if it is widely administered and accompanied by disease prevention education. Based on this premise, the FDA has indicated it will approve an HIV/AIDS vaccine at this level of efficacy.

South Africa's first large-scale HIV vaccine efficacy trial of a subtype B HIV on South Africa's predominantly subtype C patients started in 2007. It is difficult to find populations who are at high risk except for "sex workers." Rather than destroying an infection before it takes hold in the cells, the vaccine being tested would more likely "modify" the infection once it did take hold by pushing the viral set point as low as possible. This would delay the onset of symptoms and possibly make the virus less potent. Alternatively, the vaccine might reduce the initial peak point, when the probability of transmission is much greater.

Vaccine Expectations

Reasons for optimism about HIV vaccine development include the following:

1. Nonhuman primates vaccinated with products based on HIV or *simian* immunodeficiency virus have shown complete or partial protection against infection with the wild-type virus.
2. Successful vaccines have been developed against the *feline* immunodeficiency virus, also a retrovirus.
3. Almost all humans develop some form of immune response that is protective or able to control the viral infection over a long period. Some individuals remain disease free for up to 25 years, frequently with undetectable viral load levels.

Anthrax

An experimental anthrax vaccine cleared two hurdles in its first round of human tests. No safety problems emerged, and the responses suggest that people were developing immunity to anthrax. The requirement for an anthrax vaccine is being driven by the U.S. Federal Government for emergency use in the event of an anthrax-based attack on the U.S. civil population.

Avecia Biotechnology has received a $3.9-million federal grant to develop a version of Thraxine, a recombinant protective antigen (rPA)–based anthrax vaccine, with increased stability. Due for completion by April 2008, the program will develop a version of Thraxine that can be stored, transported, and used without the need for a conventional "cold chain." Improved temperature stability will simplify storage and transport and prolong shelf life, which could also reduce the overall cost of large-scale vaccine provision. This next-generation anthrax vaccine could have technologic benefits for the wider vaccines sector.

In addition, Avecia and Dstl are also collaborating on the development of a new plague vaccine (RypVax) for NIAID, using protein-based technology similar to rPA. The plague vaccine program is under a $50-million federal contract awarded to Avecia in 2004.

Cytomegalovirus

There is no available vaccine for preventing congenital CMV disease (present at birth). However, a few CMV vaccines are being tested in humans, including live, attenuated (weakened) virus vaccines and vaccines that contain only pieces of the virus.

The Institute of Medicine has ranked the development of a CMV vaccine as its highest priority because of the lives it would save and the disabilities it would prevent. An FDA-approved CMV vaccine, however, may take years. Because CMV is not spread as easily as some other diseases, even a partially effective CMV vaccine will have a large impact on the congenital CMV disease epidemic.

Hay Fever

Experimental DNA-based vaccine to protect against hay fever after just six injections is in development. Patients who received the vaccine experienced an average 60% reduction in allergy symptoms compared with those receiving placebo.

The vaccine lessens the immune system's excessive reactions to inhaled allergens by stimulating protective cells that turn off the Th2 helper cells. The Th2 cells send out signals for the body to create more immunoglobulin E (IgE), the protein largely responsible for allergy symptoms. Additionally, the vaccine may activate dendritic cells, keeping inflammation in check over the long term and breaking an otherwise self-sustaining allergic cycle.

DNA-based and cell line–based vaccines appear to be the future of immunology.

Human Papillomavirus

Cancer vaccines such as for human papillomavirus (HPV) are another form of biologic therapy currently under study. Cancer vaccines have already been developed to fight HPV-16, a common strain that causes cervical cancer.

These vaccines work by exposing the body's immune cells to weakened forms of an antigen (foreign substances) that form on the surface of an infectious agent. The immune system increases production of (1) cells that make antibodies to fight the infectious agent and (2) T cells that recognize the infectious agent. These immune cells remember the exposure, so the next time the agent enters the body, the immune system is already prepared to respond and stop the infection.

Types 16 (HPV-16) and 18 (HPV-18) cause approximately 70% of cervical cancers worldwide. A major breakthroughs in immunology recently resulted in the Gardasil vaccine (Merck, Whitehouse Station, NJ), approved by the FDA in June 2006 for girls and women age 9 to 26 years. (More than 30 countries had approved the vaccine before the FDA's approval.) The vaccine can prevent cervical cancer and vaginal and vulvar precancers caused by HPV-16 and HPV-18, as well as low-grade and precancerous lesions and genital wars caused by HPV types 6, 11, 16, and 18 in women not previously infected by one of the four covered HPV types.

More than 6 million people become infected with HPV every year in the United States, and almost 10,000 women are diagnosed with cervical cancer.

Additional products in development include vaccines covering other high-risk HPV types for broader coverage, as well as therapeutic vaccines designed to treat women who already have precancerous lesions or cancer.

Influenza

The efficacy of influenza vaccines may decline during years when the circulating viruses have "antigenically drifted" from those included in the vaccine. The World Health Organization (WHO) coordinates global influence–virus surveillance so that appropriate vaccine candidates can be identified by the WHO and national authorities, and vaccines can be reformulated each year. Vaccines viruses must be selected every year because genetic mutations arise continuously in influenza viruses, a process termed *antigenic drift* that results in the emergence of immunologically distinct variants. The process is repeated each year, which imposes severe time restrictions on all groups involved.

Influenza A (H3N2) components in both the inactived and the live, attenuated influenza vaccines were not optimally matched to the circulating strains. Researchers have studied the concept of *herd immunity* (indirect protection from influenza at community level), a different view of promoting immunity, particularly to vulnerable groups (e.g., very young, elderly).

The FDA recently approved FluLaval, an influenza vaccine, for immunizing people 18 years and older against flu. Currently, there are five FDA-licensed flu vaccines.

Leukemia

The search for cancer vaccines recently had a breakthrough with the development of a therapeutic vaccine directed at patients with acute myelogenous leukemia (AML). A pilot study to demonstrate the effectiveness and safety of an AML vaccine is under way. The phase I stage of the clinical trial with AML patients is aimed at determining if the PR1 peptide vaccine (a nine–amino acid HLA A2–restricted peptide derived from proteinase 3) can elicit T-cell immunity in leukemia patients whose disease has been resistant to treatment.

Polio

Polio has been reduced by more than 99%, and the number of countries with endemic transmission has been reduced by more than 96%.

Poliovirus persists in countries where the virus is endemic. New outbreaks are occurring in previously polio-free countries, including, most recently, Kenya's first documented wild-type poliovirus infection in 22 years. Four countries where the virus remains endemic—Nigeria, India, Pakistan, and Afghanistan—account for 93% of polio cases worldwide; unlike all other countries, they have never succeeded in interrupting the transmission of wild poliovirus.

The biologic reason is the same regardless of the location: insufficient immunity in the population to interrupt transmission. In almost all cases, the basic cause remains failure to vaccinate enough children with enough doses to ensure that they are immune to disease *and* infection.

In the past few years, the initiative to eradicate polio has faced substantial challenges. Large outbreaks associated with spread from the primary global reservoirs in Nigeria and India affected 25 countries and were controlled only after more than 2 years of effort. At the same time, the belief that wild-type 2 poliovirus was eradicated in 1999 becomes more certain.

Smallpox

Threats of bioterrorism with smallpox as a weapon have launched a high-profile discussion of the reintroduction of smallpox into the general U.S. population. Individuals in "high-risk" occupations and positions have already begun to be vaccinated.

Category A Agents

Smallpox vaccination was stopped in 1972 after the disease was eradicated in the United States. Smallpox is classified as a Category A agent by the CDC. Other category A agents include anthrax, plague, botulism, tularemia, and viral hemorrhagic fevers. These agents are believed to pose the greatest potential threat for adverse public health impact and to have a moderate to high potential for large-scale dissemination.

Smallpox Vaccine

Smallpox vaccine, a preventive vaccine, is the only way to prevent smallpox. The vaccine is made from a live virus called *vaccinia,* which is another "pox"-type virus related to smallpox but unable to cause smallpox. A "live virus" vaccine, including measles, mumps, rubella, chickenpox, and smallpox vaccines, is a vaccine that contains a "living" virus that is able to give and produce immunity, usually without causing illness. For most people with a healthy immune system, live-virus vaccines are safe and effective, but the live virus can be transmitted to other parts of the body or to other people from the unhealed vaccination site.

Vaccine Administration

The vaccine is not injected like other types of vaccines. It is given using a bifurcated (two-pronged) needle that is dipped into the vaccine solution. The needle is used to prick the skin a number of times in a few seconds. It takes about 3 weeks for the site to heal with a scar remaining. The first dose of vaccine offers protection from smallpox for 3 to 5 years, with decreasing immunity thereafter. A repeat vaccination offers longer immunity. Vaccination within 3 days of exposure completely prevents or significantly modifies smallpox in the vast majority of persons. Vaccination 4 to 7 days after exposure likely offers some protection from disease or may modify the severity of the disease.

CHAPTER HIGHLIGHTS

- Vaccines provide artificially acquired, active immunity to a specific disease.
- The Center for Biologics Evaluation and Research (CBER) regulates vaccine products. According to the CDC, vaccines have reduced preventable infectious diseases to an all-time low. Vaccine development is an important focus of research for AIDS, malaria, and other devastating diseases.
- Pathogens or pathogen products adapted for biologic warfare include smallpox, anthrax, plague, tularemia, brucellosis, Q fever, botulinum toxin, and staphylococcal enterotoxin B.
- Jenner discovered a fundamental principle of immunization with smallpox vaccine and paved the way for rabies (Louis Pasteur) and other vaccines (diphtheria, typhoid).
- Children now receive vaccines for many childhood diseases (e.g., rubella). Adults require boosters (tetanus). A recent vaccine for adults reduces the risk of shingles.
- International travelers frequently require vaccination to endemic diseases (e.g., hepatitis A) in a particular country. Health care professionals are now protected against hepatitis B through vaccines. Many adults receive the "flu" vaccine. Vaccines are given to pets and livestock as well.
- A vaccine stimulates active immunity and creates an immune memory so that exposure to the active disease microorganism will stimulate an already-primed immune system to fight the disease.
- Most vaccines can be divided into live, attenuated vaccines and nonreplicating vaccines.

- A vaccine must produce protective immunity with minimal side effects, produce a strong immune response, and be stable during its shelf life.
- Classic preventive vaccines are designed to mimic the effects of natural exposure to microbes. The earliest host response to vaccination is called the innate immune response.
- Vaccines either emphasize public health safety (anthrax) or prevent the return of epidemic disease.
- Preventive AIDS vaccines are for HIV-negative individuals, to prevent HIV infection. Therapeutic AIDS vaccines are for HIV-positive individuals, to improve the immune system.
- Anthrax vaccine is for emergency use in the event of an anthrax-based attack on the U.S. civil population.
- No available vaccine can prevent congenital cytomegalovirus (CMV) disease, although a few CMV vaccines are being tested in humans.
- Experimental DNA-based vaccine to protect against hay fever after just six injections is in development.
- Cancer vaccines such as Gardasil for human papillomavirus (HPV) work by exposing the body's immune cells to weakened forms of an antigen.
- FluLaval is a influenza vaccine for immunizing people 18 and older. FDA has licensed five flu vaccines.
- A new therapeutic vaccine is directed at patients with acute myelogenous leukemia (AML).
- Polio has been reduced by more than 99%, and the number of countries with endemic transmission has been reduced by more than 96%.
- The threat of bioterrorism with smallpox has led to high-risk individuals already being vaccinated.

REVIEW QUESTIONS

1. The Center for Biologics Evaluation and Research (CBER) regulates:
   a. Laboratory safety.
   b. Vaccine products.
   c. Personnel qualifications.
   d. Research grants.

2. Pathogens adapted for biologic warfare include:
   (1) Smallpox
   (2) *Bacillus anthracis*
   (3) Chickenpox
   (4) Q fever
   a. 1, 2, 3
   b. 1, 2, 4
   c. 2, 3, 4
   d. 1, 3, 4

3. Vaccines can be divided into _____ vaccines.
   a. live, attenuated
   b. nonreplicating
   c. naked DNA
   d. Both a and b

4. To meet FDA requirements, a vaccine must:
   a. Produce protective immunity with only minimal side effects.
   b. Be immunogenic enough to produce a strong and measurable immune response.
   c. Be stable during its shelf life.
   d. All the above.

5. The earliest host response to vaccination is a(n):
   a. Innate immune response.
   b. Memory response.
   c. Anamnestic response.
   d. Both a and b

Questions 6 and 7. Match the following.

6. _____ Preventive vaccine

7. _____ Therapeutic vaccine

   a. Given to HIV- negative individuals.
   b. For HIV-positive patients to improve immune system in order to prevent progression to AIDS.

Questions 8-12. Match the following (use an answer only once).

8. _____ Anthrax vaccine

9. _____ Cytomegalovirus vaccine

10. _____ Hay fever vaccine

11. _____ Human papillomavirus vaccine

12. _____ Influenza vaccine

   a. Protection against bioterrorism.
   b. Protection against cervical cancer.
   c. Not available for preventing congenital infection.
   d. DNA-based vaccine.
   e. Annual vaccination required.

Questions 13-15. Match the following.

13. _____ Leukemia vaccine

14. _____ Polio vaccine

15. _____ Smallpox vaccine

   a. Has reduced disease by 99%.
   b. Successful in cats.
   c. Given to high-risk individuals.

BIBLIOGRAPHY

Advance for Medical Laboratory Professionals: Clinical clips, 2002. www.advanceformlp.com/mtclinical.html.

Agosti JM, Goldie SJ: Introducing HPV vaccine in developing countries: key challenges and issues, *N Engl J Med* 356(19):1908-1910, 2007.

Arvin AM et al: Vaccine development to prevent cytomegalovirus disease: report from the National Vaccine Advisory Committee, *Clin Infect Dis* 39(2):233-239, 2004.

Avecia, *Wall St J,* Sept 28, 2006, p D6.

Baden LR et al: Human papillomavirus vaccine: opportunity and challenge, *N Engl J Med* 356(19):1990-1991, 2007.

Basu S: Hepatitis E vaccine, *N Engl J Med* 356(23):2421, 2007.

Belshe RB et al: Live attenuated virus inactivated influenza vaccine in infants and young children, *N Engl J Med* 356(7):685-695, 2007.

Bozzette SA et al: A model for smallpox vaccination policy, *N Engl J Med,* www.NEJM.org, Dec 19, 2002. Oct 10, 2007.

Centers for Disease Control and Prevention: Smallpox fact sheet, www.bt.cdc.gov/agent/smallpox, Dec 9, 2002. Oct 10, 2007.

Charo A: Politics, parents, and prophylaxis: mandating HPV vaccination in the United States, *N Engl J Med* 356(19):1905-1907, 2007.

Chaves S et al: Loss of vaccine-induced immunity to varicella over time, *N Engl J Med* 356(11):1121-1128, 2007.

Colgrove J: The ethics and politics of compulsory HPV vaccination, *N Engl J Med* 355(23):2389-2391, 2006.

Fukuda K, Kieny MP: Different approaches to influenza vaccination, *N Engl J Med* 355(24):2586-2589, 2006.

Herman D: Large-scale HIV vaccine trials to start in South Africa next year, *Immunol News* 6(4):1, 2006 (Dana Foundation).

Hoffmann P, Roumeguère T, van Velthoven R: Use of statins and outcome of BCG treatment for bladder cancer, *N Engl J Med* 355(25):2705-2706, 2006.

Institute of Medicine, Committee to Study Priorities for Vaccine Development: *Vaccines for the 21st century: a tool for decision making,* Washington, DC, 2000, National Academy Press.

Johnston MI, Fauci AS: An HIV vaccine: evolving concepts, *N Engl J Med* 356(20):2073-2080, 2007.

Ohmit SE et al: Prevention of antigenically drifted influenza by inactivated and live attenuated vaccines, *N Engl J Med* 355(24):2513-2522, 2006.

Pallansch MA, Sandhu HS: The eradication of polio: progress and challenges, *N Engl J Med* 355(24):2508-2511, 2006.

Penno KA: *Adv Med Lab Prof* 18(22):13-15, 2006.

Pulendran B: Tolls and beyond: many roads to vaccine immunity, *N Engl J Med* 356(17):1765-1778, 2007.

Schraeder TL, Campion EW: Smallpox vaccination: the call to arms, *N Engl J Med* 348(5):1-2, 2003.

Wilbur DC: Vaccines for preventing cervical cancer: where we are now, *CAP Today* 21(1):48, 2007.

CHAPTER 17

Streptococcal Infections

Etiology
  Morphologic Characteristics
  Extracellular Products
Epidemiology
Signs and Symptoms
  Upper Respiratory Infection
  Impetigo and Cellulitis
  Scarlet Fever
  Complications of S. pyogenes Infection
Immunologic Manifestations

Diagnostic Evaluation
Streptococcal Toxic Shock Syndrome
Group B Streptococcal Disease
Optical Immunoassay for Direct Detection of Group A
  Streptococcal Antigen
Case Study
Chapter Highlights
Review Questions
Bibliography

Learning Objectives

At the conclusion of this chapter, the reader should be able to:

- Describe the etiology, epidemiology, signs and symptoms, and complications of streptococcal infection.
- Discuss the immunologic manifestations and diagnostic evaluation of streptococcal infection.

- Explain the principle of the optical immunoassay diagnostic procedure.
- Analyze and apply laboratory data to a case study.

ETIOLOGY

Most streptococci that contain cell wall antigens of Lancefield group A are known as *Streptococcus pyogenes*. Members of this species are almost always beta-hemolytic. *S. pyogenes* is the most common causative agent of pharyngitis and its resultant disorder, scarlet fever, and the skin infection, impetigo. The most common type of bacteria causing necrotizing fasciitis is *S. pyogenes*.

In terms of human morbidity and mortality worldwide, however, the role of *S. pyogenes* in the subsequent development of complications such as acute rheumatic fever and poststreptococcal glomerulonephritis is more important. Other *S. pyogenes*–associated infections include otitis media in children, sinusitis in adults, and osteomyelitis, septic arthritis, neonatal septicemia, and rare cases of pneumonia.

Necrotizing fasciitis is a rare infection that can destroy skin and soft tissues, including fat and the tissue-covering muscles (fascia). Because these tissues die rapidly, a person with necrotizing fasciitis is sometimes said to be infected with "flesh-eating" bacteria. A highly invasive group A streptococcal infection is associated with toxic shock syndrome.

Morphologic Characteristics

Streptococcus pyogenes is a gram-positive coccus and the serotype most frequently associated with human infection. Lancefield divided these beta-hemolytic streptococci into serogroups A through O on the basis of the immunologic action of the cell wall carbohydrate (Figure 17-1).

Structures called **fimbriae** arise near the plasma membrane and project through the cell wall and capsule. These processes contain important surface components of the streptococcus. Lipoteichoic acid on the fimbriae is impor-

tant in the organism's adherence to human epithelium and the initiation of infection. The M and R antigens, which are structurally similar but immunologically distinct, are also found on the fimbriae. R antigen has no known biologic role.

M protein, a cell protein found in association with the hyaluronic capsule, is a major virulence factor of *S. pyogenes*. Strains of *S. pyogenes* that lack M protein cannot cause infection. M protein inhibits phagocytosis, and antibody synthesized against M protein provides type-specific immunity to group A streptococci. In addition, M protein is the basis for a subclassification of group A streptococci into more than 60 M serotypes.

Extracellular Products

Extracellular products are important in the pathogenesis of disease and in the serologic diagnosis of streptococcal disease. Antibodies produced in response to these substances provide evidence of recent streptococcal infection. Two hemolysins, with the ability to damage human and animal erythrocytes, polymorphonuclear leukocytes (PMNs), and platelets, are produced by most group A strains, as follows:

- **Streptolysin O (SLO),** an oxygen-labile enzyme, binds to sterols in the red blood cell (RBC) membrane, causing stearic rearrangement. This rearrangement produces submicroscopic holes in the RBC membrane, and hemoglobin diffuses from the cells. SLO is antigenic; the antibody response to it is the most frequently used serologic indicator of recent streptococcal infection.
- **Streptolysin S,** an oxygen-stable enzyme, is responsible for the beta (clear-appearing) hemolysis on the surface of a blood agar culture plate. Streptolysin S disrupts the

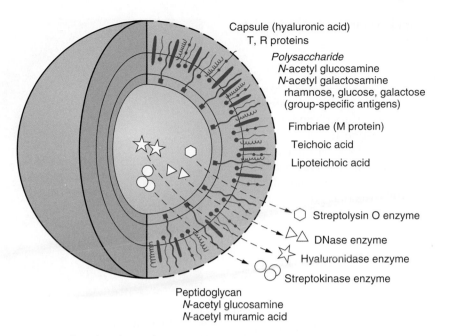

Capsule (hyaluronic acid)
T, R proteins
Polysaccharide
  N-acetyl glucosamine
  N-acetyl galactosamine
  rhamnose, glucose, galactose
  (group-specific antigens)

Fimbriae (M protein)
Teichoic acid
Lipoteichoic acid

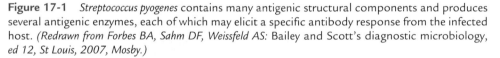

Streptolysin O enzyme
DNase enzyme
Hyaluronidase enzyme
Streptokinase enzyme

Peptidoglycan
  N-acetyl glucosamine
  N-acetyl muramic acid

Cytoplasmic membrane

Figure 17-1   *Streptococcus pyogenes* contains many antigenic structural components and produces several antigenic enzymes, each of which may elicit a specific antibody response from the infected host. *(Redrawn from Forbes BA, Sahm DF, Weissfeld AS:* Bailey and Scott's diagnostic microbiology, *ed 12, St Louis, 2007, Mosby.)*

selective permeability of the RBC membrane, causing osmotic lysis. It is not antigenic.

Other substances produced by group A streptococci presumably facilitate rapid spread through subcutaneous or deeper soft tissues and include the following:

- **Hyaluronidase,** also called "spreading factor," breaks down hyaluronic acid found in the host's connective tissue.
- Four immunologically distinct deoxyribonucleases (DNases A, B, C, and D) degrade deoxyribonucleic acid (DNA).
- **Streptokinase,** an enzyme, dissolves clots by converting plasminogen to plasmin.
- Other extracellular products that can elicit an antibody response include NADase, proteinase, esterase, and amylase.
- **Erythrogenic toxin** is elaborated by scarlet fever–associated strains and is responsible for the characteristic rash.

EPIDEMIOLOGY

Streptococcus pyogenes is one of the most common and ubiquitous of human pathogens. It is found in the respiratory tract of humans and is always considered a potential pathogen. Upper respiratory infections caused by *S. pyogenes* occur most frequently in school-age children and are uncommon in children younger than 3 years. No gender or race predilection has been described.

Infection is spread by contact with large droplets produced in the upper respiratory tract. Although not as common, food-borne and milk-borne epidemics do occur. Crowding enhances the spread of microorganisms.

A number of individuals, particularly school-age children, carry *S. pyogenes* without signs of illness. Carriers have positive cultures without serologic evidence of infection. If a person carries the organisms in the pharynx for prolonged periods after untreated infection, the number of organisms carried and their ability to produce M protein decline during carriage. This results in a progressive decline in the likelihood of spreading infection to others.

The incidence of a major complication of *S. pyogenes,* **rheumatic fever,** has decreased in the United States. It occurs primarily in the rural South and in areas of crowding and lower socioeconomic status. The incidence of rheumatic fever is 2% to 3% in epidemics and 0.1% to 1% after sporadic cases of streptococcal infection. The probability of developing rheumatic fever is age related, with younger patients more likely to develop carditis than older persons.

Rheumatic fever and resultant valvular heart disease, however, are syndromes of major importance among children in developing nations. Patients with a history of rheumatic heart disease resulting from rheumatic fever are at a significantly increased risk of developing cardiac malfunction and endocarditis later. The risk of recurrent rheumatic fever depends on factors such as the age of the patient at previous recurrences, the length of time since the last recurrence, and the presence of carditis. In addition, patients who develop streptococcal glomerulonephritis are at risk of later development of renal failure.

SIGNS AND SYMPTOMS

Streptococcus pyogenes causes a wide variety of infections, most often acute pharyngitis ("strep throat") and upper respiratory infection, as well as impetigo (pyoderma). Other manifestations of infection with *S. pyogenes* include sinusitis, otitis, peritonsillar and retropharyngeal abscess, pneumonia, scarlet fever, erysipelas, cellulitis, puerperal sepsis, and gangrene. The concern still exists that group A streptococcus may be acquiring greater virulence.

Upper Respiratory Infection

The clinical manifestations of *S. pyogenes*–associated upper respiratory infection are age dependent. In an infant or young child, the infection is characterized by an insidious onset of rhinorrhea, coughing, fever, vomiting, and anorexia. Cervical adenopathy may also be present. Rhinorrhea is sometimes purulent. This syndrome is called **streptococcosis.**

The classic syndrome of **streptococcal pharyngitis** is seen in children over 3 years old. It begins with a sudden onset of sore throat and fever, which rapidly progress in severity. Pharyngeal erythema with purulent tonsillar exudate and petechiae may be observed on the palate, posterior pharynx, and tonsils. Younger children may have abdominal pain, nausea, and vomiting. Most cases, however, do not manifest the classic syndrome. It is more common for a child with *S. pyogenes* pharyngitis to have a fever, mild sore throat, and pharyngeal erythema without exudate.

Viral pharyngitis can produce many of the same symptoms and cannot be reliably differentiated from streptococcal pharyngitis on the basis of clinical examination.

Impetigo and Cellulitis

Impetigo is a skin infection that begins as a papule (Figures 17-2 and 17-3). The lesion may itch and will eventually crust over and heal. Cellulitis caused by subcutaneous infection with group A streptococci is associated with a warm, red, tender area that may be mildly swollen. **Erysipelas,** a distinct cellulitis syndrome, usually involves the face and may be associated with pharyngitis. This syndrome is characterized by toxicity and a high fever. If left untreated, erysipelas can be fatal.

Scarlet Fever

Scarlet fever is the result of pharyngeal infection with a strain of group A streptococcus that produces erythrogenic toxin and is responsible for the characteristic rash. The signs and symptoms of scarlet fever are those of streptococcal pharyngitis with the addition of a rash. The rash usually develops on the second day of illness and results in hyperkeratosis with subsequent peeling, similar to the rash of toxic shock syndrome. About 1 week after the onset of illness, the skin of the face begins to peel, which progresses over the next 2 weeks. Exposure to erythrogenic toxin confers spe-

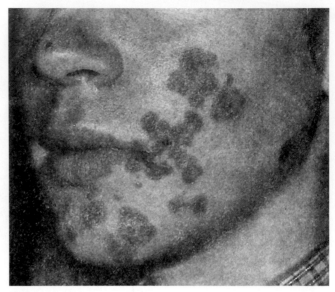

Figure 17-2 Vesicular impetigo. A thick, honey-yellow, adherent crust covers the entire eroded surface. *(From Habif TP: Clinical dermatology: a color guide to diagnosis and therapy, St Louis, 1985, Mosby.)*

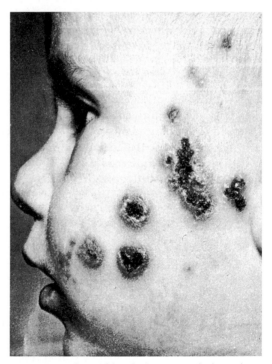

Figure 17-3 Impetigo. Older lesions are dark and encrusted. *(From Wehrle PF, Top FH: Communicable and infectious diseases, ed 9, St Louis, 1981, Mosby.)*

cific immunity, limiting to three the number of episodes of scarlet fever in a person.

Complications of *S. pyogenes* Infection

Not all infections with *S. pyogenes* lead to complications. Acute rheumatic fever, for example, occurs only after upper respiratory tract infection. In contrast, glomerulonephritis occurs after pharyngitis or skin infections (pyoderma).

Acute rheumatic fever and poststreptococcal glomerulonephritis are considered nonsuppurative because the organs themselves are not directly infected, and a purulent inflammatory response is not present in affected organs (e.g., heart, joints, blood, kidneys).

The pathogenesis of this disease process has not been fully described, but an autoimmune phenomenon may be operational. It is believed that cross-reactive antibodies, originally directed against streptococcal cell membranes, bind to myosin in human heart muscle cells. Other cross-reactive antibodies bind to components of the glomerular basement membrane and form immune complexes at the affected site. These antigen-antibody complexes attract reactive host cells and enzymes that ultimately cause the cellular damage.

All M serotypes that infect the throat appear to be capable of causing rheumatic fever. Researchers have identified a few serotypes, however, that cause a much lower proportion of rheumatic fever cases than would be expected from their frequency as a cause of pharyngitis. The incidence of rheumatic fever is directly proportional to the strength of the antibody response to SLO. Prognosis of rheumatic fever is good when carditis is absent during the initial infection.

Glomerulonephritis may follow an infection of the skin or respiratory tract with one of a limited number of nephritogenic M serotypes. These serotypes are defined by antisera against the M protein, which is also associated with virulence. Why these serotypes cause glomerulonephritis is unknown.

IMMUNOLOGIC MANIFESTATIONS

Streptococcus pyogenes is an example of a pathogen that induces production of several different antibodies. This coccus contains antigenic structural components and produces antigenic enzymes, each of which may elicit a specific antibody response from the infected host. In the course of an infection, the extracellular products act as antigens, to which the body responds by producing specific antibodies (indications of infection).

Most infected patients demonstrate increased concentration of antibody against SLO. The concentration of antibody (titer) begins to rise about 7 days after the onset of infection and reaches a maximum after 4 to 6 weeks. A rise in titer of 50 Todd units in 1 to 2 weeks is of greater diagnostic significance than a single titer. An elevated titer indicates a relatively recent infection. Peak titers are seen at the time of acute polyarthritis of acute rheumatic fever, but these titers are no longer at their peak during the carditis of acute rheumatic fever. A patient may demonstrate an elevated antibody titer for up to a year after infection; therefore the time of infection is not precisely determined by this technique. Low titers of **antistreptolysin O (ASO)** can be exhibited by apparently healthy persons because of the frequency of subclinical streptococcal infections, but persistently low titers rule out *S. pyogenes* infection.

Half the patients with *S. pyogenes*–related acute glomerulonephritis display a normal ASO titer but demonstrate an elevated titer to one of the other streptococcal substances (e.g., DNAse and NADase). **Anti–DNAse B (ADN-B)** antibody appears to be the most reliable measure of recent *S. pyogenes* skin infection. Titers of ADN-B are elevated in more than two thirds of patients with recent streptococcal impetigo. Anti-NADase antibodies are a particularly good marker in patients who develop nephritis after pharyngitis.

DIAGNOSTIC EVALUATION

In addition to throat cultures in patients with pharyngitis, antibodies to bacterial toxins and other extracellular products that display measurable activity can be tested. ASO and ADN-B are the standard serologic tests. The ability of a patient's serum to neutralize the erythrocyte-lysing capability of SLO (ASO procedure) has been used for many years as a detection method for previous streptococcal infection. After an infection such as pharyngitis with SLO-producing strains, most patients show a high titer of the antibody ASO. The use of rapid testing has replaced the use of the classic ASO procedure in many laboratories (see Optical Immunoassay procedure).

Streptococci produce the enzyme DNase B. The ADN-B neutralization test prevents the activity of this enzyme and demonstrates recent or previous *S. pyogenes* infection. Antistreptokinase and antihyaluronidase titers (AHTs) have also been used to diagnose streptococcal infection retrospectively.

Serologic testing should compare acute and convalescent sera collected 3 weeks apart. ASO becomes elevated in acute/convalescent paired specimens in 80% to 85% of patients with acute rheumatic fever. ADN-B and AHT levels are elevated in the remaining 15% to 20% of patients. In many cases, no acute serum specimen is available; therefore the antibody titer of the convalescent serum specimen is compared to a reference range value. Reference ranges vary with age, season, and geographic area. False-positive ASO results may be demonstrated because of beta-lipoprotein, contamination of the serum specimen by bacterial growth products, or oxidation of ASO. These errors are not encountered with the ADN-B procedure, which is the serologic test of choice for acute rheumatic fever and acute glomerulonephritis after *S. pyogenes* infection.

Other testing methods include the Rapid-Cycle Real Timer Polymerase Chain Reaction (Roche Diagnostics, Pleasanton, Calif), which uses LightCycler technology to copy and amplify the two DNA strands of the *S. pyogenes* gene sequence and provides results in 1½ hours. The Group A Strep Direct probe test (Gen-Probe, San Diego) is a DNA chemiluminescence probe assay targeted at group A streptococcus ribosomal ribonucleic acid (rRNA) in a specimen. These emerging technologies underscore the demand to detect group A streptococci more rapidly by replacing traditional testing methods, particularly the 48-hour throat culture, which has always been the "gold standard."

STREPTOCOCCAL TOXIC SHOCK SYNDROME

Streptococcal toxic shock syndrome (STSS) is caused by a highly invasive group A streptococcal infection and is associated with shock and organ failure.

Etiology

The portal of entry of streptococci in STSS cannot be determined in at least half the cases and can only be presumed in many others. The use of tampons has been associated with acquiring the disorder. In other patients the use of nonsteroidal antiinflammatory drugs (NSAIDs) may have either masked the early symptoms or predisposed the patient to more severe streptococcal infection and shock. Most often, STSS appears after streptococci have invaded areas of injured skin (e.g., cuts/scrapes, surgical wounds).

Immunologic Mechanisms

Pyrogenic exotoxins cause fever in humans and animals and also help induce shock by lowering the threshold to exogenous endotoxin. Streptococcal pyrogenic exotoxins A and B induce human mononuclear cells to synthesize not only tumor necrosis factor alpha (TNF-α) but also interleukin-1-beta (IL-1β) and interleukin-6 (IL-6), suggesting that TNF could mediate the fever, shock, and tissue injury observed in patients with STSS.

M protein contributes to invasiveness through its ability to impede phagocytosis of streptococci by human PMNs.

Superantigens are capable of binding to alpha/beta T-cell receptors (TCRs) and major histocompatibility complex (MHC) class II molecules. Superantigens can directly activate 1% to 2% of T cells and create high levels of cytokines in the blood. These high levels can produce "shock-like" symptoms.

Cytokine production by less exotic mechanisms also likely contributes to the genesis of shock and organ failure. Exotoxins such as SLO are also potent inducers of TNF-α and IL-1β. *Pyrogenic exotoxin B,* a proteinase precursor, has the ability to cleave pre–IL-1β to release preformed IL-1. Finally, SLO and *pyrogenic exotoxin A* together have additive effects in the induction of IL-1β by human mononuclear cells. Regardless of the mechanisms, induction of cytokines in vivo is likely the cause of shock, and exotoxins, cell wall components, and other substances are potent inducers of TNF and IL-1.

Epidemiology

The rates of STSS are highest in young children and older adults. More than half of patients have an underlying chronic illness. Streptococcal TSS is also associated with a substantial risk of transmission in households and health care institutions. Mortality following an outbreak of *S. pyogenes* that progresses to toxic shock can be as high as 70%. The illness is classified as a "rare infection" because it affects only about 300 people per year. STSS almost never follows a simple *Streptococcus* throat infection.

Signs and Symptoms

The symptoms of STSS include shock, fever, blotchy rash, and a red, swollen, and painful area of infected skin. The average incubation period for STSS is 2 to 3 days, usually after minor, nonpenetrating trauma.

Pain, the most common initial symptom of STSS, is abrupt in onset, is severe, and usually precedes tenderness or physical findings. The pain usually involves an extremity but may also mimic peritonitis, pelvic inflammatory disease, pneumonia, acute myocardial infarction, or pericarditis.

About 20% of STSS patients have an influenza-like syndrome characterized by fever, chills, myalgia, nausea, vomiting, and diarrhea. Fever is the most common early sign, although hypothermia may be present in patients with shock.

About 80% of STSS patients have clinical signs of soft tissue infection, such as localized swelling and erythema, which in 70% of one group of patients progressed to necrotizing fasciitis or myositis and required surgical debridement, fasciotomy, or amputation. An ominous sign is the progression of soft tissue swelling to the formation of vesicles, then bullae, which appear violaceous or bluish.

Laboratory Data

The case definition of STSS includes serologic confirmation of group A streptococcal infection by a fourfold rise against SLO and DNAse B. Although initial laboratory studies usually demonstrate only mild leukocytosis, the mean percentage of immature neutrophils can reach 40% to 50%. Blood cultures are positive in 60% of cases.

Renal involvement is indicated by the presence of hemoglobinuria and by serum creatinine values that are, on average, more than 2.5 times normal. Renal impairment precedes hypotension in approximately 40% to 50% of patients. Hypoalbuminemia is associated with hypocalcemia on admission and throughout the hospital course.

Treatment

Streptococcal TSS can be deadly and needs immediate treatment. Intravenous fluids and medications to maintain a normal blood pressure are required in acutely ill patients. Penicillin and other beta-lactam antibiotics are most efficacious against rapidly growing bacteria.

After recovery, the skin may peel as the rash heals. Surgery may be necessary to remove areas of dead skin and muscle around an infected wound.

GROUP B STREPTOCOCCAL DISEASE

Group B *Streptococcus agalactiae* infections cause serious disease in adults and neonates. This bacterium causes substantial morbidity and mortality in adults. The case-fatality rate ranges from 26% to 70% among men and nonpregnant women with group B streptococcal (GBS) disease. Group B streptococci are most frequently isolated from blood. The most common clinical finding is skin and soft tissue infection.

Because of the gravity of GBS disease, especially in those who are older and those who have chronic diseases, the development of a vaccine is being pursued. Determining the incidence of adult disease and groups at greatest risk helps to focus prevention efforts. Intrapartum antibiotics can prevent early-onset neonatal GBS disease, but they have not been widely used.

Optical Immunoassay for Direct Detection of Group A Streptococcal Antigen*

Principle

The new rapid surface immunoassay (Optical ImmunoAssay, OIA) allows for the direct visual detection of the physical change in thickness of thin films resulting from binding reactions between antigens and antibodies (Figure 17-4). Polyclonal anti–group A streptococcal antigen (anti-GAS) antibody is attached to a thin silicon wafer. Light reflected from the surface after passing through this thin film results in a gold color. When a liquid sample containing antigen is placed on the surface, binding occurs between the antigen and the immobilized antibody. When a substrate that binds only to the antigen-antibody complex is added, the thickness of the film increases, changing the optical path. This causes the reacted surface to appear purple. No color change occurs in the absence of antigen binding.

Specimen Collection and Preparation

A sterile swab must be used to collect a specimen properly from the throat or nasopharynx. The swab must be Dacron or rayon (synthetic) tipped on a plastic shaft.

Acceptable transport media for the swab can be either modified Stuart's liquid or semisolid medium, or Amies liquid or semisolid medium. A wet or dry swab may be transported in a paper wrapper and unrefrigerated in a dry sterile tube or in a sleeve containing acceptable transport medium. Swabs may be stored unrefrigerated and should be processed within 72 hours of collection.

*Based on STREP A Optical ImmunoAssay (OIA) kit, BioStar, Boulder, Colo, 1995. (BioStar is now Inverness Medical-BioStar.)

If a culture is to be conducted in addition to the STREP A OIA, an additional swab should be collected and handled by conventional methods for culture. If only a single swab is available, perform the culture first, then process the swab in the STREP A OIA procedure.

Handling Precautions

All throat swabs should be handled as though they were capable of transmitting disease. Observe established precautions against microbiologic hazards throughout all procedures, and dispose of swabs and reagent tubes in biohazard containers. Washing hands after performing the test is recommended.

Reagents, Supplies, and Equipment

- OIA test kit, containing reagents 1 to 5, test device, and positive control
- Transfer pipettes
- Test kit procedure insert
- Stopwatch

The test kit should be stored at 2° to 8° C. The reagent tray may be stored at room temperature for up to 12 hours and then returned to refrigeration after use. Reagents should not be used beyond the expiration date printed on the label.

Safety Precautions

The test kit is intended for in vitro diagnostic use only. Reagents are not interchangeable between lots and kits. Do not interchange caps between reagents. "Reagent 1" is an irritant.

Quality Control

A positive GAS antigen control is incorporated into each test device. This internal control appears as a small purple dot near the center of each test surface after the completion of a properly performed test.

Procedure

Follow the test procedure as described in the package insert. On completion of each test, the test surface should be examined under a bright light source. The light must be reflected off the test surface to observe test results.

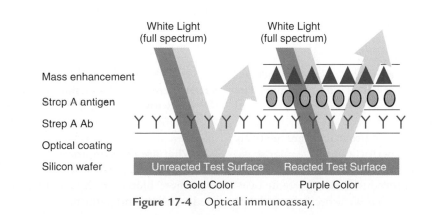

Figure 17-4 Optical immunoassay.

Reporting Results

Positive control: A small blue/purple dot in the center of the test surface on completion of each test.

Negative test: Only the internal positive control will be reactive.

Positive test: Shows the internal positive control within the reaction circle.

Strong positive test: The procedure control may be less apparent within the reaction circle.

Positive Result

A solid blue/purple reaction circle of any intensity appears in the center of the test surface.

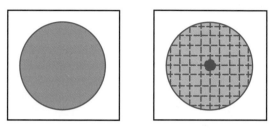

Negative Result

No blue/purple reaction circle of any intensity appears on the test surface. The positive control dot is in the center of the test surface.

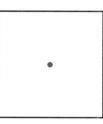

Invalid Result

No blue/purple positive control dot or solid blue/purple color appears over the test surface. The procedure should be repeated if an invalid test result occurs.

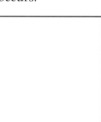

Procedural Notes

The reacted test surface and the color change associated with a positive reaction will not deteriorate over time. The test device may be considered a permanent record and should be closed for storage.

In general, direct GAS detection procedures are relatively inexpensive, rapid, and easy to perform but have poor sensitivity compared with conventional reference culture techniques. The STREP A OIA procedure has reportedly overcome related problems and now has 98% specificity and 95%

sensitivity. This exceeds the reported sensitivity of the latex agglutination ASO method (43%) and appears to be as sensitive as culture technique.

Sources of Error

Whole blood, serum, white blood cells, saliva, and sheep blood agar do not interfere with the test methodology.

Limitations

As with other diagnostic procedures, the results obtained with the STREP A OIA kit should be used as an adjunct to other clinical observations and information available to the physician. If a negative result is obtained with this assay and the symptoms persist, follow-up testing is recommended to determine other, non-GAS causes of pharyngitis. This test is not intended to differentiate carriers of group A streptococci from those with streptococcal infections.

Clinical Applications

Traditional rapid GAS antigen detection methods and culture techniques have had little influence on patient management in most clinical settings because of inherent test limitations. The OIA method appears to be a reliable and easily interpretable test for detection of GAS antigen from clinical specimens (e.g., pharyngeal swabs).

Reference

Strep A Optical Immunoassay (OIA) Kit, BioStar, Boulder, Colo, 1995.

CASE STUDY

This 19-year-old woman went to the emergency department (ED) with swelling and redness of her right leg. She had fallen down while rollerblading and had a number of abrasions on the skin of her leg. She also had a body temperature of 37.8° C. The ED physician ordered a culture of her leg wound, gave her a prescription for an antibiotic, and discharged her from treatment.

The following evening the patient collapsed onto the floor of her bedroom. Her roommate found her and called 911. On arrival, the paramedics found an unconscious female with a blood pressure of 80/40 and pronounced redness and swelling of her right leg. She was rushed to the ED and admitted to the intensive care unit, where she was immediately placed on IV fluids and medications to raise her blood pressure.

Questions and Discussion

1. Is there any relationship between this patient's problem with her leg and her collapse on the floor?

Yes; her infected wound and sudden hypotension could suggest streptococcal toxic shock syndrome (STSS).

2. What are the symptoms of STSS?

Along with the symptoms of shock, patients can manifest fever, blotchy rash, and an area of infected skin that is red, swollen, and painful.

3. What is the source of this patient's STSS?

As occurs most often with this infection, her STSS appeared after streptococci invade injured skin. It almost never follows a simple streptococcal throat infection.

4. Are there any immunologic/serologic manifestations of STSS?

Yes; serologic confirmation of group A streptococcal infection can be demonstrated by a fourfold rise against streptolysin O and DNase B.

Diagnosis

Streptococcal toxic shock syndrome.

CHAPTER HIGHLIGHTS

- Most streptococci that contain cell wall antigens of Lancefield group A are known as *Streptococcus pyogenes*. Members of this species are almost always beta-hemolytic.
- *S. pyogenes* is important in the development of complications such as acute rheumatic fever and poststreptococcal glomerulonephritis.
- Strains of *S. pyogenes* that lack M protein cannot cause infection.
- Extracellular products are important in the pathogenesis and serologic diagnosis of streptococcal disease. Antibodies produced in response to these substances indicate recent streptococcal infection.
- Substances produced by group A streptococci presumably facilitate rapid spread through subcutaneous or deeper soft tissues.

REVIEW QUESTIONS

1. *Streptococcus pyogenes* is the most common causative agent of all the following disorders and complications *except:*
   a. Pharyngitis.
   b. Gastroenteritis.
   c. Scarlet fever.
   d. Impetigo.

2. All the following characteristics are descriptive of M protein *except:*
   a. No known biologic role.
   b. Found in association with the hyaluronic capsule.
   c. Inhibits phagocytosis.
   d. Antibody against M protein provides type-specific immunity.

3. Substances produced by *S. pyogenes* include all the following *except:*
   a. Hyaluronidase.
   b. DNAses (A, B, C, D).
   c. Erythrogenic toxin.
   d. Interferon.

4. Laboratory diagnosis of *S. pyogenes* can be made by all the following *except:*
   a. Culturing of throat or nasal specimens.
   b. Febrile agglutinins.
   c. ASO procedure.
   d. Anti–DNase B.

5. False ASO results may be caused by all the following *except:*
   a. Room temperature reagents and specimens at the time of testing
   b. The presence of beta-lipoprotein
   c. Bacterial contamination of the serum specimen.
   d. Oxidation of ASO reagent caused by shaking or aeration of the reagent vial.

6. Members of the *S. pyogenes* species are almost always _____ hemolytic.
   a. alpha
   b. beta
   c. gamma
   d. alpha or beta

7. Long-term complications of *S. pyogenes* infection can include:
   a. Acute rheumatic fever.
   b. Poststreptococcal glomerulonephritis,.
   c. Rheumatoid arthritis.
   d. Both a and b.

8. Particularly virulent serotypes of *S. pyogenes* produce proteolytic enzymes that cause _____ in a wound or lesion on an extremity.
   a. necrotizing fasciitis
   b. bone degeneration
   c. burning and itching
   d. severe inflammation

Questions 9-11. Match the substances produced by group A streptococci with the appropriate description.

9. _____ Hyaluronidase

10. _____ Streptokinase

11. _____ Erythrogenic toxin
   a. Degrades DNA.
   b. Also called "spreading factor."
   c. Responsible for characteristic scarlet fever rash.
   d. Dissolves clots by converting plasminogen to plasmin.

12. All the following characteristics of *S. pyogenes* are correct *except:*
   a. It is an uncommon pathogen.
   b. It occurs most frequently in school-age children.
   c. It is spread by contact with large droplets produced in the upper respiratory tract.
   d. It has been known to cause food-borne and milk-borne epidemics.

13. The clinical manifestations of *S. pyogenes*–associated upper respiratory infection are:
    a. Mild and usually unnoticeable.
    b. Age dependent.
    c. Associated with cold sores.
    d. Difficult to detect.

14. The most reliable immunologic test for recent *S. pyogenes* skin infection is:
    a. ASO.
    b. Anti–DNAse B.
    c. Anti-NADase.
    d. Antibody to erythrogenic toxin.

Questions 15-17. Match each ASO titer situation to the appropriate description. (An answer may be used twice.)

15. _____ Rising titer

16. _____ Declining titer

17. _____ Constant (low) titer

    a. Increase in severity of infection.
    b. Not a current infection, but indicates a past infection.
    c. Trend toward recovery.
    d. No clinical significance.

18. If a streptococcal infection is suspected, but the ASO titer does not exceed the reference range, a(n) _____ should be performed.

    a. repeat titer
    b. anti–DNAse B
    c. anti-NADase
    d. throat culture

19. The classic tests to demonstrate the presence of streptococcal infection are:
    a. ASO and anti-NADase.
    b. ASO and anti–DNAse B.
    c. Anti-NADase and anti-DNAse.
    d. Both A and B.

20. The highest reported levels of sensitivity testing for group A streptococci are in:
    a. ASO titers.
    b. Direct latex agglutination tests.
    c. Surface (optical) immunoassay.
    d. Both a and b, which are equivalent.

BIBLIOGRAPHY

Anthony BF et al: Immunospecificity and quantitation of an enzyme-linked immunosorbent assay for group B streptococcal antibody, *J Clin Microbiol* 16:350-354, 1982.

Bisno AL: Group A streptococcal infections and acute rheumatic fever, *N Engl J Med* 325(11):783-793, 1991.

Davies HD et al: Invasive group A streptococcal infections in Ontario, Canada, *N Engl J Med* 335:547-554, 1996.

Farley MM et al: A population-based assessment of invasive disease due to group B streptococcus in nonpregnant adults, *N Engl J Med* 328(25): 1807-1812, 1993.

Forbes BA, Sahm DF, Weissfeld AS: *Bailey & Scott's diagnostic microbiology,* ed 12, St Louis, 2007, Mosby.

Hexter DA: Group A streptococcus septicemia in children, *JAMA* 267(1):53-54, 1992.

Hoge CW et al: The changing epidemiology of invasive group A streptococcal infections and the emergence of streptococcal toxic-shock-like syndrome, *JAMA* 269(3):384-391, 1993.

James E: Testing for strep throat, *Adv Medical Lab Prof* (online edition). www.advanceformLp.com.

Jefferson R: Rapid micro workup key to containing flesh-eating bacteria, *Adv Med Lab Prof* 7(11):6-9, 1995.

Mohle-Boetani JC et al: Comparison of prevention strategies for neonatal group B streptococcal infection, *JAMA* 270(12):1442-1448, 1993.

Schwartz B et al: Invasive group B streptococcal disease in adults, *JAMA* 266(8):1112-1114, 1991.

Smith JM, Bauman MC, Fuchs PC: An optical immunoassay for the direct detection of group A strep antigen, *Lab Med* 26(6):408-410, 1995.

Stanbio product brochure, San Antonio, Texas, 1986, Stanbio Laboratory.

Turner RB, Hendley JO: *Streptococcus pyogenes* infections. In Stein J, editor: *Internal medicine,* Boston, 1994, Little, Brown.

CHAPTER 18

Syphilis

Etiology
Epidemiology
Signs and Symptoms
   Primary Syphilis
   Secondary Syphilis
   Latent Syphilis
   Late (Tertiary) Syphilis
   Congenital Syphilis
   Neurosyphilis
Immunologic Manifestations
Diagnostic Evaluation
   Darkfield Microscopy
   Nontreponemal Methods

Treponemal Methods
   Sensitivity of Common Serologic Tests for Syphilis
Rapid Plasma Reagin Card Test
Fluorescent Treponemal Antibody Absorption Test
Case Study
Chapter Highlights
Review Questions
Bibliography

Learning Objectives

At the conclusion of this chapter, the reader should be able to:

- Describe the etiology, epidemiology, and signs and symptoms of primary, secondary, latent, and late (tertiary) syphilis.
- Describe the origin and manifestations of congenital syphilis.
- Explain the immunologic manifestations and diagnostic evaluation of syphilis.
- Discuss the principles and clinical applications of the rapid plasma reagin card test.
- Discuss the principles and clinical applications of the fluorescent treponemal antibody absorption test.

The disease syphilis was reported in the medical literature as early as 1495. In 1905 it was discovered that syphilis was caused by a spirochete type of bacteria, *Treponema pallidum* (originally called *Spirochaeta pallida*). The first diagnostic blood test, the Wassermann test, was developed in 1906. This classic procedure has subsequently been replaced by a variety of methods. In the treatment of syphilis, heavy metals, such as arsenic, were replaced by penicillin in the 1940s. Penicillin continues to remain the drug of choice in the treatment of this disease.

ETIOLOGY

Treponema pallidum is a member of the order Spirochaetales and the family Treponemataceae (Figure 18-1). The genus *Treponema* includes a number of species that reside in the gastrointestinal and genital tracts of humans. *T. pallidum*, *T. pertenue*, and *T. carateum* are human pathogens responsible for significant worldwide morbidity (Table 18-1). Direct examination of the treponemes is most often performed with darkfield microscopy. Pathogenic treponemes appear as fine, spiral (8-24 coils) organisms approximately 6 to 15 μm long. They have a trilaminar outer membrane similar to that of gram-negative bacteria.

Pathogenic treponemes are not cultivatable with any consistency in artificial laboratory media. Outside of the host, the pathogenic treponemes are extremely susceptible to a variety of physical and chemical agents. Treponemes may remain viable for up to 5 days in tissue specimens removed from diseased animals and from frozen, cryoprotected specimens.

EPIDEMIOLOGY

Pathogenic treponemes are transmitted almost uniformly by direct contact. Syphilis is a venereal disease. The three treponematoses—yaws, pinta, and bejel—are rarely seen in the United States but are prevalent in other countries. These diseases are associated with poverty, overcrowding, and poor hygiene.

Yaws, pinta, and bejel are diseases caused by bacteria closely related to *T. pallidum*. Yaws is common in the Caribbean, Latin America, Central Africa, and the Far East. Pinta is found only in Latin America, and infection is limited to the skin. Bejel is found in eastern Mediterranean countries, the Balkans, and the cooler areas of North Africa.

In these infections the skin or oral lesions contain many spirochetes that may be transmitted by personal, but not necessarily venereal, contact. These infections are generally acquired during childhood. In each of these diseases, infection elicits antibodies reactive in nontreponemal and treponemal methods.

Syphilis develops in 30% to 50% of the sexual partners of persons with syphilitic lesions. The risk of acquiring syphilis

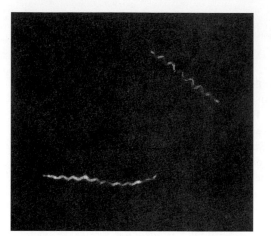

Figure 18-1 *Treponema pallidum. (From Bauer JD:* Clinical laboratory methods, *ed 9, St Louis, 1982, Mosby.)*

Table 18-1	*Treponema*-Associated Diseases in Humans
Bacteria	**Associated Disease**
Treponema pallidum	Syphilis
T. pallidum (variant)	Bejel
T. pertenue	Yaws
T. carateum	Pinta

from a single sexual exposure to an infected partner is unknown. A high percentage of partners do seek medical treatment within 90 days of contact.

Since 1999 marked changes have occurred in the epidemiology of infectious syphilis in the United States. There have been substantial reductions in diagnosed disease in women and newborn infants (congenital syphilis). Between 1991 and 2004, congenital cases declined by 92%. Rates of primary and secondary syphilis among women fell from 2.0 to 0.8 per 100,000 population.

Despite these improvements, overall rates of primary and secondary syphilis have been increasing since 2001. From 2000 to 2004, primary and secondary syphilis increased among men, particularly men who have sex with men. The incidence of syphilis per capita is higher among blacks and Hispanics than among whites.

The incidence of syphilis is highest in women age 20 to 29 years and in men 30 to 39 years. Some fundamental social problems (e.g., poverty, inadequate access to health care, lack of education) are associated with disproportionately high levels of syphilis in certain populations.

Syphilis can be acquired by kissing a person with active oral lesions. Very few cases of transfusion-acquired syphilis have been reported in recent years in the United States. During the first half of the twentieth century, however, syphilis was a major blood-borne infectious disease easily transmitted through the prevailing method of direct donor-to-patient blood transfusion. The danger of syphilis transmission still exists in tropical countries where the organization

of blood banks is deficient and where direct blood transfusion prevails in emergency situations. Refrigerated blood storage decreases accidental transmission of the microorganism because *T. pallidum* has a short survival period in stored blood. Spirochetes do not appear to survive in units of citrated blood at 4° C for more than 72 hours.

Cases have been reported of children who have acquired syphilis by sharing a bed with an infected parent. In addition, syphilis may be transmitted transplacentally to the fetus. Spirochetes can be transmitted to the fetus during the last trimester of pregnancy, before the mother manifests postpartum evidence of infection.

SIGNS AND SYMPTOMS

Untreated syphilis is a chronic disease with subacute symptomatic periods separated by asymptomatic intervals, during which the diagnosis can be made serologically.

The progression of untreated syphilis is generally divided into stages. Initially, *T. pallidum* penetrates intact mucous membranes or enters the body through tiny defects in the epithelium. On entrance, the microorganism is carried by the circulatory system to every organ of the body. *Spirochetemia* occurs very early in infection, even before the first lesions have appeared or blood tests become reactive. Before clinical or serologic manifestations develop, patients are said to be "incubating syphilis." The incubation period usually lasts about 3 weeks but can range from 10 to 90 days.

Primary Syphilis

At the end of the incubation period, a patient develops a characteristic primary inflammatory lesion called a *chancre* at the point of initial inoculation and multiplication of the spirochetes. The chancre begins as a papule and erodes to form a gradually enlarging ulcer with a clean base and indurated edge (Figure 18-2). Generally, it is relatively painless. In most cases, only a single lesion is present, but multiple chancres are not rare.

Chancres are typically located around the genitalia, but in about 10% of cases, lesions may appear almost anywhere else on the body (e.g., throat, lip, hands). In males, spirochetes are present in the lesion on the penis or discharged from deeper sites with semen. In females, infected lesions are usually located in the perineal region or on the labia, vaginal wall, or cervix. If the lesion is located inside the urethra, the only symptom may be a scanty, serous urethral discharge.

Of patients with primary syphilis of the external genitalia, 50% to 70% will subsequently develop *inguinal adenopathy*. Inguinal adenopathy, however, is less common with chancres involving the cervix or proximal part of the vagina because these sites are drained by the iliac nodes. Regional adenopathy may accompany primary inoculation at other sites; for example, cervical adenopathy may accompany a syphilitic lesion of the oral cavity.

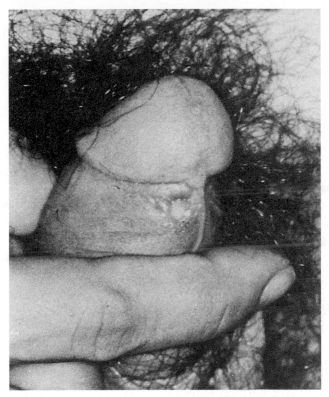

Figure 18-2   A primary chancre of syphilis. *(From Kaye D, Rose LF: Fundamentals of internal medicine, St Louis, 1983, Mosby.)*

The primary chancre will persist for 1 to 5 weeks and will heal completely in about 4 to 6 weeks, even without treatment. Regional adenopathy will also resolve itself.

Secondary Syphilis

Within 2 to 8 weeks (but occasionally as long as 6 months) after the appearance of the primary chancre, a patient may develop the signs and symptoms of secondary syphilis. In some patients, primary and secondary syphilis overlap, and the chancre is still obvious. Other patients never notice the primary chancre and initially have manifestations of secondary syphilis (Figure 18-3).

The secondary stage is characterized by a generalized illness that usually begins with symptoms suggesting a viral infection: headache, sore throat, low-grade fever, and occasionally a nasal discharge. Blood tests reveal a moderate increase in leukocytes with a relative increase in lymphocytes.

The disease progresses with the development of lymphadenopathy and lesions of the skin and mucous membranes. Approximately 75% of syphilitic patients develop generalized adenopathy. About 80% have skin lesions, which contain a large number of spirochetes and, when located on exposed surfaces, are highly contagious. Macular lesions are common, and a rash invariably involves the genitalia and often is prominent on the palms and soles. Patients may also develop *condylomata lata,* flat lesions resembling warts in moist areas of the body (e.g., around anus or vagina). These lesions do

not reflect areas of inoculation but appear to be caused by hematogeneous dissemination of spirochetes.

The central nervous system (CNS) is asymptomatically involved in about one third of patients. About 2% of cases manifest as acute syphilitic meningitis. Early CNS involvement may progress to neurosyphilis if untreated. Hepatitis and immune complex glomerulonephritis occasionally accompany secondary syphilis.

Secondary syphilis usually resolves within 2 to 6 weeks, even without therapy.

Latent Syphilis

After resolution of untreated secondary syphilis, the patient enters a latent noninfectious state in which diagnosis can be made only by serologic methods. During the first 2 to 4 years of infection, one fourth of patients will have one or more mucocutaneous relapses in which the manifestation of secondary syphilis reappears. During these relapses, patients are infectious, and the underlying spirochetemia may be passed transplacentally to the fetus. Relapses are extremely rare after 4 years of latency. About one third of patients entering latency are eventually spontaneously cured of the disease; one third will never develop further clinical manifestations of the disease; and the remaining one third will eventually develop late syphilis.

Late (Tertiary) Syphilis

The first manifestations of late syphilis are usually seen from 3 to 10 years after primary infection. About 15% of untreated syphilitic individuals eventually develop late benign syphilis, characterized by the presence of destructive

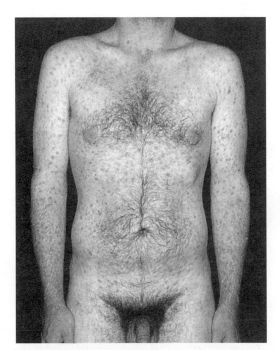

Figure 18-3   Secondary syphilis. *(From Habif TP: Clinical dermatology, ed 2, St Louis, 1990, Mosby.)*

granulomas. These granulomas, or *gummas,* may produce lesions resembling segments of circles that often heal with superficial scarring. The skeletal system is frequently affected, but treponemes are rarely seen.

Of untreated patients, 10% develop cardiovascular manifestations. *T. pallidum* may directly affect the aortic endothelium. Weakening of the blood vessels can occur as a syphilitic aneurysm, usually of the aortic arch.

In about 8% of untreated patients, late syphilis involves the CNS. Initially, CNS disease is asymptomatic and can be detected only by examination of cerebrospinal fluid (CSF). CSF should be examined in all patients being treated for syphilis of unknown duration or who have had syphilis for more than 1 year.

Meningovascular syphilis usually manifests as a seizure or cerebrovascular accident (stroke). Spirochetes may also involve the brain tissues and cause general paresis, personality changes, dementia, and delusional states. Tabes dorsalis results from involvement of the posterior columns and dorsal roots of the spinal cord and is characterized by a broad-based gait. Impotence and bladder dysfunction are common in this disorder (see Neurosyphilis).

Congenital Syphilis

Congenital syphilis is caused by maternal spirochetemia and transplacental transmission of the microorganism. The typing of congenital syphilis is according to age at diagnosis.

The *early stage* is seen in children under 2 years old who are untreated. Symptoms of the untreated early stage can include rash, condyloma latum, bone changes, hepatosplenomegaly, jaundice, or anemia.

The *late stage* is seen in children over 2 years old who are untreated. Symptoms of the untreated late stage include eighth nerve deafness, keratitis, and Hutchinson's teeth (Figure 18-4) (hutchisonian triad), as well as arthropathy and neurosyphilis. Residual stigmata can develop. Other characteristics include fissuring around the mouth and anus, skeletal lesions, perforation of the palate, and collapse of nasal bones to produce a saddle-nose deformity.

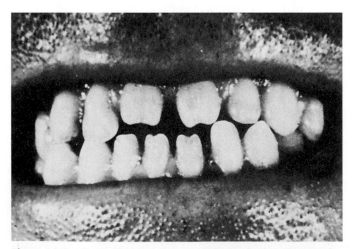

Figure 18-4   Congenital syphilis (Hutchinson's teeth). *(From Kaye D, Rose LF:* Fundamentals of internal medicine, *St Louis, 1983, Mosby.)*

Neurosyphilis

Although neurosyphilis may be asymptomatic, symptomatic forms include the following:
- Meningeal syphilis, usually less than 1 year after infection.
- Meningovascular syphilis, usually 5 to 10 years after infection.
- Parenchymatous syphilis.

Meningeal neurosyphilis involves the brain or spinal cord. Patients can suffer from headaches and a stiff neck. *Meningovascular syphilis* involves inflammation of the pia mater and arachnoid space, with focal arteritis. A stroke syndrome involving middle cerebral artery is common in young adults. *Parenchymatous neurosyphilis* manifests as general paresis, joint degeneration, and tabes dorsalis (demyelination of posterior columns, dorsal roots, and dorsal root ganglia). Tabes dorsalis is characterized by a gait disturbance and bladder symptoms.

IMMUNOLOGIC MANIFESTATIONS

In the treponemes, two classes of antigen have been recognized: (1) antigens restricted to one or a few species and (2) antigens shared by many different spirochetes. Specific and nonspecific antibodies are produced in the immunocompetent host. Specific antibodies against *T. pallidum* and nonspecific antibodies against the protein antigen group common to pathogenic spirochetes are formed. Specific *antitreponemal antibodies* in early or untreated early latent syphilis are predominantly immunoglobulin M (IgM) antibodies. The early immune response to infection is rapidly followed by the appearance of IgG antibodies, which soon become predominant. The greatest elevation in IgG concentration is seen in secondary syphilis.

Nontreponemal antibodies, often called *reagin antibodies,* are produced by infected patients against components of their own or other mammalian cells. Although almost always produced by patients with syphilis, these antibodies are also produced by patients with other infectious diseases. Infectious diseases in which reagin can be demonstrated include measles, chickenpox, hepatitis, infectious mononucleosis, leprosy, tuberculosis, leptospirosis, malaria, rickettsial disease, trypanosomiasis, and lymphogranuloma venereum. Reagin can also be exhibited by patients with noninfectious conditions such as autoimmune disorders, drug addiction, old age, pregnancy, and recent immunization.

Delayed-hypersensitivity immune mechanisms also contribute to the pathophysiology of syphilis. It is suggested that the granulomatous reactions (gummas) result from delayed hypersensitivity in the immune host. In addition, the manifestations of congenital syphilis apparently result in part from an immune-inflammatory reaction. Antigen-antibody complexes have been detected in the blood of patients with secondary syphilis and are responsible for the syphilis-associated glomerulonephritis. Suppression of the various aspects of cell-mediated immunity has been noted in syphilis and may contribute to prolonged survival of *T. pallidum*.

DIAGNOSTIC EVALUATION

The diagnosis of syphilis depends on clinical skills, demonstration of microorganism in a lesion, and serologic testing. A variety of diagnostic procedures for syphilis are available (Table 18-2). Classic serologic methods for syphilis measure the presence of the following two types of antibodies:

1. Nontreponemal methods
   - **Rapid plasma reagin (RPR)** test
2. Treponemal methods
   - **Fluorescent treponemal antibody adsorption (FTA-ABS)** test
   - **Microhemagglutination for *Treponema pallidum* (MHA-TP)** test

Darkfield Microscopy

For symptomatic patients with primary syphilis, darkfield microscopy is the test of choice. A darkfield examination is also suggested for immediate results in cases of secondary syphilis, with a titer follow-up test.

Nontreponemal Methods

The RPR is the most widely used nontreponemal serologic procedure, although the Venereal Disease Research Laboratories (VDRL) methods may be available in some clinical and reference laboratories (see EVOLVE website for traditional procedures). Each VDRL procedure is a flocculation (or agglutination) test in which soluble antigen particles coalesce to form larger particles visible as clumps when they are aggregated by antibody.

The RPR test can be performed on unheated serum or plasma using a modified VDRL antigen suspension of choline chloride with ethylenediaminetetraacetic acid (EDTA). The RPR card test antigen also contains charcoal for mac-

roscopic reading. There are three versions of the RPR test. The original RPR method used unmeasured amounts of plasma and was used as a field procedure for screening large numbers of people. The modified RPR uses the serum reagin test and is performed on measured volumes of unheated serum.

Treponemal Methods

The FTA-ABS and MHA-TP represent treponemal methods. The *T. pallidum* immobilization (TPI) test is obsolete. These two specific treponemal antigen tests can confirm reactive (positive) reagin tests but should not be used as primary screening methods. FTA-ABS and MHA-TP can be used to confirm that a positive nontreponemal test result has been caused by syphilis rather than other biologic conditions that can produce a positive serologic result. These tests also can determine quantitative titers of antibody, which is useful for following response to therapy.

An enzyme-linked immunosorbent assay (ELISA) for syphilis antibody is available, but it is not widely used at present. The ELISA method, however, does offer a sensitive and specific alternative to existing methods.

The FTA-ABS uses a killed suspension *of T. pallidum* spirochetes as the antigen. This procedure is performed by overlaying whole treponemes fixed to a slide with serum from patients suspected of having syphilis because of a previously positive syphilis serology. The patient's serum is first absorbed with non–*T. pallidum* treponemal antigens to reduce nonspecific cross-reactivity. Fluorescein-conjugated antihuman antibody reagent is then applied as a marker for specific antitreponemal antibodies in the patient's serum.

The microhemagglutination assay for *T. pallidum* is based on agglutination by specific antibodies in the patient's serum with sheep erythrocytes sensitized to *T. pallidum* antigen. The MHA-TP method uses treated red blood cells (RBCs) coated with treponemal antigens from a turkey or other animal. The presence of specific antibody produces

Table 18-2	Select Tests for Syphilis Diagnosis	
Test	**Methodology**	**Comments**
Darkfield examination	Darkfield microscopy	Use as initial diagnostic test if lesions are present.
Rapid plasma reagin (RPR)	Charcoal agglutination	Cannot be used for cerebrospinal fluid (CSF).
Treponema pallidum antibody, serum IgG by IFA	Indirect fluorescent antibody (IFA)	False positive in herpes, HIV, malaria, IV drug use, systemic lupus, rheumatoid arthritis, pregnancy, and leprosy.
T. pallidum (TP) antibody by TP-HA (MHA-TP)	Indirect hemagglutination (HA)	Cannot differentiate between IgG and IgM antibodies. Cannot be used for CSF
T. pallidum (VDRL), serum with reflex to titer	Flocculation	For serum or CSF.
T. pallidum antibody, IgM by ELISA	Enzyme-linked immunosorbent assay (ELISA)	If test results are questionable, repeat testing in 10-14 days.
T. pallidum (VDRL) CSF with reflex to titer	Flocculation	—
Treponema pallidum antibody, IgG by ELISA	ELISA	If test results are questionable, repeat testing in 10-14 days.

Modified from www.arupconsult.com, January 2007.

IgG, Immunoglobulin G; *HIV,* human immunodeficiency virus; *IV,* intravenous; *MHA,* microhemagglutination, *VDRL,* Venereal Disease Research Laboratories.

Table 18-3	Sensitivity of Common Serologic Tests for Syphilis		
	Stage		
Test*	Primary	Secondary	Late
Nontreponemal (Reagin Tests)			
Rapid plasma reagin (RPR)	80%	99%	1%†
Automated reagin test (ART)			0%
Specific Treponemal Tests			
Fluorescent treponemal antibody absorption test (FTA-ABS)	85%	100%	95%
Treponema pallidum hemagglutination assay (TP-HA; MHA-TP)	65%	100%	95%

From Tramont E: *Treponema pallidum.* In Mandell GL, Douglas RG Jr, Bennett JE, editors: *Principles and practice of infectious diseases,* ed 2, New York, 1985, Wiley & Sons.
*Percentage of patients with positive serologic tests in treated or untreated primary or secondary syphilis.
†Treated late syphilis.

RBC agglutination, demonstrated by the formation of a flat mat across the bottom of a microdilution well in which the test is performed.

Sensitivity of Common Serologic Tests for Syphilis

Detection of syphilis by serologic methods is related to both the stage of the disease and the test method (Table 18-3).

In the primary stage, about 30% of cases become serologically active after 1 week, and 90% of patients demonstrate reactivity after 3 weeks. Reagin titers increase rapidly during the first 4 weeks of infection and then remain stable for about 6 months. Patients in the secondary stage of syphilis are serologically positive.

During latent syphilis there is a gradual return of nonreactive serologic manifestations, as seen with nontreponemal methods. About one third of patients in the latent stage will remain seroreactive and presumably infectious. In late syphilis, treponemal tests are generally reactive; nontreponemal methods are nonreactive.

Rapid Plasma Reagin Card Test

Principle

The RPR test is designed to detect *reagin,* an antibody-like substance present in serum. In this procedure, serum is mixed with an antigen suspension of a carbon-particle *cardiolipin* antigen. If the specimen contains antibody, *flocculation* occurs with a coagglutination of the carbon particles of antigen. This flocculation appears as black clumps against the white background of a plastic-coated card. The cards are viewed macroscopically.

This is a nontreponemal testing procedure for the serologic detection of syphilis; however, pinta, yaws, bejel, and other treponemal diseases may produce positive results. Positive reactions are occasionally observed with other acute or chronic conditions.

Specimen Collection and Preparation

No special preparation of the patient is required before specimen collection. The patient must be positively identified when the specimen is collected. The specimen is to be labeled at the bedside and must include the patient's full name, the date the specimen is collected, and the patient's hospital identification number. The phlebotomist's initials should also appear on the label.

Blood should be drawn by an aseptic technique. The required specimen is a minimum of 2 mL of clotted blood (red-top evacuated tube). After allowing the blood to clot, centrifuge the specimen and allow the serum to remain in the original tube. Severely lipemic or hemolyzed serum is unsuitable for testing.

Note: In special situations, when nontreponemal test results are needed rapidly and the specimen is collected in EDTA anticoagulant, plasma can be used for both qualitative and quantitative procedures if the test is performed within 24 hours. Store the specimen at 2° to 8° C, and centrifuge before testing.

Reagents, Supplies, and Equipment

Note: Except for the antigen, all other components should be stored at room temperature in a dry place in the original kit packaging.

The following components are provided in Macro-Vue RPR Card Test kit*:
- RPR card test antigen

This antigen suspension is similar to VDRL antigen: cardiolipin, lecithin, cholesterol, EDTA, Na_2HPO_4, KH_2PO_4, thimerosal (preservative), charcoal, choline chloride, and distilled water.

If frozen during shipment, the ampule of antigen can be reconstituted once by warming to room temperature. Avoid repeated freezing and thawing.

Store the antigen suspension in ampules or in the plastic dispensing bottle at 2° to 8° C. Unopened ampules have a shelf life of 12 months from the date of manufacture. Before opening, shake the ampule vigorously for 10 to 15 seconds to resuspend the antigen and dispense any carbon particles that may have lodged in the neck of the ampule. Even if carbon remains in the neck of the ampule after this shaking,

---

*Macro-Vue RPR Card Test, 1.8-mm circles; Brewer Diagnostic Kit product insert, BBL Microbiology Systems, Cockneysville, Md.

make no additional effort to dislodge it; this will only tend to produce a coarse antigen.

To prepare the antigen, attach the needle to the tapered fitting on the plastic dispensing bottle. Be sure the antigen is below the break line; snap the ampule neck and withdraw all the antigen into the dispensing bottle by collapsing the bottle and using it as a suction device. Shake the card antigen dispensing bottle gently before each series of antigen droppings. The needle and dispensing bottle should be discarded when the kit reagents are depleted.

Once the antigen ampule is opened and placed in the dispensing bottle, it is stable for 3 months or the expiration date on the label (if it occurs sooner) if refrigerated at 2° to 8° C. Label dispensing bottle with antigen lot number, expiration date, and date antigen is placed in bottle.

Immediate use of refrigerated antigen may result in decreased sensitivity in testing. Allow the antigen to warm to room temperature (23°-29° C) before use. Do not use beyond expiration date. Avoid bright sunlight.
- Needle, 18 gauge, without bevel

The needles should deliver 60 ±2 drops of antigen suspension per milliliter when held in a vertical position. Take care to obtain drops of uniform size. On completion of tests, remove needle from dispensing bottle and rinse needle with distilled or deionized water. Do not wipe needle; this would remove the silicone coating and could affect the accuracy of the drop of antigen being dispensed.
- Specially prepared, plastic-coated cards, each with ten 18-mm circle spots designed for use with RPR card antigen

Take care not to finger-mark the test areas on the card; this may result in an oily deposit and improper test results. Avoid scratching the card when spreading the specimen. If the specimen does not spread to the outer perimeter of the test area, use another test area of the card.
- Dispenstirs, 0.05 mL/drop
- Capillary pipettes, 0.05-mL capacity, or one of the following pipettes:
  0.2 mL (graduated in 0.01-mL subdivisions)
  0.5 mL (graduated in 0.01-mL subdivisions)
  1.0 mL (graduated in 0.01-mL subdivisions)

Dispenstirs are provided with the kit for use with the 18-mm circle qualitative test; however, these stirrers may be used only to transfer a specimen to the card surface. New Dispenstirs or capillary tubes must be used for each specimen. Take care to avoid drawing specimen up into the rubber ball attached to the capillary tube.
- Rubber bulbs
- Stirrers

Other Supplies (not in kit)
- Rotator (100 rpm), circumscribing a circle 2 cm in diameter on a horizontal plane.
- Humidifier cover, containing a moistened sponge.
- 0.9% saline (for quantitative test). Prepare by adding 0.9 g of sodium chloride (ACS) to 100 mL of distilled water.

Quality Control
1. Controls with established patterns of graded reactivity should be included in each day's testing to confirm optimal reactivity of the antigen suspension. Control sera must be at 23° to 29° C at the time of testing.
   CAUTION: Because these are derived from human sources, control sera should be handled in the same manner as clinical serum.
   Serum that is nonreactive to syphilis in 0.9% saline is required for diluting test specimens, producing a reactive result at the 1:16 dilution.
2. A new lot of antigen should be compared with an antigen suspension of known reactivity before being used.
3. The calibration of the delivery needle is an important aspect of quality control. An 18-gauge needle delivers 60 ±2 drops/mL of reagent. Place the needle on a 2-mL syringe or a 1-mL pipette. Fill the syringe or pipette with the antigen suspension and, holding it in a vertical position, count the number of drops delivered in 0.5 mL. The needle is considered to be satisfactory if 30 ±1 drops are obtained from 0.5 mL of suspension.

Preliminary Testing of Antigen Suspension
See antigen description under Reagents, Supplies, and Equipment.
1. Attach needle hub to tapered fitting on plastic dispensing bottle. Shake antigen ampule to resuspend antigen particles, snap ampule neck at the break line, and withdraw all the RPR card antigen suspension into the dispensing bottle by suction, collapsing the bottle and using it as a bulb. Shake dispenser gently before each series of antigen drops is delivered.
2. Test control sera of graded reactivity each day.

Procedure
1. Place 0.05 mL of unheated serum on an 18-mm circle of the test card with a capillary or serologic pipette. Hold the dispensers in a vertical position directly over the card test area to which the specimen is to be delivered. Do not touch card surface.
2. Spread serum in the circle with an inverted Dispenstir (closed end), stirrer (broad end), or serologic pipette to fill the entire circle. Care must be taken not to scratch the card surface.
3. Gently shake antigen-dispensing bottle before use. Holding it in a vertical position, dispense several drops into the dispensing bottle cap to make sure the needle passage is clear. Add exactly 1 free-falling drop (1/60 mL) or RPR antigen suspension from the 20-gauge (yellow-hub) needle to each test area containing serum. Do not stir; mixing is accomplished during rotation.
4. Place card on rotator, and cover with humidifier cover.
   Note: The Macro-Vue RPR Card Test (Teardrop Qualitative) Brewer Diagnostic Kit (Hynson, Westcott & Dunning, Div. of Becton Dickinson, Baltimore) can be hand-rocked and used where laboratory equipment is not available.

5. Rotate 8 minutes at 100 rpm (95-110 rpm acceptable) on mechanical rotator. If below or above range, the clumping antigen tends to be less intense in test with undiluted specimen, so some minimal reactions may be missed.
6. Observe each specimen immediately in the "wet" state under a high-intensity incandescent lamp or strong daylight. Observation should be without magnification. It is permissible to gently rotate or tilt the card by hand (three or four times) to differentiate minimally reactive from nonreactive specimens.
7. Specimens producing questionable reactions should be retested by this method and other serologic methods.
8. When testing is completed, the work area should be cleaned. The dispensing needle should be rinsed in distilled water and air-dried. Do not wipe the needle because this will remove the silicone coating. Recap the antigen solution and store in the refrigerator.

Reporting Results

Reactive: Slight to large agglutination (black clumps).
Nonreactive: No agglutination, or very slight roughness (even light-gray color).

Procedural Notes

All reactive tests should be retested using the quantitative procedure to establish a baseline from which changes in titer can be determined, particularly for evaluating treatment. It is desirable to quantitate specimens that are nonreactive/rough so that an infrequent zonal specimen may be revealed.

18-mm Circle Quantitative Card Test

1. For each specimen to be tested, place 0.05 mL of 0.9% saline onto circle numbers 2 to 5 with a capillary or serologic pipette.
2. Pipette 0.05 mL of serum onto circle #1 and 0.05 mL of serum onto circle #2.
3. Prepare a serial twofold dilution by drawing the mixture up and down (avoid formation of bubbles). Transfer 0.05 mL of the dilution to the next circle, and repeat procedure to circle #5. Discard 0.05 mL of the dilution from circle #5.
4. Beginning with the most dilute specimen (circle #5), spread the dilution to fill the entire surface of the circle. Use a new stirrer for each circle.
5. Proceed with steps 3 through 8 in the qualitative procedure previously described.

Reporting Results

Report the highest dilution producing a minimal to moderate reaction (i.e., circle #1 = 1:1 undiluted, circle #2 = 1:2, circle #3 = 1:4, circle #4 = 1:8, and circle #5 = 1:16). If the 1:16 is reactive, prepare a 1:50 dilution with nonreactive serum in 0.9% saline. This preparation is to be used to prepare subsequent serial dilutions. Pipette 0.05 mL of 1:50 nonreactive serum into each of the circles 2 to 5, pipette 0.05 mL of the 1:16 dilution of test specimen in circle #1, and prepare and test the specimen as described in step 3 above.

Sources of Error

Error can be introduced into test results because of factors such as contamination of rubber bulbs or an improperly prepared antigen suspension.

False-positive biologic reactions have been reported with cardiolipin type of antigens in the following conditions:
- Lupus erythematosus
- Rheumatic fever
- Vaccinia and viral pneumonia
- Pneumococcal pneumonia
- Infectious mononucleosis
- Infectious hepatitis
- Leprosy
- Malaria
- Rheumatoid arthritis
- Pregnancy
- Aging individuals

False-negative reactions can result from the following:
- Poor technique
- Ineffective reagents
- Improper rotation

Again, if mechanical rotation is below or above the 95 to 110-rpm acceptable range, the clumping of the antigen tends to be less intense in procedures with undiluted specimen, and thus some minimal reactions may be missed. In quantitative tests, rotation above 110 rpm tends to produce a decrease in titer—approximately one dilution lower.

Limitations

A diagnosis of syphilis cannot be made based on a single reactive result without clinical signs and symptoms or history. Plasma specimens should not be used to establish a quantitative baseline from which changes in titer can be determined, particularly for evaluating treatment.

The RPR cards should not be used for testing CSF. Little reliance should be placed on cord blood serologic testing for syphilis. The RPR procedure has adequate sensitivity and specificity in relation to clinical diagnosis.

Clinical Applications

The purpose of the RPR procedure is to demonstrate reagin in cases of syphilis. The procedure may also be positive in treponemal diseases such as yaws and pinta. Reagin, however, is found in some patients who are not infected with treponemes, which can be partially explained by the necrotizing effect of spirochetes on tissues and in other conditions and disorders. It is important that results of the procedure be correlated with patient history, as well as with signs and symptoms.

Reference

Manual of tests for syphilis, US Public Health Service Pub No 411, 1969.

Fluorescent Treponemal Antibody Absorption Test

Principle

The FTA-ABS test is a direct method of observation. Although not recommended for screening, it is the most sensitive serologic procedure in the detection of primary syphilis.

Specimen Collection and Preparation

No special preparation of the patient is required before specimen collection. The patient must be positively identified when the specimen is collected. The specimen is to be labeled at the bedside and must include the patient's full name, date the specimen is collected, and patient's hospital identification number. The phlebotomist's initials should also appear on the label.

Blood should be drawn by aseptic technique. The required specimen is a minimum of 2 mL of clotted blood (red-top evacuated tube). The specimen should be centrifuged and the serum removed from the clot. Before testing, the serum should be heated at 56° C for 30 minutes if never inactivated, or for 10 minutes at 56° C if inactivated more than 4 hours before testing. Evidence of hemolysis or bacterial contamination makes the specimen unsuitable for testing.

Reagents, Supplies, and Equipment

- *Treponema pallidum* antigen

The antigen for this test is a suspension of *T. pallidum* (Nicols strain) extracted from rabbit testicular tissue, containing a minimum of 30 organisms per high-power dry field. The antigen may be stored at 6° to 10° C or may be processed by lyophilization. Lyophilized antigen is also stored at 6° to 10° C and is reconstituted for use according to directions when needed. Any antigen that becomes bacterially contaminated or does not give the appropriate reactions with control sera must be discarded.

T. pallidum antigen slides are prepared as follows:

1. Mix the antigen suspension with a disposable pipette and rubber bulb, drawing the suspension into and expelling it from the pipette at least 10 times to break the treponemal clumps and to ensure an even distribution of treponemes. Check by darkfield examination for even distribution. Additional mixing may be required.
2. Place one loopful of *T. pallidum* antigen suspension on a glass slide with a wire loop. Spread the suspension into a circle about 1 cm in diameter.
3. Allow to air-dry for at least 15 minutes.
4. Fix the smears in acetone for 10 minutes, and allow them to air-dry. No more than 60 slides should be fixed with each 200 mL of acetone.
5. After the slides are thoroughly dry, the smears should be stored in a freezer at −20° C or lower. Fixed, frozen smears can be used indefinitely if satisfactory results are achieved with controls. Antigen smears cannot be thawed and refrozen.

- FTA-ABS test sorbent

This is a standardized product prepared from culture of Reiter treponemes. It may be purchased lyophilized or in liquid state and should be stored according to the manufacturer's directions.

- Fluorescein-labeled antihuman globulin (conjugate)

This should be of proven quality for FTA-ABS test. Each new lot of conjugate should be tested to ensure its dependability with respect to working titer and to verify that it meets the criteria concerning nonspecific staining and standard reactivity. The lyophilized conjugate should be stored at 6° to 10° C. Rehydrated conjugate should be dispensed in not less than 0.3-mL quantities and should be stored at −38° C or lower. For practical purposes, a conjugate with a working titer of 1:400 or higher may be diluted 1:10 with sterile **phosphate-buffered saline** (PBS), containing thimerosal (Merthiolate) in a concentration of 1:5000 before storage. When conjugate is thawed for use, it should not be refrozen but should be stored at 6° to 10° C. It may then be used as long as acceptable reactivity is obtained with test controls. If a change in FTA-ABS test reactivity is noted in routine testing, the conjugate should be retitered to determine whether this is the contributing factor.

1. *Conjugate:* Prepare serial doubling dilutions of the new conjugate in PBS containing 2% Tween-80 to include the titer indicated by the manufacturer. Examples are as follows: (1) 1:2.5, 1:5, 1:10, 1:20, 1:40, 1:80, 1:160; or (2) 1:12.5, 1:25, 1:50, 1:100, 1:200, 1:400, 1:800. Prepare higher dilutions if necessary.
2. Test each conjugate dilution with the reactive (4+) control serum diluted 1:5 with PBS (follow the procedure below). Include a nonspecific staining control with each conjugate dilution. A standard conjugate, at its titer, is set up at the same time with a reactive (4+) control serum, a minimally reactive (1+) control serum, and a nonspecific staining control with PBS for the purpose of controlling reagents and test conditions. Table 18-4 outlines the titration of a new conjugate.

Table 18-4	New Conjugate Titration		
Conjugate	Nonspecific Staining Control (PBS)*	Reactive (4+) Control Serum (dilution 1:5)	Reactive (4+) Control Serum
Standard Titer			
1:400	Negative	4+	1+
New Conjugate Titer			
1:12.5	1+	4+	
1:25	Negative	4+	
1:50	Negative	4+	
1:100	Negative	4+	
1:200	Negative	4+	
1:400	Negative	4+	
1:800	Negative	3+	

*Phosphate-buffered saline.

Read slides in the following order:
a. Examine the three control slides to ensure that the reagents and testing conditions are satisfactory.
b. Examine the slides with new conjugate, starting with the lowest dilution of conjugate.
c. Record readings as graded reactions from negative to 4+.

The end point of the titration is the highest dilution giving maximal (4+) fluorescence. The working titer of the new conjugate is one doubling dilution below the end point. In Table 18-4, the dilution selected for the working titer is 1:200. The new conjugate should not stain nonspecifically at three doubling dilutions below the working titer of the conjugate. In Table 18-3 the conjugate would meet this criterion, because there is no nonspecific staining with the 1:25 dilution.

3. Dispense conjugate in not less than 0.3-mL quantities, and store at $-20°$ C or lower. For practical purposes, a conjugate with a working titer of 1:400 or higher may be diluted 1:10 with sterile PBS containing thimerosal (Merthiolate in 1:5000 concentration) before storage in the freezer. Verify the titer of the conjugate after at least 3 days of storage in the freezer.

4. Check testing. If the criterion of acceptability for the nonspecific staining has been met and a working titer has been determined, the new conjugate should be check-tested in parallel with a standard conjugate before being placed in routine use. Testing should be performed on more than one testing day with control sera, individual sera of graded reactivity, and nonreactive sera. Individual sera tested parallel with a standard and a new conjugate are read against the minimally reactive (1+) controls set up with the respective conjugates. A new conjugate is considered to be satisfactory when comparable test results are obtained with both conjugates.

- PBS, pH 7.2 ±0.1
  Prepare, per liter of distilled water, 7.65 g NaCl, 0.724 g Na_2HPO_4, 0.21 g KH_2PO_4.
- 2% Tween-80, pH 7.0 to 7.2
  Prepare/heat PBS and Tween-80 in 56° C water bath. To 98 mL of PBS, add 2 mL of Tween-80. Refrigerate to store. Discard if precipitate forms or if pH is outside the acceptable range (check pH periodically).
- Mounting medium, consisting of 1 part PBS, pH 7.2, plus 9 parts glycerin (reagent quality)
- Acetone (ACS)
- Pipettes
- 12 × 75–mm test tubes
- 35° to 37° C incubator
- Darkfield fluorescence microscope assembly
- Bibulous paper
- Slide holder
- Moist chamber
- Loop: bacteriologic, standard 2-mm, 26-gauge platinum wire loop
- Oil-immersion, low-fluorescence, nondrying microscope slides: 1 × 3 inch, with coverslips
- Dish-stains, glass or plastic with removable slide carriers
- Glass stirring rods

Quality Control

Control sera must be run concurrently with each set of patient specimens (Table 18-5). Controls should be prepared as follows: reactive (4+) control. This control should demonstrate 4+ fluorescence when diluted 1:5 in PBS and only slightly reduced fluorescence when diluted 1:5 in sorbent. These controls are prepared as follows:
1. PBS dilution. Pipette 0.2 mL of PBS into a small test tube. Add 0.2 mL of reactive (4+) control serum. Mix.
2. Sorbent dilution. Pipette 0.2 mL of sorbent into a small test tube. Add 0.2 mL of reactive (4+) control serum. Mix.

Minimal (1+) Control

Dilutions of reactive serum demonstrating the minimal degree of fluorescence report as reactive for use as a reading standard. The 4+ reactive control may be used for this control when diluted in PBS.

Nonspecific Serum Control

Use a nonsyphilis serum known to demonstrate at least 2+ nonspecific reactivity in the FTA-ABS test at a dilution of PBS of 1:5 or higher. Prepare as follows:
1. PBS dilution. Pipette 0.2 mL of PBS into a small test tube. Add 0.05 mL of nonspecific control serum. Mix.
2. Sorbent dilution. Pipette 0.2 mL of sorbent into a small test tube. Add 0.05 mL of nonspecific control serum. Mix. Nonspecific staining controls:
   a. Antigen smear treated with 0.03 mL of PBS.
   b. Antigen smear treated with 0.03 mL of sorbent.

Controls 1, 3, and 4 are included for the purpose of controlling reagents and test conditions. Control 2 (minimally reactive control serum) is included as the reading standard. *Note:* Each new lot of reagents should be tested in parallel with reagents that give satisfactory results before being used.

Table 18-5	Control Pattern Examples	
Control	**Reaction**
Reactive	
1:5 PBS dilution	Reactive (4+)
1:5 Sorbent dilution	Reactive (3+ to 4+)
Minimally Reactive (1+)	
Nonspecific serum	Reactive (1+)
1:5 PBS dilution	Reactive (2+ to 4+)
1:5 Sorbent dilution	Nonreactive
Nonspecific Staining	
Antigen, PBS and conjugate	Nonreactive
Antigen, sorbent and conjugate	Nonreactive

PBS, Phosphate-buffered saline.

Treponema pallidum Antigen

A new lot of antigen should be compared with a standard antigen before being placed in routine use. Testing should be performed on more than one testing day with control sera, individual sera of graded reactivity, and nonreactive sera.

A sufficient number of organisms should remain on the slide after staining so that tests may be read without difficulty. The antigen should not contain background material that stains so as to interfere with the reading of the tests. The antigen should not stain nonspecifically with a standard conjugate as its working titer.

Reportable test results on controls and individual sera should be comparable with those obtained with the standard antigen.

FTA-ABS Test Sorbent

A new lot of sorbent should be compared with a standard sorbent before being placed in routine use. Testing should be performed on more than one testing day with control sera, including sera of graded reactivity and nonsyphilis sera demonstrating nonspecific reactivity. The new sorbent should remove nonspecific reactivity of the nonspecific serum control. The new sorbent should not reduce the intensity of fluorescence of the reactive (4+) control serum to less than 3+. The nonspecific staining control with the new sorbent should be nonreactive.

Reportable test results on controls and individual sera should be with those obtained with standard sorbent. The sorbent should be usable when rehydrated to the indicated volume on the label or according to accompanying directions.

Fluorescein-Labeled Antihuman Globulin (Conjugate)

A satisfactory conjugate should not stain a standard antigen nonspecifically at three doubling dilutions below the working titer of the conjugate.

Reportable test results on controls and individual sera should be comparable with those obtained with the standard conjugate. Most manufacturers designate on the label the working titer of the conjugate that was determined under the testing conditions and with the equipment in their laboratories. Because conditions and equipment vary among laboratories, it is necessary to titer and check-test a new lot of conjugate with a fluorescence microscope.

Procedure

1. Label test tubes for patient and control sera.
2. Pipette 0.2 mL into each tube.
3. Using a 0.2-mL pipette, add 0.05 mL of inactivated sera to the appropriately labeled test tubes. Mix eight times.
4. Label a previously prepared antigen suspension slide for each of the patient sera and controls being tested.
5. Cover each antigen preparation with 0.03 mL of a serum dilution (i.e., patient or control).
6. Cover an antigen suspension slide with either 0.03 mL of PBS or sorbent. These are the nonspecific staining controls.
7. Place a moist chamber over the slides to prevent evaporation, and incubate at 35° to 37° C for 30 minutes.
8. Fill two staining dishes with PBS.
9. Place slides in a slide carrier, and rinse slides with running PBS for 5 seconds.
10. Place the slides in the staining dish containing PBS solution. Process for 5 minutes. After 5 minutes, dip the slides in and out of the solution at least 10 times.
11. Transfer the slide carrier to the fresh PBS solution in the second staining dish. Process for 5 minutes. After 5 minutes, dip the slides in and out of the solution at least 10 times.
12. Rinse the slides in running distilled water for 5 seconds.
13. Gently blot each smear with bibulous paper to remove all water droplets.
14. Dilute conjugate to its working titer in PBS containing 2% Tween-80.
15. Pipette 0.03 mL of diluted conjugate onto each smear. Spread the conjugate uniformly over the slide with a glass rod.
16. Repeat steps 7 through 13.
17. Mount slides immediately by placing a small drop of mounting medium on each smear, then applying a coverslip to each.
18. Microscopically examine slides as soon as possible. The microscope should be equipped with an ultraviolet light source and a high-power dry objective. A combination of BG-12 exciting filter, not more than 3 mm thick, and OG-1 barrier filter or equivalent has been found to be satisfactory. If a delay in reading is encountered, place the slides in a darkened room, and read within 4 hours.
19. Using the minimally reactive (1+) control slide as the reading standard, record the intensity of fluorescence of the treponemes, as follows:

Reading	Fluorescence Intensity	Report
0	None or vaguely visible	Nonreactive
<1	Weak reacting	Borderline
1+	Equivalent to 1+ control	Reactive
2+ to 4+	Moderate to strong	Reactive

20. Check nonreactive smears by using illumination from a tungsten light source to verify the presence of treponemes.

Reporting Results

Reading	Repeat Test	Report
0		Nonreactive
<1	Negative, <1, or 1+	Borderline
1+	Negative, <1+	Borderline
1+	1+ or greater	Reactive
2+ to 4+		Reactive

Procedure Notes

Limitations

The FTA-ABS test is recommended as a confirmatory procedure for syphilis. Its use is discouraged as a screening test. A reagin test such as the RPR is recommended for screening.

Clinical Applications

If a patient has two borderline test results, it is impossible to conclude definitively that the patient has or does not have serologic evidence of syphilitic infection. The attending physician should review the patient's history and physical findings. Diagnosis will rely on the clinical evidence in conjunction with the borderline serologic findings.

The false-positive rate of this test is very low, but it can be associated with autoimmune disorders such as systemic lupus erythematosus. False-positive FTA-ABS results occur in patients with other treponematoses (pinta, yaws, bejel) and in those who have high titer of antinuclear antibodies or rheumatoid factor. Evidence indicates that pregnant women occasionally have false-positive FTA-ABS test results.

References

Hunter EF, Deacon WE, Meyer PC: An improved test for syphilis—the absorption procedure (FTA-ABS), *Public Health Rep* 79:5, 1964.

Jaffe HW et al: Tests for treponemal antibody in CSF, *Arch Intern Med* 138:252, 1978.

Leclerc G et al: Study of fluorescent treponemal antibody test on cerebrospinal fluid using monospecific antiimmunoglobulin conjugates IgG, IgM, and IgA, *Br J Vener Dis* 54:303, 1978.

CASE STUDY

History and Physical Examination

A 25-year-old woman comes to an ambulatory center with pain in the right side of her pelvis and a slight temperature. She has a history of two episodes of chlamydial cervicitis and herpes simplex vulvitis.

Physical examination reveals abundant mucopurulent cervical discharge and a painless genital lesion. The patient also has some swelling of her inguinal lymph glands.

Laboratory Data

A "stat" pregnancy test is ordered. It is positive.

Questions and Discussion

1. What other laboratory tests would you expect to be ordered?

Cervical cultures for gonorrhea and chlamydiae would be appropriate. A direct Gram stain of gonorrhea might also be appropriate. HIV testing and testing for syphilis would also be reasonable.

2. Could this patient have syphilis?

Yes; this patient could have syphilis. This case is typical of primary syphilis with a painless, indurated ulcer on the genitals and mild inguinal adenopathy. It occurs 9 to 90 days after exposure, usually at 3 weeks.

3. If syphilis is suspected, what tests should be ordered?

The etiologic agent of syphilis, *Treponema pallidum,* cannot be easily cultured by routine methods. Diagnosis is made by a combination of clinical and laboratory methods. Microorganisms can be visualized by darkfield examination of fluid from the ulcer. Serologic testing is usually positive. This testing involves a screening nontreponemal test (e.g.,

RPR), followed by a confirmatory treponemal test (e.g., MHA-TP, FTA-ABS).

In primary syphilis, the RPR is negative, but the treponemal test is positive. Therefore, patients who are clinically suspected of having primary syphilis, but who have a negative screening test, should have the treponemal test performed anyway. Serologic follow-up testing is important. Titers of nontreponemal tests are thought to correlate with disease activity. A repeat serology at 3 and 6 months should demonstrate a fourfold drop in titer (2 dilutions). Patients who fail to demonstrate such a decrease should undergo a CSF examination to exclude neurosyphilis.

4. Is there risk of a congenital infection in this woman's unborn child?

Yes; the infant could contract congenital syphilis.

Diagnosis

Syphilis.

CHAPTER HIGHLIGHTS

- Syphilis is caused by a spirochete, *Treponema pallidum,* usually transmitted by sexual contact in humans.
- Untreated syphilis is a chronic disease with subacute symptomatic periods separated by asymptomatic intervals, during which the diagnosis can be made serologically. The progression of untreated syphilis is generally divided into stages.
- In primary syphilis the serum in about one third of cases becomes serologically reactive after 1 week and serologically demonstrable in most cases after 3 weeks. The reagin titer increases rapidly during the first 4 weeks and then stabilizes for about 6 months.
- Two to 8 weeks after appearance of the primary chancre, a patient enters the stage of secondary syphilis, usually characterized by generalized illness suggestive of a viral infection. Skin lesions contain spirochetes and are highly contagious on exposed surfaces. These lesions subside spontaneously after 2 to 6 weeks even if untreated. In this noninfectious latent stage, serologic tests for syphilis are positive.
- The late (tertiary) stage usually occurs 3 to 10 years after primary infection; gummas can appear in about 15% of untreated syphilitic persons who eventually develop late benign syphilis. Complications include nervous system lesions, causing tabes dorsalis or cardiovascular complications. The tertiary stage is asymptomatic and recognized only by serologic testing. Occasionally the lesions heal so completely that even serologic tests become nonreactive.
- Classic serologic tests for syphilis measure the presence of two types of antibodies: treponemal and nontreponemal.
- Darkfield microscopy is the test of choice for symptomatic patients with primary syphilis.

- The widely used nontreponemal serologic test is the RPR method, a flocculation method.
- Specific treponemal serologic tests include the fluorescent treponemal antibody absorption (FTA-ABS) and microhemagglutination for *T. pallidum* (MHA-TP).

REVIEW QUESTIONS

Questions 1-4. Match the *Treponema*-associated diseases *(a-d)* in humans with the respective causative organism.

1. _____ *Treponema pallidum*

2. _____ *T. pallidum* (variant)

3. _____ *T. pertenue*

4. _____ *T. carateum*

    a. Yaws
    b. Syphilis
    c. Pinta
    d. Bejel

Questions 5-8. Match the following stages of syphilis with the appropriate signs and symptoms.

5. _____ Primary syphilis

6. _____ Secondary syphilis

7. _____ Latent syphilis

8. _____ Late (tertiary) syphilis

    a. Diagnosis only by serologic methods.
    b. Presence of gummas.
    c. Development of a chancre.
    d. Hutchinsonian triad.
    e. Generalized illness followed by macular lesions in most patients.

9. A term for nontreponemal antibodies produced by an infected patient against components of their own or other mammalian cells is:
    a. Autoagglutinins.
    b. Reagin antibodies.
    c. Alloantibodies.
    d. Nonsyphilis antibodies.

Questions 10-12. Match the following.

10. _____ FTA-ABS test

11. _____ MHA-TP test

12. _____ RPR test

    a. Treponemal method
    b. Nontreponemal method

13. In the RPR procedure, a false-positive reaction can result from all the following *except:*
    a. Infectious mononucleosis.
    b. Leprosy.
    c. Rheumatoid arthritis.
    d. Streptococcal pharyngitis.

14. The first diagnostic blood test for syphilis was the:
    a. VDRL.
    b. Wassermann.
    c. RPR.
    d. Colloidal gold.

15. Syphilis was initially treated with:
    a. Fuller's earth.
    b. Heavy metals (e.g., arsenic).
    c. Sulfonamides (e.g., triple sulfa).
    d. Antibiotics (e.g., penicillin).

16. Direct examination of the treponemes is most often performed with:
    a. Light microscopy.
    b. Darkfield microscopy.
    c. VDRL test.
    d. RPR test.

17. Pathogenic treponemes _____ cultivatable with consistency in artificial laboratory media.
    a. are
    b. are not

18. In infected blood, *Treponema pallidum* does not appear to survive at 4° C for more than:
    a. 1 day.
    b. 2 days.
    c. 3 days.
    d. 5 days.

19. The primary incubation period for syphilis *(T. pallidum)* is usually about:
    a. 1 week.
    b. 2 weeks.
    c. 3 weeks.
    d. 4 weeks.

20. The stage of syphilis that can be diagnosed only by serologic (laboratory) methods is the:
    a. Incubation phase.
    b. Primary phase.
    c. Secondary phase.
    d. Latent phase.

21. Immunocompetent patients infected with *T. pallidum* produce:
    a. Specific antibodies against *T. pallidum.*
    b. Nonspecific antibodies against the protein antigen group common to pathogenic spirochetes.
    c. Reagin antibodies.
    d. All the above.

BIBLIOGRAPHY

Angell M, Kassirer JP: Sexually transmitted diseases in the 1990s, *N Engl J Med* 325(19):1368-1373, 1991.

Boyd RF, Hoerl BG: *Basic medical microbiology,* ed 3, Boston, 1986, Little, Brown.

Brown ST et al: Serologic response to syphilis treatment: a new analysis of old data, *JAMA* 253:1296-1299, 1985.

Centers for Disease Control and Prevention (CDC), Division of STD Prevention: *The national plan to eliminate syphilis from the United States,* Washington, DC, Atlanta, 2006, US Department of Health and Human Services, CDC.

Cerny EH: Adenovirus ELISA for the evaluation of cerebrospinal fluid in patients with suspected neurosyphilis, *Am J Clin Pathol* 85:505-508, 1985.

Farshy CE: Four-step enzyme-linked immunosorbent assay for the detection of *Treponema pallidum* antibody, *J Clin Microbiol* 21:387-389, 1985.

Gardner MF, Clark ME: The *Treponema pallidum* hemagglutination (TPHA) test, *WHO/VDT/Res* 75:332, 1975.

Hart G: Syphilis testing in diagnostic and therapeutic decision making, *Ann Intern Med* 104:368-376, 1986.

Hook EW, Marra CM: Acquired syphilis in adults, *N Engl J Med* 326(16): 1060-1069, 1992.

Larson SA et al: Cerebrospinal fluid serologies in syphilis: treponemal and nontreponemal test, International Conjoint STD Meeting, Abstract 166:218, Montreal, 1984.

Mandell GL, Douglas RG, Bennett JE, editors: *Principles and practice of infectious diseases,* ed 2, New York, 1985, Wiley & Sons.

Muller F: Specific immunoglobulins M and G antibodies in the rapid diagnosis of human treponemal infections, *Diagn Immunol* 4:1-9, 1986.

Muller F, Moskophidis J: Estimation of the local production of antibodies to *Treponema pallidum* in the central nervous system of patients with neurosyphilis, *Br J Vener Dis* 59:80-84, 1983.

Primary and secondary syphilis—United States, 2003-2004, *MMWR* 55(10): 269-273, 2006.

Radolf JD et al: Serodiagnosis of syphilis by enzyme-linked immunosorbent assay with purified recombinant *Treponema pallidum* antigen 4D, *J Infect Dis* 153:1023-1027, 1986.

Rutherford I, Li T: An evaluation of two hemagglutination tests as alternatives to FTA-ABS in otologic syphilis, *Lab Med* 25(1):22-24, 1989.

Sexually transmitted diseases: treatment guidelines, *MMWR* 420(RR-14): 505-535, 1993.

CHAPTER 19

Vector-Borne Diseases

Lyme Disease
  Etiology
  Epidemiology
  Signs and Symptoms
  Diagnostic Evaluation
  Treatment and Prevention
Human Ehrlichiosis
  Etiology
  Epidemiology
  Signs and Symptoms
  Diagnostic Evaluation
  Treatment and Prevention
Babesiosis
  Etiology
  Epidemiology

Signs and Symptoms
Diagnostic Evaluation
Treatment and Prevention
West Nile Virus
  Etiology
  Epidemiology
  Signs and Symptoms
  Diagnostic Evaluation
  Treatment and Prevention
Case Studies
Chapter Highlights
Review Questions
Bibliography

Learning Objectives

At the conclusion of this chapter, the reader should be able to:
- Describe the etiology, epidemiology, and signs and symptoms of Lyme disease.
- Discuss the immunologic manifestations and diagnostic evaluation of Lyme disease.
- Explain the treatment and prevention of Lyme disease.
- Describe the etiology, epidemiology, and signs and symptoms of ehrlichiosis.
- Discuss the immunologic manifestations and diagnostic evaluation of ehrlichiosis.

- Explain the treatment and prevention of ehrlichiosis.
- Describe the etiology, epidemiology, and signs and symptoms of babesiosis.
- Discuss the immunologic manifestations and diagnostic evaluation of babesiosis.
- Explain the treatment and prevention of babesiosis.
- Briefly discuss the etiology and laboratory diagnosis of West Nile virus.
- Analyze case studies of Lyme disease, ehrlichiosis, and babesiosis.

Disease-carrying vectors, such as mosquitoes and ticks, continue to be an ever-present threat worldwide (Table 19-1). The discovery and surveillance of many of these vector-borne diseases (e.g., Lyme disease) can be accomplished by serologic testing. Travelers may be at risk for exposure to vector-borne disease if they engage in recreational activities that bring them into contact with habitats that support the vectors or the animal reservoir species associated with these diseases.

LYME DISEASE

Since its original description more than 25 years ago, Lyme disease has become recognized as an important infectious disease in the United States. The infection, caused by the tick-borne spirochete *Borrelia burgdorferi,* has emerged as a major health hazard for humans and domestic animals. Currently, Lyme disease is a global illness. Cases have been reported on all continents except Antarctica. It is endemic in more than 15 states in the United States and in Europe and Asia.

Etiology

Lyme disease **(Lyme borreliosis)** is caused by a spirochete bacterium. It is a cutaneous-systemic infection generally transmitted by a hard-bodied tick (Figure 19-1) and caused by *B. burgdorferi* (Figure 19-2). The causative agent of Lyme borreliosis currently consists of three pathogenic species: *B. burgdorferi, B. afzelii,* and *B. garinii.* Only *B. burgdorferi* strains have been found in the United States. In contrast, most of the illness in Europe is caused by *B. afzelii,* which is associated with the chronic skin condition **acrodermatitis chronica atrophicans (ACA),** and *B. garinii,* which is associated with neurologic symptoms. Only these two species have been found in Asia. The complete genome of *B. burgdorferi* (strain B31) has now been sequenced.

The spirochete is transmitted by certain ixodid ticks that are part of the *Ixodes ricinus* complex. These include *I. scapularis* (formerly classified as *I. dammini*) in the northeastern and midwestern United States, *I. pacificus* in the western United States, *I. ricinus* in Europe, and *I. persulcatus* in Asia. The vector has not been identified in Australia. Ixodid ticks are also indigenous to Africa and South America. The lone

Table 19-1	Examples of Vector-Borne Diseases		
Vector	**Disease**	**Pathogen**	**Distribution**
Mosquitoes			
Aedes triseriatus	California encephalitis	Virus	United States: Upper Midwest, Appalachian region
Aedes aegypti	Dengue fever	Virus	Worldwide: tropical regions
	West Nile encephalitis	Virus	United States: spreading nationwide
	West Nile fever		Africa, Asia
Culiseta melanura	Eastern equine encephalitis	Virus	Eastern United States Central and South America, Caribbean
Culex spp.	St. Louis encephalitis	Virus	Eastern United States Central and South America
	Western equine encephalitis	Virus	Western United States Central and South America
Ticks			
Deer tick *Ixodes spp.*	Anaplasmosis (formerly human granulocytic ehrlichiosis)	Bacteria	Worldwide; Europe United States: Northeast, Upper Midwest, northern California
I. scapularis	Babesiosis	Protozoan parasite	United States: primarily northeastern states, rarely Pacific states
Lone star tick *Amblyomma americanum*	Human monocytic ehrlichiosis	Bacteria	United States: Southeast, south-central states
Dog tick *Rhipicephalus sanguineus*	Mediterranean spotted fever	Bacteria	Europe, Africa, Central Asia
Tick-borne, airborne vector	Q fever	Rickettsiae	Worldwide
Dog tick, wood tick *Dermacentor* spp.	Rocky Mountain spotted fever	Bacteria	North and South America
	Tick-associated rash/illness	Bacteria	Southern
Ticks, various	Tick-borne relapsing fever	Bacteria	Western United States (endemic*) Southern British Columbia Plateau regions of Mexico Central and South America Mediterranean, Central Asia, and much of Africa
Lice, Fleas, Mites			
Human body louse; squirrel flea and louse	Epidemic typhus	Rickettsiae	United States-Eastern
Rat flea *Xenopsylla cheopis*	Murine typhus	Bacteria	Worldwide, where rats are abundant
Cat or dog fleas	Murine typhus–like febrile disease	Rickettsiae	Worldwide
Mites (chiggers)	Scrub typhus	Rickettsiae	South Asia to Australia, East Asia in recently disturbed habitat, e.g., forest clearings or other persisting mite foci infested with rats and other rodents
Human body louse	Louse-borne relapsing fever	Bacteria	Africa
	Trench fever	Rickettsiae	Industrialized countries

*Most recent cases and outbreaks have occurred in rustic cabins at higher elevations (>8000 ft) in coniferous forests in the western United States.

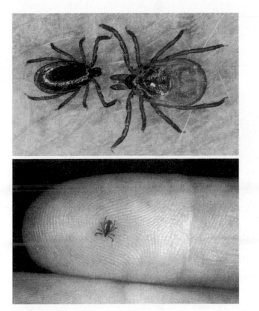

Figure 19-1 Deer tick. *(From Habif TP: Clinical dermatology, ed 2, St Louis, 1990, Mosby.)*

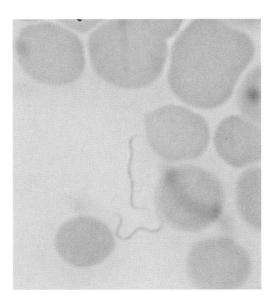

Figure 19-2 *Borrelia* organisms present in the blood of a patient with endemic relapsing fever (Giemsa stain). *(From Murray PR et al: Medical microbiology, ed 5, Philadelphia, 2005, Mosby.)*

star tick, *Amblyomma americanum*, does not transmit Lyme disease.

In the United States the preferred host for larval and nymphal stages of *I. scapularis* is the white-footed mouse, *Peromyscus leucopus*. White-tailed deer, which are not involved in the life cycle of the spirochete, are the preferred host for *I. scapularis* adult stage, and they seem to be critical to tick survival. Ixodid ticks have also been found on at least 30 types of wild animals and 49 species of birds. Illness is not known to develop in wild animals, but clinical Lyme disease does occur in domestic animals, including dogs, horses, and cattle.

Spirochetes are transmitted from the gut of the tick to human skin at the site of a bite and then migrate outwardly into the skin. This migration causes the unique expanding skin lesion, **erythema migrans (EM).** Subsequent dissemination of spirochetes to secondary sites may cause major organ system involvement in humans. In dogs the most common symptom is arthritis.

Epidemiology

In some patients, Lyme disease may be transitory and of little consequence, but in others it may become chronic and severely disabling. Accurate diagnosis is therefore essential, although better laboratory techniques are still needed.

Retrospectively, the first symptom of Lyme disease apparently was recognized as early as 1908 in Sweden. In the decades that followed, the rash produced by the disease, **erythema chronicum migrans (ECM),** was noted elsewhere in Europe, as were other symptoms that seemed to follow ECM's eruption. Secondary symptoms, such as impairment of the nervous system, were described in France, Germany, and again in Sweden.

In the United States the European rash was virtually unknown until 1969, when a case of a physician bitten by a tick while hunting in Wisconsin was reported. Although a few ECM cases were seen in Americans who had traveled to Europe, there were no further native American cases until 1975, when physicians at the U.S. Navy base in Groton, Connecticut, reported seeing four patients with a rash similar to ECM. At the same time an epidemiologist at the Connecticut State Department of Health and a rheumatologist at Yale were notified of an unusual cluster of cases of arthritis occurring in children in Lyme, Connecticut.

It was not until 1982 that Burgdorfer and Barbour isolated a previously unrecognized spirochete, now called *Borrelia burgdorferi,* from *I. scapularis* ticks, and **Lyme disease** became a recognized vector-borne, infectious disease. Two factors influence the chance that a bitten patient will contract the disease: the likelihood that local ixodid ticks carry the Lyme spirochete, and the likelihood of infection after a bite by an infected tick. The probability of infection after an ixodid tick bite in an area of endemic disease is about 3%, but it varies in different regions from less than 1% to as high as 5%. It has been suggested that HLA-DR4 and, secondarily, HLA-DR2 may increase the risk that Lyme arthritis will become chronic and fail to respond to antibiotics.

Lyme disease now accounts for more than 95% of all reported vector-borne illness in the United States. In 2006, 19,931 cases of Lyme disease were reported, yielding a national average of 8.2 cases per 100,000 persons. In the 10 states where Lyme disease is most common, the average was 30.2 cases per 100,000 persons (Figure 19-3). Persons of all ages and both genders are equally susceptible.

The majority of cases remain concentrated in the northeastern, north-central, and Pacific coastal regions (Figure 19-4). In 2006, Delaware and Connecticut continued to have the highest incidences of cases per 100,000 population. No

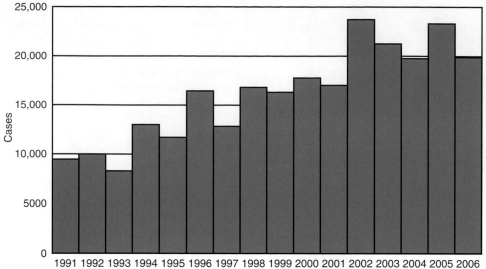

Figure 19-3 Reported cases of Lyme disease by year—United States, 1991-2006.

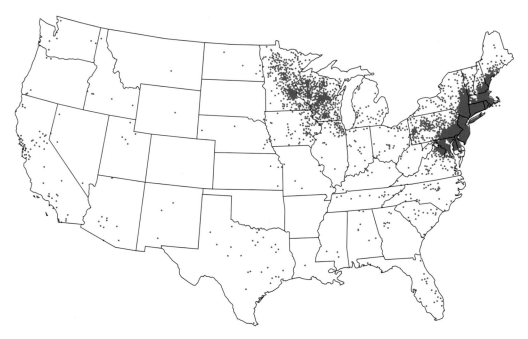

One dot placed randomly within county of residence for each reported case

Figure 19-4 Reported cases of Lyme disease—United States, 2006.

cases of Lyme disease were reported in six states: Arkansas, Colorado, Hawaii, Mississippi, Montana, and Oklahoma. Lyme disease is considered an emerging infectious disease because of the impact of changing environmental and socioeconomic factors, such as the transformation of farmland into suburban woodlots favorable for deer and deer ticks. Although pets may represent a spirochete reservoir, it is unlikely that humans can be infected directly by them. In areas of endemic Lyme disease, however, both adult and nymphal ticks, carried into the household by dogs and cats, may infest humans.

Signs and Symptoms

The basic features of Lyme disease are similar worldwide, but there are regional variations, primarily between the illness in America and that in Europe and Asia.

In at least 60% to 80% of U.S. patients, Lyme disease begins with a slowly expanding skin lesion, EM, which occurs at the site of the tick bite. The skin lesion is frequently accompanied by flulike symptoms.

The Centers for Disease Control and Prevention (CDC) clinical case definition for Lyme disease includes the presence of EM or at least one objective, late-manifesting sign of

Table 19-2	Clinical Features of Lyme Disease	
Stage	Duration	Signs and Symptoms
I	4 weeks (median) after injection	Cutaneous manifestations (erythema migrans) or other skin eruptions, flulike syndrome, neurologic symptoms.
II	Follows a variable latent period	Target organs and systems include the nervous system, heart, eyes, and skin, all of which can manifest abnormalities.
III	Weeks to years after infection	Arthritis, late neurologic complications, acrodermatitis chronica atrophicans.

musculoskeletal, neurologic, or cardiovascular disease and a positive serologic test for antibody to *B. burgdorferi*. Many misdiagnosed patients actually have chronic fatigue syndrome or fibromyalgia, both of which can cause similar symptoms, such as joint stiffness or pain, fatigue, and sleep disturbance.

Lyme borreliosis is a multisystem illness that primarily involves the skin, nervous system, heart, and joints (Table 19-2). Lyme disease usually begins during the summer months with EM and flulike symptoms and may be accompanied by right upper quadrant tenderness and a mild hepatitis (stage 1). This stage is followed weeks to months later by acute cardiac or neurologic disease in a minority of untreated individuals (stage 2), then by arthritis and chronic neurologic disease (stage 3) in many untreated patients weeks to years after disease onset. There is considerable overlap between these stages, but Lyme disease is best characterized as an illness that evolves from "early" to "late" disease without reference to an arbitrary staging system. However, a patient may have one or all of the stages, and the infection may not become symptomatic until stage 2 or 3. The majority of affected patients have EM, and one fourth manifest arthritis; neurologic manifestations and cardiac involvement are uncommon.

Arthritis

Arthralgia and myalgia are common features of early Lyme disease, but frank arthritis during EM is unusual. Arthritis is a well-described complication of Lyme disease and characteristically occurs months to years after *Borrelia* infection. Therefore, cases of Lyme arthritis occur during every month of the year. Lyme arthritis and parvovirus B19 arthritis can occur in the absence of other symptoms, such as the characteristic rash. Some suspected cases of Lyme arthritis might be caused by parvovirus B19, particularly those occurring during the parvovirus B19 season.

Arthritis in patients with chronic Lyme disease may be associated with a long-standing infiltration of the joints by *B. burgdorferi* spirochetes, along with a local inflammatory response. It may not be triggered simply by the presence of

circulating immunoglobulin G (IgG) antibodies against outer surface proteins.

Cutaneous Manifestations

Cutaneous manifestations can be demonstrated as early ECM (Figure 19-5), secondary lesions (disseminated lesions and lymphocytoma), and late lesions (ACA). Except for the late lesions, cutaneous manifestations generally resolve spontaneously over weeks to months. The red papule at the site of the tick bite is most often located on the thigh, groin, or axilla. Facial EM is seen more frequently in children.

Several days to weeks after the onset of EM, almost half of untreated patients develop secondary skin lesions. A rare early manifestation of Lyme disease is *Borrelia* lymphocytoma, a violaceous, tumorlike swelling or nodule at the base of the earlobe or the nipple caused by a dense lymphocytic infiltrate of the dermis. This lesion occurs at the site of a tick bite and in conjunction with other symptoms; it may be confused with lymphoma.

Acrodermatitis chronica atrophicans (ACA) is a late skin manifestation of Lyme disease more prevalent in Europe than in the United States. Lesions display bluish red discoloration, doughy swelling, and fibrotic nodules. Eventually, striking atrophy of skin and subcutaneous tissues follows. Polyneuropathy coexists in 30% to 45% of patients.

Cardiac Manifestations

Lyme carditis occurs in approximately 8% of untreated patients within 1 to 2 months (range, >1 week to 7 months) after the onset of infection, and it may be the initial manifes-

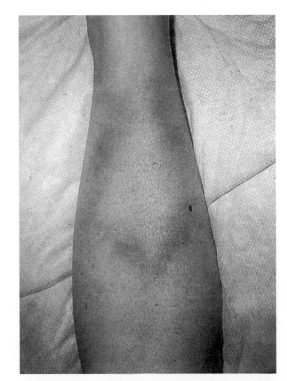

Figure 19-5 Erythema chronicum migrans. *(From Habif TP: Clinical dermatology, ed 2, St Louis, 1990, Mosby.)*

tation of Lyme disease. Cardiac features of Lyme disease usually result in a fluctuating degree of atrioventricular conduction defects (first-degree, second-degree, and complete block, as well as bundle branch and fascicular blocks) or tachyarrhythmias. Myopericarditis can occur, but symptomatic congestive heart failure is uncommon. Patients usually develop signs of lightheadedness, syncope, dyspnea, palpitations, and chest pain. Symptoms are more common in patients with more severe degrees of heart block. The carditis usually follows a self-limited and mild course, but temporary pacing may be needed in a small percentage of patients.

Neurologic Manifestations

Neurologic abnormalities occur in approximately 15% of untreated patients. These manifestations are usually observed 2 to 8 weeks after disease onset and may include aseptic meningitis, cranial nerve palsies, peripheral radiculoneuritis, and peripheral neuropathy. The predominant symptoms of Lyme meningitis are severe headache and mild neck stiffness, which may fluctuate for weeks after a post–EM latent period.

Months to years after the initial infection with *B. burgdorferi*, patients with Lyme disease may have chronic encephalopathy, polyneuropathy, or less often, leukoencephalitis. The appearance of mild encephalopathy has been seen 1 month to 14 years after the onset of disease. Encephalopathy is characterized by memory loss, mood changes, or sleep disturbance. In addition, increased cerebrospinal fluid (CSF) protein levels and evidence of intrathecal production of antibody to *B. burgdorferi* may occur. Chronic neurologic manifestations can also include polyneuropathy with radicular pain or distal paresthesias, fatigue, headache, hearing loss, and verbal memory impairment. These chronic neurologic abnormalities usually improve with antibiotic therapy.

Ocular manifestations may occur in Lyme disease and include cranial nerve palsies, optic neuritis, panophthalmitis with loss of vision, and choroiditis with retinal detachment.

Pregnancy

Transplacental transmission of *B. burgdorferi* with fetal infection has been confirmed. A uniform pattern of congenital malformations has not been identified in maternal-fetal transmission of Lyme disease.

In observed cases cited, infants succumbed shortly after birth. The mothers acquired infection during the first trimester and received inadequate or no treatment.

Immunologic Manifestations

Cellular immune responses to *B. burgdorferi* antigens begin concurrent with early clinical illness. An increase in spontaneous suppressor cell activity and reduction in natural killer (NK) cell activity have been noted. Mononuclear cell, antigen-specific responses develop during spirochetal dissemination, and humoral (antibody) immune responses soon follow.

Serodiagnostic tests are insensitive during the first several weeks of infection. In the United States, approximately 20%

to 30% of Lyme patients have positive responses, usually of the immunoglobulin M (IgM) isotype, during this period, but by convalescence 2 to 4 weeks later, about 70% to 80% have seroreactivity even after antibiotic treatment. After about 1 month, the majority of patients with active infection have IgG antibody responses. After antibiotic treatment, antibody titers slowly fall, but IgG and even IgM responses may persist for many years after treatment. An IgM response cannot be interpreted as a manifestation of recent infection or reinfection unless the appropriate clinical characteristics are present. Antibodies formed include cryoglobulins, immune complexes, antibodies specific for *B. burgdorferi*, and anticardiolipin antibodies. Elevated titers of IgM are noted in early disease. Immunoblot analysis demonstrates that IgM antibodies form initially against the flagellar 41-kilodalton (kD) polypeptide, but react later to additional cell wall antigens. An overlapping IgG response to these antigens develops in some individuals. These antigen-specific cellular and humoral responses are not known to eradicate infection in early disease or participate in disease pathogenesis.

Specific IgM or IgG antibodies against *B. burgdorferi* are usually not detectable in a patient's serum unless symptoms have been present for at least 2 to 4 weeks. In cases of Lyme arthritis, tests for serum antinuclear antibodies (ANAs), rheumatoid factor (RF), and Venereal Disease Research Laboratories (VDRL) are generally negative. However, anti-*B. burgdorferi* antibodies of the IgG type should be present in the serum of patients with Lyme arthritis.

Outer surface protein A antibodies develop late in the course of human Lyme infection, and then only in a subset of patients. A temporal association may exist between the onset of chronic Lyme arthritis in 4HLA-DR4–positive patients and the development of antibodies to the outer surface protein.

Persistent organisms and spirochetal antigen deposits elicit a vigorous immune reaction, as manifested by a tissue-rich plasma cell and lymphocytic exudate containing abundant T cells, predominantly of the helper subset, plus IgD-bearing B cells. *B. burgdorferi* antigens elicit a strong immune reaction that intensifies with chronicity of arthritis and stimulates macrophages to secrete interleukin-1 (IL-1). IL-1 is capable of stimulating synovial cells and fibroblasts to secrete collagenase and prostaglandin E_2, both of which are elevated in Lyme synovial fluid and can cause erosion of joint cartilage and bone.

Diagnostic Evaluation

The culture of *B. burgdorferi* from specimens in Barbour-Stoenner-Kelly medium permits a definitive diagnosis. With a few exceptions, positive cultures have been obtained only early in the illness, primarily from biopsy samples of EM lesions, less often from plasma samples, and only occasionally from CSF samples in patients with meningitis. Later in the infection, polymerase chain reaction testing is superior to culture in the detection of *B. burgdorferi* in joint fluid.

In the United States the diagnosis is usually based on the recognition of the characteristic clinical findings, a history

Table 19-3	Various Methods of Lyme Disease Detection
Method	**Comments**
Isolation	Successful cultures have been obtained from ticks, skin biopsies, ear punches, cerebrospinal fluid, blood, and synovial fluid; blood is not a reliable sample for culture. Isolation of spirochetes is highly variable.
Histology	Lyme spirochetes are rarely observed in blood smears; examination of tissue is usually performed, in addition to an immunologic assay such as fluorescence microscopy. The process is labor intensive; the test is of limited value.
Serology	Not sufficiently reliable to make a definitive diagnosis of Lyme disease; only IFA and EIA test systems are FDA approved.
Antigen detection systems	Screen for antigenic products rather than for the host's immune response to the infection.

IFA, Indirect fluorescent antibody; *EIA,* enzyme immunoassay; *FDA,* Food and Drug Administration.

Table 19-4	Diagnostic Criteria for Lyme Borreliosis	
Diagnostic Factor		**Relative Value**
Two or more systems (e.g., monoarthritis and facial palsy)		2
Erythema migrans, physician confirmed		7
Acrodermatitis chronica atrophicans, biopsy confirmed		7
Seropositivity		3
Seroconversion on paired sera		4
Tissue microscopy, silver stain		3
Tissue microscopy, monoclonal immunofluorescence		4
Culture positivity		4
B. burgdorferi antigen recovery		4
B. burgdorferi DNA/RNA recovery		4

From Burrascano J: *Advanced topics in Lyme disease,* ed 13, 2000, www.LymeNet.org.

of exposure in an area where the disease is endemic, and except in patients with EM, an antibody response to *B. burgdorferi* by enzyme-linked immunosorbent assays (ELISA) and Western blot. In more than half of cases, positive test results are inconsequential because physicians are comfortable making the diagnosis based on symptoms and patient history. Testing becomes important, however, when the telltale "bull's eye" rash or other symptoms characteristic of Lyme disease do not appear.

In the early phase of Lyme disease, laboratory findings are nonspecific and typically may include an elevated erythrocyte sedimentation rate (ESR), elevated serum IgM levels, and mildly elevated hepatic alanine transaminase (serum ALA, GPT) levels. Various methods for detection of disease are available (Table 19-3).

Much of the diagnostic process in late, disseminated disease often involves ruling out other illnesses and defining the extent of damage that might require separate evaluation and treatment. Consideration should be given to tick exposure, rashes (even atypical ones), evolution of typical symptoms in a previously asymptomatic individual, and results of tests for tick-borne pathogens. In late disease there may be repeatedly peaking IgM levels; therefore a reactive IgM level may not differentiate early from late disease, but it does suggest an active infection. When late cases of Lyme disease are seronegative, 36% will transiently become seropositive at the completion of successful therapy.

Lyme disease is now been diagnosed based on its relative value (Table 19-4). Lyme borreliosis is highly likely if its relative value score is 7 or greater. Lyme borreliosis is possible if its relative value is between 5 and 6, and Lyme borreliosis is unlikely if its relative value is 4 or less.

Antibody Detection
Assays for the detection of antibodies to *B. burgdorferi* are the most practical means of confirming infection. At present, rapid tests usually rely on detecting antibodies produced by

a patient. However, an antibody response may be delayed or may not occur. This leads to false-negative laboratory assay results. In addition, false-positive results can occur if an individual has been exposed to related bacteria.

The most common laboratory assays for *B. burgdorferi* antibody detection include indirect fluorescent antibody (IFA) staining methods, ELISA for total immunoglobulins or IgM and IgG antibodies, and PreVue *B. burgdorferi* Antibody Detection Assay for Lyme disease (Wampole Laboratories, Princeton, NJ). Immunoblotting techniques can be used along with ELISA to characterize immune response and for diagnosis.

Enzyme-Linked Immunosorbent Assay
The ELISA is the standard test method; it is the most widely available and frequently performed test. The sensitivities of IFA and ELISA methods are usually low during the initial 3 weeks of infection; therefore negative results are common. The most serious disadvantages of current techniques are low sensitivity and lengthy processing time. In addition, false-positive reactions can result from cross-reactivity in tests for Lyme disease. For example, tick-borne relapsing fever spirochetes, *Borrelia hermsii,* are closely related to *B. burgdorferi.* Antibodies to *B. hermsii,* an agent that coexists with the Lyme disease spirochete in portions of the western United States, strongly cross-react with *B. burgdorferi* in IFA staining and ELISA testing. Common antigens are shared among the *Borrelia* organisms and even with the treponemes. Serum from syphilitic patients reacts positively in assays for Lyme disease. Therefore, serologic test results for antibodies to *B. burgdorferi* should be considered along with clinical data and epidemiologic information when a patient is evaluated for Lyme disease.

PreVue *B. burgdorferi* Antibody Detection Assay
PreVue *B. burgdorferi* Antibody Detection Assay for Lyme disease is a CLIA-waived procedure intended to be used as the first presumptive step in testing individuals suspected of

having Lyme disease. Positive results must be confirmed with a Western blot test done by a laboratory. The CDC recommends two-stage testing. The new test uses antigenic proteins developed by recombinant DNA techniques rather than a whole-cell *B. burgdorferi* preparation. Antigenic proteins developed by recombinant DNA techniques allow for more accuracy. The "false-positive" rate is similar to that of laboratory tests for Lyme disease.

Western Blot Analysis

Western blot analysis can verify reactivity of antibody to major surface or flagellar proteins of *B. burgdorferi* (Figure 19-6). Western blot is helpful in determining "borderline" negative or weakly positive results obtained from other tests, but the values are not always reliable. This procedure is more definitive in later Lyme disease when multiple antibody bands specific for *B. burgdorferi* appear. Reported results from test done by Western blots for Lyme disease in its late phase indicates reactive bands for IgM levels. The 41-kD bands are the earliest to appear, but can cross-react with

other spirochetes. The 18-kD, 23 to 25–kD (Osp C), 31-kD (Osp A), 34-kD (Osp B), 37-kD, 39-kD, 83-kD, and 93-kD bands are the most specific, but appear later or may not appear at all.

Polymerase Chain Reaction

Polymerase chain reaction (PCR) testing can detect spirochete in the synovial fluid around the joints or in other clinical samples. PCR looks for DNA of the organism. In the past, PCR has been taken as definitive evidence that a person has an infection, but it is possible to have antigens in the presence of nonviable organism. PCR amplifies small amounts of DNA that may remain even when intact organisms are no longer present, an indication that the organism does or did exist. PCR may miss the spirochete in the blood, allowing it to move into other tissues.

The PCR technique directly identifies the pathogen instead of measuring the host's immune response to it. PCR can detect the DNA from as few as one to five organisms, even those that are nonviable. Different specific probes have been produced, and PCR has been used to detect *B. burgdorferi* DNA in a variety of body fluids. The appeal of PCR lies in its rapid turnaround time (2 days vs. 6-8 weeks for culture) and avoiding the difficulties associated with culture or immunohistochemistry. PCR has very high specificity, but the sensitivity may be as low as 70%. PCR may be useful in diagnosing early Lyme disease when the patient is still seronegative.

Other Methods Used for Antibody Detection

Cerebrospinal Fluid Analysis. Spinal taps are not routinely recommended; a negative tap does not rule out Lyme disease. Antibodies to *B. burgdorferi* can be detected in the CSF in only 20% of patients with late disease. Therefore, spinal taps are performed only on patients with pronounced neurologic manifestations. The goal is to rule out other conditions and determine if *B. burgdorferi* antigens are present. It is especially important to look for elevated protein and mononuclear cells, which would dictate the need for more aggressive therapy, as well as check the opening CSF pressure, which can be elevated and can contribute to headaches, especially in children.

Antigen Detection Systems. These systems screen for antigenic products rather than for the host's immune response to the infection. Antigen detection systems could be expected to confirm both infections in patients with depressed immune systems and early infections in patients who have not yet produced a detectable antibody response. It is presumed that clearance of such antigens from hosts would indicate successful treatment and elimination of infecting spirochetes in patients. In addition, an antigen system can detect bacteria in the tick itself.

Two categories of procedures have been developed: T-cell proliferative assays and antibody-based antigen detection systems. *T-cell proliferative assays* recognize spirochetal antigens by cloned, antigen-specific cells. When T cells bind and

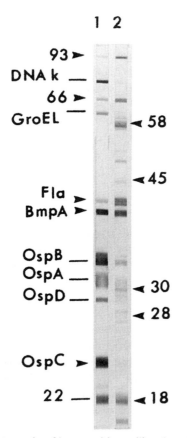

Figure 19-6 Example of immunoblot calibration. *Lane 1,* Monoclonal antibodies defining selected antigens to *B. burgdorferi* B31 separated in a linear SDS-PAGE gel Marblot (MarDx Diagnostics, Carlsbad, Calif.). *Lane 2,* Human serum (IgG) reactive with the 10 antigens scored in recommended criteria for blot scoring; lines indicate other calibrating antibodies. Molecular masses are in kilodaltons. *Osp,* Outer surface protein. *(From Detrick B et al, editors: Manual of molecular and clinical laboratory immunology, ed 7, Washington, DC, 2006, American Society for Microbiology Press, p 499.)*

recognize Lyme spirochetes in a specimen, T-cell division is induced. This division can be measured by counting T cells or by measuring the incorporation of labeled nutrients into the T cells. The T-cell proliferative assay may be a helpful diagnostic test in the small subset of patients with late Lyme disease who have negative or indeterminate antibody response by ELISA.

In 1993 the **p39 antigen,** a protein unique to *B. burgdorferi,* was first identified. A recombinant p39 antigen diagnostic test was developed, and the U.S. Food and Drug Administration (FDA) approved three p39-based test kits (one is a dipstick test kit). The tests detect antibodies to the p39 antigen, which is not found in closely related bacteria such as syphilis and tick-borne relapsing fever. Unfortunately, this procedure is of limited use because the p39 antigen is rarely found in early stages of infection, but it is a highly specific marker for late Lyme disease.

Monoclonal or polyclonal antibodies also detect specific Lyme spirochete antigens. Quantities of proteins that include flagellin, outer surface proteins A and B (OspA, OspB) are detectable. Assays based on **OspA** and **OspB,** two closely related *B. burgdorferi* proteins from the outer wall of the bacteria, are available. Both these proteins are characteristically exposed on the surface of different strains of the Lyme disease spirochete, but are not found in other species of bacterial spirochetes (e.g., syphilis). This system of antigen capture is useful for screening various fluids and tissues, including urine, blood, and CSF.

Treatment and Prevention

Treatment decisions after a tick bite are influenced by the following factors:

- Probability that the tick is a carrier of *B. burgdorferi.*
- Length of time the tick was attached.
- Chance that disease will develop without the telltale rash.
- Risk and severity of short-term and long-term sequelae.
- Accuracy of antibody tests.
- Efficacy of antibiotics at various stages of the disease.
- Risk of adverse reactions to the antibiotics.
- Patient's level of anxiety.
- Probability that the patient will comply with follow-up monitoring.
- Cost of various strategies; presence of coinfections or immunodeficiencies; prior significant steroid use while infected; age and weight; gastrointestinal (GI) function; blood levels achieved.

Antibiotics

It is unclear whether antimicrobial treatment after an *I. scapularis* tick bite will prevent Lyme disease. One study concluded that a single 200-mg dose of doxycycline given within 72 hours after an *I. scapularis* tick bite can prevent the development of Lyme disease.

Another study concluded that there is considerable impairment of health-related quality of life among patients with persistent symptoms despite previous antibiotic treatment for acute Lyme disease. In two clinical trials, however, treatment with intravenous (IV) and oral antibiotics for 90 days did not improve symptoms more than placebo.

Various types of antibiotics are in general use for *B. burgdorferi* treatment. The tetracyclines, including doxycycline and minocycline, are bacteriostatic unless given in high doses. If high blood levels are not attained, treatment failures in early and late disease are common; however, it is difficult to tolerate high doses.

Penicillins are bactericidal. As would be expected in managing an infection with a gram-negative organism such as *B. burgdorferi,* amoxicillin has been shown to be more effective than oral penicillin V. Because of its short half-life and need for high levels, amoxicillin is usually administered along with probenecid. Because of variability, blood levels are usually measured. Third-generation agents are currently the most effective of the cephalosporins because of their very low blood level counts (0.06 for ceftriaxone), and they have been shown to be effective in penicillin and tetracycline failures. Cefuroxime axetil (Ceftin), a second-generation agent, is also effective against staphylococci and thus is useful in treating atypical EM, which may represent a mixed infection containing common skin pathogens in addition to *B. burgdorferi.* Because of this agent's GI side effects and high cost, cefuroxime is not used as a first-line drug.

Preventive Practices

Note: On February 26, 2002, GlaxoSmithKline, the maker of the Lyme vaccine LYMErix, pulled the vaccine off the market.

When hiking in the woods or mountains, picnicking at local parks, or walking in tall grass in shore areas, individuals should do the following:

- Check daily for ticks.
- Wear light-colored clothing so tick viewing is easier.
- Tuck pants into socks.

HUMAN EHRLICHIOSIS

Human ehrlichiosis was first described in the United States in 1986; since then, reporting of tick-borne illnesses has increased. Unlike Lyme disease, which tends to be indolent, Rocky Mountain spotted fever and ehrlichiosis can be fatal and must be recognized and treated promptly.

Etiology

Tick-borne rickettsiae of the genus *Ehrlichia* have recently been recognized as a cause of human illness in the United States. *Ehrlichia* species belong to the same family as the organism that causes Rocky Mountain spotted fever. *Ehrlichia chaffeensis,* the novel etiologic agent of human monocytic ehrlichiosis in the United States, was demonstrated to cause disease in a patient from Arkansas with tick bites in 1987. Since then, two more *Ehrlichia* species, *E. ewingii* and an *E. phagocytophila*–like agent that differs antigenically and genetically from *E. chaffeensis,* have been identified as the cause of anaplasmosis (human granulocytic ehrlichiosis).

Epidemiology

Although the prevalence rates are low, human ehrlichiosis is endemic in the United States. Some fatalities have been reported. Incidence rates increase with age and are higher among men than women. Human ehrlichiosis occurs most frequently in the southern mid-Atlantic and south-central states during spring and summer.

The major vector for *E. chaffeensis* is the Lone Star tick, *Amblyomma americanum*. The principal reservoir for *E. chaffeensis* is the white-tailed deer, which hosts all stages of *A. americanum*. The primary tick vector for the agent of human granulocytic ehrlichiosis is *I. scapularis* in the eastern United States and *I. pacificus* in California. *Dermacentor variabilis* represents a second tick vector in the United States. The major reservoir for infection may be the white-footed mouse in the eastern United States. The onset of illness in spring and early summer for most cases parallels the time when the ticks, *A. americanum* and *D. variabilis*, are most active.

Signs and Symptoms

Ehrlichiosis is a general term for both "human granulocytic ehrlichiosis," now called **anaplasmosis,** and **human monocytic ehrlichiosis (HME).** The syndrome of human ehrlichiosis is not typically recognized by physicians, but it should be considered in patients with a history of tick exposure and acute febrile, flulike illness. Most patients are not suspected of having a rickettsial infection. Because ehrlichiosis can cause fatal infections in humans, early detection and treatment with tetracycline or chloramphenicol appear to offer the best chance for complete recovery.

Symptoms are nonspecific and include fever, chills, and headache. Fever and skin rashes are the most common physical findings. In children, fever and headache are universal. Myalgias, nausea, vomiting, and anorexia are also common.

Diagnostic Evaluation

Laboratory investigations indicate that the hematologic, hepatic, and central nervous systems are usually involved in human ehrlichiosis. Definitive diagnosis is based on inclusions in leukocytes (Figure 19-7). *Ehrlichia* species undergo three developmental stages, as follows:

1. Elementary bodies enter a leukocyte by phagocytosis and multiply rapidly.
2. After 3 to 5 days, small numbers of tightly packed elementary bodies (initial bodies) are visible.
3. During the next 7 to 12 days, the initial bodies develop into *morular,* or "mulberry," forms.

Characteristically, the presence of intracytoplasmic inclusions **(morula)** in leukocytes of patients presenting with temperature of 38.5° C or higher can be observed when a blood smear is examined by light microscopy. Careful examination should reveal morulae in 20% to 80% of acutely infected individuals. For anaplasmosis, direct observation of intraleukocytic morulae in Wright-Giemsa–stained peripheral blood or buffy coat smears is a rapid and inexpen-

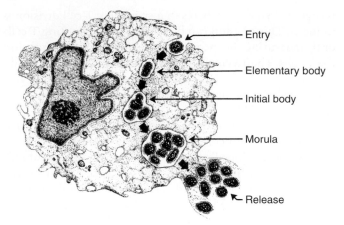

Figure 19-7   Schematic representation of the growth cycle of ehrlichiae in an infected cell. Elementary bodies (EB; individual ehrlichiae) enter the leukocyte by phagocytosis and multiply. After 3 to 5 days, small numbers of tightly packed EBs are observable and are called *initial bodies.* During the next 7 to 12 days, additional growth and replication occur, and the initial bodies develop into mature inclusions, which appear by light microscopy as mulberry (morular) forms. This morula is a hallmark of ehrlichial infection. *(From McDade J:* J Infect Dis *161:609, 1990.)*

sive laboratory test. In HME, intraleukocytic morulae are difficult to detect in peripheral blood smears. The quantitative buffy coat method can also be used for diagnosis of either HME or anaplasmosis.

In most cases reported, a lymphocytopenia is present either at diagnosis or during the illness. Early in the course of antibiotic treatment (48-72 hours), the lymphocytopenia corrects itself and is rapidly followed by a lymphocytosis of T cells that express CD3 but are negative for CD4 and CD8. Blood smears usually become negative 24 to 48 hours after the beginning of antibiotic therapy. In addition to leukopenia, thrombocytopenia is usually evident.

In anaplasmosis the diagnosis is confirmed by seroconversion or by a single serologic titer greater than 1:80 in patients with a supporting history and clinical symptoms. Seroconversion is defined as a fourfold rise in the titer of paired acute and convalescent sera. In HME the diagnosis is confirmed by seroconversion or by a serologic titer greater than 1:128 in patients with a supporting history and clinical symptoms. Serum or CSF can be analyzed for IgM and IgG antibodies to *Ehrlichia* species.

The PCR-based detection of the *E. phagocytophila*–like agent of anaplasmosis represents the most sensitive and direct approach to diagnosis. PCR detection of *E. chaffeensis* includes amplification of sequences with 16SrDNA.

Treatment and Prevention

Both HME patients and those with anaplasmosis are treated with doxycycline. No established guidelines exist for long-term therapy. Prevention consists of reducing the risk of exposure to ticks (see Lyme disease prevention).

BABESIOSIS

Etiology

Babesiosis is a rare, severe, and sometimes fatal tick-borne disease caused by various types of *Babesia,* a microscopic parasite that infects red blood cells (Figure 19-8). The causative organism of babesiosis was first described by Babes in 1888. In New England and the eastern United States, the disease is caused by *B. microti;* in California, it is caused by *B. equi.* In Europe, the disease is caused by *B. divergens* and *B. bovis. B. canis* has been found to be responsible for several cases in Mexico and France.

Epidemiology

Babesia microti is transmitted by the tick *Ixodes scapularis* in the northeastern United States. The larvae of the tick feed mainly on the white-footed mouse *(P. leucopus).* When larvae develop into nymphs and adults, they feed on the white-tailed deer *(Odocoileus virginianus),* but may also choose a human host.

Babesiosis is seen most frequently in older individuals, splenectomized patients, or immunocompromised patients. In the 1970s, cases were primarily reported during spring, summer, and fall in coastal areas in the northeastern United States, especially Nantucket Island off the coast of Massachusetts and on Long Island in New York. Cases have also been reported in Wisconsin, California, Georgia, and Missouri, as well as in some European countries. The organism has also been transmitted through blood transfusion from asymptomatic donors.

Signs and Symptoms

The incubation period is approximately 7 to 21 days. The clinical presentation is variable, ranging from asymptomatic to rapidly progressive and sometimes fatal. Infections caused by *B. divergens* tend to be more severe (frequently fatal if not appropriately treated) than those caused by *B. microti* (clinical recovery usually occurs).

The disease can cause fever, fatigue, and hemolytic anemia lasting several days to several months. It may take from 1 to 8 weeks, sometimes longer, for symptoms to appear. The disease course is characterized by high fever, massive hemolysis, hemoglobinemia, and hemoglobinuria.

Diagnostic Evaluation

Because of the hemolytic component of the disease, many patients exhibit an increased reticulocyte count, elevated lactate dehydrogenase (LDH), increased bilirubin, and decreased haptoglobin levels. Variant lymphocytes are usually present on a peripheral blood smear. The ESR is usually elevated.

Two rapid screening methods are used for the identification of *Babesia* organisms. The "gold standard" for identification of *Babesia* organisms is the visualization of the intraerythrocytic organisms in thick or thin blood films. *Babesia* organisms can be seen on Giemsa staining of peripheral blood smears. The organisms appear as intraerythrocytic oval ring structures (1-3 g) with pale-blue cytoplasm and one or two tiny red dots. As the *Babesia* organisms mature, they assume an ameboid morphology, and multiple organisms can exist inside the same cell.

The *Babesia* organism ring structures can be easily confused with the ring forms in malaria infections. Several features distinguish *Babesia* ring structures from malaria. *B. microti* occasionally have four or five rings per erythrocyte and sometimes form a tetrad, called a "Maltese cross." Because these organisms may be difficult to detect in peripheral blood, direct visualization lacks sensitivity, producing false-negative results with low-level parasitemia. The degree of parasitemia varies between 1% and 20% in patients with a normal, functioning spleen. It can be as high as 85% in splenectomized patients.

The Field's test is a rapid method performed with a thick peripheral blood film. Erythrocytes in the film are lysed and stained with methylene blue, azure B, and eosin. The method dehemoglobinizes and stains in less than 15 seconds.

This rapid screening method is being replaced by the quantitative buffy coat (QBC) method. Although initially developed for detection of malaria parasites, the QBC test can also be used as a screening test for babesiosis and is at least as sensitive as peripheral blood smear analysis. This method requires centrifuging the patient's blood in a microcapillary tube with a coating on its wall of acridine orange (AO) stain. AO stains nucleic acid. Denser, infected erythrocytes concentrate with the rest of the red blood cells (RBCs) and are detected by fluorescence microscopy.

Acute and convalescent antibody titers may be useful for diagnosis. A titer greater than 1:256 is considered diagnostic of acute infection. Only IgG antibody determinations are performed. PCR amplification can be used for diagnosis.

Molecular diagnosis can also be useful. In some infections with intraerythrocytic parasites, the morphologic

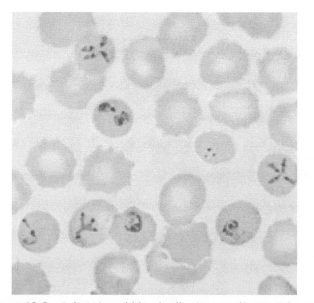

Figure 19-8 *Babesia* in red blood cells. *(From Forbes BA, Sahm DF, Weissfeld AS:* Bailey & Scott's diagnostic microbiology, *ed 12, St Louis, 2007, Mosby.)*

characteristics observed on microscopic examination of blood smears do not allow an unambiguous differentiation between *Babesia* and *Plasmodium* organisms. In these cases the diagnosis can be derived from molecular techniques such as PCR, using the appropriate primers, and single-step or the more sensitive nested-PCR technique. In addition, molecular approaches are valuable in investigations of new *Babesia* variants (or species) observed in recent human infections in the United States and Europe.

Treatment and Prevention

Standardized treatments for babesiosis have not been developed. However, some drugs used in the treatment of malaria have been found to be effective in some patients with babesiosis.

Antimicrobial therapy is recommended for splenectomized or immunodeficient patients, older patients, and patients with severe infections. The usual regimen consists of a combination of clindamycin and oral quinine. An alternative treatment option is oral azithromycin and oral atovaquone. Exchange transfusion has been effective for patients with a high level of parasites (>10%), severe disease, or massive hemolysis.

Prevention requires vigilance when in tick-infested areas (see Lyme disease prevention).

WEST NILE VIRUS

Etiology

West Nile virus (WNV) is a member of the Japanese encephalitis virus group of flaviviruses that cause febrile illness and encephalitis in humans. WNV is a mosquito-borne pathogen.

Epidemiology

The virus has been in the United States since at least the summer of 1999. Figure 19-9 shows the distribution of avian, animal, or mosquito infections and number of human cases, if any, by state as of March 4, 2008. If WNV infection is reported to CDC from any area of a state, the entire state is shaded.

Avian, animal, or mosquito WNV infections have been reported to CDC ArboNET from 39 states and Puerto Rico. Human cases have been reported in 25 states: Alabama, Arizona, Arkansas, California, Colorado, Georgia, Idaho, Illinois, Iowa, Kansas, Minnesota, Mississippi, Missouri, Montana, Nebraska, Nevada, New Mexico, North Dakota, Ohio, Pennsylvania, South Dakota, Texas, Utah, Virginia, and Wyoming.

Signs and Symptoms

West Nile virus infection is characterized by fever, headache, fatigue, aches, and sometimes a rash. Illness can last from a few days to several weeks.

Diagnostic Evaluation

Historically, flavivirus infections have been diagnosed by serologic tests or virus isolation. Several molecular techniques are available for diagnosis. Molecular detection of WNV is used for prevention of transmission by blood transfusion and transplantation. Reverse-transcription (RT) PCR is the preferred diagnostic method.

Nucleic amplification tests (NATs) include the TaqMan Assay (Roche Diagnostics), based on a real-time, quantitative RT-PCR format, and Procleix West Nile Virus Assay (Gen-Probe and Chiron). In 2003 the FDA approved two

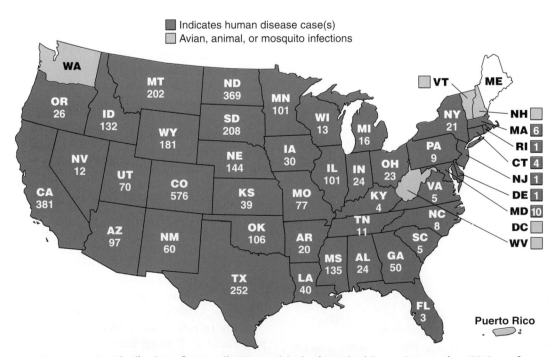

Figure 19-9 Distribution of West Nile virus activity in the United States (reported to CDC as of 3/4/08). *(Courtesy Centers for Disease Control and Prevention, Atlanta.)*

ELISA tests that detect IgG and IgM antibodies to WNV (PanBio Ltd, Australia; Focus Diagnostics, Va).

The IgM antibody is evident in most infected patients 7 to 8 days after the onset of symptoms. IgM antibody has been shown to persist for more than 500 days in approximately 60% of cases. Most patients demonstrate IgG antibody in 3 to 4 weeks after infection.

Treatment and Prevention

There is no specific treatment for WNV infection. In patients with milder disease, symptoms resolve over time, although even healthy people have been sick for several weeks. In patients with more severe disease, hospitalization is usually required for supportive treatment, including IV fluids.

Prevention consists of avoiding mosquito bites.

CASE STUDY

A 42-year-old executive lived in New York City. Her company annually sponsored a Memorial Day weekend golf outing at a Long Island club. In early June she noticed a solid, bright-red spot on her left thigh. The spot was about 2 inches wide in the bright-red area with an overall diameter of about 6 inches, including the surrounding pale area. The ensuing 11 months passed without further incident.

The following Memorial Day weekend, she was stung several times by bees. Both a systemic and a local reaction followed. About a week later, last year's red ring on the thigh reappeared. During this interval, she experienced fever, malaise, arthromyalgias, headache, and a stiff neck, but recovered completely.

In the fall the woman noticed insidiously progressive fatigue, malaise, memory deficits, irritability, and inattentiveness to the demands of her job.

She visited a physician, but no abnormalities were noted, and she was referred to a Manhattan neurologist. The patient was eventually diagnosed as having Lyme disease.

Questions and Discussion

1. Did the patient's residence or travel history suggest that she might have been exposed to Lyme disease?

Yes; although the patient did not travel far from her urban residence, she did visit a nearby endemic area. In the United States there are three major foci of infection: the northeastern coastal states from Massachusetts to Maryland, the upper midwestern states of Minnesota and Wisconsin, and portions of four western states: California, Oregon, Nevada, and Utah. In this case, Long Island happens to be a "hot spot" for Lyme disease.

2. Why did it take so long for the patient to develop symptoms of Lyme disease?

Lyme disease often has a prolonged latency period. It usually begins during the summer months with EM and flulike symptoms and may be accompanied by right upper quadrant tenderness and a mild hepatitis (stage 1). This stage is followed weeks to months later by acute cardiac or neurologic disease in a minority of untreated individuals (stage 2), then by arthritis and chronic neurologic disease (stage 3) in many untreated patients weeks to years after disease onset.

Diagnosis

Lyme disease.

CASE STUDY

This 25-year-old graduate student visited his local family physician because of episodic arthromyalgias, sporadic global headaches, fatigue, irritability, and depression. Over the last several months he had become seriously dysfunctional at work and home.

His residence and travel history revealed a week-long vacation on Cape Cod the previous summer. He could not recall any tick bites or any skin lesions fitting the description of EM.

A laboratory test revealed a positive test, and a 4-week course of doxycycline was initiated. Two weeks later he noted significant improvement in symptoms, but 3 months later his previous symptoms recurred. His laboratory test was repeated and again was positive. A month's regimen of amoxicillin and probenecid was initiated. This time there was no improvement. No neurologic findings were apparent. His joints were painful, but no overt synovitis was present. Two months after the second course of antibiotic, his Lyme test was still positive, and the patient received 2 weeks of infusion therapy with ceftriaxone. His symptoms disappeared after this treatment.

Questions and Discussion

1. Why was the treatment regimen initially unsuccessful?

For most patients with a positive Lyme antibody titer whose only symptoms are nonspecific myalgia or fatigue, the risks and costs of empirical parenteral antibiotic therapy exceed the benefits. Treatment usually fails because the patient is not suffering from Lyme disease.

2. Why did the patient demonstrate a positive laboratory result, even though the usual treatment regimen was unsuccessful?

False-positive results can occur if an individual has been exposed to a related bacteria. For example, tick-borne relapsing fever spirochetes, *B. hermsii*, are closely related to *B. burgdorferi*. Antibodies to *B. hermsii*, an agent that coexists with the Lyme disease spirochete in portions of the western United States, strongly cross-react with *B. burgdorferi* in IFA staining and ELISA testing. Common antigens are shared among the *Borrelia* and even with the treponemes. Serum from syphilitic patients reacts positively in assays for Lyme disease. Therefore serologic test results for antibodies to *B. burgdorferi* should be considered along with clinical data and epidemiologic information when a patient is evaluated for Lyme disease.

Diagnosis

Lyme disease.

CASE STUDY

A 45-year-old man from upstate New York visited his physician because of a worsening headache, myalgia, arthralgia, and generalized weakness. He had been in good health until about 1 week before the appointment. A fever and myalgia began after the patient removed a small tick from his left thigh while he was on vacation in an area in which *B. burgdorferi* is endemic. In addition, the deer tick found in locale that he visited on vacation is the vector of Lyme disease, babesiosis, and most likely, anaplasmosis.

On physical examination the patient had a slight fever. His thigh had a rash suggestive of EM. Laboratory results included a complete blood count and liver function tests. A skin scraping was obtained to culture *B. burgdorferi*. Buffy coat smears of peripheral blood were also requested.

The patient had a slight leukopenia, normal white blood cell differential, and a normal hemoglobin and hematocrit. His liver function tests were slightly abnormal. Wright-stained buffy coat smears revealed the presence of morulae of anaplasmosis. The patient was prescribed oral doxycycline twice daily for 14 days. Nine days after initiation of treatment, the patient improved greatly. Repeat laboratory tests were all within the normal reference range. His rash had resolved.

Questions and Discussion

1. Can the vector of *B. burgdorferi* and the agent of anaplasmosis be the same?

Yes; *Ixodes* ticks infected with *B. burgdorferi* and the anaplasmosis agent have been identified.

2. Is it important to determine if one or both infections are present in the same host?

Simultaneous infection with *B. burgdorferi* and the agent of anaplasmosis is important because the natural history of each disease may change in the presence of the other. Another consideration by a physician is selection of antimicrobial therapy. In addition, dual infection with *B. burgdorferi* may result in more serious disease than an infection with either agent alone.

3. How can coinfection with *B. burgdorferi* and the agent of anaplasmosis be demonstrated in the laboratory?

Coinfection with *B. burgdorferi* and anaplasmosis can be demonstrated by the isolation of both organisms from clinical specimens. Serologic evidence alone is insufficient. Among the many problems associated with a dual infection, anaplasmosis itself may produce false-positive results on serologic tests for Lyme disease. Even with PCR testing, care must be taken to avoid contamination and to use appropriately specific primers.

Diagnosis

Coinfection with *B. burgdorferi* (Lyme disease) and anaplasmosis.

CASE STUDY

This 73-year-old, previously healthy man had spent the previous summer on Martha's Vineyard. On returning to his home in Boston after Labor Day, he began to feel unusually tired and having difficulty breathing. He also reported that his urine had become dark-brown several days after returning home.

On physical examination the patient was jaundiced, and he had an enlarged spleen. A complete blood count, urinalysis, and blood chemistries were ordered. His total white blood cell count was normal, but he had an increased percentage of segmented neutrophils. His hemoglobin, hematocrit, and platelet count were all below the normal reference range. He had hematuria and proteinuria in his urine. His liver function tests were greatly elevated. His renal function assays were also elevated. A follow-up Wright-stained peripheral blood smear revealed numerous *B. microti* organisms.

The patient was treated with quinine and the antibiotics clindamycin and doxycycline. He also received 2 U of packed RBCs. Six days later the patient was discharged from the hospital.

Questions and Discussion

1. Would the patient's travel history be suggestive of malaria or another blood-borne infectious disease?

Although some of the patient's symptoms resemble malaria, it would not be associated with the area that the patient visited; however, other tick-borne illnesses (e.g., Lyme disease, babesiosis) are considerations.

2. What is the definitive diagnosis for babesiosis?

Definitive diagnosis relies predominantly on the demonstration of intraerythrocytic ring-shaped or pleomorphic parasites in Wright-Giemsa–stained blood smears.

3. What additional laboratory tests are of diagnostic value?

PCR should be used only when blood smear results are questionable or negative in patients in whom babesiosis is strongly suspected and a travel history to a malaria-endemic area is absent. In cases of diagnostic uncertainty or suspected chronic infection, serologic studies can be conducted. The method of choice is the IFA test. Western blot assay is also available.

Diagnosis

Babesiosis.

CASE STUDY

A 35-year-old field biologist from central Missouri was positive for human immunodeficiency virus (HIV). Her work required that she spend a great deal of time in the woods in the surrounding areas. Although she was in good health despite the HIV positivity, she began having back pain, fever, chills, sweats, a productive cough, and extreme tiredness before her visit to the emergency room.

She was admitted to the hospital because her laboratory results demonstrated severe leukopenia and thrombocytopenia. Her liver function tests were also extremely abnormal. Later on the day of admission, renal failure developed. The patient died the next day.

Questions and Discussion

1. What was the cause of death?

The cause of death was determined to be human monocytic ehrlichiosis (HME). The presence of inclusion, predominantly in monocytic cells, established the diagnosis.

2. What immunologic studies could be performed?

At autopsy, tissue samples from the spleen, kidneys, lymph nodes, and bone marrow were obtained for further study. These specimens were examined immunohistologically using monoclonal and polyclonal anti–*Ehrlichia chaffeensis* antibodies. The antibodies reacted strongly with the inclusions in the tissues.

3. Is human monocytic ehrlichiosis a risk in the United States?

Human ehrlichiosis is endemic in the United States. HME is seen in the south central and southeast United States. In contrast, anaplasmosis has been identified in the upper midwestern and the northeastern United States.

Diagnosis

Human monocytic ehrlichiosis.

CHAPTER HIGHLIGHTS

- Lyme disease (borreliosis) is caused by the tick-borne spirochete *Borrelia burgdorferi* and is a major health hazard for humans and domestic animals.
- Lyme disease is considered an emerging infectious disease because of the impact of changing environmental and socioeconomic factors (e.g., transformation of farmland into suburban woodlots favorable for deer and deer ticks).
- Basic features of Lyme disease are similar worldwide. In at least 60% to 80% of U.S. patients it begins with a slowly expanding skin lesion, erythema migrans (EM), at the site of the tick bite.
- Lyme borreliosis is a multisystem illness that primarily involves the skin, nervous system, heart, and joints. It usually begins during the summer months with EM and flulike symptoms.
- Cellular immune responses to *B. burgdorferi* antigens begin concurrently with early clinical illness, with increased spontaneous suppressor cell and reduced natural killer cell activity. Mononuclear cell, antigen-specific responses develop during spirochetal dissemination, and humoral (antibody) immune responses soon follow.
- Serodiagnostic tests are insensitive during the first several weeks of *Borrelia* infection. About 20% to 30% of U.S. patients have positive responses, usually of the IgM isotype, during this period, but by convalescence 2 to 4 weeks later, about 70% to 80% have seroreactivity even after antibiotic treatment. After about 1 month, most patients with active infection have IgG antibody responses. After antibiotic treatment, antibody titers fall slowly, but IgG and IgM responses may persist for years.
- Specific IgM or IgG antibodies against *B. burgdorferi* are usually not detectable in a patient's serum unless symptoms have been present for at least 2 to 4 weeks. In Lyme arthritis, tests (ANAs, RF, VDRL) are generally negative, and anti–*B. burgdorferi* antibodies (IgG) should be present.
- The most common laboratory assays for *B. burgdorferi* antibody detection include IFA, ELISA, and PreVue. Immunoblotting techniques can be used with ELISA. PreVue is the first presumptive step in testing individuals with suspected Lyme disease. Positive results must be confirmed by Western blot.
- T-cell proliferative assays and antibody-based antigen detection systems, as well as monoclonal or polyclonal antibodies, also detect specific Lyme spirochete antigens. Quantities of proteins (flagellin, OspA, OspB) are detectable. OspA and OspB are *B. burgdorferi* proteins from bacterial outer wall.
- Described first in the U.S. in 1986, tick-borne rickettsiae of the genus *Ehrlichia* cause human illness. Ehrlichiosis is a general term for both anaplasmosis and human monocytic ehrlichiosis (HME).
- Anaplasmosis diagnosis is confirmed by seroconversion (fourfold rise in acute/convalescent sera titer) or single serologic titer greater than 1:80 in patients with a history and symptoms. HME diagnosis is confirmed by seroconversion or serologic titer greater than 1:128.
- Babesiosis is a rare, severe, possibly fatal tick-borne disease caused by *Babesia*, which infects RBCs.
- *Babesia* species are visualized as intraerythrocytic organisms in thick peripheral (rapid Field's test) or thin blood films. Acute and convalescent antibody titers may be useful; titer greater than 1:256 is diagnostic of acute infection. Only IgG antibody determinations are performed. PCR amplification can be used for diagnosis.
- West Nile virus (WNV), a mosquito-borne virus present in the U.S. since at least 1999, causes febrile illness and encephalitis in humans.
- Molecular detection of WNV is used to prevent transmission by blood transfusion and transplantation. RT-PCR is the preferred diagnostic method.
- In WNV, IgM antibody is evident in most infected patients 7 to 8 days after onset of symptoms, persisting for more than 500 days in 60%. Most patients demonstrate IgG antibody in 3 to 4 weeks after infection.

REVIEW QUESTIONS

1. Common vectors of Lyme disease include all the following *except*:
   a. *Ixodes pacificus.*
   b. *I. scapularis.*
   c. *I. ricinus.*
   d. *D. variabilis.*

2. The only continent without Lyme disease is:
   a. Asia.
   b. Europe.
   c. Africa.
   d. Antarctica.

3. The primary reservoir in nature for *B. burgdorferi* is the:
   a. White-tailed deer.
   b. White-footed mouse.
   c. Lizard.
   d. Meadowlark.

4. The first *B. burgdorferi* antigen to elicit an antibody response is:
   a. Outer surface protein A.
   b. Outer surface protein B.
   c. Flagellar 41-kD polypeptide.
   d. 60-kD polypeptide.

5. The incidence of infection following an *I. scapularis* tick bite in an endemic area on average is:
   a. 1%.
   b. 3%.
   c. 5%.
   d. 10%.

6. Erythema migrans:
   a. Occurs in all patients.
   b. Harbors *B. burgdorferi* in the advancing edge.
   c. Is easily distinguished from other erythemas.
   d. Is more common in the winter months.

7. The predominant symptoms of Lyme meningitis are:
   a. Severe headache and mild neck stiffness.
   b. Aseptic meningitis and double vision.
   c. Cranial nerve palsies and blurred vision.
   d. Peripheral radiculoneuritis and peripheral neuropathy.

8. Cardiac involvement in Lyme disease may include:
   a. Murmurs.
   b. Conduction abnormalities.
   c. Congestive heart failure.
   d. Vasculitis.

9. Ocular involvement in Lyme disease includes all following *except*:
   a. Cranial nerve palsies.
   b. Conjunctivitis.
   c. Panophthalmitis with loss of vision.
   d. Choroiditis with retinal detachment.

10. Pregnancy in Lyme disease:
    a. Does not produce high fetal mortality.
    b. Has been associated with transplacental infection.
    c. Should be terminated because of maternal risk.
    d. Is not associated with congenital abnormalities.

11. The most useful test for distinguishing between true-positive and false-positive serologic tests is:
    a. Enzyme-linked immunosorbent assay.
    b. Immunofluorescence assay.
    c. Polymerase chain reaction.
    d. T-cell assay.

12. Preventive methods include all the following *except*:
    a. Wearing light-colored clothes.
    b. Removing ticks.
    c. Tucking pants into socks.
    d. Applying insect repellent to skin and clothes.

13. Lyme disease, the most common tick-borne disease in the United States, is a major health hazard for:
    a. Dogs.
    b. Horses and cattle.
    c. Humans.
    d. All the above.

14. Lyme disease is a _____ type of infection.
    a. bacterial
    b. parasitic
    c. viral
    d. fungal

15. The first case of Lyme disease occurred in:
    a. Connecticut.
    b. Wisconsin.
    c. Florida.
    d. New York.

Questions 16-19. Fill in the blanks, choosing from the following answers.

Possible answers for question 16:
   a. 3 days
   b. 1 week
   c. 4 weeks
   d. 3 months

Possible answers for question 17:
   a. Neurologic
   b. Rheumatoid
   c. Cutaneous (e.g., erythema migrans)
   d. Cardiac

Possible answers for question 18:
   a. Hours to weeks
   b. Days to weeks
   c. Weeks to months
   d. Weeks to years

Possible answers for question 19:
   a. Arthritis
   b. Lyme carditis
   c. Transplacental transmission
   d. Lymphocytoma

Clinical Features of Lyme Disease

Stage	Length of Time	Common Signs and Symptoms
I	16. _____ (median).	17. _____ manifestation after infection.
II	Follows a variable latent period.	Target organs and systems can manifest abnormalities.
III	18. _____ after infection.	19. _____, late neurologic complications.

20. Unlike some procedures, polymerase chain reaction (PCR) can be used to detect Lyme disease-causing organisms in:
    a. Urine.
    b. Cerebrospinal fluid.
    c. Synovial fluid.
    d. Blood.

Questions 21 and 22. Fill in the blanks, choosing from the possible answers (a-d).

Antigen detection systems in Lyme disease testing screen for (21) _____ rather than for (22) _____ associated with the infection.
    a. antibody
    b. microorganisms
    c. antigenic products
    d. infected tick

23. A patient who has a specific Lyme disease–associated manifestation may be treated with:
    a. Vaccination.
    b. Interferon.
    c. Antibiotic.
    d. Analgesic.

24. *Ehrlichia* species belong to the same family as the organism that causes:
    a. Lyme disease.
    b. Rocky Mountain spotted fever.
    c. Toxoplasmosis.
    d. Infectious mononucleosis.

25. One of the most common physical findings in adults with ehrlichiosis is:
    a. Hives.
    b. Fever.
    c. Erythema migrans.
    d. Nausea.

26. Definitive diagnosis of ehrlichiosis requires:
    a. A complete blood count.
    b. Detection of the presence of lymphocytopenia.
    c. Acute and convalescent serum antibody titers.
    d. Direct microscopic observation of inclusions in leukocytes.

27. In human granulocytic ehrlichiosis (anaplasmosis), the diagnosis is confirmed by seroconversion or by a single serologic titer of _____ in patients with a supporting history and clinical symptoms.
    a. 1:2
    b. 1:16
    c. 1:80
    d. 1:160

28. In the eastern United States, babesiosis is caused by:
    a. *Babesia microti.*
    b. *B. canis.*
    c. *B. bovis.*
    d. *B. equi.*

29. Babesiosis is characterized by:
    a. Fever.
    b. Fatigue.
    c. Hemolytic anemia.
    d. All the above.

30. *Babesia* organisms can be found in:
    a. Peripheral blood.
    b. Sputum.
    c. Synovial fluid.
    d. Various exudates.

31. West Nile Virus causes:
    a. Encephalitis.
    b. Polio.
    c. Measles.
    d. Arthritis.

32. West Nile virus is transmitted by:
    a. Dogs.
    b. Cats.
    c. Rats.
    d. Mosquitoes.

BIBLIOGRAPHY

Barenfanger J, Patel PG, Dumler JS, Walker DH: Identifying human ehrlichiosis, *Lab Med* 27:372-374, 1996.
Brown S et al: Role of serology in the diagnosis of Lyme disease, *JAMA* 282(1):62, 1999.
Burrascano J: *Advanced topics in Lyme disease,* ed 13, 2000, www.LymeNet.org.
Caldwell CW et al: Lymphocytosis of gamma/delta T cells in human ehrlichiosis, *Am J Clin Pathol* 103(6):761-766, 1995.
Callister SM et al: Detection of borreliacidal antibodies by flow cytometry: an accurate, highly specific serodiagnostic test for Lyme disease, *Arch Intern Med* 154(14):1625-1632, 1994.
Coon D, Versalovic J: Three tick-borne diseases in the northeastern United States: Lyme disease, babesiosis, and ehrlichiosis, *TurnAround Times Clin Lab Rev* (Mass Gen Hosp, Div Lab Med) 9:5-10, 2001.
Hazell S: West Nile virus is still with us, *Med Lab Observer* 39(4:32-33, 2007.
Klempner MS et al: Two controlled trials of antibiotic treatment in patients with persistent symptoms and a history of Lyme disease, *N Engl J Med* 345(2):85-92, 2001.
Medical Letter on Drugs and Therapeutics, 2000, website: www.medletter.com.
Nadelman RB et al: Prophylaxis with single-dose doxycycline for the prevention of Lyme disease after an *Ixodes scapularis* tick bite, *N Engl J Med* 345(2):79-84, 2001.

Nadelman RB et al: Simultaneous human granulocytic ehrlichiosis and Lyme borreliosis, *N Engl J Med* 337:27-30, 1997.

Niedrig M et al: First International Proficiency Study on West Nile Virus Molecular Detection, *Clin Chem* 52(10):1851-1854, 2006.

Pantanowitz L, Ballesteros E, DeGirolami P: Laboratory diagnosis of babesiosis, *Lab Med* 32:184-186, 2001.

Shapiro ED et al: Doxycycline for tick bites: not for everyone, *N Engl J Med* 345:133-134, 2001.

Steere AC: Lyme disease, *N Engl J Med* 345:115-123, 2001.

Sullivan E: Food and Drug Administration extends deferral period for blood donors with West Nile virus, *Lab Med* 36(11):692-693, 2005.

US Department of Health and Human Services, Centers for Disease Control and Prevention. Lyme Disease, www.cdc.gov, 2007.

US Department of Health and Human Services, Centers for Disease Control and Prevention: Lone star tick a concern, but not for Lyme disease, www.cdc.gov, 2007.

US Department of Health and Human Services, Centers for Disease Control and Prevention: Rickettsial infections, www.cdc.gov, 2007.

US Department of Health and Human Services, Centers for Disease Control and Prevention: Tick-borne relapsing fever, www.cdc.gov, 2007.

Wampole Laboratories: Wampole PreVue package insert, 2002.

Wormser GP: Early Lyme disease, *N Engl J Med* 354(26):2794-2801, 2006.

Wyeth Pharmaceutical Co: LymeVax, June 14, 2002, www.wyeth.com.

CHAPTER 20

Toxoplasmosis

Etiology
Epidemiology
    Transplacental Transmission
    Seroprevalence
Signs and Symptoms
    Acquired Infection
    Congenital Infection
Immunologic Manifestations

Diagnostic Evaluation
    Serologic Tests
    Histologic Diagnosis
    Cell Culture
Case Study
Chapter Highlights
Review Questions
Bibliography

Learning Objectives

At the conclusion of this chapter, the reader should be able to:

- Describe the etiology and epidemiology of toxoplasmosis.
- Explain the signs and symptoms of acquired and congenital toxoplasmosis infection.

- Discuss the immunologic manifestations and diagnostic evaluation of toxoplasmosis, including the quantitative determination of IgM antibodies to *Toxoplasma gondii*.

ETIOLOGY

Toxoplasmosis is a widespread disease in humans and animals. This infection is caused by *Toxoplasma gondii,* recently recognized as a tissue coccidian.

EPIDEMIOLOGY

Toxoplasma gondii was first discovered in a North African rodent and has been observed in numerous birds and mammals worldwide, including humans. It is a parasite of cosmopolitan distribution able to develop in a wide variety of vertebrate hosts. Human infections are common in many parts of the world. For unknown reasons, the incidence rates vary from place to place. The highest recorded rate (93%) occurs in Parisian women who prefer undercooked or raw meat; a 50% rate of occurrence exists in their children.

The definitive host is the house cat and certain other Felidae (Figure 20-1). Domestic cats are a source of the disease because oocysts are often present in their feces. Accidental ingestion of oocysts by humans and animals, including the cat, produces a proliferative infection in the body tissues. Fecal contamination of food or water, soiled hands, inadequately cooked or infected meat, and raw milk can be major sources of human infection.

Transfusion-transmitted toxoplasmosis has been associated with the use of leukocyte concentrates. Patients at risk are those receiving immunosuppressive agents or corticosteroids.

Transplacental Transmission

All mammals, including humans, can transmit the infection transplacentally. Transplacental transmission usually takes place in the course of an acute but inapparent or undiagnosed maternal infection. New evidence indicates that the number of infants born in the United States each year with congenital *T. gondii* infection is considerably higher than the 3000 previously estimated. It is estimated that 6 of every 1000 pregnant women in the United States will acquire primary infection with *Toxoplasma* during a 9-month gestation. Approximately 45% of the women who acquire the infection for the first time and who are not treated will give birth to congenitally infected infants. Consequently, the expected incidence of congenital toxoplasmosis is 2.7 per 1000 live births.

It is recommended that all pregnant women be tested for toxoplasmosis immunity. If a patient is susceptible, screening should be repeated during pregnancy and at delivery. Prevention of infection in pregnant women should be practiced to avert congenital toxoplasmosis (Box 20-1). To further prevent infection of the fetus, women at risk should be identified by serologic testing, and pregnant women with primary infection should receive drug therapy.

Seroprevalence

Seroprevalence (antibody to *T. gondii*) varies considerably in the general population. It ranges from 96% in Western Europe to 10% to 40% in the United States. Of those patients with acquired immunodeficiency syndrome (AIDS) who are seropositive for *T. gondii,* approximately 25% to 50% will develop toxoplasmic encephalitis (meningoencephalitis). In areas with a lower seroprevalence, such as the United States, the percentage of AIDS patients who develop toxoplasmic encephalitis is lower (5%-10%).

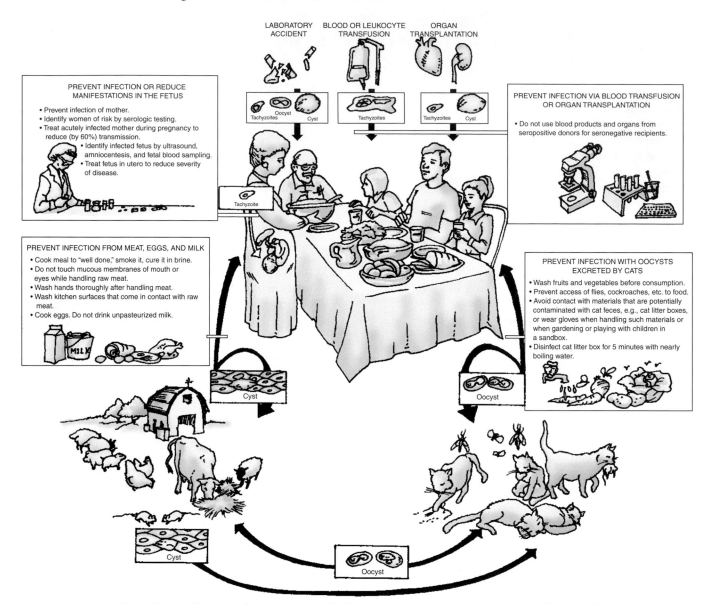

LABORATORY ACCIDENT   BLOOD OR LEUKOCYTE TRANSFUSION   ORGAN TRANSPLANTATION

PREVENT INFECTION OR REDUCE MANIFESTATIONS IN THE FETUS

- Prevent infection of mother.
- Identify women of risk by serologic testing.
- Treat acutely infected mother during pregnancy to reduce (by 60%) transmission.
  - Identify infected fetus by ultrasound, amniocentesis, and fetal blood sampling.
  - Treat fetus in utero to reduce severity of disease.

PREVENT INFECTION VIA BLOOD TRANSFUSION OR ORGAN TRANSPLANTATION

- Do not use blood products and organs from seropositive donors for seronegative recipients.

PREVENT INFECTION FROM MEAT, EGGS, AND MILK

- Cook meal to "well done," smoke it, cure it in brine.
- Do not touch mucous membranes of mouth or eyes while handling raw meat.
- Wash hands thoroughly after handling meat.
- Wash kitchen surfaces that come in contact with raw meat.
- Cook eggs. Do not drink unpasteurized milk.

PREVENT INFECTION WITH OOCYSTS EXCRETED BY CATS

- Wash fruits and vegetables before consumption.
- Prevent access of flies, cockroaches, etc. to food.
- Avoid contact with materials that are potentially contaminated with cat feces, e.g., cat litter boxes, or wear gloves when handling such materials or when gardening or playing with children in a sandbox.
- Disinfect cat litter box for 5 minutes with nearly boiling water.

Figure 20-1   Life cycle of *Toxoplasma gondii*. *(Redrawn from Krugman S et al:* Infectious diseases of children, *ed 9, St Louis, 1992, Mosby.)*

Box 20-1	Methods for Prevention of Congenital Toxoplasmosis

Avoid touching mucous membranes of the mouth and eye while handling raw meat.

Wash hands thoroughly after handling raw meat.

Wash kitchen surfaces that come in contact with raw meat.

Cook meat to >18.8° C; smoke it, or cure it in brine.

Wash fruits and vegetables before consumption.

Prevent access of flies, cockroaches, and other insects to fruits and vegetables.

Avoid contact with or wear gloves when handling materials that are potentially contaminated with cat feces (e.g., cat litter boxes) and when gardening.

SIGNS AND SYMPTOMS

In adults and children other than newborns, toxoplasmosis is usually asymptomatic. A generalized infection probably occurs. Although spontaneous recovery follows acute febrile disease, the organism can localize and multiply in any organ of the body or the circulatory system. Toxoplasmic encephalitis in AIDS patients may result in death even when treated (Figure 20-2). Persons at risk can be identified by screening patients positive for human immunodeficiency virus (HIV) for antibody to *T. gondii*.

Acquired Infection

When seen, symptoms are frequently mild. Toxoplasmosis can simulate infectious mononucleosis, with chills, fever, headache, lymphadenopathy, and extreme fatigue. Primary

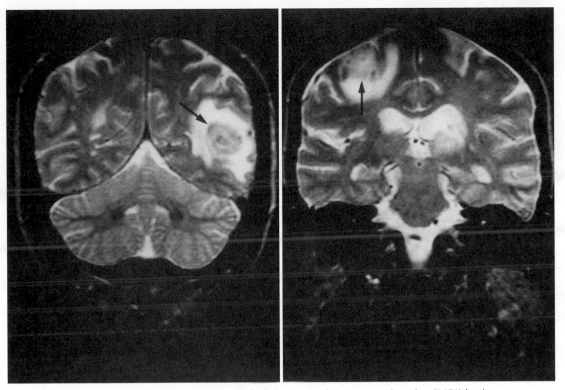

Figure 20-2 Toxoplasmic meningoencephalitis. Magnetic resonance imaging (MRI) brain scans of patients with AIDS. Arrows indicate areas infected with toxoplasmosis.

infection may be promoted by immunosuppression. A chronic form of toxoplasmic lymphadenopathy exists. *T. gondii* presents a special problem in immunosuppressed or otherwise compromised hosts. Some of these patients have experienced reactivation of a latent toxoplasmosis. These patients have included those with Hodgkin's and non-Hodgkin's lymphoma, as well as recipients of organ transplants.

Reactivation of cerebral toxoplasmosis is not uncommon in patients with AIDS, in whom toxoplasmic meningoencephalitis is almost always a reactivation of a preexisting latent infection, most often occurring when the total CD4 count falls below 100×10^9/L. *T. gondii*–seropositive, HIV-infected patients may develop toxoplasmic encephalitis because of (1) genetic susceptibility in the human immune response to *T. gondii,* (2) subtle differences in patients' immunocompromised status, (3) differences in the virulence of individual strains of *T. gondii,* (4) possible recurrent infections with different strains, and (5) variable coinfections with other opportunistic pathogens.

Congenital Infection

Congenital toxoplasmosis can result in central nervous system (CNS) malformation or prenatal mortality. In infants who are serologically positive at birth, many fail to display neurologic, ophthalmic, or generalized illness at birth. Toxoplasmosis acquired in utero can result in blindness, encephalomyelitis, mental retardation, convulsions, and death in infected neonates (TORCH syndrome).

In as many as 75% of congenitally infected newborns not serologically diagnosed at birth, the disease remains dormant, only to be discovered when other symptoms become apparent, such as chorioretinitis, unilateral blindness, and severe neurologic sequelae.

IMMUNOLOGIC MANIFESTATIONS

Both clinical and laboratory findings in toxoplasmosis resemble infectious mononucleosis. An increased number of variant lymphocytes can be seen on a peripheral blood smear.

The diagnosis can be established serologically by detecting a marked elevation of *Toxoplasma* antibodies. Antibodies are demonstrable within the first 2 weeks after infection, rising to high levels early in the infection, then falling slightly, but persisting at an elevated level for many months before declining to low levels after many years. The best evidence for current infection is a significant change on two appropriately timed specimens (paired acute and convalescent specimens), where both tests are done in the same laboratory at the same time.

If a significant level of *T. gondii* immunoglobulin M (IgM) antibody is detected, it may indicate a current or recent infection. The presence of IgM to *T. gondii* in an adult indicates an infection, but low levels of IgM antibodies occasionally may persist for more than 12 months after infection. The Centers for Disease Control and Prevention (CDC) recommends that any equivocal or positive result should be retested using a different assay from another reference laboratory specializing in toxoplasmosis testing.

DIAGNOSTIC EVALUATION

The diagnosis of toxoplasmosis can be established by the following (Table 20-1):
*   Serologic tests
*   Polymerase chain reaction (PCR)
*   Indirect fluorescent antibody (IFA)
*   Isolation of the organism

Serologic Tests

The mainstay of diagnosis of *T gondii* infection is serologic testing. A relatively high proportion of people have antibody to *T gondii*, which makes interpretation of serologic testing difficult. Assays for different isotypes of antibodies have been developed to support the diagnosis of acute or chronic *T gondii* infection.

The enzyme-linked immunosorbent assay (ELISA) is considered by many to be the method of choice for detection of IgM antibodies in toxoplasmosis (see EVOLVE website for representative procedural protocol). For the detection of IgM antibodies to *T. gondii*, indirect immunofluorescence (IFA; Figure 20-3) and ELISA tests have been developed. Indirect qualitative enzyme immunoassay for IgM or IgG, IgM (capture), microparticle enzyme immunoassay using the automated AxSYM System, and chemiluminescent immunoassay are available methods of antibody detection.

A panel of tests performed by specialized reference laboratories can determine whether an infection is consistent with a new or past infection. The **T. gondii serologic profile (TSP)** consists of the following:
*   IgM, IgA, and IgE ELISAs
*   IgE immunosorbent agglutination assay
*   Sabin-Feldman dye test (IgG)
*   Differential agglutination test (AC/HS test; IgG antibody)
*   Newer methodologies

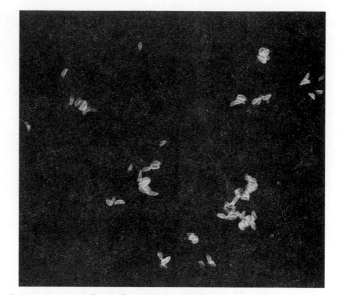

Figure 20-3   Indirect fluorescent antibody (IFA) test for *T. gondii* antibodies. *Toxoplasma* organisms affixed to the slide bind specific antibodies in the patient's serum. Antihuman antibody conjugated with fluorescein binds in turn to the bound patient's antibodies, causing the organisms to fluoresce. *(From Baron EJ, Peterson LR, Finegold SM: Bailey and Scott's diagnostic microbiology, ed 9, St Louis, 1994, Mosby.)*

IgM Antibodies

The IgM assay was widely used in the past, but this assay is not recommended for routine use in adults because it may yield frequent false-positive or false-negative results, particularly in immunocompromised patients, pregnant women, and patients from areas where *Toxoplasma* infection is highly endemic. IgM antibodies tend to appear earlier and decline more rapidly than IgG antibodies. Persistently elevated IgM-specific antibody titers after the initial infection can lead to false-positive results and difficulty in interpreting these tests.

In patients with recently acquired infection, IgM *T. gondii* antibodies are detected initially, and in most cases these titers become negative within a few months. In some patients, however, positive IgM *T. gondii*–specific titers can be observed during the chronic stage of the infection. IgM antibodies have been reported to persist as long as 12 years after the acute infection. Persistence of these IgM antibodies does not seem to be clinically relevant, and these patients should be considered chronically infected.

Clinicians should be cautious when using IgM antibody levels in prenatal screening. Any positive result in a pregnant patient confirmed positive by a second reference laboratory should be evaluated by amniocentesis and PCR testing for *T. gondii*. A negative result does not rule out the presence of PCR inhibitors in the patient specimen or *T. gondii* DNA concentrations below the level of detection of the assay.

The U.S. Food and Drug Administration (FDA) has recommended that sera with positive IgM test results obtained at nonreference laboratories should be sent to a *Toxoplasma* reference laboratory. After IgM-positive sera undergo confir-

Table 20-1	Diagnostic Evaluation of Toxoplasmosis
Test	**Recommended Use**
Toxoplasma gondii antibodies, IgG and IgM	First-line test in endemic areas for identifying *T. gondii* infection in pregnant women.
	Diagnosis of opportunistic infections in immunocompromised hosts.
T. gondii by polymerase chain reaction (PCR)	Confirmation of toxoplasmosis infection in immunocompromised hosts.
T. gondii antibody, IgM	When results from initial antibody testing are equivocal.
T. gondii antibody, IgG	When results from initial antibody testing are equivocal.

Data from ARUP Laboratories, www.arup.com, 2007.

matory testing, the results are interpreted as (1) a recently acquired infection, (2) an infection acquired in the past, or (3) a false-positive result.

IgA Antibodies

Immunoglobulin A (IgA) antibodies may be detected in sera of acutely infected adults and congenitally infected infants using ELISA or **immunosorbent agglutination assay (ISAGA)** methods. As with IgM, the IgA antibodies may persist for many months to more than 1 year and offer little additional assistance for diagnosis of the acute infection in the adult. Increased sensitivity of IgA assays over IgM assays for diagnosis of congenital toxoplasmosis represents an advance in diagnosis of the infection in the fetus and newborn.

In addition to detecting IgA specific for *T. gondii,* the avidity of IgA can be determined. This is useful during the first trimester of pregnancy in determining whether infection has occurred. ELISA rarely detects IgA antibodies in the sera of AIDS patients with toxoplasmic encephalitis.

IgE Antibodies

Immunoglobulin E (IgE) antibodies are detectable by ELISA in sera of acutely infected adults, congenitally infected infants, and children with congenital toxoplasmic chorioretinitis. The IgE ISAGA, which binds the patient's IgE to a solid surface and uses intact tachyzoites to detect IgE antibodies, is read in the same manner as the agglutination test. For the diagnosis of *T. gondii* infection in the newborn or fetus, IgE testing does not appear to be as useful as IgA testing.

The duration of IgE seropositivity is less than with IgM or IgA antibodies and appears useful as an adjunctive method for identifying recently acquired infections. IgE-specific antibodies have been detected in patients with toxoplasmic encephalitis.

IgG Antibodies

Immunoglobulin G (IgG) antibodies appear 1 to 2 weeks after the initial infection, peak after about 6 to 8 weeks, decline gradually over the next 1 to 2 years, and in some cases, persist for life. The most widely used tests to measure the IgG responses to *T. gondii* are the (1) Sabin-Feldman dye test, (2) ELISA, (3) IFA test, and (4) modified (differential) agglutination test.

Sabin-Feldman Dye Test. IgG antibodies are primarily measured by the Sabin-Feldman dye test (DT). This is considered the "gold standard." The DT is a sensitive and specific neutralization test in which live organisms are lysed in the presence of complement and the patient's IgG *T. gondii*–specific antibody. IgG antibodies usually appear within 1 to 2 weeks of the infection, peak within 1 to 2 months, fall at variable rates, and usually persist for life. The titer does not correlate with the severity of illness. This test is available mainly in reference laboratories.

A negative test result practically rules out prior *T. gondii* exposure (unless the patient is hypogammaglobulinemic).

In a small number of patients, IgG antibodies might not be detected within 2 to 3 weeks after the initial exposure to the parasite. Rare cases of toxoplasmic chorioretinitis and toxoplasmic encephalitis have been documented in immunocompromised patients negative for *T. gondii*–specific IgG antibodies.

ELISA. The ELISA-based test detects IgG antibodies to *T. gondii.* No single IgG titer can differentiate a recent infection from a previously acquired infection.

IFA Test. This test uses killed organisms as a substrate, with patient serum assayed for activity against them. IFA is used widely because it measures the same antibodies as the Sabin-Feldman DT, and results parallel DT results. False-positive results may occur with sera that contain antinuclear antibodies; false-negative results may occur when using sera from patients with low titers of IgG antibody.

Differential Agglutination Test. The differential agglutination test (also known as the "AC/HS test") uses two antigen preparations that express antigenic determinants found early after acute infection (*AC* antigen) or in the later stages of infection (*HS* antigen). Ratios of titers using AC versus HS antigen are interpreted as acute, equivocal, nonacute patterns of reactivity or nonreactive. The acute pattern may persist for 1 or more years after infection. This test has proved useful in helping differentiate acute from chronic infections but is best used in combination with a panel of other tests.

The strength of this test is helping to differentiate a recent (acute) from a remote infection in adults and older children. Agglutination titers to formalin-fixed tachyzoites (HS antigen) are compared with titers against acetone-fixed or methanol-fixed tachyzoites (AC antigen). In general, an acute pattern demonstrates high AC and HS titers, whereas a nonacute pattern demonstrates high AC titers and low HS titers. This method can differentiate an acute from a remote infection in pregnant women, whereas IgM and IgA antibodies detectable by ELISA or ISAGA are elevated for prolonged periods.

Avidity Test. The functional affinity of specific IgG antibodies is initially low after primary antigenic challenge and increases during subsequent weeks and months. Protein-denaturing reagents are used to dissociate the antibody-antigen complex. The avidity result is determined using the ratios of antibody titration curves of urea-treated and untreated serum.

The avidity test can be used as an additional confirmatory diagnostic tool in patients with a positive or equivocal IgM test or with an acute or equivocal pattern in the AC/HS test. Its highest value is observed when laboratory test results reveal high–IgG avidity antibodies and the serum is obtained during the time window of exclusion of acute infection for a particular method (range, 12-16 weeks). Low- or equivocal–IgG avidity antibody results should not be interpreted as diagnostic of recently acquired infection. These low- or equivocal-avidity antibodies can persist for months to 1 year or longer.

Studies of the avidity of IgG in pregnant women who have seroconverted during gestation have shown that women with high-avidity test results were infected with *T. gondii* at least 3 to 5 months earlier (time to conversion from low-avidity to high-avidity antibodies varies with the method used). Because low-avidity antibodies may persist for many months, their presence does not necessarily indicate recently acquired infection.

Polymerase Chain Reaction

Polymerase chain reaction (PCR) amplification is used to detect *T. gondii* DNA in body fluids and tissues. PCR can be used to detect the presence or absence of *T. gondii* DNA in fresh or frozen biopsy tissue, cerebrospinal fluid (CSF), amniotic fluid, serum, or plasma. A negative result does not rule out the presence of PCR inhibitors in the specimen or *T. gondii* DNA concentrations below the level of detection by the assay.

A PCR test performed on amniotic fluid has revolutionized the diagnosis of fetal *T. gondii* infection by enabling an early diagnosis to be made, which avoids the use of more invasive procedures on the fetus.

Lateral Blot Rapid Tests

Lateral blot Toxo IgG card tests (BioQuant, San Diego) is a chromatographic immunoassay in which a lateral-flow immunoblot assay designed for qualitative detection of IgM or IgG antibodies to *T. gondii* in human serum or plasma. *Toxoplasma* antigens are immobilized on the membrane within the test zone. Specimen applied in the membrane of the sample area migrates by capillary action through the test zone. *T. gondii*–specific IgM or IgG antibodies present in the specimen are captured by the immobilized antigens in the test zone and subsequently visualized in the form of a magenta test line by the gold–protein A conjugate applied to the test card. The absence of a test line indicates a negative test. A magenta control zone is included as a quality control measure.

Histologic Diagnosis

Demonstration of tachyzoites in tissue sections or smears of body fluid (e.g., CSF, amniotic fluid, bronchoalveolar lavage fluid) establishes the diagnosis of the acute infection. The immunoperoxidase method is applicable to unfixed or formalin-fixed paraffin-embedded tissue sections.

A rapid and technically simple method is the detection of *T. gondii* in air-dried, Wright-Giemsa–stained slides of centrifuged (e.g., cytocentrifuged) sediment of CSF or of brain aspirate or in impression smears of biopsy tissue. Multiple tissue cysts near an inflammatory necrotic lesion indicate acute infection or reactivation of latent infection.

Cell Culture

Detection of *T. gondii* in the blood could represent a major advance in the diagnosis of toxoplasmosis in patients with AIDS. A new cell culture method for the growth of *T. gondii* has been developed using monocytes. After 4 days, parasites in the culture are revealed by immunofluorescence with an anti-P30 monoclonal antibody. A quantitative and qualitative analysis by cytofluorometry can then be performed on the cultured cells.

CASE STUDY

History and Physical Examination

A 24-year-old woman with a history of AIDS presents for evaluation of left-sided weakness. She has also been experiencing headaches and seizures, and others have observed an alteration in her mental status.

The patient's medical history is notable for an episode of *Pneumocystis carinii* pneumonia, primary syphilis treated with penicillin 5 years ago, and occasional thrush. She takes zidovudine and monthly aerosolized pentamidine for *Pneumocystis* prophylaxis. An urgent computed tomography (CT) scan of the head shows two 1-cm lesions in the right basal ganglia, enhanced with intravenous contrast media.

Laboratory Data

CD4 cell count: 50×10^9/L
Rapid plasma reagin (RPR): positive at 1:2
Toxoplasmosis IgG: positive
Toxoplasmosis IgM: negative

Questions and Discussion

1. What is the most common cause of lesions in the brain?

Cerebral toxoplasmosis is the most common cause of CNS mass lesions in patients with AIDS. Lesions occur in approximately one third of AIDS patients seropositive for *T. gondii*. Other conditions that may produce CNS mass lesions in these patients include CNS lymphoma, progressive multifocal leukoencephalopathy, and more rarely, bacterial and fungal brain abscesses.

2. What is the source of this infection?

Disease is believed to occur from the reactivation of a prior infection. Initially, in cases of toxoplasmosis, accidental ingestion of oocysts by humans and animals, including cats, produces a proliferative infection in the body tissues. Fecal contamination of food or water, soiled hands, inadequately cooked or infected meat, and raw milk can be major sources of human infection. Transfusion-transmitted toxoplasmosis has been associated with leukocyte concentrates. Patients at risk are those receiving immunosuppressive agents or corticosteroids.

3. Is this a newly acquired infection?

In these cases, serologic studies usually show positive IgG and negative IgM tests, indicating the initial infection occurred in the past.

The diagnosis is established by serologically demonstrating marked elevations of *Toxoplasma* antibodies. Antibodies are demonstrable within the first 2 weeks after infection, rising to high levels early in the infection, then falling slightly, but persisting at an elevated level for months before declining to low levels after many years.

Levels of IgM and IgG antibodies to *T. gondii* can be determined serologically. The presence of IgM to *T. gondii* in an adult indicates an active infection. In the newborn, detection of IgM also suggests an active infection because IgM antibodies are not able to cross the placenta; therefore they are of fetal origin.

4. How can the patient be treated?

Lifelong therapy is needed because this infection tends to recur in those with prior disease.

5. Should pregnant women be tested for this microorganism?

It is recommended that all pregnant women be tested for toxoplasmosis immunity. If a patient is susceptible, screening should be repeated during pregnancy and at delivery. Prevention of infection in pregnant women should be practiced to avert congenital toxoplasmosis. To further prevent infection of the fetus, at-risk women should be identified by serologic testing, and pregnant women with primary infection should receive drug therapy. Treatment consists of a combination of pyrimethamine and sulfadiazine. These drugs, with leucovorin to counter the side effects, can be administered orally from midpregnancy to delivery. The newborn is treated with the same drugs for the first 2 weeks postpartum.

Diagnosis

Toxoplasmosis.

CHAPTER HIGHLIGHTS

- Toxoplasmosis is a widespread disease in humans and animals caused by *Toxoplasma gondii,* often found in cat feces.
- Fecal contamination of food or water, soiled hands, inadequately cooked or infected meat, and raw milk are sources of human infection. All mammals, including humans, can transmit the infection transplacentally.
- In adults and children other than newborns the disease is usually asymptomatic. A generalized infection probably occurs.
- Although spontaneous recovery follows acute febrile disease, the organism can multiply in any organ of the body or circulatory system.
- Congenital toxoplasmosis can result in central nervous system malformation or prenatal mortality.
- *T. gondii* is difficult to culture and diagnosis must be supported by serologic methods to determine levels of IgM and IgG antibodies to *T. gondii*. IgM to *T. gondii* in an adult indicates active infection. Detection of IgM also suggests active infection in the newborn.
- ELISA is the method of choice for detection of IgM antibodies in toxoplasmosis. Serologic tests include IFA, chemiluminescent immunoassay, and PCR.

REVIEW QUESTIONS

1. Toxoplasmosis is a _____ infection.
   a. bacterial
   b. mycotic
   c. parasitic
   d. viral

2. The definitive host of *T. gondii* is the:
   a. Horse.
   b. Pig.
   c. Dog.
   d. Domestic cat.

3. All the following are specific methods for preventing congenital toxoplasmosis *except:*
   a. Avoid touching mucous membranes while handling raw meat.
   b. Wash hands thoroughly after handling raw meat.
   c. Eliminate food contamination by flies, cockroaches, and other insects.
   d. Dispose of fecally contaminated cat litter into plastic garbage bags.

4. The presence of IgM to *T. gondii* in an adult is indicative of:
   a. Carrier state.
   b. Active infection.
   c. Chronic infection.
   d. Latent disease.

5. All the following characteristics are correct regarding toxoplasmosis *except:*
   a. It is recognized as a tissue coccidian.
   b. Domestic dogs are a source of the disease.
   c. It can be transmitted by infected blood.
   d. It can be transmitted transplacentally.

6. Toxoplasmosis is a serious health threat to:
   a. AIDS patients.
   b. Adults.
   c. Children more than 2 years old.
   d. Elderly patients.

7. Congenital toxoplasmosis can cause:
   a. Congenital heart disease.
   b. Central nervous system malformation.
   c. Urinary tract infections.
   d. Muscular disorders.

8. Antibodies to *T. gondii* are demonstrable _____ after infection.
   a. 3 to 5 days
   b. within 10 days
   c. within 2 weeks
   d. within 4 weeks

9. The method of choice for detecting IgM antibodies in toxoplasmosis is:

a. Enzyme-linked immunosorbent assay (ELISA).
b. Indirect fluorescent antibody (IFA).
c. Indirect hemagglutination (IHA).
d. Complement fixation (CF).

BIBLIOGRAPHY

Associated Regional and University Pathologists (ARUP): Reference test guide, 2002, www.aruplab.com.

Beaman MH, Luft BJ, Remington JS: Prophylaxis for toxoplasmosis in AIDS, *Ann Intern Med* 117(2):163-164, 1992.

Bruce-Chwatt LJ: Transfusion associated parasitic infections. In Bruce-Chwatt LJ: *Infection, immunity, and blood transfusion,* New York, 1985, Alan R Liss.

Forbes BA, Sahm DF, Weissfeld AS: *Bailey and Scott's diagnostic microbiology,* ed 12, St Louis, 2007, Mosby.

Hill DE, Chirukandoth S, Dubey JP: Biology and epidemiology of *Toxoplasma gondii* in man and animals, *Anim Health Res Rev* 6(1):41-61, 2005.

Jones JL, Schulkin J, Maguire JH: Therapy for common parasitic diseases in pregnancy in the United States: a review and a survey of obstetrician/gynecologists' level of knowledge about these diseases, *Obstet Gynecol Surv* 60(6):386-393, 2005.

Kravetz JD, Federman DG: Toxoplasmosis in pregnancy, *Am J Med* 118(3):212-216, 2005.

Lopez A et al: Preventing congenital toxoplasmosis, *MMWR* 49(RR-2):59-68, 2000.

Montoya JG, Kovacs JA, Remington JS: *Toxoplasma gondii.* In Mandell GL et al: *Principles and practice of infectious diseases,* ed 6, Philadelphia, 2005, Churchill Livingstone, pp 3170-3198.

Montoya JG: Laboratory diagnosis of *Toxoplasma gondii* infection and toxoplasmosis, *J Infect Dis* 185(suppl 1):S73-S82, 2002.

Montoya JG, Liesenfeld O: Toxoplasmosis, *Lancet* 363(9425):1965-1976, 2004.

Montoya JG, Rosso F: Diagnosis and management of toxoplasmosis, *Clin Perinatol* 32(3):705-726, 2005.

Tirard V et al: Diagnosis of toxoplasmosis in patients with AIDS by isolation of the parasite from the blood, *N Engl J Med* 324(9):634, 1991.

Turgeon ML: *Clinical hematology,* ed 3, Philadelphia, 2005, Lippincott–Williams & Wilkins.

CHAPTER 21

Cytomegalovirus

Etiology
Epidemiology
  Transmission
  Latent Infection
  Congenital Infection
Signs and Symptoms
  Acquired Infection
  Congenital Infection
Immunologic Manifestations
  Immune System Alterations
  Serologic Markers

Laboratory Evaluation
Passive Latex Agglutination for Detection
  of Antibodies to Cytomegalovirus
Quantitative Determination of IgG Antibodies
  to Cytomegalovirus
Case Study
Chapter Highlights
Review Questions
Bibliography

Learning Objectives

At the conclusion of this chapter, the reader should be able to:

- Discuss the etiology and epidemiology of acquired, latent, and congenital cytomegalovirus (CMV) infection.
- Explain the signs and symptoms of acquired and congenital CMV infections.
- Describe the immunologic manifestations of CMV.

- Identify and explain the serologic markers and diagnostic evaluation of CMV.
- Discuss the principles and applications of the passive latex agglutination and other quantitative determination of IgM and IgG antibodies.

ETIOLOGY

Cytomegalovirus (CMV) is a ubiquitous human viral pathogen. The first descriptive report of histologic changes characteristic of those now associated with CMV infection was originally published in 1904, when protozoan-like cells in the lungs, kidneys, and liver of a syphilitic fetus were seen. It was not until 1956 and 1957 that CMV was isolated in the laboratory. Actual isolation of the virus after transfusion, as well as observation of elevated antibody titers, occurred in 1966.

Human CMV is classified as a member of the herpes family of viruses (herpesviruses). There are presently five recognized human herpesviruses: herpes simplex I, herpes simplex II, varicella-zoster virus (VZV), and Epstein-Barr virus (EBV), and CMV. All the herpesviruses are relatively large, enveloped DNA viruses that undergo a replicative cycle involving DNA expression and nucleocapsid assembly within the nucleus. The viral structure gains an envelope when the virus buds through the nuclear membrane, which in turn is altered to contain specific viral proteins.

Although the herpesviruses produce diverse clinical diseases, they share the basic characteristic of being *cell associated*. The requirements for cell association vary, but herpesviruses may spread from cell to cell, presumably via intercellular bridges and in the presence of antibody in the extracellular phase. CMV spreads to the lymphoid tissues and proceeds to circulate to systemic lymph nodes. The virus finally comes to rest in the epithelial cells of many tissues. This common characteristic may play a role in the ability of these viruses to produce subclinical infections that can be reactivated under appropriate stimuli.

EPIDEMIOLOGY

Cytomegalovirus infection is endemic worldwide, with the majority of urban adults demonstrating evidence of infection; 50% to 80% of U.S. adults are infected with CMV by age 40. The prevalence of CMV seropositivity increases steadily with age. CMV is found in all geographic and socioeconomic groups, but in general it is more widespread in developing countries and areas of lower socioeconomic conditions.

Cytomegalovirus is a major health risk because a large proportion of women, particularly white women, entering their childbearing years lack antibody to CMV. Those at greatest risk of infection are fetuses and immunocompromised persons. CMV is the most common virus transmitted to the fetus. Approximately 1 in 150 children is born with congenital CMV infection. Approximately 8000 children each year suffer permanent disabilities caused by CMV.

Transmission

Transmission of CMV may be by oral, respiratory, or venereal routes. The virus has been isolated in urine, saliva, feces, breast milk, blood, cervical secretions, virus-infected grafts from a donor, semen, vaginal fluid, and respiratory droplets. It may also be transmitted by the transfusion of fresh blood.

Transmission of CMV appears to require intimate contact with secretions or excretions.

Peripheral blood leukocytes and transplanted tissues are strongly incriminated as sources of CMV. Transmission of CMV by transfusion of blood or blood components containing white blood cells (WBCs) is assuming increased importance in patients with severely impaired immunity who require supportive therapy. Low-birth-weight (LBW) neonates are also at high risk for CMV infection through transfusion of CMV-infected blood products. Preventive methods in these patients include effective donor screening, leukocyte-depleted blood products, and immune globulin containing passively acquired CMV antibodies.

Once in a person's body, CMV stays there for life. Most CMV infections are "silent," causing no signs or symptoms. Individuals who are CMV positive (infected with CMV in the past) usually do not have virus in urine or saliva, so the risk of acquiring a CMV infection from casual contact is negligible.

Women who are pregnant or planning a pregnancy should follow hygienic practices (e.g., careful handwashing) to avoid CMV infection. Because young children are more likely to have CMV in their urine or saliva than are older children or adults, pregnant women who have young children or work with young children should be especially careful.

Health care professionals are one of the groups becoming increasingly concerned about the risks associated with exposure to CMV. Nosocomial transmission from patients to health care workers has not been documented, but observance of good personal hygiene and handwashing offer the best measures for preventing transmission.

Latent Infection

Persistent infections characterized by periods of reactivation are frequently termed *latent infections*. CMV can persist in a latent state, and active infections may develop under a variety of conditions (e.g., pregnancy; immunosuppression; after organ, bone, or stem cell transplantation). Of immunosuppressed patients, only seronegative patients appear to be at a significant risk of developing CMV infection. Patients at the highest risk of mortality from CMV infections are allograft transplant, seronegative patients who receive tissue from a seropositive donor. The great majority of infections in allograft recipients are transmitted by a donated organ or arise from the reactivation of the recipient's latent virus.

True viral latency is defined by the presence of the genetic information in an unexpressed state in the host cell. An operational definition of *latency* can include the conditions of a dynamic relationship between the virus and the host, along with evidence of latency and reactivation of a latent infection. As with any herpesvirus, CMV reactivation is possible at any time, but rarely manifests in immunocompetent individuals.

Congenital Infection

Primary and recurrent maternal CMV infection can be transmitted in utero. Congenital CMV infection is the most common intrauterine infection, affecting 0.4% to 2.3% of all live births in the United States. The presence of maternal antibody to CMV before conception provides substantial protection against damaging congenital CMV infection in the newborn.

Primary maternal infection during pregnancy, occurring in 1% to 3% of U.S. women, is associated with more severe sequelae of congenital CMV infection. Infected infants can become severely ill, and premature infants may die. Most newborns infected with CMV survive, but they may be mentally impaired or may develop other health problems. Approximately 10% of congenitally infected infants have symptoms at birth, and of the 90% who are asymptomatic, 10% to 15% will develop symptoms over months or even years.

SIGNS AND SYMPTOMS

Acquired Infection

Acquired CMV infection is usually asymptomatic and can persist in the host as a chronic or latent infection. The incubation period is believed to be 3 to 12 weeks.

In the majority of patients, CMV infection is asymptomatic. Occasionally a self-limited, heterophile-negative, mononucleosis-like syndrome results. CMV hepatitis can occur as well.

Symptoms include a sore throat and fever, swollen glands, chills, profound malaise, and myalgia. Lymphadenopathy and splenomegaly may be observed. Infections occurring in healthy immunocompetent individuals usually result in seroconversion. Virus may be excreted in the urine during both primary and recurrent CMV infection; it can persist sporadically for months or years. Persons experiencing acquired infection, reinfection with the same or different strains of CMV, or reactivation of a latent infection can excrete the virus in titers as high as 10^6 infective units/mL in the urine or saliva for weeks or months.

Normal adults and children usually experience CMV infection without serious complications. Infrequent complications of CMV infection in previously healthy individuals, however, include interstitial pneumonitis, hepatitis, Guillain-Barré syndrome, meningoencephalitis, myocarditis, thrombocytopenia, and hemolytic anemia.

However, CMV infection can be life threatening in immunosuppressed patients. Infections in these patients may result in disseminated multisystem involvement, including pneumonitis, hepatitis, gastrointestinal (GI) ulceration, arthralgias, meningoencephalitis, and retinitis. Retinitis and encephalitis are common manifestation of disseminated CMV. Ulcerative damage of tissues (e.g., esophagus) is another demonstration of the cytopathic effect of CMV. Interstitial pneumonitis, frequently associated with CMV infection, is a major cause of death after allogeneic bone marrow transplantation. In premature infants, acquired CMV infection can result in atypical lymphocytosis, hepatosplenomegaly, pneumonia, or death.

Transfusion-acquired CMV infections may cause not only mononucleosis-like syndrome but also hepatitis and increased rejection of transplanted organs. The following three types of CMV infections are possible in blood transfusion recipients:

1. *Primary infection* occurs when a previously unexposed (seronegative) recipient is transfused with blood from an actively or latently infected donor. This type of infection is accompanied by the presence of virus in the blood and urine, an immediate antibody response, and eventual seroconversion. Patients with primary infections may be symptomatic, but the great majority are asymptomatic.

2. *Reactivated infection* can occur when a seropositive recipient is transfused with blood from either a CMV antibody–positive or –negative donor. Donor leukocytes are thought to trigger an allograft reaction, which in turn reactivates the recipient's latent infection. Such infections may be accompanied by significant increases in CMV-specific antibody. Some reactivated infections exhibit viral shedding as their only manifestation. Reactivated infections are largely asymptomatic.

3. *Reinfection* can occur by a CMV strain in the donor's blood that differs from the strain originally infecting the recipient. A significant antibody response is observed, and viral shedding occurs. Although it is difficult to differentiate a reactivated infection if both the patient and the donor are CMV antibody positive before transfusion, reinfections can be documented if isolates can be obtained from both donor and recipient.

Congenital Infection

The classic congenital CMV syndrome is manifested by a high incidence of neurologic symptoms, as well as neuromuscular disorders, jaundice, hepatomegaly, and splenomegaly (Figure 21-1). Petechia is the most common clinical sign, seen in about 50% of CMV-infected infants.

Congenitally infected newborns, especially those who acquire CMV during a maternal primary infection, are more prone to develop severe **cytomegalic inclusion disease (CID).** The severe form of CID may be fatal or can cause permanent neurologic sequelae, such as intracranial calcifi-

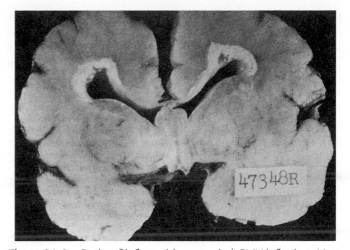

Figure 21-2 Brain of infant with congenital CMV infection. Note extensive periventricular necrosis and calcification. *(From Krugman S et al:* Infectious diseases of children, *ed 9, St Louis, 1992, Mosby.)*

cations (Figure 21-2), mental retardation, deafness, vision defects, microcephaly, and motor dysfunction. Psychomotor impairment is seen in 51% to 75% of survivors. Hearing loss is observed in 21% to 50% and visual impairment in 20% of patients. Infants without symptoms at birth may develop hearing impairment and neurologic impairment later.

IMMUNOLOGIC MANIFESTATIONS

Immune System Alterations

Cytomegalovirus infection is known to alter the immune system, as well as produce overt manifestations of infection. Infection interferes with immune responsiveness in both normal and immunocompromised individuals. This diminished responsiveness results in a decreased proliferative response to the CMV antigen, which persists for several months. In patients with CMV mononucleosis-like syndrome, alterations of T-lymphocyte subsets result, producing an increase in the absolute number of CD8+ lymphocytes and a decrease in CD4+ lymphocytes. These subset abnormalities persist for months.

Questions have been raised regarding CMV as a potentially oncogenic virus because viral antigens and nucleic acids have been found in human malignancies, which include adenocarcinoma of the colon, carcinoma of the cervix, cancer of the prostate, and Kaposi's sarcoma. CMV does have transforming properties in vitro. Although considerable circumstantial evidence exists linking CMV to human malignancies, especially Kaposi's sarcoma, a direct cause-and-effect relationship has not been established.

Serologic Markers

In cells infected by CMV, several antigens appear at varying times after infection. Before replication of viral DNA takes place, immediate-early antigens and early antigens are present in the nuclei of infected cells. *Immediate-early* antigens appear within 1 hour of cellular infection, and *early* antigens are

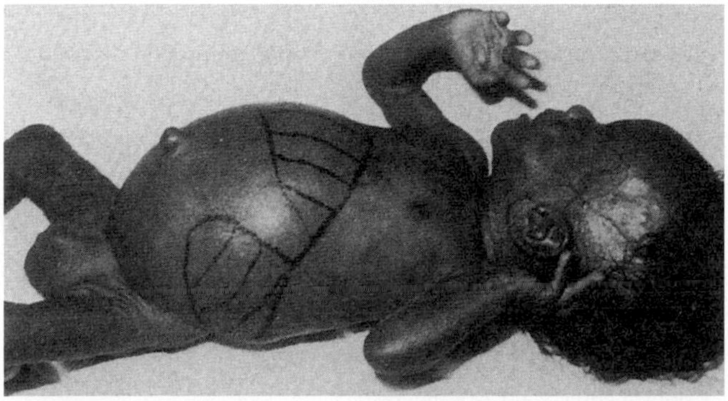

Figure 21-1 Four-month-old child with symptomatic congenital cytomegalovirus (CMV) infection manifesting severe failure to thrive, hepatitis with hepatosplenomegaly, bilateral inguinal hernia, and micropenis. *(From Krugman S et al:* Infectious diseases of children, *ed 9, St Louis, 1992, Mosby.)*

present within 24 hours. At about 72 hours after infection, or the end of the viral replication cycle, *late* antigens are demonstrable in the nucleus and cytoplasm of infected cells.

The immune antibody response to these various antigens differs in incidence and significance. The presence of antibodies against immediate-early and early antigens is associated with active infection, either primary or reactivated. New CMV infections can be identified by testing for immunoglobulin G (IgG) antibodies on blood samples taken at different times. If the first sample is negative and the second sample is positive, the patient became infected with CMV between the two blood samples. A new method, called *IgG avidity testing*, needs only one blood sample to show recent CMV infection. However, this test is currently not commercially available in the United States. A traditional test used IgM antibodies to detect recent infections. Because this test is often positive when there is no new CMV infection, it should not be used without the other tests.

Antibody to early antigen undergoes a relatively rapid decline after recovery but can persist for up to 250 days, and it may identify patients with recent, as well as active, infections. The presence of antibody to early antigen is strongly associated with viral shedding. Antibodies to late antigens persist in high titer long after the recovery from an active infection.

The incidence of viral exposure and subsequent antibody formation (seropositivity) varies greatly depending on the socioeconomic status and living conditions of the population surveyed. The prevalence of CMV antibody varies with age and geographic location but ranges from 40% to 100%.

The characteristic antibody responses associated with infection are as follows:

- *Primary infection,* demonstrated by a transient virus-specific IgM antibody response and eventual seroconversion to produce IgG antibodies to the virus.

- *Reactivation* of latent infection in seropositive (IgG) individuals, which may be accompanied by significant increases in IgG antibodies to the virus, but which elicits no detectable IgM response.
- *Reinfection* by a strain of CMV different from the original infecting strain. A significant IgG antibody response is demonstrated. It is not known whether an IgM response occurs.

There is no available vaccine for preventing congenital CMV disease (present at birth). A few CMV vaccines are being tested in humans, including live, attenuated (weakened) virus vaccines and vaccines that contain only pieces of the virus.

In CMV infection, hematologic examination of the blood usually reveals a characteristic leukocytosis. A slight lymphocytosis with more than 20% variant lymphocytes is common. CMV infection is possible in the following situations:

- The patient has mononucleosis-like symptoms but exhibits a negative EBV test result.
- The patient manifests hepatitis symptoms but does not demonstrate any positive results when tested for common hepatitis viruses.

In affected infants the most common laboratory abnormality is a low platelet count (thrombocytopenia). Clinical chemistry assays may demonstrate abnormal liver function tests. Presence of infection is also demonstrated by inclusion bodies in leukocytes in urine sediment.

LABORATORY EVALUATION

In immunocompromised patients, CMV serology is not recommended. The preferred method for diagnosis is culture of virus and/or polymerase chain reaction (PCR). A variety of methods can be used for screening purposes (Table 21-1).

Table 21-1	Laboratory Diagnosis of Cytomegalovirus (CMV) Infection*	
Target	**Test Method**	**Recommended Use**
CMV cell	Culture, immunofluorescence	Diagnose CMV infection. Gold standard test for tissue.
CMV	PCR	Rapid test for diagnosing CMV in immunocompromised patients or organ donors.
CMV DNA quantitation	PCR	Diagnose CMV infection. Monitor disease state in organ transplant and HIV patients.
CMV: whole blood or bone marrow	PCR	Diagnose CMV infection.
CMV antibodies: IgG and IgM	Latex agglutination	Screen pregnant women and infants possibly infected with CMV. Infants may test positive during first 6 months due to maternal antibodies. Discriminate between current (IgM) and prior infections (IgG).
CMV antibodies: total	Solid-phase agglutination	Screen organ donors.
CMV antibody, IgM	ELISA	Confirm equivocal CMV IgM results.
CMV antibody, IgG	Chemiluminescent immunoassay	Confirm equivocal CMV IgG results.

Modified from ARUP Laboratories, 2008, www.arup.com.
*A negative result (<2.6 log copies/mL, or <390 copies/mL) does not rule out the presence of polymerase chain reaction *(PCR)* inhibitors in the patient specimen or CMV nucleic acid in concentrations below the assay's level of detection. Inhibition may also lead to underestimation of viral quantitation.
HIV, Human immunodeficiency virus; *ELISA,* enzyme-linked immunosorbent assay.

A fourfold rise in IgG antibody titer suggests, but does not prove, recent CMV infection. The presence of IgG antibody in infants complicates the interpretation of serologic results during the first 6 months of life because the antibody may be maternal in origin.

Passive Latex Agglutination for Detection of Antibodies to Cytomegalovirus

Principle

The CMVscan Card Test* is a passive latex agglutination test for the detection of IgM and IgG CMV antibodies. It can be used as a diagnostic tool or to screen donor specimens for antibodies to CMV in human serum and plasma. This assay can be performed *qualitatively* on undiluted serum to identify antibodies to CMV and *quantitatively* using serial twofold dilutions to determine the titer of CMV antibody.

In this procedure, latex particles previously sensitized with CMV viral antigen are mixed with serum. If antibody to CMV is present, the agglutinated particles will be macroscopically visible. In the absence of specific antibody or in the event of low antibody concentration, the latex particles will not agglutinate in the reaction mixture, and the particles will appear smooth and evenly dispersed.

The absence of CMV antibodies suggests no viral exposure, whereas presence of CMV antibodies indicates previous exposure to the virus. Recurrent infection, if it occurs, may not be as severe as primary infection. Because CMV is a blood-borne pathogen, infection is of greatest concern to newborn infants requiring transfusion and immunosuppressed allograft recipients.

Specimen Collection and Preparation

No special preparation of the patient is required before specimen collection. The patient must be positively identified when the specimen is collected, and the specimen is to be labeled at the bedside. Specimen labels must include the patient's full name, the date the specimen is collected, the patient's hospital identification number, and the phlebotomist's initials.

Blood should be drawn by aseptic technique. A minimum of 2 mL of clotted blood (red-top–evacuated tube) or anticoagulated blood (lavender-top–evacuated tube) is required. The specimen should be centrifuged promptly and an aliquot of serum or plasma removed. Plasma specimens containing ethylenediaminetetraacetic acid (EDTA) or heparin as an anticoagulant can be used for qualitative or quantitative testing using the same technique as for serum samples. Plasma specimens containing citrate-phosphate-dextrose-adenine (CPDA-1) as an anticoagulant can also be used for qualitative or quantitative testing after a 1% dilution is made with the buffer.

Serum or plasma specimens may be stored for up to 1 week at 2° to 8° C or frozen at −18° C, or lower if longer storage is required. Serum specimens with obvious microbial contamination should not be used for testing. The presence of mild lipemia or hemolysis will not affect the test.

Testing of CPDA-1 plasma specimens from platelet units stored at 22° C for 5 days and from red blood cell (RBC) units prepared for transfusion stored at 2° to 6° C for 14 days has been successful.

Reagents, Supplies, and Equipment

CMVscan Card Test Kit Components (supplied with the CMVscan Kit, Franklin Lakes, NJ)
- Reagent A: CMVscan Latex Antigen

  CMV antigen–coated latex particles prepared from disrupted CMV (strain AD 169) judged to be inactivated by bioassay procedures. This preparation contains 0.02% gentamicin and 0.02% sodium azide (preservatives). Refrigerate at 2° to 8° C to store, and return to refrigerator when not in use. Do not freeze or use beyond expiration date on the label. Do not mix reagents from different kit lot numbers. Avoid microbial contamination of reagents.
- Reagent B: dilution buffer

  Phosphate-buffered saline (PBS) solution, pH 7.4, containing bovine serum albumin with 0.02% sodium azide (preservative). Refrigerate at 2° to 8° C to store, and return to refrigerator when not in use. Do not freeze or use beyond expiration date on the label.
- Test cards

  These cards must be flat for proper reactions. If necessary, flatten cards by bowing back in the direction opposite that of the curl. Do not touch test areas; fingerprints may result in an oily deposit and improper test results. Use each card once and discard. Store the cards in their original packaging in a dry area at room temperature.
- Plastic stirrers
- Dispensing needle, 21 gauge, green hub

  On completion of daily tests, remove the needle from the dispensing bottle and recap the bottle. Rinse the needle with distilled water to maintain a clear passage and accurate drop delivery. Do not wipe the dispensing needle; it is silicone coated, and wiping can remove the silicone.

Additional Required Equipment and Supplies (not supplied with kit)
- Centrifuge
- Rotator with humidifying cover

  The recommended rotation speed is 100 ±2 rpm, but rotation at 95 to 110 rpm does not significantly affect results. The rotator should circumscribe a circle approximately 2 cm in diameter in the horizontal plane. A moistened humidifier cover must be used to prevent drying of test specimens during rotation.
- High-intensity incandescent lamp
- Micropipettors, 25 μL delivery
- Vortex mixer
- General equipment necessary for preparation, storage, and handling of serologic specimens

---

*Product insert revised March 2005; Becton Dickinson, Franklin Lakes, NJ.

Quality Control

CMVscan Test Control ++ (high-reactive control): human serum with 0.1% sodium azide (preservative). This control should demonstrate agglutination when tested.

CMVscan Test Control + (low-reactive control): human serum with 0.1% sodium azide (preservative). This control should demonstrate agglutination when tested.

CMVscan Test Control − (nonreactive control): human serum with 0.1% sodium azide. This control should demonstrate no agglutination when tested.

The control serum must react appropriately.

Donor Screening (using qualitative procedure)

The CMVscan Test Control − and a 1:4 dilution of the Test Control + should be tested with each batch of patient samples. Refer to the following procedures to make a 1:4 dilution:

Option 1 (for use when testing one batch/day)

1. With a micropipettor, place 50 μL of Reagent B (dilution buffer) on circles A1 and A2.
2. Using the same tip, add 50 μL of Control + to circle A1, and mix by drawing up and down with micropipettor seven times.
3. Using the same micropipettor and tip, transfer 50 μL from circle A1 to circle A2, and mix as before. Withdraw 50 μL from circle A2 and discard.
4. The dilution in the circle is now a 1:4 dilution of the Control + and should be tested immediately using the qualitative testing procedure.

Option 2 (for use when testing more than one batch/day)

1. With a micropipettor, place 150 μL of Reagent B into a clean, dry test tube.
2. With a micropipettor, add 50 μL of Control + to the test tube.
3. Mix thoroughly by vortexing or shaking.
4. The dilution in the tube is now a 1:4 dilution of the Control + and may be used for up to 24 hours to perform quality control (QC) using the qualitative procedure.

Note: The CMVscan Test Control + and Test Control − should be tested each day of use for QC of the qualitative procedure. When using the quantitative procedure, Control ++ and Control + should be titered with each batch of patient samples. If controls do not produce appropriate reactions, the test results are invalid (see Procedure Notes).

Quality control requirements must be performed in accordance with applicable local, state, and federal regulations or accreditation requirements and an individual laboratory's standard QC procedures. It is recommended that the user refer to pertinent Clinical and Laboratory Standards Institute (CLSI) guidelines and Clinical Laboratory Improvements Amendment (CLIA) regulations for appropriate QC practices.

CAUTION: The serum controls are derived from human blood tested by an FDA-approved method for the presence of the antibody to human immunodeficiency virus (HIV) and hepatitis B surface antigen (HbsAg) and found to be nonreactive. However, the control serum is derived from human sources and should be handled in the same manner as clinical serum specimens (Standard Precautions; see Chapter 6).

WARNING: The latex reagent, controls, and buffer contain sodium azide as a preservative. Sodium azide may react with lead and copper plumbing to form highly explosive metal azides. On disposal, flush with a large volume of water to prevent azide buildup. Sodium azide is toxic if inhaled.

Procedure

Preliminary Preparation

1. Allow the reagents to come to room temperature before testing.
2. The latex reagent should be mixed for 5 to 10 seconds (use the highest setting for variable-speed mixers). Vortexing of the CMVscan Latex Antigen (Reagent A) should be performed at the beginning of each batch of specimens, even if more than one batch is tested per day.
3. Remove the cap from the latex reagent and attach the green-hub needle to the tapered fitting.
4. Label each circle of the card with the appropriate identification of patient sera and controls.

Qualitative Testing Procedure

1. Using a micropipettor, place 50 μL of each specimen (patient or controls) onto the appropriately labeled, separate circles, using a new tip each time.
2. Using a new plastic stirrer for each circle, spread the serum to fill the entire circle.
3. Hold the bottle cap over the tip of the needle, and gently invert Reagent A latex reagent dispensing bottle several times. While holding the bottle in an inverted, vertical position, dispense several drops of the latex reagent into the bottle cap until a drop of uniform size has formed. This predropped reagent may be recovered after testing by aspirating it back into the bottle.
4. Dispense one free-falling drop Reagent A (~15 μL) onto each circle containing the serum.
   Note: To ensure proper drop delivery when dispensing latex antigen, the dispensing bottle must be inverted vertically.
5. Hand-rotate the card (back and forth) three or four times to distribute the latex antigen throughout each circle. Avoid cross-contamination with adjacent circles.
6. Place the card on a rotator, and mix for 8 minutes under a moistened humidifying cover.
7. Immediately after rotation, read the card macroscopically in the wet state.

Reading of Test Results

To help differentiate weak agglutination from no agglutination, a brief hand rotation of the card (three or four back-and-forth motions) must be made after mechanical rotation. Results should be read promptly under a high-intensity incandescent lamp. Fluorescent lighting is generally insufficient to distinguish minimally reactive results. The use of magnification in reading test results is not recommended.

Note: Failure to add sample results in inability to spread the sample to fill a circle, as required in the procedure.

Reporting Results

Qualitative Method
Positive (reactive): any agglutination of the latex reagent.
Negative (nonreactive): suspension remains evenly dispersed with no agglutination.

Optional: Quantitative Method
Replace step 3 of the Qualitative Testing Procedure with the following quantitative protocol:

a. Using a micropipettor, place 50 μL of the negative control onto circle #1 in the row marked "nonreactive control." This control requires no dilution.

b. Move to a new row. With a micropipettor, place 50 μL of Reagent B (dilution buffer) into circles #2 through #7. Leave circle #1 empty.

c. Pipette 50 μL of high-reactive control (Test Control ++) onto circle #1.

d. Using the same micropipettor and tip, add an additional 50 μL of high-reactive control directly into the buffer in circle #2. Mix the serum and buffer by drawing the constituents up and down with the micropipettor seven times. The serum in this circle (circle #2) is now a 1:2 dilution.

e. Using the same micropipettor and tip, transfer 50 μL of the 1:2 dilution directly into the buffer in circle #3. Mix as in step d. Continue this method of preparing serial twofold dilutions through circle #7.

f. Withdraw 50 μL of serum-buffer dilution from circle #7 and discard. The dilution in circle #7 is now 1:64.

Note: If further dilutions are required, continue the process described in steps b through e. To continue the dilutions, 50 μL of the serum-buffer in circle #7 is transferred to the next row of circles. When the final desired dilution is prepared, discard 50 μL of the serum-buffer dilution from the last circle.

g. Repeat steps a through f for the low-reactive control (Test Control +) and each patient specimen.
Return to step 4 in the Qualitative Testing Procedure.

Quantitative Method
Report reactivity in terms of the highest dilution showing any agglutination of the latex reagent. Serum showing no agglutination at any dilution is reported as "nonreactive."

Reference Range
- The incidence of CMV infection depends on geographic and socioeconomic factors and patient age.
- Serologic studies indicate that 25% to 50% of the American population demonstrate CMV antibodies by age 15 years.
- In adult populations the incidence of antibodies to CMV ranges from 15% to 70%.

Procedure Notes

Sources of Error
Incorrect test results may be caused by a variety of factors. Specimens that are incorrectly collected or stored can produce errors in the test results. The use of components or procedures other than those previously described may also lead to erroneous results.

Limitations
Several limitations are inherent in CMV antibody detection, as follows:

1. Patients with acute infection may not have detectable antibody.

2. Seroconversion may indicate recent infection, but an increase in antibody titer by this method does not differentiate between a primary and secondary antibody response.

3. The timing of antibody response during a primary infection may differ slightly. The pattern of antibody response during a primary CMV infection has not been demonstrated.

4. Test results from neonates should be interpreted with caution because the presence of CMV antibody is usually the result of passive transfer from the mother to the fetus.

5. Although the CMV latex procedure will detect IgM and IgG antibodies, detection of IgA and IgE antibodies has not yet been demonstrated.

A negative CMV test result may be useful in excluding possible infection, but the diagnosis of an actual CMV infection should be documented by demonstrating the presence of the virus directly or by viral culture.

Clinical Applications
The CMVscan Card Test performed as a qualitative test on a single specimen is designed to detect the presence of CMV antibodies. The CMVscan Card Test will perform satisfactorily with acute-phase or convalescent-phase antibodies. Antibody present in a single specimen is evidence of prior exposure to the virus.

The quantitative test can be used to determine the relative amount of antibody in serum or plasma. When using properly paired specimens (at least 2 weeks apart), demonstration of seroconversion (fourfold or greater rise in antibody titer) may serve as evidence of recent infection. Both specimens should be tested simultaneously. The absence of a fourfold titer rise does not necessarily rule out exposure and infection.

The absence of CMV antibodies suggests that a patient has not been previously exposed to CMV. In the early stages of a primary infection, antibodies may not be detectable.

Package insert CMV Scan, Becton Dickinson Microbiology Systems, Cockeysville, Md.

The presence of CMV antibodies in qualitative testing on a single acute or convalescent specimen is an indication of previous exposure to the virus but does not indicate immunity to subsequent reinfection.

When paired specimens are tested simultaneously, the absence of a fourfold rise in titer does not definitely rule out the possibility of exposure and infection. Demonstration of seroconversion in quantitative testing (or a fourfold or greater rise in antibody titer) on paired specimens collected at least 2 weeks apart may suggest recent infection. Conversion from seronegativity to positivity or a change in antibody titer between paired specimens may occasionally be caused by influenza A or *Mycoplasma pneumoniae* infections, suggesting stress reactivation of CMV antibody.

Clinically, selection of CMV-seronegative blood donors or organs by serologic screening for antibody has reportedly been effective in reducing CMV infection in CMV-seronegative recipients. The most suitable candidates for seronegative blood for transfusion are newborn and unborn infants and immunocompromised organ transplant recipients.

Becton Dickinson, Franklin Lakes, NJ, CMVscan product insert, revised March 1, 2005.

Quantitative Determination of IgG Antibodies to Cytomegalovirus

Principle

Diluted samples are incubated in antigen-coated wells. CMV antibodies, if present, are immobilized in the wells. Residual sample is eliminated by washing and draining, and conjugate (enzyme-labeled antibodies to human IgG) is added and incubated. If IgG antibodies to CMV are present, the conjugate will be immobilized in the wells. Residual conjugate is eliminated by washing and draining, and the substrate is added and incubated. In the presence of the enzyme, the substrate is converted to a yellow end product, which is read photometrically for absorbance maximum at 405 nm. The intensity of the absorbance at 405 nm is proportional to the amount of antibody to CMV present in the sample.

Procedure Notes

The procedural protocol is posted on the EVOLVE website.

Limitations

The detection of IgM is of limited value in determining the timing of primary infection. In addition, testing results should serve only as an aid to diagnosis and should not be interpreted as diagnostic in themselves.

Clinical Applications

The serologic detection of IgM and/or IgG antibodies to CMV is a clinically useful aid in the diagnosis of CMV infection.

The presence of IgM antibodies to CMV is, in general, indicative of primary CMV infection. Specific IgM antibody, however, has been reported in reactivations and reinfec-

tions. IgM antibody may persist for as long as 9 months in immunocompetent individuals and longer in immunosuppressed patients.

The IgM responses vary among individuals. Of infants congenitally infected with CMV, 10% to 30% fail to develop IgM antibody responses. Approximately 27% of adults with primary CMV infection may not demonstrate an IgM response. In pregnant women the presence or absence of CMV IgG or IgM response is of limited value in predicting congenital CMV infection. The presence of CMV-specific IgM antibody in the circulation of the newborn is indicative of infection.

CASE STUDY

History and Physical Examination

A 35-year-old man has recently been the recipient of a kidney transplant. He had been feeling well until 2 weeks ago, when he experienced a sore throat, fever, chills, profound malaise, and myalgia. Lymphadenopathy and splenomegaly may be observed. His medications include cyclosporine.

Questions and Discussion

1. **Could this patient be suffering from an infectious disease?**

   Yes; the patient could have CMV infection, which is endemic worldwide. Dissemination of the virus may be by oral, respiratory, or venereal routes. It may also be transmitted parenterally by organ transplantation or transfusion of fresh blood.

   It has been recognized for more than 15 years that transfusion of blood from healthy, asymptomatic blood donors is occasionally followed by active CMV infection in the recipient. Strong evidence incriminates peripheral blood leukocytes and transplanted tissues as sources of CMV.

2. **Why would this patient be susceptible to an opportunistic infection?**

   By adulthood, most individuals have experienced asymptomatic contact with CMV. Because CMV can persist latently, active infections may develop under certain conditions (pregnancy, immunosuppression) or subsequent to organ or bone marrow transplantation. Only immunosuppressed patients who are seronegative appear to be at significant risk of developing CMV infection. Patients with the highest mortality risk from CMV infections are allograft transplant, seronegative patients who receive tissue from a seropositive donor. Most infections in allograft recipients are transmitted by the donor kidney or arise from reactivation of the recipient's latent virus.

   Cytomegalovirus infection can be life threatening in immunosuppressed patients; infections can result in multisystem involvement (pneumonitis, hepatitis, GI ulceration, arthralgias, meningoencephalitis, retinitis). Interstitial pneumonitis, frequently associated with CMV infection, is a major cause of death after allogeneic bone marrow transplantation.

3. How could an infection of this type be potentially eliminated?

Transmission of CMV by transfusion of blood or WBC components is receiving more critical attention, particularly as it affects patients with severely impaired immunity who require supportive therapy. Preventive methods in these patients include effective donor screening, leukocyte-depleted blood products, and immune globulin containing passively acquired CMV antibodies.

4. Are health care workers at risk for infections of this type?

Yes; health care professionals are increasingly concerned about the risks associated with exposure to CMV. Nosocomial transmission from patients to health care workers has not been documented, but good personal hygiene and handwashing offer the best measures for preventing transmission.

5. Can congenital infections of this type occur?

Both primary and recurrent maternal CMV infection can be transmitted in utero. Congenital CMV infection is the most common intrauterine infection, affecting 0.4% to 2.3% of all live births. The presence of maternal antibody to CMV before conception protects against damaging congenital CMV infection in the newborn.

Primary maternal infection during pregnancy is associated with more severe sequelae of congenital CMV infection. Most CMV-infected newborns are asymptomatic, but 1% manifest damage caused by CMV. Infected infants can become severely ill, and premature infants may die (atypical lymphocytosis, hepatosplenomegaly, pneumonia).

Congenitally infected newborns, especially those who acquire CMV during a maternal primary infection, are more prone to develop severe cytomegalic inclusion disease, which may be fatal or can cause permanent neurologic sequelae (e.g., intracranial calcifications, microcephaly), with psychomotor impairment (51%-75%), hearing loss (21%-50%), and visual impairment (20%). Infants without symptoms at birth may develop hearing and neurologic impairments later.

6. How can this disease be diagnosed?

Definitive diagnosis involves isolating CMV from urine or blood samples or demonstrating CMV-specific IgM or increased CMV-specific IgG antibody titers. Viral culture is the method of choice for confirming CMV infection.

Serologic methods to detect IgM antibodies assist in the diagnosis of primary infection detection of CMV-specific IgM can represent primary infection (or rare reactivation) of infection. False-positive results can result from other antibodies, such as rheumatoid factor. Although tests for heterophil, Epstein-Barr virus, and *Toxoplasma* antibodies are generally negative, antibody titers of several different antibodies may be elevated (ANA, RF, and nonspecific cold agglutinins). The inability to demonstrate IgM in a blood specimen can result from the presence of a large amount of virus-specific IgG. Lack of a CMV-specific IgM response is common in congenital infections. Detection of a significant increase in CMV-specific IgG antibody suggests recent infection or reactivation of latent infection.

Diagnosis

Cytomegalovirus.

CHAPTER HIGHLIGHTS

- Cytomegalovirus (CMV) is a herpesvirus. All of the herpesviruses are relatively large, enveloped DNA viruses that undergo a replicative cycle involving DNA expression and nucleocapsid assembly within the nucleus. Although the herpes family produces diverse clinical diseases, herpesviruses share the basic characteristic of being cell associated.

- CMV may produce subclinical infections that can be reactivated under appropriate stimuli. Dissemination of the virus may occur by oral, respiratory, or venereal routes, as well as parenterally by organ transplantation or by transfusion of fresh blood.

- The incidence of primary CMV infections during childhood is low. Patients at highest risk of mortality from CMV infections are allograft-transplant, seronegative patients who receive tissue from a seropositive donor. Most of these infections are transmitted by donor organ or from reactivation of the recipient's latent virus.

- Transmission of CMV through transfusion of blood and blood components containing white blood cells is increasingly important in immunocompromised patients who require supportive therapy. Low-birth-weight neonates are also at high risk from CMV infections from infected blood products.

- Persistent infections characterized by periods of reactivation of CMV (latent infections) have not been clearly defined for CMV.

- CMV is a major cause of congenital viral infections in the United States because primary and recurrent maternal CMV infection can be transmitted in utero.

- In CMV-infected cells, antigens appear at various times after infection, before replication of viral DNA. Immediate-early antigens appear within 1 hour of cellular infection and early antigens within 24 hours. At about 72 hours or the end of the viral replication cycle, late antigens appear.

- The presence of antibodies against immediate-early and early antigens is associated with active infection, primary or reactivated. The following characteristic antibody responses are associated with CMV infection:
  - Primary infection is demonstrated by a transient, virus-specific IgM antibody response and eventual seroconversion to produce IgG antibodies to the virus.
  - Reactivation of latent CMV infection in seropositive (IgG) individuals may be accompanied by significant increases in IgG antibodies to the virus, but elicits no detectable IgM response.
  - Reinfection by a different CMV strain than the original infecting strain results in a significant IgG antibody response but unknown IgM response.

- Serologic methods (e.g., EIA) to detect CMV-specific IgM can represent primary infection or rare reactivation. Detection of significant increases in CMV-specific IgG antibody suggest, but do not prove, recent infection or reactivation of latent infection.

REVIEW QUESTIONS

1. All the following describe cytomegalovirus (CMV) *except:*
   a. Herpes family virus.
   b. DNA virus.
   c. Cell-associated virus.
   d. Epidemic worldwide.

2. Because CMV can persist latently, an active infection may develop as a result of all the following conditions *except:*
   a. Pregnancy.
   b. Immunosuppressive therapy.
   c. Organ or bone marrow transplantation.
   d. Transfusion of leukocyte-poor blood.

3. CMV is recognized as the cause of congenital viral infection in what percentage of all live births?
   a. 0.1% to 0.4%
   b. 0.5% to 2.4%
   c. 2.5% to 4.9%
   d. 5.0% to 9.9%

4. Transfusion-acquired CMV infection can cause:
   a. Mononucleosis-like syndrome.
   b. Hepatitis.
   c. Rejection of a transplanted organ.
   d. All the above.

Questions 5-7. Match the three types of CMV infection with their appropriate description.

5. _____ Primary infection

6. _____ Reactivated infection

7. _____ Reinfection

   a. Significant antibody response and viral shedding are caused by different strain of virus.
   b. Seronegative recipient is transfused with blood from actively or latently infected donor.
   c. Seropositive recipient is transfused with blood from CMV antibody–positive or –negative donor.

Questions 8-10. Match the following serologic markers of CMV infection.

8. _____ Early antigens

9. _____ Immediate-early antigens

10. _____ Late antigens
    a. Appear 72 hours after infection or at end of viral replication cycle.
    b. Appear within 1 hour of cellular infection.
    c. Present within 24 hours.

11. Antibodies to immediate-early and early antigens are associated with:
    a. Primary active infection.
    b. Reactivated active infection.
    c. Latent infection.
    d. Increasing age and gender of the patient.

Questions 12-14. Match the following.

12. _____ Primary infection.

13. _____ Reactivation of latent infection in seropositive IgG patient.

14. _____ Reinfection with strain of CMV different from original strain.

    a. IgG, but IgM response unknown.
    b. Specific IgM antibody response.
    c. IgG (no detectable IgM).

15. All the herpesviruses share the characteristic of being:.
    a. RNA viruses.
    b. Small viruses.
    c. Cell-associated viruses.
    d. Nonenveloped viruses.

16. The most likely mode of CMV acquisition is:
    a. Transplantation.
    b. Blood transfusion.
    c. Venereal route.
    d. Respiratory infection.

17. Which of the following appears to be the only immunosuppressed group at significant risk of acquiring CMV infection?
    a. Transplant patients
    b. Seronegative patients
    c. Seropositive patients
    d. Health care workers

18. All the following are methods for prevention of CMV *except:*
    a. Effective donor screening.
    b. Leukocyte-depleted blood products.
    c. Immune globulin with CMV antibodies.
    d. Transfusion of fresh blood.

Questions 19-22. Indicate true statements with the letter "A," and false statements with the letter "B."

19. _____ Primary and recurrent maternal CMV infections can be transmitted in utero.

20. _____ CMV is the most common intrauterine infection.

21. _____ Few CMV-infected newborns are asymptomatic.

22. _____ Normal adults and children usually experience CMV infection without serious complications.

BIBLIOGRAPHY

Adler SP: Transfusion-associated cytomegalovirus infections, *Rev Infect Dis* 5:977-993, 1983.

Bailey TC et al: Ganciclovir for cytomegalovirus after heart transplantation, *N Engl J Med* 327(12):891, 1992.

Betts RF: The relationship of epidemiology and treatment factors to infection and allograft survival in renal transplantation. In Platkin SA et al, editors. *CMV pathogenesis and prevention of human infection,* New York, 1984, Alan R Liss.

Bowden R et al: Cytomegalovirus immune globulin and seronegative blood products to prevent primary cytomegalovirus infection after marrow transplantation, *N Engl J Med* 314:1006-1010, 1986.

Brady MT: Cytomegalovirus infections: occupational risk for health professionals, *Am J Infect Control* 14(5):197-203, 1986.

Brennan D: Dancing partners: cytomegalovirus and allograft injury, XVIII International Congress of the Transplantation Society, 2000, Rome.

Burny W et al: Epidemiology, pathogenesis and prevention of congenital cytomegalovirus infection, *Expert Rev Anti Infect Ther* 2(6):881-894, 2004.

Demmler GJ et al: Enzyme-linked immunosorbent assay for the detection of IgM-class antibodies to cytomegalovirus, *J Infect Dis* 153:1152-1155, 1986.

Dobbins JG, Stewart JA: Surveillance of congenital cytomegalovirus disease, 1990-1991, *MMWR* 41(55-2):35-44, 433-434, 1992.

Gandhi MK, Khanna R: Human cytomegalovirus: clinical aspects, immune regulation, and emerging treatments, *Lancet Infect Dis* 4(12):725-738, 2004.

Griffiths PD, Walter S: Cytomegalovirus, *Curr Opin Infect Dis* 18(3):241-245, 2005.

Hirsch MS et al: Cytomegalovirus and human herpesvirus types 6, 7, and 8. In Kasper D et al, editors: *Harrison's principles of internal medicine,* ed 16, New York, 2005, McGraw-Hill, pp 1049-1053.

Mace M et al: A serological testing algorithm for the diagnosis of primary CMV infection in pregnant women, *Prenat Diagn* 24(11):861-863, 2004.

Murph JR et al: The occupational risk of cytomegalovirus infection among day-care providers, *JAMA* 265(5):603-608, 1991.

Preiksaitis JK et al: Canadian Society of Transplantation Consensus Workshop on Cytomegalovirus Management in Solid Organ Transplantation: final report, *Am J Transplant* 5(2):218-227, 2005.

Ross SA, Boppana SB: Congenital cytomegalovirus infection: outcome and diagnosis, *Semin Pediatr Infect Dis* 16(1):44-49, 2005.

Rowshani AT et al: Clinical and immunologic aspects of cytomegalovirus infection in solid organ transplant recipients, *Transplantation* 79(4):381-386, 2005.

Schrier RD, Nelson JA, Nelson MB: Detection of human cytomegalovirus in peripheral blood lymphocytes in a natural infection, *Science* 230:1048-1051, 1985.

Schuster V et al: Detection of human cytomegalovirus in urine by DNA-DNA and RNA-DNA hybridization, *J Infect Dis* 154:309-314, 1986.

Sia IG et al: Evaluation of the COBAS Amplicor CMV Monitor test for detection of viral DNA in specimens taken from patients after liver transplantation, *J Clin Microbiol* 38(2):600-606, 2000.

Turgeon ML: *Clinical hematology,* ed 4, Philadelphia, 2005, Lippincott-Williams & Wilkins.

CHAPTER 22

Infectious Mononucleosis

Etiology
Epidemiology
Signs and Symptoms
Laboratory Diagnostic Evaluation
Immunologic Manifestations
    Heterophil Antibodies
    Epstein-Barr Virus Serology
    Early Antigen

Epstein-Barr Nuclear Antigen
Additional Testing
MonoSlide Test
Case Study
Chapter Highlights
Review Questions
Bibliography

Learning Objectives

At the conclusion of this chapter, the reader should be able to:

- Describe the etiology, epidemiology, and signs and symptoms of infectious mononucleosis.
- Explain the immunologic manifestations of infectious mononucleosis, including heterophil antibodies.
- Discuss the elements of EBV serology and the diagnostic clinical applications of the presence of each component.
- Compare the serologic procedures and clinical applications of the Paul-Bunnell, Davidsohn differential, and agglutination techniques.

ETIOLOGY

The **Epstein-Barr virus (EBV),** a human herpesvirus, was discovered in 1964 by Dr. M. Anthony Epstein and his colleague, Yvonne Barr. Subsequently, Drs. Werner and Gertrude Henle screened human serum samples for antibodies to viral capsid antigens of EBV and established the relationship of EBV to several cancers (e.g., Burkitt's lymphoma). EBV became the most intensively studied human cancer virus. The entire genome of one EBV strain was completely sequenced in 1984. The virus parasitizes every cell system: signal transduction, cell cycle control, regulation of gene expression, posttranscriptional RNA processing, protein modification and stability, and DNA replication.

Infectious mononucleosis, caused by EBV, is usually an acute, benign, and self-limiting lymphoproliferative condition. EBV is also the cause of Burkitt's lymphoma (a malignant tumor of the lymphoid tissue occurring mainly in African children), nasopharyngeal carcinoma, and neoplasms of the thymus, parotid gland, and supraglottic larynx. EBV is an important factor in the development of nasopharyngeal carcinoma, an epithelial cancer. Although nasopharyngeal carcinoma is rare in North American and European Caucasians, it is among the most common cancers in southern China and parts of Southeast Asia. Genetics and environmental factors appear to contribute to the elevated risk of nasopharyngeal carcinoma among the Chinese.

Epstein-Barr infections can result in complications involving the cardiac, ocular, respiratory, hematologic, digestive, renal, and neurologic systems. EBV-associated neurologic syndromes include Bell's palsy, Guillain-Barré syndrome, meningoencephalitis, Reye's syndrome, myelitis, cranial nerve neuritis, and psychotic disorders. Respiratory paralysis caused by bulbar involvement can be fatal.

EPIDEMIOLOGY

Epstein-Barr virus is widely disseminated. It is estimated that 95% of the world's population is exposed to the virus, which makes EBV the most ubiquitous virus known to humans. EBV is a human herpes DNA virus. In infectious mononucleosis the virus infects B lymphocytes, but the variant lymphocytes produced in response to and seen in microscopic examination of the peripheral blood have T-cell characteristics. The mononucleosis is not from stimulation of B cells by viral infection (EBV will transform cell lines in vitro) but is from a large, effective, CD8 cytotoxic T-cell (Tc) response against the EBV-infected circulating B lymphocytes. One of the habitats of the persisting viral genome in hosts with a latent infection is the B lymphocytes of the lymphoreticular system and in epithelial cells of the oropharynx.

Although transmitted primarily by close contact with infectious oral-pharyngeal secretions, EBV is reportedly transmitted by blood transfusion and transplacental routes. Under normal conditions, EBV transmission through transfusion or transplacental exposure is unlikely. In addition, EBV-associated *posttransplantation lymphoproliferative disorder* (PTLD) develops in 1% to 10% of organ transplant recipients.

The frequency of seronegative patients is almost 100% in early infancy but declines with increasing age, more or less rapidly, depending on socioeconomic conditions, to less than 10% in young adults. After primary exposure, a person is considered to be immune and generally no longer susceptible to overt reinfection. In Western societies, primary exposure to EBV occurs in two waves. Approximately half the population is exposed to the virus before age 5 years; a second wave of seroconversion occurs during late adolescence (age 15-24). Approximately 90% of adult patients demonstrate antibodies to the virus.

Individuals at risk include those who lack antibodies to the virus. EBV is only a minor problem for immunocompetent persons, but it can become a major concern for immunocompromised patients. Blood transfusion from an immune donor to a nonimmune recipient may produce a primary infection in the recipient known as *infectious mononucleosis postperfusion syndrome.* Infectious mononucleosis or infectious mononucleosis–like illness after blood transfusion often may result from a concomitant cytomegalovirus (CMV) infection rather than EBV. In addition, the association with EBV appears to be a specific finding in malignant lymphoma developing after severe immunosuppression, such as that induced by cyclosporine therapy.

A low percentage of patients experience symptomatic reactivation. Reactivation of latent EBV infection has been implicated in a persistent illness referred to as the "EBV-associated fatigue syndrome," but this phenomenon is not universally accepted.

Clinically apparent infectious mononucleosis has an estimated frequency of 45:100,000 in adolescents. In immunosuppressed patients the incidence of EBV infection ranges from 35% to 47%. As occurs with other herpesviruses, there is a carrier state after primary infection.

SIGNS AND SYMPTOMS

Although EBV infects more than 95% of the world's population, most individuals experience no adverse effects. Infants typically have asymptomatic infection. The timing of initial infection is a key indicator of the ensuing symptoms. Infectious mononucleosis is the typical illness experienced by adolescents newly infected with EBV.

The majority of individuals experience seroconversion without any significant clinical signs or symptoms of disease. Immunocompetent persons maintain EBV as a chronic latent infection. In children less than 5 years old, infection is either asymptomatic or frequently characterized by mild, poorly defined signs and symptoms. Although anyone can suffer from this viral disorder, it is typically manifested in young adults.

The incubation period of infectious mononucleosis is from 10 to 50 days; once fully developed, it lasts for 1 to 4 weeks. Clinical manifestations include extreme fatigue, malaise, sore throat, fever, and cervical lymphadenopathy. Splenomegaly occurs in about 50% of cases. Jaundice is infrequent, although the most common complication is hepatitis. A smaller percentage of patients develop hepatomegaly or splenomegaly and hepatomegaly. Because abnormal liver function is more marked with EBV-induced than in CMV-associated infectious mono-

nucleosis, EBV must be considered in the differential diagnosis of hepatitis.

A significant number of patients with infectious mononucleosis do not manifest classic signs and symptoms.

LABORATORY DIAGNOSTIC EVALUATION

In addition to clinical signs and symptoms, laboratory testing is necessary to establish or confirm the diagnosis of infectious mononucleosis (Table 22-1).

Hematologic studies reveal a leukocyte count ranging from 10 to 20 × 10⁹/L in about two thirds of patients; about 10% of the patients demonstrate leukopenia. A differential leukocyte count may initially disclose a neutrophilia, although mononuclear cells usually predominate as the disorder develops. Typical relative lymphocyte counts range from 60% to 90%, with 5% to 30% variant lymphocytes. These variant lymphocytes exhibit diverse morphologic features and persist for 1 to 2 months and as long as 4 to 6 months (Figure 22-1).

If the classic signs and symptoms are absent, a diagnosis of infectious mononucleosis is more difficult to make. A definitive diagnosis can be established by serologic antibody testing. The antibodies present in infectious mononucleosis are heterophil and EBV antibodies.

Table 22-1	Classic Laboratory Findings in Acute Infectious Mononucleosis
Assay	**Result**
Heterophil antibody test	Positive
Anti-VCA IgM	Elevated titer
Liver enzymes	Elevated
Leukocyte differential	Increased number of variant (atypical) lymphocytes

VCA, Viral capsid antigen; *IgM,* immunoglobulin M.

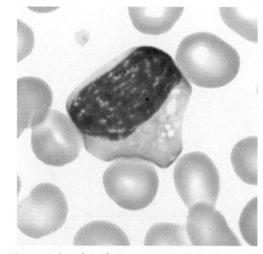

Figure 22-1 Variant lymphocytes seen in Epstein-Barr virus infection (mononucleosis). *(From Carr JH, Rodak BF: Clinical hematology atlas, ed 3, St Louis, 2009, Saunders.)*

IMMUNOLOGIC MANIFESTATIONS

Heterophil Antibodies

Heterophil antibodies are composed of a broad class of antibodies. These antibodies are stimulated by one antigen and react with an entirely unrelated surface antigen present on cells from different mammalian species. Heterophil antibodies may be present in normal individuals in low concentrations (titers), but a titer of 1:56 or greater is clinically significant in patients with suspected infectious mononucleosis.

The immunoglobulin M (IgM) type of heterophil antibody usually appears during the acute phase of infectious mononucleosis, but the antigen that stimulates its production remains unknown. IgM heterophil antibody is characterized by the following features:

- Reacts with horse, ox, and sheep erythrocytes.
- Absorbed by beef erythrocytes.
- Not absorbed by guinea pig kidney cells.
- Does not react with EBV-specific antigens.

Paul and Bunnell first associated infectious mononucleosis with sheep cell agglutination and developed a test for the infectious mononucleosis heterophil. Davidsohn modified the original Paul-Bunnell test, introducing a differential adsorption aspect to remove the cross-reacting Forssman and serum sickness heterophil antibodies (see EVOLVE website for classic procedures). Rapid slide tests are now available.

Epstein-Barr Virus Serology

Within the adult population, 10% to 20% of individuals with acute infectious mononucleosis do not produce infectious mononucleosis heterophil antibody. The pediatric population is of particular concern because more than 50% of children less than 4 years old with infectious mononucleosis are heterophil negative. In diagnostically inconclusive cases of infectious mononucleosis, a more definitive assessment of immune status may be obtained through an EBV serologic panel. Candidates for EBV serology include those who do not exhibit classic symptoms of infectious mononucleosis, who are heterophil negative, or who are immunosuppressed.

Epstein-Barr–infected B lymphocytes express a variety of "new" antigens encoded by the virus. Infection with EBV results in the expression of *viral capsid antigen* (VCA), *early antigen* (EA), and *nuclear antigen* (NA), with corresponding antibody responses. Assays for IgM and IgG antibodies to these EBV antigens are available. EBV-specific serologic studies are beneficial in defining immune status, and their time of appearance may indicate the stage of disease (Figure 22-2 and Table 22-2). This can provide important information for both the diagnosis and management of EBV-associated disease. Patients with nasopharyngeal carcinoma have elevated titers of IgA antibodies to EBV-replicative antigens, including VCA. These antibodies, which frequently precede the appearance of the tumor, serve as a prognostic indicator of remission and relapse.

Viral Capsid Antigen

Produced by infected B cells, VCA can be found in the cytoplasm. Anti-VCA IgM is usually detectable early in the course of infection, but it is low in concentration and disappears within 2 to 4 months. Anti-VCA IgG is usually detectable within 4 to 7 days after the onset of signs and symptoms and persists for an extended period, perhaps lifelong.

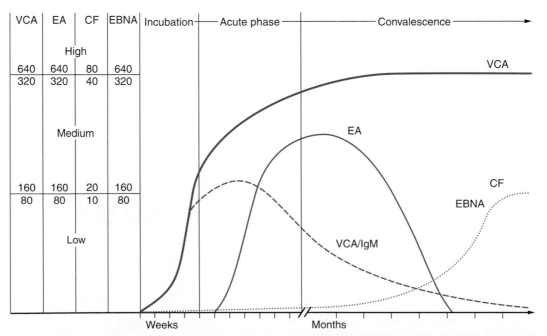

Figure 22-2   Epstein-Barr virus (EBV) antibody response during the course of infectious mononucleosis. *EA,* Early antigen; *VCA,* viral capsid antigen; *EBNA,* Epstein-Barr nuclear antigen; *CF,* complement fixation test. *(Redrawn from Krugman S et al: Infectious diseases of children, ed 9, St Louis, 1992, Mosby.)*

Table 22-2	Characteristic Antibody Formation in Infectious Mononucleosis					
	VCA IgM	VCA IgG	EA-D	EA-R	EBNA IgG	Heterophil
No previous exposure	−	−	−	−	−	−
Recent (acute) infection	+	+	+/−	−	−	+
Past infection (convalescent) period	−	+	−	−	+	−
Reactivation of latent infection	+/−	+	+/−	+/−	+	+/−

VCA, Viral capsid antigen; *EA-D,* early antigen–diffuse; *EA-R,* early antigen–restricted; *EBNA,* Epstein-Barr nuclear antigen; *IgG,* immunoglobulin G.

Early Antigen

This antigen is a complex of two components: early antigen–*diffuse* (EA-D), which is found in both the nucleus and the cytoplasm of the B cells, and early antigen–*restricted* (EA-R), usually found as a mass only in the cytoplasm.

Anti–EA-D of the IgG type is highly indicative of acute infection, but it is not detectable in 10% to 20% of patients with infectious mononucleosis. EA-D disappears in about 3 months; however, a rise in titer is demonstrated during reactivation of a latent EBV infection.

Anti–EA-R IgG is not usually found in young adults during the acute phase but may be seen in the serum of very young children during the acute phase. Anti–EA-R IgG appears transiently in the later, convalescent phase. In general, anti–EA-D and anti–EA-R IgG are not consistent indicators of the disease stage.

Epstein-Barr Nuclear Antigen

Epstein-Barr nuclear antigen (EBNA) is found in the nucleus of all EBV-infected cells. Although the synthesis of NA precedes EA synthesis during the infection of B cells, EBNA does not become available for antibody stimulation until after the incubation period of infectious mononucleosis, when activated T lymphocytes destroy the EBV genome–carrying B cells. As a result, antibodies to NA are absent or barely detectable during acute infectious mononucleosis.

Anti-EBNA IgG does not appear until a patient has entered the convalescent period. EBNA antibodies are almost always present in sera containing IgG antibodies to VCA of EBV unless the patient is in the early acute phase of infectious mononucleosis. Patients with severe immunologic defects or immunosuppressive disease may not have EBNA antibodies, even if antibodies to VCA are present.

Under normal conditions, antibody titers to NA gradually increase through convalescence and reach a plateau 3 to 12 months after infection. The antibody titer remains at a moderate, measurable level indefinitely because of the persistent viral carrier state established after primary EBV infection. Most healthy individuals with previous exposure to EBV have antibody titers to EBNA that range from 1:10 to 1:160. In EBV-associated malignancies, the levels of EBNA antibody are usually high in patients with nasopharyngeal carcinoma and can range from barely detectable to very high in patients with Burkitt's lymphoma.

Test results of antibodies to EBNA should be evaluated in relationship to patient symptoms, clinical history, and anti-

Table 22-3	Characteristic Diagnostic Profile of Epstein-Barr Virus
Stage	Description
Susceptibility	If the patient is seronegative (lacks antibody to VCA).
Primary infection	Antibody (IgM) to VCA is present; EBNA is absent. High or rising titer of antibody (IgG) to VCA and no evidence of antibody to EBNA after at least 4 weeks of symptoms.
Reactivation	If antibody to EBNA and increased antibodies to EA are present, patient may be experiencing reactivation.
Past infection	Antibodies to VCA and EBNA are present.

VCA, Viral capsid antigen; *EBNA,* Epstein-Barr nuclear antigen; *EA,* early antigen.

body response patterns to VCA and EA to establish a diagnosis (Table 22-3). The antibody profile can be especially useful. For example, a patient with an infectious mononucleosis–like illness caused by reactivation of a persistent EBV infection resulting from an immunosuppressive malignancy or nonmalignant disease can demonstrate high titers of both IgM and IgG VCA antibodies. If the antibody to EBNA is also elevated, however, a diagnosis of primary EBV infection can be excluded.

Additional Testing

A common test in the EBV serology is based on immunofluorescence. Antigen substrate slides containing EBV-infected B cells are incubated with the patient's serum. The presence of specific antibody is detected by the addition of fluorescein-conjugated antihuman IgG or IgM. The disadvantages of this type of testing are that it is time-consuming, difficult to interpret, and prone to interference from other serum components (e.g., rheumatoid factor).

Enzyme-linked immunosorbent assay (ELISA) may be used to detect antibodies to EBNA. This ELISA uses a synthetic peptide antigen to determine relative amounts of IgM and IgG antibodies in patient serum or plasma. Its sensitivity is reportedly 98.9%, with a specificity of 99.0%.

MonoSlide Test

Principle

The MonoSlide procedure is based on **agglutination** of horse erythrocytes by heterophil antibody present in infectious mononucleosis. Because horse red blood cells (RBCs) exhibit antigens directed against both Forssman and infectious mononucleosis antibodies, a differential absorption of the patient's serum is necessary to distinguish the specific heterophil antibody from those of the Forssman type.

The basic principle of the absorption steps in this procedure is comparable to that originally described by Davidsohn in his sheep agglutinin test. Serum or plasma is absorbed with both guinea pig kidney and beef erythrocyte stroma. Guinea pig kidney contains only the Forssman antigen, and beef erythrocytes contain only the antigen associated with infectious mononucleosis. Guinea pig kidney will absorb only heterophil antibodies of the Forssman type, and beef erythrocytes will absorb only the heterophil antibody of infectious mononucleosis. Agglutination of horse RBCs by the absorbed patient specimen indicates a positive reaction for heterophil antibody.

The BBLMonoSlide Test* uses a disposable card, guinea pig kidney antigen for absorption, and specially treated horse erythrocytes (color-enhanced) to increase specificity and sensitivity and to enhance readability. No special equipment is required to read the BBLMonoSlide Test.

Specimen Collection and Preparation

No special preparation of the patient is required before specimen collection. The patient must be positively identified when the specimen is collected. The specimen should be labeled at the bedside and should include the patient's full name, date the specimen is collected, patient's hospital identification number, and phlebotomist's initials.

Blood should be drawn using aseptic technique. The required specimen is a minimum of 2 mL of whole blood. Serum or plasma mixed with anticoagulants, including EDTA, sodium oxalate, potassium oxalate, sodium citrate, acid-citrate-dextrose (ACD) solution, or heparin, may be used.

Centrifuge the tube of blood and remove an aliquot of serum. Serum or plasma samples should be clear and free of particles. The presence of hemolysis makes the specimen unsuitable for testing. Inactivation of the serum is not necessary, although inactivated serum may be used. Before testing, serum or plasma may be stored at 2° to 8° C for several days after collection. If prolonged storage is desired, the serum or plasma may be frozen.

Reagents, Supplies, and Equipment

BBLMonoSlide Test Kit Components (included in kit)
- Reagent A: guinea pig antigen

A suspension of guinea pig kidney antigen preserved with 0.1% sodium azide. Store at 2° to 8° C. Do not freeze. If properly stored, the reagent is stable until the expiration date.
- Reagent B: horse erythrocytes

A suspension of stabilized horse red blood cells preserved with 0.1% sodium azide. Store at 2° to 8° C. Do not freeze. If properly stored, the reagent is stable until the expiration date. Hemolysis will indicate that the cells are deteriorating,

*BD BBLMonoSlide, Franklin Lakes, NJ.

but proper reactivity may be verified by use of the positive control serum.

WARNING: The reagents and controls contain sodium azide as a preservative. Sodium azide may react with lead and copper plumbing to form highly explosive metal azides. On disposal, flush with a large volume of water to prevent azide buildup.
- Test cards (and test disposables)

Test cards and test disposables must be stored flat in the original package in a dry area at room temperature.

Additional Required Equipment (not provided in kit)
- Stopwatch or laboratory timer
- Test tubes (13 × 75 mm)
- 0.85% sodium chloride solution
- Transfer pipettes for dilutions
- Laboratory equipment used for preparation, storage, and handling of serologic specimens

Quality Control

Positive control serum (human): contains the heterophil antibody of infectious mononucleosis, preserved with 0.1% sodium azide.

Negative control serum (human): does not contain the heterophil antibody of infectious mononucleosis, preserved with 0.1% sodium azide.

The control sera should be checked when the kit arrives and periodically during the dating period.

CAUTION: Because the control sera are derived from human sources, they should be handled in the same manner as clinical serum specimens (Standard Precautions; see Chapter 6).

Procedure

All the reagent cells should be shaken well to provide a homogeneous suspension before testing. Reagents should be kept at room temperature.

Qualitative Method
1. Place the slide on a flat surface under a direct light source.
2. Put 1 drop of thoroughly mixed guinea pig antigen (Reagent A) in the left side of the test circle on the card.
3. Put 1 drop of thoroughly mixed horse erythrocytes (Reagent B) in the circle to the right side of the test circle on the card.
4. Using a disposable plastic pipette, add 1 drop of the patient serum or plasma Reagent A on the left side of the test circle.
5. Invert the pipette, and use the paddle end to mix thoroughly (10-15 circular strokes) Reagent A (clear liquid) and sample (patient or control). Gradually mix this solution into Reagent B (reddish brown liquid, covering entire test circle).
6. Rock the card by hand slowly and gently for 1 minute about (13-16 rocks/min).
7. Immediately observe for agglutination.

Reporting Results

Qualitative Method

Positive: A positive infectious mononucleosis reaction will have dark clumps against a blue-green background, distributed uniformly throughout the test circle.

Negative: A negative reaction will have no agglutination but may have fine granularity against a brown-tan background. Peripheral color development associated with fine granularity should be interpreted as negative (e.g., giant blue-green halo on periphery of test circle should not be interpreted as a positive result).

Procedure Notes

If a positive qualitative result is demonstrated, a titration procedure may be performed to provide a quantitative indication of the level of heterophil antibody.

Titration Procedure for Semiquantitative Method

1. Serial dilutions of serum can be prepared by pipetting 0.5 mL of 0.85% saline into each of the desired number of tubes. Pipette 0.5 mL of patient serum into the first tube, mix, and transfer 0.5 mL of the diluted serum to the second tube. Repeat this process until the final tube is reached. Discard 0.5 mL of the diluted serum from the last tube.

Tube	Dilution
1	1:2
2	1:4
3	1:8
4	1:16
5	1:32
6	1:64

2. Place a titration slide on a flat surface under a direct light source. Treat each of the dilutions as if it were an individual serum, and follow the steps for the qualitative procedure for each of the appropriately labeled circles.
3. The highest dilution in which visible agglutination occurs is the *end point*. If agglutination is present in all the dilutions, extend the serial dilutions. Record the titration value.
4. A quantitative result can be approximated by multiplying the reciprocal of the highest dilution in which agglutination occurs (end point) by 28.

Although the titration value is not indicative of the severity of the disease, sequential examinations may provide information of value to the clinician.

Sources of Error

For accurate results, only clear, particle-free serum or plasma specimens should be used.

False-positive results can be caused by the following:
1. Observing agglutination after the observation time.
2. Misinterpreting agglutination.
3. Simultaneous occurrence of infectious mononucleosis and hepatitis has been reported.

A result interpreted as "false positive" may be caused by residual heterophil antibody present after clinical symptoms have subsided.

Clinical Applications

Infectious diseases such as influenza, rubella, and hepatitis may cause clinical symptoms that mimic infectious mononucleosis and present problems in diagnosis. Although the final diagnosis of infectious mononucleosis depends on clinical, hematologic, and serologic findings, a positive test result indicates the presence of the heterophil antibody specific for infectious mononucleosis.

Limitations

Diagnosis of infectious mononucleosis should be based on the results of all clinical and laboratory findings. Some segments of the population do not produce detectable heterophil antibody (e.g., ~50% of children <4 years old; 10% of adolescents). Detectable levels of heterophil antibody may persist for months, and more rarely for years, in some individuals.

Note: Other forms of rapid testing include Wampole Laboratories Colorcard Mono and Mono-plus.

Reference

BD, Franklin Lakes, NJ, BBL MonoSlide product insert, 2002.

CASE STUDY

History and Physical Examination

A female college freshman reports to the infirmary, complaining of extreme fatigue, frequent headaches, and a sore throat. A routine physical examination by the college physician shows that the patient has swollen lymph nodes (lymphadenopathy), redness of the throat, and a slightly enlarged spleen. A complete blood count (CBC), urinalysis (UA), and mononucleosis screening test are ordered.

Laboratory Data

CBC
- Hemoglobin and microhematocrit: within normal range.
- Total leukocyte count: elevated (13.5×10^9/L).
- Leukocyte differential: elevated lymphocytes (56%).
- Many variant forms of lymphocytes (25%).

Urinalysis: normal.

Mononucleosis screening test: negative.

Therapy and Follow-Up

The physician prescribes bed rest and medication for the patient's headache. A follow-up appointment is scheduled for 10 days later.

Questions and Discussion

1. **What is this patient's absolute lymphocyte count? Is this considered normal?**

   The patient's absolute lymphocyte count is 7.83×10^9/L.

This represents an increase, so a lymphocytosis is present. Lymphocytosis associated with infectious mononucleosis results from preferential infection of B cells by EBV. This infection results in a short burst of B-cell proliferation and mobilization, which produces the transient rise in the number of B cells with the variant lymphocyte structure. The altered membrane of the B cells further induces a prolonged proliferative response in T cells.

2. What is the most probable diagnosis of this disorder?

The age and physical findings in this patient are highly suggestive of infectious mononucleosis. The laboratory findings of an increase in variant lymphocytes further support the diagnosis. However, the absence of a positive heterophil screening test precludes a definitive diagnosis of infectious mononucleosis.

3. If repeat testing is performed on the patient after 10 days, could any of the results vary?

The heterophil antibody test usually becomes positive within 3 weeks after the initial symptoms.

4. Discuss the antibodies that could occur in this patient's condition.

Heterophil antibodies are the antibodies normally encountered in infectious mononucleosis. Rare cases of infectious mononucleosis have been described as "heterophil negative." The clinical manifestations of infectious mononucleosis are present in these patients, but the heterophil test result remains negative for weeks after the onset. An EBV antibody test may be helpful in distinguishing these cases from syndromes caused by other agents, such as CMV or toxoplasmosis. Occasionally, unusual antibodies occur in infectious mononucleosis; some may produce false-positive results for antinuclear antibody (ANA), rheumatoid factor (RF), and syphilis.

Anti-i can also be encountered in acquired hemolytic anemia, subsequent to infectious mononucleosis.

Heterophil antibodies make up a broad class of antibody. They are stimulated by one antigen and react with an entirely unrelated surface antigen present on cells from different mammalian species. Heterophil antibodies may be present in normal individuals in low concentrations (titers), but a titer of 56 or greater is clinically significant in suspected infectious mononucleosis.

The IgM type of heterophil antibody usually appears during the acute phase of infectious mononucleosis, but the antigen that stimulates its production remains unknown. IgM heterophil antibody reacts with horse, ox, and sheep erythrocytes and is absorbed by beef erythrocytes. It is not absorbed by guinea pig kidney cells, however, and it does not react with EBV-specific antigens.

5. What type of antigens could be tested for in the blood?

Infected B lymphocytes express a variety of "new" antigens encoded by EBV. Infection results in expression of VCA, EA, and NA, with corresponding antibody responses. Assays for IgM and IgG antibodies to these EBV antigens are available. EBV-specific serologic studies are beneficial in de-fining immune status; the time of appearance for IgM and IgG antibodies may be indicative of the stage of disease (see Table 22-2). This can provide important information for both the diagnosis and the management of EBV-associated disease.

Diagnosis

Infectious mononucleosis.

CHAPTER HIGHLIGHTS

- Epstein-Barr virus (EBV), a DNA virus, is the cause of infectious mononucleosis.
- An estimated 95% of the world's population is exposed to EBV, making it the most ubiquitous virus known. The virus infects B lymphocytes. Although transmitted primarily by infectious oral-pharyngeal secretions, EBV may also be transmitted by blood transfusion and transplacentally.
- The frequency of seronegative patients is almost 100% in early infancy but declines with increasing age, to less than 10% in young adults. After primary exposure, a person is considered immune and generally no longer susceptible to overt reinfection.
- In Western societies, primary exposure to EBV occurs in two waves among children and adolescents. EBV is only a minor problem for immunocompetent persons but can become a major concern for immunocompromised individuals.
- The antibodies present in infectious mononucleosis are heterophil and EBV antibodies.
- EBV-infected B lymphocytes express a variety of "new" antigens encoded by the virus. Infection with EBV results in the expression of viral capsid antigen (VCA), early antigen (EA), and nuclear antigen (NA), with corresponding antibody responses. Assays for IgM and IgG antibodies to these EBV antigens are available.
- EBV-specific serologic studies are beneficial in defining immune status, and their time of appearance may indicate stage of disease.

REVIEW QUESTIONS

1. The Epstein-Barr virus can cause all the following *except:*
   a. Infectious mononucleosis.
   b. Burkitt's lymphoma.
   c. Nasopharyngeal carcinoma.
   d. Neoplasms of the bone marrow.

2. The primary mode of EBV transmission is:
   a. Exposure to blood.
   b. Exposure to oral-pharyngeal secretions.
   c. Congenital transmission.
   d. Fecal contamination of drinking water.

3. Infants infected with EBV are more likely to experience symptomatic infection than are EBV-infected adolescents.
   a. True
   b. False

4. IgM heterophil antibody is characterized by all the following features *except:*
   a. Reacts with horse, ox, and sheep RBCs.
   b. Absorbed by beef erythrocytes.
   c. Absorbed by guinea pig kidney cells.
   d. Does not react with EBV-specific antigens.

5. Characteristics of EBV-infected lymphocytes include all the following *except:*
   a. B type.
   b. Expression of viral capsid antigen.
   c. Expression of early antigen.
   d. Expression of EBV genome.

6. Which of the following stages of infectious mononucleosis infection is characterized by antibody to Epstein-Barr nuclear antigen (EBNA)?
   a. Recent (acute) infection
   b. Past infection (convalescent) period
   c. Reactivation of latent infection
   d. Both b and c

7. Which of the following stages of infectious mononucleosis infection is characterized by heterophil antibody?
   a. Recent (acute) infection
   b. Past infection (convalescent) period
   c. Reactivation of latent infection
   d. Both a and c

8. What percentage of the world's population is exposed to EBV?
   a. 25%
   b. 50%
   c. 75%
   d. 95%

9. Infectious mononucleosis postperfusion syndrome is a primary infection resulting from a blood transfusion from a(n) _____ to a(n) _____ recipient.

   a. immune; nonimmune
   b. nonimmune; immune
   c. infected; nonimmune
   d. infected; immune

10. In infectious mononucleosis there is no:
    a. Acute state.
    b. Latent state.
    c. Carrier state.
    d. Reactivation.

11. The incubation period of infectious mononucleosis is:
    a. 2 to 4 days.
    b. 10 to 15 days.
    c. 10 to 50 days.
    d. 51 to 90 days.

12. The use of horse erythrocytes in rapid slide tests for infectious mononucleosis increases their:
    a. Cost.
    b. Sensitivity.
    c. Specificity.
    d. Availability.

13. EBV-infected B lymphocytes express all the following "new" antigens *except:*
    a. Viral capsid antigen (VCA).
    b. Early antigen (EA).
    c. Cytoplasmic antigen (CA).
    d. Nuclear antigen (NA).

14. Anti-EBNA IgG does not appear until a patient has entered the:
    a. Initial phase of infection.
    b. Primary infection phase.
    c. Convalescent period.
    d. Reactivation of infectious stage.

Questions 15-17. Match each procedure to the appropriate description.

15. _____ Paul-Bunnell screening test

16. _____ Davidsohn differential test

17. _____ MonoSlide agglutination test

   a. Distinguishes between heterophil antibodies; uses beef erythrocytes, guinea pig kidney cells, and sheep erythrocytes.
   b. Detects heterophil antibodies and uses horse erythrocytes.
   c. Detects heterophil antibodies and uses sheep erythrocytes.

BIBLIOGRAPHY

Akashi K et al: Severe infectious mononucleosis-like syndrome and primary human herpesvirus 6 infection in an adult, *N Engl J Med* 329(3):168-172, 1993.

Andiman W: Use of cloned probes to detect Epstein-Barr viral DNA in tissues of patients with neoplastic and lymphoproliferative diseases, *J Infect Dis* 148:967-977, 1983.

Bennett N: Laboratory-based investigations of IM and Epstein-Barr virus, *MLO* 39(1):10-14, 2007.

Horwitz CA et al: Long-term serological follow-up of patients for Epstein-Barr virus after recovery from infectious mononucleosis, *J Infect Dis* 151:1150-1153, 1985.

Lennette ET, Henle W: Epstein-Barr virus infections: clinical and serologic features, *Lab Manage* 25:23-28, 1987.

Monospot product brochures, Raritan, NJ, 1984, Ortho Diagnostics.

Mori JA et al: Monoclonal proliferation of T cells containing Epstein-Barr virus in fatal mononucleosis, *N Engl J Med* 327(1):58, 1992.

Papadopoulos EB et al: Infusion of donor leukocytes to treat Epstein-Barr virus–associated lymphoproliferative disorders after allogeneic bone marrow transplantation, *N Engl J Med* 330(17):1185-1196, 1994.

Pathmanathan R et al: Clonal proliferation of cells infected with Epstein-Barr virus in preinvasive lesions related to nasopharyngeal carcinoma, *N Engl J Med* 333(11):693-698, 1995.

Randhawa PS et al: Expression of Epstein-Barr virus–encoded small RNA (by the EBER-1 gene) in liver specimens from transplant recipients with post-transplantation lymphoproliferative disease, *N Engl J Med* 327(24): 1710-1714, 1992.

Robertson ES: Epstein-Barr virus, *N Engl J Med* 355(25):2708, 2006.

Sumaya CV: Serological testing for Epstein-Barr virus: development in interpretation, *J Infect Dis* 151:984-987, 1985.

Sumaya CV: Epstein-Barr virus serologic testing: diagnostic indications and interpretations, *Pediatr Infect Dis* 5:337-342, 1986.

Sumaya CV: Infectious mononucleosis and other EBV infections: diagnostic factors, *Lab Manage* 24:37-45, 1986.

Sumaya CV, Ench Y: Epstein-Barr virus infectious mononucleosis in children. I. Clinical and general laboratory findings, *Pediatrics* 75:1003-1010, 1985.

Turgeon ML: Leukocytes: *Clinical hematology*, ed 3, Philadelphia, 1999, Lippincott–Williams & Wilkins.

Zilmans et al: Epstein-Barr virus–associated lymphoma in a patient treated with cyclosporine, *N Engl J Med* 326(20):1362, 1992.

CHAPTER 23

Viral Hepatitis

General Characteristics of Hepatitis
  Etiology
  Incidence
  Signs and Symptoms
Hepatitis A
  Etiology
  Epidemiology
  Signs and Symptoms
  Immunologic Manifestations
  Diagnostic Evaluation
  Prevention and Treatment
Hepatitis B
  Etiology
  Epidemiology
  Signs and Symptoms
  Laboratory Assays
  Diagnostic Evaluation
  Differentiating Acute and Chronic Hepatitis
    and the Chronic Carrier State
  Prevention and Treatment
Hepatitis D
  Etiology
  Epidemiology
  Signs and Symptoms
  Immunologic Manifestations
  Diagnostic Evaluation
Hepatitis C
  Etiology
  Viral Characteristics

Epidemiology
Viral Transmission
Signs and Symptoms
Laboratory Assays
Acute Hepatitis C
Chronic Hepatitis C
Treatment
Prevention
Hepatitis E
  Etiology
  Epidemiology
  Signs and Symptoms
  Immunologic Manifestations
  Diagnostic Evaluation
  Prevention and Treatment
Hepatitis G
  Etiology
  Epidemiology
  Signs and Symptoms
  Diagnostic Evaluation
  Prevention
Transfusion-Transmitted Virus
  Etiology
  Epidemiology
  Signs and Symptoms
Case Studies
Chapter Highlights
Review Questions
Bibliography

Learning Objectives

At the conclusion of this chapter, the reader should be able to:
- Identify and describe the characteristics of the various forms of primary infectious hepatitis, including laboratory assays.
- Compare the etiology, epidemiology, signs and symptoms, laboratory evaluation, and prevention of the various types of hepatitis.
- Analyze representative case studies on viral hepatitis.

GENERAL CHARACTERISTICS OF HEPATITIS

The term *hepatitis* refers to inflammation of the liver. This chapter discusses infectious hepatitis caused by various viruses.

In the United States, acute viral hepatitis most frequently is caused by infection with hepatitis A virus (HAV), hepatitis B virus (HBV), or hepatitis C virus (HCV). These unrelated viruses are transmitted through different routes and have different epidemiologic profiles. Safe and effective vaccines have been available for hepatitis B since 1981 and for hepatitis A since 1995.

Etiology

Viral hepatitis is the most common liver disease worldwide. Approximately half the population of Western society has serologic evidence of prior infection with viral hepatitis. The viral agents of acute hepatitis can be divided into two major groups, as follows:
- Primary hepatitis viruses: A, B, C, D, E, and G.
- Secondary hepatitis viruses: Epstein-Barr virus (EBV), cytomegalovirus (CMV), herpesvirus, and others.

Table 23-1	Characteristics of Viral Hepatitis			
	Type A Travelers	Type B Hospital Personnel	Delta	Type C Posttransfusion
Agent	Hepatitis A RNA	Hepatitis B DNA	Delta agent RNA	Hepatitis C (one agent recently identified) DNA
Antigens	HA Ag	HBsAg, HBcAg, HBeAg	Delta	HCV
Antibodies	Anti-HAV	Anti-HBs, anti-HBc, anti-HBe	Antidelta	Anti-HCV
Epidemiology	Fecal-oral	Parenteral	Parenteral	Parenteral and nonparenteral
Incubation period	15-45 days	40-180 days	30-50 days	15-150 days

Incidence

Primary hepatitis viruses account for approximately 95% of the cases of hepatitis. These viruses are classified as *primary* hepatitis viruses because they attack primarily the liver and have little direct effect on other organ systems. The *secondary* viruses involve the liver secondarily in the course of systemic infection of another body system. The viruses for hepatitis types A, B, C, D, E, and G, as well as secondary viruses (e.g., EBV, CMV) have been isolated and identified (Table 23-1).

Signs and Symptoms

As a clinical disease, hepatitis can occur in acute or chronic forms. The signs and symptoms of hepatitis are extremely variable. It can be mild, transient, and completely asymptomatic, or it can be severe, prolonged, and ultimately fatal. Many fatalities are attributed to hepatocellular carcinoma in which hepatitis B and C are the primary causes. The course of viral hepatitis can take one of four forms: acute, fulminant acute, subclinical without jaundice, and chronic (Table 23-2).

Table 23-2	Forms of Hepatitis
Form	Characteristics
Acute hepatitis	Typical form with associated jaundice. Four phases: *incubation, preicteric, icteric, and convalescence* Incubation period, from the time of exposure and the first day of symptoms, ranges from a few days to many months. Average length of time is 75 days (range, 40-180) in hepatitis B virus (HBV) infection.
Fulminant acute hepatitis	Rare form of hepatitis associated with hepatic failure.
Subclinical hepatitis without jaundice	Probably accounts for persons with demonstrable antibodies in their serum but no reported history of hepatitis.
Chronic hepatitis	Accompanied by hepatic inflammation and necrosis that lasts for at least 6 months. Occurs in about 10% of patients with HBV infection.

HEPATITIS A

Etiology

The hepatitis A virus (HAV) is a small, RNA-containing picornavirus and the only hepatitis virus that has been successfully grown in culture (Figure 23-1, *A*). The structure is a simple, nonenveloped virus with a nucleocapsid designated as the *hepatitis A antigen* (HA Ag). Inside the capsid is a single molecule of single-stranded ribonucleic acid (RNA). The RNA has a positive polarity, and proteins are translated directly from the RNA. Replication of HAV appears to be limited to the cytoplasm of the hepatocyte.

The highest titers of HAV are detected in acute-phase stool samples. Human infectivity of saliva and urine from patients with acute hepatitis A does not pose a significant risk. Sexual contact has been suggested as a possible mode of transmission.

Epidemiology

Hepatitis A virus was formerly called "infectious hepatitis" or "short-incubation hepatitis." In developing countries, hepatitis A is primarily a disease of young children; the prevalence of infection, as measured by the presence of antibody (immunoglobulin G [IgG] anti-HAV), approaches 100% at or shortly after 5 years of age. The national rate of hepatitis A has declined steadily since the last peak in 1995. After asymptomatic infection and underreporting were taken into account, an estimated 32,000 new infections occurred in 2006. The incidence of hepatitis A varies by age. Historically, the highest rates were observed among children and young adults. Effective vaccines have been available since 1995. Since the issuance in 1999 of recommendations for routine childhood vaccination, rates of hepatitis A have declined. In 2005 the licensing of hepatitis A vaccines was revised to allow vaccination of children aged 12 to 23 months. Nationwide, hepatitis A vaccination of children is likely to result in lower overall rates of infection.

Susceptibility to infection is independent of gender and race. Crowded, unsanitary conditions are a definite risk factor. HAV is transmitted almost exclusively by a fecal-oral route during the early phase of acute illness; the virus is shed in feces for up to 4 weeks after infection. Large outbreaks are usually traceable to a common source, such as an infected food handler, a contaminated water supply, or the consumption of raw shellfish. Institutions and day care

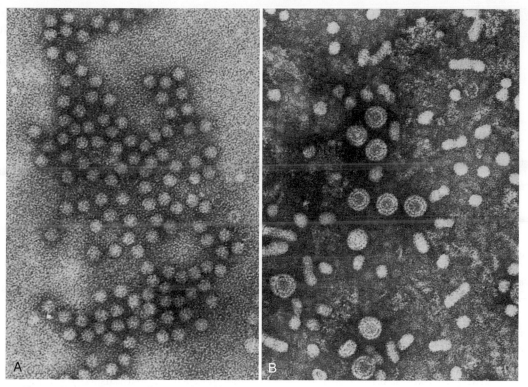

Figure 23-1   **Electron micrographs of hepatitis viruses. A,** Hepatitis A virus (HAV). **B,** Hepatitis B virus (HBV). Note Dane particles (see Figure 23-3). *(From Krugman S et al:* Infectious diseases of children, *ed 9, St Louis, 1992, Mosby.)*

centers are known to be favorable sources for transmission as well.

Hepatitis A infection is noted for occurring in isolated outbreaks or as an epidemic, but it also may occur sporadically. Although rarely a transfusion-acquired hepatitis because of its transient nature, an outbreak of HAV infection that occurred in 52 patients with hemophilia in Italy was documented to have been acquired through infusion of contaminated-factor VIII concentrate. This concentrate had been treated by a virucidal method (solvent-detergent) that ineffectively inactivates nonenveloped viruses.

Improvements in socioeconomic and sanitary conditions and declining family size may be responsible for a declining frequency of infection. The incidence of HAV infection is not increasing among health care workers or in dialysis patients. Maternal-neonatal transmission of HAV is not recognized as an epidemiologic entity. Person-to-person contact, usually among children and young adults, remains the major route of HAV infection.

In 2006, among cases for which information regarding exposures during the incubator period was collected, the most frequently identified risk factor for hepatitis A was international travel, reported for 15% of case patients overall. As in previous years, the majority of travel-related cases were associated with travel to Mexico and Central or South America (70%). As HAV transmission in the United States has decreased, cases among travelers to countries where

hepatitis is endemic have accounted for an increased proportion of all cases.

Sexual and household contact with another person with hepatitis A has been among the most frequently identified risk factors, reported for 10% of cases in 2006. In 2006 the proportion of HAV-infected persons who reported injection of street drugs was 2.1%.

Signs and Symptoms

Nonimmune adult patients infected with HAV can develop clinical symptoms within 2 to 6 weeks after exposure (average about 4 weeks). However, hepatitis A is often a subclinical disease, with many patients being anicteric. Clinically apparent cases show elevated serum liver function enzymes and bilirubin levels, with jaundice developing several days later. Viremia and fecal shedding of virus disappear at the onset of jaundice. Atypical presentations include prolonged intrahepatic cholestasis, a relapsing course, and extrahepatic immune complex deposition, all of which resolve spontaneously.

Complete clinical recovery is anticipated in virtually all patients (Figure 23-2). Hepatitis A rarely causes fulminant hepatitis, and it does not progress to chronic liver disease. Unusual clinical variants of hepatitis A include cholestatic, relapsing, and protracted hepatitis. In *cholestatic hepatitis,* serum bilirubin levels may be dramatically elevated (>20 mg/dL), and jaundice persists for weeks to months before resolution. In *relapsing hepatitis* and *protracted hepatitis,* complete resolution is anticipated.

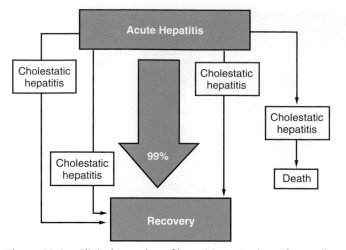

Figure 23-2   Clinical sequelae of hepatitis A. *(Redrawn from Gollan JL: Viral hepatitis. In* International Review of Internal Medicine, *Boston, 1995, Brigham and Women's Hospital, Harvard University Medical School, pp 781-792.)*

Chronic carrier state (persistent infection) and chronic hepatitis (chronic liver disease) do not occur as long-term sequelae of hepatitis A. Rarely, injection with HAV may cause fulminant hepatitis, with about 0.1% mortality. Fulminant hepatitis is the most likely complication of coinfection with other hepatitis viruses.

Immunologic Manifestations

Shortly after onset of fecal shedding, an immunoglobulin M (IgM) antibody is detectable in serum, followed within a few days by the appearance of an IgG antibody. IgM anti-HA is almost always detectable in patients with acute HAV. IgG anti-HAV, a manifestation of immunity, peaks after the acute illness and remains detectable indefinitely, perhaps lifelong.

The finding of IgM anti-HAV in a patient with acute viral hepatitis is highly diagnostic of acute HAV. Demonstration of IgG anti-HAV indicates previous infection. The presence of IgG anti-HAV protects against subsequent infection with HAV, but it is not protective against hepatitis B or other viruses.

Diagnostic Evaluation

Testing methods for HAV include the following:
- Hepatitis A antibodies (total): enzyme immunoassay (EIA), microparticle EIA.
- Hepatitis A antibody, IgM antibody.

The short period of viremia makes detection difficult. Specific IgM antibody usually appears about 4 weeks after infection and may persist for up to 4 months after onset of clinical symptoms. The presence of IgG or total (IgM and IgG) antibody indicates past infection or immunization and associated immunity. The total assay detects IgM and IgG antibodies but does not differentiate between them. The hepatitis A antibody, IgM assay is appropriate when acute HAV infection is suspected. Specific IgG antibody ap-

parently protects an individual from symptomatic infection, but specific IgM may increase with reinfection. In the acute phase of HAV liver function tests (e.g., alanine transaminase [ALT]) will be elevated and may aid in establishing the diagnosis.

Prevention and Treatment

The first effective control measures to prevent enterically transmitted viral hepatitis resulted from World War II research. In 1945 it was demonstrated that (1) infectious virus could be transmitted by contaminated drinking water, (2) treatment of the water by filtration and chlorination made it safe to drink, and (3) gamma globulin derived from convalescent-phase serum from patients with hepatitis could protect adults from clinical hepatitis. For 50 years, refining food and water preparation and establishing standards for immune globulin constituted the methods of HAV prevention. An individual who has had close contact with an HAV-infected person should receive passive immunization with immune globulin intramuscularly.

A safe, highly immunogenic, formalin-inactivated, single-dose vaccine is available (0.6 mL, 25 HAV units) to prevent HAV infection (Box 23-1). Larger doses may be required in older or heavier individuals. HAV vaccine should be targeted at high-risk groups (e.g., staff in child care centers; food handlers; international travelers, including military personnel; homosexual men; institutionalized patients).

Universal childhood vaccination may prove to be the most cost-effective method of protecting large populations both nationally and globally. Routine childhood hepatitis A vaccination is recommended.

In May 2001 the U.S. Food and Drug Administration (FDA) approved a new combination vaccine that protects individuals 18 years of age and older against diseases caused by HAV and HBV. The vaccine, called Twinrix (GlaxoSmithKline Beecham, Philadelphia), combines two already-approved vaccines, Havrix (hepatitis A vaccine, inactivated) and Engerix-B (hepatitis B vaccine, recombinant) so that people at high risk for exposure to both viruses can be immunized against both at the same time. Areas with a high rate of both HAV and HBV include Africa, parts of South America, most of the Middle East, and South and Southeast Asia. Clinical trials of Twinrix, given in a three-dose series at ages 0, 1 month, and 6 months, showed that the combination vaccine was as safe and effective as the already-licensed, separate HAV and HBV vaccines.

HEPATITIS B

Etiology

Hepatitis B virus (HBV) is the classic example of a virus acquired through blood transfusion. It serves as a model when transfusion-transmitted viral infections are considered (Figure 23-1, *B*).

The Australia antigen, now called **hepatitis B surface antigen (HBsAg),** was discovered in 1966. This discovery

Box 23-1	Hepatitis Vaccine Q & A

Hepatitis A

Who should receive hepatitis A vaccine?

Some people should be routinely vaccinated with hepatitis A vaccine:

- All children 1 year (12 through 23 months) of age.
- Persons 1 year of age and older traveling to or working in countries with high or intermediate prevalence of hepatitis A, such as those located in Central or South America, Mexico, Asia (except Japan), Africa, and eastern Europe. For more information, see www.cdc.gov/travel.
- Children and adolescents through 18 years of age who live in states or communities where routine vaccination has been implemented because of high disease incidence.
- Men who have sex with men.
- Persons who use street drugs.
- Persons with chronic liver disease.
- Persons who are treated with clotting factor concentrates.
- Persons who work with HAV-infected primates or who work with HAV in research laboratories.

Other people might receive hepatitis A vaccine in special situations:

- Hepatitis A vaccine might be recommended for children or adolescents in communities where outbreaks of hepatitis A are occurring.

At what time before anticipated exposure should the vaccine be administered?

Hepatitis A vaccine must be given at least 1 month before exposure is expected. Travelers with less than a month before a trip to an endemic area can receive vaccine and immune globulin (injected at separate anatomic sites).

How long does a vaccination last?

It appears that healthy individuals who receive at least two doses of vaccine are protected for at least 5 years and probably much longer (20 years).

If you are unvaccinated and experience an unusual exposure, what can be done to prevent transmission?

Immune globulin, 0.02 mL/kg, should be given to all close personal contacts including sexual partners and members of the household. Health care workers without unusual exposure to feces or blood do not generally need immune globulin.

Hepatitis B

Who should be vaccinated?

- All babies, at birth.
- All children 0-18 years of age who have not been vaccinated.
- People of any age whose behavior or job puts them at high risk for HBV infection (see risk factors under general information).

What are the dosages and schedules for hepatitis B vaccines?

The vaccination schedule most often used for adults and children has been three intramuscular injections, the second and third administered 1 and 6 months after the first. Recombivax HB has been approved as a two-dose schedule for ages 11-15 years. Engerix-B has also been approved as a four-dose accelerated schedule.

Can you receive one dose of hepatitis B vaccine from one manufacturer and the other doses from another manufacturer?

Yes. The immune response when one or two doses of a vaccine produced by one manufacturer are followed by subsequent doses from a different manufacturer has been shown to be comparable with that resulting from a full course of vaccination from one manufacturer.

What should be done if there is an interruption between doses of hepatitis B vaccine?

If the vaccination series is interrupted after the first dose, the second dose should be administered as soon as possible. The second and third doses should be separated by an interval of at least 2 months. If only the third dose is delayed, it should be administered when convenient.

Can other vaccines be given at the same time that hepatitis B vaccine is given?

Yes. When hepatitis B vaccine has been administered at the same time as other vaccines, no interference with the antibody response of the other vaccines has been demonstrated.

Are hepatitis B vaccines safe?

Yes. Hepatitis B vaccines have been shown to be safe when administered to both adults and children. Over 4 million adults have been vaccinated in the United States, and at least that many children have received hepatitis B vaccine worldwide.

How long does hepatitis B vaccine protect you?

Recent studies indicate that immunologic memory remains intact for at least 23 years and confers protection against clinical illness and chronic HBV infection, even though anti-HBs levels might become low or decline below detectable levels.

Can hepatitis B vaccine be given after exposure to HBV?

Yes. After a person has been exposed to HBV, appropriate treatment, given in an appropriate time frame, can effectively prevent infection. The mainstay of postexposure prophylaxis is hepatitis B vaccine, but in some settings the addition of HBIG will provide some increase in protection.

Who should receive postvaccination testing?

Testing for immunity is advised only for persons whose subsequent clinical management depends on knowledge of their immune status (e.g., infants born to HBsAg-positive mothers, immunocompromised persons, health care workers, sex partners of persons with chronic HBV infection).

When should postvaccination testing be done?

When necessary, postvaccination testing, using the anti-HBs test, should be performed 1 to 2 months after completion of the vaccine series—*except* for postvaccination testing of infants born to HBsAg-positive mothers. Testing of these infants should be performed 3 to 9 months after the completion of the vaccination series.

Who should *not* receive the vaccine?

A serious allergic reaction to a prior dose of hepatitis B vaccine or a vaccine component is a contraindication to further doses of hepatitis B vaccine. The recombinant vaccines that are licensed for use in the United States are synthesized by *Saccharomyces cerevisiae* (common baker's yeast), into which a plasmid containing the gene for HBsAg has been inserted. Purified HBsAg is obtained by lysing the yeast cells and separating HBsAg from the yeast components by biochemical.

From Centers for Disease Control and Prevention, August 2007, www.cdc.org.

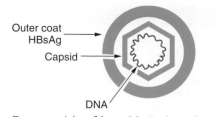

Figure 23-3 Dane particle of hepatitis B virus. *(From Bauer JD: Clinical laboratory methods, ed 9, St Louis, 1982, Mosby.)*

and its subsequent association with HBV led to the biochemical and epidemiologic characterization of HBV infection.

Hepatitis B is a complex DNA virus that belongs to the family Hepadnaviridae, genus *Hepadnavirus*. The intact virus is a double-shelled particle referred to as the **Dane particle** (Figure 23-3). It has an outer surface structure, HBsAg, and an inner core component, the **hepatitis B core antigen (HBcAg).** Inside this core is the viral genome, a single molecule of partially double-stranded deoxyribonucleic acid (DNA).

The unique structure of the DNA of HBV is one of the distinguishing characteristics of *Hepadnavirus*. The DNA is circular and double stranded, but one of the strands is incomplete, leaving a single-stranded or "gap" region that accounts for 10% to 50% of the total length of the molecule. The other DNA strand is nicked (3' and 5' ends are not joined). The entire DNA molecule is small, and all the genetic information for producing both HBsAg and HBcAg is on the complete strand. During the disease process, viral DNA of HBV is actually incorporated into the host's DNA.

Epidemiology

Hepatitis B infection has been referred to as "long-incubation hepatitis." In 2006 a total of 4713 acute, symptomatic cases of hepatitis B were reported nationwide in the United States. The overall incidence was the lowest ever recorded and represents a decline of 81% since 1990. After accounting for asymptomatic infection and underreporting, an estimated 46,000 new infections occurred in 2006.

About 1.25 million people in the United States have chronic HBV infection, 20% to 30% of whom acquired the infection in childhood. Each year about 3000 to 5000 people die from cirrhosis or liver cancer caused by HBV. The highest rate of disease occurs in those age 20 to 49 years.

The greatest decline has occurred in children and adolescents because of routine hepatitis B vaccination.

The incidence of HBV infection caused by blood transfusion is increasingly rare in developed countries. Transfusion-acquired HBV has been severely reduced because high-risk donor groups (e.g., paid donors, prison inmates, military recruits) have been eliminated as major sources of donated blood, and because specific serologic screening procedures have been instituted. This shift to an all-voluntary donor supply probably accounts for a 50% to 60% reduction of transfusion-related hepatitis. The overall incidence of HBV is high among patients who have received multiple transfusions or blood components prepared from multiple-donor plasma pools, hemodialysis patients, drug addicts, and medical personnel (see Table 23-1).

Persons at risk of exposure to HBV, including those mentioned previously, include members of the following groups:
- Heterosexual men and women.
- Homosexual men with multiple partners.
- Household contacts and sexual partners of HBV carriers.
- Infants born to HBV-infected mothers.
- Patients and staff in custodial institutions for developmentally disabled persons.
- Recipients of certain plasma-derived products (including patients with congenital coagulation defects).
- Health care and public safety workers who may be in contact with infected blood.
- Persons born in HBV-endemic areas and their children.

Hepatitis B virus does not seem capable of penetrating the skin or mucous membranes; therefore some break in these barriers is required for disease transmission. Transmission of HBV occurs via percutaneous or permucosal routes, and infective blood or body fluids can be introduced at birth, through sexual contact, or by contaminated needles. Infection can also occur in settings of continuous close personal contact. About half the patients with acute type B hepatitis have a history of parenteral exposure. Inapparent parenteral exposure involves intimate or sexual contact with an infectious individual. Transmission between siblings and other household contacts readily occurs through transmission from skin lesions such as eczema or impetigo, sharing of potentially blood-contaminated objects such as toothbrushes and razor blades, and occasionally through bites. HBV has been found in saliva, semen, breast milk, tears, sweat, and other biologic fluids of HBV carriers. Urine and wound exudate are capable of harboring HBV. Stool is not considered to be infectious.

Signs and Symptoms

Infection with HBV causes a broad spectrum of liver disease, ranging from subclinical infection to acute, self-limited hepatitis and fatal, fulminant hepatitis (Figure 23-4). Expo-

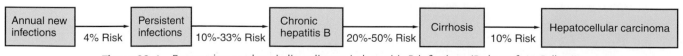

Figure 23-4 Progression to chronic liver disease in hepatitis B infection. *(Redrawn from Gollan JL: Viral hepatitis. In International Review of Internal Medicine, Boston, 1995, Brigham and Women's Hospital, Harvard University Medical School, pp 781-792.)*

Table 23-3	Serologic Markers for Hepatitis B Virus (HBV) Infection					
Marker	Early (Asymptomatic)	Acute or Chronic	Low-Level Carrier	Immediate Recovery	Long after Infection	Immunized with HBsAg
HBsAg	+	+	−	−	−	−
Anti-HBs	−	±	−	−	±	+
Anti-HBc	−	+	+	+	±	−
Anti-HBc (IgM)	−	+	−	+	−	−

Modified from Hoofnagle JH: Type A and type B hepatitis, *Lab Med* 14(11):713, 1983.
+, Positive; −, negative; ±, questionable.

sure to HBV, particularly when it occurs early in life, may also cause an asymptomatic carrier state that can progress to chronic active hepatitis, cirrhosis of the liver, and eventually hepatocellular carcinoma.

A number of factors, including the dose of the agent and an individual's immunologic host response ability, influence the clinical course of HBV infection. Extrahepatic manifestations, reflecting an immune complex–mediated, serum sickness–like syndrome, are seen in fewer than 10% of patients with acute hepatitis B and include rash, glomerulonephritis, vasculitis, arthritis, and angioneurotic edema. Manifestations such as vasculitis, glomerulonephritis, arthritis, and dermatitis are mediated by circulating immune complex deposition (HBV antigen-antibody) in blood vessels.

Infection with HBV in the adolescent or adult usually results in complete recovery. In fewer than 1% of patients with acute hepatitis B, fulminant disease develops; this complication is often fatal, but liver transplantation has dramatically increased survival. In about 5% to 10% of individuals with HBV, especially patients with immunodeficiencies (e.g., AIDS), the disease will progress to a chronic state.

Persistent infection is the usual consequence of HBV infection acquired at an early age, signaled by the prolonged presence of HBsAg. Some individuals with chronic HBV infection are asymptomatic carriers, whereas others have clinical, laboratory, and histologic evidence of chronic hepatitis that may be associated with development of postnecrotic cirrhosis. Persistent HBV infection is believed to be a precursor of primary hepatocellular carcinoma.

Asymptomatic Infection

The most frequent clinical response to HBV is an asymptomatic or subclinical infection. In patients developing clinical symptoms of transfusion-associated hepatitis B, jaundice, and abnormal serum enzyme levels (ALT/SGPT) can be manifested from a few weeks to up to 6 months after a single transfusion episode. However, in patients with a classic serologic response associated with HBV, the diagnosis is rarely in doubt, even in the absence of significant symptoms. Diagnosis is more difficult in asymptomatic patients with negative HBV serology who develop a mild elevation of ALT levels a few weeks after a transfusion. Elevated enzyme levels may persist for 1 or 2 weeks.

Laboratory Assays

Laboratory diagnosis and monitoring of both acute and chronic HBV infections involve the use of several of the following tests (Tables 23-3 and 23-4):

1. HBsAg
2. Hepatitis Be antigen (HBeAg)
3. Hepatitis B core antibody, total or IgM (anti-HBc)
4. Hepatitis Be antibody (anti-HBe)
5. Hepatitis B surface antibody (anti-HBs)
6. Hepatitis B viral DNA by polymerase chain reaction (PCR, qualitative and quantitative)

These procedures may be performed by EIA, microparticle EIA, PCR, or hybridization/chemiluminescence detection assay.

Table 23-4	Interpretation of Hepatitis B Panel	
Tests	Results	Interpretation
HBsAg	Negative	Susceptible
Anti-HBc	Negative	
Anti-HBs	Negative	
HBsAg	Negative	Immune because of natural infection
Anti-HBc	Positive	
Anti-HBs	Positive	
HBsAg	Negative	Immune because of hepatitis B vaccination
Anti-HBc	Negative	
Anti-HBs	Positive	
		Acutely infected
HBsAg	Positive	Chronically infected
Anti-HBc	Positive	
IgM anti-HBc	Negative	
Anti-HBs	Negative	
HBsAg	Negative	Four interpretations possible*
Anti-HBc	Positive	
Anti-HBs	Negative	

*As follows:
1. Might be recovering from acute HBV infection.
2. Might be distantly immune and test not sensitive enough to detect very low level of anti-HBs in serum.
3. Might be susceptible with a false-positive anti-HBc.
4. Might be undetectable level of HBsAg present in the serum, and the person is actually chronically infected.

Hepatitis B Surface Antigen

The initial detectable marker found in serum during the incubation period of HBV infection is HBsAg. HBsAg usually becomes detectable 2 weeks to 2 months before clinical symptoms, and as soon as 2 weeks after infection. This marker is usually present for 2 to 3 months. This procedure screens for the presence of the major coat-protein of the virus (HBsAg) in serum and is considered to be the most reliable method of choice for preventing the transmission of HBV via blood. The presence of HBsAg indicates active HBV infection, either acute or chronic.

The titer of HBsAg rises and generally peaks at or shortly after the onset of elevated serum enzymes (e.g., ALT/SGPT). Clinical improvement of the patient's condition and a decrease in serum enzyme concentrations are paralleled by a fall in the titer of HBsAg, which subsequently disappears. There is variability in the duration of HBsAg positivity and in the relationship between clinical recovery and the disappearance of HBsAg (Figure 23-5). About 5% of positive HBsAgs are false positive.

Among persons infected with HBV with detectable HBsAg in their serum, not all the HBsAg represents complete Dane particles. HBsAg-positive serum also contains two other viruslike structures, which are incomplete spherical and tubular forms consisting entirely of HBsAg and devoid of HBcAg, DNA, or DNA polymerase. The incomplete HBsAg particles can be present in serum in extremely high concentrations and form the bulk of the circulating HBsAg.

Test protocols for HBsAg are EIA or microparticle EIA. One of the most popular methods is the Ayszyme II EIA.

Hepatitis B–Related (HBe) Antigen

A hepatitis B–related antigen, the HBeAg, is found in the serum of some HBsAg-positive patients. HBV DNA and DNA polymerase will appear along with HBeAg. These are all indicative of active viral replication. HBeAg is rarely found in the absence of HBsAg. HBeAg appears to be associated with the HBV core; however, the relationship between HBeAg and the structure of HBV is unclear. HBeAg appears to be a reliable marker for the presence of high levels of virus and a high degree of infectivity.

Hepatitis B Core Antibody

During the course of most HBV infections, HBsAg forms immune complexes with the antibodies produced as part of the recovery process. Because the HBsAg contained in these complexes is usually undetectable, HBsAg disappears from the serum of up to 50% of symptomatic patients. During this phase an indicator of a recent hepatitis B infection is anti-HBc, the antibody to the core antigen. The time between the disappearance of detectable HBsAg and the appearance of detectable antibody to HBsAg (anti-HBs) is called the "anti-core window" or "hidden antigen" phase of HBV infection.

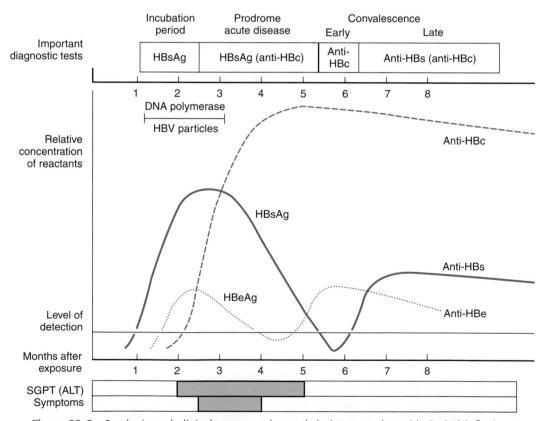

Figure 23-5 Serologic and clinical patterns observed during acute hepatitis B viral infection. *(Redrawn from Hollinger FB, Dreesman GR. In Rose RN, Friedman H, editors:* Manual of clinical immunology, *ed 2, Washington, DC, 1980, American Society for Microbiology.)*

This window phase may last for a few weeks, several months, or a year, during which anti-HBc may be the only serologic marker. Anti-HBc occurs in 3% to 5% of persons. Of 100 anti-HBc–positive persons, 97 will have anti-HBs, two will have HBsAg, and one may have only anti-HBc.

Testing for antibody to the core of the virus (anti-HBc) may provide additional advantage and lead to the identification of a person recently recovered from a HBV infection who may still be infectious. EIA or microparticle EIA is the method of choice.

An anti-HBc test is the Corzyme (Abbott Laboratories, Abbott Park, Ill) EIA. The most recent assay to be developed is the test for anti-HBc IgM. This test is considered a reliable marker during the "window" period, diagnostic of acute infection, when most other markers may be absent. The IgM anti-HBc titer rises rapidly in the acute phase and becomes negative in most patients in 3 to 9 months, although it may persist for many years.

Antibodies to HBeAg and HBsAg

Antibodies to HBeAg (anti-HBe) and HBsAg (anti-HBs) develop during convalescence and recovery from HBV infection. The development of anti-HBe in a case of acute hepatitis is the first serologic evidence of the convalescent phase. Antibody to HBsAg (anti-HBs), unlike anti-HBc and anti-HBe, does not arise during the acute disease; it is manifested during convalescence. Anti-HBs is a serologic marker of recovery and immunity. Anti-HBs is probably the major protective antibody in this disease. Thus, hepatitis B immune globulin is so named because it contains high levels of anti-HBs.

A diagnostic anti-HBs antigen assay on a random-access system has been introduced (Ortho-Clinical Diagnostics, Raritan, NJ).

Hepatitis B Viral DNA

The newest tests in the assessment of HBV infections are the qualitative and quantitative measures of HBV DNA by molecular methods (e.g., PCR). In the qualitative assay, a highly conserved region of the surface gene of HBV is detected at a level as low as 1.5×10^4 copies of the viral genome per milliliter. This assay may be of value in confirming HBV infection in patients with questionable results. A less sensitive, quantitative assay that uses an RNA probe is available for monitoring therapeutic responsiveness in chronically infected patients.

Diagnostic Evaluation

Appropriate diagnostic procedures should be ordered depending on clinical factors such as patient history, signs and symptoms being evaluated, and cases involving donated blood. The various components of HBV infection can be measured by laboratory assay.

Interrelationship of Test Results

If HBsAg is negative and anti-HBc is positive, the anti-HBs will confirm previous HBV infection or immunity. The presence of anti-HBc IgM in the absence of HBsAg in the serum indicates a recent HBV infection. An absence of IgM anti-HBc in the presence of HBsAg and HBeAg suggests high infectivity in chronic HBV disease; the presence of anti-HBe in this situation indicates low infectivity.

A vaccine-type response includes test results negative for anti-HBc and positive for anti-HBs. In evaluation of individuals before vaccination, positive results for both anti-HBc and anti-HBs should be required as proof of immunity, especially if the result for anti-HBs displays a low positive reaction. Because there is a positive relationship between the amount of HBsAg present and a positive reaction for HBeAg, testing for HBeAg is usually not necessary, except in pregnant women. A positive HBsAg during pregnancy results in an 80% to 90% risk of infection in the newborn in the absence of prophylaxis.

Differentiating Acute and Chronic Hepatitis and the Chronic Carrier State

Acute Infection

In an HBsAg-positive individual, the differential diagnosis should include acute hepatitis B, reactivation of chronic HBV infection, HBeAg seroconversion to anti-HBe flare, superinfection by other hepatitis viruses, and liver injury resulting from other causes (e.g., drug-induced, alcoholic, or ischemic hepatitis). Accurate diagnosis requires testing for serologic markers and sequential studies.

The first antibody to appear during an acute HBV infection is antibody to hepatitis B core antigen (anti-HBc). Anti-HBc becomes measurable shortly after HBsAg is detected and reaches peak levels within several weeks of onset of infection. It persists long after the disappearance of HBsAg. Initially, the predominant immunoglobulin class of anti-HBc is IgM. Early after the development of serologic tests for HBV markers, when tests for anti-HBs were less sensitive than current assays, a "window" period between the loss of HBsAg and the appearance of anti-HBs was recognized. During this infrequently encountered "window," or when levels of HBsAg do not reach detection thresholds, the detection of IgM anti-HBc is the sole marker of acute HBV infection. Over several weeks to months, the titer of IgM anti-HBc falls, tending to become undetectable after 6 months. Total anti-HBc reactivity declines at a considerably slower rate; the predominant immunoglobulin form of anti-HBc during the late recovery phase is IgG. This IgG anti-HBc persists in slowly declining titers for many years to decades after acute infection.

Within a few days to 1 or 2 weeks of the appearance of HBsAg, hepatitis Be antigen (HBeAg) also becomes detectable in the circulation of acutely infected individuals. HBeAg, a nonstructural nucleocapsid protein, is a marker of HBV replication; its presence is correlated with the presence of complete HBV particles and HBV DNA in the circulation. In acute HBV infection, patients are most infectious during that period in which HBeAg can be detected. In self-limited HBV infection, HBeAg disappears before HBsAg disappears. With the disappearance of HBeAg, its corresponding antibody, anti-HBe, becomes detectable and persists for a prolonged period.

HBV DNA, and possibly HBV virions, may persist in circulating immune complexes. The viral genome can remain in an active form in peripheral blood mononuclear cells for more than 5 years after complete clinical and serologic recovery from acute viral hepatitis B.

Chronic Infection

Hepatitis B virus can lead to chronic infection, and HBV patients have been shown to have the viral DNA actually incorporated into the DNA of their liver cells. This integration may be an important factor in the eventual development of liver cell cancer, *hepatocellular carcinoma*, a well-known long-term outcome of chronic HBV infection.

The risk of progressing to chronic infection is age dependent (2%-6% of patients older than 5 years; 30% of children 1-5 years; up to 90% of infants). People with chronic infection can infect others and are at increased risk of serious liver disease, including cirrhosis and liver cancer.

The hepatitis B virus is not directly cytopathic, and the hepatocellular necrosis results from the host immune response to the viral antigens of the replicating virus present in infected hepatocytes. Cytotoxic T cells recognize both histocompatibility and HBcAg receptors on the liver cell membrane surface. Attachment of T cells to the receptors, together with natural killer (NK) cells, results in hepatocellular necrosis; in the setting of an effective immune response, HBV replication ceases.

Studies of peripheral blood mononuclear cells have revealed that patients with acute HBV produce vigorous T-cell responses against multiple HBV antigenic determinants located on the viral core, envelope, and polymerase proteins, whereas patients with chronic infection have a very weak or undetectable cellular immune response. These findings suggest that a prompt, vigorous, and broad-based cellular immune response results in clearance of the virus from the liver, whereas a qualitatively or quantitatively less efficient or restricted immune response may permit the persistence of virus and the development of ongoing, immunologically mediated liver cell injury. In addition to a patient's immune response, viral factors (HBV genome) may also be important in determining the course of HBV infection.

Chronic HBV occurs in two phases: a more infectious *replicative* phase (high levels of circulating virions, HBV DNA, HBeAg) and a minimally infectious *nonreplicative* phase (few virions, circulating spherical and tubular forms of HBsAg, undetectable HBV DNA and HBeAg, but circulating anti-HBe and integrated HBV DNA in hepatocytes). In patients with chronic HBV infection, HBsAg remains detectable for more than 6 months, and in rare cases HBsAg persists for decades. Spontaneous HBsAg clearance in chronic infection is unusual. Clearance of the virus results in complete clinical and histologic recovery, ultimately leaving the patient with a serologic pattern characterized by hepatitis B core antibody (IgG anti-HBc) and anti-HBs, the latter conferring immunity.

Asymptomatic individuals in whom tests for HBsAg remain positive are labeled "HBsAg carriers." Other chronically infected HBsAg-positive individuals may have clinical or laboratory evidence of chronic liver disease. Anti-HBc is present in all chronic HBV infections. In most chronically infected patients, IgM anti-HBc is a minor fraction of total anti-HBc reactivity. In all patients with HBV infection, HBeAg can be detected during the early phase of infection, but in contrast to the situation with acute self-limited HBV infection, HBeAg may remain detectable in chronically infected individuals for many months to years. In these patients, HBV DNA is also readily detected in the circulation. The presence of circulating HBV DNA is highly correlated with the presence of whole-virus replication and thus with the potential infectivity of the patient. HBV DNA is also detectable in the hepatocytes of individuals with chronic HBV infection. For a variable but generally prolonged period, this hepatic HBV DNA is present in a free, episomal replicating form. In some patients, HBV DNA becomes integrated into the genome of the host hepatocyte. Viral replication may diminish spontaneously over time or after treatment, signaled by the decline or disappearance of serum HBV DNA, loss of HBeAg, and the appearance of anti-HBe in the circulation, as detected by commercial assays. Research suggests that both anti-HBe and anti-HBs may be present early in chronic hepatitis B complexed to HBeAg and HBsAg.

In 10% to 40% of patients with chronic HBV infection, anti-HBs is detected concurrently with HBsAg. Presence of anti-HBs does not signal reduced infectivity or imminent clearance of HBsAg.

There are at least six drugs used for the treatment of people with chronic hepatitis B: adefovir dipivoxil, interferon alfa-2b, pegylated interferon alfa-2a, lamivudine, entecavir, and telbivudine.

Carrier State

There are an estimated 400 to 500 million HBV carriers worldwide. In the United States, 50,000 to 100,000 people acquire HBV infection each year, even though a highly effective vaccine is available. About 5% to 10% of infected patients become long-term carriers of the virus. Immunocompromised patients, including those with human immunodeficiency virus (HIV) infection, are at increased risk for chronic HBV infection.

Age at the time of acquisition of HBV infection is a major determinant of chronicity, as reflected by the development of the HBsAg carrier state. As many as 90% of infected neonates become carriers. The rate falls progressively with increasing age at the time of infection, so that only 1% to 10% of newly infected adults fail to clear HBsAg. Another important risk factor for chronicity is the presence of intrinsic or iatrogenic immunosuppression. Immunosuppressed individuals are at increased risk of becoming carriers after HBV infection. Gender is a determinant of chronicity. Women are more likely than men to clear HBsAg; therefore men predominate in all populations of HBsAg carriers.

The prevalence of the HBsAg carrier state varies widely around the world. In the United States, as in many Western nations, carriers account for approximately 0.2% of the general population. However, among certain groups (e.g., homosexual men, intravenous drug abusers) within the general population, carrier rates 4 to 10 times greater have been identified. Carrier rates as high as 25% have been recognized among Alaskan natives in some Alaskan villages.

Perinatal transmission continues to occur. This rate should be reduced significantly by the implementation of routine screening of all pregnant women for HBsAg, followed by vaccination of their newborn. Hepatitis B vaccination is gradually being incorporated into routine infant immunization programs. A multivalent, triple-antigen HBV vaccine recently developed should have wide practical application.

Carriers can be divided into two categories based on differing infectivity, depending on the presence in their serum of another antigen, hepatitis Be antigen (HBeAg), or its antibody (anti-HBe). The types of carrier states include the following:

- The more frequently identified carriers have anti-HBe in their serum and are at a later stage of infection.
- Anti-HBe carriers are less infectious but may transmit infection through blood transfusion.
- HBsAg-positive carriers will become anti-HBe–positive carriers at a rate of about 5% to 10% per year.
- All HBsAg-positive individuals must be excluded from giving blood for transfusion.
- About one in four carriers has HBeAg in their serum. It is likely that these individuals have recently become carriers and that their blood is highly infectious.

Prevention and Treatment

Routine hepatitis B vaccination of U.S. children began in 1991. Since then, the reported incidence of acute hepatitis B among children and adolescents (younger than 15 years old) has dropped by more than 98%, and by 93% in those aged 15 to 24 years. Although not as large as the declines in younger age groups, substantial decreases also have occurred among older persons. The rates are a decrease of 78% in adults aged 25 to 44 years and 61% in adults 45 years of age or older.

The most important factors in preventing transfusion-acquired HBV are donor interviewing, screening of donor blood, use of hepatitis-free products when possible, and appropriate use of blood and blood components. In addition, the avoidance of high-risk blood components such as untreated factor VIII prepared from multiple-donor pools reduces the incidence of HBV.

Elimination of high-risk donors has accounted for at least a 50% reduction in the incidence of hepatitis, and routine testing of donated blood for HBsAg has further reduced the incidence by another 20% to 30%. Testing for anti-HBc will detect almost 100% of HBsAg-positive persons, the rare asymptomatic donor in the core window, and the large number of donors who have had subclinical hepatitis B infections and are now immune.

The use of recombinant vaccine against hepatitis B licensed in 1982 is warranted for high-risk persons, including medical personnel (see Box 23-1). HBV vaccine is administered in three doses over 7 months and is about 80% to 95% effective. The vaccine is now included in the childhood vaccination sched-

ule. Hepatitis B vaccine is also a vaccine against cancer (hepatocellular carcinoma). Vaccination offers a new approach to preventing transfusion-acquired HBV and the dependent hepatitis D virus (HDV) in patients who are likely to need ongoing transfusion therapy, such as nonimmune patients with hemophilia, sickle cell anemia, or aplastic anemia.

In cases of accidental needlestick exposure or exposure of mucous membranes or open cuts to HBsAg-positive blood, hepatitis B immune globulin (HBIG) should be administered within 24 hours of exposure and again 25 to 30 days later to nonimmunized patients. Infants born to mothers with acute hepatitis B in the third trimester or with HBsAg at delivery should be given HBIG as soon as possible and no later than 24 hours after birth. Persons who are HBsAg positive or who have anti-HBs need not be given HBIG unless the HBV titer is shown to be low or unknown.

Current FDA-approved drug treatment protocols for HBV consist of administration of interferon alfa-2b, (Intron-A; Schering-Plough, Kenilwood, NJ) and an antiretroviral nucleoside analog, lamivudine (3TC, Epivir; GlaxoSmithKline, Philadelphia). Many other drugs are in preclinical, Phase I, or Phase II trials. Bay Hep B (Bayer, Pittsburgh) and Nabi-Hb (Nabi, Boca Raton, Fla) are FDA-approved HBIG therapies. Liver transplantation is also used in some severe cases of liver disease caused by HBV, although the new organ usually becomes infected with HBV.

HEPATITIS D

Etiology

The hepatitis D virus (HDV), initially called the "delta agent" and then the "hepatitis delta virus," was first described in 1977 as a pathogen that superinfects some patients already infected with HBV (see Table 23-1). Persons with acute or chronic HBV infection, as demonstrated by serum HBsAg, can be infected with HDV. HBV is required as a "helper" to initiate infection.

The HDV is a replication defective or incomplete RNA virus that is unable by itself to cause infection. HDV consists of a single-stranded, circular RNA coated in HBsAg. HDV is interesting because it can force the host's RNA polymerase to transcribe the HDV RNA genome.

Epidemiology

Hepatitis D was originally described in Italy and appears to be most common in southern European countries. It also appears to be endemic among Indian tribes living in the Amazon basin. In the United States, Northern Europe, and Asia, infection is uncommon. In the United States, hepatitis D is seen predominantly in intravenous (IV) drug users and their sexual partners, but it has been reported in homosexual men and men with hemophilia. According to the Centers for Disease Control and Prevention (CDC), there are approximately 70,000 people with chronic HDV infection in the United States.

Hepatitis D is a severe and rapidly progressive liver disease for which no therapy has proved effective. Patients with this form of hepatitis are significantly more likely to have cirrhosis and liver failure and to require liver transplantation than patients with HBV infection alone. Chronic HDV infection is responsible for more than 1000 deaths each year in the United States. The mortality rate can be up to 20% of infected patients.

Hepatitis D virus is spread chiefly by direct contact of HBsAg carriers with HDV/HBV-infected individuals. Family members and intimate contacts of infected individuals are at greatest risk. IV drug users and individuals with multiple sex partners are two other high-risk groups. Maternal-neonatal transmission is uncommon.

Hepatitis D can be acquired either as a co–primary infection (coinfection) with HBV (e.g., after inoculation with blood or secretions containing both agents) or as a superinfection in patients with established HBV infection (HBsAg carriers or patients with chronic hepatitis B). A superinfection can make an HBV infection worse by transforming a mild infection into a persistent infection in 80% of patients. In contrast, coinfection rarely leads to a chronic condition. Although HDV is dependent on HBV for its expression and pathogenicity, replication of HDV appears to be independent of the presence of its associated hepadnavirus.

Signs and Symptoms

Hepatitis D infection may be benign and brief, but fulminant hepatitis and chronic hepatitis are being attributed with increasing frequency to HDV. Chronic HDV infection is associated with increased hepatic damage and a more severe clinical course than is expected from chronic HBV infection alone. The occurrence of sequential attacks of HBV in the same patient is probably attributable in most cases to HDV infection superimposed on a previous acute HBV infection.

Infection with HDV agent can occur in several conditions, and the symptoms would be typical of either acute or chronic hepatitis, as follows:
- Acute hepatitis D with concurrent acute hepatitis B (coinfection)
- Acute hepatitis D in a chronic HBsAg carrier
- Chronic hepatitis D in a chronic HBsAg carrier

Immunologic Manifestations

The HDV probably partially suppresses HBV replication. Hepatitis D infection is diagnosed by the appearance of HDV antigen in serum or by development of IgM or IgG HDV antibodies that appear sequentially in a time frame similar to that described for hepatitis A or B antibodies. HBsAg will be present as well.

Coinfection with HBV

In patients with acute, self-limited HDV coinfection with HBV, various serologic responses indicative of HDV infection have been identified. Serum HDV RNA and HDV antigen (HDAg) may be detected early, concurrent with detection of HBsAg. HDAg disappears as HBsAg disappears, and

seroconversion to anti–hepatitis D (anti-HD) (initially IgM and later IgG) follows. The IgM reactivity usually appears several days to a few weeks after the onset of illness, whereas IgG anti-HD appears in the convalescent phase. In about 60% of coinfections, HDAg is not detected by anti-HD, but patients can manifest both IgM and IgG antibodies. IgM anti-HD in self-limited coinfections is usually transient. IgG anti-HD often disappears as well, but occasionally persists in declining titer for many months, and may remain detectable as long as 1 to 2 years after disappearance of HBsAg. In a small number of patients, the early appearance of isolated IgM anti-HD, or its appearance during convalescence of isolated IgG anti-HD, may be the only detectable marker of HDV infection.

Superinfection of Hepatitis B Carrier

Hepatitis D superinfection of HBV (HBsAg) carriers causes the appearance of HDAg and HDV RNA, a simultaneous reduction in HBV replication, and a consequent diminution in the titer of circulating HBsAg. Termination of the HBsAg carrier state appears to occur infrequently after HDV inhibition of HBV replication. Often, HDV infection becomes chronic, and HDAg and HDV RNA may remain detectable at low levels in the serum; in persistent HDV infection, large quantities of HDAg can be detected in hepatocytes. High titers of IgM and IgG anti-HD are maintained in persistent infection, reflecting progressive HDV-induced, chronic liver disease.

Diagnostic Evaluation

The HDV appears in the circulating blood as a particle with a core of delta antigen and a surface component of HBsAg. A person with hepatitis D will have detectable antigen in the liver and antibody in the serum. Test methodologies for HDV include the following:
- Total antibody by EIA
- IgM assay by radioimmunoassay (RIA)
- Antigen detection by double immunodiffusion (DIF)
- HDV RNA hybridization
- Reverse-transcription PCR

In addition, HDV antigen can be demonstrated in liver biopsies by DIF and immunoperoxidase, and in serum by cloned DNA (cDNA). The importance of detection of antibodies to HDV is largely prognostic. Detection of IgG anti-HDV in the presence of IgM anti-HBc antibody strongly suggests simultaneous infection (coinfection). Detection of IgM anti-HDV in a patient with chronic HBV infection is evidence of HDV superinfection.

Screening for total HDV antibodies in serum is important in the identification of a subpopulation of apparently healthy HBsAg carriers whose risk of serious liver damage is fourfold higher than that of anti-HDV–negative carriers. The combined presence of total anti-HDV antibody and abnormal liver function tests in a symptom-free carrier suggests parenchymal damage and is considered an indication for liver biopsy. Hepatic lesions in anti-HDV–positive carriers often consist of chronic active hepatitis or advanced cirrhosis. A positive test result for IgM anti-HDV increases the likelihood of occult active HBV infection.

HEPATITIS C

Etiology

Hepatitis C was previously called "non-A, non-B (NANB) hepatitis," a term introduced in the 1970s. This form of hepatitis was regarded as a diagnosis of exclusion because of the absence of specific serologic markers and unknown viral origin. The hepatitis C virus (HCV) has now been identified, with immunologic assays developed for its detection. No homology exists between HAV, HBV, or HDV and HCV.

Viral Characteristics

Hepatitis C virus is a small, enveloped, single-stranded RNA virus. Because the virus mutates rapidly, changes in the envelope protein may help it evade the immune system.

There are six known major genotypes and more than 50 subtypes of HCV. The different genotypes have different geographic distributions; genotypes 1a and 1b are the most common genotypes in the United States. However, the HCV genotype does not appear to play a role in severity of disease. Knowing the genotype-specific antibodies of HCV is useful to physicians in making recommendations and counseling patients regarding therapy. Patients with genotypes 2 and 3 are more likely to respond to IFN-α treatment.

Epidemiology

An estimated 3.5 million people in the United States have chronic hepatitis C. Each year, 8000 to 10,000 chronically infected patients die of liver-related complications, and 1000 undergo liver transplantation.

In the past hepatitis C was considered a disease limited to transfusion recipients. HCV is now recognized in many other epidemiologic settings (see Table 23-1) and as a major cause of chronic hepatitis worldwide. The number of cases reported to the National Notifiable Disease Surveillance System are considered unreliable because of (1) the lack of a serologic marker for acute infection and (2) the inability of most health departments to determine if a positive laboratory result for HCV represents acute infection, chronic infection, repeated testing of a person previously reported, or a false-positive result.

During 2005-2006 the number of confirmed cases of acute hepatitis C reported increased 19%, from 671 to 802. After asymptomatic infection and underreporting were taken into account, approximately 20,000 new HCV infections occurred in 2005.

Since the mid-1990s, hepatitis C rates have declined in all age groups, with a plateau since 2003. The greatest decline has occurred among persons 25 to 39 years old, the age group traditionally with the highest rates of disease, in whom incidence has declined by 58% since 2000.

The difference in rates between men and women has declined over the decade. In 2006 the male/female ratio was the smallest since reporting began in 1966. Males have a slightly higher incidence.

Viral Transmission

Hepatitis C virus is spread primarily by percutaneous contact with infected blood or blood products. Currently, injectable drug abuse is the most common risk factor. Workers with needlestick injuries, infants born to HCV-infected mothers, individuals with multiple sexual partners, and recipients of unscreened donor blood are also at risk for contracting HCV.

Although the majority of hepatitis C patients are injectable drug abusers, many patients acquire HCV without any known exposure to blood or drug use. Sporadic or community-acquired infections without a known source occur in about 10% of acute hepatitis C cases and 30% of chronic cases.

Posttransfusion Hepatitis

After the introduction of serologic testing in the screening of blood donors, the rate of posttransfusion hepatitis C decreased from 33% to approximately 15%. Before laboratory screening, the transfusion of infected blood or blood components (e.g., factor VIII or IX) constituted a clear route of HCV transmission. The incidence of posttransfusion hepatitis C declined in the 1980s because of the effort to replace the pool of high-risk, paid donors. Also, dialysis patients now require fewer blood transfusions because recombinant erythropoietin (EPO) is used to stimulate the patient's own bone marrow to produce red blood cells.

Parenteral and Occupational Exposure

In 2006, illegal IV drug use continued to be the most frequently identified risk factor for HCV infection.

Accidental needlestick injuries also are a clearly documented route of hepatitis transmission (Figure 23-6). The Occupational Safety and Health Administration (OSHA) estimates that the general risk to health care workers of occupational transmission of HCV is 20 to 40 times higher than the risk of contracting HIV. The CDC more conservatively estimates that the average risk of HCV transmission after a needlestick injury is six times greater than the risk of HIV transmission. Because of these grim statistics, occupationally acquired HCV infection is a growing concern for health care providers.

Hepatitis C infection after accidental needlestick injury	
Donor source	Hepatitis
• Anti-HCV positive	0%-10%
• HBsAg positive	7%-30%

Figure 23-6 Hepatitis C infection after accidental needlestick injury. (Modified from Hernandez ME et al: Risk of needlestick injuries in the transmission of hepatitis C in hospital personnel, J Hepatol 16:56-58, 1992; Mitsui T et al: Hepatitis C infection in medical personnel after needlestick accident, J Hepatol 16:1109-1114, 1992.)

A person with a high level of circulating HCV may be capable of transmitting the virus by exposing others percutaneously or mucosally to small amounts of blood or other body fluids. A person with a low level of circulating HCV may be capable of transmitting the virus only by exposing others percutaneously to a large volume of blood. The threshold concentration of virus needed to transmit or cause infection is uncertain.

Sexual Transmission

Sexual transmission is believed to occur, but it is infrequent. Spouses of patients with HCV viremia and chronic liver disease have an increased risk of acquiring HCV proportional to the duration of marriage.

Other Sources

Mother-to-infant transmission has been documented. HCV is vertically transmitted from mother to infant, and the risk of transmission is correlated with the level of HCV RNA in the mother. Personal contact is thought to be a route of infection but has not been conclusively demonstrated, and the actual risk for such transmission is unknown.

Between 25% and 50% of sporadic community-acquired cases of hepatitis in the United States are of the HCV type and are unrelated to parenteral exposure. Some of these cases are believed to result from heterosexual transmission, but in approximately 40% the route of infection cannot be identified. Therefore, transmission can occur by inapparent as well as apparent parenteral routes, and this form of hepatitis cannot be distinguished from other types of viral hepatitis solely by epidemiologic characteristics.

In addition, liver disease can occur among the recipients of organs from donors with antibodies to HCV. Almost all the recipients of organs from anti-HCV–positive donors become infected with HCV. The current tests for anti-HCV antibodies may underestimate the incidence of transmission and the prevalence of HCV infection among immunosuppressed organ recipients. If the medical condition of the potential recipient is so serious that other options no longer exist, however, the use of an organ from an anti-HCV–seropositive donor should be considered.

Prognosis

The natural history and outcome of HCV infection are beginning to be understood (Figure 23-7). Several strains of HCV exist; the genotype of HCV may influence the clinical course of HCV, as well as the response to IFN treatment.

It is believed that about 50% of patients with acute hepatitis C will continue to have elevated serum ALT levels more than 6 months after the onset of illness. These patients usually have persistent HCV RNA detected in their serum, as well as evidence of chronic hepatitis on liver biopsy. Viremia, as detected by HCV RNA assay, may persist for months to years in patients in whom serum ALT levels return to normal, and liver biopsy may reveal chronic hepatitis.

Chronic hepatitis C appears to be a slowly progressive, often silent disease. In addition, HCV may be associated

Interval from posttransfusion hepatitis to liver disease	
• Liver disease	Years (mean ± SD)
• Chronic hepatitis	10 ±11.3
• Cirrhosis	21.2 ± 9.6
• HCC	29 ± 13.2

Figure 23-7 Hepatitis C infection: natural history. *HCC*, Hepatocellular carcinoma. *(Modified from Gollan JL: Viral hepatitis. In* International Review of Internal Medicine, *Boston, 1995, Brigham and Women's Hospital, Harvard University Medical School, pp 781-792.)*

with hepatocellular carcinoma predominantly, if not exclusively, in the setting of cirrhosis.

Signs and Symptoms

Although the clinical characteristics of the acute disease of both types of hepatitis C are basically indistinguishable, the chronic consequences are very different. The signs and symptoms of hepatitis C are extremely variable. It can be mild, transient, and completely asymptomatic, or it can be severe, prolonged, and ultimately fatal.

Hepatitis C more closely resembles HBV than HAV in regard to transmission and clinical features. Hepatitis C, as with HBV, can be acute and ranges from mild anicteric illness to fulminant disease. A fulminant course with a rapidly fatal outcome is rare. Most often the patient is only mildly symptomatic and nonicteric; less than 25% of patients develop jaundice. Transfusion-associated hepatitis C can be divided into short- and long-incubation types. Incubation periods for the short-duration type range from 1 or 2 to 5 weeks; the longer-duration type ranges from 7 to 12 weeks to 6 months or longer.

Hepatitis C is characterized by ALT levels in the range of 200 to 800 U/L and marked fluctuations, with intervening periods of normalcy. Mean ALT and bilirubin levels of patients with hepatitis C, however, are significantly lower than those of patients with HBV, and the extensive overlap of the ranges of elevation precludes identification of the type of viral hepatitis by the use of these assays.

The diagnosis of hepatitis C has a guarded prognosis. Although hepatitis C was initially thought to be a relatively benign disease, there is increasing evidence of progression to cirrhosis in about 20% of patients, liver failure, and even hepatoma. The hepatic damage is caused by both the cytopathic effect of the virus and the inflammatory changes secondary to immune activation. Up to 60% of patients with posttransfusion hepatitis C develop chronic liver disease, based on biopsy analysis, and up to 20% of these patients develop cirrhosis.

Posttransfusion hepatitis C affects men and women equally, but a reported 75% of patients developing chronic hepatitis were men. Patients with parenterally acquired (nontransfusion) hepatitis C, including those who have no identifiable source, have the same clinical characteristics and develop chronic liver disease with the same frequency.

Extrahepatic immunologic abnormalities have been shown to occur frequently in patients with chronic HCV infection. HCV infection has been linked with a number of extrahepatic conditions, including Sjögren's syndrome, cryoglobulinemia, urticaria, erythema nodosum, vasculitis, glomerulonephritis, and peripheral neuropathy. HCV apparently causes the cases of mixed cryoglobulinemia previously considered "essential."

Laboratory Assays

Three major types of assays are available for HCV testing: EIA, Western blot, and PCR.

Enzyme Immunoassay

The first-generation enzyme-linked immunosorbent assay (ELISA) HCV procedures, introduced in 1990, contained a single HCV recombinant antigen (c100-3). The ELISA was used for testing donated blood to reduce the incidence of posttransfusion NANB hepatitis C. In 1992 a second-generation ELISA was developed that contained recombinant antigens from the HCV nonstructural region (c100-3 and c33c) and an antigen (c22-3) from the core viral protein. This assay was more sensitive than its predecessor and became widely used as a clinical diagnostic method. More recently, the FDA has approved a third-generation ELISA with even greater sensitivity and three recombinant antigens (c22-3, c200, and NS5) for screening donated blood.

Western Blot

Western blot or **recombinant immunoblot assay (RIBA)** can be used to confirm anti-HCV reactivity. Three successive generations of RIBAs have evolved since 1990, each providing incrementally improved specificity. In this procedure, serum is incubated on nitrocellulose strips on which four recombinant viral proteins are blotted. Color changes indicate that antibodies are adhering to the proteins. An immunoblot is considered positive if two or more proteins react. The assay is considered indeterminate if only one positive band is detected.

Confirmatory testing by immunoblotting is helpful in some clinical situations (e.g., positive anti-HCV detected by EIA but negative for HCV RNA). The positive EIA anti-HCV reactivity could represent the following:

- False-positive reaction.
- Recovery from hepatitis C.
- A viral infection with levels of virus too low to be detected.

If the immunoblot test for anti-HCV is positive, the patient has most likely recovered from hepatitis C and has persistent antibody without virus. If the immunoblot test is negative, the EIA result was probably false positive.

Immunoblot tests are used routinely in blood banks when an anti-HCV–positive sample is found by EIA. Immunoblot assays are highly specific and valuable in verifying anti-HCV reactivity. Indeterminate tests require follow-up

testing, including attempts to confirm the specificity by repeat testing for HCV RNA.

The current third-generation RIBA uses three recombinant antigens (c33c, c100-3, and NS5) and one synthetic peptide from the core region. Because the RIBA is based on the same recombinant antigens and synthetic peptides as the ELISA, it is licensed as an additional, more specific test.

Polymerase Chain Reaction

The PCR amplification technique can detect low levels of HCV RNA in serum. Testing for HCV RNA is a reliable way of demonstrating that hepatitis C infection is present and is the most specific test for infection. Testing for HCV RNA by PCR is particularly useful in the following situations:

- Transaminases are normal or only slightly elevated.
- Anti-HCV is not present.
- Several causes of liver disease are possible.

The best confirmatory assay to confirm a diagnosis of hepatitis C is to test for HCV RNA using a PCR assay. In addition, HCV RNA testing is of value when EIA tests for anti-HCV are unreliable (e.g., immunocompromised patients, who may not produce sufficiently high antibody titer for detection with EIA). Immunosuppressed or immunocompetent patients pose diagnostic problems because of their inability to produce anti-HCV. HCV RNA testing may be required for the following:

- Immunosuppressed patients (e.g., recipients of solid-organ transplant).
- Patients receiving dialysis because of chronic renal failure.
- Patients taking corticosteroids.
- Patients experiencing agammaglobulinemia.

Patients exhibiting anti-HCV who have another form of liver disease (e.g., alcoholism, autoimmune disorder) can be difficult to diagnose. In these situations the anti-HCV may represent a false-positive reaction, previous HCV infection, or mild hepatitis C occurring concurrently with another hepatic abnormality. In these cases, HCV RNA testing can help to confirm that hepatitis C is contributing to the liver problem.

Hepatitis C RNA Titers in Serum

Several methods are available for measuring the titer or level of virus in serum, which is an indirect assessment of viral load. These methods include a quantitative PCR and a branched DNA test. Because these assays are not standardized, different laboratories may provide different results on the same specimen. In addition, serum levels of HCV RNA may vary spontaneously by threefold to tenfold over time. With these limitations in mind, however, carefully performed quantitative assays provide important insights into the nature of hepatitis C.

The utility of determining the viral load does not correlate with the severity of the hepatitis or with a poor prognosis, but viral load does correlate with the likelihood of a response to antiviral therapy. Monitoring viral load during the early phases of treatment may provide early information on the likelihood of a response. Rates of response to a course of IFN-α and ribavirin are higher in patients with low levels of HCV RNA. The usual definition of a low level of HCV RNA is less than 2 million copies per milliliter.

The Heptimax assay (Quest Diagnostics, Teterboro, NJ) is an ultrasensitive quantitative test that detects levels of HCV based on transcription-mediated amplification technology. Because this technology can detect minute quantities of HCV, physicians can monitor HCV infection better, demonstrate posttreatment resolution, and detect relapses with greater sensitivity.

Acute Hepatitis C

The signs and symptoms of acute hepatitis C infection usually include jaundice, fatigue, and nausea. Laboratory manifestations include a significant increase in ALT (usually greater than 10-fold) and presence or de novo development of anti-HCV.

Demonstration of HCV antibodies can be problematic because anti-HCV is not always present in the patient with symptoms. In 30% to 40% of patients, anti-HCV is not detected until 2 to 8 weeks after onset of symptoms. Acute hepatitis C can also be diagnosed by testing for HCV RNA, apparently the earliest detectable marker of acute HCV infection, preceding the appearance of anti-HCV by several weeks. The current ELISA for antibodies to recombinant HCV antigens becomes positive earlier and is more sensitive than preceding ELISAs. Another approach is to repeat the anti-HCV testing 1 month after onset of illness.

Hepatitis C viremia may persist despite the normalization of serum ALT levels. Intracytoplasmic HCV antigen has been found in the hepatocytes of acutely infected chimpanzees, and by analogy is presumed to be present in acute hepatitis C in humans. HCV antigens were not detected in hepatocyte nuclei, in Kupffer or sinusoidal lining cells, in bile duct epithelium, or in blood vessels.

Chronic Hepatitis C

Chronic hepatitis C varies greatly in its course and outcome. At one end of the spectrum are asymptomatic patients who generally have a favorable prognosis; at the other end are patients with severe hepatitis C who have symptoms, HCV RNA in their serum, and elevated serum liver enzymes. These patients typically develop cirrhosis and end-stage liver disease.

Episodic fluctuations in the serum levels of ALT appear to be a feature of chronic hepatitis C. This pattern, presumably reflecting waves of hepatocellular inflammation and necrosis, may last for months to years. Such episodes of disease activity may be related to the emergence of "HCV neutralization escape mutants," but other poorly defined mechanisms also may play a role. HCV RNA is detected in the serum by PCR in virtually all patients with chronic hepatitis C. HCV replication may be increased in advanced liver disease and may contribute to progression of disease.

At least 20% of patients with chronic hepatitis C develop cirrhosis, a process that takes 10 to 20 years. After 20 to 40 years, a smaller percentage of patients with chronic dis-

ease develop liver cancer. Liver failure from chronic hepatitis C is one of the most common reasons for liver transplants in the United States.

Chronic hepatitis C is diagnosed when anti-HCV is present and serum transaminase levels remain elevated for more than 6 months. Testing for HCV RNA by PCR confirms the diagnosis and documents that viremia is present. Most patients with chronic infection will have the viral genome detectable in serum by PCR.

Approximately one third of those infected with HCV manifest anti-HCV antibodies within several weeks; others may take months or, less often, as long as 1 year to express antibodies. The current test antigen represents only 12% of the encoding capacity of the virus.

Although good markers for chronic viremia, current assays are not comprehensive enough to detect all stages of infection. Therefore a reactive test implies infection with HCV, but not infectivity or immunity.

Treatment

The main goal of treatment of chronic hepatitis C is to eliminate detectable viral RNA from the blood. Lack of detectable HCV RNA from blood 6 months after completing therapy is known as a "sustained response" and has a very favorable prognosis that may be equivalent to a cure. Other, more subtle benefits of treatment may include slowing the progression of fibrosis in patients who do not achieve a sustained response.

All current treatment protocols for hepatitis C are based on the use of various preparations of *interferon alpha* (INF-α), a naturally occurring glycoprotein that is secreted by cells in response to viral infections. It exerts its effects by binding to a membrane receptor which initiates a series of intracellular signaling events that ultimately leads to enhanced expression of certain genes. This leads to enhancement and induction of certain cellular activities including augmentation of target cell killing by lymphocytes and inhibition of virus replication in infected cells.

Interferon alfa-2a (Roferon-A; Hoffmann-La Roche, Basel, Switzerland), IFN-alfa-2b (Intron-A; Schering-Plough), and IFN-alfacon-1 (Infergen; Intermune) are all approved in the United States for the treatment of adults with chronic hepatitis C as single agents. Treatment is administered for 6 months to 2 years. Treatment with IFN alone leads to a sustained response in less than 15% of subjects. Because of this low response rate, these IFNs alone are rarely used for the treatment of patients with chronic hepatitis C.

More recently, *peginterferon alpha,* sometimes called "pegylated IFN," has been available for the treatment of chronic hepatitis C. There are two preparations: peginterferon alfa-2b (Peg-Intron; Schering-Plough) and peginterferon alfa-2a (Pegasys; Hoffmann-La Roche). With peginterferon alfa-2a alone, approximately 30% to 40% of patients achieve a sustained response to treatment for 24 to 48 weeks. The addition of ribavirin to IFN-α is superior to IFN-α alone in the treatment of chronic hepatitis C.

Ribavirin is a synthetic nucleoside that has activity against a broad spectrum of viruses. The FDA did not approve ribavirin alone for hepatitis C, but the FDA did approve IFN-alfa-2b plus ribavirin (1998) for the treatment of individuals with chronic hepatitis C who "relapsed" after previous IFN-α therapy. "Relapsers" were defined as patients who had normal serum ALT activities at the end of up to 18 months IFN-α therapy, with abnormal ALT activities within 1 year after the end of the most recent course of therapy. Most recently, the FDA has approved the combination of peginterferon alpha plus ribavirin for the treatment of chronic hepatitis C. For eligible patients with chronic hepatitis C, a peginterferon alpha plus ribavirin is likely to be the best treatment option. Clinical trials have shown that the sustained response rate is approximately 50% of patients given this combination for 24 to 48 weeks.

Most studies indicate that genotypes 1a and 1b are more resistant to treatment with any IFN-α–based therapy than non–type 1 genotypes. For this reason, some physicians may prescribe longer durations of treatment for patients infected with viral genotype 1a or 1b. The best available current treatment for chronic hepatitis C, peginterferon alpha plus ribavirin, leads to an overall sustained response rate in more than 50% of all patients. The sustained response rates are even better for individuals infected with non–type 1 genotypes of the hepatitis C virus.

Several drugs, known as "immune modifiers" or "immunomodulators," that alter the immune response are being tested (some with IFN-α) in clinical trials for chronic hepatitis C. These drugs alter the inflammatory response against liver cells infected with the virus; however, their mechanisms of action are poorly understood. Compounds tested in humans include thymosin-alpha-1 (Zadaxin; SciClone Pharmaceuticals, San Mateo, Calif) and histamine dihydrochloride (Ceplene; Maxim Pharmaceuticals, San Diego).

New medications and approaches to treatment are needed for HCV infection. Most promising for the immediate future are newer forms of long-acting IFNs. In addition, promising molecular therapies consist of using *ribozymes,* enzymes that break down specific viral RNA molecules, and *antisense oligonucleotides,* small complementary segments of DNA that bind to viral RNA and inhibit viral replication.

Therapeutic vaccines are also being developed to enhance the immune response against the HCV. In contrast to a preventive vaccine (likely a distant development for hepatitis C), a therapeutic vaccine is administered to already-infected individuals to stimulate the immune system to fight the infection. Several therapeutic vaccines are in preclinical development for hepatitis C. The most promising of these are DNA vaccines involving injection of DNA copies of the HCV RNA genome, which are taken up by certain immune system cells. Theoretically, these cells then express viral proteins, stimulating an immune response against the virus.

Who Should or Should Not Be Treated?

Patients with anti-HCV, HCV RNA, elevated serum ALT levels, and evidence of chronic hepatitis on liver biopsy, and with no contraindications, should be offered therapy with a combination of IFN-α and ribavirin. The National Institutes of Health Consensus Development Conference Panel recommended that therapy for hepatitis C be limited to those patients who have histologic evidence of progressive disease without signs of decompensation. According to current recommendations, all patients with fibrosis or moderate to severe degrees of inflammation and necrosis on liver biopsy should be treated, and patients with less severe histologic disease should be managed on an individual basis. Patient selection should not be based on the presence or absence of symptoms, the mode of acquisition, the genotype of HCV RNA, or serum HCV RNA levels.

Interferon and combination therapy have not been shown to improve survival or the ultimate outcome in patients with preexisting cirrhosis. The benefit of treatment in patients over 60 years old has not been well documented. The role of IFN therapy in children with hepatitis C remains uncertain.

Prevention

Preventive practices among health care workers to avoid needlestick injuries should be promoted. Recent investigations have shown that removal of blood from donors with anti-HBcAg from the blood supply and use of third-generation anti-HCV testing have reduced the incidence of posttransfusion hepatitis C.

Vaccines and immunoglobulin products do not exist for prevention or treatment of hepatitis C. Development of preventive strategies appears unlikely in the near future because these products would require antibodies to all the genotypes and variants of hepatitis C; however, some type of vaccine may eventually be developed.

HEPATITIS E

Etiology

The virus that causes hepatitis E was identified only recently.

Epidemiology

Only a few cases of hepatitis E have been reported, with none originating in the United States. All have been seen in travelers returning from the Indian subcontinent, northern Africa, the Far East, portions of Russia (the former Soviet Union), and Mexico.

Hepatitis E virus (HEV) is transmitted by the fecal-oral route. Infection is usually the result of poor sanitation conditions. HEV is responsible for large, water-borne outbreaks of hepatitis in the developing world and is the most common cause of sporadic hepatitis in young adults in developing nations. Clinically apparent disease frequently is found in patients 15 to 40 years old.

The HEV infection rate among household contacts of infected patients appears to be low. The seroprevalence of HEV in blood donors is approximately 2%.

Viruslike particles have been observed in the stool from patients with HEV infection. In addition, serologic tests (IgM and IgG anti-HEV) have been developed now that the HEV genome has been cloned and sequenced.

Signs and Symptoms

The incubation period of HEV ranges from 2 to 9 weeks, with an average of 6 weeks. The symptoms of HEV infection are similar to those of other forms of viral hepatitis. HEV particles may appear in feces, inconstantly, during prodromal symptoms of hepatitis E. Fecal HEV shedding occurs predominantly during the first week after onset of jaundice and has not been identified in stool samples obtained at 8 to 15 days. Viremia may occur during the period of fecal HEV shedding.

No form of chronic liver disease has been attributable to infection by HEV. Although most acute infections are self-limited and mild, in pregnant women about 10% to 20% of HEV infections result in fulminant hepatitis, especially in the third trimester of pregnancy.

Immunologic Manifestations

A short-lived IgM anti-HEV has been found in acute-phase sera. IgG anti-HEV appears and replaces IgM anti-HEV about 2 to 4 weeks after symptoms subside. The duration of detectable IgG anti-HEV remains uncertain.

Diagnostic Evaluation

Specific serologic tests for IgM and IgG anti-HEV are available. HEV can be diagnosed by performing immunoelectron microscopy on a stool specimen. Serum ALT and aspartate transaminase (AST/SGOT) assay levels, if elevated, are indicative of the acute phase of the infection.

Prevention and Treatment

Standard gamma globulin preparations have not been shown to be effective in the prevention of viral E hepatitis. No effective vaccine has been developed. Treatment of HEV is usually supportive care.

HEPATITIS G

Etiology

Hepatitis G virus (HGV) is an RNA virus. HGV is similar to the previously identified GB-C virus and distantly related to the hepatitis C (HCV), GB-B, and GB-A viruses. In 1995 and 1996, two independent groups discovered and sequenced an agent with limited homology to HCV, named GBV-C/HGV. The viral agents have 96% amino acid identity and represent variants of HGV.

Epidemiology

Hepatitis G virus is a blood-borne agent. Transfusion recipients and IV drug abusers are at risk of infection. The virus frequently occurs as a coinfection with HCV. Prevalence patterns of GBV-C/HGV suggest that the virus is transmitted sexually.

Hepatitis G infection is common; 1% to 2% of U.S. blood donors have HGV RNA detectable in their serum. HGV is estimated to produce 900 to 2000 infections per year, most of which may be asymptomatic. Chronic infection develops in 90% to 100% of infected persons. Chronic disease is rare or may not occur at all.

Signs and Symptoms

Chronic HGV infection does not appear to be a common cause of important liver disease and does not alter the course of chronic HCV infection. The vast majority of patients with acute, non–A-E hepatitis have no evidence of HGV infection. The role of HGV (GBV-C) in human hepatitis remains unclear.

Hepatitis G may not be a significant cause of acute or chronic liver disease. In all, 15% of children with chronic hepatitis C or hepatitis B are infected with HGV. In these cases, HGV coinfection does not appear to cause more severe liver disease.

The HGV has not been proven to cause fulminant hepatitis. In fact, recent studies suggest that the virus may not even replicate in the liver. The role of HGV in acute and chronic hepatitis remains to be fully defined.

Diagnostic Evaluation

A cDNA expression library was constructed from the plasma of a patient with chronic hepatitis C. Immunoscreening of the expression library with the patient's serum identified several unique HCV and other sequences, from which an anchored PCR method was used to amplify overlapping clones for the entire viral genome. The virus was termed the "hepatitis G virus."

Prevention

Confirmation of disease association, establishment of routes of transmission, and development of serologic screening assays are necessary before preventive measures can be considered.

TRANFUSION-TRANSMITTED VIRUS

Etiology

A recent addition to the infectious hepatitis family is the transfusion-transmitted virus (TTV). TTV is an nonenveloped, single-stranded DNA virus with 3739 nucleotides. Two genetic groups have been identified, differing by 30% in nucleotide sequences. TTV was discovered in 1997 through cloning and DNA sequence analysis by Japanese scientists. This novel, single-stranded linear DNA virus has been designated "TT virus" or "TTV" after the initials of the first patient (TT) from whom the virus was isolated.

The most remarkable feature of TTV is the extraordinarily high prevalence of chronic viremia in apparently healthy people, up to almost 100% in some countries.

Epidemiology

The TTV has been associated with posttransfusion hepatitis of unknown etiology (non–A-G). The prevalence in the global population, particularly the United States, United Kingdom, Japan, Germany, and Thailand, can reach 100% in healthy people.

There is evidence that TTV may be transmitted not only by parenteral exposure to blood, but also by fecal-oral route and from mother to child.

Signs and Symptoms

Although similar to HGV, TTV may be an example of a human virus with no clear disease association. This hypothesis is supported by the fact that the high prevalence of active TTV infection in the general population, both in the United Kingdom and in Japan, is not comparable to the rate of significant liver damage.

As with HGV, the pathogenicity of TTV has not been proven.

CASE STUDY

History and Physical Examination

Several workers at a local fast-food restaurant call in sick and report to the local ambulatory clinic for treatment. All of them complain of extreme fatigue. In addition, another 26-year-old food handler, who returned from visiting his relatives in Costa Rica a month ago, is sick. Within the last 1 or 2 weeks, he has had no energy and "just doesn't feel well." When he recently visited a physician at a local ambulatory clinic, he was slightly jaundiced.

Laboratory Data

Food handler's test results: Complete blood count: normal. Serum bilirubin: slightly elevated.

Questions and Discussion

1. **What types of additional laboratory tests could be of value in determining the 26-year-old food handler's source of illness?**

Because of this patient's recent travel history, hepatitis A should be considered as the possible cause of the jaundice and abnormal bilirubin. Hepatitis A infections can be acquired by adults during travel to endemic, developing areas. A viral stool culture could be of value. If this patient has hepatitis A, the highest titers of HAV are detected in acute-phase stool samples. Serologic tests may also be of value.

2. **What are the immunologic manifestations?**

Shortly after the onset of fecal shedding, an IgM antibody is detectable in serum, followed in a few days by the appearance of IgG antibody. IgM anti-HA is almost always detectable in patients with acute HAV. IgG anti-HA peaks after the acute illness and remains detectable indefinitely, perhaps lifelong. The finding of IgM anti-HA in a patient with acute viral hepatitis is highly diagnostic of acute HAV infection. Demonstration of IgG anti-HA indicates previous infection. The presence of IgG anti-HA protects against subsequent infection with HAV, but it is not protective against HBV or other viruses.

3. **What is the prognosis in this disease?**

Complete clinical recovery is anticipated in virtually all patients; however, rare cases of fulminant and even fatal disease have been documented. Unusual clinical variants of hepatitis A include cholestatic, relapsing, and protracted hepatitis. In cholestatic hepatitis, serum bilirubin may be dramatically elevated (>20 mg/dL), and jaundice persists

for many weeks to months before resolution. In relapsing and protracted hepatitis, complete resolution is anticipated. A chronic carrier state (persistent infection) and chronic hepatitis (chronic liver disease) do not occur as long-term sequelae of hepatitis A.

4. **What are the methods of prevention and prophylaxis?**

Careful handwashing when preparing food is essential. In addition, after close personal contact with a person with hepatitis A, unvaccinated individuals should receive immune globulin intramuscularly. Unvaccinated persons who travel to or remain in an endemic area for more than 3 months should receive immune globulin injections every 5 months. Persons at risk should take advantage of the available hepatitis A vaccine.

5. **Because of this patient's occupation, could particular infectious diseases be of concern?**

Hepatitis A virus is transmitted by a fecal-oral route during the early phase of acute illness. Large outbreaks are usually traceable to a common source (e.g., infected food handler, contaminated water supply). HAV is noted for occurring in isolated outbreaks or as an epidemic, but it also may occur sporadically.

Diagnosis

Hepatitis A infection.

CASE STUDY

History and Physical Examination

A 30-year-old phlebotomist presented with fever, persistent fatigue, and joint pain. She reports that a needle in a plastic garbage bag nicked her finger about 2 months ago. Her physical examination was within normal limits.

Laboratory Data

Her laboratory data, however, revealed elevated serum ALT and total bilirubin levels. Additional laboratory data included positive HBsAg and positive IgM anti-HBc. Her IgM anti-HAV and anti-HCV tests were negative.

Questions and Discussion

1. **Does this patient have a form of infectious hepatitis? If so, what type?**

Yes; the patient's history and laboratory results support a working diagnosis of infectious hepatitis, probably type B.

2. **Can any further tests be done to confirm the diagnosis?**

Additional tests can include HBeAg testing.

3. **What is the patient's prognosis?**

Treatment with IFN-α is effective in about 50% of patients with HBV infection. However, this patient could become a carrier of HBV and could eventually develop hepatocellular carcinoma.

Diagnosis

Hepatitis B infection.

CASE STUDY

History and Physical Examination

This 75-year-old Caucasian woman had an 18-month history of right-sided abdominal pain and progressive fatigue. Her other medical problems include insulin-dependent diabetes mellitus and hypertension.

She reported no history of blood transfusion, IV drug use, or excessive alcohol use. She has no family history of liver disease. Her physical examination showed no cutaneous stigmata of chronic liver disease, hepatosplenomegaly, or ascites. Her daily medications include Humulin U-100 insulin and a drug for her high blood pressure.

Laboratory Data

Her abnormal laboratory values included elevated liver serum enzymes (ALT) and total bilirubin. She also exhibited hypergammaglobulinemia. Other relevant findings included negative HBsAg, positive anti-HCV antibody (by RIBA), and positive HCV RNA (by PCR).

Questions and Discussion

1. Does this patient have a form of infectious hepatitis? If so, what type?

This patient demonstrates clinical and laboratory findings that support a diagnosis of hepatitis C.

2. Can any further tests be done to confirm the diagnosis?

Radiologic studies were done, including abdominal ultrasound, CT scan, and upper gastrointestinal series. The results all were unremarkable. In addition, a liver biopsy specimen showed features of moderately severe chronic hepatitis.

3. What is the patient's prognosis?

The patient was treated with steroids (prednisone) and azathioprine. She responded clinically and biochemically. Her liver enzymes returned to normal 8 months after therapy began. A liver biopsy specimen obtained 3 years after treatment showed marked improvement. In addition, her hypergammaglobulinemia resolved. However, the patient remains positive for HCV RNA.

Diagnosis

Hepatitis C infection.

CASE STUDY

History and Physical Examination

A 45-year-old, previously healthy medical technologist visited her primary care physician because of increasing fatigue and loss of appetite. She has had a monogamous sexual relationship with her husband for 25 years.

Laboratory Data

After an initial workup for chronic fatigue, including a risk factor history that revealed several needlesticks on the job, she was found to be anti-HCV positive, by both EIA and RIBA, and to have an abnormal liver function profile.

Questions and Discussion

1. What is the probable source of the HCV infection?

Noting that HCV infection is a major concern among providers, the CDC estimates that the average risk of HCV transmission to a health care worker after needlestick injury is 1.8%, or six times greater than the risk of HIV transmission.

2. What steps should be taken after exposure?

Postexposure evaluation varies. Testing for HCV in the source patient depends on cost and how quickly an exposed worker wants to know his or her status. At least 15% of people with HCV do not have the virus circulating in their body. PCR, in addition to anti-HCV test, would show if the patient has circulating antibodies. If the PCR is negative, the risk of transmission in a worker would be virtually nonexistent.

Follow-up strategies include counseling. Many health care providers discourage pregnancy or breastfeeding.

3. What behavioral changes are necessary now that the patient knows that she has HCV infection?

Condoms may be suggested, although the risk of sexually transmitted HCV is low. In addition, only a few cases of provider-to-patient transmission of HCV have been noted.

Diagnosis

Hepatitis C infection.

CHAPTER HIGHLIGHTS

- Viral agents of acute hepatitis can be divided into primary hepatitis viruses: A, B, C, D, E, and G, as well as secondary hepatitis viruses, including Epstein-Barr virus, cytomegalovirus, herpesvirus, and others. Primary hepatitis viruses account for approximately 95% of the cases of hepatitis.
- As a clinical disease, hepatitis can occur in acute or chronic forms.
- Hepatitis A virus (HAV; formerly infectious or short-incubation hepatitis) is common in underdeveloped or developing countries.
- HAV is transmitted almost exclusively by a fecal-oral route during the early phase of acute illness because the virus is shed in feces for up to 4 weeks after infection occurs.
- The incidence of HAV is not increased among health care workers or in dialysis patients.
- Hepatitis B virus (HBV) is the classic example of a virus acquired through blood transfusion. Reported cases of acute hepatitis B have decreased dramatically in the United States in the last decade.
- HBV is largely spread parenterally through blood transfusion, needlestick accidents, and contaminated needles, although the virus can be transmitted in the absence of obvious parenteral exposure.

- Serologic markers for HBV infection include HBsAg, HBeAg, anti-HBc, anti-HBe, anti-HBs, and DNA analysis.
- Hepatitis D virus (HDV; initially the delta agent) super-infects some patients already infected with HBV.
- Hepatitis C virus (HCV) is prevalent in the United States and Western Europe and resembles HBV in terms of transmission characteristics. Health care workers should avoid needlestick injuries.
- Hepatitis E virus (HEV) is transmitted by the fecal-oral route and usually is caused by poor sanitation. No form of chronic liver disease has been attributable to HEV infection. Although most acute infections are self-limited and mild, in pregnant women about 10% to 20% of HEV infections result in fulminant hepatitis, especially in the third trimester of pregnancy.
- Hepatitis G virus (HGV) is a blood-borne agent. Transfusion recipients and IV drug abusers are at risk of infection. HGV frequently occurs as a coinfection with HCV. HGV is estimated to produce 900 to 2000 infections per year; most asymptomatic. Chronic disease is rare or may not occur at all.
- Transfusion-transmitted virus (TTV), a recent addition to the infectious hepatitis family. The most remarkable feature of TTV is the extraordinarily high prevalence of chronic viremia in apparently healthy people, almost 100% in some countries. As with HGV, the pathogenicity of TTV has not been proven.

REVIEW QUESTIONS

Questions 1-4. Match the following forms of hepatitis with the appropriate description (a-d), using each answer only once.

1. _____ Acute hepatitis
2. _____ Fulminant acute hepatitis
3. _____ Subclinical hepatitis without jaundice
4. _____ Chronic hepatitis

a. This rare form is associated with hepatic failure.
b. Typical form of hepatitis with associated jaundice.
c. Probably accounts for persons with serum antibodies but no history of hepatitis.
d. Accompanied by hepatic inflammation and necrosis.

Questions 5-8. Match the following (use an answer only once).

5. _____ Hepatitis A
6. _____ Hepatitis B
7. _____ Hepatitis D
8. _____ Hepatitis C

a. Intact virus is the Dane particle.
b. Transmission by both parenteral and nonparenteral routes.
c. Requires HBV as a helper.
d. Most common form of hepatitis.

Questions 9-12. Match the following (use an answer only once).

9. _____ Hepatitis A
10. _____ Hepatitis B
11. _____ Delta agent
12. _____ Hepatitis C

a. Should receive immune globulin intramuscularly after exposure.
b. Defective or incomplete RNA virus.
c. Has an epidemiology similar to HA virus.
d. Previously called Australia antigen.

Questions 13-17. Match the following serologic markers with the appropriate description.

13. _____ HBsAg
14. _____ HBeAg
15. _____ Anti-HBc
16. _____ Anti-HBe
17. _____ Anti-HBs

a. Indicator of recent HBV infection may be only serologic marker during the window phase.
b. Found in the serum of some patients who are HBsAg positive; marker for level of virus, infectivity.
c. A serologic marker of recovery and immunity.
d. Initial detectable marker found in serum during incubation period of HBV infection.
e. In the case of acute hepatitis, the first serologic evidence of the convalescent phase.

18. Of patients in the United States with chronic hepatitis B, _____ of them acquired the virus in childhood.

a. Less than 20%
b. 20% to 30%
c. 30% to 40%
d. More than 40%

19. The rate of posttransfusion hepatitis C decreased to _____ after the introduction of serologic testing in the screening of blood donors.

a. Less than 1%
b. 5%
c. 10%
d. 15%

Questions 20-22. Match the following forms of hepatitis with the correct average incubation time.

20. _____ Hepatitis A

21. _____ Hepatitis B

22. _____ Hepatitis C

   a.   5 days
   b.   25 days
   c.   50 days
   d.   75 days
   e.   150 days

23. Which form of hepatitis does not have a chronic form of the disease?
   a.   Hepatitis A
   b.   Hepatitis B
   c.   Hepatitis C

24. Another name for hepatitis B infection is:
   a.   Infectious hepatitis.
   b.   Serum hepatitis.
   c.   Australia antigen.
   d.   Dane particle.

25. The most frequent clinical response to hepatitis B virus is:
   a.   Jaundice within 75 days.
   b.   Asymptomatic infection.
   c.   Subclinical infection.
   d.   Both b and c.

26. The first laboratory screening test of donor blood was for the detection of:
   a.   HBc.
   b.   HBsAg.
   c.   HBe.
   d.   Anti-HBe.

27. Which surface marker is a reliable marker for the presence of high levels of hepatitis B virus (HBV) and a high degree of infectivity?
   a.   HBeAg
   b.   HBsAg
   c.   HBcAg
   d.   Anti-HBsAg

28. The serologic marker during the "window period" of hepatitis B is:
   a.   Anti-HBs.
   b.   Anti-HBc.
   c.   Anti-HBe.
   d.   HBsAg.

29. Which of the following is a characteristic of the delta agent?
   a.   Is a DNA virus.
   b.   Usually replicates only in HBV-infected hosts.
   c.   Infects patients who are HBcAg positive.
   d.   Is frequently found in the United States.

30. Which of the following viruses is rarely implicated in transfusion-associated hepatitis?
   a.   Hepatitis A
   b.   Hepatitis B
   c.   Hepatitis C
   d.   Cytomegalovirus

31. In health care workers, the risk of contracting hepatitis C is _____ higher than the risk of contracting AIDS.
   a.   10% to 20%
   b.   20% to 40%
   c.   40% to 80%
   d.   80% to 100%

32. The specific diagnostic test for hepatitis C is:
   a.   Absence of anti-HAV and anti-HBsAg.
   b.   Increase in serum ALT.
   c.   Detection of non-A, non-B antibodies.
   d.   Anti-HCV.

33. The earliest detectable serologic marker of acute hepatitis C is:
   a.   Anti-HCV.
   b.   Anti-HBc and ALT.
   c.   HCV-RNA.
   d.   Anti-HBs and anti-HBc.

34. *Primary* hepatitis viruses are given this name because they primarily attack:
   a.   A variety of body systems.
   b.   The liver.
   c.   The skin.
   d.   The nervous system.

35. Hepatitis A has all the following characteristics *except:*
   a.   DNA virus.
   b.   Short-incubation hepatitis.
   c.   Crowded, unsanitary conditions are risk factor.
   d.   Rare occurrence of transfusion acquisition.

36. The Australia antigen is now called:
   a.   Dane particle.
   b.   Long-incubation hepatitis.
   c.   Hepatitis B surface antigen (HBsAg).
   d.   Hepatitis B core antigen (HBcAg).

Questions 37-42. Fill in the following table, using a, b, or c, as indicated.
   a.   Positive (+)
   b.   Negative (−)
   c.   Questionable (±)

Serologic Markers for Hepatitis B Virus Infection

	Early (Asymptomatic)	Acute/Chronic	Low-Level Carrier	Immunity with HBsAg
HbsAg	37. _____	38. _____	Negative (−)	Negative (−)
Anti-HBs	Negative (−)	Questionable (±)	Negative (−)	Positive (+)
Anti-HBc	Negative (−)	39. _____	40. _____	41. _____
Anti-HBc (IgM)	Negative (−)	Positive (+)	Negative (−)	42. _____

43. Which category has the highest incidence of acute hepatitis C?
    a. Low socioeconomic status
    b. Dialysis
    c. Transfusion
    d. Drug abuse

44. Which category has the lowest incidence of acute hepatitis C?
    a. Sexual/household
    b. Dialysis
    c. Drug abuse
    d. Transfusion

Questions 45-48. Match each form of hepatitis to the appropriate mode of transmission. (You may use an answer more than once.)

45. _____ Hepatitis A

46. _____ Hepatitis B

47. _____ Hepatitis C

48. _____ Hepatitis E

    a. Fecal-oral
    b. Parenteral
    c. Parenteral and nonparenteral

49. The mean length of time from posttransfusion hepatitis to chronic hepatitis is:
    a. 2 years.
    b. 4 years.
    c. 8 years.
    d. 10 years.

50. The mean length of time from posttransfusion hepatitis to cirrhosis is:
    a. 4.8 years.
    b. 8.9 years.
    c. 21.2 years.
    d. 35.4 years.

BIBLIOGRAPHY

Aikawa T, Sugai Y, Okamoto H: Hepatitis G infection in drug abusers with chronic hepatitis C (letter), *N Engl J Med* 334:195-196, 1996.

Alter HJ: The cloning and clinical implications of HGV and HGBV-C, *N Engl J Med* 334:1536-1537, 1996.

Alter HJ et al: The incidence of transfusion-associated hepatitis G virus infection and its relation to liver disease, *N Engl J Med* 336:747-754, 1997.

Alter MJ et al: Acute non-A-E hepatitis in the United States and the role of hepatitis G virus infection, *N Engl J Med* 336:741-746, 1997.

Bean P: The use of alternative medicine in the treatment of hepatitis C, *Am Clin Lab* 21(4):19-21, 2002.

Bean P: New strategies in the treatment of hepatitis C, *Am Clin Lab* 21(3):18-20, 2002.

Bendinelli M et al: Molecular properties, biology, and clinical implications of TT virus, a recently identified widespread infectious agent of humans, *Clin Microbiol Rev* 14:98-113, 2001.

Bruno R et al: Challenges for hepatitis C patients coinfected with HIV, *Am Clin Lab* 21(4):26-29, 2002.

De Lamballerie X, Charrel RN, Bussol B: Hepatitis GB virus C in patients on hemodialysis, *N Engl J Med* 334:1549, 1996.

Changing landscape of HIV-hepatitis C virus and HIV coinfection. HIV/AIDS treatment updates, 2000, Medscape, www.medscape.com.

DiBisceglie AM: Interferon therapy for chronic viral hepatitis, *N Engl J Med* 330(2):137-138, 1994.

DiBisceglie AM: Hepatitis G virus infection: a work in progress, *Ann Intern Med* 125:772-773, 1996.

Dula WT, Anderson SM: Diagnosis and monitoring of hepatitis C infection, *ADVANCE Administrators Lab* 7(6):65-69, 1998.

Emerson SU, Purcell RH: Running like water: the omnipresence of hepatitis C, *N Engl J Med* 351(23):2367-2368, 2004.

Farci P et al: Treatment of chronic hepatitis D with interferon alfa-2a, *N Engl J Med* 330(2):88-94, 1994.

Focus: markers on hepatitis, *ADVANCE Administrators Lab,* October 2001.

Fried MW et al: Hepatitis G virus co-infection in liver transplantation recipients with chronic hepatitis C and nonviral chronic liver disease, *Hepatology* 25:1271-1275, 1997.

Gibb DM et al: Mother-to-child transmission of hepatitis C virus, *Hosp Physician* 36(11):16, 2000 (review).

Gindler J et al: Successful immunization for children and adults, *Patient Care* 31(15):124, 1997.

Gudima S et al: Origin of hepatitis delta virus mRNA, *J Virol* 74(16):7204-7210, 2000.

Gretch DR et al: Assessment of hepatitis C viremia using molecular amplification technologies: correlations and clinical implications, *Ann Intern Med* 123(5):321-336, 1995.

Heathcote EJ et al: Peginterferon alfa-2a in patients with chronic hepatitis C and cirrhosis, *N Engl J Med* 343:1673-1680, 2000.

Hepatitis, 2002, Division of Infectious Diseases, http://hopkins-id.edu/diseases/hepatitis.html.

Holst B, Ritter D: Managing viral hepatitis: a practical approach, *Clin Rev* 11(1):51-62, 2001.

Hoofnagle JH: Heptitis B: preventable and now treatable, *N Engl J Med* 354(10):1074-1078, 2006.

Ince N, Wands J: The increasing incidence of hepatocellular carcinoma (editorial), *N Engl J Med* 340(10):798-799, 1999.

Itoh K et al: Infection by an unenveloped DNA virus associated with non-A to -G hepatitis in Japanese blood donors with or without elevated ALT levels, *Transfusion* 39(5):522-527, 1999.

Jandreski MA: Hepatitis testing, *Clin Lab News* 24:10-12, 1999.

Kangxian J et al: Epidemiological survey and follow-up of transfusion-transmitted virus after an outbreak of enterically transmitted infection, *J Viral Hepat* 7(4):309, 2000.

Kew M: Viral hepatitis: diagnosis, therapy, and prevention (book review), *N Engl J Med* 341(10):770, 1999.

Koff R: The case for routine childhood vaccination against hepatitis A (editorial), *N Engl J Med* 340(8):644-645, 1999.

Lara CR et al: Detection of hepatitis C virus RNA in persons with and without known risk factors for blood-borne viral infections in Sweden and Honduras, *J Clin Microbiol* 36(1):255-257, 1998.

Lee WM: Hepatitis B virus infection, *N Engl J Med* 337(24):1733-1743, 1997.

Linnen J et al: Molecular cloning and disease association of hepatitis G virus: a transfusion-transmissible agent, *Science* 271:505-508, 1996.

Lopez-Alcorocho JM et al: Detection of hepatitis GB virus type C RNA in serum and liver from children with chronic viral hepatitis B and C, *Hepatology* 25:1258-1260, 1997.

Lucey M: Hepatitis B virus infection, American Association for the Study of Liver Disease, 51st Annual Meeting and Postgraduate Course, October 2000.

Mannucci PM et al: Transmission of hepatitis A to patients with hemophilia by factor VIII concentrates treated with organic solvent and detergent to inactivate viruses, *Ann Intern Med* 120(1):1-7, 1994.

Martinot M et al: Influence of hepatitis G virus infection on the severity of liver disease and response to interferon-alpha in patients with chronic hepatitis C, *Ann Intern Med* 126:874-881, 1997.

Masuko K et al: Infection with hepatitis GB virus C in patients on maintenance hemodialysis, *N Engl J Med* 334:1485-1490, 1996.

Mauser-Bunschoten EP: Transmission of hepatitis C virus in spouses, *Ann Intern Med* 122(2):154, 1995.

McHutchison JG et al: Interferon alfa-2b alone or in combination with ribavirin as initial treatment for chronic hepatitis, *N Engl J Med* 339(21):1485-1492, 1998.

MEDLINE plus Health Information, 2002, www.nlm.nih.gov.

Modahl LE, Lai MM: Hepatitis delta virus: the molecular basis of laboratory diagnosis, *Crit Rev Clin Lab Sci* 37(1):45-92, 2000.

Moradpour D, Wands JR: Understanding hepatitis B virus infection, *N Engl J Med* 332(16):1092-1093, 1995.

Ngo Y et al: A prospective analysis of the prognostic value of biomarkers (Fibro test) in patients with chronic hepatitis C, *Clin Chem* 52(10):1887-1896, 2006.

Pawlotsky JM: Treating hepatitis C in "difficult-to-treat" patients, *N Engl J Med* 351(5), 2004.

Pessoa MG et al: Hepatitis G virus in patients with cryptogenic liver disease undergoing liver transplantation, *Hepatology* 25:1266-1270, 1997.

Reshef RR, Sbeit W, Tur-Kaspa W: Lamivudine in the treatment of acute hepatitis B, *N Engl J Med* 343(15):1123-1124, 2000.

Sainato D: Viral testing in hepatitis, *Clin Lab News* 24:12-15, 1999.

Sato S et al: Hepatitis B virus strains with mutations in the core in patients with fulminant hepatitis, *Ann Intern Med* 122(4):241-248, 1995.

Sandler SG: Gains and strains of HCV diagnosis, *CAP Today* 16:22-28, 2001.

Sebastian J, Conrad A: Blood screening, *Adv Hepatitis* 10(10):30-35, 2001.

Sherker AH: Clinical news and views on hepatitis. Hepatitis G, 1998, www.hepnet.com.

Simons JN et al: Identification of two flavivirus-like genomes in the GB hepatitis agent, *Proc Natl Acad Sci U S A* 92:3401-3405, 1995.

Simons JN et al: Isolation of novel virus-like sequences associated with human hepatitis, *Nat Med* 1:564-569, 1995.

Tanaka E et al: Effect of hepatitis G virus infection on chronic hepatitis C, *Ann Intern Med* 125:740-743, 1996.

Tedeschim V, Seeff LB: Diagnostic tests for hepatitis C: where are we now? *Ann Intern Med* 123(5):383-384, 1995.

Terrault N, Wright T: Interferon and hepatitis C, *N Engl J Med* 332(22):1509-1511, 1995.

Thursz MR et al: Association between an MHC class II allele and clearance of hepatitis B virus in The Gambia, *N Engl J Med* 332(16):1065-1069, 1995.

Toyoda H et al: TT virus genotype changes frequently in multiply transfused patients with hemophilia but rarely in patients with chronic hepatitis C and in healthy subjects, *Transfusion* 41(9):1130-1135, 2001.

Turgeon ML: Hepatitis C: what's new? *Adv Med Lab Prof* 12(23):24,2001.

Van Der Poel CL et al: Infectivity of blood seropositive for hepatitis C virus antibodies, *Lancet* 335:558-560, 1990.

Villeneuve JP et al: Lamivudine treatment for decompensated cirrhosis resulting from chronic hepatitis B, *Hepatology* 31(1):207-210, 2000.

Wang JT et al: Incidence and clinical presentation of posttransfusion TT virus infection in prospectively followed transfusion recipients: emphasis on its relevance to hepatitis, *Transfusion* 40(5):596-599, 2000.

Wasley A, Grytdal S, Gallagher K: *MMWR* 57(5502):1-24, 2008.

Weikersheimer P: Is hepatitis C virus targeted lookback effective? *Lab Med* 31(11):600-604, 2000.

Worman HJ: Hepatitis C: current treatment, 2002, http://cpmcnet.columbia.edu.

Worman HJ: New and future treatment of chronic hepatitis C, *Viewpoints,* Spring/Summer 2001, American Liver Foundation, Greater New York, http://cpmcnet.columbia.edu, 2002.

Zeuzem S et al: Peginterferon alfa-2a in patients with chronic hepatitis C, *N Engl J Med* 343:1666-1672, 2000.

CHAPTER 24

Rubella Infection

Etiology
Epidemiology
Signs and Symptoms
  Acquired Infection
  Congenital Infection
Immunologic Manifestations
  Acquired Infection
  Congenital Rubella Syndrome

Diagnostic Evaluation
  Hemagglutination Inhibition
  Other Methods
Passive Latex Agglutination Test
Case Study
Chapter Highlights
Review Questions
Bibliography

Learning Objectives

At the conclusion of this chapter, the reader should be able to:

- Describe the etiology and epidemiology of rubella infection.
- Explain the signs and symptoms of acquired and congenital infection.
- Compare the immunologic manifestations of acquired and congenital rubella infection.

- Explain the diagnostic evaluation of rubella, including hemagglutination inhibition and passive latex agglutination for immunoglobulin G.
- Analyze a representative rubella case study.

ETIOLOGY

The rubella virus was first isolated in 1962. *Acquired rubella,* also known as *German measles* or *3-day measles,* is caused by an enveloped, single-stranded RNA virus of the Togaviridae family. Because the virus is endemic to humans, the disease is highly contagious and transmitted through respiratory secretions. Before widespread rubella immunization, this viral infection occurred most often in childhood, although it also affected adults.

EPIDEMIOLOGY

Three strains of live, attenuated rubella vaccine virus were developed and first licensed for use in the United States in 1969. Before widespread rubella immunization in the United States and Canada, rubella infections occurred in epidemic proportion at 6- to 9-year intervals. In 1964, more than 20,000 cases of congenital rubella syndrome and an unknown number of stillbirths occurred in the United States as the result of an epidemic that year.

In countries where vaccination is uncommon, the incidence of rubella infection is high and epidemics are frequent. Because vaccination programs have prevented the rubella epidemics that once gave people naturally acquired immunity, individuals who have not been vaccinated have a higher level of susceptibility to rubella infection. Primarily, two types of outbreaks have occurred in the United States in the recent past, affecting the following groups:
- Unvaccinated preschool-age children.
- Highly vaccinated school-age children.

The epidemiology of measles reveals two major impediments to measles elimination: (1) unvaccinated preschool-age children, a factor that allows large outbreaks, and (2) vaccine failures, which account for outbreaks in highly vaccinated school-age populations. On American college and university campuses, the susceptibility to rubella infection among students is estimated to be as high as 20%. Many incidences have been either unrecognized or unreported because many cases of rubella infection are mild or subclinical.

Contracting the infection and vaccinating against rubella are the only routes to developing immunity. Individuals should be immune to rubella if they have a dated record of rubella vaccination on or after their first birthday, or if they have demonstrable rubella antibody. Even when antibody titers fall to relatively low levels, previous infection or successful vaccination appears to confer permanent immunity to rubella, except in cases of congenital rubella. The only proof of immunity is a positive serologic screening test for rubella antibody. History of rubella infection, even if verified by a physician, is not acceptable evidence of immunity.

It is critical to continue to determine the rubella immune status of women of childbearing age and to vaccinate those who are not immune. Individuals requiring rubella immune status determination include those in the following groups:
- Preschool-age and school-age children.
- All females at or just before childbearing age.
- Women about to be married.
- Married women.
  If the woman is not rubella immune, she should be vaccinated and advised not to become pregnant for

3 months because of the remote possibility that the vaccination could lead to an infected fetus.

- Pregnant women.

    A positive test confirms immunity, but to rule out any possibility of unsuspected current infection, an IgM screening procedure may also be ordered. If the patient is not rubella immune, she should be cautioned to avoid exposure to rubella infection. Vaccination is contraindicated in pregnant women; however, a woman should be vaccinated immediately after termination of the pregnancy.

- Health care personnel.

    Both men and women should be vaccinated to prevent possible spread of nosocomial infection to pregnant patients.

Adverse reactions to rubella vaccine have been reported. The Institute of Medicine determined that a causal relationship exists between rubella vaccine and *acute* arthritis in adult women. Weak but consistent evidence exists for a causal relationship between rubella vaccine and *chronic* arthritis in adult women. Incidence rates are estimated to average 13% to 15% among adult women after vaccination. Much lower levels of arthritic adverse reaction were noted among children, adolescents, and adult men. Reliable estimates of excess risk of chronic arthritis after rubella vaccination are not available.

SIGNS AND SYMPTOMS

A diagnosis of acquired rubella is not based solely on clinical manifestation. The signs and symptoms of rubella vary widely from person to person and may not be recognized in some cases, especially if the characteristic rash is light or absent, as may occur in a substantial number of cases. Rubella infection also may resemble other disorders, such as infectious mononucleosis and drug-induced rashes.

Acquired Infection

The incubation period of acquired rubella infection varies from 10 to 21 days, and 12 to 14 days is typical. Infected persons are usually contagious for 12 to 15 days, beginning 5 to 7 days before the appearance (if present) of a rash. Acute rubella infection lasts from 3 to 5 days and generally requires minimal treatment. Permanent effects are extremely rare in acquired infections.

The clinical presentation of acquired rubella is usually mild. The clinical manifestation of infection usually begins with a prodromal period of catarrhal symptoms, followed by involvement of the retroauricular, posterior cervical, and postoccipital lymph nodes, and finally by the emergence of a maculopapular rash on the face and then on the neck and trunk (Figures 24-1 and 24-2). A temperature of less than 34.4° C (94° F) is usually present. In older children and adults, self-limiting arthralgia and arthritis are common.

Congenital Infection

Rubella infection is usually a mild, self-limiting disease with only rare complications in children and adults. In pregnant women, however, especially those infected in the first tri-

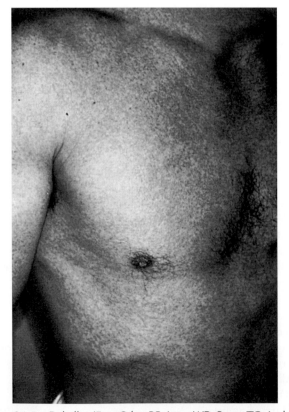

Figure 24-1   Rubella. *(From Odom RB, James WD, Berger TG:* Andrews' diseases of the skin: clinical dermatology, *ed 9, St Louis, 2000, Saunders.)*

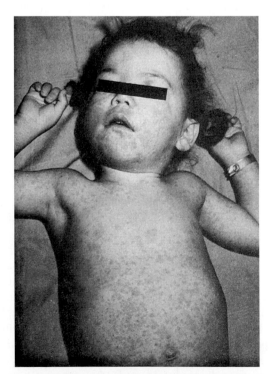

Figure 24-2   Rubella rash. *(From Krugman S et al:* Infectious diseases of children, *ed 8, St Louis, 1985, Mosby.)*

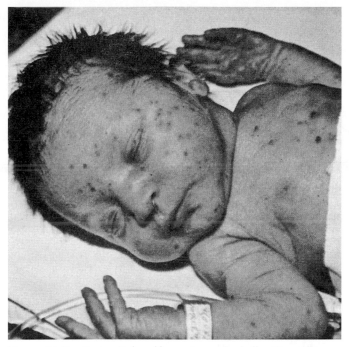

Figure 24-3   Congenital malformations of rubella. *(From Krugman S et al:* Infectious diseases of children, *ed 8, St Louis, 1985, Mosby.)*

mester, rubella can have devastating effects on the fetus (Figure 24-3). In utero infection can result in fetal death or manifest as *rubella syndrome,* a spectrum of congenital defects. About 10% to 20% of infants infected in utero fail to survive beyond 18 months.

The point in the gestation cycle at which maternal rubella infection occurs greatly influences the severity of congenital rubella syndrome (Table 24-1), and the extent of congenital anomalies varies from one infant to another. Some infants manifest almost all the defects associated with rubella, whereas others exhibit few, if any, consequences of infection. Clinical evidence of congenital rubella infection may not be recognized for months or even years after birth.

Table 24-1	Manifestation of Anomalies in Maternal Rubella
Period of Gestation	**Risk of Anomaly**
Prospective Studies	
First trimester	Approximately 25%
Second trimester	
First month	Less than 1%
Second month	25% or higher
Third month	10% or higher
Serologically Confirmed Cases of Maternal Infection	
Before 11 weeks	90%
11-12 weeks	33%
13-14 weeks	11%
15-16 weeks	24%
After 16 weeks	0%

Rubella syndrome encompasses a number of congenital anomalies. In addition to stillbirth, fetal abnormalities associated with maternal rubella infection include encephalitis, hepatomegaly, bone defects, mental retardation, cataracts, thrombocytopenic purpura, cardiovascular defects, splenomegaly, and microcephaly. Severely affected children are likely to have multiple defects in different organ systems. In neonates with congenital rubella syndrome, low birth weight and failure to thrive are common.

Rubella immunity develops in almost all children who have had congenital rubella. In late childhood, however, about one third of these patients lose antibody and become susceptible to acquired rubella. If acquired rubella occurs, it follows a typically benign course. Children with congenital rubella should be screened for rubella immunity in late childhood and vaccinated if necessary.

IMMUNOLOGIC MANIFESTATIONS

Acquired Infection

In a patient with primary rubella infection, the appearance of both immunoglobulin G (IgG) and immunoglobulin M (IgM) antibodies is associated with the appearance of clinical signs and symptoms, when present.

The IgM antibodies become detectable a few days after the onset of signs and symptoms and reach peak levels at 7 to 10 days. These antibodies persist but rapidly diminish in concentration over the next 4 to 5 weeks, until antibody is no longer clinically detectable. The presence of IgM antibody in a single specimen suggests that the patient has recently experienced a rubella infection. In most cases the infection probably occurred in the preceding month.

Production of IgG is also associated with the appearance of clinical signs and symptoms. Antibody levels increase rapidly for the next 7 to 21 days, then level off or even decrease in strength. IgG antibodies, however, remain present and protective indefinitely. Detection of IgG antibody is a useful indicator of rubella infection only when the acute and convalescent blood specimens are drawn several weeks apart. Optimum timing for paired testing in the diagnosis of a recent infection is 2 or more weeks apart, with the first *(acute)* specimen taken before or at the time signs and symptoms appear, or within 2 weeks of exposure.

Paired-specimen testing may demonstrate that the antibody levels are the same. In these cases, either the patient was previously immunized or the acute sample was taken after the antibody had already reached maximum levels. Demonstration of an unequivocal increase in IgG antibody concentration between the acute and convalescent specimens suggests either a recent primary infection or a secondary *(anamnestic)* antibody response to rubella in an immune individual. In cases of an anamnestic response, IgM antibodies are not demonstrable, but IgG production begins quickly. No other signs or symptoms of disease are exhibited.

If both IgM and IgG test results are negative, the patient has never had rubella infection or been vaccinated. Such

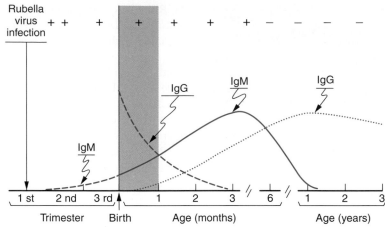

Figure 24-4   Natural history of congenital rubella: pattern of virus excretion and antibody response. *(Redrawn from Krugman S et al:* Infectious diseases of children, *ed 9, St Louis, 1992, Mosby.)*

patients are susceptible to infection. If no IgM is demonstrable but IgG is present in paired specimens, the patient is immune.

In evaluation of the immune status of patients, IgG antibodies present in a dilution of 1:8 or greater indicate past infection with rubella virus and clinical protection against future rubella infection. The clinical significance of lower levels is not currently known. Titers of 1:16, 1:64, 1:512, or greater may be found in both acute and past infections; however, diagnosis of acute infections requires an IgM antibody titer on the same specimen or a paired-specimen comparison. It should be noted that IgM also appears for a transient period after vaccination.

Congenital Rubella Syndrome

Because IgG antibody is capable of crossing the placental barrier, there is no way of distinguishing between IgG antibody of fetal origin and IgG antibody of maternal origin in a neonatal blood specimen (Figure 24-4).

Testing for IgM antibody is invaluable in the diagnosis of congenital rubella syndrome in the neonate. IgM does not cross an intact placental barrier; therefore demonstration of IgM in a single neonatal specimen is diagnostic of congenital rubella syndrome. In the newborn, serologic confirmation of rubella infection can be made by testing for IgM antibody for at least the first 6 months of life. This is especially useful when clinical evidence of congenital rubella is slow in emerging or is of uncertain origin.

DIAGNOSTIC EVALUATION

Physicians apply the results of rubella testing independently, frequently without the benefit of clinical signs and symptoms. Historically, **hemagglutination inhibition (HAI)** antibody testing has been the most frequently used method of screening for the presence of rubella antibodies. Recently, the HAI test has been replaced by more convenient assays as the screening method of choice for the determination of rubella immune (IgG) status. In some patients, such as pregnant women, it also may be necessary to determine if a recent infection has occurred. The assays for determination of immune status and evidence of recent infection are presented in Table 24-2.

Hemagglutination Inhibition

Despite wide acceptance and use of other assays, HAI testing continues to be the reference method for detection and quantitation of rubella antibody. Rubella methods vary in sensitivity and specificity when samples with antibody levels near the breakpoint of "immune versus nonimmune" are analyzed. A gray area exists around the cutoff point of any test, but marginal results may be encountered with some methods.

False-negative results with some methodologies are most frequently seen when HAI titers are at or near the cutoff antibody level of 1:8. It is important that the method used for screening demonstrates sensitivity, specificity, and reproducibility of 95% or greater based on an assay of 200 or more serum samples compared with HAI. A disadvantage of HAI, however, is that although the procedure detects a combination of IgM and IgG antibodies, it does not distinguish between them. If IgG is separated from IgM, this procedure can be used as a differential method. Separation of IgM can be by sucrose density gradient fractions, protein A–Sepharose, or an affinity column.

Table 24-2	Tests for Rubella Immune Status Serodiagnosis	
Method	**Immunity**	**Serodiagnosis**
Hemagglutination inhibition	Yes	Yes*
Fluorescent immunoassay	Yes	Yes*
Latex agglutination	Yes	No
Enzyme immunoassay, IgM	No	Yes
Enzyme immunoassay, IgG	Yes	Yes*

*Serodiagnosis may not differentiate between primary infection and reinfection. An IgM-specific procedure must be used.

Other Methods

Latex procedures provide more rapid and convenient alternatives to HAI. If more quantitative results are desired, enzyme immunoassay (EIA), chemiluminescent assay, and fluorescent immunoassay (FIA) appear to be as reliable as HAI.

An EIA can be used to measure total antibody, IgG, or IgM. IgM antibodies can be detected by EIA in 100% of patients between days 11 and 25 after onset of signs and symptoms of acquired infection, in 60% to 80% of persons at days 15 to 25 after vaccination, and in 90% to 97% of infants with congenital rubella between 2 weeks and 3 months after birth. The rubella-specific IgM often persists for 20 to 30 days after acute infection or vaccination and also in infants with congenital rubella.

Persons with infectious mononucleosis sometimes have rubella-specific IgM in low concentrations. Cross-reactions of rubella IgM-positive sera can result from parvovirus IgM. Occasionally, pregnant women will demonstrate IgM antibodies not only to rubella but also to cytomegalovirus, varicella-zoster virus, and measles virus. In these patients, diagnosis of rubella can be made only by assessment of rubella-specific IgG antibodies by HAI and EIA procedures, supported by a detailed clinical history. Rubella-specific IgG is regularly detected by EIA only later than 15 to 25 days after infection and later than 25 to 50 days after vaccination.

Passive Latex Agglutination Test

For detection and/or semiquantitation of antibodies.

Principle

Latex particles are sensitized with solubilized rubella virus antigens from disrupted virions judged to be inactivated. When the latex reagent is mixed with serum containing rubella antibodies on a dark surface, the antigen-antibody complex will form visible clumps. In the absence of antibody or if the concentration is insufficient to react, the latex particles will remain smooth and evenly dispersed. If a qualitative procedure is performed, the presence of rubella antibodies is an indication of previous infection, and presumptive immunity can be used to evaluate the immune status of that individual with regard to resistance or susceptibility to primary rubella infection.

Specimen Collection and Preparation

The protocol for specimen collection will vary depending on the testing objectives. Single specimens are required for qualitative determination of antibody levels. In suspected clinical infections or exposure, two specimens for quantitative testing should be obtained. The first should be collected within 3 days of the onset of rash or at the time of exposure and tested on arrival in the laboratory. This specimen should be frozen and stored until the second specimen is collected 7 to 21 days after the onset of the rash or at least 30 days after exposure if no clinical symptoms occur. Both specimens should be tested simultaneously.

No special preparation of the patient is required before specimen collection. The patient must be positively identified when the specimen is collected, and the specimen is to be labeled at the bedside. Specimen labels must include the patient's full name, the date the specimen is collected, the patient's hospital identification number, and the phlebotomist's initials.

Blood should be drawn by aseptic technique. A minimum of 2 mL of clotted blood (red-top evacuated tube) is required. The specimen should be centrifuged promptly and an aliquot of serum removed. Specimens may be stored up to 48 hours at 2° to 8° C. Specimens should be frozen if longer storage is required. Do not heat-inactivate the serum. The presence of particulate matter, lipemia, or hemolysis does not affect the test.

Reagents, Supplies, and Equipment

WARNING: The latex reagent, buffer, and controls contain sodium azide as a preservative. Sodium azide may react with lead and copper plumbing to form highly explosive metal azides. On disposal, flush with a large volume of water to prevent azide buildup.

RUBAscan Kit (Becton Dickinson, Franklin Lakes, NJ)

- Reagent A: Latex antigen
  This reagent contains 0.02% gentamicin and 0.2% sodium azide. Store at 2° to 8° C, and return to refrigeration when not being used. *Do not freeze.*
- Reagent B: Card dilution buffer
  Phosphate-buffered saline (PBS) solution containing bovine serum albumin with 0.02% sodium azide. Store at 2° to 8° C, and return to refrigeration when not being used. *Do not freeze.*
- Test cards
  Cards must be flat for proper reactions. If necessary, flatten cards by bowing back in a direction opposite to that of the curl. Care should be taken not to finger-mark the test areas; this may result in an oily deposit and improper test results. Use each card once and discard. Store cards in the original package in a dry area at room temperature.
- Plastic stirrers
- Dispensing needle (21 gauge, green hub)
  On completion of daily tests, remove the needle from the dispensing bottle and recap the bottle. Rinse the needle with distilled water to maintain clear passage and accurate drop delivery. Do not wipe the dispensing needle, because it is coated with silicone.

Additional Required Equipment

- Centrifuge
- Rotator
  The recommended rotation speed is 100 rpm, but rotation between 95 and 110 rpm does not significantly affect the results obtained. The rotator should circumscribe a circle approximately 2 cm in diameter in the horizontal plane. A moistened humidifying cover should be used to prevent drying of test specimens during rotation.

- Humidifying cover
- High-intensity incandescent lamp
- Micropipettors: 25 and 100 μL
- Other equipment and glassware for preparation, storage, and handling of serologic specimens

Quality Control

The following controls are provided in the RUBAscan kit:
- Control +: Low-reactive control with 0.1% sodium azide. This control is used for both the qualitative and the quantitative assay.
- Control ++: High-reactive control with 0.1% sodium azide. This control is used in the quantitative assay only.
- Control −: Nonreactive control with 0.1% sodium azide. This control is used for both the qualitative and quantitative assay.

Each of these controls must be tested with each series of unknown patient specimens.

CAUTION: Because the control sera are derived from human sources, they should be handled in the same manner as clinical serum specimens (Standard Precautions; see Chapter 6).

Procedure

Note: The test area, reagents, specimens, and test components must be at 23° to 29° C before testing. Do not mix reagents from different lot numbers. The dispensing bottle must be held vertically.

Qualitative Testing

1. Remove the cap from the bottle of latex agglutination and attach the green hub needle to the tapered fitting.
2. Mark the card to identify the low-reactive and nonreactive controls and all samples.

   With Undiluted Specimens
   a. With a micropipettor, place 25 μL of low-reactive control on the appropriately marked circle.
   b. With the same micropipettor and a clean tip each time, repeat the procedure in step a, using the nonreactive control and each specimen to be tested.

   Alternate Procedure—1:10 Specimen Dilution
   a. Using the micropipettor, add 100 μL of buffer to the appropriate squares for each control and specimen to be tested. These squares will be used to prepare the 1:5 dilution in step c below.
   b. Using the micropipettor, add 25 μL of buffer to the appropriate squares for each control and specimen to be tested. These squares will be used to prepare the 1:10 dilution in step d.
   c. With the micropipette and a clean tip, pipette 25 μL of low-reactive control directly into the buffer in the appropriately labeled circle, and mix the serum and buffer by drawing up and down with the micropipette 12 times. Caution should be exercised to avoid the formation of bubbles. The serum in this circle is now a 1:5 dilution.
   d. Using the same micropipette and tip, transfer 25 μL of the 1:5 dilution from the circle and place directly into the buffer in the corresponding numbered circle, and mix by drawing up and down with the micropipette six times. Withdraw 25 μL from the circle and discard. The serum in this circle is now a 1:10 dilution.
   e. Repeat the procedure in step c for the nonreactive control and for each specimen to be tested.
3. Using a new plastic stirrer for each circle, spread each of the specimens to be tested (either 25 μL of serum or 25 μL of 1:10 diluted serum) to fill the entire circle.
4. Place the bottle cap over the tip of the needle, and gently invert the bottle of latex reagent several times to mix.
5. While holding the latex reagent bottle in a vertical position, dispense several drops of antigen into the bottle cap until a drop of uniform size has formed. Dispense 1 free-falling drop of antigen (~15 μL) on each circle containing diluted serum. Care must be taken to avoid contamination of the bottle tip. The predropped antigen can be recovered from the bottle cap and reused.
6. Place the card on a rotator and rotate for 8 minutes under a moistened humidifying cover.
7. Immediately after mechanical rotation, read the card macroscopically in the wet state with the aid of a high-intensity incandescent lamp. A brief hand rotation of the card (three or four back-and-forth motions) must be made after mechanical rotation to help differentiate weak agglutination from no agglutination. Fluorescent lighting is generally insufficient to distinguish minimally reactive results. The use of magnification in reading test results is not recommended.
8. The reactive control should exhibit agglutination; the nonreactive control should demonstrate no agglutination.

Reporting Results

A positive reaction demonstrates agglutination.
A negative reaction demonstrates no agglutination.

Procedure Notes

A single specimen can be used to estimate the immune status of the individual, because any detectable antibody is indicative of immunity and protection against subsequent viral infection. The alternate procedure using specimens diluted 1:10 should be used when data are needed at a sensitivity level approximating that expected with HIA methods. Optimal sensitivity can be ensured by screening all serum samples undiluted and repeating negative specimens at a 1:10 dilution. The Clinical Laboratory and Standards Institute (CLSI, formerly NCCLS) advises that the specimen should not be frozen in a frost-free freezer because the freeze-thaw cycle may be detrimental to serum proteins. CLSI guidelines further suggest that frozen specimens be retained for at least 1 year for later follow-up examination, especially for women of childbearing age who are inadvertently exposed to the rubella virus.

The acute-phase specimen should be collected as nearly as possible to the time of exposure, and no later than 3 days after the onset of rash. The convalescent-phase specimen should be taken 7 to 21 days after the onset of the rash or at least 30 days after exposure if no clinical symptoms appear because of a possible inapparent infection. Both specimens should be tested simultaneously.

Sources of Error
False-negative results may occur in the following conditions:
1. Reduction in the degree of agglutination has been reported with rare high-titered specimens when the test is performed undiluted.
2. In undiluted specimens, strong reactivity may cause the center of the test circle to appear clear because agglutinated latex has migrated to the periphery.
3. If only a 1:10 dilution is used, the procedure may fail to detect a low level antibody that might have otherwise been detected with an undiluted specimen.
4. The absence of a fourfold titer rise does not necessarily rule out the possibility of exposure and infection. If the first (acute-phase) sample is taken too late or the second (convalescent-phase) sample is taken too soon, seroconversion or a fourfold rise in titer characteristic of recent infection may not be seen.

Limitations
A single specimen determines immunity; it is not a serodiagnosis of infection/reinfection.

The qualitative card test is designed to detect the presence of rubella antibody. At a single dilution, the qualitative protocol will perform satisfactorily with both acute-phase and convalescent-phase antibodies; however, when the presence or absence of a fourfold titer rise in paired specimens must be demonstrated, the quantitative protocol is required.

Clinical Applications
The presence of antibodies in a single patient specimen is an indication of previous exposure and immunity to rubella virus. Demonstration of any detectable antibody is indicative of immunity and protection against subsequent viral infection; however, a test configuration using an undiluted specimen may be preferred.

Demonstration of seroconversion, or a fourfold or greater rise in antibody titer with properly collected paired specimens, is diagnostic of a recent or current infection with rubella virus. Seroconversion means a positive test result of 1.5 or greater after an initial nonreactive result of less than 1:5.

References
RUBAscan product brochure, Becton Dickinson, Franklin Lakes, NJ. Revised July 2003.
Skendzel LP: New guidelines and standards for rubella antibody testing from NCCLS and CAP, *Lab Med* 18(7):461, 1987.

CASE STUDY

History and Physical Examination
A 20-year-old college junior comes to the student health office because she has been exposed to rubella during a recent outbreak at the college. She has been immunized as a child.

Laboratory Data
Hemagglutination inhibition test for rubella: negative.
Pregnancy test: positive.
Ultrasonography shows the fetus is in the eighth week of development.

Questions and Discussion
1. Is this woman susceptible to rubella infection?
Yes, this woman is susceptible to rubella. She has no serologic evidence of antibody formation in response to viral antigen stimulation. The only proof of immunity is a positive serologic screening test for rubella antibody (HIA). History of rubella infection, even if verified by a physician, is not acceptable evidence of immunity.

In case of a negative result, the HIA should be repeated in 3 weeks. If the antibody or HIA titer has risen, infection has occurred.

2. Is the fetus at risk of a congenital defect?
Brief exposure to a person with rubella infection does not always mean that the infection will be transmitted. Rubella infections in pregnant women, especially those infected in their first trimester of pregnancy, can have devastating effects on the fetus. In utero infection can result in fetal death or manifest as rubella syndrome. About 10% to 20% of infants infected in utero do not survive past 18 months.

The point that maternal rubella infection occurs in the gestation cycle greatly influences the severity of congenital rubella syndrome, and the extent of anomalies varies among infants. Some manifest almost all the defects associated with rubella, whereas others exhibit few, if any. Clinical evidence of congenital rubella syndrome may not be recognized for months or years after birth. In addition to stillbirth, fetal abnormalities include encephalitis, hepatomegaly, bone defects, mental retardation, cataracts, thrombocytopenic purpura, cardiovascular defects, splenomegaly, and microcephaly. Severely affected children will likely have multiple defects in different organ systems. Low birth weight and failure to thrive are common in affected neonates.

3. Is there any treatment for the infection?
Acyclovir, a common antiviral medication that inhibits DNA synthesis, has no effect on rubella virus because rubella is an RNA virus. In addition, human immune serum globulin may hide infection without protecting the fetus; it should not be given unless it is known at the outset that the mother will refuse abortion even if infection occurs. In this circumstance, immune globulin probably offers some protection against infection of the fetus.

Rubella vaccination is not effective if transmission has occurred because it is too late to prevent natural infection from the contact. The live vaccine virus theoretically could infect the fetus and cause congenital anomalies, but this situation occurs infrequently. In addition, inadvertent vaccination during pregnancy does not necessitate the termination of pregnancy.

Rubella immunity develops in almost all children who have had congenital rubella. In late childhood, however, about one third lose antibody and become susceptible to acquired rubella. If acquired rubella occurs, it follows a typically benign course. Children with congenital rubella should be screened for rubella immunity in late childhood and vaccinated, if necessary.

4. What are the immunologic manifestations of infection?

In a patient with primary rubella infection, IgG and IgM antibodies are associated with clinical signs and symptoms. IgM antibodies are detectable a few days after onset of signs and peak at 7 to 10 days. They persist but rapidly diminish over the next 4 to 5 weeks, until IgM antibody is no longer clinically detectable. The presence of IgM antibody in a single specimen suggests that the patient has recently experienced a rubella infection. Usually, the infection occurred in the preceding month.

Production of IgG also occurs as clinical signs and symptoms appear. Antibody levels increase rapidly for the next 7 to 21 days, then level off or even decrease in strength. IgG antibodies, however, remain present and protective indefinitely. IgG antibody is a useful indicator of rubella infection only when blood specimens are drawn several weeks apart (during acute and convalescent periods). Optimum timing for paired testing in diagnosing recent infection is 2 or more weeks apart, with the first (acute) specimen taken before or when symptoms appear, or within 2 weeks of exposure.

When paired-specimen testing demonstrates that the antibody levels are the same, the patient was previously immunized, or the acute sample was taken after the antibody reached a maximum titer. Unequivocal increase in IgG antibody concentration suggests a recent primary infection or a secondary (anamnestic) antibody response to rubella in an immune individual. In an anamnestic response, IgM antibodies are not demonstrable, but IgG production begins quickly, with no other signs.

Negative IgM and IgG results indicate no previous rubella infection or vaccination. Such patients are susceptible to infection. If no IgM is demonstrable but IgG is present in paired specimens, the patient is immune. IgG antibodies in a dilution of 1:8 or greater indicate past rubella infection and clinical protection against future infection. The clinical significance of lower levels is not known. Although titers of 1:16, 1:64, 1:512, or greater may be found in acute and past infections, diagnosis of acute infections requires an IgM antibody titer on the same specimen or a paired-specimen comparison. IgM also appears transiently after vaccination.

The IgG antibody can cross the placental barrier, so IgG antibody of fetal origin cannot be distinguished from that of maternal origin in a neonatal blood specimen. IgM does *not* cross an intact placental barrier, so demonstration of IgM in a single neonatal specimen is diagnostic of congenital rubella syndrome. Serologic confirmation of rubella infection can be made by testing for IgM antibody for at least the first 6 months of life, especially when clinical evidence of congenital rubella is slow in emerging or uncertain in origin.

Diagnosis

Rubella.

CHAPTER HIGHLIGHTS

- Acquired rubella (German or 3-day measles) is caused by an enveloped, single-stranded RNA virus of the Togaviridae family. It is endemic to humans, highly contagious, and transmitted through respiratory secretions.
- Contracting rubella infection and vaccinating against rubella are the only routes to developing immunity.
- A diagnosis of acquired rubella is not based solely on clinical manifestations; signs and symptoms vary widely. Although usually mild and self-limiting with rare complications in children and adults, rubella infections in pregnant women, especially in the first trimester, can result in fetal death or congenital rubella syndrome.
- In primary rubella infection, appearance of IgG and IgM antibodies is associated with clinical signs and symptoms, when present. IgM antibodies are detectable a few days after onset of symptoms, reach peak levels at 7 to 10 days, and persist but decrease rapidly in concentration over the next 4 to 5 weeks, until no longer clinically detectable.
- IgM antibody in a single specimen suggests a recent rubella infection.
- Unequivocal increase in IgG antibody concentration between the acute and convalescent specimens suggests a recent primary infection or an anamnestic antibody response to rubella in an immune individual.
- Negative IgM and IgG test results indicate the patient has never had rubella infection or been vaccinated. Such patients are susceptible to infection. If no IgM is demonstrable but IgG is present in paired specimens, the patient is immune.
- IgM does not cross an intact placental barrier, so its demonstration in a single neonatal specimen is diagnostic of congenital rubella syndrome. Rubella infection can be confirmed serologically by IgM antibody testing for at least the first 6 months of life, especially when clinical evidence of congenital rubella is slow in emerging or has an uncertain origin.
- Latex procedures provide more rapid and convenient alternatives to the classic hemagglutination inhibition assay (HAI). If more quantitative results are desired, EIA and FIA appear to be as reliable as HAI. Widespread use of EIA and chemiluminescent assay for assessment of

immune status (IgG) and recent infection (IgM) should soon result in simplification of rubella serology. EIA can be used to measure total antibody, IgG, or IgM.

REVIEW QUESTIONS

1. All the following groups of individuals should receive rubella vaccinations *except:*
   a. School-age children.
   b. Women of childbearing age.
   c. Pregnant women.
   d. Health care personnel.

2. The greatest risk of the manifestation of anomalies in maternal rubella is _____ of gestation.
   a. during the first month
   b. during the first trimester
   c. during the third month
   d. during the fourth or fifth month

3. In a patient with primary rubella infection, the appearance of _____ antibodies is associated with the clinical signs and symptoms, when present.
   a. IgG
   b. IgM
   c. IgD
   d. both a and b

4. Testing for _____ antibody is invaluable in the diagnosis of congenital rubella syndrome.
   a. IgM
   b. IgG
   c. IgD
   d. IgE

5. The reference method for detection and quantitation of rubella antibody is:
   a. Latex agglutination.
   b. Hemagglutination inhibition.
   c. Passive hemagglutination.
   d. Enzyme immunoassay.

6. Before the licensing of rubella vaccine in the United States in 1969, epidemics occurred at _____-year intervals.
   a. 2-3
   b. 5-7
   c. 6-9
   d. 10-20

7. Acute rubella infection lasts from _____ days.
   a. 1-2
   b. 2-4
   c. 3-5
   d. 7-10

8. IgM antibodies to rubella virus reach peak levels at _____ days.
   a. 2-4
   b. 3-5
   c. 5-7
   d. 7-10

9. IgG antibodies to rubella virus increase rapidly for _____ days after the acquisition of infection.
   a. 2-8
   b. 3-10
   c. 5-15
   d. 7-21

Questions 10-12. Fill in the blanks in the following table, using the letter "a" for "Yes" answers and the letter "b" for "No" answers.

Diagnostic Tests for Immune Status/Serodiagnosis

Method	Immunity	Serodiagnosis
Hemagglutination	10. _____	Yes
FIA	Yes	Yes
Latex agglutination	11. _____	12. _____
EIA-IgM	No	Yes
EIA-IgG	Yes	Yes

13. What percentage of serologically confirmed cases of maternal infection occur before 11 weeks of gestation?
   a. 11%
   b. 24%
   c. 33%
   d. 90%

BIBLIOGRAPHY

Bellamy K et al: IgM antibody capture enzyme-linked immunosorbent assay for detecting rubella-specific IgM, *J Clin Pathol* 38:1150-1154, 1985.

Chernesky MA, Mahoney JB: Rubella virus. In Rose NR, Friedman H, Fahey HJL, editors: *Manual of clinical laboratory immunology,* ed 3, Washington, DC, 1986, American Society of Microbiology.

Enders G, Knotek F, Pacher U: Comparison of various serological methods and diagnostic kits for the detection of acute, recent, and previous rubella infection, vaccination, and congenital infections, *J Med Virol* 16:219-232, 1985.

Fennes FJ, White DO: *Medical virology,* ed 2, New York, 1976, Academic Press.

Herrmann KL: Rubella virus. In Lennette EH et al, editors: *Manual of clinical microbiology,* ed 4, Washington, DC, 1985, American Society of Microbiology.

Horvath LM, LeBar WD: A comparison of methods for the determination of rubella antibody, *Am Clin Products Rev,* April 1987, pp 18-19.

Howson CP, Fineberg HV: Adverse events following pertussis and rubella vaccines, *JAMA* 267(3):392-396, 1992.

Kurtz JB, Anderson MJ: Cross-reactions in rubella and parvovirus specific IgM tests, *Lancet* 2:1356, 1985.

MMWR: Measles—United States, 1988, *JAMA* 262:13, 1989.

Morgan-Capner P, Tedder RS, Mace JE: Reactivity for rubella-specific IgM in sera from patients with infectious mononucleosis, *Lancet* 1:589, 1983.

Sever JL: *Laboratory advances in rubella diagnosis,* North Chicago, 1983, Abbott Laboratories.

Skendzel LP: New guidelines and standards for rubella antibody testing from NCCLS and CAP, *Lab Med* 18(7):461-462, 1987.

SIA rubella product brochure, St Louis, 1988, Sigma Chemical Co.

CHAPTER 25

Acquired Immunodeficiency Syndrome

Etiology
    Viral Characteristics
Epidemiology
    Incidence
    Classification System
    Infectious Patterns
    Modes of Transmission
Signs and Symptoms
    Opportunistic Infections
    Disease Progression
Immunologic Manifestations
    Cellular Abnormalities
    Alterations in Immune System
    Serologic Markers
Diagnostic Evaluation
Testing Methods
    HIV-1 Antibodies
    HIV Antigen and Genome Testing

Confirmatory Testing
    Rapid Testing
Prevention
    Reducing Viral Transmission
    Vaccines
Treatment
    Drug Therapy
    Postexposure Prophylaxis
Rapid HIV Antibody Test
Case Study
Chapter Highlights
Review Questions
Bibliography

Learning Objectives

At the conclusion of this chapter, the reader should be able to:

- Describe the etiology and viral characteristics of human immunodeficiency virus (HIV-1).
- Explain the epidemiology, including modes of transmission, and prevention of HIV-1.
- Discuss the signs and symptoms of various stages and the classification of HIV infection.

- Describe the immunologic manifestations and cellular abnormalities of HIV-1 infection.
- Explain the serologic markers and diagnostic evaluation of HIV.
- Analyze a representative HIV-1 case study.

ETIOLOGY

Human immunodeficiency virus (HIV) is the predominant virus responsible for **acquired immunodeficiency syndrome (AIDS).**

In 1983, researchers at the Pasteur Institute in Paris isolated a retrovirus, "lymphadenopathy-associated virus" (LAV), from a homosexual man with lymphadenopathy. Concurrently, an American research team headed by Dr. Robert Gallo isolated the same class of virus, which they labeled "human T-lymphotropic retrovirus" (HTLV) type III. In 1984 the Gallo team was able to demonstrate conclusively through virologic and epidemiologic evidence that HTLV-III was the cause of AIDS. When it was demonstrated that LAV and HTLV-III were the same virus, an international commission changed both names of the virus to HIV to eliminate confusion caused by the two names and to acknowledge that the virus is the cause of AIDS.

Viral Characteristics

Viral Structure

Human immunodeficiency virus is a member of the family Retroviridae, a type D retrovirus that belongs to the lentivirus subfamily. Included in this family are oncoviruses (e.g., HTLV-I, HTLV-II), which primarily induce proliferation of infected cells and formation of tumors. Since the discovery of this virus, much has been learned about the impact of HIV on human cells. Two distinct HIV viruses, types 1 and 2 (HIV-1 and HIV-2), cause AIDS. **HIV-1** is divided into nine subtypes: group M (subtypes A-H), group N, and group O. **HIV-2** is divided into two subtypes, groups A and B.

The HIV-1 virus is composed of a lipid membrane, structural proteins, and glycoproteins that protrude. The viral genome consists of three important structural components: *pol, gag,* and *env.* These gene components code for various products (Table 25-1). Long terminal redundancies border

Table 25-1	Viral Genome Components
Component	**Product**
pol	Produces DNA polymerase.
	Produces endonuclease.
gag	Codes for p24 and for proteins such as p17, p9, and p7.
env	Codes for two glycoproteins, gp41 and gp120.

Table 25-3	Encoding Genes and Antigens of AIDS Virus
Encoding Gene	**Antigen**
gag	p55
gag	p24
gag	p17
pol	p66
pol	p51
sor	p24
env	gp160
env	gp120
Env	gp41
3'*orf*	p27

these three components. HIV-2 has a different envelope and slightly different core proteins.

Cells infected with HIV can be examined with an electron microscope. The virus may appear as buds of the cell membrane particles. The virion has a double-membrane envelope and electron-dense laminar crescent or semicircular cores. An intermediate, less electron-dense layer lies between the envelope and core. In a mature, free extracellular virion, the core appears as a bar-shaped nucleoid structure in cross section. This structure appears circular and is frequently located eccentrically. It is composed of structural proteins and glycoproteins that occupy the core and envelope regions of the particle. The virion consists of knoblike structures composed of a protein called gp120, which is anchored to another protein called gp41. Each knob includes three sets of these protein molecules. The core of the virus includes a protein called p25 or p24. After human exposure, these and other viral components may induce an antibody response important in serodiagnosis (Table 25-2).

Retroviruses contain a single, positive-stranded ribonucleic acid (RNA) with the virus' genetic information and a special enzyme called **reverse transcriptase** in their core. Reverse transcriptase enables the virus to convert viral RNA into deoxyribonucleic acid (DNA). This reverses the normal process of transcription in which DNA is converted to RNA, thus the term **retrovirus.**

The genomes of all known retroviruses are organized in a similar way. In the provirus, which is formed when complementary DNA (cDNA) synthesis is completed from the retroviral RNA template, viral core protein, envelope protein, and reverse transcriptase are encoded by the *gag, env,* and *pol* genes, respectively, whereas viral gene expression is regulated by *tat, trs, sor,* and 3'*orf* gene products. The *gag* gene encodes a polyprotein found at high levels in infected cells and is subsequently cleaved to form p17 and p24, both of which are associated with viral particles. The *pol* gene encodes for

reverse transcriptase, endonuclease, and protease activities. The *sor* gene stands for "small, open-reading frame." The *sor* gene product is a protein that induces antibody production in the natural course of infection. The *tat* gene also represents a small, open-reading frame; the protein product has not been identified to date.

The *env* gene encodes for a polyprotein that contains numerous glycosylation sites. The glycoprotein gp160 is found on infected cells but is deficient on viral particles; however, gp160 gives rise to two glycoproteins, gp120 and gp41, which are associated with the viral envelope. The encoding genes and gene products, or antigens, of the AIDS virus may induce an antibody response after human exposure (Table 25-3).

Long terminal redundancies (LTRs), which exist at each end of the proviral genome, play an important role in the control of viral gene expression and the integration of the provirus into the DNA of the hosts. Although a structural similarity exists between the genomes of HIV-1 and HIV-2 (HTLV-IV), the nucleotide sequence homology is limited. There is a nucleotide sequence homology of only 60% between the *gag* genes and 30% to 40% between the remainder of the genes of HIV-1 and HIV-2.

Viral Replication

The replication of HIV is complicated and involves several steps. The HIV life cycle is that of a retrovirus (Box 25-1). Retroviruses are so named because they reverse the normal flow of genetic information. In body cells the genetic material is DNA. When genes are expressed, DNA is first transcribed into

Table 25-2		HIV Proteins of Serodiagnostic Importance	
Virus	**Protein**	**Location**	**Gene**
HIV-1	gp41	Envelope (transmembrane protein)	*env*
	gp160/120	Envelope (external protein)	*env*
	p24	Core (major structural protein)	*gag*
HIV-2	gp34	Envelope (transmembrane protein)	*env*
	gp140	Envelope (external protein)	*env*
	p26	Core (major structural protein)	*gag*

Box 25-1	Summary of HIV-1 Life Cycle

1. The virus attaches to the CD4 membrane receptor and sheds its protein coat, exposing its RNA core.
2. Reverse transcriptase converts viral RNA into proviral DNA.
3. The proviral DNA is integrated into the genome (genetic complement of host cell).
4. New virus particles are produced as the result of normal cellular activities of transcription and translation. Once the viral genome is integrated into host cell DNA, the potential for viral production always exists, and the viral infection of new cells can continue.
5. New particles bud from the cell membrane.

messenger RNA (mRNA), which then serves as the template for the production of proteins. The genes of a retrovirus are encoded in RNA; before they can be expressed, the RNA must be converted into DNA. Only then are the viral genes transcribed and translated into proteins in the usual sequence.

Target Cells. The infectious process begins when the gp120 protein on the viral envelope binds to the protein receptor, called **CD4,** located on the surface of a target cell. HIV-1 has a marked preference for the CD4+ subset of T lymphocytes (Figure 25-1). In addition to T lymphocytes, macrophages, peripheral blood monocytes, and cells in the lymph nodes, skin, and other organs also express measurable amounts of CD4 and can be infected by HIV-1. About 5% of the B lymphocytes may express CD4 and may be susceptible to HIV-1 infection. Macrophages may play an important role in spreading HIV infection in the body, both to other cells and to the target organs of HIV. Monocyte-macrophages enable HIV-1 to enter the immune-protected domain of the central nervous system (CNS), including the brain and spinal cord.

Fusion of the virus to the membrane of a host cell enables the viral RNA and reverse transcriptase to invade the cytoplasm of the cell. However, CD4 receptors are not sufficient for HIV envelope fusion with the T4 cell membrane or for HIV penetration or entry into the interior of the cell. *Chemokine coreceptors* to CD4, which HIV uses to enter a host cell after binding to it, have been identified. Beta chemokine receptors are cell surface proteins that bind small peptides. They are classified into three groups, depending on the location of

the amino acid cysteine (C) in the peptide. These receptors are identified by the individual chemokine(s) that binds to them. In essence, the reference to a specific chemokine(s) also identifies its receptor. The first example of a coreceptor was CXCKR-4 (FUSIN R-4). Other coreceptors include CCKR-2 (R-2), CCKR-3 (R-3), and CC-CKR-5 (R-5). Current research involves exploring ways to block or fill the chemokine receptors with a harmless molecule, thus blocking the binding site of the HIV on the host cell.

Although some cells do not produce detectable amounts of CD4, they do contain low levels of mRNA encoding the CD4 protein, which indicates that they do produce some CD4. Because these cells can be infected by HIV in culture, the expression of only minimal CD4 or an alternate receptor molecule may be sufficient for HIV infection to occur. These cell types include certain brain cells, neuroglial cells, a variety of malignant brain tumor cells, and cells derived from bowel cancers. Cells of the gastrointestinal system do not produce appreciable amounts of CD4, although chromaffin cells sometimes appear to be infected by HIV in vivo.

Replication. Retroviruses carry a single, positive-stranded RNA and use reverse transcriptase to convert viral RNA into DNA. The life cycle of the HIV-1 virus consists of five phases, as follows (see also Box 25-1):

1. The virus attaches and penetrates target cells (e.g., lymphocytes) that express the CD4 receptor. After penetration, the virus loses its protein coat, exposing the RNA core.

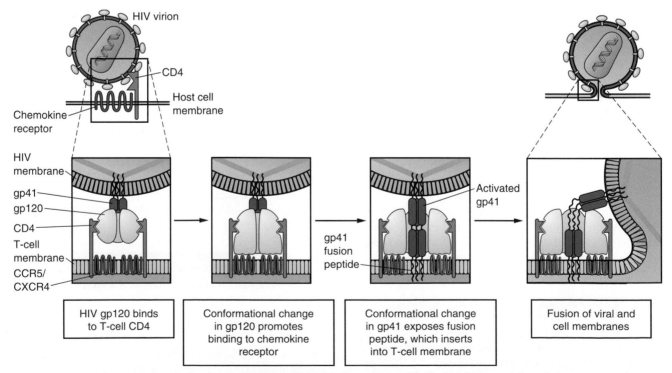

Figure 25-1 **Mechanisms of HIV entry into a cell.** In the model, depicted sequential conformational changes in gp120 and gp41 promote fusion of the HIV-1 and host cell membranes. The fusion peptide of activated gp41 contains hydrophobic amino acid residues that promote insertion into the host cell plasma membrane lipid bilayer. *(Redrawn from Abbas AK, Lichtman AH, Pillai S: Cellular and molecular immunology, ed 6, Philadelphia, 2007, Saunders.)*

2. Reverse transcriptase converts viral RNA into proviral DNA.
3. The proviral DNA is integrated into the genome (genetic complement of the host cell).
4. New virus particles are produced as a result of normal cellular activities of transcription and translation.
5. These new particles bud from the cell membrane.

Once the viral genome is integrated into host cell DNA, the potential for viral production always exists, and the viral infection of new cells can continue.

Immunologic activation of CD4+ cells latently infected with HIV induces the production of multiple viral particles, leading to cell death. The extensive destruction of cells leads to the gradual depletion of CD4+ lymphocytes. Progressive defects in the immune system include a severe B-cell failure, defects in monocyte function, and defects in granulocyte function.

EPIDEMIOLOGY

Incidence

More than 25 years after the first clinical evidence of AIDS was reported, it has become the most devastating disease humankind has ever faced. HIV/AIDS is now the leading cause of death in Sub-Saharan Africa. Worldwide, it is the fourth leading cause of death.

According to Global Health Reporting, statistics for the worldwide epidemic (or pandemic) of HIV are grim. In 2007, AIDS caused the deaths of 2.1 million adults (age ≥15 years) and children, with 1.6 million of these deaths occurring in Sub-Saharan Africa. In North America, 1.3 million adults (≥15 years) and children were living with HIV/AIDS. There were 46,000 new HIV infections diagnosed in North America and 2.5 million new HIV cases diagnosed worldwide in 2007.

Classification System

The revised definition of HIV infection, which applies to both HIV-1 and HIV-2, incorporates the reporting criteria for HIV infection and AIDS into a single case definition (Box 25-2). The revised criteria for HIV infection update the definition of HIV infection implemented in 1993; the revised HIV criteria apply to AIDS-defining conditions for adults and children that require laboratory evidence of HIV.

Infectious Patterns

Acquired immunodeficiency syndrome is present worldwide. In some countries (e.g., Sub-Saharan Africa, Thailand, India) more than 90% of HIV-1 infections are acquired through heterosexual transmission, in contrast to 10% or less in the United States and Western Europe. Subtypes A, C, and D predominate in Africa; subtypes E and B are common in Thailand; and subtype B predominates in the United States and Western Europe. HIV-1 and HIV-2 are distinct but related viruses, and both can cause AIDS. HIV-1 is responsible for the main AIDS epidemic. The discovery of HIV-2 suggests that other HIVs may also exist.

Three infection patterns of HIV have been traced worldwide, as follows:
- *Pattern 1* is found in North and South America, Western Europe, Scandinavia, Australia, and New Zealand. In these countries, AIDS is primarily a disease of homosexuals and intravenous (IV) drug abusers. In pattern 1 areas the male/female ratio of reported AIDS cases ranges from 10:1 to 15:1.
- *Pattern 2* is found in Africa, the Caribbean, and some areas of South America. In the pattern 2 areas, AIDS is primarily a heterosexual disease. The number of infected females and males is approximately equal.
- *Pattern 3* is typically demonstrated in Eastern Europe, North Africa, the Middle East, Asia, and the Pacific, excluding Australia and New Zealand. In the pattern 3 areas, relatively few cases of AIDS have been identified. Most of the affected individuals have had contact with pattern 1 or pattern 2 countries.

Human Immunodeficiency Virus Type 2

In 1986 a second virus causing AIDS was discovered. HIV-2 is endemic in parts of West Africa. Epidemiologic data indicate that the prevalence of HIV-2 infections in persons in the United States is extremely low (e.g., 94 HIV-2 infected persons had been reported to the CDC by early 2003).

The primary mode of transmission of HIV-2 is heterosexual contact, although HIV-2 infection has been reported in Europe in homosexual men, IV drug users, transfusion recipients, and men with hemophilia.

Infection with HIV-2 can cause immunosuppression and the development of AIDS. The period between infection and disease may be longer and milder for persons with HIV-2 than for those with HIV-1. HIV-2 appears to be less harmful (cytopathic) to the cells of the immune system, and it reproduces more slowly than HIV-1. Compared with persons infected with HIV-1, those with HIV-2 are less infectious early in the disease course. As the disease advances, HIV-2 infectivity seems to increase compared with HIV-1, but the duration of this increased infectivity is shorter.

In 1990 the U.S. Food and Drug Administration (FDA) licensed an enzyme immunoassay (EIA) test kit for detection of antibodies to HIV-2 in human serum or plasma. An additional combination procedure for screening for HIV-1/-2 was licensed in September 1991. The Centers for Disease Control and Prevention (CDC) does not recommend routine HIV-2 testing at HIV counseling and test sites or in settings other than blood centers. If HIV testing is to be performed, tests for antibodies to both HIV-1 and HIV-2 should be obtained if demographic or behavioral information suggests that HIV-2 infection might be present. Diagnosis of HIV-2 requires more specific supplementary tests, such as an HIV-2 Western blot assay.

Modes of Transmission

Human immunodeficiency virus enters the body in one of two ways. HIV can be transmitted as the virus itself or as a cell associated with HIV. The virus is held within leukocytes

Box 25-2   Revised HIV Classification and AIDS Surveillance Case Definition

The revised definition of HIV infection, which applies to any HIV (e.g., HIV-1 or HIV-2), incorporates the reporting criteria for HIV infection and AIDS into a single case definition.

I. In adults, adolescents, or children ≥18 months,* a reportable case of HIV infection must meet at least one of the following criteria:

Laboratory Criteria

Positive result on a screening test for HIV antibody (e.g., repeatedly reactive enzyme immunoassay), followed by a positive result on a confirmatory (sensitive and more specific) test for HIV antibody (e.g., Western blot or immunofluorescence antibody test).

OR

Positive result or report of a detectable quantity on any of the following HIV virologic (nonantibody) tests:

    HIV nucleic acid (DNA or RNA) detection (e.g., DNA PCR or plasma HIV-1 RNA).†

    HIV p24 antigen test, including neutralization assay.

    HIV isolation (viral culture).

OR

Clinical or other criteria (if the above laboratory criteria are not met).

Diagnosis of HIV infection, based on the laboratory criteria above, that is documented in a medical record by a physician.

OR

Conditions that meet criteria included in the case definition for AIDS (17-19).

II. In a child less than 18 months old, a reportable case of HIV infection must meet at least one of the following criteria:

Laboratory Criteria

Definitive

Positive results on two separate specimens (excluding cord blood) using one or more of the following HIV virologic (nonantibody) tests:

    HIV nucleic acid (DNA or RNA) detection.

    HIV p24 antigen test, including neutralization assay, in a child ≥1 month of age.

    HIV isolation (viral culture).

OR

Presumptive

A child who does not meet the criteria for definitive HIV infection but who has:

    Positive results on only one specimen (excluding cord blood) using the above HIV virologic tests and no subsequent negative HIV virologic or negative HIV antibody tests.

OR

Clinical or other criteria (if the above definitive or presumptive laboratory criteria are not met).

Diagnosis of HIV infection, based on the laboratory criteria above, that is documented in a medical record by a physician.

OR

Conditions that meet criteria included in the 1987 pediatric surveillance case definition for AIDS.

III. A child less than 18 months old born to an HIV-infected mother will be categorized for surveillance purposes as "not infected with HIV" if the child does not meet the criteria for HIV infection but meets the following criteria:

Laboratory Criteria

Definitive

At least two negative HIV antibody tests from separate specimens obtained at ≥6 months old.

OR

At least two negative HIV virologic tests‡ from separate specimens, both of which were performed at ≥1 month old and one of which was performed at ≥4 months old.

AND

No other laboratory or clinical evidence of HIV infection (i.e., has not had any positive virologic tests, if performed, and has not had an AIDS-defining condition).

OR

Presumptive

A child who does not meet the above criteria for definitive "not infected" status but who has:

    One negative EIA HIV antibody test performed at ≥6 months old and *no* positive HIV virologic tests, if performed.

OR

One negative HIV virologic test‡ performed at ≥4 months old and *no* positive HIV virologic tests, if performed.

OR

One positive HIV virologic test with at least two subsequent negative virologic tests,§ at least one of which is ≥4 months old; or negative HIV antibody test results, at least one of which is ≥6 months old.

AND

No other laboratory or clinical evidence of HIV infection (i.e., has not had any positive virologic tests, if performed, and has not had an AIDS-defining condition).

OR

Clinical or other criteria (if the above definitive or presumptive laboratory criteria are not met).

Determined by a physician to be "not infected," and a physician has noted the results of the preceding HIV diagnostic tests in the medical record.

AND

No other laboratory or clinical evidence of HIV infection (i.e., has not had any positive virologic tests, if performed, and has not had an AIDS-defining condition).

IV. A child less than 18 months old born to an HIV-infected mother will be categorized as having perinatal exposure to HIV infection if the child does not meet the criteria for HIV infection (II) or the criteria for "not infected with HIV" (III).

From Centers for Disease Control and Prevention: *MMWR* 48(RR-13):29-31, 1999.

*Children ≥18 months old but <13 years old are categorized as "not infected with HIV" if they meet the criteria in **III.**

†In adults, adolescents, and children infected by other than perinatal exposure, plasma viral RNA nucleic acid tests should *not* be used instead of licensed HIV screening tests (e.g., repeatedly reactive enzyme immunoassay). In addition, a negative (i.e., undetectable) plasma HIV-1 RNA test result does not rule out the diagnosis of HIV infection.

‡Draft revised surveillance criteria for HIV infection were approved and recommended by the membership of the Council of State and Territorial Epidemiologists at the 1998 annual meeting.

§HIV nucleic acid (DNA or RNA) detection tests are the virologic methods of choice to exclude infection in children less than 18 months old. Although HIV culture can be used for this purpose, it is more complex and expensive to perform and is less well standardized than nucleic acid detection tests. The use of p24 antigen testing to exclude infection in children less than 18 months old is not recommended because of its lack of sensitivity.

and carried in fluid (e.g., blood, semen) to the body of another person. In some cases the mode of viral transmission is associated with the viral subtype. HIV-1, subtype E, easily infects the Langerhans cells, which are abundant in the cervical mucosa. In contrast, HIV-1 subtypes E and C are associated with heterosexual sex. Transmission of HIV is believed to be restricted to intimate contact with body fluids from an infected person; casual contact with infected persons has not been documented as a mode of transmission.

Although the mode of transmission is considered to be predominantly sexual, HIV can be transmitted by contact with infected blood through blood transfusion (if not screened for HIV) or by HIV-contaminated needles. Posttransfusion AIDS is now well documented from both cellular blood components and cell-free preparations, such as unheated factor VIII concentrate and plasma.

Although injuries occur in professional football competitions, bleeding injuries, especially lacerations, occur infrequently. The estimated risk for HIV transmission during such competition is considered to be extremely remote.

Babies born to HIV-infected women may become infected before or during birth or through breastfeeding after birth. The risk of HIV infection to children born to women with HIV is 20% to 30%. HIV-2 seems to be less transmissible from an infected woman to her fetus or newborn.

Health care workers have been infected with HIV after being stuck with needles containing HIV-infected blood or, less frequently, after infected blood enters a worker's open cut or a mucous membrane (e.g., eyes, inside of nose).

The HIV virus has been isolated from blood, semen, vaginal secretions, saliva, tears, breast milk, cerebrospinal fluid (CSF), amniotic fluid, and urine. Only blood, semen, vaginal secretions, and breast milk have been implicated in the transmission of HIV to date. HIV has been found in saliva and tears in very low quantities from some AIDS patients. It is important to understand that finding a small amount of HIV in a body fluid does not necessarily mean that HIV can be transmitted by that body fluid. HIV has not been recovered from the sweat of HIV-infected persons. Contact with saliva, tears, or sweat has never been shown to result in transmission of HIV.

Sexual transmission, either heterosexual or male-male, is also a well-documented route of transmission. HIV is transmitted by infected cells and not free fluid. Relatively low levels of infective HIV particles are present in body fluids. However, genital secretion can contain substantial numbers of virus-infected cells. Up to 5% of white cells in seminal fluid can be HIV infected; approximately 10^6 mononuclear cells are found in seminal fluid. Seropositive individuals do not necessarily transmit the disease if their genital fluid does not contain a large number of infected cells.

Most transmission of HIV to organ/tissue recipients occurred before 1985, prior to implementation of donor screening recommendations. Reports of transmission from screened, HIV-antibody–negative organ or tissue donors have been rare. By early 2003, 15 women were reported to have been infected through the use of anonymous donor sperm for artificial insemination. There are no U.S. federal regulations regarding HIV testing, and only a handful of states (California, Illinois, Ohio, Michigan, and New York) require HIV testing of semen donors.

Viral transmission can result from contact with inanimate objects, such as work surfaces or equipment recently contaminated with infected blood or certain body fluids, if the virus is transferred to broken skin or mucous membranes by hand contact.

SIGNS AND SYMPTOMS

It is not known when an HIV-exposed individual becomes infectious or how soon HIV-infected individuals develop serologic markers of infection. Infection with HIV produces a chronic infection with symptoms that range from asymptomatic to the end-stage complications of AIDS.

Typically, patients in the early stages of HIV infection either are completely asymptomatic or show mild, chronic lymphadenopathy. The early phase may last from many months to many years after viral exposure. Although the course of HIV-1 infection may vary somewhat among individual patients, a common pattern of development has been recognized. The newly revised HIV classification system provides uniform and simple criteria for categorizing conditions (see Box 25-2).

During the early period after primary infection, widespread dissemination of virus occurs, with a sharp decrease in the number of CD4+ T cells in peripheral blood. The early burst of virus in the blood, *viremia*, is often accompanied by flulike symptoms that can be so severe that affected persons may seek help at a hospital emergency department. An immune response to HIV develops, with a concurrent decrease in detectable viremia. It was previously believed that the human immune system could drive the AIDS virus into a latent period that kept it inactive for years. However, this view has been replaced with the new vision of a virus that is furiously creating copies of itself throughout the disease course, even when the patient appears healthy. Even when HIV cannot be detected in the blood (viremia), it infects (in large quantities) lymphatic tissues, including the tonsils and lymph nodes throughout the body. The absence of viremia generally lasts until the end stage of the disease.

This phase is followed by a prolonged period of clinical latency (range, 7-11 years; median, 10 years). During the period of clinical latency, the patient is usually asymptomatic. Differences in the infecting virus, the host's genetic makeup, and environmental factors (e.g., concomitant infection) have been suggested as causes of the variable duration of clinical latency in persons not receiving antiretroviral therapy. Treatment with inhibitors of viral reverse transcriptase (e.g., zidovudine [Retrovir]) and prophylaxis for pneumonia caused by *Pneumocystis carinii* have increased AIDS-free time in HIV-1–infected persons.

Opportunistic Infections

Since AIDS was first recognized in the early 1980s, remarkable progress has been made in improving the quality and duration of life for HIV-infected persons in the industrialized world. During the first decade of the epidemic, this progress resulted from improved recognition of opportunistic disease processes, improved therapy for acute and chronic complications, and introduction of chemoprophylaxis against key opportunistic pathogens. The second decade of the epidemic witnessed extraordinary progress in developing **highly active antiretroviral therapy (HAART)** as well as continuing progress in preventing and treating opportunistic infections. HAART has reduced the incidence of opportunistic infections and extended life. In addition, prophylaxis against specific opportunistic infections continues to provide survival benefits even among patients receiving HAART.

The absolute number of CD4+ T lymphocytes continues to diminish as the disease progresses. When the number of cells reaches a critically low level ($<50\text{-}100 \times 10^9$/L), the risk of opportunistic infection increases. The period of susceptibility to opportunistic processes continues to be accurately indicated by CD4+ T lymphocyte counts for patients receiving HAART.

The end stage of AIDS is characterized by the occurrence of neoplasms and opportunistic infections (Box 25-3). The most common opportunistic infections are *P. jiroveci (carinii)* (Figure 25-2 and Plate 2), cytomegalovirus (CMV), *Mycobacterium avium-intracellulare, Cryptococcus, Toxoplasma, Mycobacterium tuberculosis,* herpes simplex, and *Legionella. Histoplasma capsulatum* is being recognized with increasing frequency. The most frequent malignancy observed is an aggressive, invasive variant of Kaposi's sarcoma (Figure 25-3), discovered in many cases on autopsy. Malignant B-cell lymphomas are increasingly recognized in patients with or at high risk for AIDS.

Box 25-3	Opportunistic Infections in Immunosuppressed and Immunodeficient Patients

Oral/esophageal candidiasis
Cytomegalovirus
Pneumocystis jiroveci (carinii)
Herpes simplex
Entamoeba histolytica
Giardia lamblia
Herpes zoster
Atypical acid-fast bacilli
Shigella
Campylobacter
Cryptococcus neoformans
Adenovirus
Hepatitis
Chlamydia
Salmonella
Syphilis
Anal candidiasis
Dientamoeba fragilis
Blastocystis hominis
Toxoplasma gondii

Kaposi's Sarcoma

Kaposi's sarcoma (KS) was first described in 1872 by the dermatologist Moritz Kaposi. Since then, until the AIDS epidemic, KS remained a rare tumor. Classic KS usually occurs in males. The tumor typically presents with one or more asymptomatic red, purple, or brown patches, plaque, or nodular skin lesions. The disease is often limited to single or multiple lesions, usually localized to one or both lower extremities, especially involving the ankle and soles. Classic KS most often has a relatively benign, indolent course for 10 to 15 years or more, with slow enlargement of the original tumors and gradual development of additional lesions. Up to one third of patients with classic KS develop a second primary malignancy, most often non-Hodgkin's lymphoma. An increased incidence of Hodgkin's disease occurs in HIV-infected homosexual men.

Cryptosporidiosis

Cryptosporidiosis is a disease caused by the parasite *Cryptosporidium parvum*. As late as 1976, this parasite was not thought to cause disease in humans. In 1993, more than 400,000 people in Milwaukee, Wisconsin, became ill after drinking water contaminated with the parasite. Cryptosporidiosis can be chronic and severe in immunocompromised persons. The watery diarrhea can be prolonged and debilitating and may be fatal.

Persons at risk of severe cryptosporidiosis include AIDS patients, cancer or organ/marrow transplant patients taking drugs that weaken the immune system, and persons born with genetically weakened immune systems.

Disease Progression

Although a large enough dose of the right strain of HIV-1 can cause AIDS on its own, cofactors can influence the progression of disease development. Debilitated patients, weakened by a preexisting medical condition before HIV-1 infection, may progress toward AIDS more quickly than others (Figure 25-4). Stimulation of the immune system in

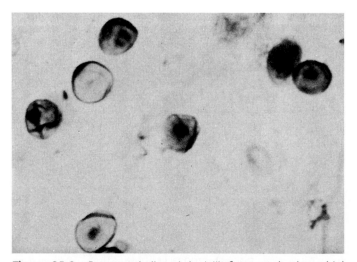

Figure 25-2 *Pneumocystis jiroveci (carinii)* from tracheobronchial aspirate; stained with methenamine silver. *(From Markell EK, Voge M: Medical parasitology, ed 5, Philadelphia, 1981, Saunders.)*

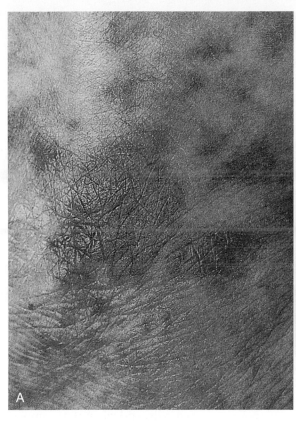

Figure 25-3 Kaposi's sarcoma. **A,** Early lesion consisting of violaceous macules and plaques. **B,** Purple nodules are seen most often on the lower legs. *(From Habif TP:* Clinical dermatology, *ed 8, St Louis, 1985, Mosby.)*

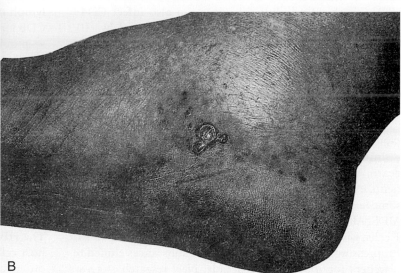

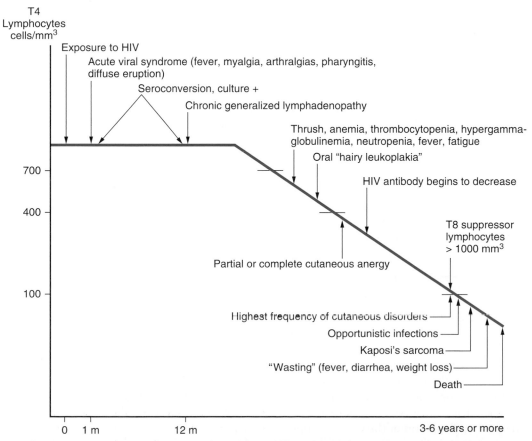

Figure 25-4 Evolution of AIDS. *(Redrawn from Habif TP:* Clinical dermatology, *ed 2, St Louis, 1990, Mosby.)*

response to later infections can also hasten disease progression. Other pathogenic microorganisms, such as a herpesvirus called "human B-cell lymphotropic virus" or *human herpesvirus 6* (HHV-6), can interact with HIV in a way that may increase the severity of HIV infection. HHV-6 is usually easily controlled by the immune system. If HIV compromises the immune system, however, HHV-6 may replicate more freely and become a health threat. The main host of HHV-6 is the B cell, but this virus can also infect CD4+ cells. If these T cells are simultaneously infected by HIV, HHV-6 can stimulate the virus, which further impairs the immune system and promotes disease progression.

The progressive decline of CD4+ cells leads to a general decline in immune function and is the primary factor in determining the clinical progression of AIDS. Plasma HIV-1 RNA is a strong, CD4+ T-cell–independent predictor of a rapid progression to AIDS after HIV-1 seroconversion.

Infection with HIV is presently considered to lead to death. When the clinically apparent disease develops, patients usually die within 2 years with current treatment, but some exposed or HIV-1–infected patients never develop AIDS. Although scientists have known since 1986 that CD8 T cells, when stimulated, could release molecules capable of suppressing HIV, the identity of these substances eluded researchers for more than a decade. New research suggests that three large proteins, identified as *alpha-defensins* 1, 2, and 3, could be major contributors to the CD8 antiviral factor that protects some patients against AIDS. In another new study, scientists at the National Institutes of Health have linked HIV resistance to a different molecule secreted by CD8 T cells, called *perforin*. More studies related to each category of molecules are needed before either of these theories is confirmed.

Another recent study at the National Institute of Allergy and Infectious Diseases examined variations in a gene called *RANTES* (regulated-on-activation normal T cells expressed and secreted) in HIV-infected and HIV-resistant individuals. This study searched for changes in a **single nucleotide polymorphism (SNP).** The results showed that one such SNP appears more often in HIV-positive than in HIV-negative persons. In addition, this particular alteration increases the activity of the RANTES gene and is associated with up to twice the risk of HIV infection. However, HIV-infected patients with this SNP take about 40% longer to develop AIDS.

IMMUNOLOGIC MANIFESTATIONS

Cellular Abnormalities

The HIV-1 virus has a marked preference for CD4+ subset of lymphocytes because the CD4 surface marker protein on these cells serves as a receptor site for the virus. Immunologic activation (e.g., participation in immune response to HIV-1 or viruses in other cells) of CD4+ cells latently infected with HIV-1 induces the production of multiple viral particles, leading to cell death. The extensive destruction of T cells leads to the gradual depletion of the CD4+ lymphocytes. The major phenotypic cell populations affected by

AIDS are CD4+ and CD8+ subsets of T lymphocytes. Normally the CD4+/CD8+ ratio is 2:1 in heterosexuals and 1.5:1 in homosexuals. A reversal of these subsets is evident in, but not diagnostic of, AIDS. In patients with AIDS the ratio is less than 0.5:1. It is important to note that this results from a marked decrease in the absolute number of circulating CD4+ cells, rather than from an absolute increase in suppressor or CD8+ cells. This abnormality exists in the lymph nodes and circulating T cells. A diminished CD4+/CD8+ ratio (altered lymphocyte subpopulation) can also be seen in individuals with other disorders, such as cutaneous T-cell lymphoma, systemic lupus erythematosus (SLE), and acute viral infections. The ratio, however, reverts back to normal after recovery from a viral infection in non-AIDS patients.

A decreased lymphocyte proliferative response to soluble antigens and mitogens exists in AIDS. Functional testing reveals a diminished response to pokeweed mitogen. This disease also demonstrates defective natural killer (NK) cell activity.

Alterations in Immune System

The HIV virus is fragile, and as the virus particle leaves its host cell, a molecule called gp120 frequently breaks off the outer coat of the virus. Glycoprotein gp120 can bind to the CD4 molecules of uninfected cells, and when that complex is recognized by the immune system, these cells can be destroyed. The lysis of infected cells and gp120-bound uninfected cells leads to the gradual depletion of the CD4+ lymphocytes. Defects in immunity are related to this T-cell depletion. Progressive defects in the immune system also include a severe B-cell failure and defects in monocyte and granulocyte function.

Although HIV-1 destroys CD4+ cells directly and hampers the immune system, this process does not cause the severe immune deficiency seen in AIDS. The severe deficiency can be explained only if the cells are also destroyed by other means. Several indirect mechanisms have been suggested. Infection by HIV can cause infected and uninfected cells to fuse into giant cells called *syncytia,* which are nonfunctional. Autoimmune responses, in which the immune system attacks the body's own tissues, may also be at work. In addition, HIV-infected cells may send out protein signals that weaken or destroy other cells of the immune system. It is possible that the binding of HIV to a target cell triggers the release of the enzyme protease. Proteases digest proteins; if released in abnormal quantities, they might weaken lymphocytes and other cells and decrease cell survival. The decline in T cells and subsequent alteration of the immune mechanism are the underlying factors in progression of HIV infection.

Serologic Markers

Detection of Core Antigen

After initial infection, the body mounts a vigorous immune response against the viremia. Immunologic activities include the production of different types of antibodies against

HIV. Some antibodies neutralize the virus, others prevent it from binding to cells, and others stimulate cytotoxic cells to attack HIV-infected cells.

The time and sequence vary for the appearance and disappearance of antibodies specific for the serologically important antigens of HIV-1 during the course of infection. A "window" period of seronegativity exists from the time of initial infection to 6 or 12 weeks or longer thereafter. Through EIA methods based on defined HIV-1 proteins produced by recombinant DNA methods, antibodies specific for gp41 are detectable for weeks or months before assays specific for p24. The appearance of antibodies specific for p24 has been shown to precede that of anti-gp41 in serum specimens undergoing Western blot analysis. This discrepancy in the sequence of antibody appearance is believed to be caused by the greater sensitivity of Western blot compared with viral lysate-based EIAs used for the detection of anti-p24. The gp41 antibodies persist throughout the course of infection. Antibodies specific for p24 not only rise to detectable levels after gp41, but also can disappear unpredictably and abruptly.

Increased production of core antigen is believed to be associated with a burst of viral replication and host cell lysis. The disappearance of antibody directed against p24 occurs concomitantly with an increase in the concentration of core antigen in the serum. This parallel activity may result from the sequestration of antibody in immune complexes, and the sudden decrease in anti-p24 is considered to be a grave prognostic sign in HIV-1–infected patients.

Antibodies to HIV-1

Antibodies to HIV-1 appear after a lag period of about 6 weeks between the time of infection and a detectable antibody response. Because of this, some virus-positive, antibody-negative individuals would be missed by initial screening assays.

In addition to a positive HIV antibody test in 85% to 90% of patients, increased antibody titers to other viruses (e.g., CMV, Epstein-Barr virus, hepatitis A/B, *Toxoplasma gondii*) and circulating immune (antigen-antibody) complexes can be found. Other ancillary findings include polyclonal hypergammaglobulinemia; elevated levels of interferon-α (IFN-α), α_1-thymosin, and β-microglobulin; and reduced levels of interleukin-1 (IL-1) or IL-2.

Specific intrathecal synthesis of HIV antibody should be assessed simultaneously with an assay for total CSF immunoglobulin M (IgM) and for intrathecal synthesis of total immunoglobulin G as well as IgG specific for an appropriate control organism (e.g., adenovirus). In progressive encephalopathy related to AIDS, an increase in HIV antibody may suggest intrathecal rather than extrathecal synthesis.

DIAGNOSTIC EVALUATION

Infection with HIV is established by detecting antibodies to the virus, viral antigens, or viral RNA/DNA or by the "gold standard," viral culture. The standard test is for antibody detection. Laboratory evaluation of asymptomatic HIV-infected patients consists of assessment of cellular and humoral components (Table 25-4).

Table 25-4	Laboratory Assessment of Asymptomatic HIV-Positive Patients
Test	**Comments**
HIV serology	Repeat test at 3- to 6-month intervals for patients with positive test results when no confirmatory assay is available, patient denies commonly accepted risk factors, assay performed with other than standard serology protocol, or other reasons (e.g., undetectable viral load and normal CD4+ lymphocyte cell count).
Complete blood count	Repeat test at 3- to 6-month intervals, or more frequently when patient has low values and is receiving bone marrow–toxic drugs.
CD4+ cell count and percentage	Repeat every 3 to 6 months, or more often if needed. CD4+ lymphocyte count is standard test to stage disease, formulate differential diagnosis, and make therapeutic decisions regarding antiviral treatment and prophylaxis for opportunistic pathogens. Also a relatively reliable indicator of prognosis that complements viral load assay. These two assays independently predict clinical progression and survival.
VDRL or RPR syphilis serology	Repeat annually.
Hepatitis serology	Anti-HBs or anti-HBc, if an HBV vaccine candidate; screen for anti-HAV (IgG), if an HAV vaccine candidate.
Cytomegalovirus (IgG)	Optional.
Toxoplasmosis (IgG)	Screen all patients; repeat if seronegative-negative, CD4+ cell count is low, and patient not receiving *P. carinii* prophylaxis, and if symptoms suggest toxoplasmosis encephalitis.
Serum chemistry	Repeat annually, or more frequently in patients with abnormal results and who are receiving hepatotoxic or nephrotoxic drugs.
G6PD assay	Optional, except in susceptible hosts, patients receiving oxidant drugs, and patients with typical symptoms of G6PD deficiency.
Lipid profile	Therapeutic monitoring recommended for patients receiving certain antiviral regimens.
PPD skin test	Repeat annually in previously negative patients.
Papanicolaou smear	Repeat at 6 months and then annually if results are normal.
Chest x-ray study	Suggested for patients with signs and symptoms of pulmonary disease or newly detected positive PPD.

From Bartlett JG, Gallant JE: *Medical management of HIV infection,* Baltimore, 2002, Johns Hopkins Press.
VDRL, Venereal Disease Research Laboratories; *RPR,* rapid plasma reagin; *G6PD,* glucose-6-phosphate dehydrogenase; *PPD,* purified protein derivative.

Table 25-5	HIV Assays and Characteristics	
Assay	Format	Target Molecule
HIV antigen assay for serum and plasma	EIA	HIV/p24 antigen
HIV antibody detection in serum or plasma	EIA (first- and second-generation testing)	Recombinant HIV-1 *env* and *gag* and HIV-2 *env* proteins *or* Purified, inactivated HIV-1 virus propagated in T-lymphocyte culture
Detection of HIV-1 groups M and O	EIA (third generation)	Purified, inactivated HIV-1 viral lysate proteins, envelope proteins, and HIV-1 group O transmembrane protein *or* Purified gp160 and p24 recombinant proteins from HIV-1, HIV-2 transmembrane gp36, and synthetic epitope of HIV-1 group O
Enzyme-linked fluorescence/p24 *or* EIA/p24	EIA (fourth generation)	HIV-1 gp160, p24 antigen, and peptides representing regions of gp41 from HIV-1 group O and gp36 from HIV-2 *or* HIV-1 antigens p31 and gp41, HIV-2 p36 recombinant protein, HIV-1 group O gp41, and anti-p24 monoclonal antibodies
HIV antibody detection in serum or plasma	Western blot	Purified and inactivated HIV-1 strain LAV grown in CEM cell line *or* Purified and inactivated HIV-1 propagated in H9/HTLV-IIIB T-lymphocyte cell line
HIV viral load assays	PCR	Reverse-transcriptase PCR *or* Nucleic acid sequence–based amplification *or* Signal amplification branched-chain DNA
Rapid testing	Rapid immunoassay	Uses recombinant proteins representing regions of HIV-1 envelope proteins *or* Uses synthetic HIV structural proteins

Modified from Zetola N, Klausner JD: *MLO* 38(9):58-62, 2006.
EIA, Enzyme immunoassay; *PCR*, polymerase chain reaction.

Screening of blood donors and patients at risk is usually done by serologic methods. In patients who have developed the signs and symptoms of AIDS, assessment of T lymphocytes and viral load concentrations are important, along with the diagnosis and treatment of opportunistic infections.

Both leukopenia and lymphocytopenia exist in the AIDS patient. Total leukocyte and absolute lymphocyte concentrations need to be periodically assessed. The common denominator of AIDS is a deficiency of a specific subset of thymus-derived (CD4+) lymphocytes. Enumeration of lymphocyte subsets is usually performed by flow cytometry (see Plate 10).

Additional testing includes viral load assay and resistance testing, an in vitro method to measure resistance of HIV to antiretroviral agents. Resistance testing can aid in antiretroviral drug selection but has limitations.

TESTING METHODS

Testing assays for HIV (Table 25-5) are categorized into the following three main classes:
1. Detection of HIV antibodies.
2. Detection of antigens, particularly p24.
3. Detection or quantification of viral nucleic acids.

HIV-1 Antibodies

Detection of HIV antibodies by EIA was the first technology developed for HIV diagnosis in 1985. Antibodies to HIV can be detected by EIA (specificity >99%, sensitivity >98%; Table 25-6) and confirmed by the immunoblot technique. The vast majority of, and probably all, seropositive patients are also infectious, as manifested by isolation of HIV from peripheral blood. The CDC estimates that one fourth of the

approximately 900,000 HIV-infected people in the United States are not aware of being infected. Antibody testing by EIA remains the standard method for screening potential blood donors. Simultaneous testing for p24 antigenemia is considered unnecessary. Third-generation serologic assays demonstrate that seroconversion typically occurs 3 to 12 weeks after infection, but significant delays can occur in some individuals.

HIV Antigen and Genome Testing

Enzyme Immunoassay: p24 Antigen
Enzyme immunoassay for HIV-1 antigen detects primarily uncomplexed p24 antigen. This procedure is applicable to blood or CSF testing as evidence of an active infection and can be diagnostic before seroconversion, can predict a patient's prognosis, and is useful for monitoring response to therapy. Disadvantages of the procedure include poor sensi-

Table 25-6	Causes of False-Positive and False-Negative HIV Enzyme Immunoassays	
False Positive	False Negative
Positive RPR (syphilis serology) test	Laboratory glove starch
Hematologic malignant disorder	Window period before seroconversion
DNA viral infections	Immunosuppressive therapy
Autoimmune disorders	Malignancies
Alcoholic hepatitis	Bone marrow transplantation
Vaccinations (e.g., hepatitis B, influenza)	Kits that mainly detect antibodies to p24
Chronic renal failure	
Renal transplantation	

Modified from Specialty Laboratories, Santa Monica, Calif.
RPR, Rapid plasma reagin; *DNA*, deoxyribonucleic acid.

tivity, the inability to detect in patients with a high titer of p24 antibody, and the failure of the method to detect HIV-2 antigen. Antibodies to p24 antigen are a better predictive marker progression than p24 antigen.

Polymerase Chain Reaction

Polymerase chain reaction (PCR) allows for the direct detection of HIV-1 by DNA amplification. This ultrasensitive PCR technique has revolutionized HIV-1 detection. In addition to confirmatory testing, DNA amplification can be used for the diagnosis of very early, postexposure HIV infection in the window period before production of antibodies.

The goal of direct detection of active virus in patient specimens by an ultrasensitive method is to detect less than 100 molecules of viral nucleic acid in the peripheral blood cells isolated from 1 mL of blood. This number is the assay target because as few as 1 in 10,000 lymphocytes express viral RNA in HIV-1–infected individuals. Therefore, of approximately 10^6 lymphocytes/mL blood, about 100 contain viral nucleic acid, corresponding to 100 to 150 copies of HIV-1 DNA. The presence of HIV-1 DNA in lymphocytes of antibody-positive, asymptomatic patients can be used to confirm exposure to the virus. The presence of viral RNA might be a sensitive indicator of viral replication and possibly of further disease progression.

The basis of PCR is amplification of minute amounts of viral nucleic acid in lymphocyte DNA. In HIV-1–infected cells, the DNA template is a provirus that exists as integrated or episomal DNA. After amplification, isotope or nonisotope methods can detect the amplified product. The most effective means of target amplification is PCR. A pair of specific oligomer primers initiate DNA synthesis in combination with heat-stable Taq I DNA polymerase. After this first round of primer extension, the material is heated to denature the product from its template and cooled to 37° C to permit annealing of the primer molecules to the original template DNA, as well as to the newly synthesized DNA fragments. Primer extension is then resumed. By repetition of these cycles of denaturation, annealing, and extension, the original DNA can be increased exponentially.

Viral RNA can also be specifically amplified with some additional steps. The *gag* region is probably the best choice of a sequence for amplification. Detection of viral RNA and DNA in clinical specimens might prove to be a better indicator of biologically active virus than DNA detection alone. The presence of both provirus and viral RNA transcriptase would be a strong indication of viral replication. Quantitation of HIV RNA in plasma is useful for determining free viral load, assessing the efficacy of antiviral therapy, and predicting progression and clinical outcome in AIDS patients.

Confirmatory Testing

Western Blot

Before an HIV result is considered positive, the results should be both reproducible and confirmable by at least one additional test. The Western blot (WB) analysis is currently

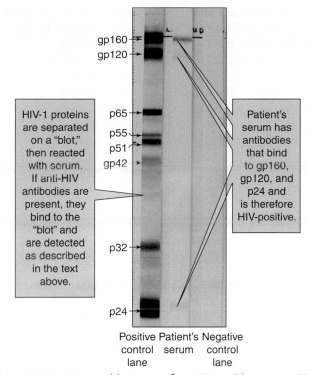

Figure 25-5 Western blot to confirm HIV-positive status. *(From Nairn R, Helbert M:* Immunology for medical students, *ed 2, Philadelphia, 2007, Mosby.)*

the standard method for confirming HIV-1 seropositivity (Figure 25-5).

The WB assay is based on the recognition of the major HIV proteins (p24, gp41, gp120/160) by fractionating them according to weight by electrophoresis, then visualizing their binding with specific antibodies over nitrocellulose sheets. If the test is positive for bands gp41 and/or p24 in conjunction with a positive EIA test, it is regarded as a confirmatory test. The WB appears to work best with samples that contain high levels of antibody. Antibody specificities against known viral components (generally the core component p24 and envelope component gp41) are considered true-positive results, whereas antibodies specific against nonviral cellular contaminants are nonspecific, false-positive results.

The WB technique is time-consuming and expensive. It is also open to considerable interpretation and has many sources of error. Variables in the test include the following:

- The technical skill and experience of the technologist performing the procedure.
- Characteristics of the technical methodology.
- General sensitivity of the WB in detecting antibodies specific for various HIV-1 antigens (especially during the window period of seronegativity).
- Frequent lack of specificity because of contamination of the viral reference preparation by histocompatibility and other antigens that electrophoretically migrate with p24 and gp41.
- Variation in band reactivity patterns in sera from an individual over the course of HIV-1 infection.

Indeterminate test results account for 4% to 20% of WB assays with positive bands for HIV-1 proteins. Indeterminate WB results can be caused by the following:

- Serologic tests in the process of seroconversion; anti-p24 is usually the first antibody to appear.
- End-stage HIV infection, usually with loss of core antibody.
- Cross-reacting nonspecific antibodies, as seen with collagen vascular disease, autoimmune diseases, lymphoma, liver disease, injection drug use, multiple sclerosis, parity, or recent immunization.
- Infection with O strain or HIV-2.
- Recipients of HIV vaccine.
- Perinatally exposed infants who are seroconverting (losing maternal antibody).
- Technical or clerical error.

In addition, nonspecific reactions producing indeterminate results in uninfected persons have occurred more frequently among pregnant women or mothers than among persons in other groups characterized by low HIV seroprevalence. The incidence of indeterminate WB results is relatively low. Immunoflourescence assay can be used to resolve an EIA-positive, WB-indeterminate sample.

The most important factor in evaluating indeterminate results is risk assessment. Patients in low-risk categories with indeterminate tests are almost never infected with HIV-1 or HIV-2; repeat testing usually continues to show indeterminate results, and the cause of this pattern is seldom established. Follow-up serology testing at 3 months is recommended to verify the previous results. Patients with indeterminate tests who are in the process of seroconversion usually have positive WB tests within 1 month; repeat tests at 1, 2, and 6 months are generally advocated, with appropriate precautions to prevent viral transmission in the interim.

False-positive WB results, especially those with a majority of bands, are extremely uncommon.

Line Immunoassay

Line immunoassay (LIA) is a popular confirmatory test. It incorporates separate HIV antigens on nitrocellulose strips, so each reaction can be visualized separately. It offers better quality control and better reproducibility than WB. The antigens are synthetic and recombinant, which decreases the background from nonspecific host proteins. This decreases the number of indeterminate results in uninfected patients.

Immunofluorescence Assay

Immunofluorescence assay (IFA) can provide a definitive diagnosis in samples that test indeterminate with other confirmatory tests. IFA is used to locate HIV-1 antigen in infected cells. Infected cells are treated with polyclonal or monoclonal antibody against p17 or p24. After being washed, the cells are incubated with fluorescein isothiocyanate or rhodamine conjugate as a secondary antibody, then are washed, mounted, and examined using a fluorescence microscope. The limitations of this technique include the

need for expensive equipment and the fact that fluorescence fades quickly.

Immunohistochemical Staining

In immunohistochemical (IHC) staining, infected cells are incubated with HIV-1 antibody. After incubation the cells are treated with an enzyme-labeled secondary antibody (usually alkaline phosphatase or horseradish peroxidase), and an appropriate substrate is added. The cells are washed and examined using simple light microscopy. IHC staining has the advantages of IFA but is simple and inexpensive and does not require extensive expertise. Morphologic changes can also be observed.

Rapid Testing

Routine HIV testing of whole blood in the emergency department has been shown to catch unidentified cases. A 2005-2006 study found that 0.8% to 1.5% of those tested were newly diagnosed with HIV infection. Two FDA-approved point-of-care test kits have a Clinical and Laboratory Standards Institute (CLIA) waiver for the detection of HIV-1 antibodies: Uni-Gold Recombigen HIV Test (Trinity Biotech USA, Berkley Heights, NJ) and OraQuick ADVANCE Rapid HIV-1/2 Antibody Test (OraSure Technologies, Bethlehem, Pa; see later procedure). OraQuick ADVANCE can screen oral fluid as well as whole blood. In 2007, Inverness (Waltham, Mass) acquired rights to market the Chembio (Medford, NY) rapid test for detection of HIV-1 and HIV-2 antibodies in fingertip blood, whole blood, serum, or plasma.

Currently, most protocols recommend confirming any positive rapid tests with WB or EIA. Follow-up with WB or EIA should be done 4 weeks later if confirmatory tests are negative or indeterminate.

PREVENTION

Reducing Viral Transmission

An estimated 250,000 Americans are unaware that they are infected with HIV. Because of this, the CDC recently issued new testing recommendations, making HIV screening a routine part of medical care for all patients 13 to 64 years old. CDC officials hope that these revised guidelines will increase early HIV diagnosis so that individuals can access treatment, know their health care status, and prevent transmission to others.

Health care personnel should assume that the blood and other body fluids from all patients are potentially infectious (Standard Precautions; see Chapter 6).

Vaccines

Types of potential HIV vaccines include the following:
- Live, attenuated vaccines
- Subunit vaccines
- DNA vaccines
- Recombinant vector vaccines

To date, the results of clinical trials have been disappointing (Box 25-4). Live, attenuated vaccines are not currently

| Box 25-4 | Clinical Trials for a Candidate HIV/AIDS Vaccine |

Phase I

Phase I trials are the first human tests of a candidate vaccine, generally conducted on small numbers (10-30) of healthy adult volunteers who are not at risk for the disease in question. The main goal is evaluation of safety and, to a lesser extent, analysis of the immune responses evoked by the vaccine and of different vaccine doses and immunization schedules. A Phase I trial usually takes 8 to 12 months to complete.

Phase II

Phase II testing involves a larger number of volunteers (50-500), usually a mixture of low-risk people and higher-risk individuals from the population where Phase III (vaccine efficacy) trials will eventually be conducted. Phase II trials generate additional safety data as well as information for refining the dosage and immunization schedule. Although not set up to determine whether the vaccine actually works, Phase II trials are sometimes large enough to yield preliminary indications of efficacy. These trials generally take 18 to 24 months, with the increase over Phase I primarily resulting from the additional time required for screening and enrolling larger numbers of trial participants.

Phase III

Phase III trials are the definitive test of whether a vaccine is effective in preventing disease. Using thousands of volunteers from high-risk populations in geographic regions where HIV is circulating, the incidence of HIV in vaccinated people is compared to that in people who receive a placebo. Successful demonstration of efficacy in a Phase III trial can then lead to an application for licensure of the vaccine.

Phase III trials of AIDS vaccines are generally expected to require a minimum of 3 years for enrollment, immunizations, and assessments of efficacy. Although there has been recent progress in increasing access to treatment and prevention programs, HIV continues to outpace the global response, with at least 80% of those in clinical need of antiretrovirals (ARVs) worldwide not receiving them. Further, although a decline in national HIV prevalence has occurred, for example, in some Sub-Saharan African countries, these trends are not strong or widespread enough to have a major impact on the epidemics.

Modified from International AIDS Vaccine Initiative, Vaccine science, www.iavi.org, December 2007.

being developed for use in humans because of safety concerns. The first AIDS vaccine using the subunit concept, AIDSVAX gp120 vaccine, failed to protect against HIV infection in an efficacy trial. Many of the current AIDS vaccines in development are DNA vaccines. DNA vaccines will not cause HIV infection because the vaccines do not contain all the genes of the live pathogen. Another common strategy in AIDS vaccine development is recombinant vector vaccines. Recombinant vector vaccines will not cause HIV infections because they contain copies of only one or several HIV genes, not all of them. The hope is that the addition of a vector will allow the vaccine to be more effective in creating an immune response than a DNA vaccine used alone.

Continued testing of vaccines is needed to determine whether they are more immunogenic in different doses, in different populations, and in combination with other candidate HIV vaccines (see Chapter 16).

More than 30 clinical trials are in progress to develop a vaccine to prevent HIV (see www.iavi.org). The first generation of successful HIV vaccines likely will offer some protection but will not be entirely protective (no vaccine is 100% effective). Future generations of a preventive HIV vaccine will become increasingly more effective over time as scientific knowledge improves. However, even partially effective vaccines could make a difference in the following ways:

1. Protecting some vaccinated individuals against HIV infection.
2. Reducing the probability that a vaccinated individual who later becomes infected will transmit the infection to others.
3. Slowing the rate of progression to AIDS for those who later become infected with HIV.

An HIV vaccine could substantially alter the course of the AIDS pandemic and reduce the number of people newly infected, even if vaccine efficacy and population coverage levels are relatively low.

TREATMENT

Despite declines in morbidity and mortality with combination antiretroviral therapy, its effectiveness is limited by adverse events, problems with patient adherence, and resistance of HIV. Episodic antiretroviral therapy, guided by the CD4+ count, significantly increases the risk of opportunistic disease or death from any cause compared with continuous antiretroviral therapy, as a consequence of lowering the CD4+ cell count and increasing the viral load. Episodic antiretroviral therapy does not reduce the risk of adverse events associated with antiretroviral therapy.

Drug Therapy

At present there are 64 HIV and HIV-related FDA-approved medicines on the market in the United States.

Traditional Therapy

Antiretroviral agents from three traditional classes of drugs are available for the treatment of HIV infection, as follows:

1. *Nucleoside analog reverse-transcriptase inhibitors* (NRTIs). The original NRTI was zidovudine (AZT), approved in March 1987. Since then, five additional NRTIs have been approved. In 2001 the first *nucleotide* analog, tenofovir, was approved for HIV treatment. It blocks HIV replication in a manner similar to the nucleoside analogs. NRTIs are potent in combination with other drugs. If used alone, resistance to HIV will develop. Some of the drugs in this class (e.g., AZT) penetrate the blood-brain barrier.
2. *Nonnucleoside analog reverse-transcriptase inhibitors* (NNRTIs). The first drug in this class, nevirapine, was approved in June 1996. NNRTIs may interact with other cytochrome P-450–processed drugs (e.g., protease inhibitors). NNRTIs have a mixed ability to penetrate the blood-brain barrier.

3. *Protease inhibitors* (PIs). The first approved drugs in this class for the treatment of HIV were ritonavir and indinavir (March 1996). PIs are very potent and may interact with other drugs using cytochrome P-450 metabolic pathways. However, poor absorption may affect potency.

New Drugs

Drugs in three new additional classes are now available, as follows:

1. *Fusion inhibitors.* The first drug in this class, pentafuside (T-20), went into Phase III clinical trials in early 2001. The mode of action of the drug is the prevention of HIV entry into the host cell.
2. *Integrase inhibitors.* The drug in this class, zintevir (AR-177), prevents HIV DNA from entering human DNA.
3. *Zinc finger inhibitors.* The drug in this class, benzamide, disrupts polyprotein formation essential for HIV replication.

New drugs are needed because resistant mutations that protect HIV against existing classes of antiretroviral drugs would be unlikely also to confer resistance to novel agents. In January 2003, 84 companies had 126 drugs and vaccines for AIDS and AIDS-related conditions in testing.

Drug discovery and FDA approval currently take an average of 12 to 15 years, and it costs about $400 million for a drug to go from laboratory to pharmacy in the United States. Drug approval requires testing in three phases of a clinical trial for safety and efficacy before approval, as follows:

- **Phase I** takes about 1 year and includes 20 to 80 healthy volunteers who are tested for the safety of a new drug.
- **Phase II** lasts about 2 years and expands the number of volunteers to 100 to 300 persons with the disease to assess the effectiveness of a drug and to observe for adverse side reactions.
- **Phase III** of a clinical trial lasts about 3 years and expands the number of patients with a specific disease to 1000 to 3000 to further verify effectiveness and to identify any specific negative side effects of the drug.

Since the FDA Regulatory Modernization Act of 1997, the FDA review process has been streamlined to hasten approval of new therapies to treat severe diseases. Phase I and Phase II are now allowed to be combined to shorten the approval process. It now takes about 18 months for a drug to go through the review process for approval by the FDA. Only about one in five medicines that enters a clinical trial is approved.

Anti-HIV drugs under development include agents that interfere with other steps in the HIV life cycle (fusion inhibitors, integrase inhibitors) and a second-generation NNRTI.

One new approach involves preventing HIV from invading the human cells in which it replicates, a concept known as **entry inhibition.** To gain entry to host cells, HIV binds to the cell's CD4 receptor in tandem with a coreceptor, usually CXCR5 or CXCR4. This process allows HIV to fuse with the cell membrane and inject its genes inside the cell. Patients with certain mutations in CCR5 are resistant to HIV infection, so drugs that block this receptor might prevent the virus from invading cells.

In addition to new studies of drugs that prevent the virus from binding to host cell receptors, Phase III clinical trials are under way for the T-20 agent, a fusion inhibitor that blocks a different event in viral invasion: the fusion of HIV with the host cell membrane. Another experimental viral entry inhibitor that appears to inhibit activity of gp120, the viral envelope protein that must interact with the host cell's CD4 receptor for HIV invasion to occur, is under development.

Also in early phases of development is an experimental agent intended to block HIV at a later stage, after it has invaded cells. The compound, S-1360, targets integrase, a viral enzyme that enables HIV to splice its DNA into the host cell's DNA. Human trials of the integrase inhibitor AR-177 are now under way.

Also on the horizon are improved versions of NNRTIs. The NNRTIs (e.g., EFV, nevirapine) target a key viral enzyme, reverse transcriptase, inhibiting its function by binding to a pocket near the enzyme's catalytic site. However, NNRTI resistance can develop when HIV acquires one or more mutations that alter the binding pocket. The drug TMC-125, given as a single agent, performed as well as the five-drug regimen containing agents from all three currently licensed classes of anti-HIV medications.

Drug Resistance

Antiviral drug resistance is defined as the reduction in the susceptibility of mutated viruses to specific antiviral drugs. An estimated 50% of patients in the United States receiving antiretroviral therapy are infected with viruses resistant to at least one of the currently available antiretroviral drugs.

The origins of drug resistance are diverse, but drug resistance is associated with the high mutation rate in the HIV genome, which is one of the key biologic characteristics of the virus. Genomic mutation is determined by the following:

- The number of mistakes per genome per replication cycle. This is extremely high in HIV because reverse transcriptase has no "proofreading" ability.
- The number of viral replications cycles per unit of time. This is reflected in an infected patient's viral load.

The relationship between resistance mutations and response to therapy is complex. Each resistance mutation is characterized by the level of associated phenotypic resistance and the specificity of the resistance mutation to one or more drugs. Either genotypic or phenotypic assays can be used to measure HIV drug resistance.

Postexposure Prophylaxis

Among health care workers exposed to HIV occupationally, prompt treatment can decrease the subsequent risk of HIV infection by more than 80%. However, treatment should begin within 1 to 2 hours after exposure. Rapid HIV testing facilitates successful treatment.

The NRTI combinations for postexposure prophylaxis (PEP) include zidovudine (ZDV) and lamivudine (3TC), 3TC and stavudine (d4T), and didanosine (ddI) and d4T. The addition of a third drug for PEP after high-risk exposures is based on demonstrated effectiveness in reducing viral burden in HIV-infected persons. Previously, indinavir or nelfinavir was recommended as the first-choice agent for inclusion in an expanded PEP regimen. In 1998 the FDA approved efavirenz (EFV), an NNRTI; abacavir (ABC), a potent NRTI; and lopinavir/ritonavir (Kaletra), a PI, for PEP. Although side effects might be common with the NNRTIs, EFV might be considered for expanded PEP regimens, especially when resistance to PIs in the source person's virus is known or suspected. ABC has been associated with dangerous hypersensitivity reactions but, with careful monitoring, may be considered as a third drug for PEP. Kaletra is a potent HIV inhibitor that, with expert consultation, may be considered in an expanded PEP regimen. Lopinavir is a newly developed inhibitor that, when formulated with ritonavir, has antiviral activity superior to that of a nelfinavir-containing regimen by itself in the initial treatment of HIV-infected adults.

Recommendations for HIV PEP include a basic 4-week regimen of two drugs (ZDV and 3TC, d4T, or ddI and d4T) for most HIV exposures. An expanded regimen includes the addition of a third drug for HIV exposures that pose an increased risk for transmission. When the source person's virus is known or suspected to be resistant to one or more of the drugs considered for the PEP regimen, the recommendation is to select drugs to which the source person's virus is unlikely to be resistant. In addition, consultation with local experts and the National Clinicians' Postexposure Prophylaxis Hotline ([PEPline] 1-888-448-4911) is advised under special circumstances (e.g., delayed exposure report, unknown source person, pregnancy in exposed person, resistance of source virus to antiretroviral agents, toxicity of PEP regimen). Occupational exposures should be considered urgent medical concerns to ensure timely postexposure management.

Failure of PEP to prevent HIV infection in health care personnel (HCP) has been reported in very few cases. Guidelines for the treatment of HIV infection, a condition usually involving a high total-body viral burden, include recommendations for the use of three drugs; however, the applicability of these recommendations to PEP remains unknown. In HIV-infected patients, combination regimens have proved superior to monotherapy regimens in reducing HIV viral load, reducing the incidence of opportunistic infections and death, and delaying onset of drug resistance. A combination of drugs with activity at different stages in the viral replication cycle theoretically could offer an additional preventive effect in PEP, particularly for occupational exposures that pose an increased risk of transmission. Although a three-drug regimen might be justified for exposures that pose an increased risk of transmission, it is uncertain whether the potential added toxicity of a third drug is justified for lower-risk exposures.

Information from the National Surveillance System for Health Care Workers and the HIV Postexposure Registry indicates that almost 50% of HCP experience adverse symptoms (e.g., nausea, malaise, anorexia, headache) while taking PEP, and that approximately 33% stop taking PEP because of adverse signs and symptoms. Some studies have shown that side effects and discontinuation of PEP are more common among HCP taking three-drug combination regimens for PEP than HCP taking two-drug regimens. Serious side effects, including nephrolithiasis, hepatitis, and pancytopenia, have been reported with the use of combination drugs for PEP. Known or suspected resistance of the source virus to antiretroviral agents, particularly to agents that might be included in a PEP regimen, is a concern. Resistance to HIV infection occurs with all the available antiretroviral agents, and cross-resistance within drug classes is common. Recent studies have demonstrated the emergence of drug-resistant HIV among source persons for occupational exposures. Despite recent studies and case reports, the relevance of exposure to a resistant virus is still not well understood.

Rapid HIV Antibody Test

OraQuick ADVANCE Rapid HIV-1/2 Antibody Test (OraSure Technologies, Bethlehem, Pa).

Principle

This point-of-care test is a manually performed, visually read, 20-minute qualitative lateral-flow immunoassay to detect antibodies to HIV-1 and HIV-2 in oral fluid and blood.

Specimen Collection and Preparation

An oral fluid specimen is collected using the flat pad on the test device, followed by the insertion of the test device into the vial of developer solution.

In the oral collection procedure, the patient being tested removes the collection device from its pouch without touching the flat pad. The flat pad is placed above the teeth against the outer gum, and the outer gums (upper and lower) are gently swabbed. Do not swab the roof of the mouth, the inside of the cheek, or the tongue.

After swabbing, the test device must be inserted into the developer solution vial within 30 minutes of collection. A test device containing an oral fluid specimen that is not inserted into the developer solution vial within 10 minutes of collection should be stored on a flat surface or returned to the divided pouch, after the desiccant has been removed from the pouch. For a 10- to 30-minute delay in insertion, return the test device containing the oral fluid specimen to the divided pouch, after the desiccant has been removed. Ensure that the divided pouch containing the test device is kept in a horizontal position until the device is inserted into the developer solution vial.

The flat pad must touch the bottom of the vial. The "Result" window on the device should be facing toward you.

A fingerstick or venipuncture whole-blood specimen or plasma specimen is collected (according to directions in package insert) and transferred into the vial of developer solution, followed by the insertion of the test device.

Once the flat pad is inserted, start timing the test. Do not remove the device from the vial while the test is running.

Pink fluid will appear and travel up the Result window. The pink fluid will gradually disappear as the test develops.

Reagents, Supplies, and Equipment

OraQuick ADVANCE Rapid Test Kit

- Divided pouches (for one-time use only)
  Each pouch contains test device, absorbent packet, and developer solution vial. Each vial contains 1 mL of a phosphate-buffered saline (PBS) solution containing polymers and an antimicrobial agent.
- Specimen collection loops
- Subject information pamphlets
- Package insert
- Customer letter

Other Required Test Materials

- Timer or watch capable of timing 20 to 40 minutes
- Clean, disposable, absorbent workspace cover
- Biohazard waste container

Additional Items

The following supplies are required for fingerstick and venipuncture whole-blood collection and plasma specimens:
- Antiseptic wipe
- Sterile lancet (fingerstick) or supplies for venipuncture
- Sterile gauze pads
- Disposable gloves
- Centrifuge (to process plasma specimen)

The OraQuick ADVANCE rapid test comprises a single-use test device and a single-use vial containing a premeasured amount of PBS developer solution. Each component is sealed in separate compartments of a single pouch. The device's plastic housing holds an assay test strip composed of several materials that provide the matrix for the immunochromatography of the specimen and the platform for indication of the test results.

The assay test strip, which can be viewed through the test device Result window, contains synthetic peptides representing the HIV envelope region and a goat antihuman IgG procedural control immobilized on a nitrocellulose membrane in the test zone and the control zone, respectively.

Quality Control

Test kit controls: HIV-1 positive control, HIV-2 positive control, and HIV negative control.

On the assay strip, a "C" zone is included. The test sample encounters this zone as it migrates up the strip. This built-in procedural control demonstrates that a specimen was added to the vial and that the fluid has migrated adequately through the test device. A reddish purple line will appear in the C zone during the performance of all valid tests, regardless of whether the sample is positive or negative for antibodies to HIV-1 and/or HIV-2.

Kit controls should be run under the following circumstances:
- A new operator, before testing patient specimens.
- A new test kit lot.

- A new shipment of test kits.
- If storage temperature of test kit falls outside the range of 2° to 27° C.
- If testing area temperature falls outside the range of 15° to 37° C.
- At periodic intervals, as dictated by the operator's facility.

Procedure

1. Open the two chambers of the OraQuick ADVANCE divided pouch by tearing at the notches on the top. To prevent contamination, leave the test device in the pouch until you are ready to use it.
2. Remove the developer solution vial from the pouch. Hold the vial firmly in your hand. Carefully remove the cap from the vial by gently rocking the cap back and forth while pulling it off. Set the cap on your workspace cover.
3. Slide the vial into the top of one of the slots in the stand. Do not force the vial into the stand from the front of the slots because splashing may occur. Make sure the vial is pushed all the way to the bottom of the slot in the stand.
   Note: do not cover the two holes in the back of device with labels or other materials. Doing so may cause an invalid result.

Reporting Results

Test results are interpreted at 20 minutes, but not more than 40 minutes, after the introduction of the test device into the developer solution containing the test specimen. Adequate lighting is required to read a test result.

Nonreactive: No reddish purple line next to the triangle labeled "T"; reddish purple line appears next to the triangle labeled "C."
- Interpreted as negative for HIV-1 and HIV-2 antibodies.

Individuals infected with HIV-1 and/or HIV-2 who are receiving highly active antiretroviral therapy (HAART) may produce false-negative results.

Reactive: Reddish purple line next to the triangle labeled T; reddish purple line appears next to the triangle labeled C. One line may be darker than the other. A test is reactive if any color appears next to the T triangle and next to the C triangle, regardless of how faint.
- Interpreted as positive for HIV-1 and/or HIV-2 antibodies.

Procedure Notes

- After collection of a specimen into the developer solution, the solution facilitates the flow of the specimen into the device and onto the test strip. As the diluted specimen flows through the device, it rehydrates the protein-A gold colorimetric reagent in the device. As the specimen continues to migrate up the strip, it encounters the "T" zone. If the specimen contains antibodies that react with the antigens immobilized on the nitrocellulose membrane, a reddish purple line will appear, qualitatively indicating the presence of antibodies to HIV-1 and/or HIV-2 in the specimen. The intensity of the line color is not directly proportional to the amount of antibody present in the specimen.

- No precision pipetting, predilutions, or special instruments are required to perform the OraQuick ADVANCE Rapid HIV-1/2 Antibody Test.
- Standard Precautions must be practiced throughout the testing procedure.
- The test should be performed at temperatures in the range of 15°-37° C. All refrigerated reagents must reach room temperature before testing.
- If the test kit is stored at temperatures outside ambient temperatures of 2° to 27° C or used outside the operating temperature of 15° to 37° C, use the kit controls to ensure performance of the test.

Reference

OraQuick ADVANCE Rapid HIV-1/2 Antibody Test product insert, OraSure Technologies, Bethlehem, Pa. Revised October 2005.

CASE STUDY

History and Physical Examination

A 40-year-old man with a history of IV drug use comes to the emergency room because of a rash and fever. In addition, the patient is complaining of a several-day history of malaise, fatigue, fever, headache, and a sore throat.

Physical examination reveals a moderately ill-appearing male with a temperature of 38.8° C. He has a blanching erythematous, macular-papular rash evident over the trunk, back, and upper and lower extremities. In addition, his throat shows enlarged tonsils and broad-based ulcerations on the buccal mucosa.

He has a history of an episode of endocarditis 2 years ago. At that time, an HIV serology was performed. It was negative.

Laboratory Data

A complete blood count and liver function tests are ordered. Results show that the patient is anemic (hematocrit 38%). He also has a severely decreased total leukocyte count and a severely decreased absolute lymphocyte count. Some of his liver function tests are abnormal.

Questions and Discussion

1. What is a likely diagnosis of this patient's condition?

The patient's history, physical examination, and laboratory data strongly suggest a diagnosis of acute HIV infection. Approximately 50% of those infected with HIV will have asymptomatic illness at the time of primary HIV infection. Acute Epstein-Barr virus (EBV) may produce an illness almost indistinguishable from acute HIV, but some of the features that suggest HIV over EBV are mucosal ulcerations,

rash, and the absence of atypical (variant) lymphocytes on the peripheral blood smear.

2. What is the natural history of this disease?

The early phase of HIV infection may last months to years after infection. Typically, patients in the early stages are either completely asymptomatic or show mild, chronic lymphadenopathy. HIV often replicates abundantly at first, and free virus appears in CSF surrounding the brain and spinal cord and in circulating blood. Within a few weeks, the viral concentration in the bloodstream and CSF drops precipitously, and the initial symptoms disappear.

An unknown number of infected patients experience a brief, infectious, mononucleosis-like or flulike illness with fever, malaise, and possibly a skin rash. Neurologic complaints may also be reported. These symptoms parallel the first wave of HIV replications and develop at about the time antibodies produced by the body against HIV are first detected, usually 2 weeks to 3 months after infection, rarely later. After HIV infection and any clinical signs and symptoms, a person may remain symptom free for years.

From 2 to 10 years after HIV infection, replication of the virus flares again, and the infection enters its final stage. An average of 8 or 9 years may pass before AIDS is fully developed. The virus behaves differently, depending on the host cell and its level of mitotic activity. In T cells, however, the virus can lie dormant indefinitely, but it can destroy the host cell in a burst of replication. HIV grows continuously, but slowly, in macrophage-monocytes. This slow growth of the virus saves the cell from destruction but probably alters its function.

Clinical symptoms of the later phase of HIV infection include extreme weight loss, fever, and multiple secondary infections. The end stage of AIDS is characterized by neoplasms and opportunistic infections. Lethal *P. carinii* pneumonia has been a hallmark of AIDS. Other opportunistic infections may coexist. Cryptosporidiosis and *H. capsulatum* are increasingly recognized.

The most common malignancy is an aggressive, invasive variant of Kaposi's sarcoma, discovered in many cases through autopsy. KS produces tumors in the skin and linings of internal organs, lymphomas, and cancers of the rectum and tongue. Malignant B-cell lymphomas are also increasingly recognized in patients with or at high risk for AIDS. Because certain lymphomas can develop early, B-cell hyperactivity may play a role in their development. Lymphomas and other cancers late in HIV disease could also result from the compromised immune system failing to recognize and destroy cancer cells.

3. What immunologic laboratory tests might be of value in establishing a diagnosis for this patient?

A screening test for infectious mononucleosis might be helpful to corroborate the absence of atypical lymphocytes on the patient's peripheral blood smear.

Approximately 7 to 14 days after exposure to HIV, a burst of viral replication leads to detectable levels of p24 antigen in the blood. Antibody is not detectable initially; therefore an HIV antibody test would be negative. Patients with acute

HIV infection will develop a positive antibody test within 6 months.

Follow-up serologic testing is important if p24 antigen testing is not done. Other tests that may be positive in this period before seroconversion are PCR and viral culture.

Diagnosis

Acquired immunodeficiency syndrome.

CHAPTER HIGHLIGHTS

- HIV-1 is the predominant virus responsible for AIDS. In addition to the original HIV-1, a second AIDS-causing virus, HIV-2, was identified in 1985.
- The HIV virus is composed of structural proteins and glycoproteins that occupy the core and envelope regions of the particle.
- Retroviruses contain a single, positive-stranded RNA with the genetic information of the virus and a special enzyme, reverse transcriptase, in their core. Reverse transcriptase enables the virus to convert viral RNA into DNA.
- HIV has a marked preference for the CD4+ subset of lymphocytes. Macrophages, as many as 40% of the peripheral blood monocytes, and cells in the lymph nodes, skin, and other organs also express measurable amounts of CD4 and can be infected by HIV. In addition, about 5% of the B lymphocytes may express CD4 and be susceptible to HIV infection.
- Transmission of HIV is believed to be restricted to intimate contact with body fluids from an infected person; casual contact with infected persons has not been documented as a mode of transmission.
- The early phase of HIV-1 infection may last months to years after initial infection. Typically, patients in the early stages of HIV-1 infection are either completely asymptomatic or show mild, chronic lymphadenopathy. HIV-1 causes a predictable, progressive derangement of immune function, and AIDS is one late manifestation of that process.
- Two to 10 years after HIV infection, replication of the virus flares again, and the infection enters its final stage. An average of 8 or 9 years may pass before AIDS is fully developed. The virus behaves differently depending on host cell and its level of mitotic activity. The end stage of AIDS is characterized by neoplasms and opportunistic infections.
- Immunologic activities associated with HIV-1 infection include the production of different types of antibodies against HIV-1. Some antibodies neutralize it, others prevent it from binding to cells, and others stimulate cytotoxic cells to attack HIV-infected cells.
- A window period of seronegativity exists from the time of initial infection to 6 or 12 weeks or longer. Using EIA methods based on defined HIV-1 proteins produced by recombinant DNA methods, antibodies specific for gp41 are detectable for weeks or months before assays specific for p24. The appearance of antibodies specific for p24 precedes that of anti-gp41 in Western blot serum specimens.
- Laboratory evaluation of HIV-infected patients consists of assessment of cellular and humoral components. Screening of blood donors and patients is usually by serologic methods. In patients with signs and symptoms of AIDS, both the assessment of cellular concentrations and function and the diagnosis and treatment of opportunistic infections become important.
- Antibodies to HIV-1 are usually detected by EIA and confirmed by Western blot, currently the standard for confirming HIV-1 seropositivity. If positive for band p41 or p24 with a positive EIA, the test is confirmatory.

REVIEW QUESTIONS

1. The major structural protein (core) of the HIV-1 virus is:
   a. gp41.
   b. p24.
   c. gp34.
   d. gp140.

2. The infectious process of AIDS begins when the gp120 protein on the viral envelope bends to the protein receptor, _____, on the surface of a target cell.
   a. CD8
   b. CD4
   c. p24
   d. p26

3. HIV can infect all of the following cells *except:*
   a. CD4+ subset of lymphocytes.
   b. Macrophages.
   c. Monocytes.
   d. Polymorphonuclear leukocytes.

4. The most rapidly growing segment of the HIV-infected population is:
   a. Homosexual males.
   b. Lesbians.
   c. Health care workers.
   d. IV drug users and their sexual partners.

5. In HIV infections, a window period of seronegativity extends from the time of initial infection up to:
   a. 2 weeks.
   b. 2 to 6 weeks or longer.
   c. 6 to 12 weeks or longer.
   d. 4 to 8 months or longer.

Questions 6 and 7. HIV antibodies are usually detected by (6) _____ and confirmed by (7) _____ .

Possible answers for question 6:
  a. latex agglutination
  b. enzyme immunoassay
  c. enzyme inhibition
  d. radioimmunoassay

Possible answers for question 7:
  a. Southern blot
  b. Northern blot
  c. Western blot
  d. DNA hybridization

8. The AIDS-causing virus HIV has also been referred to as:
  a. Human T-lymphotropic virus type III.
  b. HTLV-III.
  c. Lymphadenopathy-associated virus (LAV).
  d. All the above.

9. HTLV-I was unique when it was isolated because it was the first:
  a. Bovine infectious retrovirus.
  b. Canine infectious retrovirus.
  c. Human infectious retrovirus.
  d. Isolated AIDS virus.

Questions 10-12. Fill in the blanks in the following table with the correct letter, choosing from the following answers:
  a. Codes for p24 and for proteins such as p17, p9, and p7.
  b. Codes for two glycoproteins, gp41 and gp120.
  c. Produces DNA polymerase; produces endonuclease.

Viral Genome Structural Components

Component	Product
pol	10. _____
gag	11. _____
env	12. _____

Questions 13-17. Arrange the HIV-1 life cycle events in proper order.

13. _____
14. _____
15. _____
16. _____
17. _____

  a. Reverse transcriptase converts viral RNA into proviral DNA.
  b. New virus particles are produced as the result of normal cellular activities of transcription and translation.
  c. New particles bud from the cell membrane.
  d. Virus attaches to CD4 membrane receptor and sheds its protein coat, exposing its RNA core.
  e. Proviral DNA is integrated into the genome (genetic complement of cell).

Questions 18-20. Match the characteristics to the three infectious patterns of HIV virus.

18. _____ Pattern 1: North and South America, Western Europe, Scandinavia, Australia, New Zealand.

19. _____ Pattern 2: Africa, Caribbean, parts of South America.

20. _____ Pattern 3: Eastern Europe, North Africa, Middle East, Asia, Pacific (excluding Australia and New Zealand).

  a. Primarily a disease of heterosexuals.
  b. Few cases of AIDS.
  c. Primarily a disease of homosexuals and IV drug abusers.

21. The criteria for HIV infection for persons 13 years or older include:
  a. Repeatedly reactive screening test for HIV antibody.
  b. Specific HIV antibody identified by use of supplemental tests.
  c. Direct identification of the virus.
  d. All the above.

22. After the early period of primary HIV infection, the patient enters a period of clinical latency that lasts a median of _____ years.
  a. 5
  b. 10
  c. 15
  d. 20

23. As AIDS progresses, the quantity of _____ diminishes, and the risk of opportunistic infection increases.
  a. HIV antigen
  b. HIV antibody
  c. CD4+T lymphocytes
  d. CD8+T lymphocytes

24. The clinical symptoms of the later phase of AIDS are:
  a. Weight loss and decreased PMN cells.
  b. Extreme weight loss and fever.
  c. Multiple secondary (opportunistic) infections.
  d. Both b and c.

25. The most frequent malignancy observed in AIDS patients is:
  a. *Pneumocystis jiroveci (carinii)*.
  b. Kaposi's sarcoma.
  c. Toxoplasmosis.
  d. Non-Hodgkin's lymphoma.

26. Sources of error in the Western blot test include:
    a. Concentration of HIV antigen.
    b. Presence of other infectious agents.
    c. Technical skill and experience of the technologist performing the test.
    d. Age of the blood specimen.

27. All the following methods have been developed to detect HIV-1 antigen *except:*
    a. Transcriptase method.
    b. Synthetic peptide approach.
    c. Immunofluorescence assay.
    d. Immunohistochemical staining.

28. All the following methods have been developed to detect the presence of HIV-1 viral gene *except:*
    a. Radioimmunoassay.
    b. In situ hybridization.
    c. Southern blot analysis.
    d. DNA amplification.

BIBLIOGRAPHY

Bartlett JG, Gallant JE: *Medical management of HIV: 2001-2002,* Baltimore, 2001, Johns Hopkins Press.

Bayer R, Oppenheimer GM: Pioneers in AIDS care: reflections on the epidemic's early years, *N Engl J Med* 355(22):2273-2278, 2006.

Branca M: Chipping away at AIDS mystery, *Bio-IT World* 1:20, 2002.

El-Sadr WM et al: CD4+ count–guided interruption of antiretroviral treatment, *N Engl J Med* 355(22):2283-2294, 2006.

Gallo RC, Montagnier L: AIDS in 1988, *Sci Am* 259(4):40-51, 1988.

Global Health Reporting: Facts at a glance, December 2007, www.global healthreporting.org.

Goudsmit J et al: Expression of human immunodeficiency virus antigen (HIV-Ag) in serum and cerebrospinal fluid during acute and chronic infection, *Lancet* 2:177-180, 1986.

Goudsmit J et al: Intrathecal synthesis of antibodies to LAV/HTLV-III specific IgG in individuals without AIDS or AIDS-related complex, *N Engl J Med* 292:1231-1234, 1986.

Goudsmit J et al: Intrathecal synthesis of antibodies to HTLV-III in patients without AIDS or AIDS-related complex, *Br Med J* 192:1231-1234, 1986.

Haseltine WA, Wong-Stall F: The molecular biology of the AIDS virus, *Sci Am* 259(4):52-63, 1988.

James E: Clinical clips: FDA approves rapid HIV test, *ADVANCE Med Lab Professionals* 14(25):12, 2002.

Koziel MJ, Peters MG: Viral hepatitis in HIV infection, *N Engl J Med* 356(14):1445-1454, 2007.

McCutchan FE: *Understanding the genetic diversity of HIV-1, AIDS 2000,* Philadelphia, 2000, Lippincott–Williams & Wilkins.

McDermott D et al: Chemokine promoter polymorphism affects risk of both HIV infection and disease progression in multicenter AIDS cohort study, *AIDS* 14:2671-2678, 2000.

McDowell J: CDC revamps HIV testing recommendation to include adolescents and all adults, *Clin Lab News* 32(11), 33(1):1, 2007.

Miller LE: Effects of HIV on the immune system, *ADVANCE Med Lab Professionals,* May 1999, pp 12-17.

Montgomery KA: Taking the test, *ADVANCE Med Lab Professionals,* Feb 12, 2007, pp 27-28.

News brief: Routine HIV testing in the ED catches unidentified cases, *Clin Lab News* 33(8):1, 2007.

Redfield RR, Burke DS: HIV infection: the clinical picture, *Sci Am* 259(4):90-98, 1988.

Resnick L: Intra–blood-brain barrier synthesis of HIV specific IgG in patients with neurologic symptoms associated with AIDS or AIDS-related complex, *N Engl J Med* 313:1498-1502, 1985.

Salahuddin SZ: HTLV-III in symptom-free seronegative persons, *Lancet* 2:1418-1420, 1984.

Schim van der Loeff MF, Aaby P: *Towards a better understanding of the epidemiology of HIV-2, AIDS,* Philadelphia, 1999, Lippincott–Williams & Wilkins.

Scosyrev E: An overview of the human immunodeficiency virus featuring laboratory testing for drug resistance, *Clin Lab Sci* 19(4):231-248, 2006.

Sepkowitz KA: One disease, two epidemics: AIDS at 25, *N Engl J Med* 354(23):2411-2417, 2006.

Shaw GM et al: HTLV-III infections in brains of children and adults with AIDS encephalopathy, *Science* 227:177-182, 1985.

Smith T: Employing HIV molecular and rapid testing, *ADVANCE Admin Lab* 15(5):44-51, 2006.

Specialty Laboratories: Test information, 2002, www.specialtylabs.com.

Stephenson J: Scientists find some genes a bad omen for anti-HIV drug, *JAMA* 287(13):1637, 2002.

Stine G: *AIDS Update 2003,* Upper Saddle River, NJ, 2003, Prentice Hall.

Strategies for Management of Antiretroviral Therapy (SMART) Study Group: CD4+ count–guided interruption of antiretroviral treatment, *N Engl J Med* 355(22):2283-2296, 2006.

Turgeon ML: *Clinical hematology: theory and procedures,* ed 3, Philadelphia, 1999, Lippincott–Williams & Wilkins.

US Department of Health and Human Services, Henry J Kaiser Family Foundation: Guidelines for the use of antiretroviral agents in HIV-infected adults and adolescents, February 2002, www.hivatis.org.

US Department of Health and Human Services, Centers for Disease Control and Prevention: Cases of HIV/AIDS and AIDS, August 2007, www.cdc.gov.

Walmsley S et al: Lopinavir-ritonavir versus nelfinavir for the initial treatment of HIV infection, *N Engl J Med* 346:2039-2046, 2002.

Weber JN, Weiss RA: HIV infection: the cellular picture, *Sci Am* 259(4):100-109, 1988.

Weiss SH et al: Screening test for HTLV-III (AIDS agent) antibodies: specificity, sensitivity, and applications, *JAMA* 253:221-225, 1985.

Wong-Stall F, Gallo RC: Human T-lymphotropic retroviruses, *Nature* 317:395-403, 1985.

Wright AA, Katz IT: Home testing for HIV, *N Engl J Med* 354(5):437-442, 2006.

Zetola N, Klausner JD: HIV testing: an update, *Med Lab Observer MLO* 38(9):58-62, 2006.

PART IV

Immunologically and Serologically Related Disorders

26 Hypersensitivity Reactions
27 Immunoproliferative Disorders
28 Autoimmune Disorders
29 Systemic Lupus Erythematosus

30 Rheumatoid Arthritis
31 Solid Organ Transplantation
32 Bone Marrow Transplantation
33 Tumor Immunology

CHAPTER 26

Hypersensitivity Reactions

What is Hypersensitivity?
What is an Allergy?
Types of Antigens and Reactions
   Environmental Substances
   Infectious Agents
   Self Antigens
   Hypersensitivity Reactions
Type I Hypersensitivity Reactions
   Etiology
   Immunologic Activity
   Signs and Symptoms
   Laboratory Evaluation of Allergic Reactions
   Treatment
Type II Hypersensitivity Reactions
   Type II Antibody-Dependent, Complement-Mediated
      Cytotoxic Reactions
   Type II Antibody-Dependent, Cell-Mediated
      Cytotoxicity
   Type II Hypersensitivity and Antibodies
      That Affect Cell Function
   Testing for Type II Hypersensitivity

Type II Autoimmune Hypersensitivity
   Against Solid Tissue
Prevention and Treatment
Type III (Immune Complex) Reactions
   Mechanism of Tissue Injury
   Clinical Manifestations
   Autoimmune Disorders
   Testing for Type III Hypersensitivity Reactions
   Treatment
Type IV Cell-Mediated Reactions
   Characteristics
   Latex Sensitivity
   Testing for Delayed Hypersensitivity
   Treatment
Rapid Test for Food Allergy
Direct Antiglobulin Test
Case Studies
Chapter Highlights
Review Questions
Bibliography

Learning Objectives

At the conclusion of this chapter, the reader should be able to:

- Define the terms hypersensitivity, allergy, and sensitization/immunization.
- Identify and explain the three categories of antigens.
- Compare the basic differences among and give examples of types I, II, III, and IV hypersensitivity reactions.
- Describe the etiology, immunologic activity, signs and symptoms, laboratory evaluation, and treatment of type I hypersensitivity reactions.
- Discuss examples of type II hypersensitivity reactions, including laboratory evaluation.

- Describe the mechanism of tissue injury, clinical manifestations, and laboratory testing for type III hypersensitivity reactions.
- Describe the characteristics and laboratory evaluation of type IV hypersensitivity reactions.
- Discuss the acquisition and consequences of latex sensitivity.
- Analyze case studies related to hypersensitivity reactions.

WHAT IS HYPERSENSITIVITY?

Hypersensitivity can be defined as a normal but exaggerated or uncontrolled immune response to an antigen that can produce inflammation, cell destruction, or tissue injury.

Hypersensitivity has traditionally been classified on the basis of time after exposure to an offending antigen. When this criterion is used, the terms **immediate hypersensitivity** and **delayed hypersensitivity** are appropriate. As described in Chapter 1, immediate hypersensitivity is antibody mediated, and delayed hypersensitivity is cell mediated.

The term **immunization,** or **sensitization,** describes an immunologic reaction dependent on the host's response to a subsequent exposure of antigen. Small quantities of the antigen may favor sensitization by restricting the quantity of antibody formed. An unusual reaction, such as an allergic or hypersensitive reaction that follows second exposure to the antigen, reveals the existence of the sensitization.

WHAT IS AN ALLERGY?

Our basic understanding of allergy has evolved from the discovery in 1967 of a previously unknown antibody, **immunoglobulin E (IgE).** The most significant property of IgE antibodies is that they can be specific for hundreds of different **allergens.** Common allergens include animal dander, pollens, foods, molds, dust, metals, drugs, and insect stings.

The term **allergy** originally meant any altered reaction to external substances. A related term, **atopy,** refers to immediate hypersensitivity mediated by IgE antibodies. The terms *allergy* and *atopy* are now often used interchangeably. Atopic allergies include hay fever, asthma, food allergies, and latex sensitivity.

Allergies are very common and increasing in prevalence in the United States, Western Europe, and Australia. Allergies also occur in families, although not necessarily the same allergy.

TYPES OF ANTIGENS AND REACTIONS

Antigens that trigger allergic reactions are called *allergens.* These small-molecular-weight substances can enter the body by being inhaled, eaten, or administered as drugs.

Hypersensitivity reactions can occur in response to different types of antigen, including environmental substances, infectious agents, and "self" antigens.

Environmental Substances

Environmental substances in the form of small molecules can trigger several types of hypersensitivity reactions. Dust can enter the respiratory tract, mimicking parasites, and stimulate an antibody response. An immediate hypersensitivity reaction associated with IgE, such as **rhinitis** or asthma, can result. If dust stimulates immunoglobulin G (IgG) antibody production, it can trigger a different type of hypersensitivity reaction, such as farmer's lung. If small molecules diffuse into the skin and act as haptens, a delayed hypersensitivity reaction, such as contact **dermatitis,** will result.

Drugs administered orally, by injection, or on the skin can provoke a hypersensitivity reaction mediated by IgE, IgG, or T lymphocytes.

Metals (particularly nickel) and chemicals can cause type I hypersensitivity reactions as well. Low-molecular-weight chemicals usually act as a hapten by binding to body proteins or the major histocompatibility complex (MHC) molecules. The complex of antigen and MHC molecules is then recognized by specific T cells, which initiate the reaction.

Infectious Agents

Not all infectious agents are capable of causing hypersensitivity reactions. The influenza virus can cause hypersensitivity that results in damage to epithelial cells in the respiratory tract. Sometimes an exaggerated immune response occurs. Influenza virus, for example, can trigger high levels of cytokine secretion or what is called a "cytokine storm."

In comparison, streptococci can cause a hypersensitivity reaction termed *immune complex disease.*

Self Antigens

A very small immune response to "self" antigens is normal and exists in most people. When these become an exaggerated response, however, or when tolerance to other antigens breaks down, hypersensitivity reactions can occur (see Chapter 28).

Hypersensitivity Reactions

The four types of hypersensitivity reaction (I-IV) are defined by the principal mechanism responsible for a specific cell or tissue injury that occurs during an immune response (Table 26-1). Types I, II, and III reactions are antibody dependent, and type IV is cell mediated. Some overlapping occurs among the various types of hypersensitivity reactions, but there are major differences in how each type is diagnosed and treated.

TYPE I HYPERSENSITIVITY REACTION

Type I hypersensitivity reactions can range from life-threatening **anaphylactic reactions** to milder manifestations associated with food allergies.

Etiology

Atopic allergies are mostly naturally occurring, and the source of antigenic exposure is not always known. Atopic illnesses were among the first antibody-associated diseases demonstrating a strong familial or genetic tendency.

Several groups of agents cause anaphylactic reactions. The two most common agents are drugs (e.g., systemic penicillin) and insect stings. Insects of the order Hymenoptera (e.g., common hornet, yellow jacket, yellow hornet, paper wasp) are representative examples of insects causing the most serious reactions.

Table 26-1	Classification of Hypersensitivity Reactions			
	Type I	**Type II**	**Type III**	**Type IV**
Reaction	Anaphylactic	Cytotoxic	Immune complex	T cell dependent
Antibody	IgE*	IgG, possibly other immunoglobulins	Antigen-antibody complexes* (IgG, IgM)	None
Complement involved	No	Yes*	Yes*	No
Cells involved	Mast cells, basophils, granules (histamine)*	Effector cells (macrophages, polymorphonuclear leukocytes)*	Macrophages, mast cells	Antigen-specific T cells
Cytokines involved	Yes*	No	Yes*	Yes* (T-cell cytokines)
Comparative description	Antibody mediated, immediate	Antibody dependent; complement or cell mediated	Immune complex mediated (immune complex disease)	T cell mediated, delayed type
Mechanism of tissue injury	Allergic and anaphylactic reactions	Target cell lysis; cell-mediated cytotoxicity	Immune complex deposition, inflammation	Inflammation, cellular infiltration
Examples	Anaphylaxis	Transfusion reactions	Arthus reaction	Allergy or infection
	Hay fever	Hemolytic disease of newborn	Serum sickness	Contact dermatitis
	Asthma	Thrombocytopenia	Systemic lupus erythematosus	
	Food allergy			

*Mediator.

Immunologic Activity

Mast cells (tissue basophils) are the cellular receptors for IgE, which attaches to their outer surface. These cells are common in connective tissues, the lungs, and uterus and around blood vessels. They are also abundant in the liver, kidney, spleen, heart, and other organs. The granules contain a complex of heparin, histamine, and zinc ions, with heparin in a ratio of approximately 6:1 with histamine.

Immediate hypersensitivity is the basis of acute allergic reactions caused by molecules released by mast cells when an allergen interacts with membrane-bound IgE (Figure 26-1). Acute allergic reactions result from the release of preformed granule-associated mediators, membrane-derived lipids, cytokines, and chemokines when an allergen interacts with IgE that is bound to mast cells or basophils by the alpha chain of the high-affinity IgE receptor (FcεRI-α). This antigen receptor also occurs on antigen-presenting cells, where it can facilitate the IgE-dependent trapping and presentation of allergen to T cells.

Histamine, leukotriene C4, interleukin-4 (IL-4), and interleukin-13 (IL-13) are major mediators of allergy and asthma. All are formed by basophils and released in large quantities after stimulation with interleukin-3; IL-3's effect is restricted to basophil granulocytes. Basophil granulocytes should be considered as key effector cells in type 2 helper T (Th2)–cell immune response and allergic inflammation. IL-3 strongly induces messenger ribonucleic acid (mRNA) for granzyme B, a major effector of granule-mediated cytoxicity.

Anaphylactic Reaction

Anaphylaxis is the clinical response to immunologic formation and fixation between a specific antigen and a tissue-fixing antibody. This reaction is usually mediated by IgE antibody and occurs in the following three stages:
1. The offending antigen attaches to the IgE antibody fixed to the surface membrane of mast cells and basophils. Cross-linking of two IgE molecules is necessary to initiate mediator release from mast cells.
2. Activated mast cells and basophils release various mediators.
3. The effects of mediator release produce vascular changes; activation of platelets, eosinophils, and neutrophils; and activation of the coagulation cascade.

It is believed that physical allergies (e.g., heat, cold, ultraviolet light) cause a physiochemical derangement of proteins or polysaccharides of the skin and transform them into **autoantigens** responsible for the allergic reaction. Most, if not all, of these reactions are caused by the action of a self-directed IgE.

Anaphylactoid Reaction

Anaphylactoid reactions (anaphylaxis-like) are clinically similar to anaphylaxis and can result from immunologically inert materials that activate serum and tissue proteases and the alternate pathway of the complement system. Anaphylactoid reactions are not mediated by antigen-antibody interaction; instead, offending substances act directly either on the mast cells, causing release of mediators, or on the tissues, such as *anaphylotoxins* of the complement cascade (C3a, C5a). Direct chemical degranulation of mast cells may be the cause of anaphylactoid reactions resulting from the infusion of macromolecules, such as proteins.

Atopic Reaction

In a person with **atopy,** exposure of the skin, nose, or airway to an allergen produces allergen-specific IgG antibodies. In response to the allergen, the T cells (when tested in vitro) exhibit moderate proliferation and production of interferon gamma (IFN-γ) by type 1 helper T (Th1) cells. In comparison, individuals with atopy have an exaggerated response characterized by the production of allergen-specific IgE antibodies and positive reactions to extracts of common airborne

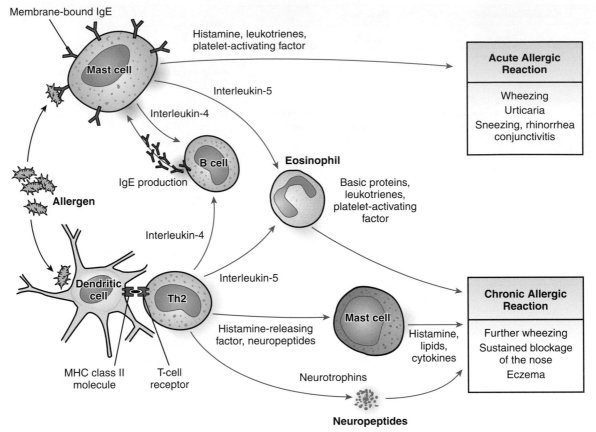

Figure 26-1 Pathways leading to acute and chronic allergic reactions. Acute allergic reactions are caused by the antigen-induced release of histamine and lipid mediators from mast cells. In the skin and upper airways, basophils (not shown) may also participate in allergic tissue reactions. Chronic allergic reactions, including the late-phase reaction, may depend on a combination of pathways, including recruitment of eosinophils, liberation of mast cell products by histamine-releasing factors, and neurogenic inflammation involving neurotrophins and neuropeptides. *Th2,* T-helper cell type 2; *MHC,* major histocompatibility complex. *(Redrawn from Kay AB:* N Engl J Med *344(1):30-38, 2001.)*

allergens when tested with a skin prick test. T cells from the blood of atopic patients respond to allergens in vitro by inducing cytokines produced by Th2 cells (e.g., IL-4, IL-5, and IL-13), rather than cytokines produced by Th1 cells (IFN-γ and IL-2).

There are always exceptions to the rule, but the immunologic hallmark of allergic disease is the infiltration of affected tissue by Th2 cells.

Signs and Symptoms

Although everyone inhales airborne allergens derived from pollen, house-dust mites, and animal dander, children and adults without atopy produce an asymptomatic, low-grade immunologic response. In a person with atopy, exposure of the skin, nose, or airway to a single dose of allergen produces symptoms (skin redness, sneezing, wheezing) within minutes. Depending on the amount of allergen, immediate hypersensitivity reactions are followed by a late-phase reaction that reaches a peak 6 to 9 hours after exposure to the allergen and then slowly subsides.

Localized Reaction

A localized reaction occurs as an immediate response to mediators released from mast cell degranulation. Local reactions can consist of **urticaria** and **angioedema** at the site of antigen exposure or angioedema of the bowel after ingestion of certain foods. Localized reactions are severe but rarely fatal. Skin reactions are characterized be the appearance of redness and itching at the site of the introduction of the allergen. This phenomenon is the principle of the skin test to diagnose an allergy or confirm sensitivity to a specific antigen.

Generalized Reaction

A generalized (anaphylactic) reaction is produced by mediators such as cytokines and vasoactive amines (e.g., histamine) from mast cells. Anaphylactic reactions are dramatic and rapid in onset. The physiologic effects of the primary and secondary mediators on the target organs, such as the cardiovascular or respiratory system, gastrointestinal (GI) tract, or the skin, define the signs and symptoms of anaphy-

Table 26-2	Mediators of Anaphylaxis
Mediator	Primary Action
Histamine	Increases vascular permeability. Promotes contraction of smooth muscle.
Leukotrienes	Alters bronchial smooth muscle and enhances the effects of histamine on target organs.
Basophil kallikrein	Generates kinins.
Serotonin	Contracts smooth muscle.
Platelet-activating factor	Enhances the release of histamine and serotonin from platelets that affect smooth muscle tone and vascular permeability.
Eosinophil chemotactic factor of anaphylaxis	Attracts eosinophils to area of activity; these cells release secondary mediators that may limit the effects of primary mediators.
Prostaglandins	Affect smooth muscle tone and vascular permeability.

Box 26-1	Common Battery of Food/Environmental Allergy Profile Testing

Childhood Allergy
Cat dander
Cockroach
Codfish
Dog dander
Egg white
House-dust mite *(Dermatophagoides farinae)*
Milk
Mold *(Alternaria alternata)*
Peanut
Soybean
Wheat
Total IgE

Adult Profile
Clam
Codfish
Corn
Egg white
Milk
Peanut
Scallop
Shrimp
Soybean
Walnut
Wheat
Total IgE

From Quest Diagnostics: ImmunoCAP methodology, www.immunocap invitrosight.com, July 2007.

laxis. Several important, pharmacologically active compounds are discharged from mast cells and basophils during anaphylaxis (Table 26-2).

Histamine release leads to constriction of bronchial smooth muscle, edema of the trachea and larynx, and stimulation of smooth muscle in the GI tract, which causes vomiting and diarrhea. The resulting breakdown of cutaneous vascular integrity results in urticaria and angioedema; vasodilation causes a reduction of circulating blood volume and a progressive fall in blood pressure, leading to shock. Kinins also alter vascular permeability and blood pressure.

The body's "natural moderators of anaphylaxis" are the enzymes that decompose the mediators of anaphylaxis. Antihistamines have no effect on histamine release from mast cells or basophils. In humans, antihistamines are effective antagonists of edema and pruritus, probably related to their blockage of a histamine-induced increase in capillary permeability but are relatively less effective in preventing bronchoconstriction.

Allergic Disease in Children

Atopic children characteristically experience a progression of allergic disease called **allergy march.** Formation of IgE antibodies begins early in life, and sensitization can be detected before clinical symptoms. Sensitization to food allergens such as cow's milk is manifested as colic or chronic otitis. The highest incidence of sensitization is at age 2 years. After 3 years of age, food sensitivities tend to decrease, and sensitization to inhalant allergens typically increases during the preschool years (Box 26-1). In most children with asthma, symptoms begin before age 5 years. Risk factors for allergic asthma include a family history of allergy, sensitization to food allergens, total serum IgE greater than 100 kU/L before age 6 years, living in an allergen-rich environment, and smoking.

Testing for Type I Hypersensitivity Reactions

Two types of testing protocols are used to confirm allergen-specific IgE antibodies in patients with suspected allergy, as follows:
- In vivo skin prick testing
- In vitro blood testing

In Vivo Skin Testing. Skin testing can be performed by:
- Skin prick test
- Intradermal test
- Skin patch test

Placing a drop of a solution containing a possible allergen on the skin is the basis of skin testing. A series of scratches or needle pricks allows the solution to enter the skin. If the skin develops a red, raised, itchy area, this is a positive reaction. A positive reaction usually means that the person is allergic to that particular allergen.

Intradermal testing involves injecting a small amount of allergen solution into the skin. An intradermal allergy test may be a follow-up to the skin prick test when a person is suspected to be allergic to a substance, but the skin prick test was negative or questionable. The intradermal test is more sensitive but may produce false-positive results.

Skin patch testing involves taping a patch that has been soaked in the allergen solution to the skin for 24 to 72 hours. This type of testing is used to detect contact dermatitis.

Skin testing is a simple outpatient technique to screen for many potential allergens, but it may not be suitable for pediatric patients, pregnant women, or other groups. The procedure carries the risk of triggering a systemic reaction (e.g., anaphylactic reaction) or initiating a new sensitivity.

Laboratory Evaluation of Allergic Reactions

Advantages of in vitro testing include the lack of risk of a systemic hypersensitivity reaction and the lack of dependence on skin reactivity, which can be influenced by drugs, disease, or the patient's age. Detection of an increased amount of either total IgE or allergen-specific IgE in serum indicates an increased probability of an allergic disorder, parasitic infection, or aspergillosis. In vitro laboratory testing can be performed by a variety of methods.

The clinical significance of serum allergen-specific IgE (sIgE) in allergic disorders has long been recognized. Quantitative measure of serum sIgE antibodies is essential for differential diagnosis and for identifying the causative allergens for proper medical treatment. The quality and availability of allergens, reagent stability, and degree of automation all influence the method of testing.

First- and Second-Generation Testing

The original **radioallergosorbent testing (RAST)** represented first-generation testing. RAST is no longer in use, partly because of the risks associated with a radioactive substance. The assay used a specific allergen bound to a solid-phase carrier, which was then incubated with a serum sample containing an unknown amount of IgE specific for the allergen. Results measured radioactive counts per second emitted from an isotopically labeled antibody. The amount of label bound is only a measure of the allergen-specific IgE in the serum.

Second-generation testing, marketed in the 1990s, improved the specificity and sensitivity of in vitro testing. However, second-generation testing created background noise that prevented the quantitative measurement of very low levels of serum IgE (<0.35 kIU/L). This presented an obstacle to further improvement in clinical sensitivity.

Third-Generation Methods

Third-generation assays offer the following major improvements:

- Detection of low levels of serum sIgE.
- Standardization of testing as a result of automation.
- Use of test antigens that are better defined and standardized.

Chemiluminescent Enzyme Immunoassay. A third-generation sIgE method (ImmunoLite 2000; Siemens Healthcare Solutions, N.J.) is a solid-phase (bead), two-step chemiluminescent enzyme immunoassay (EIA). Allergens are covalently lined to a soluble polymer–ligand matrix, allowing immunochemical reactions to occur in liquid phases for random-access automation.

Protein Microarray. An experimental protein microarray can be used for detection of specific IgE antibodies. Micro-

Test Principle

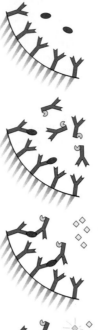

Anti-ECP covalently coupled to ImmunoCAP, reacts with the ECP in the patient serum sample.

After washing, enzyme-labeled antibodies against ECP are added to form a complex.

After incubation, unbound enzyme–anti-ECP is washed away, and the bound complex is then incubated with a developing agent.

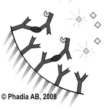

After stopping the reaction, the fluorescence of the eluate is measured. The fluorescence is directly proportional to the concentration of ECP in the serum sample. To evaluate test results, the responses for patient samples are compared directly to the responses for calibrators.

© Phadia AB, 2008

Figure 26-2 ImmunoCAP test: principle, steps, and evaluation. *ECP,* Eosinophilic cationic protein. *(Courtesy Phadia AB, Uppsala, Sweden.)*

spots are arrayed on a capillary flow membrane and contain natural allergen extracts that are covalently immobilized. Starting with 20-μL serum sample applications, a sequential series of liquid flows and assay events are induced.

ImmunoCAP. ImmunoCAP is an in vitro quantitative assay that measures allergen-specific IgE in human serum (Figure 26-2). It is intended for in vitro use as an aid in the clinical diagnosis of IgE-mediated allergic disorders, in conjunction with other clinical findings (Tables 26-3 and 26-4). ImmunoCAP assays can be performed on hundreds of allergens, such as weeds, trees, pollens, mold, food, and animal dander.

The U.S. Food and Drug Administration (FDA) has cleared the technology used in ImmunoCAP to provide quantitative measurement of IgE. The innovative ImmunoCAP technology is based on a cellulose polymer in a plastic reservoir and provides high binding capacity of clinically relevant allergen proteins, including those present in very low levels.

Table 26-3	Comparison of Tests for Specific IgE		
	Skin Prick Testing	**Intradermal Testing**	**Blood Testing (ImmunoCAP)**
Sensitivity (%)	93.6	60.0	87.2
Specificity (%)	80.1	32.3	90.5

Modified from Choo-Kang LR: *MLO* 38(3):10-14, 2006.

Table 26-4	Interpretation of Results: Specific IgE Blood Test (ImmunoCAP)	
Quantity (kU$_A$/L)	Level	Clinical Relevance
<0.35	Absent/undetectable	Consider nonallergic causes.
0.35-0.69	Low	Uncertain clinical relevance.
0.70-3.49	Moderate	Probably a contributing factor to total allergic load.
3.50-17.49	High	Clinically relevant.
17.50-49.99	Very high	Highly clinically relevant.
50.0-100.0		
>100		

From Quest Diagnostics: ImmunoCAP methodology, www.immunocap invitrosight.com, July 2007.

Eosinophilic Cationic Protein. Eosinophilic cationic protein (ECP-2) is a protein generated in certain white blood cells (WBCs) actively engaged in the immune defense system.

The clinical use of inhaled steroids is becoming increasingly popular because of their antiinflammatory effects, although overtreatment may have serious side effects. To ensure the lowest effective dosage throughout treatment, the laboratory can periodically monitor the occurrence in serum of ECP-2 released from inflammatory cells. Using a diagnostic test developed by Phadia (Portage, Mich), ECP can be detected in body fluids.

Treatment

Treatment of patients with allergies involves identifying and eliminating or avoiding possible allergens. Drug therapy and desensitization are two treatment strategies.

Drug Therapy

Drug treatments include the following:
- Epinephrine (adrenaline) can be lifesaving in anaphylaxis. Epinephrine stimulates both α-adrenergic and β-adrenergic receptors, decreases vascular permeability, increases blood pressure, and reverses airway obstruction.
- Antihistamines block specific histamine receptors and play an important role in allergies affecting the skin, nose, and mucous membranes. Antihistamines act much slower than epinephrine in treating anaphylaxis and are not very useful in asthma because histamine is not an important allergic mediator released by mast cells in the lung.
- Specific receptor antagonists block the effects of leukotrienes. One drug, montelukast, reduces the amount of airway inflammation in asthma.
- Corticosteroids, often given topically, are widely used in the prevention of symptoms in patients with allergy.
- Other drugs in development aim to block the Th2 cytokine pathway or prevent IgE binding to FcεR.

Desensitization

Desensitization, or **immunotherapy,** is a well-established technique to improve allergy symptoms caused by specific allergens (e.g., hay fever) (Figure 26-3). If a patient has a history of life-threatening conditions, and if other treatment alternatives are unsatisfactory, desensitization is used to prevent anaphylaxis resulting from insect stings (e.g., yellow jackets). It is best if only one allergen is incriminated.

Specific immunotherapy is associated with downregulation of the cytokines produced by Th2 cells, upregulation of cytokines produced by Th1 cells, and the induction of regulatory T (Treg) cells. These changes in produce inhibition of allergic inflammation, increases in cytokines that control the production of IgE (INF-γ and IL-12), production of blocking antibodies (IgG), and release of cytokines involved in allergen-specific hyporesponsiveness (IL-10 and transforming growth factor β).

Different routes of desensitization induce different T-cell populations: Th1 and Treg cells in the case of subcutaneous administration and Th2 cells in the case of a sting on the skin.

For desensitization to insect venom, venom is injected subcutaneously in increasing doses at fixed intervals of time. Treatment starts with very small doses of venom because there is a risk of inducing anaphylactic shock. Over time the patient receives injections with increasing quantities of venom, eventually corresponding to the amount of venom in an insect sting. Once desensitization has been carried out, high levels of allergen-specific IgG will bind venom and prevent it from cross-linking IgE on mast cells. After following the prescribed treatment protocol, more than 90% of patients will *not* develop anaphylaxis if they are stung again.

TYPE II HYPERSENSITIVITY REACTIONS

Type II hypersensitivity reactions are a consequence of IgG or IgM binding to the surface of cells. Three different mechanisms of antibody-mediated injury exist in type II hypersensitivity, as follows:

1. *Antibody-dependent, complement-mediated cytotoxic reactions* are characterized by the interaction of IgG or IgM antibody to cell-bound antigen. This binding of an antigen and antibody can result in the activation of complement and destruction of the cell (cytolysis) to which the antigen is bound. Erythrocytes, leukocytes, and platelets can be lysed by this process. Examples of antibody-dependent, complement-mediated cytotoxic reactions include immediate (acute) transfusion reactions and immune hemolytic anemias (e.g., hemolytic disease of the newborn).

2. *Antibody-dependent, cell-mediated cytotoxicity* depends on initial binding of specific antibodies to target cell surface antigens. The antibody-coated cells are lysed by effector cells, such as natural killer (NK) cells and macrophages, expressing Fc receptors. The Fc receptors of these effector cells attach to the Fc portion of the anti-

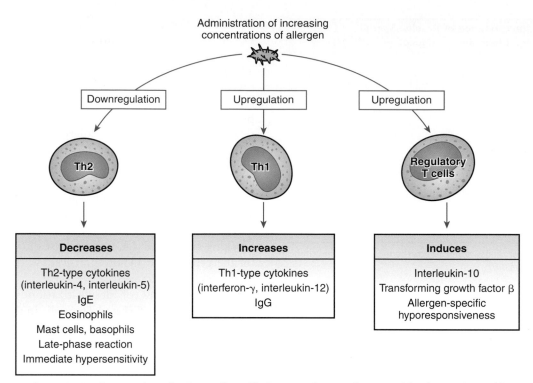

Figure 26-3   Proposed mechanisms of specific immunotherapy (hyposensitization or desensitization). Specific immunotherapy is associated with downregulation of the cytokines produced by Th2 cells, upregulation of cytokines produced by Th1 cells, and induction of regulatory T cells. These changes in turn lead to inhibition of allergic inflammation, increases in cytokines that control production of IgE (interferon-γ and interleukin-12) and "blocking" antibodies (IgG), and release of cytokines involved in allergen-specific hyporesponsiveness (interleukin-10 and transforming growth factor β). *(Redrawn from Kay AB:* N Engl J Med *344(2):109-113, 2001.)*

body that is coating the target cell. Target cell destruction occurs when cytotoxic substances are released by the effector cells. This is the mechanism of injury in antibody-mediated glomerulonephritis and many other diseases. Antibody binding damages solid tissues, where the antigen may be cellular or part of the extracellular matrix (e.g., basement membrane).

3. *Antireceptor antibodies* disturb the normal function of receptors. Less often, antibodies may modify the function of cells by binding to receptors for hormones (autoimmune hypersensitivity against solid tissue), as illustrated by autoimmune thyroid disease (see Chapter 28). Hyperacute graft rejection is also an example of type II hypersensitivity (see Chapter 31).

Type II Antibody-Dependent, Complement-Mediated Cytotoxic Reactions

Transfusion Reactions

Transfusion reactions are examples of antibody-dependent, complement-mediated cytotoxic reactions. The term *transfusion reaction* generally refers to the adverse consequences of incompatibility between patient and donor erythrocytes. Transfusion reactions can include hemolytic (RBC-lysing) reactions occurring during or shortly after a transfusion, shortened posttransfusion survival of red blood cells (RBCs), an allergic response, or disease transmission.

Transfusion reactions can be divided into hemolytic and nonhemolytic types. *Hemolytic reactions* are associated with the infusion of incompatible erythrocytes. These reactions can be further classified into acute (immediate) or delayed in their manifestations (Box 26-2). Several factors influence whether a transfusion reaction will be acute or delayed, including the following:

- Number of incompatible erythrocytes infused.
- Antibody class or subclass.
- Achievement of the optimal temperature for antibody binding.

Immediate Hemolytic Reactions. The most common cause of an acute hemolytic transfusion reaction is the transfusion of ABO-group incompatible blood. In patients with preexisting antibodies resulting from prior transfusion or pregnancy, other blood groups may be responsible.

Epidemiology. Acute hemolytic reactions are the most serious and potentially lethal transfusion reactions. Most fatalities resulting from acute hemolytic transfusion reactions occur in anesthetized or unconscious patients, with the immediate cause of death being uncontrollable hypotension.

Signs and Symptoms. Reactions can occur with the infusion of as little as 10 to 15 mL of incompatible blood. The most common initial symptoms are fever and chills, which mimic a febrile, nonhemolytic reaction caused by leukocyte incompatibility. Back pain, shortness of breath, pain at the infusion site, and hypotension are additional symptoms. In addition to shock, the release of thromboplastic substances into the circulation can induce disseminated intravascular coagulation and acute renal failure.

Immunologic Manifestations. Acute hemolytic reactions occur during infusion or immediately after blood has been infused. Infusion of incompatible erythrocytes in the presence of preexisting antibodies initiates an antigen-antibody reaction, with activation of the complement, plasminogen, kinin, and coagulation systems. Other initiators of acute hemolytic reactions include bacterial contamination of blood or infusion of hemolyzed erythrocytes. Many reactions demonstrate both extravascular and intravascular hemolysis. If an antibody is capable of activating complement and is sufficiently active in vivo, intravascular hemolysis occurs, producing a rapid increase of free hemoglobin in the circulation. Although uncertain, the cause of the immediate clinical symptoms may be products released by the action of complement on the erythrocytes, which triggers multiple shock mechanisms.

Delayed Hemolytic Reaction. A delayed reaction may not manifest until 7 to 10 days after transfusion. In contrast to an immediate reaction, a delayed reaction occurs in the extravascular spaces. These reactions are associated with decreased RBC survival because of the coating of the RBCs (positive direct antiglobulin test), which promotes phagocytosis and premature removal of RBCs by the mononuclear phagocyte system. If an antibody does not activate complement or activates it very slowly, extravascular hemolysis occurs. Most IgG antibody–coated erythrocytes are destroyed extravascularly, mainly in the spleen.

A delayed hemolytic transfusion reaction may be of two types. It may represent an **anamnestic** antibody response in a previously immunized recipient on secondary exposure

to transfused erythrocyte antigens, or it may result from primary **alloimmunization.** In an anamnestic response the antibodies are directed against antigens to which the recipient has been previously immunized by transfusion or pregnancy.

Hemolytic Disease of the Newborn

Hemolytic disease of the newborn (HDN), previously called "erythroblastosis fetalis," results from excessive destruction of fetal RBCs by maternal antibodies. HDN in the fetus or neonate is clinically characterized by anemia and jaundice. If the hemoglobin breakdown product that visibly produces jaundice (bilirubin) reaches excessive levels in the newborn's circulation, it will accumulate in lipid-rich nervous system tissue and can result in mental retardation or death.

Etiology. Antigens possessed by the fetus that are foreign to the mother can provoke an antibody response in the mother. Any blood group antigen that occurs as an IgG antibody is capable of causing HDN.

Although anti-A and anti-B are present in the absence of their corresponding antigens as environmentally stimulated (IgM) antibodies, infrequent IgG forms may be responsible for HDN because of ABO incompatibility. High titers of anti-A/B of the IgG type in group O mothers often cause mild HDN. Anti-A and anti-B antibodies are usually 19S (IgM) in character and as such are unable to pass through the placental barrier. In addition, the A and B antigens are not fully expressed on the erythrocytes of the fetus and newborn. In a survey of antibodies that have caused HDN, more than 70 different antibodies were identified.

Epidemiology. The incidence of HDN resulting from ABO incompatibility ranges from 1 in 70 to 1 in 180, with an estimated average of 1 in 150 births. The most frequent form of ABO incompatibility occurs when the mother is type O and the baby is type A or type B, usually type A.

Until the early 1970s, the Rh antibody anti-D was the most frequent cause of moderate or severe forms of HDN. Anti-D occurred either alone or in combination with another Rh antibody such as anti-C. Anti-D accounted for approximately 93% of the cases of non-ABO HDN. Since the development of modern treatment to prevent primary immunization to the D antigen, the frequency of HDN caused by anti-D has significantly decreased.

Signs and Symptoms. Hemolytic disease resulting from ABO incompatibility is usually mild because of fewer A and B antigen sites on the fetal/newborn erythrocytes, weaker antigen strength of fetal/newborn A and B antigens, and competition for anti-A and anti-B between tissues and erythrocytes. The number and strength of A and B antigen sites on fetal erythrocytes are less than on adult RBC membranes. In addition, A and B substances are not confined to the RBCs, so only a small fraction of IgG anti-A and anti-B that crosses the placenta combines with the infant's erythrocytes.

Manifestations of HDN caused by other antibodies can range from mild to severe. In addition to possible death in utero, newborns may demonstrate severe anemia and an increase in RBC breakdown products such as bilirubin. Accumulation of bilirubin causes jaundice and may result in mental retardation if methods are not applied to clear bilirubin from the infant's body.

Immunologic Mechanism. For antibody formation to take place, the mother must lack the antigen, and the fetus must express the antigen (gene product). The fetus would inherit the gene for antigen expression from the father. HDN results from the production of maternal antibodies that have been stimulated by the presence of these foreign fetal antigens. The actual production of antibodies depends on a variety of factors: the genetic makeup of the mother, the antigenicity of a specific antigen, and the actual amount of antigen introduced into the maternal circulation.

Transplacental hemorrhage (TPH) can occur at any stage of pregnancy. Immunization resulting from TPH can result from negligible doses during the first 6 months in utero; however, significant immunizing hemorrhage usually occurs during the third trimester or at delivery. Fetal erythrocytes can also enter the maternal circulation as the result of physical trauma from an injury, abortion, ectopic pregnancy, amniocentesis, or normal delivery. Abruptio placentae, cesarean section, and manual removal of the placenta are often associated with a considerable increase in TPH.

An example of the normal pattern of immunization is demonstrated by the case of an Rh (D)–negative mother whose primary immunization (sensitization) was caused by either a previously incompatible Rh (D)-positive pregnancy or a blood transfusion, which stimulates the production of low-titered anti-D, predominantly of the IgM class. Subsequent antigenic stimulation, such as fetal-maternal hemorrhage during pregnancy with an Rh (D)-positive fetus, can elicit a secondary (anamnestic) response, characterized by the predominance of increasing titers of anti-D of the IgG class.

Immune antibodies subsequently react with fetal antigens. Erythrocytic antigens, as well as leukocyte and platelet antigens, can induce maternal immunization by the formation of IgG antibodies. In HDN the erythrocytes of the fetus become coated with maternal antibodies that correspond to specific fetal antigens. Antibodies to IgG, the only immunoglobulin that is selectively transported to the fetus, are transferred from the maternal circulation to the fetal circulation through the placenta. The mechanism by which IgG passes through the placenta has not been definitively established. Most research on transplacental passage supports the hypothesis that all IgG subclasses are capable of crossing the placental barrier between mother and fetus.

When the antigen and its corresponding antibody combine in vivo, increased lysis of RBCs results. Because of this hemolytic process, the normal 45- to 70-day life span of the fetal erythrocytes is reduced. To compensate for RBC loss, the fetal liver, spleen, and bone marrow respond by increasing production of erythrocytes. Increased RBC production outside the bone marrow, *extramedullary hematopoiesis,* can result in enlargement of the liver and spleen and premature release of nucleated erythrocytes from the bone marrow into the fetal circulation. If increased RBC production cannot compensate for the cell being destroyed, a progressively severe anemia develops that can cause the fetus to develop cardiac failure with generalized edema and death in utero. Less severely affected infants continue to experience erythrocyte destruction after birth, which generates large quantities of unconjugated bilirubin. Bilirubin resulting from excessive hemolysis can produce the threat of accumulation of free bilirubin in lipid-rich tissue of the central nervous system.

Diagnostic Evaluation. The following procedures are generally used in the prenatal or postnatal diagnostic evaluation of HDN:

- ABO blood grouping
- Rh testing
- Screening for irregular antibodies; identification and titering of any antibodies
- Amniocentesis (prenatal)
- Serum bilirubin of cord or infant blood
- Direct antiglobulin test of cord or infant blood
- Peripheral blood smear
- Kleihauer-Betke test

Prevention. Three independent research teams showed that a passive antibody, Rh IgG, could protect most Rh-negative mothers from becoming immunized after the delivery of Rh (D)–positive infants or similar obstetric conditions. In 1968, Rh IgG was licensed for administration in the United States. Since that time, the incidence of HDN caused by anti-D has decreased dramatically, although complete elimination may never occur because of the cases in which anti-D is formed before delivery. All pregnant Rh-negative women should receive Rh IgG, even if the Rh status of the fetus is unknown, because fetal D antigen is present on fetal erythrocytes as early as 38 days from conception.

Autoimmune Hemolytic Anemia

Autoimmune hemolytic anemia is an example of a type II hypersensitivity reaction directed against "self" antigens on RBCs. It can take two forms: cold **autoagglutinins** and warm autoagglutinins.

Cold autoimmune hemolytic anemia. Cold autoagglutinins, usually IgM, represent about one third of cases of immune hemolytic anemia. Cold agglutinins react best at room temperature or lower.

Warm autoimmune hemolytic anemia. In contrast to the cold form, warm autoagglutinins, usually IgG, represent the majority of cases of autoimmune hemolytic anemia. Although the source of antigen exposure may be unknown, antibodies can be formed to microorganisms or drugs. Warm autoagglutinins react best at 37° C.

Type II Antibody-Dependent, Cell-Mediated Cytotoxicity

Autoantibodies can also attack and damage components of solid tissues, as in Goodpasture's syndrome. In this disorder, IgG autoantibodies bind a glycoprotein in the basement membrane of the kidney's glomeruli and the lungs. Anti–basement membrane antibody activates complement that can trigger an inflammatory response. This group of diseases can be detected by demonstrating autoantibody.

Type II Hypersensitivity and Antibodies That Affect Cell Function

In another type II hypersensitivity reaction, antibodies bind to cells and affect their function. These antibodies simply stimulate the target organ function without causing organ damage. In some situations, such as Wegener's granulomatosis, stimulation of cells by autoantibody leads to tissue damage.

Testing for Type II Hypersensitivity

The **direct antiglobulin test (DAT)** is performed to detect transfusion reactions, hemolytic disease of the newborn, and autoimmune hemolytic anemia (see later procedure). Polyspecific anti–human globulin, a mixture of antibodies to IgG and complement components (e.g., C3d), is used for preliminary screening. If positive, the DAT can be repeated using monospecific anti-IgG and anti-C3d reagents for more exact determination. If an autoimmune hemolytic anemia caused by IgM exists, only the C3d assay would be positive.

The **indirect anti–human globulin (AHG) assay** is used to determine the presence of an unexpected antibody.

Platelet agglutination assays may be of value if **idiopathic thrombocytopenic purpura** is suspected. If Goodpasture's syndrome is suspected, direct fluorescent examination of a renal tissue biopsy would be helpful.

Type II Autoimmune Hypersensitivity Against Solid Tissue

Autoantibodies can also attack and damage components of solid tissues. These antibodies can simply stimulate the target organ function without causing much target organ damage, as in Graves' disease. In other situations, stimulation of cells by autoantibody leads to tissue damage. As noted earlier, Goodpasture's syndrome involves IgG autoantibodies and a glycoprotein in the basement membrane of the lung and glomeruli. Anti–basement membrane antibody activates complement, which can trigger an inflammatory response. Goodpasture's syndrome can be diagnosed by finding antibodies to glomerular basement membrane in patient serum on indirect immunofluorescence (Figure 26-4) and autoantibodies in serum (see Appendix B).

Prevention and Treatment

Checking the donor and recipient and providing immunization to prevent HDN are two prevention strategies. Immunosuppressive drugs can reduce B-cell autoantibody secretion. **Plasmapheresis** is a method of reducing the quantity of antibody in a patient's circulating blood.

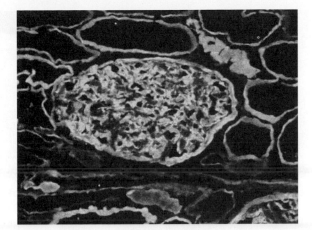

Figure 26-4 Indirect immunofluorescence used to detect autoantibodies in patient with Goodpasture's syndrome. Kidney tissue is used as the target antigen for this test. Linear staining along the glomerular basement membrane appears to be "lit up" compared with the renal tubules in the background. *(From Nairn R, Helbert M: Immunology for medical students, ed 2, St Louis, 2007, Mosby.)*

TYPE III (IMMUNE COMPLEX) REACTIONS

Type III hypersensitivity reactions are caused by the deposition of immune complexes in blood vessel walls and tissues. Repeated antigen exposure leads to sensitization with the production of an insoluble antigen-antibody complex. As these complexes are deposited in tissues, the complement system is activated, macrophages and leukocytes are attracted, and immune-mediated damage occurs. Common skin conditions in this category include allergic vasculitis and erythema nodosum. Pulmonary reactions include hypersensitivity pneumonitis, characterized best by **farmer's lung,** which is a reaction to thermophilic actinomycetes found in moldy hay. Chemicals such as toluene diisocyanate, phthalic anhydride, and trimetallic anhydride can cause bathtub refinisher's lung, epoxy resin lung, and plastic worker's lung, respectively.

Farmer's lung and the **Arthus reaction** (Figure 26-5) are examples of local immune complex disease. Poststreptococcal glomerulonephritis is an example of circulating-immune complex disease, as in systemic lupus erythematosus (SLE; Chapter 29). Immune complexes are lattices of antigen and antibody that may be localized to the site of antigen production or may circulate in the blood. Immune complexes are produced as part of the normal immune response and are usually cleared by mechanisms involving complement. However, immune complexes cause disease in various situations. Failure to clear immune complexes can result from saturation of mechanisms involving excessive ongoing production of immune complexes, as well as antigenemia caused by chronic infection.

The formation of immune complexes under normal conditions protects the host because these complexes facilitate the clearance of various antigens and invading microorganisms by the mononuclear phagocyte system. In immune

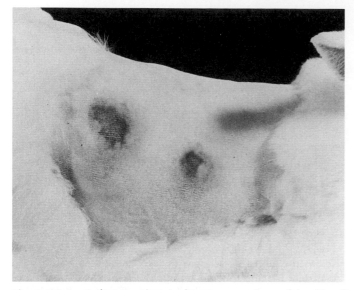

Figure 26-5   **Arthus reaction.** In these two reactions of the skin of a rabbit, the larger reaction has an extensive zone of erythema and edema surrounding its necrotic center. *(From Markell EK, Voge M: Medical parasitology, ed 5, Philadelphia, 1981, Saunders.)*

complex reactions (disease), antigen-antibody complexes form in the soluble or fluid phase of tissues or in the blood and assume unique biologic functions, such as interaction with complement and with cellular receptors.

Other type III (immune complex) reactions include serum sickness and certain aspects of autoimmune disease (e.g., glomerulonephritis in SLE). Circulating soluble immune complexes are responsible for or associated with a variety of human diseases in which both exogenous and endogenous antigens can trigger a pathogenic immune response and result in immune complex disease (Table 26-5).

Mechanism of Tissue Injury

Type III reactions are caused by IgG, IgM, and possibly other antibody types. Immune complexes can exhibit a spectrum of biologic activities, including suppression or augmentation of the immune response by interacting with B and T cells; inhibition of tumor cell destruction; and deposition in blood vessel walls, glomerular membranes, and other sites. These de-

Table 26-5	Diseases Associated with Immune Complexes
Type	**Examples**
Autoimmune diseases	Rheumatoid arthritis, systemic lupus erythematosus, Sjögren's syndrome, mixed connective tissue disease, systemic sclerosis, glomerulonephritis
Neoplastic disease	Solid and lymphoid tumors
Infectious disease	Bacterial infective endocarditis, streptococcal infection, viral hepatitis, infectious mononucleosis

posits interrupt normal physiologic processes because of tissue damage secondary to the activation of complement and resulting activities such as mediating immune adherence and attracting leukocytes and macrophages to the sites of immune complex deposition. The release of enzymes and possibly other agents damages the tissues. The three general anatomic sites of antigen-antibody interactions are as follows:

1. Antibody can react with soluble antigens in the circulation and form immune complexes that may disseminate and lodge in any tissue with a large filtration area and cause lesions of immune complex disease.
2. Antibody can react with antigen secreted or injected locally into the interstitial fluid. The classic example is the experimental *Arthus reaction,* the basic model of local immune complex disease (see Figure 26-5).
3. Antibody can also react with structural antigens that form part of the cell surface membranes or with fixed intercellular structures such as the basement membranes. The systemic immune complex disease *serum sickness* is an example of soluble and tissue-fixed antigen involvement.

Clinical Manifestations

The persistence of immune complexes in the blood circulation is not inherently harmful. Immune complex disease develops when these circulating complexes are not cleared from the circulation by phagocytosis and subsequently deposited in certain tissues.

Serum Sickness

Acute serum sickness develops within 1 to 2 weeks after initial exposure or repeated exposure by injection of heterologous serum protein. There is no preexisting antibody, and the disease appears as antibody formation begins. The hallmark of serum sickness is the protracted interaction between antigen and antibody in the circulation with the formation of antigen-antibody complexes in an environment of antigen excess. Chronic serum sickness can be experimentally induced if small amounts of antigen are given daily and represent just enough antigen to balance antibody production.

Autoimmune Disorders

Systemic lupus erythematosus (SLE) is an autoimmune disorder characterized by autoantibodies that form immune complexes with autoantigens, which are deposited in the renal glomeruli (see Chapter 29). As a consequence of this type III hypersensitivity reaction, **glomerulonephritis** (inflammation of capillary vessels in the glomeruli) develops.

Testing for Type III Hypersensitivity Reactions

Specific autoimmune disorders, such as rheumatoid arthritis (see Chapter 30), have specific assays for detection and monitoring the autoimmune disorder. Common assays use latex agglutination, nephelometry, and chemiluminescence techniques.

Fluorescent staining of tissue biopsy specimens can be used to observe deposition of immune complexes in the tissues. Staining patterns and affected tissue can assist in disease diagnosis and prognosis.

Another laboratory assay used in assessment is the quantitation of complement (C3 and C4 components).

Treatment

The most direct treatment is avoidance of the offending antigen. Corticosteroids block some of the damage caused by effector cells. Cyclophosphamide is an alkylating agent that impairs DNA synthesis and prevents rapid proliferation of cells (e.g., lymphocytes reduce B-cell proliferation).

TYPE IV CELL-MEDIATED REACTIONS

Type IV cell-mediated immunity consists of immune activities that differ from antibody-mediated immunity. Cell-mediated immunity is moderated by the link between T lymphocytes and phagocytic cells (i.e., monocyte-macrophages). Lymphocytes (T cells) do not recognize the antigens of microorganisms or other living cells but are immunologically active through various types of direct cell-to-cell contact and by the production of soluble factors.

Characteristics

Type IV **delayed-type hypersensitivity (DTH)** involves antigen-sensitized T cells or particle remains phagocytized in a macrophage and encountered by previously activated T cells for a second or subsequent time. T cells respond directly or by the release of lymphokines, to exhibit contact dermatitis and allergies of infection (Figure 26-6).

Cell-mediated immunity is responsible for the following immunologic events:

- Contact sensitivity
- Delayed hypersensitivity
- Immunity to viral and fungal antigens
- Immunity to intracellular organisms
- Rejection of foreign tissue grafts
- Elimination of tumor cells bearing neoantigens
- Formation of chronic granulomas

Under some conditions, the activities of cell-mediated immunity may not be beneficial. Suppression of the normal adaptive immune response (immunosuppression) by drugs or other means is necessary in conditions such as organ transplantation, hypersensitivity, and autoimmune disorders.

Delayed hypersensitivity can be a physiologic reaction to pathogens that are difficult to clear, such as hepatitis B virus and *Mycobacterium tuberculosis*. This triggers the most extreme DTH reactions, characterized by granuloma formation, extensive cell death, and the appearance of caseous necrosis. Delayed hypersensitivity can also occur in response to innocuous environmental antigens (e.g., nickel). Antigens must have a low molecular weight to enter the body.

Delayed hypersensitivity reactions also take place against autoantigens. In insulin-dependent (type 1) diabetes, T cells respond to pancreatic islet cell antigens, damaging the islets and eventually preventing insulin secretion.

Delayed hypersensitivity reactions are initiated when tissue macrophages recognize the presence of danger signals and initiate the inflammatory response. Dendritic cells loaded with antigen migrate to local lymph nodes, where they present antigen to T cells. Specific T-cell clones proliferate in response to antigens and migrate to the site of inflammation. T cells and macrophages stimulate one another through the cytokine network. Tumor necrosis factor alpha (TNF-α) is secreted by both macrophages and T cells and stimulates much of the damage in DTH reactions. Because of the need for antigen presentation by T cells, DTH reactions are often associated with specific human leukocyte antigen (HLA) alleles.

The hallmark of occupational type IV hypersensitivity is allergic *contact dermatitis* caused by metals (e.g., nickel, mercury, copper), sunscreen agents, disinfectants, perfumes and fragrances, and pesticides. Pulmonary hypersensitivity can be caused by inorganic dust particles, hard metal, and beryllium. Hard-metal exposure involves cobalt from the grinding of steel.

Latex Sensitivity

In the health care setting, natural latex can be an allergen in personnel who have significant cumulative exposure. Since 1985, policies of "universal standards" have resulted in an exponential increase in the use of latex gloves. The use of latex condoms has also increased. The increase in total exposure to latex and variations in manufacturing apparently have led to an increase in the number of persons with latex sensitivity.

Once sensitized, an individual may experience allergic symptoms when exposed to any product containing latex. At-risk groups sensitized to natural rubber latex include 8% to 17% of health care workers, as well as children who have repeated surgeries. Less than 1% of the general U.S. population (~3 million) demonstrate latex sensitivity.

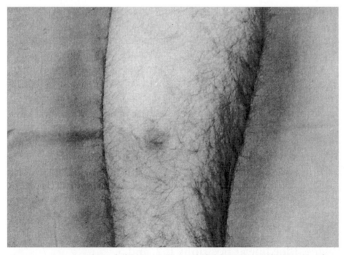

Figure 26-6 Delayed skin reaction exhibiting an erythematous but nonedematous zone 15 mm in diameter at 48 hours. A control site, inoculated higher on the forearm, shows no reaction at this time. *(From Barrett JT: Textbook of immunology, ed 5, St Louis, 1988, Mosby.)*

Latex contains low-molecular-weight soluble proteins that cause IgE-mediated allergic reactions. Latex allergy can give rise to a broad range of symptoms. Glove wearers may experience type IV, or delayed-hypersensitivity, contact dermatitis that ranges from nonspecific pruritus to eczematous, red, weepy skin. These symptoms and the irritant contact dermatitis are caused by the accelerators and chemicals used in glove manufacturing, not by the latex itself. Avoidance of latex gloves is often sufficient to prevent these symptoms.

Anaphylactic reactions to latex have been reported in persons who previously had experienced only irritant or allergic contact dermatitis. Direct skin contact with latex may cause a type I, or immediate-hypersensitivity, IgE-mediated reaction within 30 to 60 minutes of exposure. Urticaria may be local or generalized, and the spectrum of progression is notably unpredictable; some persons have experienced anaphylactic reactions after having minimal or no previous symptoms.

Certain fruits, such as bananas, chestnuts, kiwi, avocados, and tomatoes, show cross-reactivity, perhaps because of a similarity to a latex protein component. These foods have been responsible for anaphylactic reactions in latex-sensitive persons. Many other foods, including figs, apples, celery, melons, potatoes, papayas, and pitted fruits (e.g., cherries, peaches), have caused progressive symptoms beginning with oral itching. Persons with a history of reactions to these foods are at increased risk of developing latex allergy, and those who are sensitive to latex should avoid foods to which they have had previous reactions.

Testing for Delayed Hypersensitivity

The skin test for testing of exposure to tuberculosis is a classic example of a delayed-hypersensitivity reaction. The test is based on the principle that soluble antigens from *Mycobacterium tuberculosis* induce a reaction in individuals who have acquired or been exposed to the tuberculosis microorganism or a related organism at some time. It does not mean that the person has tuberculosis.

A small amount of antigen is injected under the skin (intradermally) with a fine-needle syringe. The site is observed at 48 and 72 hours for the presence of induration (lesion at least 10 mm in diameter).

Other antigens that can be skin-tested include diphtheria toxoid, tetanus toxoid, fungal antigens (e.g., trichophyton, histoplasmin), and *Candida albicans.*

In cases of persistent dermatitis, a patch test may be performed. An adhesive patch containing the suspected allergen is applied to the skin. The skin is checked for redness with papules or tiny blisters, indicating a positive test, over 48 hours.

Diagnosis of latex allergy is determined by the patient history and immunologic testing. FDA-approved in vitro tests to measure latex-specific IgE are available (Pharmacia CAP, Pharmacia-UpJohn Diagnostics, Kalamazoo, Mich; AlaSTAT, Diagnostic Products, Los Angeles). The low specificity of these tests, which have a false-negative rate of at least 20% and thus unclear positive predictive value, limits clinical usefulness. Negative serologic testing with a strongly positive history would suggest the value of skin prick testing to confirm the diagnosis.

Treatment

Strategies to avoid a DTH reaction include avoiding antigen exposure. Antiinflammatory drugs or corticosteroids may be useful. In some patients, TNF monoclonal antibodies and recombinant interferon-β may be administered.

Rapid Test for Food Allergy

Principle

The RAPID 3-D Casein Test utilizes a three-line diagnostic dry-strip format. When a food extract containing casein is extracted and applied to a collector comb, blue latex particles coated with antibodies to casein are mobilized. These particles bind casein in the sample and flow along the test strip, where they are trapped by a second, immobilized casein antibody, revealing a blue line.

Specimen Collection and Preparation

Cooked or uncooked food ingredients (e.g., chocolate, cereal, infant formulas) or environmental swabs are tested in a manufacturing or industrial food preparation plant or for food-labeling enforcement testing to determine whether adulteration, unintentional inclusion, or contamination has occurred.

Reagents, Supplies, and Equipment

BioKits RAPID 3-D Casein Test (902075M).

Quality Control

The presence or absence of lines at all positions provides information on casein content in the sample. Position 2 is unique to the BioKits RAPID 3-D range and ensures against excess sample/matrix interference, which could result in false-negative results. Position 3 is a control ensuring the device has worked and the sample has been successfully processed for analysis.

Procedure

1. Weigh or estimate a representative amount of food sample.
2. Add sample to extraction buffer 1 and mix.
3. Add extraction buffer 2 and mix.
4. Correctly apply extracted sample to collector "comb."
5. Insert comb into test device.
6. Read test results in 5 minutes.

Reporting Results

Positive: Blue line at positions 1, 2, and 3.

Negative: No blue line at position 1, but blue lines at positions 2 and 3.

Very high or overload casein content: Blue line at position 3 only, or at position 3 with a thin blue line at position 1.

Procedure Notes

RAPID 3-D kits are available for gluten, peanuts, almonds, hazelnuts, and shellfish.

Limitations

The testing kit is not suitable for the testing of foods consumed at home or in a restaurant by allergic persons.

Clinical Applications

Casein, a protein naturally present in milk, is one of the eight major food allergens, which can initiate reactions ranging from urticaria to anaphylactic shock (type I to type IV hypersensitivity reactions).

Identification of casein minimizes the risks posed by food allergens by identifying cross-contamination of ingredient supplies or inadequate cleaning between production batches.

Reference

RAPID 3-D Casein Test, Tepnel Biosystems, Stamford, Conn, 2007.

Direct Antiglobulin Test

Principle

The direct antiglobulin test (DAT) is based on the principle that antiglobulin antibodies induce in vitro agglutination of erythrocytes with immunologically bound antibodies. After erythrocytes (RBCs) are washed to remove free plasma protein from the test mixture, they are tested directly with polyspecific reagents containing anti-IgG and anti-C3d. The DAT procedure is clinically important in the diagnosis of conditions such as hemolytic anemia, including hemolytic disease of the newborn.

Specimen Collection and Preparation

No special preparation of the patient is required before specimen collection. After proper identification of the patient, blood should be drawn by aseptic technique and the specimen tested as soon as possible. The specimen can be a clotted blood sample or an EDTA anticoagulated sample. Newborn or infant samples may be from a cord blood sample.

Reagent, Supplies, and Equipment

- Disposable test tubes (10 × 75 mm)
- Disposable pipettes (4⅝-inch plastic or Pasteur)
- Normal saline (0.9%)
- Antiglobulin reagent antisera*
- Check cells (IgG-sensitized cells)*
- Test tube rack
- Centrifuge
- High-intensity lamp or optical magnifying lens
- Cell washer (optional)

---

*Should be refrigerated when not in use.

Quality Control

In addition to the daily reagent quality assessment check, each test must have a saline control run concurrently to rule out autoagglutination. Control check cells must be added to each test that does not exhibit agglutination. Agglutination of check cells verifies the reactivity of the AHG antiserum.

Procedure

1. Prepare a 2% suspension of the patient's RBCs.
2. Label one test tube as "DAT." Label a second test tube as "DAT Control."
3. Using a disposable pipette, add 1 drop of the RBC suspension to each tube.
4. Wash the contents of both tubes three times. If they are washed by hand, fill both tubes with saline, resuspend the RBCs, centrifuge at 3400 rpm for 30 seconds, and decant. Repeat three times. Be sure saline is completely decanted after the final wash.
   Note: Washing should be rapid to prevent elution of the antibody into the saline.
5. Add 2 drops of AHG reagent to the tube labeled DAT.
6. Add 2 drops of saline to the tube labeled DAT Control.
7. Resuspend RBCs complete in both tubes, and mix well.
8. Centrifuge at 3400 rpm for 15 seconds.
9. Gently resuspend RBCs, and examine macroscopically and microscopically for agglutination. Grade the reaction and record results. The DAT Control tube should demonstrate no agglutination (negative reaction).
   Note: Following addition, the test should be spun and read immediately.
10. Verify the AHG activity if the DAT tube demonstrated no agglutination:
    a. Add 1 drop of control check cells to the DAT tube.
    b. Centrifuge at 3400 rpm for 15 seconds.
    c. Gently resuspend RBCs, and examine macroscopically and microscopically for agglutination.
    d. Agglutination must be present. If agglutination is not present, the test is invalid and must be repeated.

Reporting Results

Negative test: Absence of agglutination in DAT test tube.
Positive test: Presence of agglutination.

Sources of Error

False-positive results in the DAT can be caused by:
- Contamination of AHG antisera or supplies.
- Overcentrifugation.
- Bacterial contamination of specimen or reagents.
- Fibrin clot in cell suspension.
- Overzealous reading of serum-cell mixture.

False-negative results usually results from technical error. Common causes of false-negative reactions include:
- Failure to add AHG reagent.
- Inadequate washing of RBCs.
- Weak or inactive AHG.

Reference

Turgeon ML: *Fundamentals of immunohematology*, ed 2, Philadelphia, 1995, Williams & Wilkins, pp 354-356.

CASE STUDY

Mr. R.M., a 60-year-old Caucasian, was stung by a bee while gardening. He had been stung once before earlier in the summer. Within a few seconds, his hand began to itch, and he began to experience abdominal cramping. He subsequently had difficulty breathing. Fortunately, he was able to reach a first-aid kit in his garage. Inside the kit was an EpiPen (injectable epinephrine) for his wife because she was allergic to bee venom. He used the pen and began to feel somewhat better. He immediately had his wife drive him to the hospital.

He was asymptomatic on arrival at the hospital. R.M. had no history of adverse reactions to bee venom or antibiotics. Because of the nature of the incident, a diagnosis of anaphylactic shock caused by bee venom sensitivity was made. An IgE level was ordered. The results indicated a level more than twice the (normal) reference range value. In addition, a follow-up skin test was performed. The patient was extremely positive for bee venom.

Questions and Discussion

1. What is the mechanism involved in anaphylaxis?

The term *anaphylaxis* is used to describe a systemic clinical syndrome caused by IgE-mediated degranulation of tissue basophils (mast cells) and peripheral blood basophils. Susceptible individuals exposed to a sensitizing antigen produce specific IgE antibodies that bind to high-affinity IgE receptors found on mast cells and basophils. The receptor binds the Fc portion of the antibody, leaving the Fab binding sites available to interact with antigen. The avidity of this Fc binding reaction is high; the dissociation of IgE from the receptors is slow. If a repeat exposure occurs, the antigen is bound by the IgE receptor complexes, which causes receptor-mediated activation of the cells with release of mediators. The rapid release of massive amounts of mediators is responsible for the clinical manifestations of anaphylaxis.

2. What types of agents can induce anaphylactic shock?

The IgE-mediated mast cell degranulation can be triggered by a variety of agents: antibiotics (e.g., penicillins, cephalosporins), pharmacologic agents (e.g., streptokinase, vaccines), foods (e.g., peanuts, shellfish), and foreign proteins (e.g., latex, bee venom).

Mast cell degranulation can also occur by IgE-independent pathways. In this situation, prior exposure is not a prerequisite because specific IgE antibodies are not involved. Three putative mechanisms of anaphylactoid reactions are blood, blood products, and immunoglobulins; certain therapeutic and diagnostic agents; and reaction to nonsteroidal antiinflammatory drugs (NSAIDs).

Blood, blood products, and immunoglobulins can cause an anaphylactoid reaction because of the formation of immune complexes with subsequent complement activation

and production of C3a and C5a. C3a and C5a are capable of degranulating mast cells directly and increase vasopermeability, which can induce hypotension and shock.

Certain therapeutic and diagnostic agents (e.g., opiates, muscle relaxants, radiographic contrast media) are also capable of directly causing mast cell degranulation and anaphylaxis.

Reaction to NSAIDs (e.g., aspirin) can be observed in a minority (5%-10%) of patients with asthma. The ability of these agents to cause anaphylaxis appears to correlate with their unknown mode of action in inhibiting prostaglandin synthesis.

Diagnosis

Type I hypersensitivity reaction.

CASE STUDY

Mrs. C.C., a 35-year-old gravida 4 para 1+2, was seen by her gynecologist when she was 8 weeks pregnant. Her first pregnancy 4 years ago was unremarkable. The patient reported that her second and third pregnancies had resulted in a stillbirth at 36 weeks and a spontaneous abortion at 10 weeks of gestation. Her medical history revealed no history of blood transfusions. She remembered being vaccinated for rubella. Her medical records had been destroyed in a fire at the clinic. Repeat blood grouping and Rh testing and an irregular antibody screen were ordered (see Box 26-3).

Mrs. C.C. returned in 2 weeks for a repeat anti-D titer. The titer had risen to 1:16. At 17 weeks' gestation an amniocentesis was performed. Severe hemolysis was demonstrated, and an intrauterine transfusion of the fetus was carried out using fresh, washed, cytomegalovirus screening test–negative, group O, Rh (D)–negative blood. Because of the continuing risk to the fetus, a cesarean section was performed at 36 weeks' gestation. On delivery the baby was noted to be jaundiced and pale. The first of three exchange transfusions was performed. Phototherapy was also used to degrade the bilirubin deposited in the skin. The baby made an uneventful recovery with no signs of kernicterus and was discharged from the hospital 5 days after birth.

Questions and Discussion

1. What is the mechanism of hemolytic disease of the newborn (HDN)?

Destruction of fetal RBCs can occur when maternal IgG specific for antigens on the baby's RBCs cross the placental barrier. The cells become coated by the antibody in vivo and

Box 26-3	Case Study Laboratory Results	
Mrs. C.C.	Group A; Rh (D) negative	Irregular antibody screen: positive anti-D (1:8)
Mr. C.C.	Group A; Rh (D) positive	(CDe/CDe)

are destroyed by the fetal phagocytic system. Unborn babies can die in utero, or live-born babies can present with symptoms of anemia, jaundice, or cardiac failure at birth.

Before the availability of prophylactic therapy for Rh disease caused by the D antigen, most severe cases of HDN were attributable to the D antigen of the Rh blood group system. The mother lacks the D antigen; the baby possesses the D antigen. Initial maternal exposure to fetal RBCs causes a primary IgM antibody response, which often results from transplacental hemorrhage at birth. The first child is not usually affected. Subsequent Rh (D)–positive children are at risk from the antibodies because they are of the IgG class and thus cross the placenta freely.

Many D-negative mothers do not become sensitized to the D antigen of the fetus because of maternal-fetal ABO incompatibility. The most common examples occur if the mother is group O and the baby is group A. If such an incompatibility exists, fetal RBCs entering the maternal circulation will be coated with the mother's isoantibody and destroyed before they have a chance to provoke a D-antigen–specific antibody response. Many cases of ABO incompatibility occur with group O mothers who have an increased incidence of IgG anti-B and anti-A antibodies. Most infants with ABO HDN are mildly affected. Phototherapy normally resolves the jaundice, with less than 0.05% of babies requiring exchange transfusions.

2. What prophylactic measures are used to prevent HDN caused by the D antigen?

Anti-D antibodies are administered to eligible Rh (D)–negative women immediately after birth of an Rh (D)–positive child. The perceived prevention mechanism is that the injected antibody coats the baby's D-positive cells circulating in the mother's blood. The coated cells are removed by the mononuclear phagocyte system, and no immunologic exposure to the D antigen occurs.

Diagnosis

Type II hypersensitivity reaction.

CASE STUDY

Z.Z.'s medical history included frequent sore throats as a child. He had been treated with antibiotics, particularly penicillin. Eventually he developed a rash. He was told that he had developed an allergy to penicillin and that he should not have it again.

A decade later he developed a urinary tract infection. He was treated with an antibiotic, trimethoprim, for 8 days. A few days after completing the regimen, he developed a headache and some itchy bumps on his skin. The next day he had sore and swollen joints. His physician confirmed that the rash was urticaria. Z.Z. also had an elevated temperature and swollen glands in his neck. The diagnosis of a drug allergy was made. The patient was given antihistamines. If this medication failed to alleviate the symptoms, more aggressive steroid therapy would be pursued.

Z.Z.'s symptoms did not improve, and he was started on an oral corticosteroid, prednisone. Three weeks later, the patient returned to his physician. He was asymptomatic.

Questions and Discussion

1. What is the likely mechanism of this reaction?

The symptoms of rash, headache, and joint pain are the hallmarks of an allergic drug response. A delayed onset reflects the need for antigen to remain in the circulation for a prolonged period in order for a sufficient amount of antibody to be synthesized. Once an adequate titer of antibody has been produced, circulating antigen-antibody complexes are formed, which "precipitate" out in various target tissues. Wherever the complexes are located, complement can be fixed, and local damage can manifest as joint and skin inflammation. Anaphylatoxins (C3a and C5a) can directly release histamine from mast cells. This activity can lead to a confusing picture of a type III hypersensitivity reaction presenting clinically as anaphylactic shock.

2. What types of agents can lead to drug reactions?

A variety of drugs can cause reactions by activating effector pathways by nonimmunologic means. Opiates, for example, can cause the release of mediators from mast cells by direct action on the cell without the involvement of IgE. Other agents leading to drug reactions include x-ray contrast media, which activates the alternative pathway of complement and can produce anaphylatoxins (C3a and C5a) and lead to anaphylactic shock.

Drugs (e.g., aspirin, NSAIDs) alter arachidonic acid pathways and can produce anaphylactic shock.

Diagnosis

Type III hypersensitivity reaction.

CASE STUDY

A 19-year-old college student went to the Student Health Services because she had a slowly developing rash on both earlobes, the hands and wrist, and around her neck.

Her medical history revealed that she had eczema in childhood. During her early teens she had facial acne, for which she was given tetracycline. Physical examination revealed a rash of erythema and small blisters, with marked excoriation because of the itching. Her hands were red, scaly, and dry. The rash on her hands looked different than the eruptions on her neck and ears. A contact hypersensitivity was suspected.

Follow-up patch tests included a standard battery of agents: rubber, cosmetics, plant extracts, perfumes, nickel, and makeup. Strongly positive reactions for rubber and nickel were observed.

The student was advised to eliminate contact with rubber (e.g., rubber gloves) used at home or on the job. Her jewelry probably contained nickel and was believed to be the source of the irritation to her earlobes, neck, and wrists. She was advised to wear only nickel-free jewelry. A mild corticosteroid cream was prescribed for use until her symptoms disappeared.

Questions and Discussion

1. Why did the jewelry cause a rash?

A contact allergy is a classic example of type IV hypersensitivity. The reaction involves eczema where the external agent comes into contact with the skin. The most common causative agents are *haptens* (e.g., metals such as nickel, chemicals, poison ivy/oak). Topically applied drugs can also be a source of contact dermatitis.

Haptens are small molecules that are too small themselves to elicit an immunologic response. When these small molecules penetrate the epidermis, however, they form covalent bonds with body proteins and produce the immunogenic hapten-carrier complex.

2. What is the mechanism of type IV hypersensitivity involvement in contact eczema?

There are two main phases of a contact hypersensitivity reaction:

- *Sensitization* is the first phase and can take up to 2 weeks. During this stage the hapten has combined with the carrier protein and has been processed by Langerhans cells in the epidermis. These cells migrate to the paracortical area of the draining lymph node, where MHC class II molecules present the antigen to CD4+ lymphocytes, leading to clonal expansion.
- *Elicitation* is the phase that involves the Langerhans cells. After application of the contact agent to the skin, the resident population of Langerhans cells in the epidermis decreases. Presentation of the antigen occurs in the skin and local lymph node with the release of cytokines from many types of cells. There is also evidence of mast cell degranulation after contact with the allergen. This leads not only to mediator release but to further production of cytokines as well. Tumor necrosis factor alpha and interleukin-1 induce adhesion molecules on endothelial cells, which produce the signal for mononuclear cell migration into the skin, peaking at 48 to 72 hours.

Diagnosis

Type IV hypersensitivity reaction.

CASE STUDY

A 35-year-old woman reported that she had experienced three bouts of urticaria of unknown origin about 10 years ago. The urticaria affected her mucous membranes and skin.

She experienced similar symptoms after repair of a fractured femur caused by a skiing accident. These symptoms were attributed to an antibiotic reaction.

As an emergency room nurse, she observed occasional localized hives following the use of latex gloves. Even when she used hypoallergenic latex gloves, she continued to have hives every few months. Increased urticaria, at times generalized, continued to occur.

Within 30 minutes of having a routine vaginal examination performed by a health care provider wearing latex gloves, she had an anaphylactic reaction that required resuscitation and hospitalization. One week later, a vaginal biopsy required a latex-free environment for her safety.

A short time later, she was forced to retire from nursing because of symptoms of asthma. She has also developed food allergies to shellfish.

Questions and Discussion

1. What are the most likely type and mechanism of the urticarial hypersensitivity reaction?

Patients can experience either irritant contact dermatitis (nonimmune) or allergic contact dermatitis (type IV hypersensitivity).

Irritant contact dermatitis (nonimmune) has a gradual onset over days. This type of reaction can be caused by hand-washing, occlusion, antiseptics, and glove chemicals. The symptoms include redness, cracks, fissures, and scaling.

With *allergic contact dermatitis,* or type IV (delayed-type) hypersensitivity, the onset of symptoms occurs 6 to 48 hours after contact. Symptoms include erythema, vesicles, papules, pruritus, and blisters.

2. What are the most likely type and cause of the anaphylactic reaction?

Immediate hypersensitivity, or type I reactions, can occur within minutes, rarely longer than 2 hours, after exposure to latex. Direct skin contact with latex may cause a type I, IgE-mediated reaction within 30 to 60 minutes of exposure. Urticaria may be local or generalized, and the spectrum of progression is notably unpredictable; some persons have experienced anaphylactic reactions after minimal or no previous symptoms.

Symptoms include local and generalized urticaria, feeling of faintness, feeling of impending doom, angioedema, nausea, vomiting, abdominal cramps, rhinoconjunctivitis, bronchospasm, and anaphylactic shock.

Diagnosis

Type I hypersensitivity reaction to latex.

CHAPTER HIGHLIGHTS

- The term *immunization,* or *sensitization,* is used to describe an immunologic reaction dependent on the response of the host to a subsequent exposure of antigen.
- Hypersensitivity has traditionally been classified as *immediate* and *delayed* based on time after exposure to an offending antigen.
- Type I hypersensitivity reactions can range from life-threatening anaphylactic reactions to milder manifestations associated with food allergies. This reaction is usually mediated by IgE antibody.
- In vitro evaluation of type I hypersensitivity reactions involves various methods. The advantages of in vitro testing include no risk of a systemic hypersensitivity reaction and no dependence on skin reactivity influenced by drugs, disease, or age.
- Type II cytotoxic reactions are characterized by the interaction of IgG or IgM antibody to cell-bound antigen.

This binding of an antigen and antibody can result in activation of complement and destruction of the cell (cytolysis) to which the antigen is bound. Erythrocytes, leukocytes, and platelets can be lysed by this process.

- Examples of type III reactions include the Arthus reaction, serum sickness, and certain aspects of autoimmune disease.
- Type IV cell-mediated immunity consists of immune activities that differ from antibody-mediated immunity. Cell-mediated immunity is moderated by the link between T lymphocytes and phagocytic cells and is responsible for contact sensitivity, delayed hypersensitivity, immunity to viral and fungal antigens, immunity to intracellular organisms, rejection of foreign tissue grafts, elimination of tumor cells bearing neoantigens, and formation of chronic granulomas.

REVIEW QUESTIONS

Questions 1-4. Match the following types of hypersensitivity with their respective type of reaction.

1. _____ Type I hypersensitivity
2. _____ Type II hypersensitivity
3. _____ Type III hypersensitivity
4. _____ Type IV hypersensitivity

   a. Cytotoxic reaction
   b. Cell-mediated reaction
   c. Immune complex reaction
   d. Anaphylactic reaction

5. With which cell type are anaphylactic reactions associated?
   a. T lymphocyte
   b. B lymphocyte
   c. Monocyte
   d. Mast

6. Type III reactions are exemplified by all the following *except:*
   a. Arthus reaction.
   b. Serum sickness.
   c. Glomerulonephritis.
   d. Shingles.

7. Type IV reactions are responsible for all the following *except:*
   a. Contact sensitivity.
   b. Delayed hypersensitivity.
   c. Immunity to viral and fungal antigens.
   d. Immunity to bacteria.

8. Type I hypersensitivity reactions can be associated with:
   a. Food allergies.
   b. Hay fever.
   c. Asthma.
   d. All the above.

9. The most common agents that cause anaphylactic reactions are:
   a. Drugs and food.
   b. Drugs and insect stings.
   c. Poison ivy and insect stings.
   d. Food and insect stings.

Questions 10-12. Arrange the sequence of events in anaphylaxis in the proper sequence.

10. _____ a. The effects of mediator release produce vascular changes; activation of platelets, eosinophils, and neutrophils; and activation of the coagulation cascade.
11. _____ b. The offending antigen attaches to the IgE antibody fixed to the surface membrane of mast cells and basophils.
12. _____ c. Activated mast cells and basophils release various mediators.

Questions 13-18. Complete the table, choosing from the possible answers provided.

Mediators of Anaphylaxis

Mediator	Primary Action
Histamine	13. _____
Leukotrienes	14. _____
Serotonin	15. _____
Platelet-activating factor	16. _____
Eosinophil chemotactic factors of anaphylaxis	17. _____
Prostaglandins	18. _____

Possible answers to questions 13-15
   a. Enhances the effects of histamine on target organs.
   b. Increases vascular permeability and promotes contraction of smooth muscle.
   c. Generates kinins.
   d. Contracts smooth muscle.

Possible answers to questions 16-18
   a. Affects smooth muscle tone and vascular permeability.
   b. Enhances the release of histamine and serotonin.
   c. Attracts cells to area of activity; these cells release secondary mediators that may limit the effects of primary mediators.
   d. Alters bronchial smooth muscle.

19. In vitro evaluation of type I hypersensitivity reactions can include:
    a. RIST.
    b. Skin testing.
    c. Neither a nor b.
    d. Both a and b.

20. Cytotoxic reactions are characterized by interaction of:
    a. IgG to soluble antigen.
    b. IgG to cell-bound antigen.
    c. IgM to soluble antigen.
    d. IgM or IgG to cell-bound antigen.

21. An example of a delayed nonhemolytic (type II hypersensitivity) reaction is:
    a. Febrile reaction.
    b. Graft-versus-host disease.
    c. Urticaria.
    d. Congestive heart failure.

22. Under normal conditions, immune complexes protect the host because they:
    a. Facilitate the clearance of various antigens.
    b. Facilitate the clearance of invading microorganisms.
    c. Interact with complement.
    d. Both a and b.

27. Immune complexes can:
    a. Suppress or augment the immune response by interacting with T and B cells.
    b. Inhibit tumor cell destruction.
    c. Be deposited in blood vessel walls.
    d. All the above.

24. The general anatomic sites of antigen-antibody interaction are:
    a. Tissues with a large filtration area.
    b. Interstitial fluids.
    c. Cell surface membranes or fixed intercellular structures.
    d. All the above.

25. Type IV hypersensitivity reactions are responsible for all the following *except:*
    a. Contact sensitivity.
    b. Elimination of tumor cells.
    c. Rejection of foreign tissue grafts.
    d. Serum sickness.

BIBLIOGRAPHY

Altman LC, editor: *Clinical allergy and immunology,* Boston, 1984, GK Hall.
American Latex Allergy Association: Latex allergy statistics, www.latexallergyresources.org, November 2006.
Anderson DC, Stiehm R: Immunization, *JAMA* 268(20):2959-2963, 1992.
Bach J: The effect of infections on susceptibility to autoimmune and allergic diseases, *N Engl J Med* 347(12):911-920, 2002.
Bochner BS, Lichtenstein LM: Anaphylaxis, *N Engl J Med* 324(25):1785-1790, 1991.
Choo-Kang LR: Specific IgE testing: objective laboratory evidence supports allergy diagnosis and treatment, *Med Lab Observer MLO* 38(3)10-14, 2006.
Choo-Kang LR: The progression of allergic disease, *Med Lab Observer MLO* 38(3):18, 2006.
Creticos PS et al: Immunotherapy with a ragweed–toll-like receptor 9 agonist vaccine for allergic rhinitis, *N Engl J Med* 355(14):1445-1454, 2006.
Faix JD et al: Multiplexed chemiluminescent immunoassay of specific IgE antibody for in vitro diagnosis of allergic disorders, AACC Annual Meeting, July 2006 (abstract).
Fu P, Zic V: Specific IgE assay on the ImmunoLite 2000 analyzer, AACC Annual Meeting, July 2004 (abstract).
Gardner P, Schaffner W: Immunization of adults, *N Engl J Med* 328(17):1252-1258, 1993.
Gold DR, Fuhlbrigge AL: Inhaled corticosteroids for young children with wheezing, *N Engl J Med* 354(19):2058-2062, 2006.
Homburger HA: The laboratory evaluation of allergic diseases. Part I, *Lab Med* 22(11):780-782, 1991.
Homburger HA: The laboratory evaluation of allergic diseases. Part II, *Lab Med* 22(12):845-848, 1991.
Ishizaka K: Regulation of IgE biosynthesis, *Hosp Pract* 20:53-41, 1989.
Kaitin KI: Graft-versus-host disease, *N Engl J Med* 325(5):357-358, 1991.
Kay AB: Allergy and allergic disease, *N Engl J Med* 344(1-2):30-38, 109-113, 2001.
Kay AB: Natural killer T cells and asthma, *N Engl J Med* 354(11):1186-1188, 2006.
Kirchner DB: The spectrum of allergic disease in the chemical industry, *Int Arch Occup Environ Health* 75(suppl):107-112, 2002.
Lundin P: Evaluation of technical performance of four immunoassay systems for allergy testing: ImmunoCAP 1000, ImmunoCAP 250, Advia Centaur, and Immulite 2000, AACC Annual Meeting, July 2005 (abstract).
Mardis CT, Bal T, Levy R: The masks of allergy undone by IVT, *Med Lab Observer MLO* 39(6):12-21, 2007.
Nairn R, Helber M: *Immunology for medical students,* ed 2, St Louis, 2007, Mosby.
Nystrand M et al: A multiplexed immunoassay for rapid detection of specific IgE in allergy diagnosis, www.gesim.de, July 2007.
Ollert M et al: Allergen-specific IgE measured by a continuous random-access immunoanalyzer: interassay comparison and agreement with skin testing, *Clin Chem* 51(7):1241-1249, 2005.
Peter G: Childhood immunizations, *N Engl J Med* 327(25):1794-1800, 1992.
Quest Diagnostics: ImmunoCap: specific IgE blood test, www.questdiagnostics.com, November 2006.
Reedy S: Latex allergy, *Am Fam Physician* 57(1):1-14, 1998. www.aafp.org.
Sussman GL, Tarlo S, Dolovich J: The spectrum of IgE-mediated responses to latex, *JAMA* 265(21):2844-2847, 1991.
Tepnel Biosystems: How long before you discover a better way to test? November 2006.
Tschopp CM et al: Granzyme B, a novel mediator of allergic inflammation: its induction and release in blood basophils and human asthma, *Blood* 108(7):2290-2298, 2006.
Turgeon ML: *Fundamentals of immunohematology,* ed 2, Baltimore, 1995, Williams & Wilkins.
US Department of Health and Human Services: Radioallergosorbent test (RAST) methods for allergen-specific immunoglobulin E (IgE): final guidance for industry and FDA, August 2001.
Valentine MD: Anaphylaxis and stinging insect hypersensitivity, *JAMA* 268(20):2830-2833, 1992.
Walker RH: *AABB technical manual,* ed 11, Bethesda, Md, 1993, American Association of Blood Banks.

CHAPTER 27

Immunoproliferative Disorders

General Characteristics of Monoclonal Gammopathies
General Characteristics of Polyclonal Gammopathies
Multiple Myeloma
    Etiology
    Pathophysiology
    Epidemiology
    Signs and Symptoms
    Immunologic Manifestations
    Diagnostic Evaluation
    Prognosis
    Treatment
Waldenström's Primary Macroglobulinemia
    Etiology
    Epidemiology
    Signs and Symptoms

    Immunologic Manifestations
    Diagnostic Evaluation
    Treatment
Other Monoclonal Disorders
    Monoclonal Gammopathy of Undetermined
      Significance
    Light-Chain Disease
    Heavy-Chain Disease
    Gammopathies with More Than One Band
Bence Jones Protein Screening Procedure
Case Study
Chapter Highlights
Review Questions
Bibliography

Learning Objectives

At the conclusion of this chapter, the reader should be able to:

- Compare the general characteristics of monoclonal and polyclonal gammopathies.
- Describe and compare the etiology, epidemiology, signs and symptoms, immunologic manifestations, diagnostic evaluation, and treatment of multiple myeloma and Waldenström's primary macroglobulinemia.

- Explain and contrast the characteristics of other monoclonal disorders, such as monoclonal gammopathy of unknown significance.
- Analyze a representative case study.

A small number of long-lived plasma cells in the bone marrow (<1% of mononuclear cells) produce most of immunoglobulins G and A (IgG and IgA) in normal adult serum. These well-differentiated cells do not divide and have a characteristic phenotype: CD38^{bright}, syndecan-1^{bright}, CD19+, and CD56$^{weak/-}$. Their precursors are slowly proliferating **plasmablasts,** which migrate to the marrow from lymph nodes after stimulation by antigens and cytokines from helper T (Th) cells in the germinal centers. Events in germinal centers initiate somatic mutations of the immunoglobulin genes of B cells and a switch from the production of immunoglobulin M (IgM) to production of IgG or IgA. After the activated B cells enter the bone marrow, they stop proliferating and differentiate into plasma cells, under the influence of adhesion molecules and factors such as interleukin-6. Normal plasma cells die by **apoptosis** after several weeks or months.

Hypergammaglobulinemias are either monoclonal or polyclonal in nature. A **monoclonal gammopathy,** which can be either a benign or a malignant condition, results from a single clone of lymphoid-plasma cells producing elevated levels of a single class and type of immunoglobulin, referred to as a **monoclonal protein, M protein,** or **paraprotein.** Disorders in this category of plasma cell dyscrasias include

multiple myeloma (MM), Waldenström's macroglobulinemia (WM), monoclonal gammopathy of undetermined significance (MGUS), light-chain deposition disease, and heavy-chain diseases. In comparison, a **polyclonal gammopathy** is classified as a secondary disease and characterized by the elevation of two or more immunoglobulins by several clones of plasma cells.

GENERAL CHARACTERISTICS OF MONOCLONAL GAMMOPATHIES

Monoclonal gammopathies are characterized by the production of monoclonal immunoglobulin and are associated with suppressed, uninvolved immunoglobulins and dysfunctional T-cell responses.

Although MM is the prototypic monoclonal gammopathy, the most common plasma cell disorder is the premalignant precursor of myeloma, MGUS.

Serum and urine electrophoresis and other immunoglobulin assays can demonstrate strikingly abnormal results in disorders such as MM and WM. The gamma region of the electrophoretic pattern can show a dense, highly restricted band from uncontrolled proliferation of one cell clone, whereas the other, normal immunoglobulins are deficient.

Clinical interpretation of some patterns can be difficult. In contrast, some symptomatic patients do not exhibit the characteristic monoclonal band or spike in their serum protein patterns. This is often the case with **light-chain disease (LCD),** where only kappa (κ) or lambda (λ) monoclonal light chains are synthesized by the clone. These low-molecular-weight immunoglobulin fragments are filtered through the glomerulus and into the urine, producing a serum electrophoretic pattern that suggests hypogammaglobulinemia, with either a very faint monoclonal band or no band at all. These light chains also suggest the presence of a nonsecretory clone, which produces no monoclonal immunoglobulins and frequently demonstrates hypogammaglobulinemia because of the inhibition of normal clones.

GENERAL CHARACTERISTICS OF POLYCLONAL GAMMOPATHIES

A polyclonal gammopathy is a common protein abnormality. It is defined as an increase in more than one immunoglobulin and involves several clones of plasma cells. In contrast to a monoclonal protein, a polyclonal protein consists of one or more heavy-chain classes and both light-chain types. Polyclonal increases are exhibited as secondary manifestations of infection or inflammation. They are often seen in chronic infections; chronic liver disease, especially chronic active hepatitis; rheumatoid connective tissue (autoimmune) diseases; and lymphoproliferative disorders.

A polyclonal protein is characterized by a broad peak or band, usually of gamma mobility, on electrophoresis; by a thickening and elongation of all heavy-chain and light-chain arcs on immunoelectrophoresis; and by the absence of a localized band on immunofixation. A polyclonal gammopathy therefore resembles a normal pattern, with the serum staining more intensely. A selective polyclonal increase is of special interest because only one class of immunoglobulin is significantly elevated; however, the increase is polyclonal because immunoglobulin is produced by several clones of plasma cells, and both kappa and lambda types are produced. Quantitation by specific assay procedures of the immunoglobulins demonstrates which immunoglobulin is increased. Immunofixation is not recommended in cases of polyclonal gammopathy because it presents no additional information.

MULTIPLE MYELOMA

Multiple myeloma is a plasma cell neoplasm characterized by the accumulation of malignant plasma cells within the bone marrow. Normal bone marrow has about 1% plasma cells, but in MM the plasma cell concentration can rise to 90%. Bone marrow identification of monoclonal plasma cells by histology is an essential part of MM diagnosis and is frequently based on identifying intracellular κ and λ using direct immunofluorescent techniques.

Plasma cells produce one of five heavy-chain types together with κ and λ molecules. There is approximately 40%

excess production of free light chain over heavy-chain synthesis, to allow proper conformation of the intact immunoglobulin molecules.

Etiology

The cause of MM is unknown. Radiation may be a factor in some cases, and a viral cause has been suggested. Other factors may include environmental stimulants, such as exposure to asbestos, benzene, or industrial toxins. The likelihood of a genetic factor in some cases is supported by well-documented reports of familial clusters with MM.

Pathophysiology

In contrast to normal plasma cells, myeloma cells are often immature and may have the appearance of plasmablasts. These cells usually are CD19-CD56[bright], CD38, and syndecan-1, and they produce very low amounts of immunoglobulins.

Most patients demonstrate complex karyotype abnormalities with chromosomal gains, deletions, and translocations, some of which are identical to those observed in certain B-cell lymphomas. Many numerical and structural abnormalities occur, mainly on chromosomes 13 (13q−) and 14 (14q+). These genetic abnormalities may prevent the differentiation and apoptosis of myeloma cells, which continue to proliferate and accumulate in the bone marrow. Chromosomal aberrations are of sufficient number to be detected on flow analysis of DNA content, which is aneuploid in about 80% of patients.

Most patients exhibit a slight nuclear DNA excess of 5% to 10%; hypoploidy is observed in only 5% to 10% of patients and is strongly associated with resistance to standard chemotherapy. Deletions of chromosomes 13 and 17 have been observed. The morphologic immaturity, hypodiploidy, and 13q− and 14q+ abnormalities correlate with the resistance to treatment and short survival that are characteristic of aggressive disease.

The somatic mutations of the immunoglobulin genes of myeloma cells indicate that the putative myeloma cell precursors are stimulated by antigens and are either memory B cells or migrating plasmablasts.

Myeloma cells proliferate slowly in the marrow (Figure 27-1 and Table 27-1). Less than 1% divide at any one time, and myeloma cells do not differentiate. The absolute number of these cells correlates with disease activity and predicts the progression of disease in **smoldering multiple myeloma.** Circulating myeloma cells may disseminate the tumor within the bone marrow and elsewhere.

Interleukin-6 (IL-6) is essential for the survival and growth of myeloma cells, which express specific receptors for this cytokine. Initially identified as a growth factor for myeloma cells, IL-6 was recently shown to promote the survival of myeloma cells by preventing spontaneous or dexamethasone-induced apoptosis. An increased level of IL-6 in the serum of patients with MM can be explained by the overproduction of IL-6 in the marrow. The IL-6 system also has a role in the pathogenesis of bone lesions in MM. IL-6, solu-

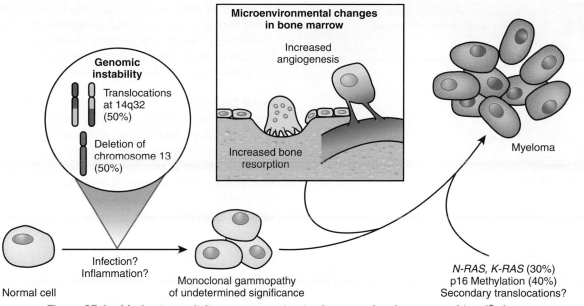

Figure 27-1 Mechanisms of disease progression in the monoclonal gammopathies. *(Redrawn from Kyle RA, Rajkumar SV: N Engl J Med 351(18):1860-1871, 2004.)*

Table 27-1	Three Phases of Disease Progression in Multiple Myeloma		
Variable	**Initial Phase**	**Medullary Relapse**	**Extramedullary Relapse**
Site of myeloma-cell accumulation or proliferation	Bone marrow	Bone marrow	Blood, pleural effusion, skin, many other sites
Growth fraction*	<1%	≥1% (1%-95%)	≥1% (1%-95%)
Genetic or oncogenic events	Deregulation of *c-myc* Illegitimate switch recombinations	N-*ras* and K-*ras* point mutations	p53 point mutations
Phenotypic changes	CD19 loss CD56 overexpression	CD28 expression LFA-1 and VLA-5 loss	CD28 expression CD56 loss
Cytologic changes	Detectable plasmablastic compartment in 15% of cases	Plasmablastic compartment growing	Major plasmablastic compartment
Circulating malignant plasma cells	<1%	Increasing	Increasing

From Bataille R, Harousseau JL: Medical progress: multiple myeloma, *N Engl J Med* 336(23):1657, 1997.
*Growth fraction is the rate of atypical cells proliferating in the bone marrow.

ble IL-6 receptor alpha (sIL-6Rα), and interleukin-1 beta (IL-1β) activate osteoclasts in the vicinity of myeloma cells and thus initiate bone resorption. IL-6 may account for MM-associated anemia and for the lack of thrombocytopenia because of its stimulation of megakaryopoiesis.

Epidemiology

Multiple myeloma is the most common form of dysproteinemia. It accounts for 1% of all types of malignant diseases and 10% of hematologic malignancies. The general incidence is estimated to be 4 cases per 100,000 population per year in the United States. About 10,000 Americans die each year from MM.

Onset of MM is between ages 40 and 70 years, with a peak incidence in the seventh decade. It is uncommon (<2% of cases) in patients less than 40 years old. In general, patients with LCD and with IgD myeloma are younger than those with IgG or IgA myeloma and have a poorer prognosis because of their high incidence of nephropathy. Males are af-

fected in approximately 62% of cases; the male/female ratio is 1.6:1. In addition, African Americans are affected twice as often as Caucasians.

Immunoglobulin G myeloma is the most common form of MM (Table 27-2). Four subtypes of IgG heavy chains are known to exist among patients with IgG myeloma. Cases of IgG myeloma are distributed as follows: 65% are gamma G1, 23% gamma G2, 8% gamma G3, and 4% gamma G4 subclass. The only subclass-dependent difference is the greater propensity for patients with IgG3 myeloma to experience hyperviscosity syndrome, similar to the manifestation in WM.

Multiple myeloma runs a progressive course, with most patients dying within 1 to 3 years. The beta-2 microglobulin level at initial evaluation has been adopted as a predictor of outcome. If the serum β_2-microglobulin level is elevated at the start of therapy, the prognosis is less favorable. The major causes of death are overwhelming infection (sepsis) and renal insufficiency. In patients with sepsis, mortality exceeds 50% despite antibiotic therapy.

Table 27-2	Distribution of Immunoglobulin Types in Patients with Multiple Myeloma
Type of Protein	Multiple Myeloma (%)
IgM	12
IgG	52
IgA	22
IgD	2
IgE	Rare
Light chains (kappa or lambda)	11
Heavy chains	Rare
Monoclonal proteins	<1
Nonsecretory myeloma	1

Signs and Symptoms

The signs and symptoms of MM include bone pain, typically in the back or chest, and weakness, fatigue, and pallor associated with anemia or abnormal bleeding. In all, 20% of patients exhibit hepatomegaly and 5% demonstrate splenomegaly. In some cases the major manifestations of disease result from acute infection, renal insufficiency, hypercalcemia, or amyloidosis. Weight loss and night sweats are not prominent until the disease is advanced. Bone pain, anemia, and renal insufficiency constitute a triad of signs and symptoms strongly suggestive of MM.

In 1975 a staging system for myeloma was developed. This system defines "indolent" versus "severe" disease and determines a basis for therapy. Patients are divided into three groups, with classification based on production of IgG by plasma cells and the total quantity of IgG in the body. The number of abnormal plasma cells is correlated with hemoglobin, serum calcium, serum IgG peak, and the presence or absence of lytic bone lesions. Renal function is also considered an important factor, not only because it is essential to survival, but also because IgG light chains can damage the kidneys.

Some physicians use a simpler system of staging based on serum albumin, hemoglobin, and β_2-microglobulin.

Skeletal Abnormalities

About 90% of patients with MM have broadly disseminated destruction of the skeleton, which is responsible for the predominance of bone pain. These abnormalities consist of punched-out lytic areas (Figure 27-2), osteoporosis, and fractures in about 80% of patients. The vertebrae, skull, thoracic cage, pelvis, and proximal humeri and femurs are the most frequent sites of involvement.

Hematologic Features

Diagnosis of MM depends on the demonstration of an increased number of plasma cells in a bone marrow aspirate and/or biopsy and supporting laboratory results (see Diagnostic Evaluation). Although the bone marrow is typically involved, the disorder may involve other tissues. For example, a positive correlation exists between the production of osteoclast-activating factor by bone marrow cells and the

extent of skeletal destruction. Other hematologic factors contributing to the signs and symptoms of pallor and anemia include bleeding, qualitative platelet abnormalities, inhibition of coagulation factors by M protein, and thrombocytopenia. Intravascular coagulation may occur.

Renal Disorders

Acute renal failure (ARF) occurs in about 5% to 10% of patients. Although ARF may occur at any time in the course of myeloma, it can be the initial manifestation of disease. ARF has been observed after infection, hypercalcemia, dehydration, and intravenous urography. Serum creatinine levels are elevated in about half these patients, and approximately one third have hypercalcemia.

Chronic renal failure is a common development in MM patients. As many as two thirds of patients display serum creatinine levels greater than 1.5 mg/dL, and 10% to 20% may develop end-stage renal disease (ESRD). Patients with IgD or light-chain myeloma are much more likely to develop renal failure than those with IgG or IgA myeloma. Proteinuria is a common finding, with over half of all MM patients excreting abnormal amounts of **Bence Jones (BJ) protein** (light chains). Patients with BJ proteinuria are much more likely to have renal tubular defects than those without BJ proteinuria.

Studies suggest that BJ proteins have a deleterious effect on renal function through at least two mechanisms. First, renal failure may result from intratubular precipitation of BJ protein and subsequent intrarenal obstruction. When the distal collecting tubules become obstructed by large casts consisting mainly of BJ protein, the disorder may be referred to as "myeloma kidney." The second mechanism of renal failure may be a function of direct tubular cell injury. As a result of these tubular defects, abnormalities in urine concentrating ability and renal acidification are observed. Although the presence of a large concentration of BJ proteinuria is usually associated with some degree of renal dysfunction, some patients excrete large amounts of BJ protein for years and maintain renal function.

Lambda light chains have been implicated in nephrotoxicity, but their role has not been firmly established.

Neurologic Features

Pain is a common characteristic of MM, often caused by compression of the spinal cord or nerves. Compression produces back pain, with weakness or paralysis of the lower extremities and bowel or bladder incontinence.

Infectious Diseases

The most frequent cause of death is infection. Patients with MM have increased susceptibility to infectious microorganisms because of an inability to cope with bacterial infections and certain viral diseases. Increased susceptibility principally results from defective antibody synthesis caused by the crowding out and suppression of normal plasma cell precursors.

Repeated bouts of sepsis, often resulting from recurrent infection by microorganisms such as pneumococci or gram-

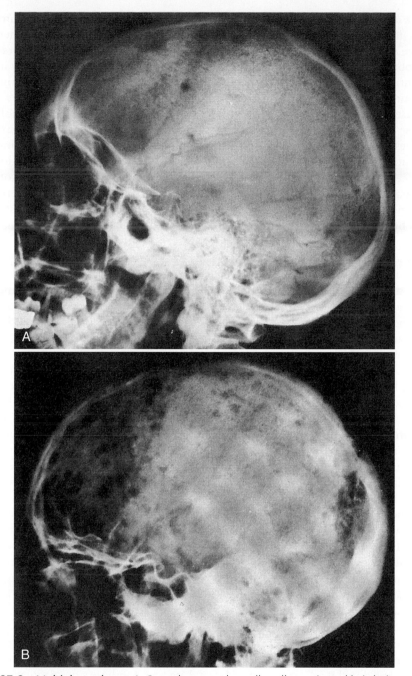

Figure 27-2   Multiple myeloma. A, Several scattered, small, well-marginated lytic lesions appear in calvarium, located in normally mineralized bone. Multiple lytic lesions can also be seen in the mandible. **B,** Multiple circumscribed lytic lesions crowd bones throughout skull. Lesions are still discrete, and margins of most are fairly sharp. *(From Newton TH, Potts DG:* Radiology of the skull and brain, *St Louis, 1971, Mosby.)*

negative bacteria, are common. Pneumonia, pyelonephritis, meningitis, and arthritis are the leading forms of sepsis; when bacteremia ensues, mortality is high.

Immunologic Manifestations

In approximately 20% of patients, multiple myeloma is diagnosed by chance in the absence of symptoms, usually after screening laboratory studies have revealed an increased serum protein concentration. MM cells express not only cytoplasmic immunoglobulins, the hallmark of plasma cells, but early B, T, natural killer (NK), myeloid, erythroid, and megakaryocytic cell markers as well. These phenotypic features are consistent with the hypothesis that MM may originate from a transformed early hematopoietic progenitor cell, which explains the occasional coexistence of MM and acute myelogenous leukemia (AML).

Patients with MM have defects in humoral but not cellular immunity. Humoral immunity is disrupted because plasma cell tumors induce suppression of antibody synthesis by normal immunoglobulin-secreting cells, and the production of antiidiotype antibodies declines proportionately. In addition, selective impairment occurs in the formation of normal antibodies because of increased immunoglobulin catabolism and the release of a protein that incites macrophages to suppress synthesis of normal immunoglobulins by myeloma cells. Depression of normal humoral immunity accounts for the high susceptibility of MM patients to bacterial infection. The normal functioning of cellular immunity is demonstrated by normal resistance to fungal and most viral infections and by normal delayed-type hypersensitivity to skin-testing antigens.

Initially, in vivo myeloma clones are subject to control by the immune network through specific idiotype-antiidiotype mechanisms. Each of the million or more potential immunoglobulin variants in every individual carries singular determinants of designated idiotypes. Antiidiotypic antibodies directed against autologous immunoglobulin are elicited during a normal immune response. The presumed mission of antiidiotypic antibodies is to help terminate the immune response by binding complementary idiotypes to form endogenous immune complexes that are removed from the circulation. The antiidiotypic antibodies in turn stimulate production of antibodies to antiidiotype, and so on, to create a modulating network that includes T cells, which recognize idiotype antigens through unique antigen receptors. Antiidiotype- and idiotype-sensitized T cells collaborate most efficiently during highly restricted responses, during which both antibodies and lymphocytes that specifically recognize the dominant idiotype are activated. These can either inhibit or enhance the response of lymphocytes to receptors expressing the idiotype. The overall net direction of the response is determined by the functional influence of T cells linked by antiidiotype receptor interactions to their molecular targets on B cells. In MM, idiotype expression is carried to an extreme. Monoclonal paraprotein secreted by plasma cell tumors induces many immunologic responses capable of acting in concert to contain or modulate tumor growth.

The earliest detectable monoclonal B cell, as identified by idiotypic structures of the myeloma protein, is the transitional form, bearing surface IgM, IgD, and IgG. This and the finding that precursor (early) B cells destined to become myeloma cells possess surface IgG (sIgG) indicate that the myeloma tumor clone includes memory B cells that can mature into plasma cells. Use of antiidiotypic antibodies in identifying IgA myeloma clones has revealed clonal expression at the pre-B state, a finding supported by the observation that B cells in the circulation of myeloma patients are clonally frozen at the pre-B stage. As maturing B-cell members of the malignant clone differentiate in the marrow, they lose IgD and IgM, in that order, accumulate sIgG, and finally shed sIg to become IgG-producing mature plasma cells, as programmed by the mutant precursor cell. Thus the mature myeloma cell contains abundant cytoplasmic (secretory) IgG but no sIgG. IgA myeloma cells proceed along the same normal differentiation scheme of B-cell maturation. Although MM-associated tumors disseminate widely, the disease is spread through release into the blood circulation of clonal precursors that show lymphoid rather than plasma cell morphology.

The most consistent immunologic feature of multiple myeloma is the incessant synthesis of a dysfunctional single monoclonal protein or of immunoglobulin chains of fragments, with concurrent suppression of the synthesis of normal functional antibody. In 99% of myeloma patients, an M component is usually found in serum, urine, or both. Different types of M components are associated with various clinical syndromes.

Diagnostic Evaluation

Hematologic Assessment

A normochromic, normocytic anemia is present in about two thirds of patients at diagnosis. In part, anemia is related to the hypervolemia caused by the increase in plasma volume because of monoclonal protein production. Rouleaux formation is a common finding on peripheral blood smears. The leukocyte count can be normal, although about one third of patients have leukopenia. Relative lymphocytosis is usually present. If lymphocyte subsets are examined, a reduction in CD4+ (helper) and an increase in CD8+ (suppressor/cytotoxic) blood lymphocytes can be noted. Defects in the proliferative responses of lymphocytes to mitogens or antigens are explained by the large portion of B cells in MM that originate from the malignant stem cell clone. Few mature plasma cells are seen in the circulation except at the terminal phase of the disease, but the covert presence of the malignant B-cell clone can be unmasked by the laboratory use of monoclonal antibodies (MAbs) or by transforming agents such as phorbol esters. In rare cases, in the terminal stages, plasmablasts and proplasmacytes may amount to 50% of the leukocytes in the peripheral blood.

Bleeding is common. Platelet abnormalities, impaired aggregation of platelets, and interference with platelet function by the abnormal monoclonal protein contribute to bleeding. Inhibitors of coagulation factors and thrombocytopenia from marrow infiltration of plasma cells or chemotherapy may also contribute to bleeding. Some patients have a tendency toward thrombosis, which may manifest as a shortened coagulation time, and increased fibrinogen and factor VIII.

Diagnosis of MM, however, depends on the demonstration of an increased number (>10%) of plasma cells in a bone marrow aspirate (Figure 27-3 and Plate 11) and/or biopsy and supporting laboratory results.

Bence Jones Proteins

Bence Jones protein has been an important diagnostic marker for MM for 160 years (see Bence Jones Protein Screening Procedure). In about 10% of MM patients, only BJ proteins are produced, with no complete IgM, IgG, or IgA.

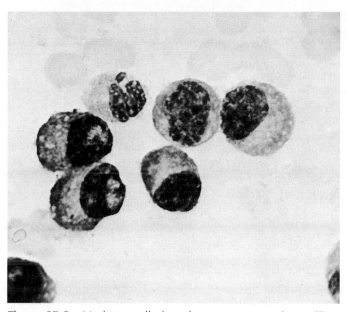

Figure 27-3 Myeloma cells in a bone marrow aspirate. *(From Bauer JD: Clinical laboratory methods, ed 9, St Louis, 1982, Mosby.)*

BJ proteins are single-peptide chains with a molecular weight of 20,000 or 22,000 daltons (D), but dimerization occurs spontaneously to form molecules of 40,000 or 44,000 D.

Bence Jones proteins are monoclonal κ or λ immunoglobulin free light chains (FLCs) not attached to the heavy chain portion of the immunoglobulin molecule. BJ proteins are seen in two types of syndromes, as follows:
- With a typical monoclonal gammopathy
- In free LCD

Serum concentrations of FLCs depend on the balance between production by plasma cells and their precursor and on renal clearance. If there is increased polyclonal immunoglobulin production and/or renal impairment, both κ and λ FLC concentrations can increase 30% to 40%. Serum FLC tests are assuming an increasing role in the detection and monitoring of monoclonal gammopathies. Serum FLCs have a short half-life in the blood (κ, 2-4 hours; λ, 3-6 hours), compared with 21 days for IgG molecules. FLC concentrations allow more rapid assessment of the effects of chemotherapy than does monoclonal IgG.

Very small amounts of BJ protein in serum can be associated with significant clinical problems, especially pathologic renal changes. FLCs filter through the glomeruli almost without obstruction because of their small molecular size and accumulate in the tubules. Renal impairment can result from the toxicity of FLCs. Pathologic changes can range from relatively benign tubular proteinuria to ARF or amyloidosis.

Bence Jones protein can be detected in serum, urine, or both. The level of monoclonal light chains in serum or urine is related to filtration, resorption, or catabolism of the protein by the kidneys. During the early stages of renal disease, when the kidneys are only mildly affected, excretion and reabsorption continue normally, but only partial catabolism occurs. At this point, BJ protein may be detected in the serum but not in the urine. Progressive renal involvement impairs reabsorption, and diminished reabsorption with decreased catabolism results in FLCs in both serum and urine. Later, as resorption is totally blocked, FLCs are present in urine only. In terminal stages of renal disease, uremia occurs, renal clearance is affected, and BJ protein again appears in the serum.

Bence Jones proteins are unusual in their response to heating. They are soluble at room temperature, become insoluble near 60° or 70° C, then resolubilize at 80° C. This pattern reverses when the temperature is lowered, which is unique to BJ protein.

Serologically, all BJ proteins are not identical, although κ and λ types exist. BJ proteins will react with antisera to the λ chains of IgG, and λ chains react with antisera to BJ protein.

Approximately 80% of patients with MM produce intact immunoglobulin monoclonal proteins, of which 46% have excess monoclonal FLCs in the urine by immunofixation electrophoresis. Serum protein electrophoresis is positive less often because of low serum concentrations of FLCs. From 3% to 4% of MM patients have nonsecretory disease. These patients have no detectable monoclonal proteins with serum and urine electrophoretic testing because their tumor cells produce small amounts of monoclonal protein. Their FLC concentrations are below the sensitivity of serum electrophoretic tests and below the threshold for clearance into the urine. These patients can be monitored by serum FLC tests rather than repeated bone marrow biopsies or whole-body scans.

Free Light Chains

Free light chains are incorporated into immunoglobulin molecules during B-lymphocyte development and are expressed initially on the surface of immature B cells. Production of FLCs occurs throughout the rest of B-cell development and in plasma cells, where secretion is highest. Tumors associated with the different stages of B-cell maturation will secrete monoclonal FLCs into the serum, where they may be detected by FLC immunoassays (Box 27-1 and Table 27-3).

Box 27-1	**Benefits of Serum FLC Immunoassays**

- Better sensitivity and precision than current electrophoretic assays.
- Numerical results for disease monitoring.
- Convenience of serum as a test medium.
- Identification of AL amyloidosis and NSMM patients who have detectable monoclonal proteins by conventional tests.
- More accurate marker of complete disease remission than existing assays.
- Short half-life marker for rapid assessment of treatment responses.
- Identification of progression risk in individuals with MGUS.
- Better screening of symptomatic patients.

From Bradwell AR: *Serum free light chain analysis,* Birmingham, UK, 2006, Binding Site, p 4.
FLC, Free light chain; *AL,* immunocyte derived; *NSMM,* nonsecretory multiple myeloma; *MGUS,* monoclonal gammopathy of undetermined significance.

Table 27-3	Assays for Free Light Chains (FLCs)	
Assay	Advantages	Disadvantages
Total urine protein	Simple, inexpensive, widely used.	Inadequate sensitivity for FLC detection.
Urine dipstick	Simple, inexpensive, widely used.	Inadequate sensitivity for FLC detection.
Serum protein electrophoresis	Simple, manual/semi-automated method.	Insensitive (<500-2,000mg/L).
	Well established, inexpensive.	Cannot detect FLCs at low concentration.
	Monoclonal bands observed.	Subjective interpretation of results.
	Quantitative results with scanning.	
Urine protein electrophoresis	Simple, manual/semi-automated method.	Subjective interpretation of results.
	Well established, inexpensive.	Urine may require concentration with possible protein loss
	Monoclonal bands observed.	False bands from concentrating urine.
	Sensitive in concentrated urine (10 mg/L).	Heavy proteinuria obscures results.
	Quantitative results with scanning.	Cumbersome 24-hour urine collection.
Immunofixation electrophoresis (IFE) on serum and urine	Well established.	Nonquantitative.
	Good sensitivity for serum and very sensitive for concentrated urine (5-30 mg/L).	Serum sensitivity (150-500 mg/L) inadequate for normal serum FLC levels.
		Rather laborious to perform.
		Visual interpretation may be difficult.
		Expensive use of antisera.
		Cannot be used to quantify monoclonal immunoglobulins because of precipitating antibody.
Capillary zone electrophoresis	Automated technology.	Less sensitive (400 mg/L) than IFE for serum FLCs.
	Quantitative.	Can fail to detect 5% of positive sample "false negative."
Total serum κ and λ assays	Automated immunoassay.	Not sensitive enough for routine testing.
		Specificity inadequate for detecting many patients with light-chain multiple myeloma.

Modified from Bradwell AR: *Serum free light chain analysis,* Birmingham, UK, 2006, Binding Site, pp 23, 47-52.

Production of FLCs in normal individuals is approximately 500 mg/day from bone marrow and lymph node cells. The molecules enter the blood and are readily partitioned between the intravascular and extravascular compartments. In normal individuals, serum FLCs are rapidly cleared and metabolized by the kidneys, depending on their molecular size.

Immunologic Testing

Traditionally, laboratories have detected the monoclonal immunoglobulins by protein electropheresis, which began in the 1930s, and have characterized the proteins by immunofixation electrophoresis (IFE), which was established in the 1980s.

Identification of κ and λ molecules has been accomplished with the use of antibodies specific for each type of protein. Immunodiffuison was initially used, followed by immunoelectrophoresis in 1953, radial immunodiffusion, and ultimately nephelometry and turbidimetry. Automated nephelometric assay described in 2001 represented a major breakthrough. This methodology allows for the quantitation of both κ free light chains and λ free light chains, and can be performed on automated instruments (e.g., Dade Behring, Beckman Coulter, Roche/Hitachi, Olympus) (see Chapter 13).

Each monoclonal protein (M protein or paraprotein) consists of two heavy-chain polypeptides of the same class and subclass and two light-chain polypeptides of the same type. The different monoclonal proteins are designated by capital letters corresponding to the class of their heavy chains,

which are designated by Greek letters: gamma (γ) in IgG, alpha (α) in IgA, mu (μ) in IgM, delta (δ) in IgD, and epsilon (ε) in IgE. The subclasses are IgG1, IgG2, IgG, and IgG4, or IgA1 and IgA2, and their light-chain types are κ and λ. A monoclonal protein is characterized by a narrow peak or a localized band on electrophoresis; by a thickened, bowed arc on immunoelectrophoresis; and by a localized band on immunofixation. Many different entities are associated with M proteins (monoclonal gammopathies) (Box 27-2).

Electrophoresis of the serum or urine reveals a tall, sharp peak on the densitometer tracing or dense localized band in a majority of cases of multiple myeloma (Figure 27-4). A monoclonal protein is demonstrable in the serum and urine in 90% of patients. In all, 60% of patients exhibit IgG, 20% IgA, 10% light chain only (BJ proteinemia), and 1% IgD. Electrophoresis of urine shows a globulin peak in 75% of

Box 27-2	Monoclonal Gammopathies

I. Malignant monoclonal gammopathies
  A. Multiple myeloma (IgG, IgA, IgD, IgE, and free light chains)
  B. Plasmacytoma
  C. Malignant lymphoproliferative diseases
  D. Heavy-chain diseases
  E. Amyloidosis
II. Monoclonal gammopathies of undetermined significance
  A. Benign (IgG, IgA, IgD, IgM, and rarely, free light chains)
  B. Associated with neoplasms of cell types not known to produce monoclonal proteins
  C. Biclonal gammopathies

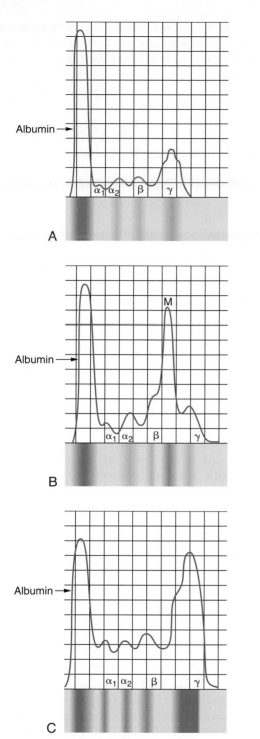

Figure 27-4 Serum electrophoretic patterns. **A,** Normal patient. **B,** Patient with multiple myeloma. **C,** Patient with Waldenström's macroglobulinemia.

Table 27-4	Suggested Sequence of Immunologic Testing for Monoclonal Proteins
M Spike on Serum Protein Electrophoresis	
Serum	**Urine**
Immunoelectrophoresis	Screening of urine for increased protein, (e.g., sulfosalicylic acid)
Immunofixation	Total protein assay of a 24-hour urine specimen
Quantitation of immunoglobu-lins by radial immunodiffu-sion or nephelometry	Urinary protein electrophoresis
Screening for cryoglobulins	Urinary immunoelectrophoresis
Determination of serum viscos-ity, if IgM, IgA, or IgG, or signs and symptoms sugges-tive of hyperviscosity	Immunofixation

method of determining the blood levels of three major immunoglobulins—IgM, IgG, and IgA—based on their combined electrophoretic and immunologic properties (see Chapter 11).

Immunoelectrophoresis is also used frequently to diagnose MM, which affects the bone marrow. Drugs that may cause increased immunoglobulin levels include therapeutic gamma globulin, hydralazine, isoniazid, phenytoin (Dilantin), procainamide, oral contraceptives, methadone, steroids, and tetanus toxoid and antitoxin. The laboratory should be notified if the patient has received any vaccinations or immunizations in the 6 months before the test. Prior immunizations lead to increased immunoglobulin levels, resulting in false-positive results.

Because immunoelectrophoresis is not quantitative, it is being replaced by **immunofixation,** which is more sensitive and easier to interpret.

Prognosis

The CD200 membrane glycoprotein imparts an immuno-regulatory signal that leads to the suppression of T-cell–mediated immune responses. Patients with CD200[absent] MM cells have an increased event-free survival of 24 months; patients with CD200[present] demonstrate an event-free survival of 14 months after high-dose therapy and stem cell transplantation. The presence or absence of CD200 expression in MM cells is considered a predictor of event-free survival for patients that is independent of the stage of disease or β_2M serum levels. This marker could be a new therapeutic target for MM.

Treatment

One treatment for myeloma is chemotherapy. Thalidomide has gained in popularity recently. Radiation therapy (high-energy, penetrating x-rays) may also be given. If a patient undergoes chemotherapy, the number of myeloma cells in the bone marrow and the amount of monoclonal protein in the blood and urine are closely monitored. A stable monoclonal protein level indicates that the disease is stable, often

cases, mainly albumin in 10% of patients, and a normal pattern in 15%. When an M spike is observed on serum protein electrophoresis, the suggested sequence of testing includes testing by immunoelectrophoresis and immunofixation (Table 27-4). Screening for cryoglobulins and viscosity may also be warranted.

Immunoelectrophoresis, also called gamma globulin electrophoresis or immunoglobulin electrophoresis, is a

the result of effective treatment. The monoclonal protein rarely disappears completely from blood and urine.

Other possible treatments include peripheral stem cell transplantation (see Chapter 32). This involves the use of high-dose chemotherapy or radiation therapy and the transfusion of previously collected immature, or "young," blood cells to replace diseased or damaged marrow. The proper role for peripheral stem cell transplantation in treating MM is being investigated.

Vaccination with the myeloma idiotype of a monoclonal immunoglobulin is a potential means of immunotherapy. DNA hybridization or blotting technology is the newest technology available and can be used to detect abnormal gene arrangements and mutations in cellular oncogenes. Although the gene product of MAbs is the method of detection, DNA probes that can detect the abnormal gene are now available. Blotting techniques may replace the current approach to the laboratory evaluation of monoclonal gammopathies.

WALDENSTRÖM'S PRIMARY MACROGLOBULINEMIA

Etiology

Waldenström's primary macroglobulinemia (WM), or simply *macroglobulinemia,* is a B-cell disorder characterized by the infiltration of lymphoplasmacytic cells into bone marrow and the presence of an IgM monoclonal gammopathy. WM is considered to be a *lymphoplasmacytic lymphoma,* as defined by the Revised European American Lymphoma (REAL) and World Health Organization (WHO) classification systems. WM is a malignant lymphocyte–plasma cell proliferative disorder that exhibits abnormally large amounts of immunoglobulin of the 19S IgM type. The cause of WM is unknown, but a possible genetic predisposition may exist. A greater frequency of IgM monoclonal proteins, as well as quantitative abnormalities, has been observed in some relatives of patients with WM.

Because WM is a malignant offshoot of B-cell development before the myelomas, the sole gene product is IgM. Patients with WM have chromosomal rearrangements characteristic of B-cell neoplasia, including t(8:14) and trisomy 12.

Epidemiology

Waldenström's macroglobulinemia occurs about one-tenth as frequently as multiple myeloma. WM has an age-specific incidence; it is most often found in older individuals, with a mean age of onset of 60 to 64 years. No significant gender differences exist in the incidence of WM. Disease onset is usually insidious, and the median survival is approximately 3 years after diagnosis.

Signs and Symptoms

The signs and symptoms of WM have an indolent progression over many years. Initially, disease onset is slow and insidious, with the pace of manifestations determined by the rate of proliferation of the IgM-secreting clone. Most clinical signs and symptoms of disease stem from intravascular accumulation of high levels of IgM macroglobulin. When the IgM is precipitable at cold temperatures, as it is in 37% of cases, clinical manifestations of cold sensitivity such as Raynaud's phenomenon, arthralgias, purpura of the extremities, renal insufficiency, and peripheral vascular occlusions may develop. Cold hypersensitivity can occur when serum IgM levels exceed 2 to 3 g/dL and the protein precipitates at temperatures exceeding 20° C.

Although the patient experiences weakness and fatigue, it is usually the onset of bleeding from the gums or nose that arouses concern. Patients undergo weight loss, and the incidence of infection is twice the normal rate. As the disease progresses, about 40% of patients develop hepatomegaly, splenomegaly, and lymphadenopathy. Occasionally the clinical manifestations may simulate diffuse lymphoma. Specific dysfunctions and abnormalities occur in a variety of body systems.

Skeletal Features

In contrast to multiple myeloma, bone pain is virtually nonexistent in WM. Diffuse osteoporosis may be seen, but bone lesions are extremely rare.

Hematologic Abnormalities

Patients with WM usually have chronic anemia and bleeding episodes. Bleeding problems in the form of bruising, purpura, and bleeding from the mouth, gums, nose, and gastrointestinal tract are common. The quantities of circulating platelets may be normal or decreased, but the most notable alteration is a disturbance in platelet function. Therefore, thrombocytopenia or hyperviscosity may contribute to the bleeding disorder.

In addition to anemia caused by chronic or recurrent bleeding, the decrease in red blood cells (RBCs) becomes more severe as the disease progresses because of a dilutional effect caused by increased immunoglobulin production. In addition, the presence of macroglobulin also produces an increased erythrocyte sedimentation rate (ESR). Microscopic examination of a peripheral blood smear usually reveals normocytic and frequently hypochromic RBCs with striking rouleaux (rolled-coin) formation. The total blood leukocyte count is either normal or slightly decreased because of moderate neutropenia. In a terminal patient the blood may be inundated with malignant lymphoplasmacytic cells.

Renal Dysfunction

Renal function becomes mildly or moderately impaired in about 15% of WM patients. Nephrosis is uncommon. BJ proteinuria, however, is present in about 70% of WM patients, although the quantity of light chains excreted is much less than in multiple myeloma.

Glomerular lesions are the predominant form of renal injury. IgM collects on the endothelial side of the basement membrane of the kidney, and sometimes these macroglobulin accumulations obstruct glomerular capillaries.

Ocular Manifestations

Blurred vision is a frequent abnormality of WM. Rouleaux induced by elevations of IgM causes distention of veins and capillaries; retinal oxygenation diminishes as rouleaux-inducing IgM rises. As a result of increased IgM levels, retinal hemorrhage, exudate formation, and varicosities develop, which can lead to more permanent retinal damage unless IgM levels are lowered by therapy.

Neuropsychiatric Problems

The most common serious neurologic consequence of the slowed cerebral perfusion caused by macroglobulinemia is acute cerebral malfunction, beginning with headache, fluctuating confusion, forgetfulness, and slowed mentation. This can progress to somnolence, stupor, and coma–diffuse brain syndrome, sometimes called "coma paraproteinaemicum." Neurologic abnormalities can be improved by reduction of plasma viscosity.

Polyneuropathy affects 5% to 10% of patients with WM. This condition is associated with an increase in spinal fluid protein and deposits of monoclonal IgM on myelin sheaths. Monoclonal IgM found in the plasma and attached to damaged nerves has been shown in some cases to share idiotypic determinants. This suggests that polyneuropathy of WM may be an autoimmune process caused by monoclonal IgM possessing antibody activity for a component of nerve tissue.

Cardiopulmonary Abnormalities

Congestive heart failure becomes a serious problem in patients with chronic, uncontrolled WM. About 90% of IgM remains trapped in the circulating plasma and exerts an unbalanced transendothelial osmotic effect sufficient to cause marked expansion of the plasma volume. This in turn creates a dilutional anemia and augments cardiac filling and cardiac output. As a result, increased cardiac output and blood viscosity overwork the myocardium.

About 10% of patients develop pulmonary lesions. Pulmonary tumors, diffuse infiltrates, and pleural involvement are all about equally represented. The signs and symptoms of pulmonary dysfunction include coughing and dyspnea.

Cutaneous Manifestations

Cold sensitivity is a frequent manifestation of WM; however, skin lesions are uncommon. A small number of patients develop flat, violaceous, macular skin lesions resulting from dense infiltration by lymphoplasmacytoid cells. Pink, pearly-looking papules caused by dense deposits of IgM may be seen.

Immunologic Manifestations

The basic abnormality in this macroglobulinemia is uncontrolled proliferation of B lymphocytes and plasma cells. As a result, there is a heavy accumulation of monoclonal IgM in the circulating plasma and plasmacytoid lymphocytes in the bone marrow.

In many cases, WM is associated with mixed cryoglobulinemia, which reflects the binding of IgG or IgA antiidiotypic antibody to the mutant IgM. In a small number of patients, dysplastic tumor cells secrete 7S IgM monomers, μ chains, or other monoclonal immunoglobulins or fragments. Therefore the major IgM production indicates that the immunoglobulin (gene) lesion sometimes degenerates and codes for more than one M component.

Diagnostic Evaluation

Hematologic Assessment

Microscopic examination of a bone marrow aspirate reveals that the lymphoplasmacytic cells vary morphologically from small lymphocytes to obvious plasma cells. Frequently the cellular cytoplasm is ragged and may contain material staining positive on periodic acid–Schiff (PAS) stain, probably identical to the circulating macroglobulin.

The total peripheral blood leukocyte count is usually normal, with an absolute lymphocytosis. Moderate to severe degrees of anemia are frequently observed on peripheral blood smears, as well as rouleaux formation. The patient's plasma volume may be greatly increased, and ESR is also increased.

Platelet counts are usually normal. Faulty platelet aggregation and release of platelet factor 3 are caused by nonspecific coating of platelets by IgM. The most common coagulation defect is a prolonged thrombin time, resulting from the binding of M component to fibrin monomers and consequent gel clotting of IgM-coated fibrin. Bleeding abnormalities can be demonstrated by the following:

- Faulty platelet adhesiveness
- Defective platelet aggregation
- Abnormal release of platelet factor 3
- Impaired clot retraction
- Prolonged bleeding time
- Positive tourniquet test
- Prolonged thrombin/prothrombin time test
- Decreased levels of factor VIII

Immunologic Assessment

Serum electrophoresis usually demonstrates the overproduction of IgM (19S) antibodies. Diagnosis is made by demonstration of a homogeneous M component composed of monoclonal IgM. Quantitation of immunoglobulins reveals IgM levels ranging from 1 to 12 g/dL (usually >3 g/dL), accounting for 20% to 70% of total protein. Characteristically, blood samples are described as having "hyperviscosity."

In addition, cryoglobulins can be detected in the patient's serum. *Cryoglobulins* are proteins that precipitate or gel when cooled to 0° C and dissolve when heated. In most cases, monoclonal cryoglobulins are IgM or IgG. Occasionally the macroglobulin is both cryoprecipitable and capable of cold-induced, anti-i–mediated agglutination of RBCs. IgM may also occasionally be a *pyroglobulin,* which precipitates on heating to 50° to 60° C but does not redissolve on cooling or intensified heating, as do typical BJ pyroglobulins. Many cryoglobulins have the ability to fix complement and initiate an inflammatory reaction similar to antigen-antibody complexes. Cryoglobulins have been classified into the following three types:

- *Type I* is composed of a single class. IgM and IgG classes are most common; IgA or light-chain, single cryoglobulins are seen less frequently. Type I constitutes about 25% of cryoglobulins and is generally associated with multiple myeloma, macroglobulinemia, and other, rarer neoplastic proliferations of plasma cells and lymphocytes.
- *Type II* cryoglobulins consist of two forms. The monoclonal form always has rheumatoid factor activity and usually is an IgM with κ light chains. The second form is polyclonal IgG, which reacts with the monoclonal IgM rheumatoid factor.
- *Type III* is a mixed cryoglobulin in which both constituent immunoglobulins are polyclonal. More than 90% of type III cryoglobulins contain IgM rheumatoid factor and IgG. Type III cryoglobulins are seen in a variety of autoimmune, systemic rheumatic diseases and persistent infections with immune complexes (e.g., bacterial endocarditis).

Treatment

Current treatment of WM includes single-agent alkylator, nucleoside analog, or standard-dose rituximab therapy. New studies suggest that extended-dose rituximab as well as other treatment options were likely to yield as good or even better results than currently recommended therapy. These options include therapy with either nucleoside analogs or alkylator agents; rituximab in combination with nucleoside analogs; nucleoside analogs plus alkylator agents; and combination chemotherapy (e.g., cyclophosphamide, doxorubicin, vincristine, prednisone; CHOP) or cyclophosphamide and dexamethasone.

OTHER MONOCLONAL DISORDERS

Monoclonal Gammopathy of Undetermined Significance

Monoclonal gammopathy of undetermined significance (MGUS) represents the presence of a monoclonal protein in patients with no features of multiple myeloma or related malignant disorders (e.g., WM, B-cell lymphoma, chronic lymphocytic leukemia). MGUS was originally considered a benign monoclonal gammopathy, but it is now known that this disorder can evolve into a malignant monoclonal gammopathy.

The International Myeloma Working Group has established the differences between MGUS and plasma cell neoplasms (Table 27-5).

Characteristics of MGUS include the following:
- Serum monoclonal protein concentration less than 3 g/dL
- Fewer than 10% plasma cells in the bone marrow
- Absence of lytic bone lesions
- Anemia
- Hypercalcemia
- Renal insufficiency
- No clinical signs or symptoms related to the monoclonal gammopathy

In terms of incidence, half the patients with a monoclonal gammopathy have MGUS, and 15% to 20% have multiple myeloma. The incidence of MGUS increases with age. The median age at diagnosis is about 70 years. MGUS occurs more frequently in men than women and more often in blacks than in whites. IgG is the most common immunoglobulin affected, followed by IgM. The cause is unknown.

The monoclonal gammopathies are characterized by a rearrangement of immunoglobulin genes that result in the production of a monoclonal protein. There are two populations of plasma cells in patients with MGUS: (1) normal and polyclonal (CD38+, CD56+, CD19−) and (2) clonal with an abnormal immunophenotype (CD38+, CD56+, CD19−). The plasma cell clone and associated monoclonal protein concentrations usually remain stable for many years. After a prolonged period, a substantial number of patients with MGUS progress to a malignant plasma cell disorder (e.g., MM, B-cell lymphoma, chronic lymphocytic leukemia).

Recommended laboratory testing includes the following:
- Hemoglobin concentration
- Serum calcium
- Creatinine concentrations
- Bone marrow aspiration examination
- Total serum protein concentration and serum electrophoresis (serum monoclonal protein concentration)
- 24-hour urine protein excretion concentration and urine electrophoresis (urine monoclonal protein concentration)

Table 27-5	Diagnostic Criteria for MGUS,* Multiple Myeloma, and Waldenström's Macroglobulinemia			
	MGUS	Smoldering Multiple Myeloma	Multiple Myeloma	Waldenström's Macroglobulinemia
Bone marrow plasma cells	<10% *and*	≥10% *and/or*	≥10% *and/or*	>10% *and* <10% lymphoplasmacytoid cells *and*
Circulating monoclonal protein	<3 g/dL	≥3 g/dL	≥3 g/dL	>3 g/dL
Clinical signs and symptoms	Absent	Absent	Present	Present

Modified from International Myeloma Working Group: Criteria for the classification of monoclonal gammopathies, multiple myeloma and related disorders, *Br J Haematol* 121:749-757, 2003.
*Monoclonal gammopathy of undetermined significance.

- Serum and urine immunofixation (type of monoclonal protein)
- Determination of serum FLC ratio (κ and λ FLCs), particularly for the assessment of prognosis

Light-Chain Disease

Light-chain disease represents about 10% to 15% of monoclonal gammopathies, ranking behind IgG and IgA myelomas, which represent about 60% and 15%, respectively. LCD occurs about as frequently as WM. In LCD, only κ or λ monoclonal light chains or BJ proteins are produced.

Diagnostic evaluation of suspected LCD is similar to the protocol for any lymphoproliferative disorder, but certain changes in approach are necessary because of the low levels of paraprotein that can be involved. Agarose high-resolution protein electrophoresis of serum and urine should be done to determine the total protein concentration. A 24-hour urine specimen should be examined electrophoretically because almost all the protein may be BJ protein. Visual examination of the electrophoretic pattern is essential because a small light-chain band frequently does not exhibit a significant peak on densitometric scanning. Serum protein electrophoretic patterns from patients with monoclonal gammopathies may demonstrate the following:
- Typical well-defined monoclonal band
- Somewhat broad, diffuse band caused by polymerization of monoclonal protein
- Normal gamma region
- Hypogammaglobulinemia

Heavy-Chain Disease

As the name implies, heavy-chain disease is characterized by the presence of monoclonal proteins composed of the heavy-chain portion of the immunoglobulin molecule. The term *Franklin's disease* is synonymous with gamma heavy-chain disease. Alpha heavy-chain disease is the most common of the heavy-chain gammopathies and is frequently seen in men of Mediterranean descent. Mu heavy-chain disease is rare.

Heavy chains may be detected in serum or urine, or both (depending on the class of heavy chain involved). When heavy-chain disease is suspected, nonspecific anti-Fab antisera should be used for definitive testing. The serum sample should also be diluted and retested with κ and λ light-chain antisera to rule out prozoning caused by antigen excess.

Gammopathies with More Than One Band

In some cases, more than one monoclonal band is produced. Although gammopathies with two bands may represent a true biclonal condition, routine laboratory techniques cannot distinguish between the various mechanisms that could produce two or more monoclonal bands. Therefore a serum specimen with an IgG κ and an IgA λ band should be appropriately reported as a gammopathy with IgG κ and IgA λ monoclonal bands.

The appearance of more than one band on electrophoresis is often associated with an advanced gammopathy, in which the asynchronous production of the components of the immunoglobulin molecule occurs. In such cases, synthesis of an intact monoclonal immunoglobulin and an excess of monoclonal light chains may be observed. An example of the demonstration of more than one band on electrophoresis can include cases in which the pentameric IgM breaks down into 7S subunits, which appear on electrophoresis as one or more "extra" monoclonal bands. In addition, monoclonal IgA molecules tend to dimerize, and the resulting dimer often has a different mobility than the monomer parent molecule.

Bence Jones Protein Screening Procedure

Principle

Heat solubility is used to detect Bence Jones (BJ) protein, the urinary protein characteristic of multiple myeloma (MM). BJ protein is soluble in urine at room and body temperature. When the urine is heated to 40° C, a white cloud appears. A distinct precipitate forms at 60° C. The precipitate dissolves again at around 100° C (boiling) but reappears on cooling. The minimal detectable concentration of BJ protein is about 30 mg/dL. Excessive amounts of acid or salt will prevent the appearance of the precipitate.

Specimen Collection and Preparation

A random or a 24-hour urine specimen is collected in a clean container. The specimen can be refrigerated to prevent bacterial growth.

Reagents, Supplies and Equipment

- Heat block or boiling-water bath
- Acetate buffer, 2 mol/L, pH 4.9 (or 10% aqueous solution of acetic acid)

  Prepare by adding 4.1 mL of glacial acetic acid to 17.5 g of sodium acetate trihydrate, and then add distilled water to a total volume of 100 mL.
- Test tubes

Procedure

1. Measure 4 mL of clear urine into a test tube. Add 1 mL of acetate buffer (or acetic acid) and mix.
2. Place the urine-buffer solution into a heat block or boiling-water bath at 56° C for 15 minutes.
3. If the solution develops turbidity (cloudiness), transfer the test tube to a 100° C heat source, (e.g., boiling-water bath) for 3 minutes.
4. Examine the urine solution for turbidity.
5. Filter the urine solution immediately after removing it from the boiling-water bath.
6. Examine the solution for turbidity as it cools; reexamine for turbidity as the solution reaches room temperature.

Reporting Results

If BJ proteins are present in the urine, the solution will become cloudy as it cools and become clear as it reaches room temperature.

Procedure Notes

If the precipitate is heavy, it is best to dilute the urine (1:2) and repeat the procedure.

Clinical Applications

Bence Jones protein is found in urine in many patients with MM, osteogenic sarcoma, osteomalacia, and carcinomatosis.

Reference

Modified from Bradwell AR: *Serum free light chain analysis,* Birmingham, UK, 2006, Binding Site, p 9.

CASE STUDY

History and Physical Examination

A 58-year-old nuclear power plant worker sees his family physician because of increasing fatigue and weakness. He also reports pain in his lower back and arms when he walks. Physical examination reveals that the man has pale mucous membranes and hepatosplenomegaly. The physician orders a complete blood count (CBC) and urinalysis (UA). A follow-up appointment is scheduled for the following week.

Laboratory Data

The CBC reveals that the patient has anemia. His leukocyte count and differential count are normal, except for a rouleaux (rolled-coin) appearance of the RBCs. The UA is normal. The patient is called and requested to return to the laboratory for additional tests. The physician orders ESR, kidney screening profile, liver blood profile, and radiographic skeletal survey, with the following results:

ESR: 50 mm/hr
Kidney profile: normal
Liver profile: normal, except for increased globular protein
Skeletal survey: bone lesions in various sites

Questions and Discussion

1. **What follow-up laboratory tests might be ordered to assist in establishing a definitive diagnosis?**

In this patient, further investigation of the increased serum globular protein is ordered. Serum electrophoresis and immunoelectrophoresis reveal the presence of an abnormal protein, 7S immunoglobulin. A monoclonal gammopathy, which can be either a benign or malignant condition, results from a single clone of lymphoid-plasma cells, producing elevated levels of a single class and type of immunoglobulin. The elevated immunoglobulin is referred to as a monoclonal protein, M protein, or paraprotein. Disorders in this category of plasma cell dyscrasias include MM, WM, LCD, and heavy-chain diseases.

Serum and urine electrophoretic patterns and other Ig assays can demonstrate strikingly abnormal results in such disorders as MM and WM.

2. **What is the nature of the protein found in the urine?**

BJ protein is identified in the urine. BJ protein precipitates when heated to 56° C, dissolves when heated to boiling, and reprecipitates with cooling. On electrophoresis, BJ protein will reflect its monoclonal nature and appear in the beta or gamma region.

3. **What is the most significant laboratory finding in this disorder?**

The presence of increased plasma cells is significant in establishing the diagnosis. Laboratory tests, particularly serum and urine electrophoresis, are important adjuncts.

4. **What type of immunologic defect exists in this disease process?**

Patients with MM have defects in humoral, but not cellular, immunity. Humoral immunity is disrupted because plasma cell tumors induce suppression of antibody synthesis by normal Ig-secreting cells; the production of antiidiotypic antibodies decreases proportionally. In addition, selective impairment occurs in the formation of normal antibodies because of increased Ig catabolism and the release of a protein that incites macrophages to suppress synthesis of normal immunoglobulins by myeloma cells. Depression of normal humoral immunity accounts for the high susceptibility of these patients to bacterial infection. The normal functioning of cellular immunity, however, is demonstrated by normal resistance to fungal and most viral infections and normal delayed-type hypersensitivity to skin-testing antigens.

5. **Does this patient have a risk of occupational exposure?**

Yes. Nuclear plant workers have an increased likelihood of developing MM. Older workers, especially 45 years and older, with cumulative radiation doses of 5 rem (roentgen equivalent man) or more were found to have almost 3.5 times the chance of dying from MM than workers at the same plants with cumulative doses less than 1 rem. A rem represents a dosage of radiation that has the same biologic effect as 1 roentgen of x-radiation or gamma radiation.

Reference

Bureau of National Affairs: *BNA's Safety Net* 3(8):57, 2000.

Diagnosis

Multiple myeloma.

CHAPTER HIGHLIGHTS

- Hypergammaglobulinemias are either monoclonal or polyclonal.
- A monoclonal gammopathy can be benign or malignant and results from a single clone of lymphoid-plasma cells producing elevated levels of a single class and type of immunoglobulin referred to as a monoclonal protein, M protein, or paraprotein. Such disorders include multiple myeloma (MM) and Waldenström's macroglobulinemia (WM). MM is the most common form of dysproteinemia.

- A polyclonal gammopathy is classified as a secondary disease and is characterized by the elevation of two or more immunoglobulins produced by several clones of plasma cells. Polyclonal protein consists of one or more heavy-chain classes, and both light-chain types increase as secondary manifestations of infection or inflammation.
- The cause of MM is unknown, but radiation may be a factor; a viral cause has also been suggested. Other etiologic factors may include environmental stimuli or genetic factors.
- Signs and symptoms of MM include bone pain (back or chest), weakness, fatigue, and pallor associated with anemia or abnormal bleeding.
- Proteinuria is a common finding in more than half of patients excreting abnormal amounts of Bence Jones (BJ) protein (light chains). Patients have defects in humoral but not cellular immunity.
- Laboratory diagnosis of MM includes electrophoresis of the serum or urine. A monoclonal protein is seen in the serum and urine in 90% of patients. DNA hybridization or blotting technology can be used to detect abnormal genes in B cells. Although the gene product of monoclonal antibodies (MAbs) is the method of detection, DNA probes that detect the abnormal gene are now available. Blotting techniques may replace current laboratory evaluation of monoclonal gammopathies.
- WM is a malignant cell disorder that exhibits abnormally large amounts of 19S IgM. The cause is unknown, but a genetic predisposition may exist.
- WM has an indolent progression over many years. The basic abnormality is uncontrolled proliferation of B lymphocytes and plasma cells.
- Laboratory diagnosis of WM involves serum electrophoresis showing a homogeneous M component composed of monoclonal IgM. Blood samples characteristically display hyperviscosity. In addition, cryoglobulins can be detected.
- Other monoclonal disorders include light-chain disease (LCD), which represents about 10% to 15% of monoclonal gammopathies. In LCD, only kappa or lambda monoclonal light chains or BJ proteins are produced. A 24-hour urine specimen should be examined electrophoretically because almost all the protein may be BJ.
- Heavy-chain disease is characterized by monoclonal proteins composed of the heavy-chain portion of the immunoglobulin molecule. Alpha heavy-chain disease is most common.

REVIEW QUESTIONS

1. Polyclonal gammopathies can be exhibited as a secondary manifestation of all the following *except:*
   a. Chronic infection.
   b. Chronic liver disease.
   c. Multiple myeloma.
   d. Rheumatoid connective disease.

2. What is the most frequent cause of death in a patient with multiple myeloma?
   a. Skeletal destruction
   b. Chronic renal failure
   c. Neurologic disorders
   d. Infectious disease

3. Patients with multiple myeloma have defects in:
   a. Cellular immunity.
   b. Humoral immunity.
   c. Synthesis of normal immunoglobulins.
   d. Both b and c.

4. What is the most consistent immunologic feature of multiple myeloma?
   a. Synthesis of dysfunctional single monoclonal proteins
   b. Synthesis of Ig chains or fragments
   c. Presence of M protein in serum and/or urine
   d. All the above

Questions 5 and 6. Fill in the blanks, choosing the correct temperature *(a-d).*

Bence-Jones proteins are soluble at room temperature, become insoluble near (5) _____, and then resolubilize at (6) _____.

   a. 37° C
   b. 50° C
   c. 65° C
   d. 80° C

7. M proteins are associated with all the following malignant conditions *except:*
   a. Multiple myeloma.
   b. Plasmacytoma.
   c. Malignant lymphoproliferative diseases.
   d. Lymphoma.

8. Cryoglobulins are proteins that precipitate or gel at:
   a. −18° C.
   b. −4° C.
   c. 0° C.
   d. 4° C.

9. Monoclonal gammopathy involves elevated levels of a single class and type of immunoglobulin referred to as:
   a. Monoclonal protein.
   b. M protein.
   c. Paraprotein.
   d. All the above.

Questions 10 and 11. Fill in the blanks, choosing from the following answers:

In light-chain disease only (10) _____ or (11) _____ monoclonal light chains are synthesized by a one-cell clone.

Possible answers to question 10:
a. beta
b. gamma
c. kappa
d. alpha

Possible answers to question 11:
a. lambda
b. alpha
c. beta
d. gamma

12. Multiple myeloma is also referred to as:
    a. Plasma cell myeloma.
    b. Kahler's disease.
    c. Myelomatosis.
    d. All the above.

13. Most patients with multiple myeloma manifest:
    a. Bone pain.
    b. Acute renal failure.
    c. No symptoms.
    d. Hepatomegaly and splenomegaly.

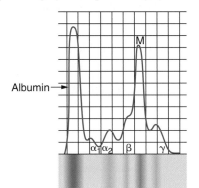

14. The figure above represents the serum electrophoresis of a patient with:
    a. Waldenström's macroglobulinemia.
    b. Multiple myeloma.
    c. No protein abnormality.
    d. Polyclonal gammopathy.

15. Patients with Waldenström's macroglobulinemia exhibit abnormally large amounts of:
    a. IgM.
    b. IgG.
    c. IgE.
    d. IgA.

16. Monoclonal gammopathy of undetermined significance (MGUS) represents a:
    a. Monoclonal protein in patients with no features of multiple myeloma or related malignant disorders.
    b. Disorder that can evolve into a malignant monoclonal gammopathy.
    c. Serum monoclonal protein concentration less than 3 g/dL.
    d. All the above.

17. MGUS is characterized by all the following *except:*
    a. Fewer than 10% plasma cells in the bone marrow.
    b. Presence of lytic bone lesions.
    c. Anemia.
    d. Hypercalcemia.

18. Light-chain disease represents about _____ of monoclonal gammopathies.
    a. 5% to 10%
    b. 10% to 15%
    c. 15% to 25%
    d. 25% to 50%

BIBLIOGRAPHY

Alexanian R, Dimopoulos M: The treatment of multiple myeloma, *N Engl J Med* 330(7):484-489, 1994.

American Cancer Society: How is multiple myeloma diagnosed? www.cancer.org, May 2006.

Aucouturier P et al: Heavy-chain deposition disease, *N Engl J Med* 329(19): 1389-1393, 1993.

Barlogie B et al: Thalidomide and hematopoietic-cell transplantation for multiple myeloma, *N Engl J Med* 543(10):1021-1029, 2006.

Blade, J. Monoclonal gammopathy of undetermined significance, *N Engl J Med* 355(26):2765-2670, 2006.

Bradwell AR: *Serum free light chain analysis,* ed 4, Birmingham, UK, 2006, Binding Site.

Caroscio JT: Quantitative CSF IgG measurements in multiple sclerosis and other neurologic diseases, *Arch Neurol* 40:409-413, 1983.

Hoffman EG: Laboratory evaluation of monoclonal gammopathies, *Can J Med Technol* 49(2):99-115, 1987.

Jandl JA: Multiple myeloma and other differentiated B cell malignancies. In Jandl JA: *Blood,* Boston, 1988, Little, Brown.

Joshua DE, editor: *Thalidomide in the treatment of multiple myeloma,* Vol 1, No 11, Pavia, Italy, 2005, Ferrata-Storti Foundation.

Keren DF, Morrison N, Gulbranson R: Evolution of a monoclonal gammopathy, *Lab Med* 25(5):313-317, 1994.

Keshgegian AA, Coblentz J, Lisak RP, editor: Oligoclonal immunoglobulins in cerebrospinal fluid in multiple sclerosis, *Clin Chem* 26(9):1340-1345, 1980.

Killingsworth LM: Clinical applications of protein determination in biological fluids other than blood, *Clin Chem* 28(5):1093-1258, 1982.

Killingsworth LM, Warren BM: *Immunofixation for the identification of monoclonal gammopathies,* Beaumont, Texas, 1986, Helena Laboratories.

Konrad RJ et al: Myeloma-associated paraprotein directed against the HIV-1 p27 antigen in an HIV-1-seropositive patient, *N Engl J Med* 328(25):1817-1819, 1993.

Kyle A et al: Prevalence of monclonal gammopathy of undetermined significance, *N Engl J Med* 354:1362-1369, 2006.

Kyle RA, Rajkumar SV: Multiple myeloma, *N Engl J Med* 351(18):1860-1871, 2004.

Lab tests at a glance, www.labtestsonline.org, May 2006.

Mayo Clinic, Myeloma Amyloidosis Monoclonal Gammopathy Group, www.mayo.edu.

Moreaux J et al: CD200 is a new prognostic factor in multiple myeloma, *Blood* 108(13):4194-4197, 2006.

Othman Y: Protein bands in all lanes of the immunofixation electrophoresis pattern of serum from a 50-year-old Saudi woman, *Lab Med* 37(3):152-154, 2006.

Papadopoulos NM et al: A unique protein in normal human cerebrospinal fluid, *Clin Chem* 29(10):1842-1844, 1983.

Prabhala RH et al: Dysfunctional T regulatory cells in multiple myeloma, *Blood* 107(1):301-304, 2006.

Ritzmann EE: Immunoglobulin abnormalities. In Ritzmann S, editor: *Serum protein abnormalities: diagnostic and clinical aspects,* Boston, 1976, Little, Brown.

Smolens P, Stein JH: Renal manifestations of dysproteinemias. In Stein J, editor: *Internal medicine,* ed 2, Boston, 1987, Little, Brown.

Treon SP et al: Update on treatment recommendations from the Third International Workshop on Waldenström's Macroglobulinemia, *Blood* 107(9):3442-3446, 2006.

Turgeon ML: *Clinical hematology: theory and procedures,* ed 4, Philadelphia, 2004, Lippincott–Williams & Wilkins.

CHAPTER 28

Autoimmmune Disorders

What Is Autoimmunity?
Spectrum of Autoimmune Disorders
Factors Influencing Development of Autoimmunity
 Genetic Factors
 Patient Age
 Exogenous Factors
Immunopathogenic Mechanisms
Self-Recognition (Tolerance)
Major Autoantibodies
Organ-Specific and Midspectrum Disorders
 Cardiovascular Disorders
 Collagen Vascular Disorders
 Endocrine Gland Disorders
 Pancreatic Disorders

Reproductive Disorders
Exocrine Gland Disorder
Gastrointestinal Disorders
Autoimmune Hematologic Disorders
Neuromuscular Disorders
Neuropathies
Renal Disorders
Skeletal Muscle Disorders
Skin Disorders (Bullous Disease and Other Conditions)
Case Studies
Chapter Highlights
Review Questions
Bibliography

Learning Objectives

At the conclusion of this chapter, the reader should be able to:
- Describe the nature of autoimmune disorders.
- Compare organ-specific and organ-nonspecific characteristics.

- Describe organ-specific and midspectrum disorders.
- Analyze representative case studies.

WHAT IS AUTOIMMUNITY?

Autoimmunity represents a breakdown of the immune system's ability to discriminate between "self" and "nonself." The term **autoimmune disorder** refers to a varied group of more than 80 serious, chronic illnesses that involve almost every human organ system. In all these disorders the underlying problem is similar: the body's immune system becomes misdirected, attacking the organs it was designed to protect.

Autoimmune disorder remains among the most poorly understood and poorly recognized of any category of illnesses. Individually, autoimmune disorders occur infrequently, except for thyroid disease, diabetes, rheumatoid arthritis, and systemic lupus erythematosus. Overall, autoimmune disorders represent the fourth-largest cause of disability in Europe and the United States.

The term autoimmune disorder is used when demonstrable immunoglobulins **(autoantibodies)** or cytotoxic T cells display specificity for "self" antigens, or **autoantigens,** and contribute to the pathogenesis of the disorder (Table 28-1). Autoimmune disorders are characterized by the persistent activation of immunologic effector mechanisms that alter the function and integrity of individual cells and organs. The sites of organ or tissue damage depend on the location of the immune reaction. The variety of signs and symptoms seen in patients with autoimmune disorders reflects the various forms of the immune response.

Table 28-1	Examples of Autoimmune Disorders and Associated Abnormalities	
Clinical Diagnosis		**Autoantigen**
Addison's disease		P-450 enzymes
Crohn's disease		p-ANCA, pancreatic acinar cells
Ovarian failure/infertility		P-450 enzymes
Pernicious anemia		Parietal cells
Ulcerative colitis		p-ANCA

It is also important to note that autoantibodies may be formed in patients secondary to tissue damage or when no evidence of clinical disease exists. Unlike autoimmune disorder, autoantibodies can occur as immune correlates of conditions such as blood transfusion reactions. In addition, autoantibodies can be demonstrated in hemolytic disease of the newborn and graft rejection and can result from disorders such as serum sickness, anaphylaxis, and hay fever, when the immune response is clearly the cause of the disease.

SPECTRUM OF AUTOIMMUNE DISORDERS

Many disorders are believed to be related to immunologic abnormalities, and additional diseases are continually identified (Box 28-1). Autoimmune disorders exhibit a full spectrum of tissue reactivity (Figure 28-1). At one extreme are

Active chronic hepatitis
Addison's disease
Autoimmune atrophic gastritis
Autoimmune hemolytic anemia
Dermatomyositis
Discoid lupus erythematosus
Goodpasture's syndrome
Hashimoto's thyroiditis
Idiopathic thrombocytopenic purpura
Insulin-dependent ("juvenile," type 1) diabetes mellitus

Multiple sclerosis
Myasthenia gravis
Pemphigus vulgaris
Pernicious anemia
Primary biliary cirrhosis
Primary myxedema
Rheumatoid arthritis
Scleroderma
Sjögren's syndrome
Systemic lupus erythematosus
Thyrotoxicosis

organ-specific disorders such as Hashimoto's disease of the thyroid; at the other extreme are disorders that manifest as organ-nonspecific diseases such as systemic lupus erythematosus (SLE; Chapter 29) and rheumatoid arthritis (RA; Chapter 30) (Table 28-2).

In organ-specific disorders, both the lesions produced by tissue damage and the autoantibodies are directed at a single target organ (e.g., thyroid). Midspectrum disorders are characterized by localized lesions in a single organ and by organ-nonspecific autoantibodies. For example, in primary biliary cirrhosis the small bile duct is the main target of inflammatory cell infiltration, but the serum autoantibodies are mainly mitochondrial antibodies and are not liver specific.

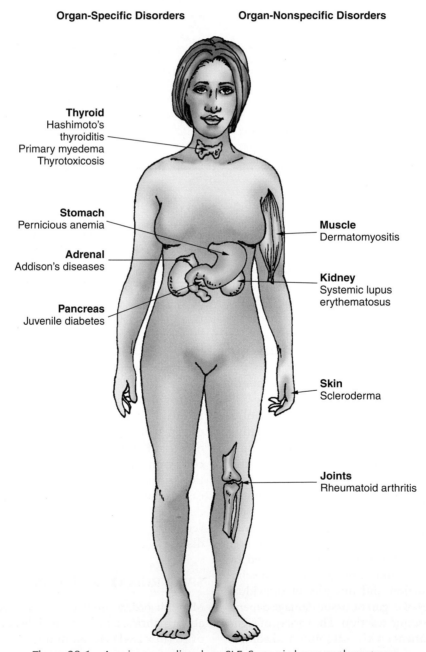

Organ-Specific Disorders　　　**Organ-Nonspecific Disorders**

Thyroid
Hashimoto's thyroiditis
Primary myedema
Thyrotoxicosis

Stomach
Pernicious anemia

Adrenal
Addison's diseases

Pancreas
Juvenile diabetes

Muscle
Dermatomyositis

Kidney
Systemic lupus erythematosus

Skin
Scleroderma

Joints
Rheumatoid arthritis

Figure 28-1　Autoimmune disorders. *SLE,* Systemic lupus erythematosus.

Table 28-2	Summary of Organ-Specific and Organ-Nonspecific Disorders

Similarities

1. Circulating autoantibodies react with normal body constituents.
2. Increased immunoglobulin concentration in serum often found.
3. Antibodies may appear in each of the main immunoglobulin classes.
4. Disease process not always progressive; exacerbations and remissions occur.
5. Autoantibody tests of diagnostic value.

Differences

Organ Specific	*Organ Nonspecific*
Antibodies and lesions are organ specific.	Antibodies and lesions are organ nonspecific.
Clinical and serologic overlap (e.g., thyroid, stomach, adrenal glands, kidney).	Overlap of SLE, RA, and other connective tissue disorders.
Antigens only available to lymphoid system in low concentrations.	Antigens accessible at higher concentrations.
Antigens evoke organ-specific antibodies in normal animals with complete Freund's adjuvant.	No antibodies produced in animals with comparable stimulation.
Familial tendency to develop organ-specific autoimmunity.	Familial tendency to develop connective tissue disease.
	Questionable abnormalities in immunoglobulin synthesis in relatives.
Lymphoid invasion, parenchymal destruction by questionable cell-mediated hypersensitivity or antibodies.	Lesions caused by deposition of antigen-antibody (immune) complexes.
Tendency to develop cancer in the organ.	Tendency to develop lymphoreticular neoplasia.

SLE, Systemic lupus erythematosus; *RA,* rheumatoid arthritis.

Organ-nonspecific disorders are characterized by the presence of both lesions and autoantibodies not confined to any one organ.

FACTORS INFLUENCING DEVELOPMENT OF AUTOIMMUNITY

Autoimmunity begins with an abnormal interaction of T and B lymphocytes with autoantigens. No single theory or mechanism has been identified as a cause. The potential for autoimmunity, if given appropriate circumstances, is constantly present in every immunocompetent individual because lymphocytes that are potentially reactive with "self" antigens exist in the body. Antibody expression appears to be regulated by a complex set of interacting factors; influences include genetic factors, patient age, and exogenous factors.

Genetic Factors

Although a direct genetic etiology has not been established in autoimmune disease, there is a tendency for familial aggregates to occur. In addition, there is a tendency for more than one autoimmune disorder to occur in the same individual. For example, patients with Hashimoto's disease have a higher incidence of pernicious anemia than would be expected in a random population matched for age and gender.

Another factor related to genetic inheritance is that autoimmune disorders and autoantibodies are found more frequently in women than in men.

The presence of certain human leukocyte antigens (HLAs) is also associated with an increased risk of certain autoimmune states.

Patient Age

Autoantibodies are manifested infrequently in the general population. The incidence of autoantibodies, however, increases steadily with age, reaching a peak at around 60 to 70 years.

Exogenous Factors

Ultraviolet radiation, drugs, viruses, and chronic infectious disease may all play a role in the development of autoimmune disorders. These factors may alter antigens, which the body then perceives as "nonself" antigens.

IMMUNOPATHOGENIC MECHANISMS

Autoimmune disorder is usually prevented by the normal functioning of immunologic regulatory mechanisms. When these controls dysfunction, antibodies to "self" antigens may be produced and bind to antigens in the circulation to form circulating immune complexes or to antigens deposited in specific tissue sites.

The mechanisms governing the deposition in one organ or another are unknown; however, several mechanisms may be operative in a single disease. Wherever antigen-antibody complexes accumulate, complement can be activated, with the subsequent release of mediators of inflammation. These mediators increase vascular permeability, attract phagocytic cells to the reaction site, and cause local tissue damage. Alternatively, cytotoxic T cells can directly attack body cells bearing the target antigen, which releases mediators that amplify the inflammatory reaction. Autoantibody and complement fragments coat cells bearing the target antigen, which leads to destruction by phagocytes or antibody-seeking K-type lymphocytes.

An individual may develop an autoimmune response to a variety of immunogenic stimuli (Table 28-3). These responses may be caused by the following:

- Antigens that do not normally circulate in the blood. The "hidden-antigen" (sequestered-antigen) theory is one of the earliest views of organ-specific antibodies. Antigens are sequestered within the organ, and because of the lack of contact with the mononuclear phagocyte system, they fail to establish immunologic tolerance. Any conditions producing a release of antigen would then provide an opportunity for autoantibody formation. This situation occurs when sperm cells or lens and heart tissues are released directly into the circulation, and autoantibodies are formed. Unmodified extracts of tissues involved in organ-specific autoimmune disorders, however, do not readily elicit antibody formation.
- Altered antigens that arise because of chemical, physical, or biologic processes (e.g., hapten complexing, physical denaturation, mutation).
- A foreign antigen that is shared or cross-reactive with self antigens or tissue components.
- Mutation of immunocompetent cells to acquire a responsive to self antigens.
- Loss of the immunoregulatory function by T-lymphocyte subsets.

Understanding the mechanism of autoimmunity requires an understanding of the regulation of the immune response. The immune response involves interaction of cellular elements such as lymphocytes and macrophages, antigen, antibody, immune complexes, and complement.

Table 28-3	Examples of Antigens Implicated in Autoimmune Endocrine Diseases
Disorder	**Antigen**
Hashimoto's disease	Thyroglobulin
	Thyroid peroxidase
	Thyrotropin receptor
Graves' disease	Thyrotropin receptor
	Thyroid peroxidase
	Thyroglobulin
	64-kilodalton (kD) antigen
	70-kD heat shock protein
Type 1 diabetes	Insulin/proinsulin
	Insulin receptor
	Glutamic acid decarboxylase
	B cell release granule
	Pancreatic cytokeratin
	64-kD antigen
	Glucagon
	65-kD heat shock protein
Addison's disease	Adrenal cortical cells
	55-kD microsomal antigen
Idiopathic hypoparathyroidism	200-kD and 130-kD antigens
	Endothelial antigen
	Mitochondrial antigen

SELF-RECOGNITION (TOLERANCE)

In the initial stage of some diseases, infiltration by T lymphocytes may induce inflammation and tissue damage, leading to alterations in self antigens and production of autoantibodies. In other diseases, only production of autoantibodies is noted with tissue damage. These autoantibodies attack cell surface antigens or membrane receptors or combine with antigen to form immune complexes that are deposited in tissue, subsequently causing complement activation and inflammation.

An immune response requires presentation of a foreign antigen by an antigen-presenting cell (APC) and another signal from the appropriate major histocompatibility complex (MHC) molecule on the host's cells. Both are needed for an immune response. **Tolerance** is the lack of immune response to self antigens and is initiated during fetal development (central tolerance) by elimination of cells with the potential to react strongly with self antigens. **Peripheral tolerance** is a process involving mature lymphocytes and occurs in the circulation. **Central tolerance** develops in the thymus during fetal life. Self antigens are presented by dendritic cells to self-reactive T cells that are responsible for both positive selection and negative selection of specific lymphocytes. The ultimate goal is to remove T lymphocytes that respond strongly to self antigens. As genes rearrange and code for antigen receptors, the T-cell receptors (TCRs) that are produced may or may not be specific for the MHC expressed on that individual's cells. Positive-selection cells that have TCRs capable of responding with self antigens (low-level MHC affinity) are selected for continued growth.

Self-recognition (tolerance) is induced by at least two mechanisms involving contact between antigen and immunocompetent cells, as follows:

- Elimination of the small clone of immunocompetent cells programmed to react with the antigen (Burnet's clonal selection theory).
- Induction of unresponsiveness in the immunocompetent cells through excessive antigen binding to them and triggering of a suppressor mechanism. The normal immune response is modulated by both antigen-specific and nonspecific suppressor cell activity.

MAJOR AUTOANTIBODIES

Major autoantibodies can be detected in different disorders. Many diagnostic laboratory tests are based on detecting these autoimmune responses. Common autoantibodies include thyroid, gastric, adrenocortical, striated muscle, acetylcholine receptor, smooth muscle, salivary gland, mitochondrial, reticulin, myelin, islet cell, and skin. Antibodies to antinuclear antibodies (ANAs) include deoxyribonucleic acid (DNA), histone, and nonhistone protein antibodies. The action of specific autoantibodies and their use in medical diagnosis are listed next.

Acetylcholine receptor (AChR)–binding antibody measures antibody to AChRs at neuromuscular junctions of skeletal muscle; useful in the diagnosis of myasthenia gravis.

Acetylcholine receptor (AChR)–blocking antibody measures antibodies to AChRs; found in about one third of patients with myasthenia gravis.

Antiadrenal antibody measures antibodies to adrenal cortex cells. High antibody titers are characteristic of autoimmune hypoadrenalism in about three fourths of cases, but are not found in tuberculous Addison's disease.

Anticardiolipin antibody. Antibodies directed to cardiolipin are present in patients with SLE associated with arterial and venous thromboses and in those with placental infarcts in early pregnancy with or without SLE. Elevation may be predictive of risk of thrombosis or recurrent spontaneous abortions of early pregnancy. Cardiolipin antibodies are also called *lupus anticoagulants* and *phospholipid antibodies.*

Anticentriole antibody measures antibodies to cellular ultrastructures, the centrioles. The appearance of these antibodies is unusual but can be demonstrated in systemic sclerosis.

Anticentromere antibody measures anticentromere (antikinetochore) to chromosomal centromeres. Most patients with calcinosis, Raynaud's phenomenon, esophageal dysfunction, sclerodactyly, and telangiectasia (CREST) syndrome demonstrate these antibodies. They can also be exhibited by about one third of patients with Raynaud's disease and approximately 10% of patients with systemic sclerosis.

Anti-DNA antibody measures antibody to DNA. Increased amounts (>25% by membrane assay) and decreased quantities of the C4 complement component confirm the diagnosis of SLE. These tests are also useful in monitoring the activity and exacerbations of SLE. The absence of anti-DNA is demonstrated in about one fourth of patients with SLE.

Anti–glomerular basement membrane antibody measures the amount of antibody to glomerular basement membrane (anti-GBM). High titers are suggestive of Goodpasture's disease or anti-GBM nephritis. The test is also useful for monitoring anti-GBM nephritis. Negative results, however, do not rule out Goodpasture's disease.

Anti–intrinsic factor antibody measures antibody to intrinsic factor (IF). The presence of IF-blocking antibodies is diagnostic of pernicious anemia and found in approximately 60% of cases.

Anti–islet cell antibody measures antibody to the islet cells of the pancreas. This test is useful as an early marker of beta pancreatic cell destruction.

Anti–liver-kidney microsomal (anti-LKM) antibody measures antibody to components of renal and hepatic microsomes. The presence of a high titer is diagnostic of hepatic disease and suggests aggressive disease.

Antimitochondrial antibody measures antibody to cellular ultrastructures, the mitochondria. A high titer strongly suggests primary biliary cirrhosis (PBC); the absence of mitochondrial antibodies is strong evidence against PBC. Other forms of liver disease frequently exhibit low mitochondrial antibody titers.

Antimyelin antibody measures antibody to components of the myelin sheath of nerves or myelin basic protein. Antibodies to myelin are associated with multiple sclerosis (MS) or other neurologic diseases. Myelin antibodies are not detectable in the cerebrospinal fluid (CSF) of MS patients.

Antimyocardial antibody measures antibody to components of the myocardium. The presence of myocardial antibodies is diagnostic of Dressler's (cardiac injury) syndrome or rheumatic fever.

Antineutrophil antibody is an autoantibody producing a characteristic granular cytoplasmic staining pattern (c-ANCA) to cytoplasmic constituents of neutrophilic granulocytes. Antineutrophil cytoplasmic antibody has been described as a sensitive and specific marker for active Wegener's granulomatosis, a systemic vasculitis. Antibody producing a perinuclear staining of neutrophils (p-ANCA) occurs in a wide range of diseases.

Antinuclear antibody (ANA) measures antibody to nuclear antigens. ANAs are found in 99% of patients with untreated SLE.

Anti–parietal cell antibody measures antibody to parietal cells (large cells on margin of peptic glands of stomach). About 80% of patients with pernicious anemia have parietal cell antibodies. In their presence, gastric biopsy almost always demonstrates gastritis. Low antibody titers to parietal cells are often found with no clinical evidence of pernicious anemia or atrophic gastritis and are sometimes seen in elderly patients.

Antiplatelet antibody measures immunologically attached IgG on platelets. The presence of platelet antibodies, measured indirectly, is associated with immune thrombocytopenia SLE.

Antireticulin antibody measures antibody to reticulin, an albuminoid or scleroprotein substance present in the connective framework of reticular tissue. About 80% of patients with childhood gluten-sensitive enteropathy demonstrate reticulin antibodies. These antibodies can also be found in dermatitis herpetiformis, adult gluten-sensitive enteropathy, and about one fifth of patients with chronic heroin addiction.

Anti–rheumatoid arthritis nuclear antigen (anti-RANA; RA precipitin) measures an antibody to a component of the Epstein-Barr virus (EBV). The antibody is found in most patients with RA and in about 15% of patients with SLE. Anti-RANA is not useful in diagnosis or differential diagnosis of arthritis.

Antiribosome antibody measures the presence of antibody to the cellular organelles, ribosomes. Ribosomal antibodies are found in about 10% of patients with SLE.

Anti–nuclear ribonucleoprotein (anti-nRNP) antibody measures an ANA, nuclear ribonucleoprotein. A high titer of this antibody is characteristic of mixed connective tissue disease (MCTD) or undifferentiated connective tissue disease. In MCTD, anti-nRNP is found in the absence of various other ANAs. Low titers of anti-nRNP are seen in about one third of patients with SLE and are typically found in association with other ANAs such as anti-DNA or anti-Sm.

Anti-Scl antibody or **anti–Scl-70 antibody** measures an antibody to a basic nonhistone nuclear protein. The presence of anti-Scl is diagnostic of systemic sclerosis (SSc); however, it is demonstrable in only about one fifth of SSc patients.

Antiskin (dermal-epidermal) antibody measures antibody to the basement membrane area of the skin. Antibodies are present in more than 80% of patients with bullous pemphigoid, but the absence of antibodies does not rule out the disorder.

Antiskin (interepithelial) antibody measures antibody to intercellular substance of the skin. Antibodies can be detected in 90% of patients with pemphigus; the absence of demonstrable antibody usually excludes the diagnosis. The presence of antibodies is also useful in evaluating blistering disease. A rising antibody titer may indicate an impending relapse of pemphigus, and a falling titer is suggestive of effective control of the disease.

Anti-Sm antibody measures Sm (Smith) antibody to acidic nuclear protein. Sm antibody is demonstrated by about one third of patients with SLE. Presence of the antibody confirms the diagnosis of SLE, but the absence of antibody does not exclude the diagnosis.

Anti–smooth muscle antibody measures antibody to components of smooth muscle. A high and persistent titer is suggestive of the autoimmune form of chronic active hepatitis. Anti–smooth muscle antibodies are also seen in viral disorders such as infectious mononucleosis.

Antisperm antibody evaluates the presence of sperm antibodies. Half of vasectomized men demonstrate the antibody, as well as 40% of men and women with fertility problems.

Anti–SS-A (SS-A precipitin; anti-Ro) antibody detects the presence of antibody to acidic nucleoprotein of human spleen extract. SS-A precipitins are demonstrable in more than 70% of patients with Sjögren's syndrome-sicca complex and are often found in a subset of these patients at risk for vasculitis. The antibody is also found in one third of patients with SLE and in those with Sjögren's syndrome–RA or the annular variety of subacute cutaneous lupus erythematosus. In neonatal lupus erythematosus autoantibodies to SS-A, discoid skin lesions and congenital heart block are common.

Anti–SS-B (SS-B precipitin, anti-La) antibody is demonstrated by most patients with Sjögren's syndrome–SLE. One half to three fourths of patients with Sjögren's syndrome have the antibody; it is frequently found in a subset of these patients at risk for vasculitis.

Antistriational antibody measures antibody to components of striated muscle. Antibodies to striated muscles may be detected in patients with myasthenia gravis or thymoma or in those undergoing penicillamine treatment. Absence of the antibody in patients with myasthenia gravis generally rules out the presence of thymoma.

Antithyroglobulin and antithyroid microsome antibody evaluates the presence of antibodies to the thyroid components: *thyroglobulin,* an iodine-containing protein secreted by the thyroid gland and stored within its colloid substance, and *thyroid microsomes,* particles derived from the endoplasmic reticulum. The presence of microsome antibodies is considered predictive of an elevated thyroid-stimulating hormone (TSH) level. A positive thyroid antibody test and an elevated TSH titer are associated with a risk of hypothyroidism. Absence of both antibodies is strong evidence against autoimmune thyroiditis.

Histone-reactive antinuclear antibody (HR-ANA) measures the presence of HR-ANA. A high titer of HR-ANA is highly suggestive of drug-induced (e.g., hydralazine) lupus erythematosus. HR-ANA may occasionally be demonstrated in patients with SLE.

Jo-1 antibody detects precipitins to an acidic nuclear protein from calf thymus. Approximately one third of patients with uncomplicated polymyositis and some patients with dermatomyositis demonstrate Jo-1 antibody.

Ku antibody detects precipitins to an acidic nuclear protein from calf thymus. About half of patients with overlapping signs and symptoms of scleroderma and polymyositis demonstrate Ku precipitins.

Mi-1 antibody detects antibodies to an acidic nuclear protein from calf thymus. Some patients with dermatomyositis and polymyositis demonstrate Mi-1 antibodies.

PM-1 antibody detects antibodies to an acidic nuclear protein from calf thymus. These precipitins are found in 87% of patients with polymyositis-scleroderma. More than half the patients with polymyositis demonstrate PM-1 antibody, but it is detected in less than one fifth of patients with dermatomyositis.

ORGAN-SPECIFIC AND MIDSPECTRUM DISORDERS

Cardiovascular Disorders

The primary immunologic diseases of the blood vessels are termed *vasculitis;* those of the heart are called *carditis.*

Vasculitis

Deposition of circulating immune complexes is considered directly or indirectly responsible for many forms of vasculitis. The inflammatory lesions of blood vessels produce variable injury or necrosis of the blood vessel wall. This may result in narrowing, occlusion, or thrombosis of the lumen or aneurysm formation or rupture. Vasculitis occurs as a primary disease process or as a secondary manifestation of another disease (e.g., RA).

Vasculitis is characterized by inflammation within blood vessels, which often results in a compromise of the vessel

Box 28-2 Examples in Classification of Vasculitic Syndromes

Systemic necrotizing arteritis
   Polyarteritis nodosa
   Allergic angiitis and granulomatosis
   Overlap syndrome
Hypersensitivity vasculitis
   Henoch-Schönlein purpura
   McDuffie's syndrome
Wegener's granulomatosis
Lymphomatoid granulomatosis
Giant cell arteritis
   Takayasu's arteritis
Mucocutaneous lymph node syndrome (Kawasaki's disease)
Behçet's disease
Thromboangiitis obliterans
Central nervous system vasculitis
Miscellaneous
   Cogan's syndrome
   Eales disease
   Hypereosinophilic syndrome with vasculitis

lumen with ischemia. Ischemia causes the major manifestations of the vasculitic syndromes and determines the prognosis. Any size and type of blood vessel may be involved. Therefore the vasculitic syndromes are a heterogeneous group of diseases (Box 28-2).

Antibody specific to endothelial cells also contributes to immune vasculopathy. Antiendothelial antibodies are autoantibodies directed against antigens in the cytoplasmic membrane of endothelial cells.

Carditis

The heart shares with other organs a susceptibility to immune-mediated injury. Numerous cardiac diseases are characterized by the presence of inflammatory cells within the myocardium resulting from immune sensitization to endogenous or exogenous cardiac antigens. The consequent reaction of cardiac myocytes to immune injury can range from reversible modulation of their electrical and mechanical capabilities to cell death. Carditis can be caused by a variety of conditions, including acute rheumatic fever, Lyme disease, and cardiac transplant rejection.

Myocardial contractility can be impaired by cell-mediated injury or local release of cytokines. The study of immune cardiac disease has entered a period of rapid expansion. *Primary idiopathic myocarditis* is an autoimmune disease characterized by infiltration of the heart by macrophages and lymphocytes. Studies involving the mechanisms by which immune cells and factors localize in the myocardium, modulate myocyte function, and remodel myocardial architecture are under way.

A diagnosis of acute rheumatic fever requires differentiation from other immunologic and infectious diseases. The immunologic basis for rheumatic heart disease has long been suspected. Patients with rheumatic heart disease exhibit antimyocardial antibodies that bind in vitro to foci in the myocardium and heart valves. These antibodies may be responsible for the deposition of immunoglobulin and complement components found in the same area of rheumatic heart disease tissues at autopsy.

Antimyocardial antibodies appear to be strongly cross-reactive with streptococcal antigens, but they are not toxic to heart tissue unless the latter is damaged previously by some other cause. Because antimyocardial antibodies are often found in patients with a recent myocardial infarction or streptococcal infection without cardiac sequelae, detection of these antibodies has not been a particularly useful differential diagnostic test for cardiac injury. The presence of myocardial antibodies, however, is diagnostic of Dressler's syndrome (cardiac injury) or rheumatic fever.

Collagen Vascular Disorders

Progressive Systemic Sclerosis (Scleroderma)
Scleroderma is a collagen vascular disease of unknown etiology that assumes various forms. *Eosinophilic fasciitis* may be a variant of scleroderma.

Development of scleroderma has been associated with a number of occupations and with drugs such as bleomycin sulfate, tryptophan, and carbidopa. Occupational exposure to vinyl chloride, vibratory stimuli, and silicosis have been associated with subsequent development of scleroderma.

Epidemiology. Scleroderma occurs in all races and three times more frequently in women than men.

Signs and Symptoms. Scleroderma is characterized by fibrosis in skin and internal organs and by arterial occlusions with a distinct proliferative pattern. Initial symptoms usually appear in the third decade of life. Raynaud's phenomenon is the most frequent manifestation. The disease is slowly progressive and chronically disabling, but it can be rapidly progressive and fatal.

Immunologic Manifestations. Idiopathic scleroderma is considered an autoimmune disease because of the associated autoantibodies and the overlapping syndromes of scleroderma-polymyositis and scleroderma-SLE.

Antinuclear antibodies are formed in 40% to 90% of patients to (1) extractable nuclear antigens, (2) the nucleolus, (3) the centromere, and (4) Scl-70. The anticentromere antibody is sensitive and is specific for patients with a subset of scleroderma with CREST syndrome.

In addition, T-cell hyperactivity correlates with disease activity. Activated T cells can result in both the vascular changes and the increased collagen production in scleroderma. It is now thought that both the vascular disorder and the fibrosis result from this cellular immune activation. Vascular injury could be mediated by cytokines or direct cell-cell interaction by activated lymphocytes and endothelial cells.

Signs and Symptoms. Systemic sclerosis is a chronic, multisystem disorder that causes thickening of the skin (**scleroderma**) and involves other organ systems.

In more than half of patients, Raynaud's phenomenon occurs before the onset of other manifestations. Skin manifestations can proceed through the stages of pitting edema, a sclerotic "hidebound" stage, and a final stage of atrophy or softening and a return toward normal. Articular complaints are common. Hypomotility of the gastrointestinal tract is the second most common clinical feature.

Eosinophilia-Myalgia Syndrome

Many people exposed to the agent causing eosinophilia-myalgia syndrome (EMS) may develop illness. Patients develop severe myalgia. More than half of patients with EMS develop scleroderma-like manifestations.

The most important predictor of EMS is ingestion of contaminated L-tryptophan. The association of ingestion of L-tryptophan with a systemic disease now called EMS was first observed in 1989. Some patients have died from the L-tryptophan.

L-Tryptophan was widely used after it was introduced in 1974 as an over-the-counter nostrum for various ailments (e.g., insomnia, premenstrual syndrome, anxiety). Medical professionals also recommended its use for neuropsychiatric or fibromyalgia disorders.

Endocrine Gland Disorders

Numerous endocrine gland disorders are attributable to an autoimmune process. Several of the classic and more common disorders are discussed in this section.

Thyroid

The clinical spectrum of autoimmune thyroid disease is very broad. There are two major forms of autoimmune thyroid disease: chronic autoimmune thyroiditis and Graves' disease. Lymphoid (Hashimoto's) chronic thyroiditis is a classic example of an organ-specific autoimmune disorder.

Other autoimmune disorders affecting the thyroid gland include transient thyroiditis syndrome and idiopathic hypothyroidism.

Lymphoid (Hashimoto's) Chronic Thyroiditis

Etiology. The exact mechanism is unknown but is believed to be related to an autoimmune process in which the development of circulating cytotoxic antibodies eventually destroys the thyroid gland, producing hypothyroidism. This disorder is associated with the presence of HLA-DR4 and DR5. However, these associations are not consistent in different races and ethnic groups.

Epidemiology. Lymphoid thyroiditis can occur at any age but is first diagnosed most often in the third to fifth decade of life and is much more common in women than in men. The fibrous variant of the disease is more often present in middle-age and older patients.

The mode of inheritance is unknown. However, a genetic tendency to inherit the trait for the development of antibodies against the thyroid gland is highly possible. It is common to have multiple members of a family develop the same disease (e.g., Graves' disease, lymphoid thyroiditis).

Signs and Symptoms. Lymphoid thyroiditis is believed to be the most common cause of sporadic goiter. Characteristically, there is a firm, diffusely enlarged, nontender thyroid gland that may be lobulated. Hypothyroidism, however, is a common late sequela of lymphoid thyroiditis, and patients are usually euthyroid when first seen by a physician. Some individuals have clinical and pathologic evidence of the coexistence of both Graves' disease and lymphoid (Hashimoto's) thyroiditis. Histologically, Hashimoto's thyroiditis is characterized by diffuse lymphocytic infiltration (Figure 28-2).

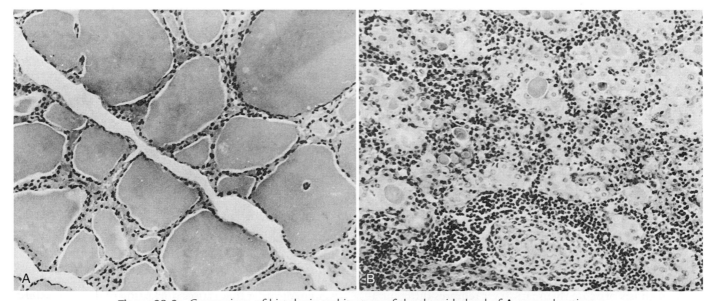

Figure 28-2   Comparison of histologic architecture of the thyroid gland of **A,** normal patient, and **B,** patient with Hashimoto's disease. In the normal thyroid, colloid fills the vesicles, but in a diseased gland, only isolated deposits of colloid are seen. The cell infiltrate is lymphoid in nature. Note germinal center in *B,* lower middle. *(From Anderson JR, Buchanan WW, Goudie RB: Autoimmunity, Springfield, Ill, 1967, Charles C Thomas.)*

Immunologic Manifestations

Patients with lymphoid thyroiditis, as well as other autoimmune thyroid disorders, can demonstrate histologic and immunologic manifestations of the disease. Antibodies to thyroid constituents may be observed in these patients. Antibodies to the following constituents may be demonstrated serologically:

- Thyroglobulin
- Thyroid microsome
- Second colloid antigen (CA2 antigen)
- Thyroid membrane receptors
- Thyronine (T_4) and triiodothyronine (T_3)

Thyroglobulin. Antithyroglobulin (TgAb) was the first antibody discovered against a thyroid protein, thyroglobulin. Immunofluorescent laboratory methods using fluorescein-labeled anti–human globulin can demonstrate the binding of antithyroglobulin antibody to thin sections of thyroid tissue in abnormal conditions or in approximately 4% of the normal population. the frequency of positive titers gradually increases in the female population with aging. The absence of antithyroglobulin antibodies, however, does not exclude the diagnosis of Hashimoto's thyroiditis; conversely, the presence of antibodies does not establish the diagnosis because it can be positive in Graves' disease and is occasionally positive in thyroid cancer and subacute thyroiditis. Testing for antibody may also be used to monitor patients with thyroid cancers.

Thyroid Microsomes. Antibodies directed against thyroid microsomes, antithyroid microsomal antibodies or antithyroperoxidase antibodies (TPO Abs) can be detected in about 7% of the population, with titers ranging from 1:100 to 1:1600. Even a low titer of antithyroid antibodies correlates with a degree of thyroid involvement by an autoimmune process. The absence of antibodies has been documented in diagnosed cases of autoimmune thyroiditis, which may be explained by special characteristics of the antibody, or because it forms complexes with thyroglobulins in the circulation and escapes detection. The presence of such circulating complexes has been documented in patients with thyroid autoimmune disorders.

Second Colloid Antigen. CA2 antigen is directed against a colloid protein and can be detected by immunofluorescent examination. Antibody to CA2 is present in about 50% of patients who have subacute thyroiditis, and it is detectable in some patients with Hashimoto's thyroiditis whose sera show no other evidence of abnormal antibodies.

Thyroid Membrane Receptors. The thyroid membrane receptors are a group of immunoglobulin G (IgG) antibodies that interact with receptors on thyroid membranes. They often produce hyperthyroidism that manifests itself clinically, chemically, and histologically. At present, classification of these IgG antibodies is operational, based on their method of detection. *Long-acting thyroid stimulator* (LATS) and *long-acting thyroid stimulator protector* (LATS-P) assays are of importance.

Thyronine and Triiodothyronine. Antibodies to T_4 and T_3 have been found in several patients, most of whom had evidence of a thyroid autoimmune process such as goiter or hypothyroidism. In these cases the underlying autoimmune process is most likely responsible for the hypothyroidism rather than hormone binding by the circulating antithyronine antibodies.

Diagnostic Evaluation

Fine-needle aspiration biopsy of the thyroid is useful in conjunction with clinical evaluation and serologic studies in the diagnosis of lymphocytic thyroiditis.

Histologic examination of thyroid tissue demonstrates variable infiltration of the entire gland with lymphocytes. Germinal lymphoid centers are characteristic, and destruction and distortion of normal thyroid follicles are apparent. The thyroid cells remain intact but are hypertrophied, although the usual heterogeneity of small, enlarged thyroid follicles, some containing flat epithelium, also can be seen. In advanced cases, there is almost complete destruction of normal thyroid tissue, with replacement by lymphocytes or fibrous tissue.

When the disease produces hypothyroidism, a slight increase in the plasma TSH concentration can usually be demonstrated in the early phase, followed by a fall in serum T_4 and eventually by a fall in serum T_3. Antithyroglobulin and/or antithyroid microsomal antibodies are found in moderate to high titers in more than 50% of patients, but the presence of antimicrosomal antibodies is considered to be more diagnostic.

Antibodies directed against thyroid microsomal antigen (thyroid peroxidase antibody [anti-TPO]) can be detected by various techniques (Table 28-4). Chemiluminescent immunoassay is typically performed to detect anti-TPO autoantibodies. TPO plays a significant role in the biosynthesis of

Table 28-4	Antithyroid Antibody Tests
Antigen	**Test To Identify Antibody**
Thyroglobulin	Indirect immunofluorescence on fixed thyroid tissues
	Tanned red blood cell (RBC) hemagglutination
	Immunometric assays (IMAs) or sandwich methods
	Radioimmunoassay (RIA)
Microsomal antigen	Enzyme-linked immunosorbent assay (ELISA)
Second colloid antigen (CA2)	Indirect immunofluorescence
Thyroid membrane receptors	Long-acting thyroid stimulator (LATS)
	Long-acting thyroid stimulator protector (LATS-P)
	In vitro assays for thyroid-stimulating immunoglobulin (TSI) or thyroid-stimulating hormone (TSH)–binding inhibition (TBI)
Triiodohyronine (total T_3)	RIA using different separation methods
	Electrophoresis with radioactive-labeled thyronines

thyroid hormones by catalyzing both the iodination of tyrosyl residues in thyroglobulin and the coupling of the iodotyrosyl residues to form T_4 and T_3. Autoantibodies produced against TPO are capable of inhibiting the enzyme activity. They are also complement-fixing antibodies that can induce cytotoxic changes in cells and consequently cause thyroid dysfunction. More than 90% of patients with autoimmune thyroiditis (Hashimoto's thyroiditis) have anti-TPO. Antibodies to TPO have also been found in most patients with idiopathic hypothyroidism (85%) and Graves' disease (50%).

Pancreatic Disorders

Insulin-Dependent Diabetes Mellitus

Etiology. Insulin-dependent diabetes mellitus (IDDM), or type 1 diabetes mellitus, is a disorder of deficient insulin production caused by immune destruction of the B cells of the pancreatic islets. The only definitively identified environmental factor causing IDDM is congenital rubella infection. Reports of an association between diabetes and infection with coxsackievirus B and several other viruses suggest other triggers for the disease.

Genetic susceptibility factors have been identified. IDDM is associated with HLA-DR3, DR4, DQ2, and DQ8 antigens. About 90% of Caucasian patients with IDDM have either one or both DR antigens. The presence of both DR3 and DR4 antigens yields an even higher risk of disease development than the additive susceptibility from either antigen, suggesting that other MHC-related genes may be involved in pathogenesis. Another HLA antigen, DR2, is found less frequently in people with diabetes than in the general population, indicating that this antigen is associated with some type of protective effect. HLA-DQw8 is associated with a twofold to sixfold increased risk for diabetes. Several lines of investigation have implicated the CD4+ T lymphocyte as central in the immune process that leads to the development of diabetes.

Epidemiology. IDDM was previously called "juvenile-onset diabetes" because of the time of life in which it often presents; 10% of people with diabetes have IDDM, and approximately 10,000 new cases are diagnosed each year. Most patients develop IDDM in childhood or early adolescence, but it may occur at any age. Approximately 95% of patients who develop clinical diabetes before age 30 years have IDDM.

Signs and Symptoms. The central clinical feature is the requirement for exogenous insulin to maintain euglycemia.

Immunologic Manifestations. T cells of the CD4+ type are responsible for initiating the immune response to the islets that results in islet cell autoantibodies and B-cell destruction. Patients with IDDM have the following types of autoantibodies:

- Antiinsulin (IAA)
- Anti–glutamic acid decarboxylase (GAD)
- Anti–islet cell antigen 2 (IA-2)

Antibodies reacting with the cells of the pancreatic islets have been found in patients with diabetes accompanying autoimmune endocrine disorders. Autoantibodies to islet-related antigens precede the development of clinical IDDM by a prolonged period, often several years. A higher incidence of these anti–islet cell antibodies, however, has been demonstrated in patients with IDDM.

An immunoglobulin in the sera of patients with insulin-resistant diabetes appears to bind to a tissue receptor for insulin, which prevents some of the biologic effects of insulin. In addition, antibodies that bind to and possibly kill pancreatic islet cells have been found in most young patients with IDDM.

A small subgroup of patients with IDDM has demonstrated antireceptor antibody (InR), an IgG class of antibodies directed against the insulin receptor. Antibodies to InR may be directed to the binding site or to determinants away from the binding site for insulin. This condition is predominant in non-Caucasian females of all ages.

Anti–islet cell antigen 2 (IA-2) is directed against a phosphatase-type transmembrane 37-kD islet beta-cell antigen (ICA512).

Autoimmune Pancreatitis

Autoimmune pancreatitis is a heterogeneous disease. This type of chronic pancreatitis is characterized by an autoimmune inflammatory process in which prominent lymphocyte infiltration with associated fibrosis of the pancreas causes organ dysfunction.

Etiology. Although the cause of the disorder is unknown, it is thought to be a systemic autoimmune disorder. It is frequently associated with other autoimmune disorders (e.g., RA).

Epidemiology. Autoimmune pancreatitis is rare, but an increasing number of cases has been reported in the last decade. Although this condition can occur in both genders, it is at least twice as common in men as women. Most patients are older than 50 years at diagnosis.

Signs and Symptoms. Symptoms vary. Many patients have jaundice; some have abdominal pain. Histologic examination of pancreatic tissue reveals a collarlike periductal infiltrate composed of lymphocytes and plasma cells. Computed tomography (CT) typically reveals a diffuse enlargement of the pancreas with a halo around the peripheral rim of the organ. Various findings on imaging radiography are correlated with serologic and histologic analysis. It is important to diagnose autoimmune pancreatitis correctly on the basis of imaging, histology, and serology because it can mimic pancreatic cancer.

Immunologic Manifestations. In the Japanese population, an association between HLA haplotype DRB1*0405-DQB1*0401 has been observed. Immunologic abnormalities include the following:

- Hypergammaglobulinemia (elevated serum IgG or gamma globulin level) in patients with enhanced peripheral rim "halo" of the pancreas on CT scan.
- Elevated serum IgG4 concentrations in patients with a diffusely enlarged pancreas.
- Autoantibodies against carbonic anhydrase II (ACA II), lactoferrin (antilactoferrin antibody, ALA), anti–smooth

muscle antibody (ASMA), or antinuclear antibody (ANA).
- Increased number of CD4+ T lymphocytes in peripheral blood.

Adrenal Glands

Idiopathic adrenal atrophy is the primary cause of *Addison's disease*. It is believed that many of these cases are autoimmune in etiology. Women are afflicted twice as often as men. The disease usually presents in the third or fourth decade of life. Although a great potential exists for morbidity, it has a relatively low incidence. The adult form of Addison's disease is associated with HLA class II antigens DR3 and DR4.

Idiopathic Addison's disease is usually diagnosed in patients because of low serum cortisol levels in the presence of elevated levels of corticotropin. Approximately 80% of patients manifest serum antibodies against cortical elements, probably microsomal. Some cases demonstrate antibodies against adrenal cell surfaces. These antibodies generally bind to components in the adrenal cortex but affect only individual zones. Antibodies are generally low in titer and are not a direct reflection of adrenal cell damage. In women with premature ovarian failure, autoimmune destruction of the ovarian stroma has been observed.

Pituitary Gland

Sheehan's syndrome, lymphocytic adenohypophysitis, is a disorder that causes rapid decline in pituitary function. This disorder is most frequently seen in postpartum women. Antibodies against pituitary cells are observed in some patients. The disorder is distinguished by a mononuclear infiltrate of the pituitary gland and hypophysis.

Parathyroid Gland

Idiopathic hypoparathyroidism occurs both as a childhood disorder in type I polyglandular syndrome, and less often as an isolated disorder in adults. It is associated with complement-mediated cytotoxicity of parathyroid cells, indicating a specific immune response to the parathyroid. Several antigens have been associated with this disorder, including endothelial cell proteins and mitochondria.

Polyglandular Syndromes

Three syndromes of associated endocrinopathies have been defined as the "polyglandular syndromes." *Type I polyglandular syndrome* involves mucocutaneous candidiasis and associated endocrinopathies that begin in early childhood. Patients initially develop candidiasis and hypoparathyroidism, but more than half also develop Addison's disease. Gonadal failure, alopecia, and chronic hepatitis are also seen. Patients have organ-specific autoantibodies and poorly defined defects in cell-mediated immunity.

Type II polyglandular syndrome involves the combined occurrence of either IDDM or autoimmune thyroid disease with Addison's disease. It is also called *Schmidt's syndrome.* This type of disorder is seen primarily in women in the second or third decades of life. Most cases are familial, but the mode of inheritance is unknown. There is a strong association with HLA-DR3.

Type III polyglandular syndrome is defined as autoimmune thyroid disease occurring with two other autoimmune disorders, including IDDM, pernicious anemia, or a nonendocrine, organ-specific autoimmune disorder such as myasthenia gravis. These patients do not have Addison's disease. The HLA-DR3 allele is present in more than 50% of cases. Patients in this category are overwhelmingly female.

Reproductive Disorders

Antibodies against cytoplasmic components of different cells of the ovary have been demonstrated in Addison's disease and in premature ovarian failure, which may be an immune disorder causing reproductive failure and eventually early menopause. A prevalence of smooth muscle antibody, ANA, and antiphospholipid antibodies has been found in women with unexplained infertility. In addition, autoantibodies to the ovary and gonadotropin receptors are measured in many women with polyendocrinopathies.

Patients with endometriosis have a defect in natural killer (NK) cell activity. This results in decreased cytotoxicity for autologous endometrial cells. Reduced T lymphocyte–mediated cytotoxicity to endometrial cells has also been found.

A sizable proportion of pregnancy losses may be caused by immunologic factors. The fetus is an immunogenic allograft that evokes a protective immune response from the mother, which is necessary for implantation and growth. The mechanism of pregnancy loss is hypothesized to involve two antiphospholipid antibodies. Lupus anticoagulant and anticardiolipin antibodies are directed against platelets and vascular endothelium. This causes vascular destruction and thrombosis, leading to fetal death and abortion. There is no evidence of a direct immunologic attack on the embryo. A human fetus is capable of survival in utero if it does not share a significant number of maternal MHC antigens, especially HLA-B and HLA-DR and DQ loci.

Antisperm antibodies have been detected in the serum of both men and women, in cervical mucus of women, in seminal fluid of men, and attached to sperm cells. In seminal fluid the immobilizing antibodies to sperm are usually of the IgG class, and the agglutinating antibodies are IgA. Elevated levels of antibodies to sperm have been found in more than 40% of men after vasectomy but only occasionally in men with primary testicular agenesis. Allergy-like reactions to seminal fluid have also been observed. These reactions range from local reactions to systemic reactions, including life-threatening anaphylaxis. The allergen is usually one or more prostatic proteins, but it can include IgE to spermatozoa.

Exocrine Gland Disorder

Sjögren's Syndrome

Etiology. Sjögren's syndrome is a chronic inflammatory disease of unknown etiology that affects lacrimal, salivary, and other excretory glands. It results in keratoconjunctivitis sicca and xerostomia.

As with RA and SLE, etiologic factors include infection, abnormalities of immune regulation, and genetic factors. Development of Sjögren's syndrome is strongly associated with HLA-B8 and HLA-DR3. Infectious origin is suggested. Clear evidence for excessive B-cell activity has been demonstrated, but it is not known whether this is caused by B- or T-cell abnormalities.

Epidemiology. A primary form is not associated with other diseases; a secondary form is associated with RA and other connective tissue diseases. About 90% of patients are women. A 44-fold increased incidence of lymphoma has been noted in patients with Sjögren's syndrome.

Signs and Symptoms The main clinical manifestations of Sjögren's syndrome are dry eyes, dry mouth, and recurrent salivary gland pain and swelling (Table 28-5). Hoarseness, chronic cough, and increased incidence of infection have been observed. Dryness of the vagina leads to dyspareunia and itching. Dysphagia and atrophic gastritis can also be present. Extraglandular involvement results in interstitial pneumonitis and fibrosis. Renal tubular acidosis and vasculitis involving peripheral nerves and the central nervous system (CNS) can also result from Sjögren's syndrome.

Immunologic Manifestations. The immunologic characteristics of Sjögren's syndrome include hypergammaglobulinemia, ANAs, rheumatoid factor, autoantibodies to salivary duct and other antigens, and lymphocyte and plasma cell infiltration of involved tissue. Antibodies are usually polyclonal and may result in the hyperviscosity syndrome and hypergammaglobulinemic purpura. Speckled or homogeneous ANA patterns are present in 65% of patients and are present more frequently in primary Sjögren's syndrome. Antibodies to Sjögren's syndrome–A antigen have been associated with vasculitis in primary Sjögren's syndrome. Antibodies to Sjögren's syndrome–B antigen are almost always found in association with Sjögren's syndrome–A antigen and only occur in SLE and Sjögren's syndrome. Rheumatoid factor is found in 90% of cases. A novel autoantibody, anti–alpha-Fodrin, has been found in the sera of a majority of patients with primary Sjögren's syndrome. This antibody may be pathophysiologically associated with some extra-glandular manifestations characteristically seen in patients with Sjögren's syndrome.

Autoantibodies to salivary duct antigens are frequently detected in patients with secondary Sjögren's syndrome. They are also common in one fourth of patients with RA without Sjögren's syndrome. Mitochondrial antibodies are detected in 10% of patients with primary Sjögren's syndrome and rarely in patients with secondary Sjögren's syndrome and RA. Patients with primary Sjögren's syndrome also have higher levels of antibodies to the thyroid gland, gastric parietal cells, pancreatic epithelial cells, and smooth muscle. Lymphocytic infiltration of the exocrine glands of the eyes, mouth, nose, lower respiratory tract, gastrointestinal (GI) tract, and vagina occurs. The infiltrate is composed of B and T cells. In tissue culture these cells produce large amounts of IgM and IgG. T cells are predominantly helper cells.

Gastrointestinal Disorders

Atrophic Gastritis and Pernicious Anemia

A malfunctioning immune system can target the stomach lining, resulting in autoimmune gastritis, characterized by chronic inflammation of the gastric mucosa. Persons with autoimmune gastritis may progress to pernicious anemia (PA). Autoimmune gastritis is characterized by the presence of serum autoantibodies against gastric parietal cells, H^+/K^+-ATPase (proton pump), and the cobalamin-absorbing protein, intrinisic factor.

Immunologic Findings. Antibodies against a lipoprotein cytoplasmic component of gastric parietal cells can be detected by immunofluorescence in up to 90% of PA patients and in about 60% of patients with atrophic gastritis without hematologic abnormalities. These antibodies may also be demonstrated in patients with other autoimmune diseases such as thyroiditis. In addition, antibodies can be found in asymptomatic patients and in persons more than 60 years old.

Histologic Findings. Atrophic gastritis, which almost always accompanies PA, is characterized by destruction of the gastric mucosa with lymphocytic infiltration and the absence of parietal and chief cells. The lesions are associated with decreased synthesis of gastric acid and intrinsic factor. Intrinsic factor normally binds ingested vitamin B_{12} at one site and binds to receptors in the distal ileum at another site. Therefore, vitamin B_{12} transport across the ileum is affected.

Vitamin B_{12} (Cobalamin) Transport. Cobalamin transport is mediated by three different binding proteins capable of binding the vitamin at its required physiologic concentrations: intrinsic factor, transcobalamin II, and the R proteins (Table 28-6).

Intrinsic factor (IF), a glycoprotein, is synthesized and secreted by the parietal cells of the mucosa in the fundus region of the stomach in several mammalian species, including humans. In a healthy state, the amounts of IF secreted by the stomach greatly exceed the quantities required to bind ingested cobalamin in its coenzyme forms. At a very

Table 28-5	Criteria for Diagnosis Sjögren's Syndrome

Four or More of the Following Criteria Must Be Present

Ocular symptoms	Dry eyes daily for 3 months, sand or gravel feeling in eyes
Oral symptoms	Dry mouth daily for 3 months or recurrent or persistent swollen glands
Ocular signs	Post-Schirmer test or rose bengal score >4
Histopathology	Aggregates of ≥50 mononuclear cells/4 mm² of glandular tissue
Autoantibodies	Presence of anti-Ro (SS-A), anti-La (SS-B), or antinuclear antibodies (ANAs), or rheumatoid factor

From Vitali C: Preliminary criteria for the classification of Sjögren's syndrome: results of a prospective concerted action supported by the European community, *Arthritis Rheum* 36:36, 1993.

Table 28-6	Vitamin B$_{12}$ (Cobalamin)–Binding Proteins		
	Intrinsic Factor	**Transcobalamin II**	**R Proteins**
Source	Stomach	Liver, other tissues	Leukocytes, ? other tissues
Function	Intestinal absorption	Delivery to cells	Excretion storage
Membrane receptors	Ileal enterocytes	Many cells	Liver cells

acidic pH, cobalamin splits from dietary protein and combines with IF to form a vitamin-IF complex. Binding by IF is extraordinarily specific and is lost with even slight changes in the cobalamin molecule. This complex is stable and remains unabsorbed until it reaches the ileum. In the ileum the vitamin-IF complex attaches to specific receptor sites present only on the outer surface of microvillus membranes of ileal enterocytes.

The release of this complex from the mucosal cells, with subsequent transport to the tissues, depends on **transcobalamin II (TCII).** TCII is a plasma polypeptide synthesized by the liver and probably several other tissues. TCII, which turns over very rapidly in the plasma, acts as the acceptor and principal carrier of the vitamin to the liver and other tissues, as with IF. Receptors for TCII are observed on the plasma membranes of a wide variety of cells. TCII is also capable of binding a few unusual cobalamin analogs. TCII also stimulates cobalamin uptake by reticulocytes.

The **R proteins** compose an antigenically cross-reactive group of cobalamin-binding glycoproteins. The R proteins bind cobalamin and various cobalamin analogs. Their function is unknown, but they appear to serve as storage sites and as a means of eliminating excess cobalamin and unwanted analogs from the blood circulation through receptor sites on liver cells. R proteins are produced by leukocytes and perhaps other tissues. They are present in plasma as transcobalamin I and transcobalamin III, as well as in saliva, milk, and other body fluids. Transcobalamin I probably serves only as a backup transport system for endogenous cobalamin. Endogenous vitamin is synthesized in the human GI tract by bacterial action, but none is adsorbed.

Autoimmune Liver Disease

Autoimmune processes are believed to be the possible cause of chronic liver disease. Hypergammaglobulinemia, prominent lymphocyte and plasma cell inflammation of the liver, and the presence of one or more circulating tissue antibodies are typically manifested. These manifestations suggest an organ-localized autoimmune pathogenesis.

Chronic active hepatitis, for example, is an inflammatory condition most common in young women. It is characterized by prominent lymphocyte and plasma cell inflammatory changes, which start in the portal tracts. In some patients this condition results from a chronic viral infection or inflammation, but in others a number of immunologic abnormalities are present to varying degrees, in addition to hypergammaglobulinemia and an elevated erythrocyte sedimentation rate (ESR). A defect in immunoregulation is often

demonstrated, which may lead to unrestrained immunoglobulin production. These patients display ANAs and anti-smooth muscle antibodies. A high and persistent titer of antismooth antibodies is suggestive of the autoimmune form of chronic active hepatitis or viral disorders such as infectious mononucleosis.

In some cases this disease is referred to as *lupoid hepatitis.* Patients with aggressive chronic active hepatitis have a poor prognosis, and a significant rate of mortality is reported 5 years after diagnosis.

Idiopathic Biliary Cirrhosis

Idiopathic biliary cirrhosis is a slowly progressive disease that starts as an apparently noninfectious inflammation in the bile ducts of young to middle-age women. An increased familial incidence has been noted.

Patients exhibit increased serum immunoglobulin M (IgM); depression of cellular immunity, with prominent decreases in suppressor T cells common; and associated autoimmune disorders. It is believed that tissue damage results from an unmodulated attack against host tissue antigens. Antimitochondrial antibodies directed against the cellular ultrastructures, mitochondria, can be displayed. A high titer of antimicrobial antibody strongly suggests primary biliary cirrhosis (PBC); an absence of mitochondrial antibodies is strong evidence against PBC. Other forms of liver disease, however, frequently exhibit low mitochondrial antibody titers.

Inflammatory Bowel Disease

Inflammatory bowel disease (IBD) is the collective name given to **Crohn's disease** (CD) and **ulcerative colitis** (UC). A major gene has been identified in these disorders. The Centers for Disease Control and Prevention (CDC) estimates that IBD, which is more common among Ashkenazi Jews than other groups, affects more than 1 million Americans. When researchers have examined more than 300,000 single nucleotide polymorphisms (SNPs), the variations that occur when a nucleotide, a molecular subunit of DNA, is altered, it was discovered that the frequency of variations in the receptor gene for interleukin-23 (IL-23) was significantly different for persons with IBD. A coding variant that apparently protects against IBD is found less frequently in patients with IBD than in healthy patients.

Many factors (e.g., genetic susceptibility, diet) affect onset and development of IBC. The crux of the disease is an abnormal immune response to harmless bacteria in the gut that benefit the host by providing energy and nutrient. In IBC patients, these microorganisms become a target for attack by the immune system. Inflammation seen in IBD patients has been linked to the following:

- Presence of increased levels of inflammation-promoting cytokines.
- Protein molecules used by cells of the immune system to communicate with each other.

Studies suggest that one cytokine, IL-12, is a crucial mediator of this disease. IL-12 causes inflammation by activating a class of different immune cells, type 1 helper T (Th1) cells, which in turn secrete proinflammatory molecules such as interferon gamma (IFN-γ) and tumor necrosis factor alpha (TNF-α). These pathways have been suggested as new therapeutic targets for human IBD.

The discovery of IL-23 has led some to question the central role of IL-12 and Th1 cells in IBD. New information reveals that IL-12 and IL-23 are closely related molecules that share a common subunit known as p40. IL-23 has been associated with the activation of a new class of proinflammatory T cells called Th17. These cells secrete the proinflammatory cytokine IL-17, which mediates the inflammatory response in organs such as the brain and joints. Intestinal inflammation is still associated with large increases in IL-17 production in the intestine. Innate immune cells present in inflamed intestine (e.g., granulocytes, monocytes) have been found to contribute to increased production of IL-17.

Immune Markers. The following serologic markers have been found to be useful in the diagnosis and differentiation of CD and UC:

- Deoxyribonuclease (DNase I)–sensitive perinuclear antineutrophil cytoplasmic autoantibody (p-ANCA). IBC-associated p-ANCA defines an antibody to a nuclear antigen that is sensitive to DNase I.
- Anti–*Saccharomyces cervisiae* antibody (ASCA), present in the serum of up to 70% of CD patients.
- Pancreatic antibody, observed in approximately 30% percent of CD patients.
- Anti–outer membrane porin from *Escherichia coli* (anti-OmpC). An IgA response to OmpC is observed in 55% of CD patients.

Celiac Disease

Celiac disease is a lifelong autoimmune intestinal disorder found in individuals who are genetically susceptible. Damage to the mucosal surface of the small intestine is caused by an immunologically toxic reaction to the ingestion of gluten and interferes with the absorption of nutrients. Celiac disease is unique in that a specific food component, *gluten,* has been identified as the trigger. Gluten is the common name for the offending proteins in specific cereal grains that are harmful to persons with celiac disease. These proteins are found in all forms of wheat (e.g., durum, semolina, spelt, kamut, einkorn, faro) and related grains (rye, barley, triticale) and must be eliminated.

Other Immunologic Disorders of Gastrointestinal Tract

Examples of other immunologic disorders related to the GI and hepatobiliary tracts include GI allergy, Whipple's disease, immunoproliferative intestinal disease (alpha heavy-chain disease), and infectious hepatitis (see Chapter 23). Allergy of the GI tract is an IgE-mediated hypersensitivity to food substances that involves the GI tract and in some cases the skin and lungs. Examples of systemic autoimmune disease caused by mucosal immune abnormalities are IgA nephropathy (Berger's disease), Henoch-Schönlein purpura, and diseases associated with circulating IgA complexes in the kidney and vasculature. Immunoproliferative intestinal disease is characterized by monoclonal B cells that produce an aberrant alpha heavy chain.

Autoimmune Hematologic Disorders

Various hematologic conditions can be caused by alloantibodies and autoantibodies (Table 28-7).

Autoimmune Hemolytic Anemia

Autoimmune hemolytic anemia can be classified into the following four groups:

- Warm-reactive autoantibodies (most common)
- Cold-reactive autoantibodies (<20% of cases)
- Paroxysmal cold hemoglobinuria (rare)
- Drug-induced hemolysis (<20% of cases)

Warm Autoimmune Hemolytic Anemia. This anemia is associated with antibodies reactive at warm temperatures (i.e., 37° C). In more than three fourths of cases, the erythrocytes are coated with both IgG and complement, although some may demonstrate coating with IgG alone or less often with complement coating. In warm autoimmune hemolytic anemia, negligible serum autoantibody exists because the antibody reacts optimally at 37° C and is being continuously adsorbed by red blood cells (RBCs) in vivo. Elution of the antibody from the RBCs (mechanical removal of anti-

Table 28-7	Immunohematologic Diseases
Category	**Examples**
Immune hemolysis	Warm autoimmune hemolytic anemia
	Cold agglutinin disease
	Paroxysmal cold hemoglobinuria
	Drug-induced hemolytic anemias
	Hemolytic disease of the newborn
Immune thrombocytopenia	Idiopathic (autoimmune) thrombocytopenic purpura
	Neonatal alloimmune thrombocytopenia
Immune neutropenia	Autoimmune neutropenia
Immune-mediated transfusion reactions	Acute hemolytic transfusion reaction
	Febrile reactions
	Pulmonary hypersensitivity reaction
	Allergic reactions
	IgA-deficient recipient
	Delayed hemolytic reactions
	Posttransfusion purpura
	Transfusion-associated graft-versus-host disease
Anemias	Pernicious anemia
Deficiency of hemostasis and coagulation	Autoimmune protein S deficiency

bodies) can demonstrate an autoantibody, but testing for specificity is not routinely necessary.

Cold Autoimmune Hemolytic Anemia. Cold hemagglutinin disease (CHAD), whether acute or chronic, is the most common type of hemolytic anemia associated with cold-reactive autoantibodies. The acute form is often secondary to *Mycoplasma pneumoniae* infection or lymphoproliferative disorders such as lymphoma. The chronic form is seen in older patients and produces mild to moderate hemolysis. In addition, Raynaud's phenomenon and hemoglobinuria occur in cold weather.

In CHAD a cold-reactive IgM autoantibody reacts with RBCs in the peripheral circulation when the body temperature falls to 32° C or below and binds complement to the cells. Therefore, complement is the only globulin detected on the erythrocytes. Elutions prepared from RBCs collected at 37° C will not demonstrate antibody reactivity in the eluate.

Paroxysmal Cold Hemoglobinuria. Previously associated with syphilis, paroxysmal cold hemoglobinuria is now seen more often as an acute transient condition secondary to viral infections, particularly in young children. It may also occur as an idiopathic chronic disease in older people.

The autoantibody is an IgG protein that reacts with RBCs in colder parts of the body; this produces complement components C3 and C4 to bind irreversibly to the erythrocytes. At warmer temperatures, RBCs are hemolyzed, and the antibody elutes from the cells. Eluates are also nonreactive. This IgG autoantibody, a biphasic hemolysin, can be demonstrated by performing the Donath-Landsteiner test. The autoantibody has anti-p specificity and reacts with all except the rare p or p^k phenotypes. Exceptions that include examples with anti-IH specificity have been described.

Drug-Induced Hemolysis. Coating of RBCs demonstrated by a positive direct anti–human globulin test (DAT) may be drug induced and accompanied by hemolysis (Table 28-8). The mechanisms of reactivity have been described as being caused by four basic mechanisms: (1) drug adsorption, (2) immune complex mechanism, (3) membrane modification, and (4) autoantibody formation.

Drug Adsorption. Penicillin is a representative example of an agent that displays drug adsorption. In this type of mechanism the drug strongly binds to any protein, including RBC membrane proteins. This binding produces a drug-RBC-hapten complex that can stimulate antibody formation. The antibody is specific for this complex, and no reactions will take place unless the drug is adsorbed on erythrocytes. Massive doses of intravenous penicillin are needed to coat the erythrocytes sufficiently for antibody attachment to occur.

Approximately 3% of affected patients will demonstrate a positive DAT, and less than 5% will develop hemolytic anemia because of the drug. The hemolysis of RBCs is usually extravascular and occurs slowly. It is not life threatening and will abate when penicillin is discontinued. There appears to be no connection between this type of antibody production and allergic penicillin sensitivity caused by IgE production.

Other drugs that display drug adsorption are cephalothin derivatives (e.g., cephalothin [Keflin], quinidine).

Immune Complex Mechanism. Immune complexing is associated with a variety of drugs, including phenacetin, quinine, rifampin, and stibophen. In this interaction the drug and antibody form a complex in the serum and attach nonspecifically to the RBCs. Once attached, this complex initiates the complement cascade, which culminates in intravascular hemolysis. The immune complex may dissociate from the RBC membrane after complement activation and attach to another erythrocyte. This action allows a small amount of drug to produce a severe anemia. When the offending drug is discontinued, the hemolytic process disappears quickly.

Membrane Modification. Drugs of the cephalosporin type (e.g., cephalothin) occasionally cause a positive DAT with polyspecific and monospecific anti–human globulin antisera by membrane modification. In this type of mechanism, the drug alters the membrane so that there is nonspecific absorption of globulins, including IgG, IgM, IgA, and complement. Hemolysis is not a common complication in this type of membrane augmentation.

Autoantibody Formation. Drugs such as methyldopa (Aldomet), levodopa, and mefenamic acid (Ponstel) have been implicated in positive DATs caused by autoantibody formation. The autoantibody formed recognizes a part of the RBC and therefore reacts with most normal RBCs. Some drug-induced autoantibodies have been shown to have specificities that appear to be of the Rh type, but most have

Table 28-8	Drug-Induced Positive Direct Antiglobulin Test			
	Drug Adsorption	**Immune Complex**	**Membrane Modification**	**Autoantibody Formation**
Common cause	IgG	Complement	Nonserologic	IgG
Antibody screening	Negative*	Positive†	Negative	Variable‡
Eluate reactivity with reagent red blood cells (RBCs)	Nonreactive	Nonreactive	Nonreactive	Reactive§
Penicillin-treated RBCs	Reactive with patient's serum and eluate	Nonreactive	Nonreactive	Nonreactive

*Unless irregular antibodies are present in the sample.
†If the drug and complement are present in the test system.
‡If the autoantibody is high enough in titer, screening tests may be positive with all cells tested.
§Will react with all normal cells tested, occasionally showing Rh-like specificity.

no apparent specificity. Antibody production ceases with withdrawal of the drug.

Idiopathic Thrombocytopenic Purpura

Idiopathic thrombocytopenic purpura is now also known as *immunologic* thrombocytopenic purpura (ITP). Patients with ITP usually demonstrate petechiae, bruising, menorrhagia, and bleeding after minor trauma. ITP may be either acute or chronic. Children are most often affected with the acute type, whereas adults predominantly experience the chronic type. This common disorder may complicate other antibody-associated disorders such as SLE.

Thrombocytopenia, a condition of absent or severely decreased platelets ($<10\text{-}20 \times 10^9/L$), may result from a wide variety of conditions, such as after extracorporeal circulation in cardiac bypass surgery or from alcoholic liver disease. However, most thrombocytopenic conditions can be classified into the following three major categories:

- Decreased production of platelets
- Disorders of platelet distribution
- Increased destruction or use of platelets

Decreased platelet production may result from invasion of the bone marrow by neoplastic cells and is usually not associated with an immunologic cause. Disorders of platelet distribution are associated with a sequestering of platelets in the spleen for various nonimmunologic reasons. Increased destruction or use of platelets, however, is associated with immunologic mechanisms. These mechanisms of destruction are caused by antigens, antibodies, or complement.

Drugs or foreign substances that can cause platelet destruction include quinidine, sulfonamide derivatives, heroin, morphine, and snake venom. Sulfonamide derivative reactions involve the interaction of platelet antigens with drug antibodies. Morphine reactions involve the activation of complement.

Bacterial sepsis causes increased destruction of platelets resulting from the attachment of platelets to bacterial antigen-antibody immune complexes. Certain microbial antigens may initially attach to platelets, followed by specific antibodies to the microorganism. This mechanism has been reported to cause the thrombocytopenia that frequently complicates *Plasmodium falciparum* malaria.

Antibodies of either autoimmune or isoimmune origin may produce increased destruction of platelets. Examples of thrombocytopenias of isoimmune origin include posttransfusion purpura and isoimmune neonatal thrombocytopenia. Neonatal autoimmune thrombocytopenia is a condition caused by immunization of a pregnant female by a fetal platelet antigen and by transplacental passage of maternal IgG platelet antibodies. The antigen is inherited by the fetus from the father and is absent on maternal platelets. Posttransfusion purpura is a rare form of isoimmune thrombocytopenia.

Pernicious Anemia

Pernicious anemia is a megaloblastic anemia characterized by a variety of hematologic and chemical manifestations (Table 28-9). PA is caused by a deficiency of vitamin B_{12} that

Table 28-9	Hematologic and Chemical Findings in Pernicious Anemia	
Assay	**Finding**
Hematologic Indices	
Hemoglobin (Hb)	Severely decreased
Hematocrit (Hct)	Severely decreased
Erythrocyte (RBC) count	Decreased
Leukocyte (WBC) count	Slightly decreased
Platelet count	Slightly decreased or normal
Mean corpuscular volume (MCV)	Increased
Chemical Indices	
Serum iron	Increased
Total iron-binding capacity (TIBC)	Normal or decreased
Percentage of iron (Fe) saturation	Increased
Serum ferritin	Increased

results from the patient's inability to secrete intrinsic factor. In most cases of PA, anti-IF or antiparietal antibodies have been reported. Most authorities consider the demonstration of these antibodies to support the theory that PA is an autoimmune disorder.

Assays for anti-IF measure antibodies to IF. The presence of IF-blocking antibodies is diagnostic of PA. Antibodies can be demonstrated in about 60% of cases. Antiparietal cell assays measure antibodies to parietal cells (large cells on margin of peptic glands of stomach). Most (80%) patients with PA have parietal cell antibodies. In the presence of these antibodies, gastric biopsy almost always demonstrates gastritis. Low antibody titers to parietal cells are often found with no clinical evidence of PA or atrophic gastritis and are sometimes seen in older patients.

Neuromuscular Disorders

Several important neurologic disorders are related to the immune system. The immune system may play an important role in the pathogenesis and etiology of myasthenia gravis and multiple sclerosis. In addition, amyotrophic lateral sclerosis (ALS) has become one of the prime subjects of modern neurologic research.

Amyotrophic Lateral Sclerosis

Along with Alzheimer's disease and Parkinson's disease, ALS is one of the so-called degenerative diseases of the aging nervous system. The immune system has been implicated in ALS. Monoclonal paraproteinemia seems to be disproportionately frequent among patients with ALS. It has also been suggested that ALS patients have a higher incidence of lymphoproliferative disease–lymphoma, Waldenström's macroglobulinemia, and myeloma. There also seems to be an increased frequency of antibodies to a neuronal ganglioside, GM-1.

Inflammatory Polyneuropathies

This group of idiopathic disorders, which includes the acute disorder *Guillain-Barré syndrome* (GBS), is characterized clinically by the subacute onset of generally symmetric weakness, ranging from modest lower-extremity weakness to total, life-threatening involvement of motor and even cranial nerves. Sensory symptoms are less prominent. Unstable blood pressure and potentially fatal arrhythmias have also been observed. Progression of GBS can be rapid; however, most patients do recover.

The etiology of GBS is unknown, but it is likely that an abnormal immune response against the peripheral nervous system (PNS) is involved. This may be triggered by an antecedent viral infection. There is infiltration of the PNS with lymphocytes and macrophages and patchy myelin destruction. Some patients display deposition of IgG, IgM, and IgA in PNS tissues. Greatly elevated immunoglobulin levels in the CSF, sometimes with oligoclonal bands, suggests locally altered immunoregulation. The antigenic targets of such immunoglobulins remain unknown.

Myasthenia Gravis

Myasthenia gravis is a disorder of the neuromuscular junction characterized by neurophysiologic and immunologic abnormalities (Box 28-3). A postsynaptic defect is caused by a decrease in receptors for acetylcholine and frequently an anatomic defect in the neuromuscular junction plate. AChR-binding antibody is directed against acetylcholine receptors at neuromuscular junctions of skeletal muscle and AChR-blocking antibodies. The ligand bungarotoxin or acetylcholine is important in producing a neuromuscular block. About one third of patients with myasthenia gravis demonstrate AChR-blocking antibodies.

The role of these antibodies in producing disease is unclear. Complement-mediated, antibody-determined damage may be an important mechanism in myasthenia gravis because IgG, C3, and C9 can be demonstrated at the neuromuscular junction, and the motor endplate is often abnormal. This suggests that antibody to AChR is capable of increasing the normal rate of degradation, resulting in fewer available receptors.

Multiple Sclerosis

Multiple sclerosis (MS) is the most common demyelinating disorder of the CNS related to abnormalities of the immune system. It is characterized by regions of demyelinization of varying size and age scattered throughout the white matter of the CNS. Demyelinization "plaques" have a propensity to form in the cerebrum, optic nerves, brainstem, spinal cord, and cerebellum.

Box 28-3	Abnormalities Associated with Myasthenia Gravis

- Thymic hyperplasia with germinal follicles
- Increase in thymic B cells
- Thymoma
- Expression of acetylcholine receptor (AChR)–binding antibody and AChR-blocking antibody
- Associated with other autoimmune diseases

Etiology. After a century of study, the cause of MS remains unknown. Although research studies support both genetic and environmental components of susceptibility, epidemiologic findings are most consistent with an environmental influence against a background of genetic susceptibility as the cause of MS. There is little evidence for a single or unique environmental cause. Viral infection (e.g., human herpesvirus type 6 [HHV-6]) is highly suspected but unconfirmed. In addition, EBV, which causes infectious mononucleosis and is associated with other diseases, may increase the risk of MS.

Epidemiology. The incidence, prevalence, and mortality rates of MS vary with latitude. MS is rare in tropical and subtropical areas. The higher risk for MS in Europeans and in relatives of patients with MS and the existence of MS-resistant ethnic groups (e.g., Eskimos, Norwegian Lapps, Australian aborigines) support genetic predisposition to MS. A low prevalence of MS occurs in Africa, India, China, Japan, and Southeast Asia. In the United States the incidence is 1 in 1000 individuals.

Multiple sclerosis is the major acquired neurologic disease in young adults. Most patients develop symptoms between ages 18 and 50 years. Women are more often affected than men (2:1 ratio). Approximately 1 in 1000 persons of northern European origin who reside in temperate climates will develop prototypical MS in their lifetime. Up to 350,000 people in the United States have MS.

Pathophysiology. MS results from T-cell–dependent inflammatory demyelination of the CNS. Inflammatory demyelination caused by T lymphocytes induces B lymphocytes to produce antimyelin antibodies.

The ongoing pathologic process involves the formation of CNS lesions, called *plaques,* characterized by inflammation and demyelination. Plaques result from a localized inflammatory immune response, initiated by the entry of activated blood T cells into the CNS. These T cells cross the blood-brain barrier by binding to endothelial cells in blood vessels via reciprocal adhesion molecules. The release of enzymes, called *matrix metalloproteinases* (MMPs), allows them to penetrate the basement membrane and extracellular matrix. At the same time, other blood immune system cells penetrate the CNS, causing additional local synthesis and release of damaging inflammatory mediators. The net result is destruction of myelin sheaths, injury to axons and glial cells, and formation of permanent scar tissue.

Research studies have demonstrated that osteopontin, which is known to play a role in enhancing inflammation, may play a critical role in the immune attack in MS and its progression. Osteopontin has been found to be very active in areas of myelin damage, both during relapse and remission, and both in myelin-making cells and in nerve cells. More research is required to determine the exact role of this protein, as well as the therapeutic possibilities it presents.

Signs and Symptoms. MS begins as a relapsing illness with episodes of neurologic dysfunction lasting several weeks, followed by substantial or complete improvement (relapsing-remitting MS). Initial signs of MS are difficulty walking, abnormal sensations (e.g., numbness, possible pain, ineffective vision). Primary symptoms caused by demyelination include fatigue, bladder and bowel dysfunction, loss of balance, loss of memory, slurred speech, difficulty swallowing, and seizures. Depression is a common symptom.

Relapsing MS is the most common form; 85% of patients are symptomatic at onset. The other forms of MS are as follows:

- Primary progressive
- Secondary progressive
- Progressive relapsing

Primary progressive MS advances insidiously from onset, with or without occasional plateaus and minor improvements. Secondary progressive MS develops in about half of relapsing MS patients about 10 years into the disease. Progressive relapsing is the rarest form of the disease. Patients begin with primary progression but subsequently experience one or more relapses.

Diagnostic Methods. Magnetic resonance imaging (MRI) is a key test in establishing a diagnosis of MS. No single laboratory test confirms a diagnosis, but appropriate laboratory tests must be evaluated carefully. Conditions that need to be excluded include collagen vascular disease, vitamin B_{12} deficiency, and endocrine disorders (e.g., thyroid and adrenal gland disease). It is also important to rule out infectious diseases (e.g., Lyme disease, syphilis, HTLV-1 infection). Analysis of CSF may identify the following:

- Oligoclonal IgG band pattern by CSF electrophoresis.
- Quantification of CSF IgG and albumin concentrations.
- Interpretation of CSF indices (e.g., albumin index, IgG index, IgG synthesis rate, local IgG synthesis).

Immunologic Manifestations. Box 28-4 presents immunologic manifestations of MS suggestive of its autoimmune nature. Antimyelin antibodies directed against components of the myelin sheath of nerves or myelin basic protein can be demonstrated in patients with MS or other neurologic diseases. However, myelin antibodies are not detectable in the CSF of MS patients.

Detection of Oligoclonal Bands. Oligoclonal immunoglobulins may be seen in both serum and CSF. An oligoclonal immunoglobulin pattern consists of multiple, homogeneous, narrow, and probably faint bands in the gamma zone on electrophoresis.

Electrophoresis on cellulose acetate will rarely resolve an oligoclonal pattern. Therefore, electrophoretic media with greater resolution, such as agar or agarose gel, are required, and both require the use of concentrated CSF. It is important to perform electrophoresis a serum specimen concurrently with the CSF specimen to ensure that the demonstrated homogeneous bands are present only in the CSF, which implies endogenous synthesis rather than serum band that might appear secondarily in the CSF. Infrequently, if a prominent CSF band is present, it may appear in the serum as a homogeneous band. This situation is most often encountered in subacute sclerosing panencephalitis.

High-resolution electrophoresis attempts to achieve better resolution of proteins beyond the classic five-band pattern. The primary reason for performing high-resolution protein electrophoresis is to detect oligoclonal bands in CSF to increase the diagnostic usefulness of protein patterns. About 80% of CSF proteins originate from the plasma. The electrophoretic pattern of normal CSF is similar to a normal serum protein pattern; however, several differences are detectable, including a prominent prealbumin band and two transferrin bands.

Immunofixation has been used in some research studies to show that the oligoclonal bands seen in CSF protein patterns are made up primarily of IgG. Although this may be of academic interest, characterization of the immunoglobulin bands does not significantly improve the diagnostic usefulness of the procedure. Isoelectric focusing, however, is becoming the method of choice for oligoclonal band detection.

Significance of Oligoclonal Bands. If oligoclonal bands are present in CSF but not in the serum, they are the result of increased production of IgG by the CNS. CNS production of IgG occurs in the subarachnoid space of the brain in conjunction with the local accumulation of immunocytes. Each has its own specificity that gives rise to oligoclonal bands. Although the immunoglobulin is IgG, it is polyclonal in nature, with several groups of cells producing it. Oligoclonal bands are therefore defined as "discrete populations of IgG," with restricted heterogeneity demonstrated by electrophoresis.

One procedure for confirming local CNS production of oligoclonal IgG is to assay a matched serum specimen diluted 1:100 concurrently with an unconcentrated CSF sample. Oligoclonal bands present in CSF, but not in the serum, indicate CNS production. This matched sample procedure is especially useful if damage to the blood-brain barrier is suspected because of acute or chronic inflammation, such as meningitis, intracranial tumor, or cerebrovascular disease.

Serum oligoclonal bands may represent immune complexes and are associated with diseases such as Hodgkin's or a nonspecific early immune response to a number of diseases (Box 28-5).

Clinical Findings. Total CSF protein in patients with MS is usually normal or slightly elevated. In general, patients with no neurologic disease have IgG concentration of less than 10% of the total CSF proteins. Almost 70% of MS patients typically have IgG concentration of 11% to 35% of total CSF proteins.

Box 28-4	Immunologic Manifestations of Multiple Sclerosis

- Antimyelin antibodies
- Myelinotoxicity and glial toxicity of serum and cerebrospinal fluid in vitro
- In vitro cell-mediated immunity by blood and cerebrospinal fluid cells to myelin components
- Oligoclonal increase in cerebrospinal fluid immunoglobulin
- Increase in certain HLA and Ia antigens (HL-A A3, B7, DW2, and DRW2)

Box 28-5	Conditions Associated with Oligoclonal Cerebrospinal Fluid Gamma Globulins

- Multiple sclerosis
- Neurosyphilis-paresthesia
- Paraneoplastic syndrome–subacute sclerosing panencephalitis
- Chronic mycobacterial and fungal meningitis
- Chronic viral meningitis and meningoencephalitis (uncommon)
- Acute viral meningitis (uncommon)
- Primary optic neuritis
- Acute disseminated encephalomyelitis
- Primary optic neuritis
- Peripheral neuropathy
- Guillain-Barré syndrome
- Burkitt's lymphoma
- Psychoneurosis
- Cerebral infarction

Oligoclonal bands in serum are not absolutely indicative of MS, and their presence should be used in conjunction with the clinical evaluation and other diagnostic procedures. Although oligoclonal bands can be present in more than 90% of MS patients at some time during the course of their disease, the presence of bands does not correlate with the activity of the disease. The exact number of bands present in MS varies; some studies have demonstrated 7 to 15 bands.

Treatment. Corticosteroid therapy (e.g., methylprednisolone and prednisone) is a common symptomatic treatment for disease relapses. The relapsing form of MS can be treated with the immunomodulators: interferon beta-1b (Betaseron), interferon beta-1a (Avonex), and glatiramer acetate (Copaxone). All these drugs are approved by the U.S. Food and Drug Administration (FDA) for use in relapsing forms of MS. Possible future therapeutic strategies may include combination therapies using existing therapies, standard immunosuppressive drugs, and new immunomodulating agents. Autologous bone marrow transplantation, plasma exchange, TCR peptide vaccine, and gene therapy are other possibilities.

The Myeline Project Cell Culture Units at the University of Wisconsin–Madison and at Sweden's University of Lund are developing an immortal line of human cells, oligodendrocyte precursors, to repair myelin lesions in MS and the leukodystrophies. Studies have demonstrated that myelin produced as a result of transplantation is capable of restoring nerve conduction. The feasibility of transplanting glial cells derived from human tissue into the CNS is being explored.

French researchers have demonstrated that progesterone promotes remyelination by activating genes that control the synthesis of important myelin proteins.

Neuropathies

A **neuropathy** is a derangement in the function and structure of peripheral motor, sensory, or autonomic neurons. Autoimmune disorders constitute one of the disease categories causing neuropathy. In many cases, evidence supports autoimmune pathogenesis. Demonstration of the relationships between specific neuropathic syndromes and antibodies directed against glycolipid and neural antigens are important recent scientific advances.

In the autoimmune neuropathies, antibodies directed against peripheral nerve components are associated with specific clinical syndromes (Table 28-10). Knowledge of these syndromes and antibody tests can be used to identify a treatable neuropathy. In addition, many autoimmune neuropathic syndromes are associated with malignancies, which they often precede. Recognition of these syndromes can lead to early identification and treatment.

Most antibodies implicated in the development of autoimmune-mediated neuropathies are directed against carbohydrate epitopes of glycoproteins or glycolipids. Glycolipids are concentrated in neural membranes, where the lipid portion is immersed in the membrane bilayer and the carbohydrate portion is exposed extracellularly. The extracellular domain of the carbohydrate epitopes makes them vulnerable to antibody binding.

Systemic sclerosis (scleroderma) is an autoimmune disease characterized by a wide spectrum of clinical, pathologic, and serologic abnormalities. More that 90% of patients with systemic sclerosis spontaneously produce ANA. The structure and function of the intracellular antigens to which these ANAs are directed have been characterized. These serum autoantibodies are helpful markers because they correlate with certain clinical features of systemic sclerosis (Table 28-11). A new marker autoantibody, **anti–RNA polymerase III antibody,** has been identified in many

Table 28-10	Neuropathy Syndromes Associated with Antibodies Directed against Peripheral Nerve Components
Clinical Syndrome	**Antibodies**
Chronic sensorimotor demyelinating neuropathy	Antimyelin-associated glycoprotein
Chronic axonal sensory neuropathy	Antisulfatide or anti–chondroitin sulfate
Multifocal motor neuropathy	Anti-GM1 (IgM)
Acute axonal motor neuropathy	Anti-GM1 (IgG)
Fisher syndrome	Anti-GQ1b
Guillain-Barré syndrome	Anti-LM1, GD1b, GD1A, GT1b, sulfatide, B tubulin
Large-fiber sensory neuropathy with ataxia	Anti-GQ1b, GD3, GD1b, GT1b
Subacute sensory neuropathy/encephalomyelitis	Antineuronal nuclear antibody type 1 (anti-Hu)

From Cohen B, Mitsumoto H: Neuropathy syndromes associated with antibodies against the peripheral nerve, *Lab Med* 26(7):459-463, 1995.

Table 28-11	Clinical Types of Systemic Sclerosis (SSc) and Associated Antibody Markers
Clinical Type	**Antibodies**
SSc with diffuse cutaneous involvement (dcSsc)	Anti–RNA polymerase I, anti–topoisomerase I
SSc with limited cutaneous involvement (lcSSc)	Anti–Th ribonucleoprotein anticentromere antibody
SSc-polymyositis overlap syndrome	Anti–PM-Scl

patients who have systemic sclerosis with diffuse or extensive cutaneous involvement.

Renal Disorders

It is generally accepted that most immunologically mediated renal diseases fall into several categories (Box 28-6).

Renal Disease Associated with Circulating Immune Complexes

Renal diseases associated with circulating immune complexes are caused by nonrenal antigens and their corresponding antibodies (see Box 28-6). These complexes are deposited in one or more of several loci in the glomerulus. Deposition may depend on the size and other characteristics of the complex. Recent evidence suggests that potentially damaging immune complexes may be formed in situ and involve antigens already present or fixed in the glomerulus. In addition, immune complex activation of complement in the glomerular basement membrane may be augmented by the presence of cells with receptors for C3 located in that area. Activation probably releases biologically active products such as chemotactic substances and causes an inflammatory type of tissue injury. A renal complication of this type can be manifested in SLE.

Membranoproliferative Glomerulonephritis

Another type of glomerular disease, membranoproliferative glomerulonephritis, is believed to be caused by nonimmunologically activated complement. Activation is thought to be analogous to the alternate pathway activation of C3 by certain bacterial products and polysaccharides.

Renal Disease Associated with Anti–Glomerular Basement Membrane Antibody

Anti-GBM antibodies are directed against the glomerular basement membrane of the glomerulus of the kidney (Figure 28-3). These antibodies are induced in vivo against the basement membrane of the glomerulus and possibly that of the renal tubule or lung. The factors that stimulate antibody production are not well defined, but it appears likely that binding of drugs (e.g., methicillin), certain infectious agents, or renal damage caused by other immune mechanisms may lead to an immune antibody response. The end result may be direct damage to the bone marrow with or without complement activation. Production of anti–bone marrow antibodies, however, appears to be self-limited and lasts for several weeks to months after removal of the inciting agent (i.e., by the kidney).

High antibody titers of anti-GMB are suggestive of Goodpasture's disease, early SLE, or anti-GBM nephritis. The

Box 28-6	Categories of Immunologic Renal Disorder

Associated with Circulating Immune Complexes
Systemic lupus erythematosus
Certain vasculitis
Infections
Tumors (possibly)
Immunoglobulins and antiimmunoglobulins

Membranoproliferative Glomerulonephritis
Activation of alternate complement pathway
Possible genetic factors

Associated with Anti–Glomerular Basement Membrane Antibody
Most cases of Goodpasture's syndrome
Some rapidly progressive glomerulonephritides
Membrane altered by virus or drugs (possibly)

Tubulointerstitial Nephritis
Associated with immune complex-mediated disease
Drugs and possibly infection
Involvement of transplanted kidneys

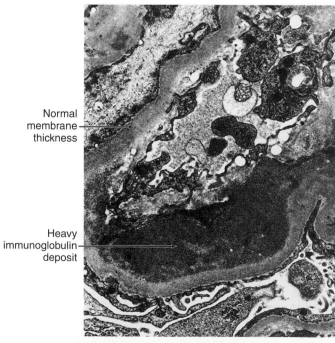

Normal membrane thickness

Heavy immunoglobulin deposit

Figure 28-3   Electron photomicrograph demonstrating an immunoglobulin deposit in the basement membrane of a patient with systemic lupus erythematosus (SLE). *(From Barrett JT:* Textbook of immunology, *ed 5, St Louis, 1988, Mosby.)*

absence of antibodies, however, does not rule out Goodpasture's disease. This type of renal disease represents less than 5% of glomerular disorders.

Tubulointerstitial Nephritis
Tubulointerstitial nephritis involving the renal tubules has been associated with a variety of causes, including immune complex–mediated disease. Precipitating factors can include drugs and possibly infection, as well as the involvement of transplanted kidneys.

Skeletal Muscle Disorders

Inflammatory Myopathy
Polymyositis and dermatomyositis are the most common expressions of a group of chronic inflammatory disorders that can be subclassified into the following six categories:
- Primary idiopathic polymyositis
- Primary idiopathic dermatomyositis
- Polymyositis or dermatomyositis associated with neoplasia
- Childhood polymyositis or dermatomyositis
- Dermatomyositis or polymyositis associated with collagen vascular disease
- Polymyositis or dermatomyositis associated with infections

All these disorders have skeletal muscle damage by a lymphocyte inflammatory process resulting in symmetric weakness, predominantly of proximal muscles.

Polymyositis may be accompanied by inflammation at other sites, especially in the joints, lungs, and heart. The term *dermatomyositis* is used for the disorder when the clinical features of disease are accompanied by characteristic inflammatory manifestations in the skin.

The causes of these disorders remain unknown, but they may develop in genetically susceptible persons after exposure to environmental agents that induce immune activation and inflammation. Infection is the most likely initiating event. As part of the inflammatory response to the infection, susceptible individuals develop a persistent cell-mediated immune attack that continues to destroy muscle after the acute infection is eradicated.

Both polymyositis and dermatomyositis are more common in females, with peaks of occurrence in childhood and the fifth decade. Clinically these disorders present with proximal muscle weakness, sometimes associated with pain, fatigue, and low-grade fever, and lead to atrophy in progressive disease.

Evidence suggests the polymyositis and dermatomyositis result from immune destruction. Muscle biopsies in patients with dermatomyositis have shown vasculitis, with IgG and complement deposition in the vessel walls in children and infrequently in adults. There is a preponderance of B lymphocytes and increased CD4+/CD8+ T-cell ratio. An increased frequency of activated T cells has been noted in both polymyositis and dermatomyositis.

Patients with myositis have many immunologic abnormalities. One unique immunologic feature is the targeting

Box 28-7 Myositis-Specific Autoantibodies

Antisynthetases
Anti–Jo-1
Anti–PL-7
Anti–PL-12 (1)
Anti–PL-12 (II)
Anti-OJ
Anti-EJ

Anti-SRP

Anti–MI-2

Others
Anti-FER
Anti-KJ
Anti-MAS

by autoantibodies of certain cytoplasmic proteins and ribonucleic acids (RNAs) involved in the process of protein synthesis. These autoantibodies are found only in patients with myositis and are known as the *myositis-specific autoantibodies* (MSAs) (Box 28-7). The MSAs are antigen driven, arise months before the onset of myositis, correlate in titer with disease activity, disappear after prolonged complete remission, and bind to and inhibit the function of targeted human autoantigenic enzymes on in vitro assays.

Skin Disorders (Bullous Disease and Other Conditions)
A wide variety of autoimmune disorders are associated with skin manifestations (Box 28-8).

Two immunologic assays that can be used in conjunction with other clinical information include measurement of antibodies to the basement membrane area of the skin and of antibodies to intercellular substance of the skin.

Antiskin (dermal-epidermal) antibodies are present in more than 80% of patients with bullous pemphigoid, but the absence of antibodies does not rule out the disorder. Antiskin (interepithelial) antibodies can be detected in 90% of patients with pemphigus. A rising antibody titer may

Box 28-8 Autoimmune Disorders Associated with Skin Manifestations

- Discoid lupus
- Bullous pemphigoid
- Pemphigus group
- Dermatitis herpetiformis

Skin may be involved in the autoimmune reaction in at least three ways:
1. Inflammatory involvement of cutaneous vessels with secondary effects (e.g., some lesions in systemic lupus erythematosus, hypersensitivity angiitis, and syndrome of urticaria and palpable purpura with or without mixed cryoglobulinemia).
2. Deposition of putative circulating immune complexes in the skin (e.g., systemic lupus erythematosus).
3. Localized autoreactivity against skin components (e.g., primary skin disorders).

indicate an impending relapse of pemphigus, and a falling titer suggests effective control of the disease. The absence of demonstrable antibody usually excludes the diagnosis.

Autoimmune Enzyme Immunoassay ANA Screening Test

Refer to Chapter 12, pp. 161-163, for a description of the Autoimmune Enzyme Immunoassay ANA screening test.

Clinical Applications

As with other antinuclear antigen (ANA) diagnostic tests, the results are to be used as an aid in diagnosis. Confirmative testing for specific antibodies should be run if a positive assay is obtained. A positive result suggests certain diseases and should be confirmed by clinical findings.

CASE STUDY

History and Physical Examination

Z.A., a 50-year-old Caucasian woman, visited her primary care provider because of extreme fatigue. She also reported experiencing mild pain in her abdominal region.

Physical examination revealed slight hepatomegaly. Her physician ordered a complete blood count and urinalysis.

Laboratory Data

	Patient's Results	Reference Range
Complete Blood Count		
Hemoglobin (Hb)	6.2 g/dL	11.5-16.0 g/dL
Hematocrit (Hct)	0.22 L/L	0.37-0.47 L/L
Red blood cell (RBC) count	1.7×10^{12}/L	$4.2\text{-}5.4 \times 10^{12}$/L
White blood cell (WBC) count	3.8×10^9/L	$4.5\text{-}11.0 \times 10^9$/L

Blood Smear Comments

3+ macrocytic RBCs, polychromatophilia, a few nucleated RBCs.

RBC Indices

Mean corpuscular volume (MCV)	129.4 fL	80-96 fL
Mean corpuscular hemoglobin (MCH)	36.5 pg	27-32 pg
Mean corpuscular hemoglobin concentration (MCHC)	28%	32%-36%

Questions and Discussion

1. What chemical and immunologic assays would be helpful in establishing a diagnosis for this patient?

A vitamin B_{12} assay and a folic acid assay are essential chemical tests. The immunologic assays of value are: anti–intrinsic factor and an anti–parietal cell assay.

2. What is the prevalence of anti–intrinsic factor in patients with pernicious anemia?

About 60% of patients with pernicious anemia exhibit intrinsic factor antibodies.

3. What is the prevalence of parietal cell antibodies in patients with pernicious anemia?

About 80% of patients with pernicious anemia exhibit parietal cell antibodies.

Diagnosis

Pernicious anemia.

CASE STUDY

History and Physical Examination

D.D. is a right-handed 25-year-old woman with no significant medical history. She came to the emergency department because of a sudden onset of slurred speech.

She reported being in excellent health until a month ago, when she began to notice weakness and numbness in her right hand and leg. She felt unsteady when walking and experienced urinary urgency.

Physical examination revealed an overweight young female with a right facial droop. In addition, she staggered on turning around and had difficulty walking in a straight line. A spinal tap and MRI were ordered.

Laboratory and Medical Imaging Data: Laboratory Findings

Cerebrospinal Fluid Examination		
Assay	Patient Results	Reference Range
Color/clarity	Clear, colorless	Clear, colorless
Total cells	6	0-8
Nucleated cells	2	0-2
Differential, lymphocytes (%)	75	40-60
CSF protein (mg/dL)	125	20-40
CSF glucose (mg/dL)	70	40-80
CSF IgG (mg/dL)	8.5	0-33
Serum albumin (g/dL)	4.2	3.5-5.0
Serum IgG (mg/dL)	941	700-1450
CSF Profile		
CSF:serum IgG index	1.2	0-0.7
CSF IgG:albumin ratio	0.28	0-0.23
Albumin index	7.38	0-7.0
CNS IgG synthesis rate (mg/dL)	22.65	0-2.8

Additional Notes

CSF agarose electrophoresis: Positive for oligoclonal bands (reference range negative).

CSF isoelectric focusing: Positive for oligoclonal bands (reference range negative).

Serum protein electrophoresis interpretation: No apparent monoclonal peak (reference range no apparent monoclonal peak).

Serum immunofixation: No paraprotein detected (reference range no paraprotein detected).

Medical Imaging

MRI scan revealed a masslike lesion in the region of the corpus callosum with extensions into the right and left hemispheres of the brain. The location of the lesion was consistent with the patient's presenting symptoms.

A follow-up biopsy of the brain was ordered. Histologically, a biopsy of white matter demonstrated sheets of macrophages, clumps of lymphocytes and plasma cells, and myelin debris.

Questions and Discussion

1. What is the etiology of the patient's symptoms?

Symptoms such as those demonstrated by this patient are caused by the formation of demyelinating lesions in the white matter of the CNS. Lesions are associated with mononuclear infiltrates of macrophages and T lymphocytes. The severity of symptoms depends on the location of the lesions in the brain.

2. Does the patient's age provide a clue to the diagnosis?

Multiple sclerosis should be suspected in females age 20 to 40 years who experience recurrent episodes of neurologic dysfunction (e.g., brain, spinal cord, optic nerve). MS is the most common, nontraumatic cause of neurologic disability in young and middle-age adults in the United States.

3. What is the significance of the laboratory analysis of the CSF?

Laboratory analysis of intrathecal immunoglobulin synthesis is important in cases of suspected MS. Electrophoresis of CSF for detection of oligoclonal bands is a classic measurement to determine intrathecal IgG synthesis. Electrophoretic separation of paired CSF and serum samples for detection of oligoclonal bands in the gamma region.

Laboratory analysis of CSF, patient history and physical examination, MRI examination, and electrophysiologic studies help to establish a clinical diagnosis of MS.

Follow-Up

Although the patient immediately began treatment with corticosteroid therapy and more recently Avonex, she has demonstrated worsening symptoms over the last 10 years.

Diagnosis

Multiple sclerosis.

CHAPTER HIGHLIGHTS

- Autoimmunity represents a breakdown of the immune system in its ability to discriminate between self and nonself.
- Autoimmune disorder is used when demonstrable immunoglobulins, autoantibodies, or cytotoxic T cells display a specificity for "self" antigens and contribute to disease pathogenesis.
- At one extreme are organ-specific disorders; at the other end of the spectrum are disorders that manifest as organ-nonspecific diseases. Midspectrum disorders are characterized by localized lesions in a single organ and autoantibodies that are organ nonspecific.
- The potential for autoimmunity is constantly present in every immunocompetent individual because lymphocytes that are potentially reactive with self antigens exist in the body.
- Antibody expression appears to be regulated by complex interactions that include genetic factors, patient age, and exogenous factors.
- Self-recognition (tolerance) is induced by at least two mechanisms: elimination of small clone of immunocompetent cells programmed to react with antigen (Burnet's clonal selection theory), or induction of unresponsiveness in immunocompetent cells through excessive antigen binding to them and through triggering of a suppressor mechanism.
- Major autoantibodies can be detected in different disorders. Many diagnostic laboratory tests are based on detecting these autoimmune responses.

REVIEW QUESTIONS

1. All the following characteristics are common to organ-specific and organ-nonspecific disorders *except:*
   a. Autoantibody tests are of diagnostic value.
   b. Antibodies may appear in each of the main immunoglobulin classes.
   c. Antigens are available to lymphoid system in low concentrations.
   d. Circulatory autoantibodies react with normal body constituents.

2. Antibody expression in the development of autoimmunity is regulated by all the following factors *except:*
   a. Genetic predisposition.
   b. Increasing age.
   c. Environmental factors (e.g., UV radiation).
   d. Active infectious disease.

3. The mechanism responsible for autoimmune disorder is:
   a. Circulating immune complexes.
   b. Antigen excess.
   c. Antibody excess.
   d. Antigen deficiency.

4. One of the mechanisms believed to induce self-tolerance is:
   a. Induction of responsiveness in immunocompetent cells.
   b. Elimination of clone programmed to react with antigen.
   c. Decreased suppressor cell activity.
   d. Stimulation of clones of immunocompetent cells.

Questions 5-8. Match the following (use an answer only once).

5. _____ Acetylcholine receptor–blocking antibodies

6. _____ Anticardiolipin antibody

7. _____ Anti-DNA antibodies

8. _____ Anti–glomerular basement membrane antibodies
   a. Helpful in monitoring Addison's disease.
   b. Found in one third of patients with myasthenia gravis.
   c. Useful in monitoring the activity and exacerbations of SLE.
   d. Suggestive of Goodpasture's disease.
   e. Present in SLE and associated with arterial and venous thrombosis.

Questions 9-12. Match the following.

9. _____ Antinuclear ribonucleoprotein

10. _____ Anti-Scl

11. _____ Anti-Sm

12. _____ Anti–smooth muscle

   a. Antibody to basic nonhistone nuclear protein, diagnostic of systemic sclerosis.
   b. Present in bullous pemphigoid.
   c. Presence of antibody confirms diagnosis of SLE.
   d. Seen in viral disorders.
   e. Characteristic of mixed connective tissue disease.

Questions 13-15. Match the following.

13. _____ Anti SS-A

14. _____ Histone-reactive antinuclear antibody

15. _____ PM-I antibody

   a. Detectable in patients with myasthenia gravis.
   b. Demonstrable in Sjögren's syndrome–sicca complex.
   c. Highly suggestive of drug-induced lupus erythematosus.
   d. Found in one third of patients with uncomplicated polymyositis and some patients with dermatomyositis.
   e. Found in majority of patients with polymyositis.

16. The term *autoimmune disorder* is used when:
   a. Demonstrable immunoglobulins display specificity for "self" antigens.
   b. Cytotoxic T cells display specificity for self antigens.
   c. Cytotoxic T cells contribute to the pathogenesis of the disease.
   d. All the above.

Questions 17-21. Indicate true statements with the letter "A," and false statements with the letter "B."

17. _____ The presence of autoantibodies are only associated with autoimmune disease.

18. _____ In organ-specific disorders, antigens are only available to the lymphoid system in low concentrations.

19. _____ There is a familial tendency to develop organ-specific disorders.

20. _____ In organ-specific disorders, lesions are caused by deposition of antigen-antibody complexes.

21. _____ In organ-specific disorders a tendency to develop cancer exists.

22. Self-recognition (tolerance) is induced by:
   a. Burnet's clonal selection theory.
   b. Elimination of the small clone of immunocompetent cells programmed to react with the antigen.
   c. Induction of unresponsiveness in the immunocompetent cells through excessive antigen binding.
   d. All the above.

Questions 23-26. Match each term below with the correct description.

23. _____ Acetylcholine receptor (AcHR)

24. _____ Anticentromere antibody

25. _____ Antiintrinsic factor antibody

26. _____ Antimitochondrial antibody antibody

   a. Strongly suggestive, in a high titer, of primary biliary binding antibody cirrhosis.
   b. Useful in the diagnosis of myasthenia gravis.
   c. Demonstrated in most patients with CREST syndrome.
   d. Found in 60% of patients with pernicious anemia.

Questions 27-30. Match each term below with the correct description.

27. _____ Antimyelin antibody

28. _____ Antimyocardial antibody

29. _____ Antineutrophil antibody (c-ANCA)

30. _____ Antinuclear antibody (ANA)

   a. Associated with multiple myeloma.
   b. Marker for Wegener's granulomatosis.
   c. Characteristic of untreated systemic lupus erythematosus.
   d. Diagnostic of Dressler's syndrome or rheumatic fever.

Questions 31-34. Match each organ in the illustration with the appropriate disease.

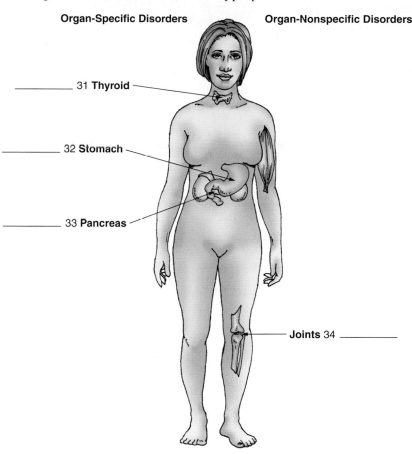

Organ-Specific Disorders   Organ-Nonspecific Disorders

_____ 31 **Thyroid**

_____ 32 **Stomach**

_____ 33 **Pancreas**

Joints 34 _____

Possible answers to question 31.
a. Takayasu arteritis
b. Behçet's disease
c. Graves' disease
d. Scleroderma

Possible answers to question 32.
a. Eosinophilia-myalgia
b. Hashimoto's thyroiditis
c. Raynaud's phenomenon
d. Pernicious anemia

Possible answers to question 33.
a. Addison's disease
b. Sheehan's syndrome
c. Insulin-dependent diabetes
d. Sjögren's syndrome

Possible answers to question 34.
a. Idiopathic biliary cirrhosis
b. Crohn's disease
c. Rheumatoid arthritis
d. Multiple sclerosis

35. The immunologic manifestations of multiple sclerosis include all the following *except:*
a. Antimyelin antibodies.
b. An oligoclonal increase in CSF immunoglobulin.
c. In vitro antibody-mediated immunity.
d. An increase in certain HLA and Ia antigens.

36. Most immunologically mediated renal diseases fall into one of the following categories, except for:
a. Association with circulating immune complexes.
b. Association with circulating antigen.
c. Association with anti–glomerular basement membrane antibody.
d. Membranoproliferative glomerulonephritis.

37. Polymyositis and dermatomyositis are the most common expressions of:
a. Rheumatoid heart disease.
b. Skeletal muscle disorders.
c. Rheumatoid arthritis.
d. Either a or b.

Questions 38-40. Indicate whether each of the following statements is true (T) or false (F) regarding the epidemiology of *autoimmune pancreatitis.*

38. _____ It is more common in women than men.

39. _____ Most patients are younger than 50 years of age at diagnosis.

40. _____ The number of reported cases has been decreasing over the last decade.

41. The immunologic abnormality associated with auto-immune pancreatitis in the Japanese population is:
   a. Autoantibodies against carbonic anhydrase.
   b. HLA haplotype.
   c. Hypogammaglobulinemia.
   d. Elevated serum IgE levels.

BIBLIOGRAPHY

Ahern P: Gut reactions: study reveals new causes of bowel disease, *Dana Foundation Immunol News* 6(4):7-8, 2006.

Ahmed AEE: Cellular immunology of autoimmune diseases, *ADVANCE,* March 1998.

Ascherio A: Epstein-Barr virus antibodies and risk of multiple sclerosis: a prospective study, *JAMA* 286(24):3083-3088, 2001.

Bach J: The effect of infections on susceptibility to autoimmune and allergic diseases, *N Engl J Med* 347(12):911-919, 2002.

Bakalar N: Crohn's disease and colitis are linked to mutant gene, *Dana Foundation Immunol News* 6(4):1-2, 2006.

Black A: Antiphospholipid syndrome: an overview, *Clin Lab Sci* 19(3):144-147, 2006.

Bridges AJ et al: Antinuclear antibody testing in a referral laboratory, *Lab Med* 24(6):345-349, 1993.

Caroscio JT: Quantitative CSF IgG measurements in multiple sclerosis and other neurologic diseases, *Arch Neurol* 40:409-413, 1983.

Celiac Disease Foundation, www.celiac.org, January 2007.

Chang A et al: Research results on myelin repair in long-standing MS brain, *N Engl J Med* 346(3):165-173, 2002.

Coles AJ et al: Pulsed monoclonal antibody treatment and autoimmune thyroid disease in multiple sclerosis, *Lancet* 354:1691-1695, 1999.

Condemi JJ: The autoimmune diseases, *JAMA* 268(20):2888-2892, 1992.

Davidson A, Diamond B: Autoimmune disease, *N Engl J Med* 345(5):340-350, 2001.

Dyment DA, Ebers GC: An array of sunshine in multiple sclerosis, *N Engl J Med* 347(18):1445-1447, 2002.

Eastwood A: Information resource center and library of the National MS Society, 2001, www.nmss.org.

Finkelberg D, Sahani D, Deshpande V, Brugge WR: Autoimmune pancreatitis, *N Engl J Med* 355(25):2670-2676, 2006.

Foley KF, Kao P: Biomarkers for inflammatory bowel disease, *Clin Lab Sci* 20(2):84-88, 2007.

Freedman J et al: Hemolytic warm IgM autoagglutinins in autoimmune hemolytic anemia, *Transfusion* 27(6):464-467, 1987.

Frohman EM, Racke MK, Raine CS: Multiple sclerosis—the plaque and its pathogenesis, *N Engl J Med* 354(9):942-954, 2006.

Hochberg EP, Gilman MD, Hasserjian RP: Case 17-2006: a 34-year-old man with cavitary lung lesions, *N Engl J Med* 354(23):2485-2492, 2006.

Hogancamp WE, Rodriguez M, Weinshenker BG: The epidemiology of multiple sclerosis, *Mayo Clin Proc* 72:871-878, 1997.

IMMCO Diagnostics: Autoimmune gastritis and pernicious anemia, Buffalo, NY, July 2006.

IMMCO Diagnostics: Autoimmunity, Buffalo, NY, July 2006.

Kahn AI, Susa J, Ansari Q: Systemic sclerosis (scleroderma), *Lab Med* 36(11):723-728, 2005.

Kamb ML et al: Eosinophilia-myalgia syndrome in L-tryptophan–exposed patients, *JAMA* 267(1):77-82, 1992.

Kappos L et al: Oral fingolimod (FTY 720) for relapsing multiple sclerosis, *N Engl J Med* 355(11):1124-1138, 2006.

Keren DF: Anti-ss DNA not useful, withdrawn from survey, *CAP Today,* November 2000, p 86.

Keshgegian AA, Coblentz J, Lisak RP: Oligoclonal immunoglobulins in cerebrospinal fluid in multiple sclerosis, *Clin Chem* 26(9):1340-1345, 1980.

Killingsworth LM: Clinical applications of protein determination in biological fluids other than blood, *Clin Chem* 28(5):1093-1258, 1982.

King D: Experts predict advances in autoimmune disease testing, *Adv Med Lab Prof* 13(4):8-11, 2001.

Krawitt EL: Autoimmune hepatitis, *N Engl J Med* 354(1):54-64, 2006.

Kuhle J et al: Lack of association between antimyelin antibodies and progression to multiple sclerosis, *N Engl J Med* 356(4):371-378, 2007.

Lange LG, Schreiner GF: Immune mechanisms of cardiac disease, *N Engl J Med* 330(16):1129-1135, 1994.

Link H, Kostulas V: Utility of IEF of CSF and serum on agarose evaluated from neurological patients, *Clin Chem* 29(5):810-815, 1983.

Malnick SDH, Sthoeger ZM: Autoimmune protein S deficiency, *N Engl J Med* 329(25):1898, 1993.

Mannon PJ et al: Anti-interleukin-12 antibody for active Crohn's disease, *N Engl J Med* 351(20):2069-2078, 2004.

Miller FW: Myositis-specific autoantibodies, *JAMA* 270(15):1846-1849, 1993.

Mooney B: Diagnosing pediatric autoimmune diseases, *Adv Med Lab Prof* 4(5):13-14, 26, 2002.

Multiple Sclerosis Foundation: MS information, 2002, www.msfacts.org.

Nakamura RM: Human autoimmune diseases: progress in clinical laboratory tests, *Med Lab Observer MLO,* October 2000, pp 32-47.

Nakamura RM: Serologic markers in inflammatory bowel disease (IBD), *Med Lab Observer MLO* 33(11):8-15, 2001.

Nimmo M: Celiac disease: an update with emphasis on diagnostic considerations, *Lab Med* 36(6), 2005.

Noseworthy JH: Multiple sclerosis, *N Engl J Med* 343(13):938-952, 2000.

Okano Y, Steen VD, Medsger TA: Autoantibody reactive with RNA polymerase III in system sclerosis, *Ann Intern Med* 119(10):1005-1013, 1993.

Oksenberk J: Immune protein may play role in MS attacks and progression, *Science* 294(5547):1613, 2001.

Pagano JS: Amyotrophic lateral sclerosis and autoimmunity, *N Engl J Med* 327(4):1752-1753, 1992.

Phelps RG, Rees AJ: The HLA complex in Goodpasture's disease: a model for analyzing susceptibility to autoimmunity, *Kidney Int* 56:1638-1653, 1999.

Pizarro TT, Kam L, Cominelli F: Interleukin-1 and interleukin-1 antagonism in inflammatory bowel disease, *Prog Inflamm Bowel Dis* 14(3):7-11, 1993.

Podolsky DK: Inflammatory bowel disease, *N Engl J Med* 347(6):417-428, 2002.

Ramsery MK, Owens D: Wegener's granulomatosis: a review of the clinical implications, diagnosis and treatment, *Lab Med* 37(2):114-116, 2006.

Rees-Smith B: Autoantibodies to the thyrotropin receptor, *Endocr Rev* 9(1):106-121, 1988.

Robert C, Kupper TS: Inflammatory skin disease, T cells, and immune surveillance, *N Engl J Med* 341:1817-1827, 1999.

Rosenwasser LJ, Joseph BZ: Immunohematologic diseases, *JAMA* 268(20):2940-2945, 1992.

Rutgeerts P et al: Infliximab for induction and maintenance therapy for ulcerative colitis, *N Engl J Med* 353(23):2462-2473, 2005.

Salama AD et al: Goodpasture's disease, *Lancet* 358:917, 2001.

Salama AD et al: In Goodpasture's disease, CD4+ T cells escape thymic deletion and are reactive with the autoantigen α3(IV)NC1, *J Am Soc Nephrol* 12:1908-1915, 2001.

Schwartz RS: Autoimmune folate deficiency and the rise and fall of "horror autotoxicus," *N Engl J Med* 352(19):1948-1950, 2005.

Scully RE et al: Case 3-1991, *N Engl J Med* 324(3):180-188, 1991.

Sloan EM et al: Preferential suppression of trisomy 8 compared with normal hematopoietic cell growth by autologous lymphocytes in patients with trisomy 8 myelodysplastic syndrome, *Blood* 106:841-851, 2005.

Smiroldo J, Coyle PK: Advances in the treatment of multiple sclerosis, *Patient Care* 33(11):88-106, 1999.

Smith LA: Autoimmune hemolytic anemias: introduction, *Clin Lab Sci* 12(2):109-124, 1999.

Smith RG et al: Serum antibodies to l-type calcium channels in patients with amyotrophic lateral sclerosis, *N Engl J Med* 327(4):1721-1728, 1992.

Tan FK: Autoantibodies against PDGF receptor in scleroderma, *N Engl J Med* 354(25):2709-2711, 2006.

Torassa U: Odd illnesses, strong clues: autoimmune woes target women, *San Francisco Chronicle,* Feb 18, 2001, p 69.

Turgeon ML: *Fundamentals of immunohematology,* ed 2, Baltimore, 1995, Williams & Wilkins.

Turgeon ML: *Clinical hematology: theory and procedures,* ed 4, Philadelphia, 2004, Lippincott–Williams & Wilkins.

Utiger RD: The pathogenesis of autoimmune thyroid disease, *N Engl J Med* 325(4):278-280, 1991.

Voulgarelis M et al: Malignant lymphoma in primary Sjögren's syndrome, *Arthritis Rheum* 42:1765-1772, 1999.

Watanabe T et al: Anti-alpha-Fodrin antibodies in Sjögren syndrome and lupus erythematosus, *Arch Dermatol* 135:535-539, 1999.

Wright MZ, Dearing LD: The role of HLA testing in autoimmune disease, *Adv Med Lab Prof* 13:81-84, 2001.

Winter WE: Diabetes disease management, *Clin Lab News* 31(7), 2005.

Yorde L: Diagnosing thyroid disorder, *Adv Med Lab Prof* 12(12):17, 2000.

Zeher M et al: Correlation of increased susceptibility to apoptosis of CD4+ T cells with lymphocyte activation and activity of disease in patients with primary Sjögren's syndrome, *Arthritis Rheum* 42:1673-1681, 1999.

Ziadie M, Wians FH: A guide to the interpretation of CSF indices, {AU: Journal} 36(9):558-562, 2005.

Zinkernagel RM: Maternal antibodies, childhood, infections, and autoimmune diseases, *N Engl J Med* 345(18):1331-1335, 2001.

CHAPTER 29

Systemic Lupus Erythematosus

Different Forms of Lupus
Etiology
    Hormonal Influences
    Genetic Predisposition
    Environmental Factors
Epidemiology
Signs and Symptoms
    Infection
    Cutaneous Features
    Renal Characteristics
    Lymphadenopathy
    Serositis
    Cardiopulmonary Characteristics
    Gastrointestinal Manifestations
    Musculoskeletal Features
    Neuropsychiatric Features
    Late-Onset Lupus

Immunologic Manifestations
    Cellular Aspects
    Humoral Aspects
    Immunologic Consequences
Diagnostic Evaluation
    Histologic Changes
    Hematologic and Hemostatic Findings
    Serologic Findings
    Laboratory Evaluation
Treatment
    Clinical Trials
Antinuclear Antibody Visible Method
Rapid Slide Test for Antinucleoprotein Factors
Case Studies
Chapter Highlights
Review Questions
Bibliography

Learning Objectives

At the conclusion of this chapter, the reader should be able to:

- Compare the different forms of lupus, citing manifestations, incidence, and other features.
- Name the two most common drugs that can cause drug-induced lupus.
- Explain the epidemiology and signs and symptoms of SLE.
- Describe the immunologic manifestations of SLE, including diagnostic evaluation.
- Discuss the laboratory evaluation of antinuclear antibodies.
- Analyze selected SLE case studies.

Systemic lupus erythematosus (SLE) is the classic model of autoimmune disease. SLE is a systemic rheumatic disorder and the term used most often for the group of disorders that includes SLE and other abnormalities involving multiple systems (e.g., joints, connective tissue, collagen vascular system) in the disease process. Table 29-1 defines American College of Rheumatology criteria for classification of SLE.

DIFFERENT FORMS OF LUPUS

There are several forms of lupus, including discoid, systemic, drug-induced, and neonatal lupus.

Discoid (cutaneous) lupus is always limited to the skin and is identified by biopsy of the rash that may appear on the face, neck, and scalp. Discoid lupus does not generally involve the body's internal organs, but it can evolve into the systemic form of the disease even if treated. Evolution to systemic lupus cannot be predicted or prevented. The **antinuclear antibody (ANA)** test may be negative or positive at a low titer. Discoid lupus accounts for approximately 10% of all cases of lupus.

Systemic lupus is usually more severe than discoid lupus and can affect the skin, joints, and almost any organ or body system, including the lungs, kidneys, heart, and brain. Systemic lupus may include periods in which few, if any, symptoms are evident *(remission)* and other times when the disease becomes more active *(flare)*. Most often when people mention "lupus," they are referring to the systemic form of the disease. Approximately 70% of lupus cases are systemic. In about half these cases, a major organ will be affected.

Drug-induced lupus occurs after the use of certain prescribed drugs (Box 29-1). The most frequently used drugs associated with drug-induced lupus are *hydralazine hydrochloride* and *procainamide hydrochloride*. Factors such as the rate of drug metabolism, the drug's influence on immune regulation, and the host's genetic composition are all believed to influence pathogenesis. Some drugs (e.g., oral contraceptives, isoniazid) induce serum antinuclear antibodies (ANAs) without symptoms. High antibody titers may exist for months without the development of clinical symptoms.

Procainamide-induced disease does not induce antibodies to double-stranded deoxyribonucleic acid (dsDNA). The ANAs in the drug-induced syndromes are histone

Table 29-1	American College of Rheumatology (ACR) 1982 Revised Criteria for Classification of Systemic Lupus Erythematosus*
Criterion	**Definition**
1. Malar rash	Fixed erythema, flat or raised, over the malar eminences, tending to spare the nasolabial folds.
2. Discoid rash	Erythematous raised patches with adherent keratotic scaling and follicular plugging; atrophic scarring may occur in older lesions.
3. Photosensitivity	Skin rash as a result of unusual reaction to sunlight, by patient history or physician observation.
4. Oral ulcers	Oral or nasopharyngeal ulceration, usually painless, observed by physician.
5. Arthritis	Nonerosive arthritis involving two or more peripheral joints, characterized by tenderness, swelling, or effusion.
6. Serositis	a. Pleuritis—convincing history of pleuritic pain or rubbing heard by a physician, or evidence of pleural effusion. OR b. Pericarditis—documented by electrocardiogram (ECG) or rub or evidence of pericardial effusion.
7. Renal disorder	a. Persistent proteinuria greater than 0.5 g/day, or greater than 3+ if quantitation not performed. OR b. Cellular casts—may be red cell, hemoglobin, granular, tubular, or mixed.
8. Neurologic disorder	a. Seizures—in the absence of offending drugs or known metabolic derangements (e.g., uremia, ketoacidosis, or electrolyte imbalance). OR b. Psychosis—in the absence of offending drugs or known metabolic derangements (e.g., uremia, ketoacidosis, or electrolyte imbalance).
9. Hematologic disorder	a. Hemolytic anemia—with reticulocytosis. OR b. Leukopenia—$<4000/mm^3$ total on two or more occasions. OR c. Lymphopenia—$<1500/mm^3$ on two or more occasions. OR d. Thrombocytopenia—$<100,000/mm^3$ in the absence of offending drugs.
10. Immunologic disorder	a. Positive LE cell preparation. OR b. Anti-DNA: antibody to native DNA in abnormal titer. OR c. Anti-Sm: presence of antibody to Sm nuclear antigen. OR d. False-positive serologic test for syphilis known to be positive for at least 6 months and confirmed by *Treponema pallidum* immobilization or fluorescent treponemal antibody absorption test.
11. Antinuclear antibody	An abnormal titer of antinuclear antibody by immunofluorescence or an equivalent assay at any point in time and in the absence of drugs known to be associated with "drug-induced lupus" syndrome.

From Tan EM et al: The 1982 revised criteria for the classification of systemic lupus erythematosus, *Arthritis Rheum* 25:1271-1277, 1982.

Updating ACR Revised Criteria for Classification of Systemic Lupus Erythematosus

Note: The ACR Diagnostic and Therapeutic Criteria Committee reviewed the 1982 revised criteria for SLE and recommended the following revisions to criterion number 10 ("Immunologic disorder"), which were approved by the Council on Research and the Board of Directors:

1. Delete item 10(a) ("Positive LE cell preparation"), and
2. Change item 10(d) to "Positive finding of antiphospholipid antibodies based on
   (1) an abnormal serum level of IgG or IgM anticardiolipin antibodies,
   (2) a positive test result for lupus anticoagulant using a standard method, or
   (3) a false-positive serologic test for syphilis known to be positive for at least 6 months and confirmed by *Treponema pallidum* immobilization or fluorescent treponemal antibody absorption test."

Standard methods should be used in testing for the presence of antiphospholipid.

From Hochberg MC. Updating the American College of Rheumatology revised criteria for the classification of systemic lupus erythematosus (letter), *Arthritis Rheum* 40:1725, 1997.

*The proposed classification is based on 11 criteria. For the purpose of identifying patients in clinical studies, a person shall be said to have SLE if any 4 or more of the 11 criteria are present, serially or simultaneously, during any interval of observation.

Box 29-1	Drugs That Can Produce Clinical and Serologic Features of Systemic Lupus Erythematosus (SLE)

Antiarrhythmics (e.g., procainamide hydrochloride)
Anticonvulsants (e.g., phenytoin)
Antihypertensives (e.g., hydralazine hydrochloride)
Miscellaneous (e.g., chlorpromazine, isoniazid, penicillin, sulfonamides)

dependent, and they are never the only ANAs present in the blood. Even with discontinuation of the drug, antibody titers usually remain elevated for months or years.

Only about 4% of patients who take these drugs will develop the antibodies suggestive of lupus. Of those 4%, only an extremely small number will develop overt drug-induced lupus. The symptoms of drug-induced lupus are similar to those of systemic lupus, but milder. Patients with drug-related lupus have a predominance of pulmonary and polyserositic signs and symptoms. Patients with drug-induced lupus have no associated renal or central nervous system (CNS) disease. In addition, lupus-inducing drugs do not appear to exacerbate idiopathic SLE. The symptoms usually fade when the medications are discontinued.

Neonatal lupus is a rare condition acquired from the passage of maternal autoantibodies, specifically anti-Ro/SS-A or anti-La/SS-B, that can affect the skin, heart, and blood of the fetus and newborn. Neonatal lupus is associated with a rash that appears within the first several weeks of life and may persist for about 6 months before disappearing. Congenital heart block can occur but is much less common than a rash. Neonatal lupus is not systemic lupus.

ETIOLOGY

The cause of SLE is unknown (idiopathic). Although no single etiologic agent has been identified, a primary defect in the regulation of the immune system is considered important in the pathogenesis of the disorder. Genetic predisposition can be a factor. Hormones and environmental factors that may trigger the disease include infections, antibiotics (especially sulfonamides and penicillin derivatives), ultraviolet (UV) light, extreme stress, and certain drugs. A combination of these factors may be synergistic.

Antibodies directed against T lymphocytes, including the membrane molecules that mediate their responses, are regularly detected in patients with SLE. Their role in the pathogenesis of autoimmunity is still unclear.

Hormonal Influences

Hormonal factors may explain why lupus occurs more frequently in women than in men. Lupus is often called a "woman's disease" because a disproportionate number of females between puberty and menopause suffer from SLE. The increase in disease symptoms may be caused by hormones, particularly estrogen. There is a risk that the disease will worsen during pregnancy and the immediate postpartum period. In addition, postmenopausal therapy is associated with an increased risk for developing SLE. The exact reason for the greater prevalence of lupus in women, and the cyclic increase in symptoms, is unknown.

A condition called the **antiphospholipid syndrome** can be secondary to lupus and may complicate pregnancy. Antibodies against specific autoantigens often present on coagulation factors can cause blood to clot faster than normal or in some cases, not at all. Antiphospholipid antibodies can be found in many patients with lupus and pose a particular risk to pregnant lupus patients because their presence is often associated with miscarriages.

Both the developing fetus and the pregnant mother with lupus are at increased risk of various complications during and after pregnancy. Passive placental transfer of maternal antibodies can produce transient abnormalities such as hepatosplenomegaly, cytopenia, and a photosensitive rash in the newborn. These conditions do resolve themselves in the newborn after the antibody titer declines (see previous discussion on neonatal lupus).

Genetic Predisposition

Lupus is known to occur within families, but there is no identified gene or genes associated with lupus. Previously, genes on chromosome 6 called "immune response genes" were associated with the disease. The recent discovery of a gene on chromosome 1 has been associated with lupus in certain families. Only 10% of lupus patients will have a parent or sibling who already has or may develop lupus. Statistics show that only about 5% of the children born to individuals with lupus will develop the illness.

Environmental Factors

Various factors, including UV light and bacterial and viral infections, are capable of inducing or exacerbating the signs and symptoms of SLE. These factors may act in different ways. For example, UV light may cause DNA to form thymine dimers, which significantly alters the antigenicity of DNA and could result in the formation of anti-DNA.

EPIDEMIOLOGY

Lupus can occur at any age and in either gender, although it occurs 10 to 15 times more frequently among adult females than among adult males after puberty. The Lupus Foundation of America estimates that approximately 1.4 million Americans have a form of lupus. The overall incidence of SLE is estimated to be 50 to 70 new cases per year per 1 million population.

Racial groups such as African Americans, Native Americans, Puerto Ricans, and Asians (particularly Chinese) demonstrate an increased frequency of SLE. Lupus is two to three times more prevalent among people of color. The incidence of SLE in African-American women between the 20 and 64 years old is 1 in 245. The reasons for ethnic differences are not clear.

The prevalence rate, based on a total population, is 1 in 2000, but it is 1 in 700 for women between 20 and 64 years old; 80% of those with systemic lupus develop it between ages 15 and 45 years.

Survival is estimated to be greater than 90% at 10 years after diagnosis. The highest mortality rate is in patients with progressive renal involvement or CNS disease. The two most frequent causes of death are renal failure and infectious complications.

SIGNS AND SYMPTOMS

Systemic lupus erythematosus is a disease of acute and chronic inflammation. Symptoms of SLE often mimic other, less serious illnesses. Fever is one of the most common clinical manifestations of SLE. Disease activity accounts for more than 66% of febrile episodes in patients with SLE. Antibodies with elevated titers that are characteristic of lupus disease activity rather than infection include anti-dsDNA and anti–ribosomal P antibodies, as well as reduced levels of complement and leukopenia.

Many of the clinical manifestations of SLE are a consequence of tissue damage from vasculopathy mediated by

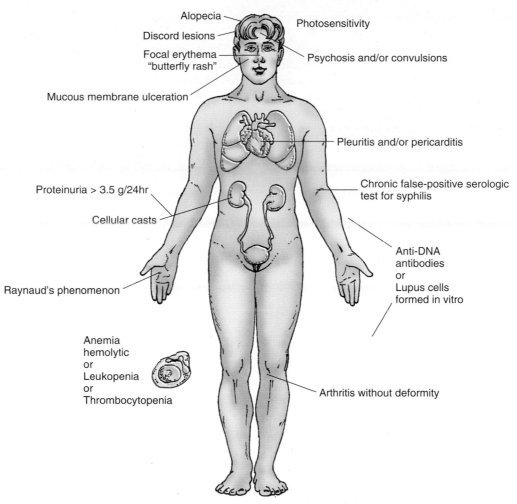

Figure 29-1   Signs and symptoms of systemic lupus erythematosus (SLE).

immune complexes. Other conditions (e.g., thrombocytope-nia, antiphospholipid syndrome) are the direct effects of antibodies to cell surface molecules or serum components.

Manifestations of the disease range from a typical mild illness limited to a photosensitive facial rash and transient diffuse arthritis to life-threatening involvement of the CNS or renal, cardiac, or respiratory system (Figure 29-1). In the early phases, it is often difficult to distinguish SLE from other systemic rheumatic disorders, such as progressive systemic sclerosis (PSS), polymyositis, primary Sjögren's syndrome, primary Raynaud's phenomenon, and rheumatoid arthritis. Polyarthritis and dermatitis are the most common clinical manifestations.

The course of the disease is highly variable. It usually follows a chronic and irregular course with periods of exacerbations and remissions. Clinical signs and symptoms can include fever, weight loss, malaise, arthralgia (joint pain) and arthritis (inflammation of the joints), and the characteristic erythematous, maculopapular ("butterfly") rash over the bridge of the nose (Table 29-2). In addition, there is a tendency toward increased susceptibility to common and

Table 29-2	Systemic Lupus Erythematosus Symptoms (Percentage of Cases)
Symptom	**%**
Achy joints (arthralgia)	95
Frequent fevers of more than 37.8° C	90
Arthritis (swollen joints)	90
Prolonged or extreme fatigue	81
Skin rashes	74
Anemia	71
Kidney involvement	50
Pain in the chest on deep breathing (pleurisy)	45
Butterfly-shaped rash across the cheek and nose	42
Sun or light sensitivity (photosensitivity)	30
Hair loss	27
Abnormal blood clotting problems	20
Raynaud's phenomenon (fingers turning white and/or blue in the cold)	17
Seizures	15
Mouth or nose ulcers	12

From www.lupusfoundation.org, April 2007.

opportunistic infections. Multiple organ systems may be affected simultaneously.

The onset of lupus can be caused by sun exposure, resulting in sudden development of a rash and then possibly other symptoms. In some patients an infection, even a cold, does not improve, and then complications arise. These complications may be the first signs of lupus. In some women the first symptoms develop during pregnancy or soon after delivery.

Infection

About one fifth of episodes of fever are caused by infections in patients with SLE. Infections are the leading cause of death in hospitalized patients. Infections can be caused by bacterial, viral, fungal, or parasitic pathogens. Immunosuppression produced by treatment (e.g., steroids) can interfere with host defense against opportunistic infections (e.g., *Mycobacterium tuberculosis, Histoplasma capsulatum, Listeria monocytogenes*).

Cutaneous Features

Approximately 20% to 25% of patients with SLE develop dermal disorders as the initial manifestation of the disease. As many as 65% of patients will develop a cutaneous abnormality during the course of the disease. The characteristic erythematous, maculopapular "butterfly rash" across the nose and upper cheeks is the cutaneous feature for which the disease is named, **lupus erythematosus,** the "red wolf" (Figure 29-2). This rash may also be observed on the arms

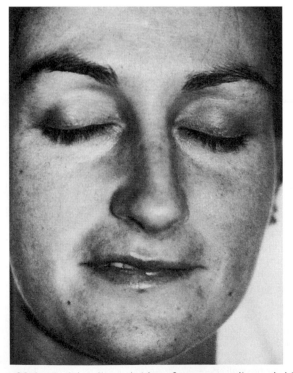

Figure 29-2 Facial rash over bridge of nose, upper lip, and chin in patient with active SLE. *(From Kaye D, Rose LF:* Fundamentals of internal medicine, *St Louis, 1983, Mosby.)*

and trunk. Exposure to UV light will worsen erythematous, as well as other types of, cutaneous lesions.

The spectrum of cutaneous abnormalities includes urticaria, angioedema, nonthrombocytopenic purpura associated with the presence of cryoglobulins, scale formation, and ulcerations of oral and genital mucous membranes. Although neither the collection of immunoglobulins and complement at the dermal-epidermal junction nor the presence of specific antibody nuclear ribonucleoprotein (RNP), Sm, native DNA, and single-stranded DNA appears to play a direct role in the pathogenesis of cutaneous lupus lesion, Ro (SS-A) and perhaps La (SS-B) antibodies may be prominent factors.

Diffuse or patchy alopecia is also a common cutaneous manifestation. Hair loss is caused by pustular lesions of the scalp and is most often related to the stress of the disease process. Although the cause of pustular lesions is unknown, these inflammatory infiltrates are characterized by the presence of predominantly Ia-positive (activated) T lymphocytes with both CD4+ and CD8+ phenotypes.

Approximately 2% to 3% of SLE patients demonstrate lupus panniculitis. This condition is characterized by tender or nontender subcutaneous nodules that sometimes ulcerate and discharge a yellowish lipid material. In addition, various nonspecific skin changes are observable secondary to vascular insults. **Raynaud's phenomenon** is demonstrated by approximately one third of patients with SLE and appears to be increased in those who have antibodies to nuclear RNP in their serum.

The presence of lesions does not distinguish between the limited cutaneous (discoid lupus erythematosus) and the cutaneous manifestation of SLE. The term **discoid lupus** is used to differentiate the benign dermatitis of cutaneous lupus from the cutaneous involvement of SLE. In discoid lupus the round lesion is an erythematous, inflammatory dermatosis. These lesions are primarily located in light-exposed areas of the skin.

Renal Characteristics

Complement-mediated injury to the renal system is a usual consequence of the high levels of immune complexes in the blood that are deposited in tissues such as the kidneys. Renal disease progression is highly unpredictable. It may be acute, but more typically it progresses slowly. As the kidneys degenerate, the urinary sediment is typical of acute glomerulonephritis and later of chronic glomerulonephritis. Acute glomerulonephritis is characterized by the presence of erythrocytes, leukocytes, and granular and red blood cell (RBC) casts in urinary sediment. The presence of proteinuria may lead to nephrotic syndrome. If end-stage renal disease (renal failure) occurs, it can be managed by dialysis or allograft transplantation.

The systemic necrotizing vasculitis of SLE involves small blood vessels and leads to renal involvement. The most common method of classification of the renal involvement of SLE is the World Health Organization (WHO) system, which is based on histopathologic criteria. The stages of renal disease range from the earliest and least severe form, class II, characterized by mesangial deposits of immunoglobulin and C3, to class V, the most severe form of involvement.

Lymphadenopathy

Enlargement of peripheral and axial lymph nodes and splenomegaly both occur in patients with SLE; however, these conditions are usually transient. Patients with SLE may be at greater risk of developing lymphoma than the general population, especially those with secondary Sjögren's syndrome.

Serositis

Serositis is an inflammation of the membrane consisting of **mesothelium,** a thin layer of connective tissue that lines enclosed body cavities. Mesothelium, a type of epithelium, is originally derived from the mesoderm lining the primitive embryonic body cavity. It becomes the covering of the serous membranes of the body surfaces such as the peritoneum, pleura, and pericardium. Inflammation of these serosal surfaces leads to sterile peritonitis, pleuritis, or pericarditis and is frequently accompanied by severe pain. Serositis is associated with an increased frequency of thrombophlebitis, which may lead to pulmonary embolization.

Cardiopulmonary Characteristics

Inflammation of the myocardium in patients with SLE can produce persistent tachycardia and, occasionally, intractable congestive heart failure. Ischemic disease or, more often, atherosclerotic coronary disease may occur. Patients with severe nephrosis or those treated with corticosteroids for a prolonged time are at an increased risk for developing atherosclerosis.

Pulmonary function studies reveal occult diffusion and obstructive abnormalities in a high proportion of SLE patients, but clinical problems secondary to pulmonary involvement are unusual. Massive hemoptysis may result from acute alveolar hemorrhage. This particular complication occurs in the absence of any detectable bleeding diathesis and is associated with a high rate of mortality.

Gastrointestinal Manifestations

Nonspecific gastrointestinal symptoms are relatively common in patients with SLE, but acute abdominal crises caused by visceral and peritoneal vasculitis are less common. Infarction and perforation of the bowel and viscera are associated with a high rate of mortality. Acute and chronic pancreatitis may also develop as a secondary complication of acute lupus or as a complication during therapy.

Musculoskeletal Features

A characteristic arthritis of SLE is a transient and peripheral polyarthritis with symmetric involvement of both small and large joints. Chronic arthritis can result in disability and deformity in SLE patients. Rheumatoid-like hand deformities develop in about 10% of patients. Osteonecrosis develops in one fourth of all SLE patients. Arthropathy of osteonecro-

sis, or *avascular necrosis,* is often initially detected in weight-bearing joints such as the hips and knees.

Neuropsychiatric Features

In SLE, various neuropsychiatric manifestations develop secondary to involvement of the central and peripheral nervous systems. CNS involvement in SLE includes inflammation of the brain or intracranial blood vessels (vasculitis) and ischemic complications of vasculitis.

The most common abnormalities are disturbances of mental function, ranging from mild confusion, with memory deficiency and impairment of orientation and perception, to psychiatric disturbances such as hypomania, delirium, and schizophrenia. The most common manifestations are cognitive dysfunction, headache, seizures, and psychiatric conditions. Aseptic meningitis, stroke, encephalopathy, movement disorders, and myelopathy can be observed.

Seizures of the grand mal type may be the initial manifestation of SLE and may be present long before the multisystem disease develops. In addition, some patients may have epilepsy and severe headaches.

Anti–ribosomal P antibodies have been detected in patients with lupus who have psychosis or depression.

Late-Onset Lupus

Lupus can occur at any age, in either gender, in any race. The average age of onset is 59 years; average age at diagnosis is 62 years. Late-onset lupus affects women eight times more often than men. Late-onset lupus is found primarily in Caucasians, but it occurs in all races.

Symptoms in most cases are relatively mild, but symptoms of lupus in older people can mimic other diseases (e.g., rheumatoid arthritis, Sjögren's syndrome, polymyalgia rheumatica). Distinguishing among these disorders can be difficult and may result in a delayed or missed diagnosis. Drug-induced lupus occurs more often in older people because they are more likely to have conditions (high blood pressure, heart disease) that require treatment that may cause the symptoms of lupus. Symptoms generally fade when the medication is discontinued. Patients with late-onset lupus have a good survival rate and rarely die of the disease or complications of therapy when treated conservatively.

IMMUNOLOGIC MANIFESTATIONS

Patients with SLE are known to produce multiple autoantibodies. There are two leading hypotheses, not mutually exclusive, as to why so many different antibodies develop. One hypothesis supports the belief that antibody-forming B lymphocytes are stimulated in a relatively nonspecific manner, so-called polyclonal B-cell activation. The second hypothesis is that the immune response in SLE is specifically stimulated by antigens. The most compelling evidence in its favor is that the antibody molecules formed over time show evidence of the gene rearrangement and somatic mutation characteristic of an antigen-driven response.

Laboratory features of SLE are the presence of ANAs, immune complexes, decreased complement level, tissue deposition of immunoglobulins and complement, circulating anticoagulants, and other autoantibodies. The human **antineutrophil cytoplasmic antibodies (ANCAs),** described for the first time in 1982, are directed against antigenic components mainly present in primary granules of neutrophils. ANCAs are serologic markers of primary necrotizing systemic vasculitis, particularly in Wegener's granulomatosis. In addition, these antibodies have a prognostic interest because, in most cases, their titer is correlated to clinical activity during the disease.

Cellular Aspects

Systemic lupus erythematosus is a disease that results from defects in the regulatory mechanism of the immune system. Studies of the immunopathogenesis of lupus nephritis have demonstrated a variety of aberrations in T-cell and B-cell function. It is uncertain if the disease represents a primary dysfunction of T cells or B cells, but alterations in function do result. Lymphocyte-subset abnormalities are a major immunologic feature of SLE. Among the T-cell subsets, a lack of or reduced generalized suppressor T-cell function and hyperproduction of helper T cells occurs. The formation of lymphocytotoxic antibodies with a predominant specificity for T lymphocytes by patients with SLE at least partially explains the interference with certain functional activities of T lymphocytes associated with SLE. Lymphocytotoxic antibodies are capable of both destroying T lymphocytes in the presence of complement and coating peripheral blood T cells.

The regulation of antibody production by B lymphocytes, ordinarily a function of the subpopulation of suppressor T cells, appears to be defective in patients with SLE. Although no single cause can be implicated in the pathogenesis of SLE, patients exhibit a state of spontaneous B-lymphocyte hyperactivity with ensuing uncontrolled production of a wide variety of antibodies to both host and exogenous antigens. Host response to some antigens, such as vaccination with influenza, is normal in many instances, and the patient manifests a specific, well-controlled humoral immune response.

Humoral Aspects

Circulating immune complexes are the hallmark of SLE. Patients with SLE exhibit multiple serum antibodies that react with native or altered "self" antigens. Demonstrable antibodies include antibodies to the following:
- Nuclear components.
- Cell surface and cytoplasmic antigens of polymorphonuclear and lymphocytic leukocytes, erythrocytes, platelets, and neuronal cells.
- Immunoglobulin G (IgG).

Systemic lupus erythematosus is characterized by autoantibodies to almost any organ or tissue in the body. These antibodies may not be specifically diagnostic for SLE. In addition, some may have pathologic significance.

Antibodies to host antigens, particularly nuclear antigens such as DNA, are the principal type of antibody produced in SLE. ANAs are a heterogeneous group of antibodies produced against a variety of antigens within the cell nucleus. ANAs may be found in diseases other than SLE (e.g., other rheumatic or nonrheumatic diseases), as well as in some patients undergoing specific drug therapy and in healthy older individuals. The absence of ANAs virtually excludes the diagnosis of SLE unless the patient is being chemically immunosuppressed. ANA titers and specific anti-DNA antibodies fluctuate during the course of the disease. In some cases a rise in titer may forewarn of an impending disease flare-up.

Antigens to which antibodies are formed are present on nucleic acid molecules (DNA and RNA) or proteins (histones and nonhistones) and on determinants consisting of both nucleic acid and protein molecules. Drug-induced cases of lupus have a high incidence of antibodies to histones. Some of these antibodies are directed against the double-stranded helical DNA (*native DNA* or dsDNA). The presence of anti–native DNA (anti-nDNA) antibodies was reported in 1957. High titers of dsDNA are seen primarily in SLE and closely parallel disease activity. Most SLE patients simultaneously demonstrate antibodies to nucleoprotein and native DNA.

Other nuclear antibodies are directed at the determinants of single-stranded DNA (ssDNA). Antibody titers of 1:32 or greater indicate a substantial concentration of antibody in an autoimmune response. Antibody to the Smith (Sm) antigen, a nuclear acidic protein extractable by aqueous solution, is considered a marker for SLE because anti-Sm has been found almost exclusively in patients with SLE. The presence of anti-Sm is seen in 25% to 30% of patients with SLE, but it rarely occurs in other systemic rheumatic (collagen) diseases.

The ANA antideoxyribonucleoprotein (anti-DNP) gives rise to the *LE cell,* which is found in more than 90% of untreated patients with active SLE (Figure 29-3). SLE patients with serositis may form LE cells in vivo. The LE cell testing procedure is now an obsolete test. In SLE patients with serositis, LE cells formed in vivo may be observed in aspirate fluid (e.g., pleural fluid). LE cells have been shown to be an expression of the interaction between IgG antibodies and deoxyribonucleohistones (DNP). Anti-DNP is referred to as the "LE serum factor."

Antibodies to the Robert (Ro) soluble substance-A (SS-A) nuclear antigens are associated with SLE skin disease and the neonatal SLE syndrome. Antibodies to the Lane soluble substance-B (SS-B) antigens are associated with SLE and with primary and secondary forms of Sjögren's syndrome. Their presence with SS-A antigen in SLE indicates mild disease. When present as the only antibody, SS-B is associated with primary Sjögren's syndrome.

Autoantibodies to RBCs result in hemolytic anemia and can be detected by the anti–human globulin (AHG) test. Membrane-specific autoantibodies to neutrophils and platelets and autoantibodies to lymphocytes (cold-reactive type) are specific for SLE. Antibody titers correlate with disease activity.

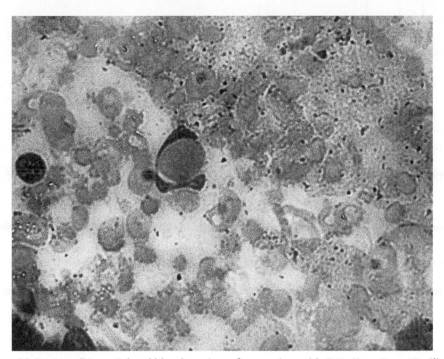

Figure 29-3   LE cell in peripheral blood specimen from patient with SLE. *(From Bauer JD:* Clinical laboratory methods, *ed 9, St Louis, 1982, Mosby.)*

Immunologic Consequences

Antibodies combine with their corresponding antigens to form immune complexes. When the mononuclear phagocyte system is unable to eliminate these immune complexes completely, immune complexes accumulate in the blood circulation. These circulating immune complexes are deposited in the subendothelial layers of the vascular basement membranes of multiple target organs, where they mediate inflammation. The sites of deposition are determined in part by the following physiochemical properties of the particular antigens or antibodies involved:

- Size
- Molecular configuration
- Immunoglobulin class
- Complement-fixing ability

After deposition, the immune complexes seem to initiate a localized inflammatory response that stimulates neutrophils to the site of inflammation, activates complement, and results in the release of kinins and prostaglandins. These activities become the basis of antibody-dependent, cell-mediated tissue injury.

DIAGNOSTIC EVALUATION

The manifestations of SLE expressed in laboratory findings are numerous. Histologic, hematologic, and serologic abnormalities reflect the multisystem nature of this disease.

Histologic Changes

The earliest pathologic abnormalities are those of acute vasculitis. Supportive tissue becomes edematous, initially infiltrated with neutrophils and later with plasma cells and lymphocytes. Persistent inflammation results in local deposition of a cellular homogeneous material, histologically similar to fibrin. Nuclear debris from resulting cellular necrosis reacts with ANAs (discussed later in this section) to form hematoxylin bodies. The presence of immunoglobulins, predominantly IgM and IgG, in vascular lesions can be demonstrated by indirect immunofluorescence.

Renal pathology can also be observed in SLE. The two basic renal abnormalities that manifest are (1) proliferative glomerulonephritis, which resembles the renal changes in immune complex nephritis, and (2) membranous nephritis.

Hematologic and Hemostatic Findings

In SLE a moderate anemia (normocytic normochromic anemia) representing chronic disease is a consistent factor. Some patients display coating of erythrocytes, which can be demonstrated by a positive AHG test, but actual hemolysis is infrequent. Lymphocytopenia is common and often reflects disease activity. Thrombocytopenia (50-100 $\times$ 10^9/L) may also be seen.

Hemostatic Testing

Lupus anticoagulants, antiphospholipid antibodies, are often seen in association with SLE. Antiphospholipid antibodies develop in up to 20% of patients with SLE. These form a group of antibodies detected by tests for lupus anticoagulant and anticardiolipin antibodies.

Circulating anticoagulants are believed to be associated with the presence of false-positive serologic test results for syphilis. Because of the presence of lupus anticoagulant, patients with SLE frequently demonstrate prolonged prothrombin time (PT) and partial thromboplastin time (PTT) results, but lupus anticoagulant rarely causes hemostatic problems. Inhibitors are not necessarily associated with bleeding unless some other defect is present. Because lupus anticoagulant is an inhibitor or a prothrombin activator, it is often associated with excessive thrombosis rather than with bleeding. Patients with SLE have a high incidence of thrombotic episodes. Although less common, specific coagulation factor antibodies directed against coagulation factors VIII, IX, XI, and XII have been described. Thrombocytopenia can also occur because of removal of antiphospholipid antibody–coated platelets.

Serologic Findings

Serologic testing frequently reveals high levels of anti-DNA antibodies, reduced complement levels, and the presence of complement breakdown products of C3 (C3d and C3c). In addition, cryoglobulins, which in some cases represent immune complexes, are frequently present in the serum of patients with SLE. Because monoclonal gammopathies have occasionally been described, a marked increase in gamma globulins may result in a hyperviscosity syndrome or renal tubular acidosis. Serum cryoglobulins of a mixed IgG-IgM type are found in patients with hypocomplementemia. The level of cryoglobulin correlates well with the severity of SLE. The following procedural results are helpful in assessing renal disease:

- Antibody to double-stranded DNA.
- Levels of C3 and C4 (with C4 probably being the most sensitive result).
- Cryoglobulin levels.

A general correlation exists between abnormal results in each of these procedures and disease activity in many patients, but considerable disagreement surrounds the usefulness of such measurements in predicting renal disease activity. The best laboratory procedures for monitoring the activity of renal disease are serum creatinine, urinary protein excretion, and careful examination of urine sediment.

Complement

Inherited deficiencies of several complement components are associated with lupuslike illnesses. Some, but not all, deficiencies are coded for by autosomal recessive genes of the sixth chromosome, which are in linkage disequilibrium with HLA-DRw2. The association of complement deficiencies with SLE may represent the fortuitous association of linked HLA-D region genes, rather than some unusual susceptibility induced by the complement deficiency.

Serum levels of complement typically are reduced, particularly during states of active disease. Deficiencies involving both classic and alternative pathway complement components in SLE patients have resulted from consumption of components at the tissue sites of immune complex deposition, impaired synthesis, or both. A depressed level of complement is not specific for the diagnosis of SLE, but it is a helpful guide in treating patients. Levels of complement (C3, C4) are generally reduced in relationship to disease activity, and the fluctuation in these levels is often used to monitor disease activity. Patients with decreased levels are at risk for renal and CNS involvement. Deficiencies of C1, C3, and C4 are associated with SLE and other rheumatic diseases.

Antibodies

Nonspecific elevation in immunoglobulin levels, particularly IgM and IgG, frequently occurs in SLE. An actual deficiency of IgA appears to be more common in SLE than in normal individuals.

The ANA procedure (discussed in detail in the next section) is a valuable screening tool for SLE; it has virtually replaced the LE cell test because of its wider range of reactivity with nuclear antigens, as well as its greater sensitivity and quality control characteristics.

Antinuclear Antibodies

Characteristics and Implications. ANAs are a heterogeneous group of circulating immunoglobulins that include IgM, IgG, and IgA. These immunoglobulins react with the whole nucleus or nuclear components (e.g., proteins, DNA, histones) in host tissues; therefore they are true autoantibodies. Generally, ANAs have no organ or species specificity and are capable of cross-reacting with nuclear material from humans (e.g., human leukocytes) or various animal tissues (e.g., rat liver, mouse kidney). ANAs are found in other diseases (e.g., rheumatoid arthritis), are associated with certain drugs, and are found in aging persons without disease (Table 29-3). Thus, assays for ANAs are not specific for SLE. ANAs are present in more than 95% of SLE patients. Because the detection of ANAs is not diagnostic of only SLE, their presence cannot confirm the disease, but the absence of ANAs can be used to help rule out SLE. The significance of the presence of ANAs in a patient's serum must be considered in relation to the patient's age, gender, clinical signs and symptoms, and other laboratory findings.

Systematic Classification. ANAs can be divided into four groups to provide a systematic classification: antibodies to DNA, antibodies to histone, antibodies to nonhistone proteins, and antibodies to nucleolar antigens.

Antibodies to DNA. Antibodies to DNA can be divided into two major groups: (1) antibodies that react with native

Table 29-3	Antibodies in Systemic Rheumatic Diseases		
Systemic Lupus Erythematosus (SLE)	**Progressive Systemic Sclerosis (PSS)**	**Polymyositis**	**Rheumatoid Arthritis (RA)**
Antinuclear antibodies	Antinuclear antibodies	Antinuclear antibodies	Antinuclear antibodies
Anti–native DNA	Anti–Scl-1	Anti–Jo-1	Rheumatoid factors
Anti-Sm			

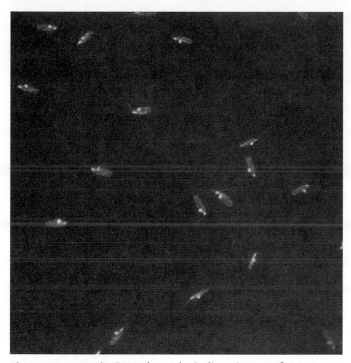

Figure 29-4 Anti-nDNA shown by indirect immunofluorescence. Staining of both the small kinetoplast and the adjacent larger nucleus of *Crithidia luciliae* occurs simultaneously. *(From Bauer JD: Clinical laboratory methods, ed 9, St Louis, 1982, Mosby.)*

Table 29-4	Immunologic Assays for Detection and Monitoring of SLE
Name of Assay	**Reference Range**
Antibodies	
Anti–double-stranded (ds) DNA antibody	Negative (1:10)
Anti-La (SS-B) antibody	Negative
Anti–liver cytosol antibody	<15 U/mL
Anti–liver-kidney microsomal (LKM) antibody	<1:40
Antimitochondrial antibody	Negative
Antinuclear antibody	Negative (1:40)
Anti–ribosomal P protein antibody	<20 U/mL
Antiribonucleoprotein (anti-RNP) antibody	Negative
Anti-Ro (SS-A) antibody	Negative
Anti-Smith IgG	Negative
Anti–soluble liver antigen antibody	<5 U/mL
Complement	
Total complement	63-145 U/mL
C3	86-145 mg/dL
C4	20-58 mg/dL

(double-stranded) DNA, and (2) antibodies that recognize denatured (single-stranded) DNA only.

Antibodies that react with native DNA appear to interact with antigenic determinants present on the deoxyribose-phosphate backbone of the beta helix of DNA. These autoantibodies characteristically stain the kinetoplast of the hemoflagellate *Crithidia luciliae,* a substrate used to detect anti–native DNA antibodies by indirect immunofluorescence (Figure 29-4). Antibodies reactive with denatured DNA probably react with the purine and pyrimidine bases of DNA. These bases are readily accessible on ssDNA; they are buried within the beta helix of dsDNA and are therefore inaccessible. Anti–denatured DNA antibodies are unable to cross-react with native DNA. Conformational changes in the deoxyribose-phosphate backbone of denatured DNA appear to be important for antigenicity.

Antibodies to Histones. Antibodies to histones have been shown to react with all major classes of histones: H1, H2A, H2B, H3, and H4. Antihistone antibodies can be induced by drugs such as procainamide and hydralazine. Procainamide-induced lupus erythematosus is characterized by IgG antibodies against the histone complex H2A-H2B in symptomatic patients with SLE. In asymptomatic patients the antibody may be restricted to the IgM class. Antibodies specific to other nuclear antigens are usually absent in drug-induced lupus, in contrast to patients with SLE, who have ANAs of multiple specificity.

Patients with SLE are characterized by the presence of antibodies to multiple antigens, including Sm, RNP, dsDNA, chromatin, and SS-A/Ro (Table 29-4). There are 11 criteria for the diagnosis of SLE, and for a definitive diagnosis, patients must meet at least four of these criteria (see Table 29-1). Two of the criteria are a positive ANA and the detection of antibodies to Sm, dsDNA, or cardiolipin. Antibodies to Sm are detected in 20% to 30% of SLE patients, and antibodies to dsDNA may occur in up to 60% of patients. Antibodies to Sm and RNP typically occur together because they react with different proteins that are associated in an RNP particle called a "spliceosome." A positive Sm indicates a high probability of SLE.

Presence of antibodies to dsDNA is one of the criteria for the diagnosis of SLE, and these antibodies are associated with active disease. The presence of dsDNA is a major concern in patients with SLE. Formation and deposition of immune complexes in various organ systems can affect various organ systems. Antibodies to dsDNA have recently been reported in rheumatoid arthritis patients being treated with the new tumor necrosis factor alpha (TNF-α) inhibitors as well. Patients with SLE have antibodies to chromatin more often than antibodies to dsDNA. These chromatin antibodies are also associated with glomerulonephritis and have been identified, along with dsDNA antibodies, in immune complexes eluted from patients' kidneys. Patients with drug-induced lupus develop antibodies to chromatin and in some cases to the histone component of chromatin, but not to dsDNA.

Demonstration of only antihistone antibodies may be useful in distinguishing drug-induced lupus from SLE.

Antibodies to Nonhistone Proteins. Another primary class of ANAs in systemic autoimmune disorders is characterized by reactivity with soluble nonhistone nuclear protein and RNA-protein complexes. Clinically important antibodies that react with nuclear nonhistone proteins are listed in Table 29-5.

Table 29-5	Antibodies to Nonhistone Proteins (NhP) and NhP-RNA Complexes in Systemic Rheumatic Diseases	
Antibody	**Disease**	**Incidence (%)**
Centromere/kinetochore	CREST variant of progressive systemic sclerosis (PSS)	70-90
	Diffuse scleroderma	10-20
Jo-1	Polymyositis	31
Ki antigen	Systemic lupus erythematosus (SLE)	20
Ku	Polymyositis/scleroderma overlap	55
Ma antigen	SLE	20
Mi-I	Dermatomyositis	11
NuMa (nuclear mitotic apparatus) antigen	Rheumatoid arthritis (RA)	
	Sjögren's syndrome	
	Carpal tunnel syndrome	
	SLE	3
Proliferating cell nuclear antigen (PCNA)	RA	90
RANA (RA-associated nuclear antigen)	PSS	20
Scl-70	SLE	30
Sm (Smith)	Sjögren's syndrome	70
SS-A/Ro	SLE	50
	Other connective tissue diseases	
	Sjögren's syndrome	40-50
SS-B/La	SLE	15
	Mixed connective tissue disease	>95
UI-RNP	SLE	35

Modified from Reimer G, Tan E: Antinuclear antibodies. In Stein J, editor: *Internal medicine,* Boston, 1987, Little, Brown.
CREST, Calcinosis, Raynaud's phenomenon, esophageal motility abnormalities, sclerodactyly, and telangiectasia.

Antibodies to Nucleolar Antigens. The antibodies to nucleolar antigens are as follows:

- U3-RNA-protein complex (enzyme-transcribing ribosomal genes in nucleolus)
- 7-2-RNP
- RNA polymerase I
- PM-Scl

These antinucleolar antibodies are primarily associated with polymyositis-scleroderma overlap, where they have the highest incidence and titers. However, they are rarely demonstrated in PSS, dermatomyositis, or scleroderma.

Laboratory Evaluation

Demonstrable antibodies include antibodies to nuclear components; cell surface and cytoplasmic antigens of polymorphonuclear and lymphocytic leukocytes, erythrocytes, platelets, and neuronal cells; and IgG. The detection of ANAs is a valuable screening tool for SLE.

Immunofluorescence is extremely sensitive and may show positive results in cases where procedures for ANAs (e.g., complement fixation or precipitation) give negative results. At present, immunofluorescence is the most widely used technique for ANA screening. Serologic testing frequently reveals high levels of anti-DNA antibodies, reduced complement levels, and the presence of complement breakdown products of C3 (C3d, C3c).

In addition, cryoglobulins, which may represent immune complexes, are frequently present in the serum of patients with SLE. The level of cryoglobulins correlates well with the severity of SLE. Assays helpful in assessing renal disease associated with SLE are antibody to dsDNA, levels of C3 and C4, and cryoglobulins.

Indirect Immunofluorescent Tests for Antinuclear Antibody

Indirect immunofluorescent tests for ANA are based on the use of fluorescein-conjugated antiglobulin. These methods are extremely sensitive. In one assay the serum specimen is delivered into a well on a microscope slide that contains a mouse liver substrate. Substrates of rat or mouse liver or kidney, or cell-cultured fibroblasts, can also be used as the antigen and are fixed to the slides. If antibody is present in the serum of the patient, the unlabeled antibody will attach to the nuclei of the cells in the substrate. After the substrate is washed in buffer, the slide is incubated with fluorescein-labeled goat anti–human immunoglobulin (AHG). If the patient antibodies have attached themselves to the nuclear antigens in the substrate, the fluorescein-tagged goat AHG will attach to these antibodies. Fluorescence will be seen microscopically using UV light. The slides should be examined as soon as possible. If immediate examination is not possible, the slides can be stored in the dark at 4° C for up to 48 hours before being read.

Several different patterns of fluorescence reactivity are seen, depending on whether the ANAs have reacted with the whole nucleus or with nuclear components such as the nuclear proteins, DNA, or histone (a simple protein). This difference in nuclear fluorescence pattern reflects specificity for various diseases. Patterns are described as being diffused or homogeneous, peripheral, speckled, or nucleolar fluorescence. Nuclear rim (peripheral) patterns correlate with antibody to native DNA and DNP and bear correlation with SLE, SLE activity, and lupus nephritis. Homogeneous (diffused) patterns suggest SLE or another connective tissue disorder. Speckled patterns are found in many diseases, including SLE. Nucleolar patterns are seen in patients with progressive systemic sclerosis (PSS) and Sjögren's syndrome.

After ensuring that the results for positive and negative control specimens are providing the expected reactions, the results for the patient are reported. Results from the screening tests are reported as positive or negative. The normal person is expected to give a negative reaction: no green or gold fluorescence is observed. The degree of positive fluorescence may be semiquantitated on a scale of 1+ to 4+. Positive samples give a green-gold fluorescence of a characteristic pattern (homogeneous, peripheral, speckled, or nucleolar).

Indirect Immunofluorescent Technique

Detection of autoantibodies by immunofluorescence has become an extremely valuable tool. This method is extremely sensitive and may be positive in cases where procedures for ANAs, such as complement fixation or precipitation, are negative. At present, the indirect immunofluorescent method on a Hep-2 cell substrate is the primary screening test for diagnosis of systemic rheumatic diseases (SRDs). A negative indirect immunofluorescence result virtually rules out a diagnosis of SLE, but the patterns observed on Hep-2 slides can provide a key to the diagnosis of other SRDs.

Principle of the Procedure. The antigen in the substrate tissue is fixed to a slide for testing. ANA is not specific for a particular organ; therefore any tissue containing nuclei may be used as substrate. The tissues most often used are rat or mouse liver or kidney, or cell-cultured fibroblasts grown on slides. If antibody is present in a patient's serum, the unlabeled antibody will attach to the nuclei in the substrate. After the substrate is washed in buffer, it is incubated with fluorescein-tagged goat AHG. If patient antibodies have affixed themselves to the nuclear antigens of the substrate, the fluorescein-tagged goat AHG will attach to these antibodies. When the slide is examined microscopically, fluorescence will be visible on UV light.

Interpretation of Staining Patterns of Major Rheumatic Autoantibodies

- Double-stranded DNA (dsDNA)
- Chromatin, Sm
- RNP, SS-A/Ro
- SS-B/La
- Scl-70
- Centromere
- Jo-1, cyclic citrullinated peptide (CCP)

Because ANAs react with the whole nucleus or with nuclear components (e.g., proteins, DNA, histone), reaction patterns reflect the distribution of the various antigens within the nuclei. Major ANAs are detected on all Hep-2 slides, but detection of antibodies to SS-A/Ro varies due to the fixation method. Alcohol diminishes or destroys the SS-A/Ro speckled ANA pattern, leading to a negative ANA. It is important always to include a control for antibodies to

Table 29-6	Antinuclear Antibody (ANA) Patterns and Disorders	
ANA Staining Pattern	**Antibody Specificities**	**Related Disorders**
Homogeneous	nDNA	Systemic lupus erythematosus (SLE)
	dsDNA	
	ssDNA	Rheumatoid arthritis (RA)
	DNP	Sjögren's syndrome
	Histones	Mixed connective tissue disease (MCTD)
Peripheral or rim	nDNA	Active SLE
	dsDNA	Sjögren's syndrome
	DNP	
Speckled	Smith (Sm)	SLE
	RNP	RA
		Sjögren's syndrome
		Progressive systemic sclerosis (PSS)
		MCTD
Nucleolar	4-6S RNP	Scleroderma
		Sjögren's syndrome
		Undiagnosed illnesses manifesting Raynaud's phenomenon
Discrete, speckled	Centromere DNA, RNA, ENA	CREST variant of PSS

CREST, Calcinosis, Raynaud's phenomenon, esophageal motility abnormalities, sclerodactyly, and telangiectasia.

SS-A/Ro. Several patterns of reactivity can be observed when a slide is examined in the ANA procedure (Table 29-6).

Diffused or Homogeneous Pattern. The diffused or homogeneous pattern (Plates 3 and 4) characterizes anti–DNA-nucleoprotein antibodies (i.e., antibodies to nDNA, dsDNA, ssDNA, DNP, or histones). Antibodies to DNP have been shown to have the same specificity as the LE factor. Although vacuoles may be seen, the whole nucleus fluoresces evenly. This pattern is typically seen in rheumatoid disorders. High titers of homogeneous ANA suggest SLE, whereas low titers may be found in SLE, rheumatoid arthritis (RA), Sjögren's syndrome, and mixed connective tissue disease (MCTD).

Peripheral Pattern. The peripheral (marginal or rim) pattern results from antibodies to DNA (i.e., nDNA, dsDNA, or DNP). The central protein of the nucleus is only lightly stained or not stained at all, but the nuclear margins fluoresce strongly and appear to extend into the cytoplasm. This pattern is associated with SLE in the active stage of the disease and in Sjögren's syndrome.

Speckled Pattern. The speckled pattern (Plate 5) occurs in the presence of antibody to any extractable nuclear antigen devoid of DNA or histone. The antibody is detected against the saline extractable nuclear antigens: anti-RNP and anti-Sm. A grainy pattern with numerous round dots of nuclear fluorescence, without staining of the nucleoli, is seen in this pattern type.

Antibodies to Sm antigen have been shown to be highly specific for patients with SLE and appear to be "marker" antibodies. Anti-RNP has been found in patients with a wide variety of rheumatic diseases, including SLE, RA, Sjögren's syndrome, PSS, MCTD, and dermatomyositis.

Nucleolar Pattern. The nucleolar pattern (Plate 6) reflects an antibody to nucleolar RNA (4-6S RNP). A few round, smooth nucleoli that vary in size will fluoresce when examined under UV light. The nucleolar pattern is present in about 50% of patients with scleroderma (PSS), in Sjögren's syndrome, and in SLE. This pattern can also be observed in undiagnosed illnesses manifesting Raynaud's phenomenon.

Centromere. The anticentromere antibody reacts with centromeric chromatin of metaphase and interphase cells. The particular pattern on tissue culture cells is discrete and speckled (Plate 7). This antibody appears to be highly selective for the CREST variant of PSS. The CREST syndrome is a variant of systemic sclerosis characterized by the presence of calcinosis, Raynaud's phenomenon, esophageal motility abnormalities, sclerodactyly, and telangiectasia. This antibody is found infrequently in the serum of patients with SLE, MCTD, and PSS.

Rapid Slide Test for Antinucleoprotein

The SLE latex test provides a suspension of polystyrene latex particles coated with DNP (see later procedure). When the latex reagent is mixed with serum containing the ANAs, binding to the DNP-coated latex particles produces macroscopic agglutination. The procedure is positive in SLE and SRDs (e.g., RA, scleroderma, Sjögren's syndrome).

Autoimmune Enzyme Immunoassay

Autoimmune enzyme immunoassay (EIA) provides a qualitative screening test for the presence of ANAs. The assay collectively detects, in one well, total ANAs against dsDNA (nDNA) histones, SS-A/Ro, SS-B/La, Sm, Sm/RNP, Scl-70, Jo-1, and centromeric antigens, along with sera positive for immunofluorescent assay (IFA) Hep-2 ANAs. This assay serves as an alternative to the IFA for screening patient's serum for ANAs.

TREATMENT

For most patients with lupus, effective treatment and prevention methods can minimize symptoms, reduce inflammation, and maintain normal body functions. For photosensitive patients, avoidance of (excessive) sun exposure and the regular application of sunscreens will usually prevent rashes. Regular exercise helps prevent muscle weakness and fatigue. Immunization protects against specific infections. Support groups and counseling can help alleviate the effects of stress. Lupus patients should avoid smoking, excessive consumption of alcohol, overuse or underuse of prescribed medication, and postponing regular medical checkups.

Medications are often prescribed for patients with lupus, depending on the organ(s) involved and the severity of involvement. Common medications include the following:

- *Nonsteroidal antiinflammatory drugs.* NSAIDs are prescribed for a variety of rheumatic diseases, including lupus.

Examples include acetylsalicylic acid (aspirin), ibuprofen (Motrin), and naproxen (Naprosyn). These drugs are usually recommended for muscle and joint pain, and arthritis. Newer NSAIDs contain a prostaglandin in the same capsule (Arthrotec). The other NSAIDs work in the same way as aspirin, but may be more potent.

- *Acetaminophen.* Acetaminophen (Tylenol) is a mild analgesic that can often be used for pain. It has the advantage of causing less stomach irritation than aspirin, but it is not nearly as effective at suppressing inflammation as aspirin.

- *Corticosteroids.* Steroids (e.g., prednisone) are used to reduce inflammation and suppress activity of the immune system. Side effects occur more frequently when steroids are taken over long periods at high doses (e.g., 60 mg prednisone daily for more than 1 month). Such side effects include weight gain, a round face, acne, easy bruising, "thinning" of the bones (osteoporosis), high blood pressure, cataracts, onset of diabetes, increased risk of infection, stomach ulcers, hyperactivity, and increased appetite.

- *Antimalarials.* Chloroquine (Aralen) or hydroxychloroquine (Plaquenil), typically used to treat malaria, may also be useful in some individuals with lupus. Antimalarials are most often prescribed for skin and joint symptoms of lupus.

- *Immunomodulating drugs.* Azathioprine (Imuran) and cyclophosphamide (Cytoxan), cytotoxic drugs, act similar to the corticosteroids in that they suppress inflammation and tend to suppress the immune system. Other agents (e.g., methotrexate, cyclosporin) can be used to control the symptoms of lupus. Some of these agents are used in conjunction with *apheresis*, a blood-filtering treatment. Apheresis has been tried by itself in an effort to remove specific antibodies from the blood, but the results have not been promising.

Recent studies suggest that immunosuppressive therapy targeted against the calcineurin pathway of T-helper (Th) cells, such as tacrolimus, may be effective in the treatment of primary membranous nephropathy.

Newer agents are directed toward specific cells of the immune system. These include agents that block the production of anti-DNA or agents that suppress the manufacture of antibodies through other mechanisms. Examples are intravenous (IV) immunoglobulin injections, which are given on a regular basis to increase platelet numbers.

- *Anticoagulants.* Anticoagulants range from aspirin at very low dose to heparin/coumadin. Generally, such therapy is lifelong in people with lupus and follows an episode of embolus or thrombosis.

Clinical Trials

New drugs are being investigated as therapy for SLE. A projection calls for quadruple the number of drugs to treat SLE by 2015.

LymphoStat-B is a human monoclonal antibody that specifically recognizes and inhibits the biologic activity of

B-lymphocyte stimulator (BlyS). BLyS is a naturally occurring protein discovered by human genome sciences that is required for B lymphocytes to develop into mature plasma B cells, which produce antibodies, the body's first line of defense against infection. Retrospective and prospective studies have shown elevated levels of BLyS in the blood of many SLE patients and in the blood and joint fluid of RA patients. In lupus, RA, and certain other autoimmune diseases, elevated BLyS levels are believed to contribute to the production of autoantibodies. Preclinical and clinical studies demonstrate that B-cell antagonists can reduce autoantibody levels and help control autoimmune disease activity.

Antinuclear Antibody Visible Method

Principle

This test is an indirect immunoenzyme method that uses tissue culture cells (human epithelial cells) as a substrate for the detection and titration of circulating antinuclear antibodies (ANAs) in human serum. Patient serum samples are diluted in buffer and added to microscope slide wells with Hep-2 (human epithelial) cells cultured in them. Hep-2 cells are characterized by extremely large nuclei and the presence of mitotic figures to aid in detection. If specific antibodies are present, stable antigen-antibody complexes are formed that bind anti–human globulin (AHG) labeled with horseradish peroxidase (HRP). The presence of HRP is indicated by a reaction with 3,3′-diaminobenzidine stain. The resulting dark-brown to black staining patterns of the nuclei can be seen with a light microscope. The presence of one or more types of circulating autoantibodies is the hallmark of systemic rheumatic diseases (SRDs).

Specimen Collection and Preparation

The patient should be in a fasting state before specimen collection. The patient must be positively identified when the specimen is collected, and the specimen is to be labeled at the bedside. Specimen labels must include the patient's full name, the date the specimen is collected, the patient's hospital identification number, and the phlebotomist's initials.

Blood should be drawn by aseptic technique. A minimum of 5 to 8 mL of clotted blood (red-top evacuated tube) is required. Allow the blood to clot at room temperature. The specimen should be centrifuged promptly, and the serum should be separated from the red cells immediately. Serum specimens may be stored at 2° to 8° C if tested within 24 to 48 hours. If the specimen cannot be tested within this period, it should be stored frozen at −20° C or below. Do not freeze and thaw sera more than once. Allow serum specimens to reach room temperature before testing. Avoid the use of sera exhibiting a high degree of lipemia, hemolysis, or microbial growth, because these characteristics may result in increased background staining, a decrease in titers, and unclear staining patterns.

Reagents, Supplies, and Equipment

System components provided in ImmunoConcepts Colorzyme ANA Test System (Sacramento, Calif):
- Reactive reagents
  a. Substrate slides

  Each Hep-2 slide well contains Hep-2 cells grown and fixed on the slide. The slides are stable until the labeled expiration date when stored at −20° C and if the pouch appears to be inflated with inert nontoxic gas.

  b. Homogeneous positive control
  c. Speckled positive control
  d. Nucleolar positive control
  e. Centromere positive control
  f. Titratable control serum
  g. Negative control serum
  h. Enzyme antibody reagent (goat anti–human IgG conjugated to HRP)
  i. Color reagent

  Dissolve contents of one pouch in 150 mL of deionized or distilled water. Mix well until completely dissolved. This color reagent is stable for 30 days or until any color change or precipitate is visible.
- Nonreactive reagents
  a. Phosphate-buffered saline (PBS) powder

  Dissolve one pouch of buffer powder in 1 L of deionized or distilled water, cover, and store refrigerated at 2° to 10° C for up to 4 weeks or until signs of contamination or other visible changes occur.

  b. Semipermanent mounting medium
  c. Coverslips

Additional Required Equipment

- 12 × 75–mm test tubes and rack
- Pasteur and calibrated pipettes
- Staining dish or Coplin jar
- Moist chamber for incubation
- Volumetric flask for PBS
- Distilled or deionized water: CAP Type 1 or equivalent, pH 6.0-7.0
- Forceps
- Wash bottle
- Blotting or bibulous paper
- Light microscope

Quality Control

Note: These controls are commercially prepared and included in the test kit.

Positive Control Serum

The ANA-positive (homogeneous) control is a ready-to-use human serum in a dropper vial containing ANAs demonstrating a staining reaction. Sodium azide (0.1% w/v) is added as a preservative. The positive control serum is stable until the labeled expiration date when stored at 2° to 8° C. The ANA-positive control should demonstrate homogeneous staining in the nuclei of the Hep-2 cells.

Negative Control Serum

The ANA-negative control is a ready-to-use human serum in a dropper vial containing no detectable autoantibodies. Sodium azide (0.1% w/v) is added as a preservative. The negative control serum is stable until the labeled expiration date when stored at 2° to 8° C. The ANA-negative control serum should demonstrate little or no nuclear staining.

The control serums must be examined before any patient specimens are examined. The control results must provide the correct positive and negative reactions to validate procedural results. Controls that do not give expected reactions are considered unsatisfactory, and patient test results should not be reported. If the controls do not produce the expected results, the test procedure must be repeated.

CAUTION: Because the control serum is derived from human sources, it should be handled in the same manner as clinical serum specimens (Standard Precautions; see Chapter 6).

Procedure

Allow serum specimens to reach room temperature before testing. Do not interchange components from other sources.

1. Prepare sample by diluting each serum 1:40 in PBS. If a serum has previously tested positive, it should be titered to the end point.
2. Prepare slides by removing a sufficient number of slides from storage. Allow them to equilibrate to room temperature (15-30 minutes); remove from envelope and label. Handle envelope and slide by edges only.
3. Apply samples and controls. Use 1 drop of the screening dilution or titration dilution per well. Apply 1 drop of the positive control and 1 drop of the negative control to the appropriate wells on at least one slide of each test run.
   Note: From this step on, the slides must remain wet.
4. Incubate the slides in a covered moist chamber at room temperature for 30 minutes.
5. Remove the slides from the chamber, and rinse briefly with a gentle stream of PBS. Direct the stream away from wells.
6. Place the slides in a Coplin or staining jar filled with PBS for 10 minutes to wash. Occasionally, agitate the slides initially, at midpoint, and before removal. Repeat this wash process with fresh PBS.
7. Remove the slides one at a time from the wash solution; drain the excess PBS. If blotting is preferred, blot gently around slide periphery only, with the edge of blotting or bibulous paper. Do not blot directly over the wells. Return to moist chamber.
8. Apply enzyme antibody reagent. Cover the wells with 12 to 14 drops.
9. Incubate the slides in a moist chamber at room temperature for 30 minutes. Protect from excess light.
10. Remove the slides from the moist chamber, and rinse briefly with a gentle stream of PBS. Direct the stream away from the wells.
11. Place the slides in a Coplin or staining jar filled with PBS to wash. Leave the slides in the PBS for 5 minutes with occasional agitation (initially, at midpoint, and before removing the slides from the wash). Repeat this washing process once with fresh PBS.
12. Reconstitute with 10 mL of distilled water. Add the contents of one vial of 0.3% H_2O_2 immediately before use. Mix well by gentle inversion or agitation.
13. Remove the slides from the wash buffer, drain the excess PBS, and return to the moist chamber. Flood the wells with the stain reagent. Do not allow wells to dry. Discard any unused reconstituted stain.
14. Incubate the slides for 15 minutes in a covered moist chamber at room temperature. Protect from light.
15. Remove the slides from the moist chamber, and rinse with a gentle stream of PBS. Place the slides in a Coplin or staining jar filled with PBS for 10 minutes. Agitate at entry, midpoint, and before removal.
16. Remove the slides (one at a time) from the wash buffer, and drain excess PBS by gently tapping the horizontal edge of the slide. If blotting is preferred, see directions in step 7.
17. Apply 1 small drop of mounting medium in each specimen well. Gently apply coverslip without pressure.
18. Examine the slides with a light microscope using high (×40) magnification.

Reporting Results

Negative: No cytoplasmic or nuclear-specific stain is observed. The cells may be slightly colored because of some nonspecific reaction of the peroxidase stain reagent.

Positive: Serum is considered positive if the nuclei of the cells stain more intensely than the negative control well and there is a clearly discernible pattern of colorations.

A grading scale similar to the one shown in Box 29-2 may be helpful in establishing the criteria for each laboratory. Positive specimens should be confirmed by repeating the test with twofold dilutions of serum. All positive ANA patterns should be titered to end point dilution to detect possible mixed antinuclear reactions that may not be apparent when interpreting a single screening dilution. The end point titer is the last serial dilution in which 1+ coloration with a clearly discernible pattern is detected.

Box 29-2	Grading Reactions
Negative	No cytoplasmic or nuclear specific stain observed. The cells may be slightly colored because of some nonspecific reaction of the peroxidase staining reagent.
Borderline ±	Beige-specific stain
Positive	
1+	Tan
2+	Light brown
3+	Medium brown
4+	Dark-chocolate brown to black

Procedure Notes

The indirect immunofluorescence test and the immunoenzyme methods are probably the most practical ways of screening for ANA in the clinical laboratory. The peroxidase enzyme-conjugated antibody method, which is comparable in sensitivity and patterns of reactivity to fluorescent methods, has certain advantages. The HRP technique has the advantages of resulting in a permanent slide and requiring only a conventional light microscope with no special equipment.

Sources of Error

False-negative results can occur if the ANA happens to be specific for an antigen other than the one used in the procedure. False-negative results may also occur if the substrate is fixed in acetone and is inadequately washed. Without fixation, however, some soluble nuclear antigen may be lost. False-negative results may also be related to the binding of antinuclear factor to circulating immune complexes and to a low antibody titer.

False-positive interpretations may occur because of nonspecific staining, which may resemble a speckled pattern of reactivity. These staining reactions occur whenever the conjugate or the serum contains antibodies to other tissue antigens. Careful rinsing and removal of excess fluoresceinated conjugate minimizes the risk of some nonspecific staining reactions.

Limitations

No diagnosis should be based solely on the results of laboratory testing. Clinical data, antibody titers, and other laboratory findings should all be reviewed before a definitive diagnosis is established.

Clinical Applications

In the evaluation of patients with connective tissue disease, the ANA must be interpreted with caution. Under proper testing conditions, a negative ANA generally rules out SLE. A negative ANA result can result from autoimmune disease in remission or nuclear autoantibodies not detectable with indirect immunofluorescent or peroxidase immunoenzyme procedures.

The significance of a positive ANA depends on the titer and to a lesser extent on the observed pattern (see Table 29-6). There is no general agreement on the significance of the various patterns, and it should be noted that some patterns may mask other patterns in high concentration. Interpretation of ANA patterns can provide additional information about the type of nuclear component reacting.

Because of the sensitivity of the Hep-2 cell substrate, some apparently normal individuals may show a low degree of staining at the 1:40 screening dilution. ANA titers of 1:10 to 1:80 usually have little significance but may be seen in patients with RA or scleroderma. ANAs are known to be gender and age dependent; therefore a positive low-titer result may be "normal" for certain individuals in the absence of other clinical signs and symptoms. If a specimen is positive at a 1:10 dilution, it should be retested at dilutions from 1:20 to 1:320. The higher the antibody titer, the more likely is the diagnosis of connective tissue disorder. Changes in the antibody titer can also be used to observe disease activity.

If the ANA test is positive, additional immunologic evaluation is necessary to determine the specificity of the reaction. These evaluations include double immunodiffusion, counterimmunoelectrophoresis, passive hemagglutination, radioimmunoassays, and identification of nuclear antigens by immunoprecipitation or immunoblotting. Such evaluations may demonstrate the presence of more than one ANA specificity reaction in the serum. An LE cell preparation is not useful because it is positive in only 75% of patients with confirmed SLE.

Reference

ImmunoConcepts Colorzyme ANA Test System product insert, Sacramento, Calif, 2003.

Rapid Slide Test for Antinucleoprotein

Remel SeraTest* SLE Rapid Latex Test Kit (Fisher Scientific).

Principle

The SLE latex test provides a suspension of polystyrene latex particles coated with deoxyribonucleoprotein (DNP). When the latex reagent is mixed with serum containing the ANAs, binding to the DNP-coated latex particles produces macroscopic agglutination. The procedure is positive in SLE and SRDs (e.g., RA, PSS, Sjögren's syndrome, MCTD, drug-induced lupus).

Specimen Collection and Preparation

No special preparation of the patient is required before specimen collection. The patient must be positively identified when the specimen is collected, and the specimen is labeled at the bedside. Specimen labels must include the patient's full name, date the specimen is collected, patient's hospital identification number, and phlebotomist's initials.

Blood should be drawn by aseptic technique. A minimum of 2 mL of clotted blood (red-top evacuated tube) is required. The specimen should be centrifuged promptly and an aliquot of serum removed.

Use fresh serum. If the test cannot be performed immediately, refrigerate the specimen at 2° to 8° C for no longer than 72 hours after collection. Freeze the serum if testing is postponed for more than 72 hours.

Reagents, Supplies, and Equipment

The following components and controls are available in the Remel SeraTest* SLE Rapid Latex Test Kit:

- SLE reagent

This contains a suspension of DNP extracted from calf thymus that is coated on polystyrene latex in a stabilized buffer (one 2.5-mL bottle). Refrigerate the latex reagent at 2° to 8° C. It is stable until the expiration date on the kit la-

bel. Do not use the reagent if it becomes grossly contaminated, or if evidence of freezing is apparent.
- Disposable pipette/stir sticks
- Glass slide

It is essential that the glass slide is clean. Before use, wash it thoroughly with mild detergent, rinse several times with distilled water, and dry.

Additional Required Equipment
- Timer or stopwatch.

Quality Control

Positive Control (Human)
The positive control must be tested with each set of tests. The positive control and SLE reagent should form a visible agglutination pattern distinctly different from the slight granularity that may be observed with the negative control. If agglutination is not visible with the positive control, the patient's test is invalid. Control contains 0.1% sodium azide as a preservative.

Negative Control (Human)
The reaction between the negative control and SLE reagent should produce a smooth or slightly granular appearance after 2 minutes of testing. If agglutination is observed, the patient's test is invalid. Control contains 0.1% sodium azide as a preservative.

CAUTION: Because the control sera are derived from human sources, they should be handled in the same manner as clinical serum specimens (Standard Precautions; see Chapter 6).

WARNING: The latex reagent and controls contain 0.1% sodium azide as a preservative. Sodium azide may react with lead and copper plumbing to form highly explosive metal azides. On disposal, flush with a large volume of water to prevent azide buildup.

Procedure

Note: All reagents, controls, and test sera must be at room temperature before testing.
1. Check the slide for cleanliness.
2. Place 1 drop (50 μL) of the positive control onto the first field of the slide. Repeat this procedure for the negative control onto the second field and subsequent fields for patient specimens. Retain the pipette/stir stick for the mixing step.
3. Resuspend the latex reagent by gently mixing it. Add 1 drop of the SLE reagent to each of the divisions containing a serum specimen and the positive and negative controls. Using separate applicator sticks for each control or specimen, mix each control or specimen with the SLE reagent in a circular manner over the entire area within the division of the slide.
4. Slowly tilt the slide back and forth for 3 minutes. Observe for agglutination. Agglutination reactions with the SLE reagent are similar to those observed in blood grouping and typing reactions and should be read using a good source of indirect light.

Reporting Results
Positive: Agglutination. Proceed with semiquantitative procedure.
Negative: No agglutination.

Procedure Notes

Sources of Error
Failure to observe the test mixture at the appropriate time can yield false results.

Limitations
No one test has been shown to be completely reliable for the diagnosis of SLE because many of the ANAs accompanying this disease are also demonstrated in other SRDs (e.g., RA, Sjögren's syndrome, PSS).

Clinical Applications
Sera from patients with SLE have been shown to contain several ANAs, as determined by a wide variety of laboratory tests. A specific diagnosis depends on the evaluation of test results and clinical manifestations.

Reference
Remel SeraTest* SLE Rapid Latex Test Kit.

Autoimmune Enzyme Immunoassay ANA Screening Test

Refer to Chapter 12, pp. 161-163, for a description of the Autoimmune Enzyme Immunoassay ANA screening test.

Clinical Applications
As with other ANA diagnostic tests, the results are to be used as an aid in diagnosis. Confirmative testing for specific antibodies should be run if a positive assay is obtained. A positive result suggests certain diseases and should be confirmed by clinical findings.

CASE STUDY

A 39-year-old African-American woman with SLE was diagnosed with the illness 20 years ago. Her initial manifestations of illness developed during the postpartum period of her second pregnancy. The pregnancy had been complicated by proteinuria, believed to be caused by toxemia of pregnancy.

The patient had polyarthralgia, alopecia, and erythematous rashes of the face, arms, and legs. A renal biopsy was performed because her urinalysis revealed proteinuria and RBC casts. The renal biopsy revealed diffuse, proliferative glomerulonephritis. In addition to abnormal laboratory results related to renal function, she manifested ANA (titer 1:1280) and antibodies to DNA and the C3 component of complement.

Questions and Discussion

1. Are the antibodies manifested by the patient typical of SLE?

Yes; immunologic tests have a significant diagnostic impact. Systemic illnesses associated with ANAs, antibodies to

DNA or ribonucleoproteins, and hypocomplementemia, regardless of the clinical features, have come to be diagnosed as SLE. Also, this patient is more likely to have SLE because the incidence of SLE in African-American women between ages 20 and 64 years is 1 in 245.

2. Do patients with SLE have significant morbidity?

Yes; several of the chronic manifestations of SLE may be responsible for significant morbidity. Discoid skin lesions can produce severe scarring and disfigurement. A rheumatoid arthropathy of the hands can develop. In addition, chronic scarring of the kidneys leads to renal failure. Infections resulting from compromised immune function secondary to SLE are responsible for significant morbidity and mortality.

Diagnosis

System lupus erythematosus.

CASE STUDY

History and Physical Examination

A 27-year-old female Caucasian seeks medical attention because of persisting pain in her wrists and ankles and an unexplained skin irritation on her face. On physical examination, swelling of the joints of the hands and ankles is evident, along with erythema of the skin over the bridge of the nose and the upper cheeks. The patient has a slightly elevated temperature.

Laboratory Data

Complete blood count, urinalysis (UA), and rheumatoid arthritis (RA) screening test are ordered, with the following results:

- Hemoglobin and hematocrit: normal.
- Total leukocyte count: 7.0×10^9/L.
- Differential leukocyte count: normal.
- Gross and microscopic UA: normal.
- RA screening test: positive.

Follow-up

An ANA screening test is ordered. The results are positive.

Questions and Discussion

1. What is the most probable diagnosis in this case?

The patient's symptoms are all highly suggestive of a collagen-type disease, such as one of the rheumatoid disorders. A positive ANA test result is highly suggestive of SLE.

Manifestations of the disease range from a typical mild illness that is limited to a photosensitive facial rash and transient diffuse arthritis to life-threatening involvement of the renal, cardiac, respiratory, or central nervous system. In the early phases, it is often difficult to distinguish SLE from other SRDs (e.g., PSS, polymyositis, primary Sjögren's syndrome, primary Raynaud's phenomenon, RA).

2. Does this patient fit into the general characteristics of patients with this disease?

Yes; this disorder is approximately eight times more common in females than in males. It is most common in females during the reproductive years and may be present for years before diagnosis. The prevalence rate, based on a total population, is 1 in 2000, but it is 1 in 700 for women between 20 and 64 years old.

3. What is the principle of the ANA test?

Antibodies to DNA with high titers of dsDNA are seen primarily in SLE. ANA testing may be by fluorescent antibody technique or radioimmunoassay. The fluorescent technique uses a substrate that contains only dsDNA. Titers of 1:32 or greater indicate substantial antibody.

Diagnosis

Systemic lupus erythematosus.

CHAPTER HIGHLIGHTS

- Systemic lupus erythematosus (SLE) is the classic model of autoimmune disease.
- No single cause of SLE has been identified, but a primary defect in immune system regulation is considered important in its pathogenesis. Other influences include the effect of estrogens, genetic predisposition, and extraneous factors.
- SLE is a disease of acute and chronic inflammation. Lymphocyte-subset abnormalities are a major immunologic feature of SLE. Regulation of antibody production of B lymphocytes, ordinarily a function of the subpopulation of T suppressor cells, appears defective in SLE.
- Circulating immune complexes are the hallmark of SLE. Patients exhibit multiple serum antibodies that react with native or altered "self" antigens. Demonstrable antibodies include antibodies to nuclear components; cell surface and cytoplasmic antigens of polymorphonuclear and lymphocytic leukocytes, erythrocytes, platelets, and neuronal cells; and IgG.
- Antibodies also combine with their corresponding antigens to form immune complexes. When the mononuclear phagocyte system is unable to entirely eliminate them, these immune complexes accumulate in the blood circulation. These circulating immune complexes are deposited in the subendothelial layers of the vascular basement membranes of multiple target organs, where they mediate inflammation.
- The antinuclear antibody (ANA) procedure is a valuable screening tool for SLE. Demonstration of ANAs can indicate various systemic autoimmune connective tissue disorders, characterized by antibodies that react with different nuclear components, such as double-stranded DNA, single-stranded DNA, and Sm antigen. ANAs can be found in SLE, MCTD, PSS (or scleroderma), Sjögren's syndrome, polymyositis/dermatomyositis, and RA. A small percentage of patients with neoplastic diseases may also demonstrate the presence of ANAs.
- ANAs are classified into antibodies to DNA, antibodies to histones, antibodies to nonhistone proteins, and an-

tibodies to nuclear antigens. Antibodies to DNA can be divided into two major groups:
- Antibodies that react with native (double-stranded) DNA.
- Antibodies that recognize denatured (single-stranded) DNA only.
- Detection of autoantibodies by immunofluorescence is extremely sensitive and may show positive results when ANA procedures (e.g., complement fixation or precipitation) give negative results. At present, immunofluorescence is the most widely used technique for ANA screening.

REVIEW QUESTIONS

1. SLE is more common in:
   a. Female infants.
   b. Male infants.
   c. Adolescent through middle-age women.
   d. Adolescent through middle-age men.

2. One of the most potent inducers of abnormalities and clinical manifestations of SLE is:
   a. Hydralazine hydrochloride.
   b. Procainamide hydrochloride.
   c. Isoniazid.
   d. Penicillin.

3. The cellular aberrations in SLE include:
   a. B-cell depletion.
   b. Deficiency of suppressor T-cell function.
   c. Hyperproduction of helper T cells.
   d. Both b and c.

4. The principal demonstrable antibody in SLE is antibody to:
   a. Nuclear antigen.
   b. Cell surface antigens of hematopoietic cells.
   c. Cell surface antigens to neuronal cells.
   d. Lymphocytic leukocytes.

5. The sites of immune complex deposition in SLE are influenced by all the following factors *except:*
   a. Molecular size.
   b. Molecular configuration.
   c. Immune complex specificity.
   d. Immunoglobulin class.

6. Renal disease secondary to SLE can be assessed by:
   a. Antibody to native dsDNA.
   b. Levels of C3 and C4.
   c. Levels of ANA.
   d. All the above.

7. SLE is a classic model of autoimmune disease and is a(n):
   a. Abnormality of the joints.
   b. Systemic rheumatoid disorder.
   c. Abnormality of connective tissue.
   d. All the above.

8. The overall incidence of SLE has an increased frequency among:
   a. African Americans.
   b. Native Americans.
   c. Puerto Ricans.
   d. All the above.

9. Patients with SLE characteristically manifest:
   a. Butterfly rash over the bridge of the nose.
   b. Skin lesions on the arms and legs.
   c. Ulcerations on the trunk.
   d. Photophobia.

10. Laboratory features of SLE include:
    a. The presence of ANAs.
    b. Circulating anticoagulant and immune complexes.
    c. Decreased levels of complement.
    d. All the above.

11. Laboratory procedures that are helpful in assessing renal disease include:
    a. Antibody to double-stranded DNA.
    b. Levels of C3 and C4.
    c. Cryoglobulin assay.
    d. All the above.

12. Antinuclear antibodies (ANAs) are always indicative of SLE.
    a. True
    b. False

Questions 13-16. Match the appropriate antibody and disease.

13. _____ Jo-1

14. _____ Mi-I

15. _____ SS-B/La

16. _____ RANA

    a. Systemic lupus erythematosus
    b. Dermatomyositis
    c. Progressive systemic sclerosis
    d. Polymyositis

Questions 17 and 18. Match the interpretation of the ANA staining pattern to its respective antibody.

17. _____ Diffused or homogeneous pattern

18. _____ Speckled pattern

    a. Anti–DNA-nucleoprotein antibody.
    b. Antibody to nucleolar RNA.
    c. Antibody to any extractable nuclear antigen devoid of DNA or histone.
    d. Anticentromere antibody.

BIBLIOGRAPHY

Boumpas DT et al: Systematic lupus erythematosus: emerging concepts, *Ann Intern Med* 123(1):42-53, 1995.

Bridges AJ et al: Antinuclear antibody testing in a referral laboratory, *Lab Med* 24(6):345-349, 1993.

CenterWatch Clinical Trials Listing Service, 2002, www.centerwatch.com.

Cha J et al: Case 39-2006: a 24-year-old woman with systemic lupus erythematosus, seizures, and right arm weakness, *N Engl J Med* 355(25):2978-2989, 2006.

Condemi JJ: The autoimmune diseases, *JAMA* 298(20):2882-2888, 1992.

Couser WG: Glomerular involvement in systemic diseases. In Stein J, editor: *Internal medicine,* ed 4, Boston, 1994, Little, Brown.

Fritzler MJ, Tan EM: Antibodies to histones in drug-induced and idiopathic lupus erythematosus, *J Clin Invest* 62:560, 1978.

Greenwals CA, Peebles CL, Nakamura RM: Laboratory tests for antinuclear antibody (ANA) in rheumatic disease, *Lab Med* 9:19-27, 1978.

Hammersburg G, Keren DF: Detection of antineutrophil cytoplasm antibodies in Wegener's granulomatosis, *Lab Med* 22(11):783-786, 1991.

Holborow EJ: Autoantibodies in rheumatic diseases. In Scott JT, editor: *Copeman's textbook of the rheumatic diseases,* ed 6, New York, 1986, Churchill Livingstone.

Hughes GVR: Systemic lupus erythematosus. In Scott JT, editor: *Copeman's textbook of the rheumatic diseases,* ed 6, New York, 1986, Churchill Livingstone.

Kallenberg C et al: Antineutrophil cytoplasmic antibodies: a still-growing class of autoantibodies in inflammatory disorders, *Am J Med* 93:675-682, 1992.

Karsh J et al: Anti-DNA, anti-deoxyribonucleoprotein and rheumatoid factor measured by ELISA in patients with systemic lupus erythematosus, Sjögren's syndrome and rheumatoid arthritis, *Int Arch Allergy Appl Immunol* 68:60, 1982.

Katan MB: Answers to the antiphospholipid antibody syndrome, *N Engl J Med* 33(15):1025, 1995.

Khamashta M et al: The management of thrombosis in the antiphospholipid-antibody syndrome, *N Engl J Med* 332(15):993-997, 1995.

Klippel JH: Systemic lupus erythematosus, *JAMA* 293(13):1812-1815, 1990.

Klippel JH, Decker JL: Systemic lupus erythematosus. In Stein JH, editor: *Internal medicine,* ed 4, Boston, 1994, Little, Brown.

Lockshin M: Therapy for systemic lupus erythematosus, *N Engl J Med* 324(3):189-192, 1991.

Lupus Foundation, 2002, website: www.lupus.org.

Marshall E: Drug market to treat systemic lupus erythematosus will quadruple by 2015, December 2006, http://www.decisionresources.com/.

Metzger AL et al: In vivo LE cell formation in peritonitis due to systemic lupus erythematosus, *J Rheum* 1(1):130-133, 1974.

Mills JA: Systemic lupus erythematosus, *N Engl J Med* 330(29):1871-1879, 1994.

Pandya MR: In vivo L phenomenon in pleural fluid, *Arthritis Rheum* 19(5):962-963, 1976.

Peebles CL: Antinuclear antibody profiles, *Clin Lab News* 31(1):10-12, 2005.

Persellin RH, Takeuchi A: Antinuclear antibody-negative systemic lupus erythematosus: loss in body fluids, *J Rheum* 7(4):547-550, 1980.

Provost TT, Alexander EL: Cutaneous manifestations of connective tissue disease. In Stein JH, editor: *Internal medicine,* ed 4, Boston, 1994, Little, Brown.

Sanchez-Guerrero J et al: Postmenopausal estrogen therapy and the risk for developing systemic lupus erythematosus, *Ann Intern Med* 122(6):430-433, 1995.

Steinberg AD: Systemic lupus erythematosus, *Ann Intern Med* 115(7):548-559, 1991.

CHAPTER 30

Rheumatoid Arthritis

Etiology
Epidemiology
Signs and Symptoms
Anatomy and Physiology of Joints
Immunologic Manifestations
Diagnostic Evaluation
    Rheumatoid Factor
    Cyclic Citrullinated Peptide Antibodies
    Other Markers
    Immune Complexes
    Complement Levels
    Antinuclear Antibodies
Felty's Syndrome
Juvenile Rheumatoid Arthritis
    Etiology
    Epidemiology

Signs and Symptoms
Immunologic Manifestations
Treatment
    Nonsteroidal Antiinflammatory Drugs
    Corticosteroids/Glucocorticosteroids
    Disease-Modifying Antirheumatic Drugs
    Other Drugs
Diagnostic Procedures
Rapid Latex Agglutination
Case Studies
Chapter Highlights
Review Questions
Bibliography

Learning Objectives

At the conclusion of this chapter, the reader should be able to:
- Describe the etiology, epidemiology, and signs and symptoms of rheumatoid arthritis.
- Discuss the immunologic manifestations and diagnostic evaluation of rheumatoid arthritis.

- Briefly describe Felty's syndrome and juvenile rheumatoid arthritis.
- Explain diagnostic procedures used in the identification and evaluation of rheumatoid arthritis.
- Analyze representative rheumatoid arthritis case studies.

ETIOLOGY

The etiology of rheumatoid arthritis (RA) remains unknown. Genetic factors are important, as are hormonal and psychosomatic factors. Evidence indicates that immunologic factors are involved in both the articular and the extraarticular manifestations of the disease. RA may represent an unusual host response to one or perhaps many etiologic agents. An infectious etiology is possible, although this has not been established.

EPIDEMIOLOGY

Rheumatic diseases are among the oldest diseases recognized. Arthritis and osteoarthritis are among the most prevalent chronic conditions. Rheumatoid arthritis has an estimated incidence of 1% to 2% worldwide. The incidence of RA in the United States has an average of about 70 per 100,000 population annually. RA affects all races, but the incidence varies across racial and ethnic groups, which reflects the prevalence of predisposing genes (e.g., HLA-DR4 allele).

This disease can begin at any age, but it initially occurs most frequently between ages 30 and 50 years. The incidence of RA is greater than 10% in people older than 65 years. Older age and overweight are recognized risk factors for arthritis. Analysis precludes determination of whether overweight precedes or results from arthritis; however, overweight has been established as a risk factor for osteoarthritis of the knee.

The female/male ratio of RA patients is 2.5:1. The National Health Interview Survey provides estimates of the prevalence and impact of arthritis among women age 15 years and older. For women over age 45, arthritis is the leading cause of activity limitation. An estimated 4.6 million (4.6%) women reported arthritis as a major or contributing cause of activity limitation from 1989 to 1991, and an estimated 22.8 million (22.7%) women self-reported arthritis from 1989 to 1991. The prevalence of self-reported arthritis increased directly with age and was 8.6% for women age 15 to 44 years, 33.5% for women age 45 to 64 years, and 55.8% for women 65 and older. Rates were higher for women who were overweight (28.9%), had 11 or fewer years of education (30.0%), and resided in households with an annual income of less than $20,000 (29.9%). Adjusted rates of activity limitation were higher for African Americans and American Indians/Alaskan Native women than for Caucasian women.

Rheumatoid arthritis occurs worldwide, but no definite geographic or climatic variation in incidence has been established. Although no specific genetic relationship has been established, a small increase in incidence has been noted in first-degree relatives of patients with RA. Persons with the HLA-DR4 haplotype do have a significantly higher incidence of RA.

Patients with RA have a shortened life span. The most frequent cause of death is cardiovascular disease. The increased prevalence of atherosclerosis in RA patients is suspected to be related to atherogenic side effects of some antirheumatic medications, the effects of chronic systemic inflammation on the vascular endothelium, or shared mechanisms between RA and atherosclerosis.

Complications resulting from an increased frequency of local or extraarticular infections in RA patients have been demonstrated. Mortality may result from conditions such as septicemia, pneumonia, lung abscess, or pyelonephritis. In the past decade the pharmacotherapy of RA has been improved by the development of more effective medications.

SIGNS AND SYMPTOMS

The term *rheumatic disease* does not have a clear boundary; more than 100 different conditions are labeled as rheumatic diseases, including RA, osteoarthritis, and autoimmune disorders such as systemic lupus erythematosus (SLE) and scleroderma, as well as osteoporosis, back pain, gout, fibromyalgia, and tendonitis.

Rheumatoid arthritis is a chronic, multisystemic, autoimmune disorder and a progressive inflammatory disorder of the joints. It is, however, a highly variable disease that ranges from a mild illness of brief duration to a progressive, destructive polyarthritis associated with a systemic vasculitis (Figure 30-1).

Box 30-1	Extraarticular Manifestations of Rheumatoid Arthritis (RA)

Constitutional manifestations (e.g., weight loss, fatigue)
Subcutaneous rheumatoid nodules
Ocular abnormalities (e.g., inflammatory lesions of episclera and sclera)
Vasculitis
Neuropathy (e.g., mononeuritis multiplex)
Myopathy
Cardiac manifestations (e.g., pericarditis)
Pulmonary manifestations (e.g., pleural effusion)
Osteoporosis
Felty's syndrome—a complex of chronic RA, splenomegaly, anemia, thrombocytopenia, and neutropenia

The pathogenesis of RA has the following three distinct stages:
1. Initiation of synovitis by the primary etiologic factor.
2. Subsequent immunologic events that perpetuate the initial inflammatory reaction.
3. Transition of an inflammatory reaction in the synovium to a proliferative destructive process of tissue.

Rheumatoid arthritis often begins with prodromal symptoms such as fatigue, anorexia, weakness, and generalized aching and stiffness not localized to articular structures. Joint symptoms usually appear gradually over weeks to months. The patient may display a wide variety of extraarticular manifestations (Box 30-1).

The revised American Rheumatism Association's criteria for diagnosis of RA are presented in Box 30-2. If these conditions are present for at least 6 weeks, the patient is designated as having classic RA. Prognostic markers such as a persistently high number of swollen joints, high serum lev-

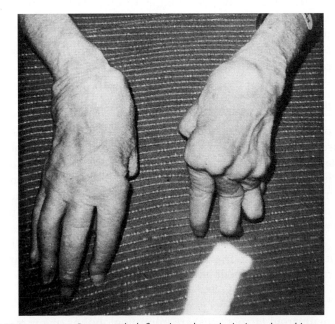

Figure 30-1 Swan-neck deformity, ulnar deviation, dorsal interosseous atrophy, and swelling of wrist—characteristics of rheumatoid arthritis. *(From Kaye D, Rose LF: Fundamentals of internal medicine, St Louis, 1983, Mosby.)*

Box 30-2	Classification of Rheumatoid Arthritis

Four of the following criteria must be present, with 1 through 4 present a minimum of 6 weeks.
1. Morning stiffness in and around the joints that lasts for at least 1 hour.
2. Arthritis of three or more joint areas; at least three joints have soft tissue swelling or fluid. The 14 possible areas are right or left posterior interphalangeal (PIP), metacarpophalangeal (MCP), wrist, elbow, knee, ankle, and metatarsophalangeal joints.
3. Arthritis of wrist, MCP, or PIP joint.
4. Symmetric involvement of joints; simultaneous involvement of the same joint areas, as defined in criterion 2 on both sides of the body.
5. Rheumatoid nodules over bony prominences, or extensor surfaces, or in juxtaarticular regions.
6. Positive serum rheumatoid factor.
7. Radiographic changes, including erosions or bony decalcification localized in or adjacent to the involved joints.

From Arnett FC et al: The American Rheumatism Association 1987 revised criteria for the classification of rheumatoid arthritis, *Arthritis Rheum* 31:315-324, 1988.

els of acute-phase reactants of immunoglobulin M (IgM) rheumatoid factor, early radiographic and functional abnormalities, and the presence of certain HLA class II alleles may help identify patients with more severe RA who are still in the early stages of the disease.

ANATOMY AND PHYSIOLOGY OF JOINTS

Diarthrodial joints are lined at their margins by a synovial membrane (*synovium*) with synovial cells lining this space. The lining cells synthesize protein as well as being phagocytic. Synovial (joint) fluid is a transparent, viscous fluid. Its function is to lubricate the joint space and transport nutrients to the articular cartilage. Mechanical, chemical, immunologic, or bacteriologic damage may alter the permeability of the membrane and capillaries to produce varying degrees of inflammatory response. In addition, inflammatory joint fluids contain lytic enzymes that produce depolymerization of hyaluronic acid, which greatly impairs the lubricating ability of the fluid.

A variety of disorders produces changes in the number and types of cells and chemical composition of the fluid. Analysis of synovial fluid plays a major role in the diagnosis of joint diseases. *Arthrocentesis* constitutes a liquid biopsy of the joint. It is a fundamental part of the clinical database, together with the medical history, physical examination, and plain radiographic films. Analysis of aspirated synovial fluid is essential in the evaluation of any patient with joint disease because it is a better reflection of the events in the articular cavity than abnormal blood tests. For example, abnormal test results such as **antinuclear antibody (ANA),** increased erythrocyte sedimentation rate (ESR), elevated uric acid, and **rheumatoid factor (RF)** can be seen in normal individuals or in unrelated joint diseases.

Disorders such as gout, calcium pyrophosphate dihydrate deposition disease, and septic arthritis can be diagnosed definitively by synovial fluid analysis and may allow for consideration or exclusion of RA and SLE. Synovial fluid analysis can also support a diagnosis of diseases as disparate as amyloidosis, hypothyroidism, ochronosis, hemochromatosis, or even simple edema. In addition, arthrocentesis may alleviate elevated intraarticular pressure. Removal of fluid will relieve symptoms and potentially decrease joint damage. Removal of the products of inflammation is an important component in the treatment of infectious arthritis and may be beneficial in other forms of arthritis.

Routine analysis of synovial fluid should include wet preparation examination for cell count and differential, crystals, Gram's stain, and microbiologic culture. Very turbid fluids, or if septic arthritis is considered for other reasons, should be sent for Gram staining and culture. Gram's stain is needed if a high likelihood of infection exists. Other observations and procedures can include volume and appearance, viscosity, mucin test, chemical analysis for protein, and glucose.

When examined by the immunofluorescent technique, the rheumatoid synovium can be seen to contain large amounts of immunoglobulin G (IgG) and IgM, alone or together. Immunoglobulins can also be seen in synovial lining cells, blood vessels, and interstitial connective tissues. B cells make immunoglobulin in the synovium of patients with RA. As many as half of the plasma cells that can be located in the synovium secrete an IgG RF that combines in the cytoplasm with similar IgG molecules (self-associating IgG).

IMMUNOLOGIC MANIFESTATIONS

The current model of the pathogenesis of RA proposes that an infective agent or other stimulus binds to receptors on dendritic cells (DCs), which activates the innate immune system (Figure 30-2). DCs migrate into lymph nodes, presenting antigen to T lymphocytes, which are activated by two signals: the presentation of antigen and costimulation through CD28. Activated T lymphocytes proliferate and migrate into the joint. Subsequently, T lymphocytes produce interferon gamma (IFN-γ) and other proinflammatory cytokines. This in turn stimulates macrophages and other cells, including B lymphocytes. B cells appear to be pivotal in the pathogenesis of RA because they can be 10,000 times as potent as DCs in presenting antigen.

Stimulated macrophages and fibroblasts release cytokines, including tumor necrosis factor alpha (TNF-α), a central component in the cascade of cytokines. This results in production of additional inflammatory mediators and further recruitment of immune and inflammatory cells into a joint. Anti–TNF-α treatment strategies (e.g., monoclonal) prevent interaction with receptors on cell surfaces.

The **leukotrienes** play a major role in the inflammatory response to injury. This class of biologically active molecules has been implicated in the pathogenesis of RA as well as in other inflammatory diseases (e.g., asthma, psoriasis, inflammatory bowel disease). Leukotrienes are major constituents of a group of oxygenated fatty acids that are synthesized de novo from membrane phospholipid through a cascade of enzymes. Current research is focused on these molecules because leukotriene inhibitors and antagonists will probably become important agents in the group of antiinflammatory drugs (see Treatment).

DIAGNOSTIC EVALUATION

Low serum iron and a normal or low iron-binding capacity are common features in RA. The ESR is elevated to a variable degree in most RA patients and roughly parallels the level of disease activity. Serum protein electrophoresis may demonstrate elevations in the alpha-2 and gamma globulin fractions, with a mild to moderate decrease in serum albumin. The gamma globulin increase is polyclonal.

Immunologic features of RA include RF, anti–cyclic citrullinated peptide (anti-CCP), immune complexes, characteristic complement levels, and ANAs.

Rheumatoid Factor

Rheumatoid factors (RFs) are immunoglobulins of any isotype with antibody activity directed against antigenic sites on the Fc region of human or animal IgG. RFs have been associated with three major immunoglobulin classes: IgM, IgG, and IgA. IgM and IgG RFs are the most common.

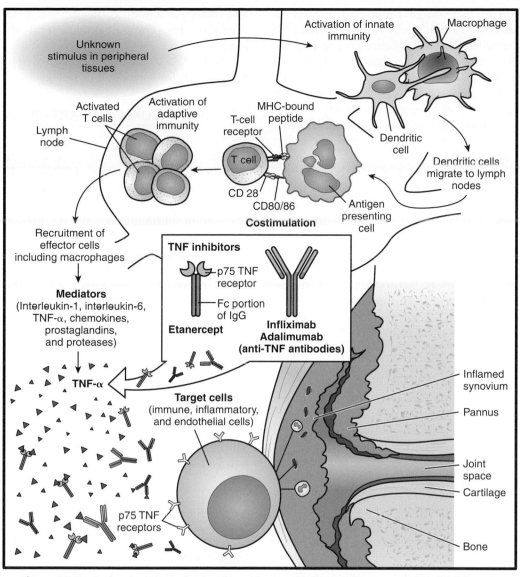

Figure 30-2 Pathophysiological role of cytokines and other mediators and their inhibitors in rheumatoid arthritis. *MHC,* Major histocompatibility complex; *TNF,* tumor necrosis factor. *(Redrawn from Scott DL, Kingsley GH:* N Engl J Med *355(7):704-712, 2006.)*

Immunoglobulin M rheumatoid factor is manifested in approximately 70% of adults, but it is not specific for RA. Being RF positive correlates with the following:
- Severity of the disease (in general)
- Nodules
- Other organ system involvement (e.g., vasculitis, Felty's syndrome, Sjögren's syndrome)

Agglutination tests for RF, such as the sensitized–sheep cell test and latex agglutination, generally detect IgM RFs. Latex agglutination is sensitive but can produce a fairly high number of false-positive results. Because conventional procedures are semiquantitative, they may be insensitive to changes in titer and may detect only those RFs that agglutinate. Newer, more sensitive methods, such as nephelometric and turbidometric assays and enzyme-linked immunosorbent assays (ELISAs), have been developed. The nephelometry and ELISA methods have the advantage of objective instrument measurement on a single sample dilution.

Rheumatoid factor has been associated with some bacterial and viral infections, including hepatitis and infectious mononucleosis, and some chronic infections, such as tuberculosis, parasitic disease, subacute bacterial endocarditis, and cancer. Elevated values may also be observed in the normal elderly population.

The concentration of RF tends to be highest when the disease peaks and tends to decrease during prolonged remission.

Cyclic Citrullinated Peptide Antibodies

Cyclic citrullinated peptide (CCP) antibodies are a highly specific indicator for RA. Antibodies to CCPs (anti-CCP1) were first described in 1998, and following the introduction of commercial ELISA products employing the so-called second-generation peptides (CCP2), there has been increased interest in using this marker in the diagnosis of early RA.

The CCP assays are increasingly being used in conjunction with tests for RF to help diagnose RA. Compared with other sensitive assays for RF, CCP is considered to be more sensitive. This antibody is reported to have high specificity (>95%) and sensitivity (80%) for RA. Together, these assays improve chances of an accurate early diagnosis and effective treatment during an early window of opportunity for controlling this autoimmune disease. Antibodies are detected in serum from individuals up to 14 years before the first clinical symptoms of RA.

Anti-CCP semiquantitative and qualitative ELISAs have been approved by the U.S. Food and Drug Administration (FDA), including the Diastat Anti-CCP kit and EliA CCP. The EliA CCP assay (Phadia US) is the first fully automated assay for the measurement of CCP.

Other Markers

Antibodies to anti–perinuclear factor (APF) and keratin (AKA) are highly specific for RA. Antibodies to APF are reported to be present in the sera of 49% to 91% of RA patients, with specificity greater than 70%.

Immune Complexes

Soluble, circulating immune complexes and cryoprecipitable proteins consisting of immunoglobulins, complement components, and RFs are demonstrable in the serum of some patients with RA. Anti–gamma globulins of the IgG and IgM classes are an integral part of these complexes.

The IgA, IgM, and IgG isotypes of RF are detected years before any symptoms of RA become apparent. The various vascular and parenchymal lesions of RA suggest that the lesions result from injury induced by immune complexes, especially those containing antibodies to IgG. Vasculitis is associated with complexes made up of IgG and 7S IgM RFs. A positive laboratory assay for mixed cryoglobulins indicates the presence of a large number of immune complexes and is associated with an increased incidence of extraarticular manifestations, particularly vasculitis.

Complement Levels

Serum complement levels are usually normal in patients with RA, except in those with vasculitis. Hemolytic complement levels are reduced in the serum of less than one third of patients, especially in patients with very high levels of RF and immune complexes. Levels of C4 and C2 are most profoundly depressed in these patients.

Antinuclear Antibodies

Antinuclear antibodies have been found in 14% to 28% of RA patients, who usually have advanced disease. However, disease manifestation is the same in both ANA-positive and ANA-negative patients.

FELTY'S SYNDROME

Felty's syndrome is the association of RA with splenomegaly and leukopenia. This syndrome almost always develops in patients with a high-titer RF assay, a positive ANA assay, and rheumatoid nodules. In addition, patients have a high titer of immune complex and low total serum complement levels.

The HLA-DR4 allele is found in 95% of patients who have a propensity for bacterial infections.

JUVENILE RHEUMATOID ARTHRITIS

Etiology

Juvenile rheumatoid arthritis (JRA) is a condition of chronic synovitis beginning during childhood. The etiologic hypotheses are similar to those proposed for adult RA. The etiology is expected to be multiple and includes factors such as infection, autoimmunity, and trauma. Research at Tulane University Medical Center suggests that JRA may be associated with a retroviral particle called *human intracisternal A-type particle* (HIAP). Antibodies to this particle have been found in a very high percentage of patients with JRA. These antibodies have also been found in a very high percentage of patients with three other autoimmune disorders: SLE, Sjögren's syndrome, and Graves' disease. Researchers believe that these four disorders may result from the presence of HIAP, together with genetic factors and some internal or external stimulus, which all combine to dictate the specific symptomatology.

Epidemiology

The incidence of JRA in pediatric populations is between 0.1 and 1.1 per 1000 children in the United States.

Signs and Symptoms

Diagnostic criteria include onset before age 16 years, presence of arthritis (i.e., joint swelling for 6 consecutive weeks or longer), and exclusion of other conditions known to cause or mimic childhood arthritis.

Several distinct subgroups of JRA vary in signs and symptoms and immunologic manifestations (Table 30-1). These

Table 30-1	Apparent Subgroups of Juvenile Rheumatoid Arthritis (JRA)	
Subgroup	Age at Onset	Immunologic Manifestations
Systemic onset (Still's disease)	Any	ANA = Negative RF = Negative
RF-negative polyarthritis	Any	ANA = 25% positive RF = Negative
RF-positive polyarthritis	Older	ANA = 50% positive RF = 100% positive HLA-DR4
Pauciarticular I	Younger	ANA = 60% positive HLA-DR5, HLA-DR6, and HLA-DRw8
Pauciarticular II	Older	HLA-B27

From Rheuma-Fac Rheumatoid Arthritis Test (Latex) product insert, Fountain Valley, Calif, July 1987, ICL Scientific (with permission); and Sigma Diagnostics product brochure, Procedure No. SIA 107.
RF, Rheumatoid factor; *ANA*, antinuclear antibody.

disorders include Still's disease, polyarticular onset, pauci-articular onset, and RA.

Still's Disease
One fifth of patients with JRA have Still's disease. These patients tend to be HLA-DR5 positive.

Systemic manifestations occur early and are present with a variety of signs and symptoms. These abnormalities include high intermittent fever with a rash, serositis, lymphadenopathy, hepatosplenomegaly, leukocytosis, and anemia. The diagnosis is frequently one of exclusion because polyarthritis and arthralgia are not prominent in the early stage. Arthritis occurs late in the course of the disease and rarely leads to chronic polyarthritis.

Polyarticular Onset
Polyarthritis begins in five or more joints and occurs in about 40% of patients. HLA-DR6 has been correlated with this abnormality.

Pauciarticular Onset
Arthritis involving four or fewer joints occurs in 40% of patients. Two distinctive subgroups have been identified. The first group is populated by girls who are younger than 6 years, are ANA positive, and have iridocyclitis (which can lead to blindness). This subgroup is associated with HLA-Dw5 and HLA-DR5. The other subgroup is populated by boys younger than 6 years with bilateral sacroiliitis. This subgroup is associated with HLA-B27.

Rheumatoid Arthritis
The remaining 20% of children meet the criteria for RA as defined by the American Rheumatism Association's criteria. Children in this group are HLA-DR4 positive.

Immunologic Manifestations
Immunologic features of JRA include RF, immune complexes, and ANAs.

Rheumatoid Factors
Approximately one fifth of children are positive for RF. Most patients who are positive for RF probably represent adult RA occurring in childhood. Detection of "hidden" RF can be detected in 65% of children with negative latex fixation tests. Children in this category do not develop the clinical manifestations of adults with RA.

Immune Complexes
Soluble immune complexes may be detected in patients with Still's disease and active synovitis. Monitoring of these complexes is not useful for diagnosis, prognosis, or monitoring of patients.

Antinuclear Antibodies
Antinuclear antibodies are detectable in very few patients with JRA. The exception is that most girls with pauciarthritis and chronic iritis demonstrate a positive ANA test.

TREATMENT
The major goals of treatment of arthritis are (1) to reduce pain and discomfort, (2) to prevent deformities and loss of joint function, and (3) to maintain a productive and active life. Inflammation must be suppressed and mechanical and structural abnormalities corrected or compensated for with assistive devices. Treatment options include reduction of joint stress, physical and occupational therapy, drug therapy, and surgical intervention.

The general classes of drugs typically used in the treatment of RA are nonsteroidal antiinflammatory drugs (NSAIDs), corticosteroids, disease-modifying antirheumatic drugs (DMARDs), and biologics.

A new class of agents for treatment of RA, *recombinant fusion proteins,* selectively modulates the CD80 or CD86-CD28 costimulatory signal required for full T-cell activation. Other drugs may also be used for treatment.

Nonsteroidal Antiinflammatory Drugs
Traditional treatment of RA consists of NSAIDs (e.g., salicylates, ibuprofen). The major effect of these agents is to reduce acute inflammation. Aspirin is the oldest drug of the nonsteroidal class, but the use of aspirin as the initial choice of drug therapy has largely been replaced by the newer NSAIDs.

Prostaglandins are a group of related compounds that are important mediators of a wide variety of physiologic processes, including immunomodulation. Prostaglandins are derived primarily from arachidonic acid via the cyclooxygenase enzymes (COX) pathway. NSAIDs inhibit prostaglandin synthesis by blocking two isoforms of COX, COX-1 and COX-2. Newer NSAID agents (e.g., Vioxx, Celebrex) selectively block the COX-2 enzyme that is primarily upregulated in response to tissue damage during inflammation but preserves COX-1 activity and enhances the safety profile.

Corticosteroids/Glucocorticoids
Corticosteroids (e.g., cortisone and prednisolone [prednisone]) have both antiinflammatory and immunoregulatory activity. Glucocorticosteroids pass through the cell membrane into the cytoplasm and activate the cytoplasmic glucocorticosteroid receptor, which represses gene expression through the transcriptional interference of activator protein 1 (AP-1) and nuclear factor kappa B (NF-κB). The proteins inhibited by glucocorticosteroids include interleukin-1 (IL-1), IL-2, IL-6, IL-8, TNF-α, and IFN-γ. Glucocorticosteroids were the original selective COX-2 inhibitors. Oral corticosteroids can produce a variety of complications, including high blood pressure, increased susceptibility to infection, and osteoporosis.

Disease-Modifying Antirheumatic Drugs
The DMARDs include methotrexate, intramuscular gold salts, hydroxychloroquine and sulfasalazine, D-penicillamine, and immunosuppressive and other cytotoxic drugs (e.g., cyclosporin A, cyclophosphamide, azathioprine). Newer drugs for the treatment of RA include leflunomide, etanercept,

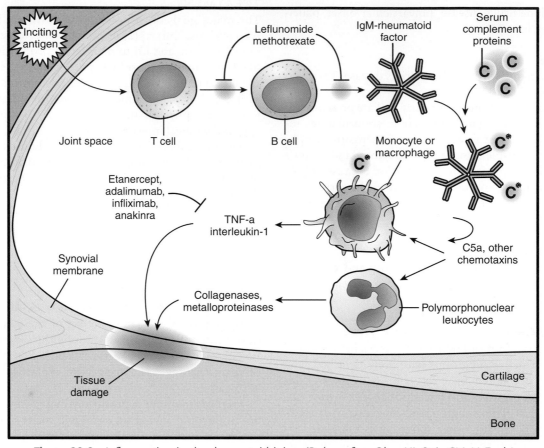

Figure 30-3   Inflammation in the rheumatoid joint. *(Redrawn from Olsen NJ, Stein CM:* N Engl J Med *350(21):2167-2179, 2004.)*

adalimumab, infliximab (Remicade), and anakinra (Figure 30-3; see Table 30-2 for primary mode of action). Antimalarials may be used as well.

Methotrexate has become the most popular DMARD because of its early onset of action (4-6 weeks), good efficacy, and ease of administration and high patient tolerability. Methotrexate is a folic acid antagonist. The immunosuppressive and cytotoxic effects of methotrexate are caused by the inhibition of dihydrofolate reductase.

Immunosuppressive and cytotoxic drugs other than methotrexate are used only in patients who have aggressive disease or extraarticular manifestations such as systemic vasculitis. The most common drugs are azathioprine (Imuran), cyclophosphamide (Cytoxan), and cyclosporin A. Because of the potential for high toxicity, these agents are used for life-threatening extraarticular manifestations or severe articular disease refractory to other therapy.

- Azathioprine is a purine analog that can cause severe bone marrow suppression, particularly in patients with renal insufficiency or when used concomitantly with allopurinol or angiotensin-converting enzyme (ACE) inhibitors.
- Cyclophosphamide is an alkylating agent associated with serious toxicities, including bone marrow suppression, hemorrhagic cystitis, premature ovarian failure, infection, and secondary malignancy, particularly an increased risk of bladder cancer. For these reasons, cyclophosphamide is not used in the treatment of uncomplicated RA.
- Cyclosporine (cyclosporin A) is an immunosuppressive agent approved for use in preventing renal and liver allograft rejection. Cyclosporine inhibits T-cell function by inhibiting transcription of IL-2.

Other Drugs

Antimalarial drugs are rapidly absorbed, relatively safe, well tolerated, and often effective remittive agents in the treatment of RA, particularly mild to moderate disease. The

Table 30-2	New Drugs for Treatment of Rheumatoid Arthritis
Drug	**Primary Action**
Leflunomide	Inhibits pyrimidine synthesis.
Etanercept	Binds TNF-α and TNF-β.
Adalimumab	Human anti–TNF-α antibody
Infliximab	Chimeric anti–TNF-α antibody
Anakinra	Interleukin-1 receptor antagonist

Modified from Olsen JJ, Stein CM: *N Engl J Med* 350(21):2169, 2004. *TNF,* Tumor necrosis factor.

mechanism of action of antimalarial drugs in the treatment of patients with RA is unknown.

Recombinant fusion proteins represent a new class of drugs selectively modulate specific cell surface receptors, CD80 or CD86, on the surface of an antigen-presenting cell binds to CD28 on the T cell. A recombinant fusion protein, abatacept, has been modified to prevent complement fixation. It competes with CD28 for CD80 and CD86 binding and can be used to selectively modulate T-cell activity. This selective costimulation modulator has been proposed to be useful for patients who have an inadequate response to anti–TNF-α therapy.

DIAGNOSTIC PROCEDURES

Diagnostic testing for RA primarily involves rheumatoid factor (RF) assays (see Rapid Latex Agglutination procedure).

Rapid Latex Agglutination*

Principle

The RA agglutination test is based on the reaction between patient antibodies in the serum, known as the "rheumatoid factor," and an antigen derived from human gamma globulin (IgG). Latex reagent consists of a stabilized latex suspension coated with albumin and chemically bonded with denatured human gamma globulin. This reagent serves as an antigen in the procedure. If RFs are present in the serum, macroscopic agglutination will be visible when the latex reagent is mixed with the serum. The determination of RFs is important in the prognosis and therapeutic management of rheumatoid arthritis; however, positive test results may be observed in a variety of disorders, such as SLE, Sjögren's syndrome, syphilis, and hepatitis.

Specimen Collection and Preparation

No special preparation of the patient is required before specimen collection. The patient must be positively identified when the specimen is collected, and the specimen is to be labeled at the bedside. Specimen labels must include the patient's full name, the date the specimen is collected, the patient's hospital identification number, and the phlebotomist's initials.

Blood should be drawn by aseptic technique. A minimum of 2 mL of clotted blood (red-top evacuated tube) is required. The specimen should be centrifuged promptly and an aliquot of serum removed. No special preparation of the serum is required.

If the test cannot be performed immediately, the specimen should be refrigerated (2°-8° C) for no longer than 24 hours. If additional delay occurs, the serum should be frozen at −20° C or below. Repeated freezing and thawing must be avoided. If turbidity is apparent upon thawing, the specimen should be clarified by centrifugation before use.

WARNING: Do not use specimens showing gross hemolysis, lipemia, or turbidity.

Preliminary Patient Specimen Preparation

Dilute specimen 1:20 with the prepared diluent (e.g., 0.1 mL of serum and 1.9 mL of diluent), and thoroughly mix the tube contents.

Reagents, Supplies, and Equipment

The following components are commercially available in kit form (Inverness Medical).

- Rheumatex: Latex reagent with dropper assembly

This is a suspension of latex particles sensitized with human IgG; contains buffer and preservative (sodium azide 0.1%). *Shake well before using.*

Note: Store at 2° to 8° C. Do not freeze latex reagent. Properly stored reagent is stable until expiration date indicated on the label. Do not use after the expiration date. Reagent that does not produce appropriate quality control results should be discarded after verification by repeat testing. The reagent should be a uniform, milky suspension of latex particles. If clumping cannot be removed after gentle vortex mixing, the reagent should be discarded.

- Concentrated diluent 20× (glycine-saline buffer)

This contains the preservative sodium azide 2.0%. Prepare a 1:20 dilution of the concentrated diluent by mixing the contents of the concentrated diluent vial with 190 mL of distilled water.

Note: Store the prepared diluent at 2° to 8° C. Properly stored reagent is stable until expiration date indicated on the kit. Reagent that does not produce appropriate quality control results should be discarded after verification by repeat testing. Discard if contaminated (i.e., evidence of cloudiness or particulate material in solution).

ADVISORY NOTE: Do not interchange reagents from different kits because the reagents from each kit have been assayed as a unit for proper sensitivity.

The reagents in the kit contain sodium azide. See Material Safety Data Sheet WM109ver.3 (prepared 6/1/99) for identity, physicochemical characteristics, fire/explosion hazard data, reactivity data, toxicology/health effects, first aid, precautions for safe handling, and control measures.

- Glass slide

Additional Required Equipment and Supplies

- Stopwatch or timer
- 37° C water bath
- 12 × 75–mm test tubes
- Serologic pipettes (1-mL graduated) and safety pipette
- Centrifuge (capable of 1000 μL × g)
- Light source
- Capillary pipettes (50 μL)
- Applicator sticks
- Distilled water

---

*Rheumatex (a modification of the Singer and Plotz procedure), Wampole Laboratories, Cranbury, NJ.

Quality Control

A positive control and a negative control must be tested with each unknown patient specimen.

Positive Control

Rheumatoid Factor Positive Serum (Human); contains buffer, stabilizer, and preservative (sodium azide 0.1%). This serum is provided in the Rheumatex kit. Store at 2° to 8° C.

Note: Failure to observe a positive reaction (agglutination) with this serum is indicative of deterioration of the latex reagent and/or positive control. The solution should be clear solutions; do not use if cloudy or obviously contaminated. Do not dilute the control. Observe results *immediately* at 1 minute. The positive control must show agglutination.

Negative Control

Rheumatoid Factor Negative Serum (Human); contains buffer, stabilizer and preservative (sodium azide 0.1%). This serum is provided in the Rheumatex kit. Store at 2° to 8° C.

Note: The solution should be clear solutions; do not use if cloudy or obviously contaminated. Do not dilute the control. Observe results *immediately* at 1 minute. If agglutination is exhibited with this control, the test should be repeated. If repeat testing produces the same results, the reagents should be replaced. The negative control should appear uniformly turbid.

CAUTION: Because the control sera are derived from human sources, they should be handled in the same manner as clinical serum specimens (Standard Precautions; see Chapter 6). Each donor unit used in the preparation of the positive and negative controls and the latex reagent was tested for hepatitis B surface antigen (HBsAg), human immunodeficiency virus (HIV-1, HIV-2), and hepatitis C virus (HCV) by an FDA-approved method and found to be nonreactive. However, handle all materials as if capable of transmitting disease (Biosafety Level 2).

Procedure

Note: All reagents and specimens must be at room temperature before testing.

Qualitative Slide Test

1. Prepare a 1:20 dilution of patient serum in with the prepared diluent.
2. Using a clean capillary pipette, place 1 free-falling drop of the diluted serum from the perpendicularly held pipette to the center of division of the slide.
3. Add 1 drop of positive control and 1 drop of negative control on either side section of the slide.
4. Mix the latex reagent, and add 1 drop of reagent to the patient specimen and to each of the controls.
5. Mix each specimen with a separate applicator stick. All the contents of the mixtures are to spread evenly over the entire area of their respective divisions on the slide.
6. Tilt the slide back and forth, gently and evenly, for 1 minute, at a rate of 8 to 10 times per minute.
7. Observe for agglutination immediately at 1 minute, using an indirect oblique light source.
8. Positive sera exhibit readily visible agglutination. A weakly positive serum may exhibit very fine granulation or partial clumping. Negative sera appear uniformly turbid.

WARNING: The latex reagent, controls, and buffer contain 0.1% sodium azide as a preservative. Sodium azide may react with lead and copper plumbing to form highly explosive metal azides. On disposal, flush with a large volume of water to prevent azide buildup.

Reporting Results

Positive reaction: Positive sera exhibit readily visible agglutination. A weakly positive serum may exhibit very fine granulation or partial clumping.

Negative reaction: Negative sera appear uniformly turbid.

Procedure Notes

Latex slide and tube tests demonstrate slightly greater sensitivity than sensitized sheep cells. The specificity of latex tube tests is comparable to sensitized–sheep cell procedures.

Specimen collection and handling are important to the quality of the test. Strict adherence must be paid to technique, with a special emphasis on drop size, complete mixing, reaction time, and temperature of reagents.

The strength of a positive reaction may be graded as follows:

1+ Very small clumping with opaque fluid background
2+ Small clumping with slightly opaque fluid background
3+ Moderate clumping with fairly clear fluid background
4+ Large clumping with clear fluid background

Quantitative Slide Procedure

If a patient serum exhibits a positive reaction, it is recommended that a quantitative test be performed. The serum may be serially diluted with diluent to determine a quantitative estimate of the RA level.

1. Serum to be titrated should be serially diluted (e.g., 1:20, 1:40) with prepared diluent. At least six dilutions should be prepared.
2. Place 1 drop of each specimen dilution onto successive sections of the slide.
3. Test each specimen dilution as described under Qualitative Slide Test, steps 3 to 7.

Quantitative Tube Test

1. Label eleven 12 × 75–mm test tubes (1 to 11) and place in a test tube rack.
2. Pipette 1.9 mL of prepared diluent into tube 1; 1.0 mL of prepared diluent into tubes 2 to 9; and 0.8 mL of prepared diluent into tubes 10 and 11.
3. Add 0.1 mL of specimen to tube 1. Mix the contents, and transfer 1.0 mL of prepared diluent into tubes 2 to 9 and 0.8 mL of prepared diluent into tubes 10 and 11.
4. Pipette 0.2 mL of the positive control into tube 10 and 0.2 mL of the negative control into tube 11.

5. The concentrations of the dilutions are:

Tube Number	Dilution	Serum Concentration (IU/mL)
1	1:20	60
2	1:40	120
3	1:80	240
4	1:160	480
5	1:320	960
6	1:640	1920
7	1:1280	3840
8	1:2560	7680
9	1:5120	
10	Positive control	
11	Negative control	

6. To each tube, add 1 drop of well-mixed latex reagent.
7. Shake all tubes thoroughly, and incubate at 37° C for 15 minutes.
8. After incubation, centrifuge all tubes at $1000 \times g$ for 2 minutes.
9. Gently shake each tube to resuspend the precipitate until an even suspension is achieved. Do not use automatic mixing devices.
10. Examine each tube for the presence of macroscopic agglutination by observing against a dark or black background under an oblique light.

Reporting Results

In the slide and tube quantitative procedures, the highest dilution at which agglutination can still be observed is considered the titer. If there is no agglutination at 1:20, the specimen is considered negative for RFs even if a subsequent dilution shows agglutination. When using RF latex tube titration procedures, a titer of 80 or greater is generally considered a positive reaction, and titers of 20 or 40 are considered weakly positive reactions. The tube titration procedure is more sensitive than the slide procedure. Consequently, differences in the raw titers will be seen between the tube titration and slide procedures.

Sources of Error

False-positive results may be observed if:
• Serum specimens are lipemic, hemolyzed, or heavily contaminated with bacteria.
• The reaction time is longer than 2 minutes; a false-positive result may also be produced as a result of a drying effect.

Biologic false-positive results can be manifested by disorders such as SLE, Sjögren's syndrome, syphilis, and hepatitis. A low rate of positive reactions has been observed in abnormalities such as periarteritis nodosa, rheumatic fever, osteoarthritis, tuberculosis, cancer, some diseases of viral origin, osteoarthrosis, arthritis type undetermined, myositis, and polymyalgia rheumatica. Circulating RF appears to represent a phenomenon of aging independent of disease.

Clinical Applications

Rheumatoid factor is present in the serum of approximately 70% to 80% of patients with clinically diagnosed RA. Almost all patients with variants of RA (e.g., Felty's or Sjögren's syndrome) demonstrate positive results. The highest titers are often found in severe cases of RA. Although the latex agglutination procedure has a 95% correlation with a clinical diagnosis of probable or definite RA, RF is not exclusively limited to patients with RA.

In using latex tests for the detection of RF, a positive result can be expected in less than 5% of healthy individuals. In patients 60 years and older, as many as 30% may be seropositive.

Limitations

As in the case of other diagnostic procedures, the results obtained by this kit yield valuable data that must be evaluated as a component of the total clinical information obtained by the physician.

Approximately 25% of patients with definite RA may exhibit negative results for serum RF. Specimens from patients with JRA are usually negative for circulating RF.

The strength of the agglutination reaction in the qualitative procedure is not indicative of the actual titer. Weak reactions may occur with either slightly elevated or greatly elevated concentrations.

The Rheumatex test is classified as "moderately complex" under the Clinical Laboratory Improvement Amendments of 1988 (CLIA '88) regulations.

References

Galen RS, Gambino SR: *Beyond normality: the predictive value and efficiency of medical diagnosis,* New York, 1975, John Wiley & Sons.
Jones WL, Wiggins GL: A study of rheumatoid arthritis latex kits, *Am J Clin Pathol* 60:703-706, 1973.
Mackay IR, Burnett FM, editors: *Autoimmune disease: serologic reactions in rheumatoid arthritis,* Springfield, Ill, 1964, Charles C Thomas.
Rheumatex product insert, Cranbury, NJ, 1997, Wampole Laboratories.
Roose JC, Oster AJ: A new approach to drug development, *N Engl J Med* 355(7)2046-2047, 2006.
Scott DL, Kingsley GH: Tumor necrosis factor inhibitors for rheumatoid arthritis, *N Engl J Med* 355(7):704-712, 2006.
Singer JM, Plotz CM, Goldberg R: The detection of antiglobulin factors utilizing pre-coated latex particles, *Arthritis Rheum* 8:194-201, 1965.

CASE STUDY

History and Physical Examination

A 62-year-old woman has been experiencing pain in her left knee unrelated to trauma. The pain occurs primarily with weight-bearing. She is currently being treated for hypertension, but is otherwise healthy.

She is obese. An examination of her knee shows tenderness over the medial epicondyle superior to the joint margin. There is a small effusion in her left knee.

Laboratory Data

Her laboratory data are normal, including RF assay, except for an elevated uric acid level. An x-ray film of her knee was read as normal.

Questions and Discussion

1. What is the cause of her painful knee?

Because her serum uric acid is high, this patient is probably suffering from gouty arthritis rather than rheumatoid arthritis.

2. What might the effusion in her left knee demonstrate microscopically?

Uric acid crystals might be seen.

3. Would a restricted diet be of value?

Red meat should be restricted in patients suffering from gout.

Diagnosis

Arthritis.

CASE STUDY

A.D., age 31 years, was referred to a rheumatologist with increasing pain and stiffness in her fingers and wrists. Before her last pregnancy 3 years earlier, she had experienced similar symptoms, but these had gone away. Since the birth of her last child, she has found it progressively more awkward to carry out a variety of work tasks and hobbies such as needlepoint. The symptoms were worse in the morning. She had no trouble with her other joints.

Her family history revealed that her mother had RA. On physical examination the patient was pale. She had bilateral and symmetric, tender swelling of her wrists and proximal to the joints of her hands. She had normal range of movement. Her other body systems appeared to be within normal limits.

Laboratory Data

Laboratory assays were ordered (Table 30-3).

A diagnosis of early RA was made. The patient was advised to take one aspirin daily. This initially provided some relief of her symptoms.

She returned to her physician 4 months later with worsening symptoms in her hands and pain in both knees. Synovial fluid was removed from her knees. A diagnosis of progressive RA was made.

Table 30-3	Case Study Laboratory Data
Assay	**Result (Reference Range)**
Erythrocyte sedimentation rate (ESR)	53 mm/hr
C-reactive protein (CRP)	4+
IgM rheumatoid factor (RF)	Positive
Antinuclear antibody (ANA)	Negative
Antibodies to extractable nuclear antigens	Negative
Double-stranded DNA (dsDNA)–binding activity	15%
Serum Complement	
C3	1.1 (0. 75-1.65)
C4	0.4 (0.20-0.65)

Questions and Discussion

1. Do genetic associations exist with RA?

Rheumatoid arthritis is an autoimmune disease associated with the HLA-DR4 and DRI haplotypes.

2. Is RA more common in women?

There is a 3:1 female/male ratio in cases of RA. Estrogens may play a role in the pathogenesis of RA. It is known that pregnancy produces a protective effect.

3. What is the immunopathogenesis of RA?

The specificity of the T-cell response in RA is unknown. The antigen may be a "self" antigen, a modified self antigen, a foreign antigen, or a superantigen. From 70% to 90% of RA patients have antibodies to a protein from the Epstein-Barr virus (EBV). These antibodies, named **rheumatoid arthritis precipitin,** cross-react with a protein found in RA patients called **rheumatoid arthritis nuclear antigen.** RA patients also have elevated frequencies of EBV-infected B cells compared with normal subjects.

4. What is rheumatoid factor?

Rheumatoid factors are autoantibodies that are able to bind IgG. RF exists in all five immunoglobulin classes, although the best characterized are IgG and IgM RF. Approximately 70% of RA patients are RF seropositive. This group tends to develop a more aggressive disease. RF appears to be a marker of disease activity, with reduced levels associated with RA remission found during pregnancy.

Diagnosis

Rheumatoid arthritis.

CHAPTER HIGHLIGHTS

- Immunologic factors may be involved in both the articular and the extraarticular manifestations of rheumatoid arthritis.
- Rheumatoid arthritis is a chronic, usually progressive inflammatory disorder of the joints, ranging from mild illness to a progressive, destructive polyarthritis associated with a systemic vasculitis.
- Two pathogenic mechanisms for RA have been hypothesized:
  - The extravascular immune complex hypothesis proposes an interaction of antigens and antibodies in synovial tissues and fluid.
  - An alternative hypothesis is that cell-mediated damage occurs because of accumulation of lymphocytes, primarily T cells, in the rheumatoid synovium, resembling a delayed-type hypersensitivity reaction. The presence of cytokines, which affect both articular inflammation and destruction, supports this hypothesis.
- Immunoglobulins can also be observed in synovial lining cells, blood vessels, and interstitial connective tissues. As many as half the plasma cells that can be located in the synovium secrete IgG. The serum of most RA patients has detectable soluble immune complexes. Rheumatoid factors (RFs) have been associated with IgM, IgG, and IgA.

- Cyclic citrullinated peptide (CCP) antibodies are a highly specific RA indicator.
- Felty's syndrome is RA with associated splenomegaly and leukopenia. High-titer RF, positive antinuclear antigen (ANA) assay, and rheumatoid nodules are frequently found in patients with Felty's syndrome.
- Juvenile rheumatoid arthritis is a condition of chronic synovitis, beginning during childhood. Subgroups of JRA include Still's disease, polyarticular onset, pauciarticular onset, and RA.

REVIEW QUESTIONS

1. Rheumatoid arthritis most frequently develops in:
   a. Adolescent females.
   b. Adolescent males.
   c. Middle-age females.
   d. Middle-age males.

2. In the United States the incidence of rheumatoid arthritis is:
   a. 1% to 2%.
   b. 2% to 4%.
   c. 5% to 10%.
   d. More than 10%.

3. Women are _____ likely than men to develop rheumatoid arthritis.
   a. less
   b. equally
   c. two to three times more
   d. 10 to 20 times more

4. Rheumatoid factor is defined as:
   a. Antigens with specificity for antibody determinants on the Fc fragment of human or certain animal IgG.
   b. Antibodies with specificity for antigen determinants on the Fc fragment of human or certain animal IgG.
   c. Antigens with specificity for antibody determinants on the Fc fragment of human or certain animal IgD.
   d. Antibodies with specificity for antigen determinants on the Fc fragment of human or certain animal IgD.

Questions 5 and 6. The principle of the latex agglutination test is based on the reaction of patient (5) _____ and (6)_____ derived from gamma globulin.

   a. antigen
   b. antibody
   c. complement levels
   d. leukocytes

Questions 7-9. Arrange the steps in the pathogenesis of rheumatoid arthritis in the proper order.

7. _____   a. Immunologic events perpetuate the initial inflammatory reaction.
8. _____   b. The primary etiologic factor initiates synovitis.
9. _____   c. An inflammatory reaction in the synovium develops into a proliferative destructive process of tissue.

10. All the following are criteria for rheumatoid arthritis *except:*
    a. Morning stiffness.
    b. Evening stiffness.
    c. Rheumatoid nodules.
    d. Radiographic changes.

11. RF correlates with all the following *except:*
    a. The severity of the disease in general.
    b. The presence of nodules.
    c. Other organ system involvement (i.e., vasculitis).
    d. Age of the patient.

12. In RA, vascular and parenchymal lesions suggest that lesions result from injury induced by immune complexes, especially those containing antibodies to:
    a. IgM.
    b. IgG.
    c. IgE.
    d. IgD.

13. Serum complement levels are usually _____ in patients with rheumatoid arthritis.
    a. normal
    b. decreased
    c. increased
    d. a or b

14. Still's disease occurs in _____ of patients with juvenile RA.
    a. 10%
    b. 20%
    c. 30%
    d. 50%

15. In the RF latex agglutination procedure, a false-negative result may be observed in undiluted serum specimens because of:
    a. Complement interference.
    b. High levels of C-reactive protein (CRP).
    c. Antigen excess.
    d. Both b and c.

16. In the indirect enzyme immunoassay (EIA) procedure for RF, biologic false-positive results can be caused by a variety of disorders, including:
    a. Infectious mononucleosis.
    b. Hepatitis.
    c. Systemic lupus erythematosus.
    d. Polymyositis.

BIBLIOGRAPHY

American College of Rheumatology Ad Hoc Committee on Clinical Guidelines: Guidelines for the management of rheumatoid arthritis, *Arthritis Rheum* 39:713, 1996.

Borque L et al: Turbidimetry of rheumatoid factor in serum with a centrifugal analyzer, *Clin Chem* 32:124, 1986.

Breedveld FD: New perspectives on treating rheumatoid arthritis, *N Engl J Med* 333(3):183, 1995.

Bridges AJ et al: Antinuclear antibody testing in a referral laboratory, *Lab Med* 24(6):345-349, 1993.

Cash JM, Klippel JH: Second-line drug therapy for rheumatoid arthritis, *N Engl J Med* 330(19):1368-1376, 1994.

Cohen MD: Update: treatment of rheumatoid arthritis, *Arthritis Care Res* 45:530-532, 2001.

Condemi JJ: The autoimmune diseases, *JAMA* 268(20):2885-2888, 1992.

Conn DL: Resolved: low-dose prednisone is indicated as a standard treatment in patients with rheumatoid arthritis, *Arthritis Care Res* 45:462-467, 2001.

Del Rincon I et al: High incidence of cardiovascular events in a rheumatoid arthritis cohort not explained by traditional cardiac risk factors, *Arthritis Rheum* 44(12):2737-2745, 2001.

Fantini F: New drugs and treatment strategies for rheumatoid arthritis, *Rec Prog Med* 94(9):361-379, 2003.

Genovese M et al: Abatacept for rheumatoid arthritis refractory to tumor necrosis factor α inhibition, *N Engl J Med* 353(11):1114-1123, 2005.

Henderson WR: The role of leukotrienes, *Ann Intern Med* 121 (9):684-696, 1994.

Jones WL, Wiggins GL: A study of rheumatoid arthritis latex kits, *Am J Clin Pathol* 60:703-706, 1973.

Liang H: Board review: rheumatology, *Int Rev Intern Med* 41:1467-1473, 1995.

Linker JB III, Williams RC Jr: Tests for detection of rheumatoid factors. In Rose NR, Friedman H, Fahey JL, editors: *Manual of clinical laboratory immunology,* ed 3, Washington, DC, 1986, American Society for Microbiology.

Mackay IR, Burnett FM, editors: *Autoimmune disease: serologic reactions in rheumatoid arthritis,* Springfield, Ill, 1964, Charles C Thomas.

Matsumoto AK: Rheumatoid arthritis: treatments, 2002, www.hopkins.som.jhmi.edu.

Olsen NJ, Stein CM: New drugs for rheumatoid arthritis, *N Engl J Med* 350(21):2167-2179, 2004.

Pinals RS: Polyarthritis and fever, *N Engl J Med* 330(11):769-774, 1994.

Prevalence of arthritis, *MMWR* 43(17):305-309, 1994.

Prevalence and impact of arthritis among women—United States, 1989-1991, *MMWR* 44(17):329-334, 1995.

Sangha O: Epidemiology of rheumatic diseases, *Rheumatology* 39(suppl.2):3-12, 2000.

Singer JM, Plotz CM, Goldberg R: The detection of antiglobulin factors utilizing precoated latex particles, *Arthritis Rheum* 8:194-201, 1965.

Sullivan et al: Rheumatoid arthritis: test for anti-CCP antibodies joining RF test as key diagnostic tools, *Lab Med* 37(1):17-19, 2006.

Tive L: Celecoxib clinical profile, *Rheumatology* 39(suppl.2):21-28, 2000.

Turgeon ML: Synovial fluid. In *Clinical hematology: theory and procedures,* ed 4, Philadelphia, 2004, Lippincott–Williams & Wilkins.

Vasishta A: Anti-CCP antibodies: early onset marker in RA, *Adv Admin Lab* 11(8):66, 2002.

Wernick R et al: IgG and IgM rheumatoid factors in rheumatoid arthritis: quantitative response to penicillamine therapy and relationship to disease activity, *Arthritis Rheum* 26:593, 1983.

Wong JB, Ramey DR, Singh G: Long-term morbidity, mortality, and economics of rheumatoid arthritis, *Arthritis Rheum* 44(12):2746-2749, 2001.

CHAPTER 31

Solid Organ Transplantation

Histocompatibility Antigens
Nomenclature of HLA Alleles
Major Histocompatibility Complex Regions
Classes of HLA Molecules
Role of MHC/HLAs
Human Leukocyte Antigen Applications
Laboratory Evaluation of Potential Transplant
Recipients and Donors
Facts about Solid Organ Transplantation
Transplantation Terminology
Types of Transplants
Kidney
Heart Valves
Heart
Cornea
Skin
Liver
Lung
Pancreas
Bone
Graft-versus-Host Disease
Etiology
Epidemiology
Signs and Symptoms

Immunologic Manifestation
Diagnostic Evaluation
Prevention
Immunologic Tolerance
Immune Response Gene–Associated Antigens
Graft Rejection
First-Set and Second-Set Rejection
Hyperacute Rejection
Accelerated Rejection
Acute Rejection
Chronic Rejection
Mechanisms of Rejection
General Characteristics
Role of T Cells
Antibody Effects
Immunosuppression
Immunosuppressive Protocols
Post–Organ Transplant Complications
Xenotransplantation
Biomarkers for Rejection
Case Study
Chapter Highlights
Review Questions
Bibliography

Learning Objectives

At the conclusion of this chapter, the reader should be able to:
- Identify and describe the histocompatibility antigens.
- Explain the clinical applications of histocompatibility antigens and human leukocyte antigens.
- Identify and describe several laboratory methods for evaluating potential transplant recipients and donors.
- List frequently used terms in transplantation.
- Identify various types of transplants.
- Define graft-versus-host disease.

- Explain the etiology, epidemiology, signs and symptoms, manifestations, diagnosis, and prevention of graft-versus-host disease.
- Describe the types of graft rejection.
- Briefly explain the mechanism of organ or tissue rejection.
- Identify and explain some methods of immunosuppression.
- Analyze a representative transplantation case study.

The first organ transplant, a kidney from an identical twin, was performed in 1954 by Dr. Joseph Murray at Peter Bent Brigham Hospital in Boston. The recipient survived for 9 years. Dr. Murray was ultimately recognized for his work by receiving the Nobel Prize in Medicine in 1990.

At present, a variety of tissues and organs are transplanted in humans, including bone marrow, peripheral stem cells, bone matrix, skin, kidneys, liver, cardiac valves, heart, pancreas, corneas, and lungs. Transplantation is one of the areas, in addition to hypersensitivity (Chapter 26) and autoimmunity (Chapter 28), in which the immune system functions in a detrimental way.

Early in the history of transplantation, tissue antigens were recognized as important to successful grafting. If significantly different foreign antigens were introduced into an immunocompetent host, the transplanted tissue or organ would undoubtedly fail. Currently, tissue (histocompatibility) matching with concomitant immunosuppression of the host in many cases is used to enhance the probability of success in organ and tissue transplantation.

Transplantation presents the following two basic problems.
- Genetic variation between donor and recipient.
- Recognition of genetic differences by a transplant recipient's immune system that causes rejection of a transplanted organ.

HISTOCOMPATIBILITY ANTIGENS

The **major histocompatibility complex (MHC)** is a cluster of genes found on the short arm of chromosomes 6 at band 21 (6p21) (Figure 31-1). These genes code for proteins that have a role in immune recognition.

The MHC encodes the **human leukocyte antigens (HLAs),** which are the molecular basis for T-cell discrimination of "self" from "nonself." The HLA complex contains over 200 genes, more than 40 of which encode leukocyte antigens, with the rest an assortment of genes not directly related to the HLA genes. Many genes within this complex have no role in immunity.

Transplanted tissue may trigger a destructive mechanism, **rejection,** if the recipient's cells recognize the MHC protein products on the surface of the transplanted tissue as "foreign," or if immunocompetent cells transplanted on the donor tissue target the foreign cells of the recipient for elimination.

Nomenclature of HLA Alleles

Each HLA allele has a unique four-, six-, or eight-letter/digit name (Table 31-1). The length of the allele designation depends on the sequence of the allele and that of its nearest relative. All alleles receive a four-letter/digit name; six- and eight-digit names are only assigned when necessary.

The first two digits describe the type, which often corresponds to the serologic antigen carried by an allotype. The third and fourth digits are used to list the subtypes, with numbers assigned in the order in which DNA sequences have been determined.

Alleles whose numbers differ in the first four digits must differ in one or more nucleotide substitutions that change the amino acid sequence of the encoded protein. Alleles that differ only by "synonymous" nucleotide substitutions (also called "silent" or "noncoding" substitutions) within the coding sequence are distinguished by the use of fifth and sixth digits. Alleles that only differ by sequence polymorphisms in the introns or in the 5′ or 3′ untranslated regions that flank the exons and introns are distinguished by the use of seventh and eighth digits.

In addition to the unique allele designation, optional suffixes may be added to an allele to indicate its expression status. Alleles shown not to be expressed, termed *null* alleles, have been given the suffix N. Alleles shown to be alternatively expressed may have the suffix L, S, C, A, or Q.

The suffix L is used to indicate an allele shown to have "low" cell surface expression compared with normal levels. The S suffix is used to denote an allele specifying a protein that is expressed as a soluble "secreted" molecule but that is not present on the cell surface. A C suffix indicates an allele product that is present in the "cytoplasm" but not on the cell

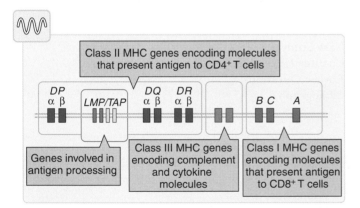

Figure 31-1 Genetic organization of major histocompatibility complex *(MHC)*/HLA antigen. *LMP,* Large multifunctional protease; *TAP,* transporter associated with antigen presentation. *(From Nairn R, Helbert M: Immunology for medical students, ed 2, St Louis, 2007, Mosby.)*

Table 31-1	HLA Naming System*
Nomenclature	**Indicates**
HLA	Human leukocyte antigen (HLA) region and prefix for an HLA gene.
HLA-DRB1	Particular HLA locus (e.g., DRB1).
HLA-DRB1*13	Group of alleles that encode the DR13 antigen.
HLA-DRB1*1301	Specific HLA allele.
HLA-DRB1*1301N	Null allele.
HLA-DRB1*130102	Allele that differs by a synonymous mutation.
HLA-DRB1*13010102	Allele that contains a mutation outside the coding region.
HLA-A*2409N	Null allele.
HLA-A*3014L	Allele encoding a protein with significantly reduced or "low" cell surface expression.
HLA-A*24020102L	Allele encoding a protein with significantly reduced or "low" cell surface expression, where the mutation is found outside the coding region.
HLA-B*44020102S	Allele encoding a protein that is expressed as a "secreted" molecule only.
HLA-A*3211Q	Allele that has a mutation previously shown to have a significant effect on cell surface expression, but where this has not been confirmed and its expression remains "questionable."

*As of June 2007, no alleles have been named with the "C" or "A" suffixes.

surface. An *A* suffix indicates "aberrant" expression, where there is some doubt as to whether a protein is expressed. A *Q* suffix is used when the expression of an allele is "questionable," given that the mutation seen in the allele has previously been shown to affect normal expression levels.

Major Histocompatibility Complex Regions

The MHC is divided into four major regions: D, B, C, and A. The A, B, and C regions are the classic or class Ia genes that code for class I molecules. The D region codes for class II molecules. Class I includes HLA-A, B, and C. The three principal loci (A, B, and C) and their respective antigens are numbered 1, 2, 3, etc. The class II gene region antigens are encoded in the HLA-D region and can be subdivided into three families, HLA-DR, HLA-DC (DQ), and HLA-SB (DP).

Classes of HLA Molecules

Structurally there are two classes of HLA molecules: class I and class II (Table 31-2). Both classes are cell surface heterodimeric structures. Class I HLA molecules consist of an alpha chain, a highly polymorphic glycoprotein, encoded within the MHC on chromosome 6. This alpha chain noncovalently associates with beta-2 microglobulin, a nonpolymorphic glycoprotein, encoded by a non-HLA gene on chromosome 15. Class II HLA molecules are composed of alpha chains and beta chains that are encoded within the MHC. The conformation of class I and class II HLA molecules provides each with a groove in which linear peptides, consisting of 8 to 25 peptides, are displayed for recognition by the cell surface expression on lymphocytes of a transmembrane heterodimeric receptor. All nucleated cells of the body display transmembrane class I HLA molecules in association with the nontransmembrane beta-2 microglobulin molecule.

The class I major transplantation antigens have been serologically defined (see http://www.anthonynolan.com for a complete list of serologically defined HLA specificities).

Class I and class II antigens can be found on body cells and in body fluids. Class I and class II molecules are surface membrane proteins. Class I molecules are transmembrane glycoproteins, but the class II dimer molecule differs from class I in that both dimers span the cell membrane. Class I and class II gene products are biochemically distinct, although they appear to be distantly related through evolution. Class III gene products such as C2, C4A, C4B, and Bf complement components are incomplete; but these structures are defined by genes lying between or very near the HLA-B and HLA-DR loci.

Multiple alleles occur at each locus. Genes of class I, II, and III antigens at each locus are inherited as codominant alleles. Inheritance within families closely follows simple mendelian dominant characteristics. Conservation of entire haplotypes through generation after generation is the general rule. Very strong linkage disequilibrium is displayed between several HLA loci, creating super or extended haplotypes that may differ from race to race. For example, the most frequent Caucasoid superextended haplotype, AL, Xw7, BB, BfS, C2-1, C4AQOB1, DR3, is virtually absent in Asians.

Role of MHC/HLAs

The histocompatibility complex that encodes cell surface antigens was first discovered in graft rejection experiments with mice. When the antigens were matched between donor and recipient, the ability of a graft to survive was remarkably improved. A comparable genetic system of alloantigens was subsequently identified in humans.

The presence of HLA was first recognized when multiple-transfused patients experienced transfusion reactions despite proper cross matching. It was discovered that these reactions resulted from leukocyte antibodies rather than from antibodies directed against erythrocyte antigens. These same antibodies were subsequently discovered in the sera of multiparous women.

The MHC gene products have an important role in clinical immunology. For example, transplants are rejected if performed against MHC barriers; thus immunosuppressive therapy is required. These antigens are of primary importance and are second only to the ABO antigens in influencing the genetic basis of survival or rejection of transplanted organs.

Although HLA was originally identified by its role in transplant rejection, it is now recognized that the products of HLA genes play a crucial role in our immune system. T cells do not recognize antigens directly but do so when the antigen is presented on the surface of an antigen-presenting cell (APC), the **macrophage.** In addition to presentation of the antigen, the macrophage must present another molecule for this response to occur. This molecule is a cell surface glycoprotein coded in each species by the MHC. T cells are able to interact with the histocompatibility molecules only if they are genetically identical (MHC restriction).

Both class I and class II antigens function as targets of T lymphocytes that regulate the immune response. Class I molecules regulate interaction between cytolytic T cells and target cells, and class II molecules restrict the activity of regulatory T cells (helper, suppressor, and amplifier subsets). Thus, class II molecules regulate the interaction between helper T cells and APCs. Cytotoxic T cells directed against class I antigens are inhibited by CD8 cells; cytotoxic T cells directed against class II antigens are inhibited by CD4 cells.

Table 31-2	Comparison of MHC Class I and Class II	
	Class I	Class II
Loci	HLA-A, B, and C	HLA-DN, DO, DP, DQ, and DR
Distribution	Most nucleated cells	B lymphocytes, macrophages, other antigen-presenting cells, activated T lymphocytes
Function	To present endogenous antigen to cytotoxic T lymphocytes.	To present endogenous antigen to helper T lymphocytes.

MHC, Major histocompatibility complex.

Many of the genes in both class I and class II gene families have no known functions.

The class I and class II molecules can also bind to "self" antigens that are produced in the normal process of cellular protein degradation. Usually, these are not recognized by the TCR **(tolerance).** In transplant patients, most immune responses are generated not from bacterial antigens, viral antigens, or self antigens, but from presentation of **alloepitopes** derived from the transplanted tissue to circulating T lymphocytes. Two types of alloepitopes are present on transplanted tissue: private and public. Cross-reactive groups have been defined that categorize the cross-reactive alleles of HLA-A and HLA-B.

Class III molecules bear no clear relation to class I and II molecules aside from their genetic linkage (presence of the gene in or near the MHC complex). Class III molecules are involved in immunologic phenomenon because they represent components of the complement pathways.

Human Leukocyte Antigen Applications

HLA matching is of value in organ transplantation, as well as in the transplantation of bone marrow. The most important HLA antigens are HLA-A, B, and DR. Everyone has two types of each of these three HLA antigens; there are many different subtypes of HLA-A, etc. The best possible match is 6/6; the worst possible match is 0/6.

In kidney allografts the method of organ preservation, the time elapsed between harvesting and transplanting, the number of pretransplantation blood transfusions, the recipient's age, and the primary cause for kidney failure are all important determinants of early transplant success or failure. HLA compatibility, however, exerts the strongest influence on long-term kidney survival. The 1-year survival for kidneys transplanted from an HLA-identical sibling approaches 95%. Approximately 50% to 65% of cadaver kidneys mismatched for all four HLA-A and B antigens function for 6 months but deteriorate thereafter with time. Only 15% to 25% of these mismatched cadaver kidneys remain functioning 4 years after transplantation.

It is obligatory to select HLA-identical donors for bone marrow transplantation to reduce the frequency of graft-versus-host disease (GVHD; discussed later in this chapter). A new method, however, that depletes donor marrow T cells capable of recognizing foreign host antigens has greatly reduced the incidence of GVHD.

HLA-matched platelets are useful to patients who are refractory to treatment with random donor platelets. In paternity testing, HLA typing is used, along with the determination of ABO, Rh, MNSs, Kell, Duffy, and Kidd erythrocyte antigen. In the past, most laboratories involved in testing individuals in disputed parentage cases used only the ABO, Rh, and MNSs systems. The chances of identifying a falsely accused man with these tests were 58%. Additional testing for Kell, Duffy, and Kidd erythrocyte antigens and for HLA typing has an exclusion rate estimated at 92%.

HLA typing is also useful in forensic medicine, anthropology, and basic research in immunology. In studies of racial

Box 31-1	Relationship of Certain Human Leukocyte Antigens and Diseases
Ankylosing spondylitis	B27
Reiter's syndrome	B27
Psoriasis vulgaris	Cw6
Rheumatoid arthritis	DR4
Behçet's disease	B5 (Bw51)
Type 1 diabetes	DR3
Gold-induced nephropathy	DR5
Congenital adrenal hyperplasia	B47
Chronic lymphatic leukemia	DR5
Kaposi's sarcoma (Mediterranean)	DR5

ancestry and migration, some antigens are virtually excluded or confined to a race (e.g., A1 and B8 are rarely detected in Mongoloids, and Bw57 is uncommon in Caucasians and African Americans). These distinctions allow for precise conclusions to be drawn regarding origin and ancestry.

HLA testing is increasingly being used as a diagnostic and genetic counseling tool. Knowledge of HLA antigens and their linkage is becoming important because of the recognized association of certain antigens with distinct immunologic-mediated reactions, autoimmune diseases, some neoplasms, and other disorders (Box 31-1); these disorders, although nonimmunologic, are influenced by non-HLA genes also located within the major MHC region.

The estimated relative risks or chances of developing a disease if a given antigen is present may be elevated in individuals bearing certain HLA antigens compared to individuals who lack the antigen (Table 31-3). The HLA-B27 antigen, however, is the only HLA antigen with a disease association strong enough to be useful in differential diagnosis. Although the degree of association between HLA antigens and other diseases may be statistically significant, it is not strong enough to be of diagnostic or prognostic value.

Although only 8% of normal Caucasians carry HLA-B27 antigen, 90% of patients with either ankylosing spondylitis (AS) or spondylitis in association with Reiter's syndrome are positive for the antigen. An elevated percentage of HLA-B27–positive patients is also observed in juvenile chronic arthritis with spinal involvement. Therefore the major indication for screening for HLA-B27 test is to rule out AS when back pain develops in relatives of patients with the disease and to help distinguish incomplete Reiter's syndrome from gonococcal arthritis, or chronic or atypical Reiter's syndrome from rheumatoid arthritis. A negative test for HLA-B27, however, does not exclude the diagnosis of AS or Reiter's syndrome.

Laboratory Evaluation of Potential Transplant Recipients and Donors

Systems developed to ascertain compatibility between donor and recipient include HLA typing and screening of the potential recipient's serum for the presence of antibodies

Table 31-3	Relationship of Human Leukocyte Antigens to Risk of Disease	
Antigen Present	**Related Disease**	**Risk***
B27	Ankylosing spondylitis	100×†
	Reiter's syndrome	40×
	Anterior uveitis	25×
	Arthritic infection with *Yersinia* or *Salmonella*	20×
	Psoriatic arthritis with spinal involvement	11×
	Spondylitis associated with inflammatory bowel disease	9×
	Juvenile chronic arthritis with spinal involvement	5×
B8	Celiac disease	9×
	Addison's disease	6×
	Myasthenia gravis	5×
	Dermatitis herpetiformis	4×
	Chronic active hepatitis	4×
	Sjögren's syndrome	3×
	Diabetes mellitus (insulin dependent)	2×
	Thyrotoxicosis	2×
B5	Behçet's syndrome	6×
BW38	Psoriatic arthritis	7×
BW15	Diabetes mellitus (insulin dependent)	3×
DR2	Goodpasture's syndrome	16×
	Multiple sclerosis	4×
DR3	Gluten-sensitive enteropathy	21×
	Dermatitis herpetiformis	14×
	Subacute cutaneous lupus erythematosus	12×
	Addison's disease	11×
	Sjögren's syndrome (primary)	10×
DR4	Pemphigus‡	32×
	Giant cell arthritis	8×
	Rheumatoid arthritis	6×
	"Juvenile" (insulin-dependent) diabetes mellitus	5×
DR5	Pauciarticular juvenile arthritis	5×
	Scleroderma	5×
	Hashimoto's thyroiditis	3×

Modified from Ashman RF: Rheumatic diseases. In Lawlor GJ, Fischer TJ, editors: *Manual of allergy and immunology*, ed 2, Boston, 1998, Little, Brown.
*Increased risk of developing the disease over a lifetime.
†Varies with ethnic group (e.g., 3× for Pima Indians and 300× for Japanese).
‡Jewish persons.

associated with rejection. Graft success is generally correlated with the presence of a compatible crossmatch, although some transplant teams are proceeding despite a positive (incompatible) crossmatch.

HLA Typing

A potential recipient needs to have HLA typing (Figure 31-2, *A*). A family search may be conducted for a suitable donor. If a suitable match is not found, the patient is placed on a waiting list (Figure 31-2, *B*). When an organ becomes available, the donor is HLA-typed, and a computerized search is made for a suitable recipient (Figure 31-2, *C*).

A newer method of HLA typing is polymerase chain reaction (PCR) amplification of DNA, followed by probing with sequence-specific oligonucleotide probes (SSOPs) and PCR amplification of alleles at loci using allele-specific primers. A simple computer program has been developed to assign the alleles and genotypes based on the probe hybridization pattern.

The difference between HLA-genotyped and zero mismatches reflects the imperfection of the HLA-typing process. "HLA genotype matched" means HLA-identical sibling, when all alleles are truly identical. A "zero mismatched" unrelated donor may be mismatched because typing does not distinguish between very closely related alleles. In addition, there may be some effect of non-HLA loci because HLA-identical siblings will share only 50% of their minor histocompatibility loci. The degree of donor-recipient mismatch is somewhat obvious, even in the first year.

Histocompatibility Testing

Because different individuals in a species carry different HLA antigens on their cell surfaces, introduction of foreign antigens can stimulate T cells. These T cells are prominently implicated in graft rejection, and they can also stimulate antibody formation under certain circumstances. Histocompatibility crossmatching is performed to rule out preexisting antibodies capable of causing hyperacute rejection (Figure 31-2, *D*).

Complement-Mediated Cytotoxicity

Class I antigens are determined by several techniques; the popular classic method is the "lymphocyte microcytotoxicity method" (complement-mediated cytotoxicity). With this technique, a battery of reagent antisera and isolated target cells are incubated with a source of complement under oil to prevent evaporation. If a specific alloantibody and a cell membrane antigen combine, complement-mediated damage to the cell wall allows for penetration of a vital dye, and the cells are killed. Cell death is determined by staining. A stain such as trypan blue will penetrate dead cells but not living cells. Unaffected cells remain brilliantly refractile when observed microscopically.

This assay can be insensitive, and scoring is subjective. Test sensitivity can be enhanced by the addition of anti–human globulin (AHG) antibody. This assay is used for pretransplant crossmatching and for antibody specificity analysis. For HLA class I typing or anti–class I antibody identification, a purified T-cell population is preferred because human T lymphocytes express class I but not class II molecules. Conversely, B lymphocytes are required for class II typing or antibody identification because human B cells express class II and class I HLA molecules.

Class II HLA-DR and HLA-DQ specificities are also recognized by similar serologic methods, except that isolated B cells are the usual target cells because their surface is rich in these molecules, as well as in class I determinants. At present, HLA-Dw and HLA-DP cannot be serologically defined, and their detection relies on the ability of these molecules to stimulate newly synthesized DNA when added to primary mixed lymphocyte (HLA-Dw) or when re-added to secondary primary lymphocyte (HLA-DP) in vitro cultures.

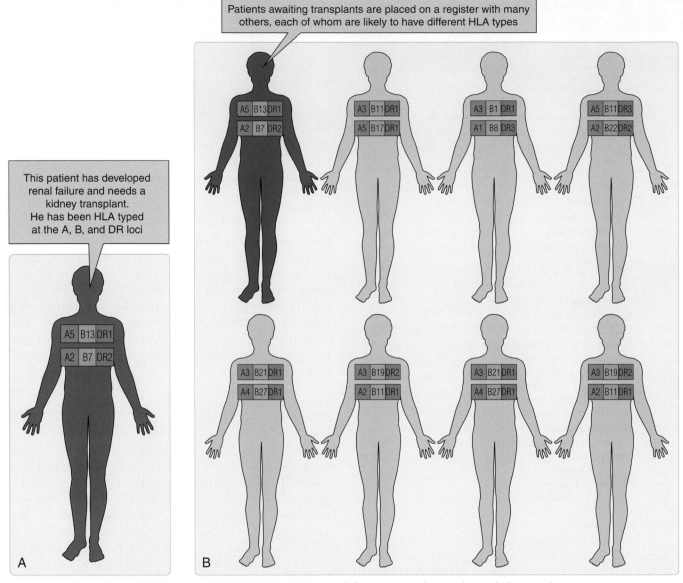

Figure 31-2 Patients (recipients) requiring a solid organ transplant such as a kidney are human leukocyte antigen (HLA)–typed **(A)** and then placed on a transplant registry waiting list **(B).** *(From Nairn R, Helbert M: Immunology for medical students, ed 2, St Louis, 2007, Mosby.)*

Class III complement specificities are recognized by the availability of diagnostic reagents, but reagents remain scarce.

Solid-Phase Enzyme-Linked Immunosorbent Assay

Enzyme-linked immunosorbent assay (ELISA) is available for **panel-reactive antibody (PRA)** determination and antibody-specificity analysis. ELISA-based HLA tests are considered reproducible, sensitive, and objective. Newer assays use pure HLA antigens produced by recombinant technology to improve specificity analysis.

Flow Cytometery

Single-cell analysis by flow cytometry is the most sensitive method for crossmatching and antibody identification (see Chapter 13). Tagged T or B lymphocytes are incubated with the patient's serum to allow formation of antigen-antibody complexes on the cell surface. Unbound proteins are washed away, and the bound antibodies are detected with a second antibody, anti–human immunoglobulin G (IgG) labeled with a chromophore. An alternative flow cytometry format uses microparticles coated with HLA antigens of known specificity (obtained through recombinant technique) instead of lymphocytes.

FACTS ABOUT SOLID ORGAN TRANSPLANTATION

Organ transplantation is widely viewed as the preferred treatment for end-stage organ failure because of the quality of life the treatment offers for patients and because of the long-term cost benefits. The increased demand for organ transplantation is fueled by the transplant success rate. Worldwide, the demand for transplant operations is increasing by about 15% per year, but the number of donated organs has remained static.

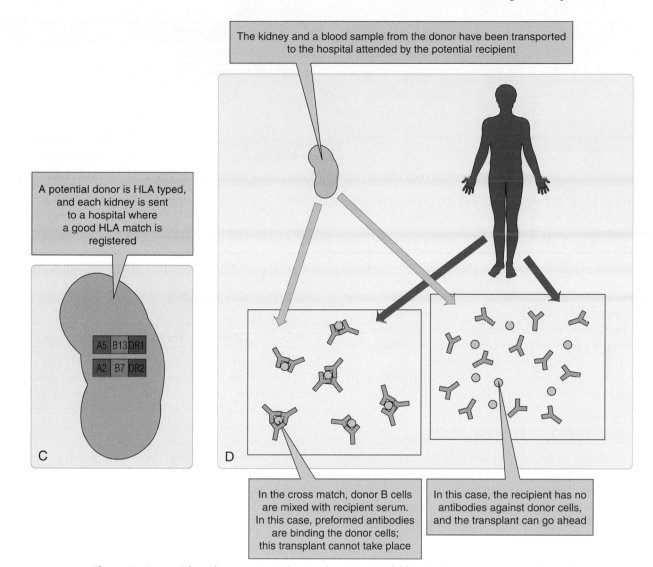

The kidney and a blood sample from the donor have been transported to the hospital attended by the potential recipient

A potential donor is HLA typed, and each kidney is sent to a hospital where a good HLA match is registered

A5 B13 DR1
A2 B7 DR2

C

D

In the cross match, donor B cells are mixed with recipient serum. In this case, preformed antibodies are binding the donor cells; this transplant cannot take place

In this case, the recipient has no antibodies against donor cells, and the transplant can go ahead

Figure 31-2, cont'd When a potential organ becomes available, the donor is HLA-typed **(C).** If the donor and recipient demonstrate a suitable match by computer, a blood sample is procured from the donor and cross-matched with the recipient's blood to determine compatibility. If no HLA antibodies are detected against the donor cells, the organ is harvested and transplanted to the recipient **(D).**

The waiting time for allergenic organ transplantation varies widely for many reasons. Each patient's situation is different. Some patients are more ill than others when they are put on the transplant waiting list. Some patients become sick more quickly than others or respond differently to treatments. Patients may have medical conditions that make finding a good match more difficult.

How long a patient waits for a transplant depends on the following factors:

- Blood type (Some are rarer than others.)
- Tissue type
- Height and weight of transplant candidate
- Size of donated organ
- Medical urgency
- Time on the waiting list
- Distance between donor's hospital and potential donor organ

- Number of donors in local area over time
- Transplant center's criteria for accepting organ offers

Depending on the kind of organ needed, some factors are more important than others.

In 1984 the U.S. Congress passed the National Organ Transplant Act. The goal of this legislation is to match a low supply of organs with the most critically ill patients, regardless of where they reside. About 56 patients receive an organ transplant every day in the United States. In 2006, more than 23,000 patients received an organ transplant.

On August 14, 2007, the United Network for Organ Sharing patient waiting list contained 96,991 names. The list continues to grow because of the scarcity of organs (Box 31-2). Most of these registrants are waiting for a kidney transplant, followed by those wanting a liver transplant and a heart transplant. Other transplant registrants are waiting for lung, kidney and pancreas, pancreas, pancreatic islet cell, heart and

Box 31-2	Factors Contributing to the Scarcity of Organs

Demand for transplantation has increased because more patients are considered eligible.
Age limits for heart and liver transplants eligibility have increased.
Diabetes is no longer an absolute contraindication for transplant eligibility.
The number of donors has shown little growth.

www.upenn.edu/ldi/issuebrief2_5.html.

lung, and intestine. Approximately 25% of patients waiting for a liver transplant are children under 10 years old.

The most common reasons for needing a transplant vary by the type of organ. Kidney recipients usually have diabetes, glomerulonephritis, hypertensive nephrosclerosis, or polycystic kidneys. Liver-recipient transplant patients typically have noncholestatic cirrhosis, cholestatic liver disease, biliary atresia, acute hepatic necrosis, or hepatitis C infection. Patients with cardiomyopathy, congenital heart disease, valvular heart disease, or coronary artery disease are the most frequent heart transplant recipients.

The number of patients living with a functioning graft has increased since 1996 (Figure 31-3).

TRANSPLANTATION TERMINOLOGY

The transplanting or grafting of an organ or tissue ranges from self-transplantation, such as skin grafts from one part of the body to another to correct burn injuries, or hair transplants from one area of the scalp to another to correct pattern baldness, to the grafting of a body component from

Table 31-4	Transplantation Terms
Term	**Definition**
Autograft	Graft transferred from one position to another in the same individual (e.g., skin, hair, bone).
Syngraft	Graft transplanted between different but identical recipient and donor (e.g., kidney transplant between monozygous twins).
Allograft (homograft)	Graft between genetically different recipient and donor of the same species; the grafted donor tissue or organ contains antigens not present in the recipient.
Xenograft (heterograft)	Graft between individuals of different species (e.g., pig heart valve to a human heart).

one species to another, such as transplanting a pig's heart valve to a human. Table 31-4 defines the most recent terms used in transplantation.

TYPES OF TRANSPLANTS

Eleven different organs or human body parts can be transplanted: corneas, middle ear, lung, heart, blood vessels, liver, pancreas, kidneys, bone, skin, and bone marrow/peripheral stem cells (see Chapter 32). Successful organ transplants have increased since the advent of the immunosuppressive drug *cyclosporine* (cyclosporin A).

Living-donor transplants have attracted significant media attention in the last few years. According to the United Network for Organ Sharing and the Health Resources and Services Administration of the U.S. Department of Health and Human Services, a living donor may donate a single

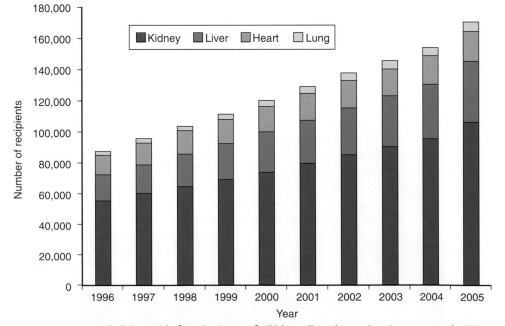

Figure 31-3 People living with functioning graft (kidney, liver, heart, lung) at year end, 1996–2005. *(From OPTN/SRTR: 2006 annual report, Table 1.14.)*

kidney, segment of the liver, portion of the pancreas, or the lobe of a lung.

Kidney

The first successful human kidney transplant was performed in 1954 between monozygotic twins. Induction of tolerance (discussed later in this chapter) was attempted through the use of sublethal total body irradiation and allogeneic bone marrow transplantation, followed by renal transplantation. By 1960, renal transplantation was firmly established as a viable treatment for end-stage renal disease. Because of the continuing problems associated with total-body irradiation, chemical immunosuppression became the mode of treatment. The criteria for recipients of renal allografts generally exclude elderly patients and patients with a history of malignancy. In addition, patients with active sepsis or patients in whom chronic infection may be reactivated by treatment with steroids or immunosuppressive therapy are also not considered transplant candidates.

Traditionally, kidney donations are not accepted from individuals over 65 years old because of a decreased likelihood of recipient survival. Donors are excluded if chronic renal disease or sepsis is present. Donations are usually not accepted from individuals with generalized or systemic diseases such as diabetes mellitus, hypertension, and tuberculosis. Because of the severe shortage of donor kidneys, organs from donors older than 55 years of age or from donors with a history of hypertension or diabetes mellitus are being used with increasing frequency. Young trauma victims are the most desirable source of cadaver organ transplants, including the kidneys. Cadaver organs are not accepted from donors with a history of any malignancy other than that involving the central nervous system.

In addition to compatibility of ABO blood group systems, newer methods of harvesting kidneys have reduced the sensitizing effect related to "passenger" leukocytes against transplantation antigens borne on these cells. HLA-A and HLA-B loci matches have the best chance for long-term survival of the graft and the recipient. The increased survival rate with HLA-A and HLA-B matches is determined not as much by class I compatibility as by the HLA-D region–related antigens associated with these regions. The strongest association between transplant survival and tissue antigens is with the D region–related antigens (DR, MB, MT). Lewis antigens on the erythrocytes and H-Y antigens associated with X and Y chromosomes are among the other antigen systems that demonstrate a reasonably significant association with graft survival.

Heart Valves

Xenogenic valve replacements are a standard modality for the treatment of aortic and mitral valve defects. Sources of these xenogenic valves are either bovine (cow) or porcine (pig), and the valves are chemically or physically modified to reduce antigenicity.

Patients receiving xenoallografts of heart valves are not immunosuppressed after surgery because only minimal or nonexistent graft rejection reactions take place in these modified valves.

Heart

The first successful allograft cardiac transplant was performed in 1967 by Dr. Christian Barnard in Cape Town, South Africa. The criteria for selecting the donor and recipient combination for cardiac transplantation are essentially the same as those used for cadaver renal transplantation. The most significant exclusion for cardiac transplantation, however, is the presence of an active infection. Cardiac transplantation donors must have sustained irreversible brain death, but near-normal cardiac function must be maintained. Prophylactic antibiotics and cytotoxic drugs are given to the donor just before harvesting of the heart. Because of the urgency of most situations, most grafts are performed despite multiple HLA incompatibilities. Transplantation recipients are maintained on immunosuppressive therapy, anticoagulants, and antithrombotic agents, as well as on low-lipid diets.

Cornea

Corneal transplants have been a common form of therapy for many years. The first human corneal eye bank was established in New York City in 1944. This type of transplantation has an extremely high success rate because of the ease in obtaining and storing viable corneas.

Corneal grafts are generally performed to replace nonhealing corneal ulcerations. Graft rejection is minimal because of (1) the **avascularity** (lack of blood vessels) of this tissue, (2) a reasonably low concentration of class I transplantation antigens, and (3) an essential absence of class II antigens. To prevent rejection, grafts are made as small as possible and are placed centrally to avoid contact with the highly vascularized limbic region. Eccentrically placed grafts are subject to a high rate of immunologic failure because vascularity will allow for lymphocyte contact. Immunosuppression is not routinely administered.

Skin

The development of nonimmunogenic skin replacement materials has lowered the demand for allografts of skin. Skin allografts elicit the rejection phenomenon because skin has an extremely high density of MHC class I antigens. Therefore, sensitization and recognition of antigenic differences are likely, with resultant rejection of the grafted skin. If done, skin allografts are performed and supported with immunosuppressive therapy.

Liver

Potential liver transplant recipients must have no extrahepatic disease or infection present. The largest group of transplant recipients has been those with congenital biliary atresia. Patients with cirrhosis may also be good candidates. HLA crossmatching appears to increase the rate of graft survival, but the influence of tissue typing is somewhat unclear. Immunosuppressive regimens such as azathioprine and corticosteroids or cyclosporin A increase survival. Major complications of this procedure have been biliary tract fistulae or leaks, which have occurred in 30% to 50% of patients.

Lung

Successful lung transplants have been difficult to achieve because of technical, logistic, and immunologic problems. Technically, lung donor and recipient must have essentially identical bronchial circumferences to obtain a good match. An additional technical problem is that the lungs are extremely sensitive to ischemic damage, and successful preservation after harvesting has been unsuccessful. Occasionally, lung-heart combination transplants have been attempted. The combined procedure is less difficult than single-organ transplant.

The lungs are susceptible to infection; sepsis is very common among potential donors. Severe rejection is common because of the high density of Ia-positive cells in the vasculature and the high concentration of passenger leukocytes trapped in the alveoli and blood vessels. Intensive immunosuppressive therapy is needed to maintain the graft. Many lung recipients have died from massive infection and sepsis.

Pancreas

New modes of transplantation include full pancreatic or isolated islet cell transplantation. Pancreatic grafts have been successful for only a short period because of a high rate of technical failure or irreversible rejection. Transplantation of small quantities of isolated islet cells into the retroperitoneal space, however, has demonstrated a reasonably good success rate.

Pancreatic islet transplants are risky and experimental, with about 50% of patients achieving insulin dependency after 1 year.

Bone

Bone matrix autografts or allografts are common. Transplantation of bone matrix is used after certain limb-sparing tumor resections and to correct congenital bone abnormalities. The major criteria for bone donation are a lack of infection, no history of intravenous drug use, and no history of prolonged steroid therapy or human growth hormone treatment. Bone can be easily harvested and frozen. Freezing not only preserves the bone but offers the additional benefit of concomitant diminution of histocompatibility antigens.

The major technical requirement for allograft transplantation is maintaining the periosteal sheath of the recipient bone in order to strip the donor bone completely of all periosteal elements. Transplantation of bone is an easy procedure. Processed bone lacks significant quantities of immunogenic substances; therefore the need for immunosuppression is almost completely eliminated.

GRAFT-VERSUS-HOST DISEASE

Graft-versus-host disease (GVHD) can be an unintentional consequence of blood transfusion or transplantation in severely immunocompromised or immunosuppressed patients. The degree of immunodeficiency in the host, rather than the number of transfused immunocompetent lymphocytes, determines whether or not GVHD will occur.

Etiology

When immunocompetent T lymphocytes are transfused from a donor to an immunodeficient or immunosuppressed recipient, the transfused or grafted lymphocytes recognize that the antigens of the host are foreign and react immunologically against them (Table 31-5). Instead of the usual transplantation reaction of host against graft, the reverse graft-versus-host reaction occurs and produces an inflammatory response.

In a normal lymphocyte transfer reaction, the results of a GVHD are usually not serious because the recipient is capable of destroying the foreign lymphocytes. However, engraftment and multiplication of donor lymphocytes in an immunosuppressed recipient are a real possibility because lymphocytes capable of mitosis can be found in stored blood products. If the recipient cannot reject the transfused lymphocytes, the grafted lymphocytes may cause uncontrolled destruction of the host's tissues and eventually death. A patient can develop acute or chronic GVHD. The stronger the antigen difference, the more severe is the reaction.

Epidemiology

It is now accepted that GVHD can occur whenever immunologically competent allogeneic lymphocytes are transfused into a severely immunocompromised host. Patients at risk include those who are immunodeficient or immunosuppressed with severe lymphocytopenia and bone marrow suppression. Despite chemotherapy at the time of bone marrow transplantation, patients are highly likely to develop acute GVHD, and some of these immunocompromised patients will die of GVHD or associated infections.

Chronic GVHD affects 20% to 40% of patients within 6 months after transplantation. Two factors closely associated with the development of chronic GVHD are increasing age and a preceding episode of acute GVHD.

Cases of transfusion-related GVHD have increased significantly in the past two decades. This reaction has been reported subsequent to blood transfusion in bone marrow transplant recipients after total-body irradiation, and in adults receiving intensive chemotherapy for hematologic

Table 31-5	Requirements for Potential Graft-versus-Host Disease	
Factor	**Comments**
1. A source of immunocompetent lymphocytes	Blood products, bone marrow transplant, organ transplant.
2. Human leukocyte antigen differences between patient and recipient	The stronger the antigen difference, the more severe the reaction.
3. Inability to reject donor cells	Patients are severely immunocompromised or immunosuppressed.

malignancies. GVHD has also occurred in infants with severe congenital immunodeficiency and in those who have received intrauterine transfusions followed by exchange transfusion. Almost 90% of patients with posttransfusion GVHD will die of acute complications of the disease. The usual cause of death is generalized infection.

Signs and Symptoms

Graft-versus-host disease causes an inflammatory response. Posttransfusion symptoms begin within 3 to 30 days after transfusion. Because of lymphocytic infiltration of the intestine, skin, and liver, mucosal destruction results, including ulcerative skin and mouth lesions, diarrhea, and liver destruction. Other clinical symptoms include jaundice, fever, anemia, weight loss, skin rash, and splenomegaly.

In bone marrow transplant patients, acute GVHD develops within the first 3 months of transplantation. The initial manifestations are lesions of the skin, liver, and gastrointestinal tract. An erythematous maculopapular skin rash, particularly on the palms and soles, is usually the first sign of GVHD. Disease progression is characterized by diarrhea, often with abdominal pain, and liver disease. Other signs and symptoms of complications related to therapy include fever, granulocytopenia, and bacteremia. Interstitial pneumonia, frequently associated with cytomegalovirus (CMV), can also occur.

Chronic GVHD resembles a collagen vascular disease, with skin changes such as erythema and cutaneous ulcers, and a liver dysfunction characterized by bile duct degeneration and cholestasis. Patients with chronic GVHD are susceptible to bacterial infections. For example, increasing age and preexisting lung disease increase the incidence of interstitial pneumonia.

Immunologic Manifestation

In immunocompromised patients the transfused or grafted lymphocytes recognize the antigens of the host as foreign and react immunologically against them. Instead of the usual transplantation reaction of host against graft, the reverse GVHD occurs.

Diagnostic Evaluation

Laboratory evidence of immunosuppression or immunodeficiency, such as a decreased total lymphocyte concentration, suggests that a patient may develop GVHD. Evidence of inflammation, such as increased C-reactive protein (CRP), elevated leukocyte count with granulocytosis, and increased erythrocyte sedimentation rate (ESR), may suggest that GVHD has developed in GVHD candidates. Complications of anemia and liver disease, characterized by increased bilirubin and blood enzymes (e.g., transaminases, alkaline phosphatase), and the presence of opportunistic pathogens (e.g., CMV) can further support the diagnosis.

Pathologic features include lymphocytic and monocytic infiltration into perivascular spaces in the dermis and dermoepidermal junction of the skin and into the epithelium of the oropharynx, tongue, and esophagus. Infiltration can also be observed into the base of the intestinal crypts of the small and large bowel and into the periportal area of the liver, with secondary necrosis of cells in infiltrated tissues.

Prevention

The incidence of GVHD can be minimized by depletion of mature lymphocytes from the marrow by using monoclonal antibodies or physical methods. The risk of GVHD can be minimized if not eliminated by irradiation of the marrow transplant or blood products. Blood product irradiation is believed to be the most efficient and probably the most economical method available for prevention of posttransfusion GVHD.

No cases of posttransfusion GVHD have been reported after administration of blood products irradiated with at least 1500 rad. The recommended radiation dose ranges from a minimum of 1500 to 3000 rad as an effective and appropriate radiation dose.

Several categories of patients possess the clinical indications for irradiated products.

High-Risk Patients
Patients at the highest risk with an absolute need for irradiated blood products include:
- Recipients of autologous or allogeneic bone marrow grafts. Recipients of autologous bone marrow may be expected to have the same risk of posttransfusion GVHD as patients receiving allogeneic bone marrow.
- Children with severe congenital immunodeficiency syndromes involving T lymphocytes. The degree of immunodeficiency in the host, rather than the number of transfused immunocompetent cells, determines whether GVHD will occur.

Intermediate-Risk Patients
Patients considered to be at less of a risk of developing GVHD include:
- Infants receiving intrauterine transfusions, followed by exchange transfusions, and possibly infants receiving only exchange transfusions. The immune mechanism of the fetus and newborn may not be sufficiently mature to reject foreign lymphocytes, and prior transfusions may induce a state of immune tolerance in the newborn. Transfused lymphocytes may continue to circulate for a prolonged time in some immunologically tolerant hosts without the development of GVHD. There is insufficient evidence to recommend irradiation of blood given to all premature infants.
- Patients receiving total-body radiation or immunosuppressive therapy for disorders such as lymphoma and acute leukemia. Although routine irradiation of blood products given to these patients can be justified, it cannot be regarded as absolutely indicated because the risk of developing GVHD is so small. Blood product irradiation, however, is advised for selected patients with hematologic malignancies, especially when transfusions are given during or near the time of sustained and severe therapy-induced immunosuppression.

Low-Risk Patients

Patients also at risk but considered the least susceptible include:

- Patients with solid tumors. The incidence of the development of GVHD is difficult to determine. However, it has developed in nonhematologic malignancies such as neuroblastoma. In one case, GVHD developed after infusion of a single unit of packed red blood cells (RBCs).
- Patients with aplastic anemia receiving antithymocyte globulin theoretically may be at increased risk of posttransfusion GVHD during therapy-induced periods of lymphocytopenia.
- Although a theoretic risk of posttransfusion GVHD may exist in patients with acquired immunodeficiency syndrome (AIDS), the disease has not actually been observed in this disorder. The routine use of irradiated blood is not recommended.

Effects of Radiation on Specific Cellular Components

Lymphocytes. Ionizing radiation is known to inhibit lymphocyte mitotic activity and blast transformation. Irradiation of normal donor lymphocytes with 1500 rad from a cesium-137 source results in a 90% reduction in mitogen-stimulated ^{14}C-thymidine incorporation. An 85% reduction in mitogen-induced blast transformation after exposure to 1500 rad and a 97% to 98.5% reduction in mitogenic response have been noted after exposure to 5000 rad.

Granulocytes. Ionizing radiation may impair granulocyte function in a dose-dependent manner. The degree of actual damage to granulocytes is controversial. Chemotactic activity decreased linearly with increasing doses of irradiation from 500 to 120,000 rad, but the reduction only reached statistical significance at 10,000 rad. A linear dose-response curve demonstrates that granulocyte locomotion is affected by very small doses of irradiation. A dose of 2000 rad is likely to eliminate lymphocytic mitotic activity and prevent GVHD without causing significant damage to granulocytes or altering their chemotactic or bactericidal ability. Irradiation before transfusion has been demonstrated to contribute to defective oxidative metabolism, but this effect is highly variable.

Mature Red Blood Cells. Mature RBCs appear to be highly resistant to radiation damage. After RBCs were exposed to 10,000 rad, ^{52}Cr-labeled in vivo RBC survival was the same as that of untreated controls. Stored erythrocytes can be treated with up to 20,000 rad without changing their viability or in vitro properties, including adenosine triphosphate (ATP) and 2,3-diphosphoglycerate (2,3-DPG) levels, plasma hemoglobin (Hb), and potassium ions (K^+).

Platelets. Ionizing radiation may impair platelet function. Although this impairment is dose dependent, the effects of irradiation on platelets have been difficult to characterize. Several studies have demonstrated unchanged in vivo platelet survival after exposure to 5000 to 75,000 rad. A 33% decrease in the expected platelet count increase was noted after transfusion of platelets exposed to 5000 rad, and similarly irradiated autologous platelets had a diminished ability to correct the bleeding times in a small number of volunteers who had consumed aspirin. In one study, platelet aggregation was not affected by exposure to 5000 rad, although an impaired response to collagen was noted.

Immunologic Tolerance

The importance of tolerance to self antigens was recognized very early in the study of immunology. Immunologic tolerance is the acquisition of nonreactivity toward particular antigens. Self-recognition (tolerance) is a critical process, and the failure to recognize self antigens can result in autoimmune disease (see Chapter 28).

Various pathways to immunologic tolerance have been recognized. It has been suggested that both T and B cells are affected independently and differently and may be tolerated under certain circumstances. Several mechanisms may operate simultaneously in a single host. During fetal development of the immune system and during the first few weeks of neonatal life, none of the cells of the immune system has reached maturity. For this reason, the entire immune system is particularly susceptible to tolerance induction at this stage of development.

T-Cell Tolerance

T cells do not show a marked difference in tolerance at different stages of maturation. The antigen required to produce tolerance and the circumstance of its presentation are specific for each individual T-cell subset. At least three pathways have been recognized for T-cell tolerance, as follows:

1. *Clonal abortion.* Immature T-cell clones may be aborted in a manner similar to B cells.
2. *Functional deletion.* The subsets of a mature T cell may be individually deleted, leading to the loss of only one of the functions of the T-cell group.
3. *T-cell suppression.* T-cell suppressors actively suppress the actions of other T-cell subsets or B cells.

B-Cell Tolerance

As a B cell matures, it becomes less susceptible to tolerization. In addition, during B-cell maturation, the forms of antigen presentation that will produce tolerance also vary. Four pathways have been established for the induction of B-cell tolerance. Therefore the mode of tolerance depends on the maturity of the cell, the antigen, and the manner of antigen presentation to the immune system.

The pathways of B-cell tolerance are as follows:

1. *Clonal abortion.* A low concentration of multivalent antigen may cause the immature clone to abort. Tolerance of immature B cells by this mechanism is high.
2. *Clonal exhaustion.* Repeated antigen challenge with a T-independent antigen may remove all mature functional B-cell clones. Tolerance of mature B cells is moderate.

3. *Functional deletion.* The combined absence of the T-helper subset and presence of T-dependent antigen (or with T-suppressor cells), or an excess of T-independent antigen, prevents mature B cells from functioning normally. The ability to tolerize B cells by this mechanism is moderate.
4. *Antibody-forming cell blockade.* An excess of T-independent antigen interferes with the secretion of antibody by antibody-forming cells. B-cell tolerance by this mechanism is low.

Immune Response Gene–Associated Antigens

The specific immune responses to a variety of antigenic substances are now known to be regulated by an immune response (Ir) gene. Ir gene control is considered genetically dominant. The homology of the HLA-D region with the animal I region suggests that the human Ir gene might be linked to the HLA complex. Evidence for the existence of the Ir gene is obtained from family and population studies. Additional evidence for the presence of Ir genes comes from HLA-linked disease susceptibility genes and HLA-disease associations. It is believed that individuals who lack this gene are unresponsive.

The generally accepted concept is that the Ir gene is responsible for the interaction of T cells with both B cells and macrophages, which are necessary for T-cell activation. Activation of T cells is required for the following:
- Conversion to active helper function
- Production of lymphokines

Mediation of delayed and contact hypersensitivity, as the proliferative response to antigen, depends on the interaction of a T cell with an APC, usually macrophage-monocytes. Helper function also depends on T-cell interaction with precursors of antibody-secreting cells. T cells interact with these cells by recognizing specific antigen bound to macrophages or to B cells and the I-region gene products expressed on the surface of these cells. T cells are able to recognize the precise details of antigen structure and distinguish between two closely related Ir gene–associated molecules expressed on the surface of these APCs or on the B cell.

GRAFT REJECTION

Organs vary with respect to their susceptibility to rejection based on inherent immunogenicity (Box 31-3), which is influenced by factors such as vascularity.

The role of sensitized lymphocytes and antibodies in graft rejection differs and is influenced by the type of organ transplanted. Lymphocytes, particularly recirculating small lymphocytes, are effective in shortening graft survival. Cell-mediated immunity is responsible for the rejection of skin and solid tumors. However, humoral antibodies can also be involved in the rejection process. The complexity of the action and interaction of cellular and humoral factors in grafts is considerable. Five possible categories of graft rejection have been demonstrated in human kidney transplant rejection: hyperacute, accelerated, acute, chronic, and immunopathologic (Table 31-6 and Plate 8).

First-Set and Second-Set Rejection

Skin transplantation is the most common experimental model for transplantation research (Figure 31-4). Rejection of skin and solid tumors can be divided into first-set and second-set rejection. Activation of cellular immunity by T cells is the predominant cause of the *first-set* allograft rejection. Lymphocytes can directly attack cellular antigens to which they are sensitized by previous exposure or by cyto-

Box 31-3	Immunogenicity of Different Transplant Tissues

Most Immunogenic
Bone marrow
Skin
Islets of Langerhans
Heart
Kidney
Liver
Bone
Xenogeneic valve replacements

Least Immunogenic
Cornea

Table 31-6	Categories and Characteristics of Graft Rejection Based on Immune Destruction of Kidney Grafts		
Type	Time of Tissue Damage	Predominant Mechanism	Cause
Hyperacute	Within minutes	Humoral	Preformed cytotoxic antibodies to donor antigens
Accelerated	2-5 days	Cell mediated	Previous sensitization to donor antigens
Acute	7-21 days	Cell mediated (possibly antibody cell-mediated cytotoxicity)	Development of allogeneic reaction to donor antigens
Chronic	Later than 3 months	Cell mediated	Disturbance of host/graft tolerance
Immunopathologic damage to the new organ	Later than 3 months	1. Immune complex disorder 2. Complex formation with soluble antigens	Immunopathologic mechanisms related to circumstances necessitating transplant

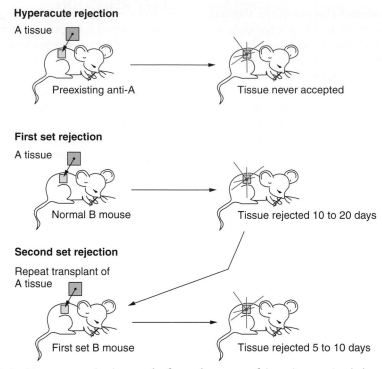

Figure 31-4 Hyperacute rejection results from placement of tissue in an animal already possessing antibodies to antigens of grafted tissue. Second-set rejection is an accelerated first-set reaction and is seen in animals that have already rejected tissue at least once. *(Redrawn from Barrett JT: Textbook of immunology, ed 5, St Louis, 1988, Mosby.)*

toxic lymphokines. The primary role of lymphocytes in first-set rejection is consistent with the histology of early reaction and shows infiltration by mononuclear cells with very few polymorphonuclear leukocytes or plasma cells. Sensitization occurs within the first few days of transplantation, and the tissue is lost in 10 to 20 days.

When sensitized lymphocytes are already present because of prior graft rejection, an accelerated rejection of tissue results from regrafting, called *second-set* rejection. Lymphocytes from a sensitized animal transferred to a first-graft recipient will accelerate rejection of the graft. Graft rejection is primarily a T-cell function, with some assistance from antibodies.

Hyperacute Rejection

Hyperacute reactions are caused entirely by the presence within the host of preformed humoral antibodies, which react with donor tissue cellular antigens. These antibodies are usually anti-A–related or anti-B–related antibodies to the ABO blood group systems or antibodies to class I MHC antigens (hypersensitivity type II). Potential recipients harboring antibodies to HLA-A, HLA-B, and HLA-C (class I) but not HLA-DR (class II) antigens are at high risk for this process.

The interaction of cellular antigens with antibodies activates the complement system and leads to grafted cell lysis and clotting within the grafted tissue. Kidney allografts can be rejected by the hyperacute rejection process within min-

utes of transplantation. The irreversible kidney damage of hyperacute rejection is characterized by sludging of erythrocytes, development of microthrombi in the small arterioles and glomerular capillaries, and infiltration of phagocytic cells.

Genetically altered pig organs could be available for transplantation into humans within 2 years, but it is likely to be at least 5 years before full-scale studies can begin. Future xenotransplantation will depend on overcoming problems of hyperacute rejection. In hyperacute rejection, the recipient of the organ produces xenoreactive antibodies, which lodge on the cells lining the blood vessels of the new organ and trigger the release of complement. This release triggers inflammation, swelling, and ultimately blockage of the blood vessels, leading to death of the organ.

Accelerated Rejection

Accelerated rejection is comparable to the second-set rejection phenomenon observed in animal models. In these cases, retransplantation is less severe than hyperacute rejection and is considered to be accelerated rejection. Accelerated rejection is caused by activation of the T-cell–mediated response.

Acute Rejection

Acute rejection can result after the first exposure to alloantigens. In this reaction, donor antigens select reactive T-cell clones and initiate visible manifestation of rejection within

6 to 14 days. The early processes in acute rejection appear to be T-cell mediated; however, later aspects may involve antibodies and complement.

Acute rejection is equivalent to a first-set allograft rejection in experimental animals and is primarily mediated by cells, as in accelerated rejection. Immunopathologic changes include the presence of immune complex deposition and other hypersensitivity reactions already present in the recipient.

Acute rejection takes place when there is HLA incompatibility. Recipient T cells can respond to donor peptides presented by recipient major MHC or to donor MHC molecules themselves. The better the HLA match, the more successful are the prospects for nonrejection. Because of the shortage of organs and the huge demand for organs, partially mismatched organs (e.g., kidneys) may be used. The survival of the kidney is related to the degree of mismatching, especially at the HLA-DR loci. Despite mismatching, 1-year survival with five mismatches was almost 80% because of the effect of potent immunosuppressive drugs.

A recipient may respond to *minor* histocompatibility antigens. Minor antigens are encoded by genes outside the HLA. These minor histocompatibility antigen mismatches are not detected by standard tissue-typing techniques but may cause rejection despite a good HLA match. Up to one third of transplants can be rejected because of minor antigens.

Acute *early* rejection, which occurs up to about 10 days after transplantation, is histologically characterized by dense cellular infiltration and rupture of peritubular capillaries. It appears to be a cell-mediated hypersensitivity reaction involving T cells. In comparison, acute *late* rejection occurs 11 days or more after transplantation in patients suppressed with prednisone and azathioprine. In kidney allografts, acute late rejection is probably caused by the binding of immunoglobulin, presumably antibody and complement, to the arterioles and glomerular capillaries, where they can be visualized by immunofluorescent techniques. These immunoglobulin deposits on the vessel walls include platelet aggregates in glomerular capillaries, which cause acute renal shutdown. The possibility of damage to antibody-coated cells through **antibody-dependent, cell-mediated cytotoxicity** (ADCC) may also take place.

Chronic Rejection

Chronic rejection occurs in most graft recipients. The process results in a slow but continual loss of organ function over months or years. However, chronic rejection is often responsive to various immunosuppressive therapies.

In kidney allografts, this insidious rejection is associated with subendothelial deposits of immunoglobulin and the C3 component of complement on the glomerular basement membranes. This may occasionally be an expression of an underlying immune complex disorder that may have originally necessitated the transplant, or it may result from complex formation with soluble antigens derived from the grafted kidney.

MECHANISMS OF REJECTION

General Characteristics

Variations in the expression of class II histocompatibility antigens by different tissues and the presence of APCs in some tissues greatly influence the success of a transplant. APCs that enter the graft through the donor's circulation are likely to elicit graft rejection. If these "passenger lymphocytes" leave the graft after transplantation and enter the draining lymphatic system, they are particularly effective in sensitizing the host.

Rejection of a graft displays the following two key features of adaptive immunity:
- Memory
- Specificity

Only sites accessible to the immune system in the recipient are susceptible to graft rejection. Certain "privileged" sites in the body allow allogeneic grafts to survive indefinitely.

Role of T Cells

Graft rejection is primarily regulated by the interaction of the host's T cells with the antigens of the graft. Unmodified rejection, however, results from the destructive effects of cytotoxic T (Tc) cells, activated macrophages, and antibody.

In tissue transplants the graft consists of tissue cells that carry class I antigens (HLA-A, HLA-B, and HLA-C) and of lymphocytes that carry both class I and class II antigens (HLA-D and related antigens of associated Ir gene). Activated T cells specific for class I antigens have the potential to express cytotoxic activity, which damages both the endothelium and the parenchymal cells of the graft. Binding of these cells to the class I antigens on target cells of the donor organ triggers the release of lymphokines and subsequently activates a nonspecific inflammatory response in the allograft.

T cells specific for class II antigens of the donor tissue are unable to react directly with the parenchymal cells of the graft not expressing class II antigens. However, these cells can activate lymphocytes in the transplant through lymphocyte release. Therefore, damage to the graft can result from a cytotoxic reaction directed against cells of the transplanted organ or from a severe nonspecific inflammatory response, or both.

Activation of T-helper (Th) cells by class II antigens such as HLA-DR probably stimulates the release of interleukin-1 (IL-1). IL-1 subsequently stimulates the release of various lymphokines from Th cells, which in turn activate macrophages, Tc cells, and antibody-releasing B cells, as well as increase the immunogenicity of the graft. In addition, macrophages and other accessory cells are subsequently stimulated by T-cell products and release IL-1, which in turn stimulates formation of interleukin-2 (IL-2) receptors, as well as the release of IL-2 by Th cells. IL-2 interacts with specific IL-2 receptors expressed on activated Th and Tc cells. This interaction stimulates the initiation of DNA synthesis and the eventual clonal proliferation of IL-2 receptor–bearing cells. IL-2 also causes the release of interferon gamma (IFN-γ), which activates macrophages and stimulates the release of

B-cell differentiation factors required for the proliferation of antigen-activated B cells. The release of IL-2–dependent IFN-γ by activated T cells may initiate a vicious circle, because IFN-γ induces the expression of class II molecules on endothelial cells, as well as the expression of certain class II–negative macrophages.

Histologic examination of an allogenic skin graft during the process of rejection demonstrates that the dermis becomes infiltrated by mononuclear cells, many of which are small lymphocytes. This accumulation of lymphocytes precedes the destruction of the graft by several days. Although this graft rejection process is caused by Tc cells, in some cases Th cells are also elicited by MHC gene differences. Graft rejection may be a special form of response related to delayed hypersensitivity reactions, in which case the ultimate effectors of graft destruction are the monocyte-macrophages recruited to the site. It is debatable whether the macrophages seen in grafts are effectors of graft destruction or arrive only as a consequence of the inflammatory process and cell damage.

Antibody Effects

Cell-mediated immunity is the major effector mechanism in graft rejection. Antibodies, however, can also be involved in graft rejection. Antibodies can cause rapid (hyperacute) graft rejection, but they are usually less significant than cell-mediated immunity. Exceptions include cases in which the recipient has been previously sensitized to a particular antigen, reactions occur to hematopoietic cells, or the graft is directly connected to the host's blood circulation (e.g., kidney allograft).

In dispersed cellular grafts such as infusion of erythrocytes, leukocytes, and platelets, antibodies (humoral immunity) may dominate the rejection process because antigens are fully exposed to a preexisting or a developing antibody response. Cells are highly susceptible to complement-activated membrane damage. If cytolysis does not occur immediately, antibodies may function as opsonins to encourage phagocytic destruction of transfused cells.

Humoral immunity is suspected of playing a major role in the rejection of xenografts. Xenografts possess a large number of antigens shared between donor and recipient. One species can possess agglutinins for cells of distantly related species, which can attack the xenogenic tissue as soon as it is transplanted.

Immunosuppression

For most patients who receive a donated organ, immunosuppressant drug therapy and monitoring of the concentration of immunosuppressants play a critical role in the success of the transplant. Laboratory methods for measuring immunosuppressant drug concentrations in blood include immunoassay, high-performance liquid chromatography (HPLC), and liquid chromatography with mass spectrometry (LC/MS). Clinical laboratories are increasingly using LC/MS for routine measurement of immunosuppressants.

Box 31-4	Immunosuppression in Human Organ Transplantation
	Research on antimetabolites, including 6-mercaptopurine azathioprine and corticosteroids, used to improve kidney graft survival.
Late 1960s	Antilymphocyte globulin proved successful.
1976	Cyclosporine developed.
1983	Cyclosporine approved by FDA.
1984	OKT3 (Muromonab-CD3) approved by FDA.
1994	Tacrolimus (FK-506) approved by FDA.
1995	Mycophenolic acid approved by FDA (almost 30 years after development).
1996	Cyclosporine microemulsion (Neoral) approved by FDA.
1997	Antithymocyte globulin approved by FDA. Dacliximab (Zenapax) approved by FDA.
1999	Sirolimus (Rapamune) approved by FDA.
2004	Enteric-coated mycophenolic acid approved by FDA.

FDA, US Food and Drug Administration.

Immunosuppression is used for the following:
- Induction (intense immunosuppression in the initial days after transplantation)
- Maintenance of transplant
- Reversal of established rejection

Forms of immunosuppression include chemical (Box 31-4), biologic, and irradiation of the lymphoid system or the donated organ. The immunosuppressive activities of therapeutic agents used in transplantation directly interfere with the allograft rejection response. The problem arising from all immunosuppressive techniques is that the individual is more susceptible to infection. If infection occurs, immunosuppression must be suspended, at which time allogeneic reactions frequently develop.

Immunosuppressive measures may be antigen specific or antigen nonspecific (Table 31-7). Antigen-nonspecific immunosuppression includes drugs and other methods of specifically altering T-cell function. Many cytotoxic drugs are primarily active against dividing cells and therefore have some

Table 31-7	Types of Immunosuppressive Treatment
Antigen Nonspecific	**Antigen Specific**
Drugs	
Azathioprine	Neonatal tolerization
Steroids	
Cyclosporine	
Other Methods	
Antilymphocyte globulin	Enhancing (antiallogenic) antibodies
Radiation	Antiidiotype antibodies to receptors on T cells
	Blood transfusion in human kidney transplant

functional specificity for any cells activated to divide by donor antigens. The use of these drugs is limited by the toxic effects they may have on other dividing cells or on the physiologic functioning of organs such as the liver.

Antigen-specific immunosuppression is an ideal form of immunosuppression. Antigen-specific tolerance is that induced by the infusion of donor cells. This is generally impractical in transplantation, but it may be useful in the phenomenon of "immunologic enhancement." Enhancement of tolerance has been attempted in renal allograft patients. In a donor-specific blood transfusion program, the patient is transfused several times before elective transplantation with blood from the prospective kidney donor. The overall effect of these transfusions appears to be a tolerance of the recipient to donor transplantation antigens other than those in the HLA-linked regions, such as minor histocompatibility loci, RBC loci, and leukocyte surface antigens. This treatment has greatly prolonged graft survival in these patients.

Cytotoxic Drugs

Cytotoxic drugs are the most common form of therapy and most frequently include alkylating agents, purine and pyrimidine analogs (Figure 31-5), folic acid analogs, or the alkaloids. The drugs of choice, excluding alkylating drugs, are azathioprine, 6-mercaptopurine, 6-thioguanine, 5-fluorouracil, cytosine arabinoside, methotrexate and aminopterin, and vinblastine and vincristine.

Most immunosuppressive drugs administered alone cannot produce antigen-specific tolerance because they act equally on all susceptible clones. Except for certain drugs (e.g., cyclosporin A), most immunosuppressive agents can be rendered antigen specific only by including an antigen-specific element in the tolerizing regimen. In these cases the drugs act as cofactors in *tolerogenesis*. Experimental evidence suggests that these regimens may act as follows:

- Lowering the threshold for tolerance induction.
- Blocking the differentiation sequence in cells triggered by antigen.

Azathioprine

Since its introduction in 1961, azathioprine, an oral purine analog that is an antimetabolite with multiple activities, has been the mainstay of antirejection therapy. Azathioprine requires activation to 6-mercatopurine, which is further metabolized to active 6-thioguanine nucleotides. Metabolites of azathioprine, such as the in vivo metabolite, 6-mercaptopurine, are incorporated into cellular DNA. This inhibits purine nucleotide synthesis and metabolism and alters the synthesis and function of ribonucleic acid (RNA). Therefore, azathioprine acts at an early stage in either T-cell or B-cell activation during the proliferative cycle of effector lymphocyte clones. Azathioprine is useful in preventing acute rejection because it inhibits the primary immune response; however, it has little or no effect on secondary responses. Adverse effects include bone marrow suppression, myopathy, alopecia, pancreatitis, and hepatitis. A drug interaction can occur with allopurinol.

Corticosteroids

Corticosteroids can be used in conjunction with azathioprine or another immunosuppressant such as cyclosporine. Corticosteroids directly inhibit antigen-driven T-cell proliferation. Steroids do not directly act on the IL-2–producing

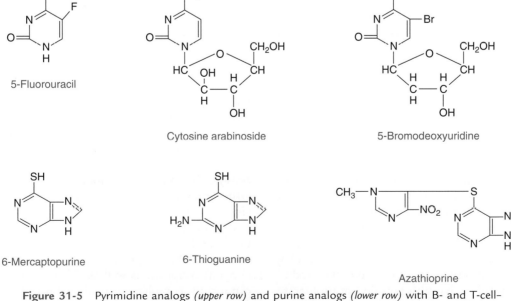

Figure 31-5 Pyrimidine analogs *(upper row)* and purine analogs *(lower row)* with B- and T-cell–suppressing activity. A large number of similar compounds are available for human use. *(Redrawn from Barrett JT: Textbook of immunology, ed 5, St Louis, 1988, Mosby.)*

T cell. They do, however, inhibit production of lymphokines by preventing monocytes from releasing IL-1, thereby blocking IL-1–dependent release of IL-2 from antigen-activated T cells. Other activities of monocytes, such as inhibition of chemotaxis, are also likely to be important in the immunosuppressive process.

High doses of corticosteroids are used to treat acute rejection. In addition, steroids probably reverse in vivo rejection episodes by preventing the production of IL-2, which would inhibit activated T cells as an essential trophic factor.

Cyclosporine (Cyclosporin A)

Cyclosporine, isolated in 1971 from the fungus *Tolypocladium inflatum,* has become the mainstay of immunosuppressive therapy in transplantation. Cyclosporine affects T cells preferentially by inhibiting the induction of cytotoxic T cells. Unlike corticosteroids, cyclosporine does not inhibit the capacity of all accessory cells to release IL-1. Cyclosporine blocks calcineurin to the IL-2 gene transcription pathway and the release of certain other lymphokines (e.g., IFN-γ). Cyclosporine binds to cyclophilin, and the complex binds to and inhibits calcineurin (a protein phosphatase). This prevents activation of the IL-2 transcription factor.

The secretion of B-cell growth and differentiation factors by activated T cells is also inhibited by cyclosporin A. Therefore, under the influence of cyclosporin A, helper T (Th) cell–dependent B cells are not fully activated because of a lack of necessary Th-cell stimulation. In pharmacologic doses, however, cyclosporin A does not grossly interfere with the activation and proliferation of suppressor T cells. Recent data indicate prolonged renal allograft survival with cyclosporin A despite potential mismatches of the HLA system. Adverse effects of corticosteroids include fluid retention, electrolyte abnormalities, hyperglycemia, hypertension, peptic ulcer disease, osteoporosis, and adrenal insufficiency. Hepatotoxicity has been observed in 4% to 7% of patients. Drug interactions can occur with grapefruit juice, erythromycin, oral contraceptives, and a variety of other drugs. Drug monitoring is critical because of the narrow therapeutic range.

A newer cyclosporine microemulsion offers the advantage of improved trough measurement correlation with the actual patient circulating concentration.

Tacrolimus

Tacrolimus (FK-506), a macrolide with mechanisms similar to that of cyclosporine, is derived from a fungus, *Streptomyces tsukub,* found in soil samples in Japan. FK-506 is 50 to 100 times more powerful than cyclosporine. Its primary target appears to be the Th lymphocytes, with little effect on other aspects of the immune response. FK-506 acts early in the process of T-cell activation and inhibits the production of IL-2. As a result, T lymphocytes do not proliferate, secretion of IFN-γ is inhibited, MHC class II antigens are not induced, and further activation of macrophages does not occur.

Because FK-506 is a more potent immunosuppressant than cyclosporine, patient recovery time is faster. FK-506 has higher toxicity compared to cyclosporine. Nephrotoxicity, hyperkalemia, hypokalemia, hypomagnesemia, hypertension, and other side effects may occur, but FK-506 causes no serious side effects (e.g., kidney damage, elevated blood pressure, mood swings). Patients receiving FK-506 have increased susceptibility to infections (e.g., CMV) and an increased risk of developing lymphoma or posttransplant lymphoproliferative diseases. Inhibitors and inducers of P-450 3A4 may demonstrate an altered rate of metabolism that requires an adjustment in drug dose.

Sirolimus

Sirolimus (Rapamune), previously referred to as "rapamycin," was under development for more than 20 years before gaining approval by the U.S. Food and Drug Administration (FDA). Sirolimus is derived from the fungi *Streptomyces hygroscopicus,* from the soil of Easter Island. Structurally, sirolimus resembles tacrolimus and has the same intracellular binding protein or immunophilin, known as FKBP-12, but sirolimus has a novel mechanism of action. Sirolimus is a substrate for P-450 3A4 and inhibits the activation and proliferation of T lymphocytes and subsequent production of IL-2, IL-4, and IL-15. Sirolimus also inhibits antibody production. Sirolimus is approved as an adjunctive agent (in combination with steroids) for the prevention of acute renal allograft rejection. The main side effects include increased risk of infections and lymphoma, hypercholesterolemia and hypertriglyceridemia, interstitial pneumonitis, insomnia and tremor, and thrombocytopenia.

Mycophenolate Mofetil

Mycophenolate mofetil (RS-61443) inhibits de novo guanosine synthesis by inhibiting inosine monophosphate dehydrogenase. This drug inhibits T- and B-lymphocyte proliferation and antibody formation by B lymphocytes and has been efficacious as both prophylactic and rescue therapy in refractory renal allograft rejection in clinical trials. Findings suggest that mycophenolate is effective in preventing acute rejection and may also slow the progression to chronic rejection. Possible toxic effects of drug therapy can include nausea and vomiting, abdominal pain, gastrointestinal hemorrhage, anemia, and neutropenia.

Antilymphocyte (Antithymocyte) Globulin

Other immunosuppressive measures directed at T cells include the use of antilymphocyte (antithymocyte) globulin (ATG), an IgG polyclonal antibody, at the time of transplantation and use of lymphoid irradiation before transplantation. Use of ATG in preventing or reversing rejection in renal allograft recipients is well established. Adverse side effects can include complement-mediated lysis of lymphocytes, serum sickness, leukopenia, and thrombocytopenia.

Among patients at high risk for acute rejection or delayed graft function who received a kidney transplant from a cadaver donor, induction therapy consisting of a 5-day course of antithymocyte globulin, as compared with basiliximab, reduced the incidence and severity of acute rejection but not the incidence of delayed graft function.

A regimen of total-lymphoid irradiation plus antithymocyte globulin decreases the incidence of acute GVHD and allows graft antitumor activity in patients with lymphoid malignant diseases or acute leukemia treated with hematopoietic cell transplantation.

Monoclonal Antibodies

Monoclonal antibody (Muromonab-CD3 [OKT2], Oerthoclone [OKT3]) is used because the CD3 surface membrane marker is found on all mature postthymic T cells. Interaction between OKT3 and the surface of mature T lymphocytes produces T-cell depletion. The use of OKT3 reverses almost all acute renal transplant rejection and is indicated for treatment of steroid-resistant rejection. A side effect of this drug is *cytokine-release syndrome,* a condition of flulike symptoms, dyspnea, aseptic meningitis, and pulmonary edema.

Dacliximab (Zenapax) is a recently approved humanized monoclonal antibody to the alpha subunit of the IL-2 receptor. A decreased incidence of renal allograft rejection has been observed with triple- and/or double-immunosuppressive regimens.

Immunosuppressive Protocols

Protocols for immunosuppression of transplant recipients vary widely depending on the transplant center, type of organ transplanted, after transplantation, underlying etiology of organ failure, and preexisting conditions (Box 31-5). Protocols are becoming more complex because of more immunosuppressive drug choices. In general, protocols include the following:
- Lymphokine synthesis inhibitors (e.g., cyclosporine, tacrolimus).
- Nucleoside synthetase inhibitors (e.g., azathioprine, mycophenolate mofetil).
- Steroids (e.g., prednisone).
- Induction or pretransplant therapy may include antithymocyte globulin, CD3 or CD25, or dacliximab).

Box 31-5	Example Protocol (Liver)
Intra-op	Methylprednisolone, 1 g ×1
Day 0	Methylprednisolone, 1 g ×1
Day 1	Prednisolone, 200 mg/day (qid)
Day 2	Taper
Day 0-5	Antilymphocyte globulin (ATG), 15 mg/kg IV; given until adequate cyclosporin A levels obtained.
Day 0-5	Azathioprine, 1 mg/kg/day IV
Day 6	Azathioprine, 2 mg/kg/day PO
Day ?	Cyclosporin A, 10-15 mg/kg/day (bid); adjust to level.

From Tsunoda S: *Update on immunosuppression,* Boston, 2000, Tufts University School of Medicine Transplant Teleconference Series.

New Approaches in Immunosuppression

New suggested strategies include the following:
- Cellular transplants
- **Transgenic** organs
- Development of **chimerism**
- Localized immunosuppression
- Prevention of chronic rejection

Post–Organ Transplant Complications

Because complications are associated with transplantation, their early diagnosis and treatment are essential. The primary risks of transplantation are rejection and infection. Five other major complications of organ transplantation are cancer, osteoporosis, diabetes, hypertension, and hypercholesterolemia.

Infectious Diseases

Infections can be viral, such as CMV (80%), Epstein-Barr virus (20%-30%), hepatitis B, or hepatitis C. Even rabies has been associated with organ transplantation. Other pathogens include *Pneumocystis carinii.* Organisms associated with central nervous system infection in renal transplant recipients, in decreasing order of frequency, are *Listeria, Cryptococcus, Mycobacterium, Nocardia, Aspergillus, Mucor, Toxoplasma,* and *Strongyloides.* Recently published guidelines advise transplant teams to do the following to minimize transplant risk:
1. Screen for infectious disease agents in both the donor and the recipient before transplantation.
2. Culture and identify known and novel pathogens in recipients after transplantation.
3. Archive serologic samples before transplantation for identification of new infections later.

Cancer

Organ transplant recipients have a 20% greater risk of the development of cancer. The incidence of non-Hodgkin's lymphoma is increased by 40%. The greatest risk for lymphoma is within the first 6 to 12 months after transplant. Transplant recipients also have a greater risk of skin cancer and a slightly increased risk of cervical cancer. An increased risk of the development of cancer may be as the result of chemotherapy and radiation therapy.

Osteoporosis

In the general population, osteoporosis affects 1 in 4 women and 1 in 8 men. The general risk factors are age, postmenopausal state, sedentary lifestyle, and inadequate calcium intake. Transplant recipients are at an increased risk of developing osteoporosis because of pretransplant immobility and the long-term effects of steroid therapy. Regular bone density scanning should be a routine component of posttransplant care.

Diabetes

Diabetes mellitus is a concern in two risk groups: patients with preexisting diabetes (25%) and those who develop diabetes after transplantation (20%). Patients with preexisting diabetes may require increased doses of insulin until stabilized on medications. Posttransplant steroid-induced hyperglycemia can produced physiologic conditions that negatively affect a graft. Steroid medication might aggravate a familial tendency toward diabetes. Steroids produce decreased use of insulin by peripheral tissues, eventual insulin resistance with decreasing receptor sites, reduction in insulin production, and accelerated glycogenolysis by the liver to assist in glucose availability. These metabolic activities perpetuate hyperglycemia. In addition to threatening graft survival, diabetes can produce other negative health consequences: adult blindness, vasculopathy, neuropathy, retinopathy, bladder infections, and a shortened life span.

Hypertension

An abnormal increase in blood pressure is usually a preexisting medical condition in transplant recipients. This condition is often associated with renal failure. Hypertension can negatively affect the patient's general health and graft survival.

Hypercholesterolemia

Increased blood cholesterol is a serious posttransplant concern because of long-term vascular effects to the patient and engrafted organ. Hypercholesterolemia can result from the return of the patient's appetite and the lifting of dietary restrictions.

Xenotransplantation

Xenotransplantation is the logical next step in transplantation (Box 31-6). There is a worldwide shortage of organs for clinical transplantation. Pig heart valves are already used to repair human hearts, and porcine pancreatic islet cells are used to treat diabetes, so it is not a big leap to envision transspecies, whole-organ transplants. Pigs are considered the most likely organ transplant donors for humans because their organs are similar in size to human organs; they are easy to breed; and the extensive biologic differences between pigs and humans make it unlikely for porcine diseases to infect humans.

Another application of cross-species organ use was successfully demonstrated in a Phase I clinical trial that used transgenic pig livers as an ex vivo (outside the body) support system for patients with acute liver failure. The pig liver was used to bridge the gap between organ failure and obtaining an appropriate human liver for transplantation in these patients. New protocols are being developed for a Phase I in vivo (inside the body) clinical trial.

Other procedures, some in clinical trials, use cells or tissues from other species to treat life-threatening illnesses such as cancer, AIDS, diabetes, liver failure, and Parkinson's disease. Even if whole organs are not transplanted, animal cells or tissues will likely be used to treat many diseases. In 1995, physicians in California transplanted bone marrow from a baboon into an AIDS patient in a highly controversial procedure that prompted the creation of strict guidelines for transplantation by the FDA, National Institutes of Health (NIH), and Centers for Disease Control and Prevention (CDC).

Ethical and medical concerns surround xenotransplantation. One very real risk is that the transplanted tissue may carry unknown latent infections that, once introduced into the recipient, could be activated and give rise to infection. In addition, an optimal antirejection drug protocol is not yet known.

BIOMARKERS FOR REJECTION

Emerging technologies, such as gene expression profiling, proteomics, metabolomics, and genomics, are rapidly advancing the pace of discovery of new biomarkers for rejection. These approaches are expected to generate improved diagnostic tests as well as knowledge that will lead to more effective therapies.

One of the most promising areas of transplant research, especially kidney transplantation, is the recent discovery of biomarkers for rejection that are detectable in blood and urine. Biopsy-confirmed rejection, the current "gold standard" for diagnosis of allograft rejection, is invasive and subject to sampling errors. Development of noninvasive assays that detect molecular biomarkers for rejection could revolutionize management of transplant recipients by:
- Detecting a prerejection profile that will allow therapeutic interventions before rejection causes graft dysfunction.
- Improving the sensitivity and specificity of rejection diagnosis.
- Developing new classification systems for rejection that will improve prognosis.
- Providing information for designing individualized immunosuppressive regimens that could prevent rejection while minimizing drug toxicity.

By studying concentrations of particular messenger RNAs (mRNAs) or proteins associated with immune activation or tissue stress, several gene products with altered expression in blood, urine, and biopsy tissue during rejection episodes were identified. Urine concentrations of *FOXP3* mRNA, a member of the "forkhead family" of cell differentiation genes and a lineage-specific transcript for graft-protecting regulatory T cells, can predict reversal of acute renal allograft rejection with very high sensitivity and high specificity.

Box 31-6	Milestones in Xenotransplantation
1963–1964	Chimpanzee-to-human renal transplants.
1964	Pig heart valve transplant.
1968	Sheep heart transplant.
1984	"Baby Fae" transplanted with a baboon heart.
1992	Baboon-to-human liver transplant.
1994	Pig pancreatic islets transplanted to insulin-dependent patients.
1995	Neuronal cells from a fetal pig transplanted to patients with Parkinson's disease.
1996	Baboon bone marrow transplanted to AIDS patient.

Modified from Wilde M: *Adv Med Lab Prof* 21:11, 1997.

Measurement of the products of individual genes such as *FOXP3* probably will not supplant conventional biopsies for diagnosis of rejection, but the development of panels of informative gene products in blood and urine, coupled with renal function and immune response markers, ultimately should achieve the sensitivities and specificities required for diagnosis and clinical management of kidney rejection.

Analysis of more than 1300 genes that were differentially expressed in kidney allografts revealed three distinct molecular signatures of acute rejection that were more predictive of allograft survival than was traditional histologic analysis. These data have also generated new hypotheses for the molecular mechanisms of rejection. For example, B-cell infiltration is characteristic of aggressive acute rejection.

A new gene expression test, AlloMap (XDx, San Francisco), is being tested to explore its ability to predict acute cardiac allograft rejection. The test appears to detect the absence of moderate to severe cellular rejection, which might reduce the need for frequent biopsies.

CASE STUDY

Forty-year-old C.G. was seen by her family physician after several episodes of painless hematuria. On direct questioning, she complained of worsening malaise and swelling of her legs and hands over the previous 2 weeks. She also reported that despite a high fluid intake, she was urinating much less frequently than normal. She had no significant medical history.

On examination, the patient was pale and had generalized swelling of her extremities. Her temperature was 38.5° C, and her blood pressure was 160/110 mm Hg. She had no palpable masses or hepatosplenomegaly.

A diagnosis of idiopathic and rapidly progressive glomerulonephritis was made. She was given antihypertensive agents, corticosteroids, and azathioprine for 2 weeks, but her renal function deteriorated, and end-stage renal failure was diagnosed. Hemodialysis was initiated.

In preparation for a possible renal transplant, she was tissue-typed for MHC antigens using anti-HLA antibodies. She was found to be HLA-A10, A28, B7, Bw52, Cw2, Cw6, DR2, DRw10, and blood group B positive. A suitable cadaveric kidney was found from a donor of HLA-A9, A28, B7, B17, Cw2, Cw6, DR2, DR4, and blood group B positive. A crossmatch of the patient's serum with donor lymphocytes was satisfactory.

She underwent successful kidney transplantation. Her posttransplant treatment was a combined triple-immunosuppressive regimen of prednisolone, cyclosporin A, and azathioprine. She progressed well immediately after transplant.

Twelve days after engraftment, the patient developed a fever and was noted to be lethargic. Physical examination revealed generalized edema. Her blood pressure was 165/110 mm Hg. Her urine output had dropped significantly. A renal biopsy was performed. Histologic examination demonstrated significant interstitial mononuclear cell infiltration. This finding was consistent with the diagnosis of acute graft rejection. She was immediately treated with parenteral methylprednisolone. This treatment failed to improve her renal function, and an antilymphocyte monoclonal antibody was administered. Her renal function improved, and she was eventually discharged receiving cyclosporin A therapy.

Questions and Discussion

1. What factors are important in matching donor to recipient in renal transplantation?

Two groups of antigens are important in renal transplantation: the ABO blood group system and the MHC/HLA system. It is essential that the ABO grouping is compatible between the donor and recipient. Donor and recipient must be HLA compatible. Donor lymphocytes are incubated with recipient serum to detect antibodies to MHC class I and II molecules. HLA matching focuses on MHC class II molecules.

2. How does this patient's graft rejection compare with other types of graft rejection?

Renal transplant rejection is classified according to the timing of the episode. Hyperacute rejection occurs minutes to hours after transplantation, because the patient has antibodies to either MHC class I or ABO blood group antigens, both of which are expressed on the renal epithelium. Blood transfusions, previous transplantation, or pregnancy can presensitize a patient. Accelerated rejection occurs 3 to 5 days after transplantation. Presensitized cytotoxic T lymphocytes or non–complement-binding antibodies may be responsible. The latter mediate an antibody-dependent, cell-mediated cytotoxic reaction against the graft by binding to Ec receptors. Vascular endothelium is often targeted because it expresses MHC I and II molecules. Histologically, the graft is infiltrated with mononuclear cells. Immunosuppressive agents may save the graft.

Acute rejection, which takes place 7 days to 3 months after transplantation, accounts for 85% of all rejection episodes. Cellular rejection is a T-cell–mediated (type IV) phenomenon characterized histologically by edema and cellular infiltration. In addition, varying degrees of vascular rejection are present, initiated by IgG or IgM antibodies to vascular wall components (a type II reaction). Grafts may be saved with high-dose methylprednisolone or, as in this case, by ATG therapy.

Chronic rejection manifests several months to years after transplantation. It appears to be an immune complex–mediated phenomenon. Immunosuppressive therapy is usually ineffective.

CHAPTER HIGHLIGHTS

- All vertebrates capable of acute rejection of foreign skin grafts possess a localized complex involving many genes that exert major control over the organism's immune reactions.
- Some of these antigens are much more potent than others in provoking an immune response and therefore are called the major histocompatibility complex (MHC).

In humans the MHC is referred to as human leukocyte antigens (HLAs).

- The MHC is divided into four major regions: D, B, C, and A. The A, B, and C regions code for class I molecules, whereas the D region codes for class II molecules.
- Class I and class II antigens can be found on surface membrane proteins of body cells and in body fluids.
- The MHC gene products have an important role in clinical immunology. For example, transplants are rejected if performed against MHC barriers; thus immunosuppressive therapy is required. These antigens are of primary importance in influencing the genetic basis of survival or rejection of transplanted organs.
- Although HLA was originally identified by its role in transplant rejection, it is now recognized that the products of HLA genes play a crucial role in our immune system. T cells do not recognize antigens directly but do so when the antigen is presented on the surface of an antigen-presenting cell (APC), the macrophage. In addition to presenting the antigen, the macrophage must present another molecule for this response to occur. This molecule is a cell surface glycoprotein coded in each species by the MHC.
- T cells are able to interact with the histocompatibility molecules only if they are genetically identical (MHC restriction). Both class I and class II antigens function as targets of T lymphocytes that regulate the immune response.
- Class I molecules regulate interaction between cytolytic T cells and target cells, and class II molecules restrict the activity of regulatory T cells (helper, suppressor, and amplifier subsets).
- Class II molecules regulate the interaction between helper T cells and APCs.
- HLA matching is of value in organ transplantation, as well as in the transplantation of bone marrow.
- Transplantation is one of the areas (in addition to hypersensitivity and autoimmunity) in which the immune system functions in a detrimental way. Tissues and organs transplanted include peripheral stem cells or bone marrow, bone matrix, skin, kidneys, liver, cardiac valves, heart, pancreas, corneas, and lungs.
- Host immunity to the donor can cause graft-versus-host disease (GVHD), believed to result from the patient being sensitized to unshared HLA antigens before transplantation or transfusion. When allogenic T lymphocytes are transfused from donor to recipient with a graft or blood transfusion, the patient can develop acute or chronic GVHD. Patients at risk for GVHD include those who are immunodeficient or immunosuppressed with severe lymphocytopenia and bone marrow suppression.
- Immunologic tolerance is the acquisition of nonreactivity toward particular antigens. Self-recognition (tolerance) is a critical process, and the failure to recognize self antigens can result in autoimmune disease.
- Immunosuppressive measures may be antigen specific or antigen nonspecific. Antigen-nonspecific immuno-suppression includes drugs and other methods of specifically altering T-cell function. Immunosuppressive measures directed at T cells include the use of ATG at the time of transplantation and of lymphoid irradiation before transplantation.

REVIEW QUESTIONS

Questions 1-4. Match the following items.

1. _____ Autograft
2. _____ Syngraft
3. _____ Allograft (hemograft)
4. _____ Xenograft

a. Graft transplanted between different but identical recipient and donor.
b. Graft transferred from one position to another in the same individual.
c. Graft between genetically different recipient and donor of the same species.
d. Graft between individuals of different species.

5. Graft-versus-host disease is most frequently associated with which transplant?
   a. Cornea
   b. Bone marrow
   c. Bone matrix
   d. Lung

Questions 6-9. Match the following types of graft rejection.

6. _____ Hyperacute
7. _____ Accelerated
8. _____ Acute
9. _____ Chronic

a. Caused by preformed cytotoxic antibodies.
b. An immunopathologic mechanism.
c. Caused by previous sensitization to donor antigens.
d. Disturbance of host/graft tolerance.
e. Development of allogeneic reaction to donor antigens.

10. The immune system functions in a detrimental way in:
    a. Hypersensitivity reactions.
    b. Autoimmunity.
    c. Transplantation.
    d. All the above.

11. The probability of success in organ and tissue transplantation increases as a result of:
    a. Histocompatibility testing.
    b. Immunosuppression.
    c. Surgical technique.
    d. Both a and b.

12. The D region of the major histocompatibility complex (MHC) codes for class _____ molecules.
    a. I
    b. II
    c. III
    d. IV

13. Class I includes HLA-_____ antigens.
    a. A, B, and C
    b. B, C, and D
    c. DR, DC(DQ), and A
    d. DR, DC(DQ), and SB

14. Class I molecules:
    a. Regulate interaction between cytolytic T cells and target cells.
    b. Restrict activity of regulatory T cells and target cells.
    c. Regulate interaction between helper T cells and antigen-presenting cells.
    d. Represent components of the complement pathways.

15. The 1-year survival for kidney transplantation from HLA-identical siblings approaches:
    a. 50%.
    b. 75%.
    c. 95%.
    d. 100%.

Questions 16-19. Match the following to show the relationship between certain HLA antigens and diseases.

16. _____ Ankylosing spondylitis   a. B8

17. _____ Type I diabetes   b. B27

18. _____ Myasthenia gravis   c. DR2

19. _____ Multiple sclerosis   d. DR3

20. The most common form of bone marrow transplant is:
    a. Allogeneic.
    b. Autologous.
    c. Xenograft.
    d. Syngraft.

21. Potential GVHD has all the following characteristics *except:*
    a. Source of immunocompetent T lymphocytes.
    b. Source of immunocompetent B lymphocytes.
    c. HLA differences between patient and recipient.
    d. Inability to reject donor cells.

22. In GVHD posttransfusion, symptoms begin within _____ day(s) after transfusion.

    a. 1
    b. 2 to 4
    c. 3 to 5
    d. 3 to 30

23. GVHD can be prevented by:
    a. Irradiating the patient pretransfusion.
    b. Irradiating the blood component pretransfusion.
    c. Administering antibiotics pretransfusion.
    d. Administering steroids posttransfusion.

24. The mainstay of immunosuppression therapy in transplantation is:
    a. Azathioprine.
    b. Corticosteroids.
    c. Cyclosporine.
    d. Antilymphocyte globulin.

BIBLIOGRAPHY

Baxter-Lowe LA, Busch MP: DNA microchimerism and organ transplant rejection, *Clin Chem* 52(4):559-560, 2006.

Brennan DC et al: Rabbit antithymocyte globulin versus basiliximab in renal transplantation, *N Engl J Med* 355(19):1967-1977, 2006.

Burckart G: Overview of organ transplantation, May 2002, www.pitt.edu.

Clinical Clips: Cell transplants help brain repair after stroke, *Adv Med Lab Prof* 13:35, 2001.

Dantal J, Soulillou JP: Immunosuppressive drugs and the risk of cancer after organ transplantation, *N Engl J Med* 353(13):1371-1372, 2005.

Delmonico FL, Burdick JF: Maximizing the success of transplantation with kidneys from older donors, *N Engl J Med* 354(4):411-412, 2006.

Gadi VK et al: Soluble donor DNA concentrations in recipient serum correlate with pancrease-kidney rejection, *Clin Chem* 52(3):379-382, 2006.

Halloran PF: Immunosuppressive drugs for kidney transplantation, *N Engl J Med* 351(26):2715-2726, 2004.

Ingelfinger JR: Risks and benefits to the living donor, *N Engl J Med* 353(5):447-449, 2005.

Janin A et al: Fasciitis in chronic graft-versus-host disease, *Ann Intern Med* 120(12):993-998, 1994.

Kirkpatrick CH, Rowlands DT Jr: Transplantation immunology, *JAMA* 268(20):2952-2958, 1992.

Kobashigawa JA et al: Effect of pravastatin on outcomes after cardiac transplantation, *N Engl J Med* 333(10):621-633, 1995.

Lowsky R et al: Protective conditioning for acute graft-versus-host disease, *N Engl J Med* 353(13):1321, 2005.

Markin RS, McPherson RA: Laboratory support for organ transplantation. Part II, *Lab Med* 22(5):319-324, 1991.

McPherson RA, Markin RS: Laboratory support for organ transplantation. Part I, *Lab Med* 22(4):243-252, 1991.

Mehltretter S: Clinical cytogenetics, *Adv Med Lab Prof* 7(13):6-9, 20, 1995.

Nehlsen-Cannarella SL: HLA and disease, *Complements* 3(1):2, 1983.

Opelz G, Wujciak T: The influence of HLA compatibility on graft survival after heart transplantation, *N Engl J Med* 330(12):816-817, 1994.

Plath KB, Talmon GA, Stickle DF: Immunosuppressant drugs, *Clin Lab News* 32(5):10-12, 2006.

Remuzzi G et al: Long-term outcome of renal transplantation from older donors, *N Engl J Med* 354(4):343-352, 2006.

Sayegh MH, Carpenter CB: Transplantation 50 years later: progress, challenges, and promises, *N Engl J Med* 351(26):2761-2766, 2004.

Shelton C: Post–organ transplantation complications, Toronto, 1999 (workshop handout).

Titus K: Steering the straits of transplant testing, *CAP Today* 20(6):68-72, 2006.

Tsunoda SM: *Update on immunosuppression*, Boston, 2000, Tufts University School of Medicine Transplant Teleconference Series.

Turgeon ML: *Fundamentals of immunohematology*, ed 2, Baltimore, 1995, Williams & Wilkins.

United Network for Organ Sharing: Critical data: U.S. facts about transplantation, August 2007, www.unos.org.

Upton H: Origin of drugs in current use: the cyclosporin story, October 2002, www.oldkingdom.org.

Venkataramanan R et al: Clinical utility of monitoring tacrolimus concentrations in liver transplant patient, *J Clin Pharmacol* 10:51, 2001.

Wilde M: Rejection, retroviruses: major barriers to xenotransplantation, *Adv Med Lab Prof* 9:14-19, 1997.

CHAPTER 32

Bone Marrow Transplantation

Cancers Treated with Progenitor Cell Transplants
   Leukemia
   Non-Hodgkin's and Hodgkin's Lymphoma
What Are Progenitor Blood Cells?
Types of Transplants
Traditional Treatment Options
   Chemotherapy
   Radiotherapy
Evaluation of Candidates for PBSC/Bone Marrow
   Transplant
Obtaining Cells for Transplant
   Bone Marrow
   Peripheral Blood Progenitor Cells

Transplantation
   Transplant-Related Complications
   Graft Manipulation and Storage
   Cell Infusion
Transplants from Unrelated Donors
Current Directions
Future Directions
Case Study
Chapter Highlights
Review Questions
Bibliography

Learning Objectives

At the conclusion of this chapter, the reader should be able to:

- Identify and discuss various types of cancer treated with progenitor cell transplants.
- Define the term *progenitor cell.*
- Name three types of stem cell transplants.
- Discuss available treatment options for cancer.
- Discuss the evaluation of candidates for transplant.
- Describe the process of obtaining blood stem cells.
- Discuss the transplantation protocol, related complications, graft manipulation and storage, and cell infusion.

- Compare at least three current directions in bone marrow transplantation.
- Identify and discuss four future directions in bone marrow transplantation.
- Analyze laboratory and clinical data of the cited case study, and apply these concepts to the field of bone marrow transplantation.

Stem cell transplantation is currently being used to treat patients with malignant and nonmalignant diseases (e.g., chronic myelogenous leukemia, severe combined immunodeficiency disease, non-Hodgkin's lymphoma). The goal of transplanting bone marrow or peripheral blood progenitor cells is to achieve a potential cure or to help patients recover from high-dose chemotherapy that has destroyed stem or marrow cells, a condition known as **myeloablation.**

CANCERS TREATED WITH PROGENITOR CELL TRANSPLANTS

Leukemia

In most types of leukemia, the body produces large numbers of immature white blood cells (WBCs) that do not function properly. Under appropriate conditions, bone marrow transplantation may be useful in treating certain types of leukemia (Box 32-1).

Acute lymphoblastic leukemia is the most common type of leukemia in young children but may also affect adults, especially those age 65 and older. It is a rapidly progressive malignant disorder involving the production of immature WBCs (blasts), which often results in the replacement of normal bone marrow with blast cells. Acute myeloid leukemia, also referred to as "nonlymphoblastic leukemia," occurs in both adults and children.

Although chronic lymphocytic leukemia most often affects adults over age 55, sometimes occurs in younger adults, but rarely affects children. Chronic myeloid leukemia occurs mainly in adults and affects a very small number of children.

Non-Hodgkin's and Hodgkin's Lymphoma

In Hodgkin's disease and non-Hodgkin's lymphoma, cells in the lymphatic system become abnormal. They divide too rapidly and grow without any order or control, and old cells do not die as cells normally do. Because lymphatic tissue is present in many parts of the body, Hodgkin's disease and non-Hodgkin's lymphoma can start almost anywhere. These diseases may occur in a single lymph node, in a group of lymph nodes, or sometimes in other parts of the lymphatic system (e.g., bone marrow, spleen).

For patients with lymphoma, chances of survival depend on the grade and stage of cancer, overall patient health, and

Box 32-1	Diseases Treatable by Stem Cell Transplantation

Acute Leukemia
Acute lymphoblastic leukemia
Acute myelogenous leukemia

Chronic Leukemias
Chronic myelogenous leukemia
Chronic lymphocytic leukemia

Myelodysplastic Syndromes
Refractory anemia
Refractory anemia with ringed sideroblasts
Refractory anemia with excess blasts
Chronic myelomonocytic leukemia

Stem Cell Disorders
Aplastic anemia
Fanconi's anemia
Paroxysmal nocturnal hemoglobinuria

Myeloproliferative Disorders
Acute myelofibrosis
Polycythemia vera

Lymphoproliferative Disorders
Non-Hodgkin's lymphoma
Hodgkin's disease

Phagocyte Disorders
Chédiak-Higashi syndrome
Chronic granulomatous disease

Immunodeficiencies
Severe combined immunodeficiency

Inherited Platelet Abnormalities
Congenital thrombocytopenia

Plasma Cell Disorders
Multiple myeloma
Plasma cell leukemia
Waldenström's macroglobulinemia

Other Malignancies
Breast cancer
Ewing's sarcoma
Neuroblastoma
Renal cell carcinoma

Inherited Erythrocyte Abnormalities
Beta-thalassemia major
Pure red cell aplasia
Sickle cell disease

Liposomal Storage Diseases
Mucopolysaccharidoses
Hurler's syndrome
Gaucher's disease
Niemann-Pick disease

response to treatment. Hodgkin's lymphoma is one of the most curable forms of cancer. Patients diagnosed with stage I disease have more than a 90% chance of living 10 years or more. Of interest, higher-grade aggressive types are more likely to be cured with chemotherapy. Lower-grade lymphoma often can have longer average survival times, with a mean survival of 10 years in some cases. Most children respond well to treatment, even though children tend to have the higher grades of lymphoma. From 70% to 90% of these children survive 5 years or more (Table 32-1).

WHAT ARE PROGENITOR BLOOD CELLS?

Progenitor cells have the ability to evolve into different types of cells. Bone marrow and peripheral blood progenitor cells are capable of reconstituting a person's immune system because they contain the precursor to the cells that make up the blood: lymphocytes, granulocytes, macrophages, and platelets. Some progenitor cells circulate in the bloodstream and are called **peripheral blood stem cells (PBSCs).** PBSCs are found in much smaller quantities in the circulating blood than in the bone marrow.

The hematopoietic stem cell population is not fully characterized, but the CD34 antigen identifies a population of stem cells that can reconstitute hematopoiesis after *myeloablative* chemotherapy. The required minimal dose of CD34+ cells is difficult to define, but most transplant centers will infuse a minimal dose of 2×10^6 CD34+ cells/kg patient weight in the autologous and allogeneic PBSC setting.

Table 32-1	Estimated 5-Year Survival Rates after Transplantation	
Disease	Allogeneic (%)	Autologous (%)
Severe combined immunodeficiency	90	N/A
Aplastic anemia	90	N/A
Thalassemia	90	N/A
Acute myeloid leukemia		
First remission	55-60	50
Second remission	40	30
Acute lymphocytic leukemia		
First remission	50	40
Second remission	40	30
Chronic myeloid leukemia		
Chronic phase	70	ID
Blast crisis	15	ID
Chronic lymphocytic leukemia	50	ID
Myelodysplasia	45	ID
Multiple myeloma	30	35
Non-Hodgkin's lymphoma		
First relapse/second remission	40	40
Hodgkin's disease		
First relapse/second remission	40	50

These estimates are based on data reported by the International Bone Marrow Transplant Registry.
N/A, Not applicable; *ID,* insufficient data.

Historically, the dose of bone marrow has been based on the **nucleated cell (NC)** count (i.e., 2 to 4 $\times$ 10^8 NC/kg recipient weight). There is no established amount of CD34+ bone marrow stem cells to infuse because there may be more primitive cells, thus likely to be CD34−, in the marrow that are capable of reconstituting the recipient's marrow.

TYPES OF TRANSPLANTS

There are three major types of transplants, as follows:
- Allogeneic
- Syngeneic
- Autologous

In an **allogeneic** setting, a person receives bone marrow or PBSCs from a related or an unrelated donor, depending on the availability of a good human leukocyte antigen (HLA) match. Because HLA tissue types are inherited, patients are more likely to find a matched donor from within their own family, racial, or ethnic group. In **syngeneic** transplants, patients receive stem cells from their identical twin. Patients who undergo an **autologous** transplant have donated their own cells after PBSC mobilization with granulocyte colony-stimulating factor (G-CSF) or granulocyte-macrophage colony-stimulating factor (GM-CSF).

TRADITIONAL TREATMENT OPTIONS

To understand why bone marrow and PBSCs are used and how they work, it is helpful to understand how chemotherapy and radiation therapies affect these cells. Chemotherapy and radiation target rapidly dividing cells. These therapies are used to treat cancers because cancer cells divide more rapidly than healthy cells. Bone marrow cells also divide at a rapid rate and can be severely damaged or destroyed by high-dose treatments. Without healthy bone marrow, the patient cannot make the blood cells that are able to fight off infections, carry oxygen, or prevent bleeding. Bone marrow and PBSC transplants can replace abnormal as well as normal blood cells that were destroyed during treatment.

Treatment for cancer includes chemotherapy, radiation therapy, surgery, hormone therapy, or immunotherapy. These therapies may be administered alone or in combination to eliminate malignant cells most effectively.

Chemotherapy

Chemotherapy may involve one drug, or a combination of two or more drugs, depending on the type of cancer and its rate of progression.

Chemotherapeutic drugs can be divided into (1) agents that are active against both dividing and nondividing cells, (2) drugs that are active against dividing cells and that affect a particular phase of cell division, and (3) agents that affect all or most of the phases of the cell cycle (Box 32-2).

Whatever the mode of action of these drugs, an important finding is that they destroy malignant cells according

Box 32-2	Cancer Chemotherapy Agents
Direct DNA-Interacting Agents	**Indirect DNA-Interacting Agents**
Alkylators	*Antimetabolites*
Cyclophosphamide	Deoxycoformycin
Chlorambucil	6-Mercaptopurine
Melphalan	2-Chlorodeoxyadenosine
BCNU (carmustine)	Hydroxyurea
CCNU (lomustine)	Methotrexate
Ifosfamide	5-Fluorouracil (5-FU)
Procarbazine	Cytosine arabinoside (ARA-C)
Cisplatin	Gemcitabine
Carboplatin	Fludarabine phosphate
	Asparaginase
Antitumor Antibiotics	
Bleomycin	*Antimitotic Agents*
Actinomycin D	Vincristine
Mithramycin	Vinblastine
Mitomycin C	Paclitaxel
Etoposide (VP-16)	Estramustine phosphate
Topotecan	
Doxorubicin and daunorubicin	
Idarubicin	
Mitoxantrone	

to *first-order kinetics.* In other words, the same proportion of cells is killed for each dose of chemotherapeutic agent.

Alkylating Agents, Antimetabolites, and Alkaloids

The first chemotherapeutic agents to be used in a bone marrow transplant were *alkylating agents* such as cyclophosphamide and busulfan. Their common mechanism of action is that on entering the cells, the alkyl groups bind to the electrophilic sites in DNA and other biologically active molecules. This bifunctional alkylation of DNA results in efficient cross-linking of the DNA, leading to strand breakage and ultimately cell death.

Antimetabolites such as 5-fluorouracil (5-FU), cytarabine, and fludarabine induce cytotoxicity by serving as false substrates in biochemical pathways. Many are nucleoside analogs that are incorporated into DNA and RNA and therefore inhibit nucleic acid synthesis. They are cell-cycle active and are specific mainly for cells in S phase.

The *vinca alkaloids,* vincristine and vinblastine, which were isolated from the periwinkle plant, inhibit microtubule assembly by binding to tubulin. This microtubule stabilization prevents the cells from dividing, and thus these alkaloids are cytotoxic predominantly during the M phase of the cell cycle. Bleomycin, an antitumor antibiotic, induces single-strand and double-strand breaks through free-radical generation and is cytotoxic mainly during the G2 and M phases of the cell cycle.

Radiotherapy

Radiotherapy uses large doses of high-energy beams or particles to destroy cancer cells in a specifically targeted area. Radiation damages DNA and keeps the cells from dividing.

Radiotherapy is most often used on localized solid tumors and on cancers such as leukemia and lymphoma that affect the bloodstream. More than 50% of patients with cancer undergo radiation therapy; for some it will be the only cancer treatment they need. Radiation is often used in combination with other treatments to shrink the tumor or to make surgery or chemotherapy more effective. Used after chemotherapy or surgery, radiation destroys any cancer cells that might remain. Normal cells that may be affected by radiotherapy will usually repair themselves.

EVALUATION OF CANDIDATES FOR PBSC/BONE MARROW TRANSPLANT

Factors that influence the eligibility for a bone marrow transplant include age, disease status, performance status for the recipient, organ function (i.e., heart, lung, liver, kidney function), infectious disease status, compatibility of the donor and recipient, and psychosocial status. Patients who undergo high-dose chemotherapy and hematopoietic stem cell transplantation require a careful evaluation of all body systems to ensure they are able to tolerate the aggressive therapy as well as the isolation of their hospital stay, which can last days to months.

Pretransplant evaluation and testing may include HLA tissue typing, bone marrow biopsy and aspiration, electrocardiogram (ECG), echocardiogram, complete history and physical examination, chest x-ray study, pulmonary function tests, dental cleaning, blood tests such as complete blood count (CBC) and blood chemistries, and screening for viruses such as hepatitis, human T-lymphotropic virus I/II, cytomegalovirus (CMV), herpes, and human immunodeficiency virus (HIV) (Figure 32-1).

At some point before transplant, a central venous catheter is usually placed in a large vein to help in drawing blood samples, infusing medications during and after the transplant, and performing the actual infusion of bone marrow or PBSCs.

OBTAINING CELLS FOR TRANSPLANT

Bone Marrow

In the procedure for "harvesting" bone marrow, the donor is given general or regional anesthesia, and marrow is usually aspirated with large needles from the posterior iliac crest; the anterior crest can also be used in certain cases (Figure 32-2). The goal of the procedure is to collect 10 to 15 mL of marrow per kilogram of recipient weight. Approximately 600 to 900 mL of marrow is collected. The aspirated marrow is collected in bags containing a buffered isotonic solution and heparin to prevent coagulation.

After the marrow has been collected, it is filtered to remove any bone chips, fat, and clots that may have been collected or formed during the procedure. The bone marrow is frequently processed to remove undesired volume and cells. If the marrow is matched and no further manipulation is needed, it is transfused within 12 to 24 hours after collection, depending on the location of the recipient. If it is not transfused within 24 hours, it is cryopreserved.

Peripheral Blood Progenitor Cells

Peripheral blood progenitor cells are increasingly being used in place of bone marrow as a source of stem cells for allogeneic transplants. Reasons for this trend are the large amount of hematopoietic stem cells that can be collected, more rapid hematologic recovery, elimination of the surgical procedure and anesthesia risk for the donor, and reduced transplant costs. However, a patient who receives allogeneic peripheral blood progenitor cells may be at a greater risk for chronic *graft-versus-host disease* (GVHD; see following discussion and Chapter 31), possibly because of the high amount of lymphocytes in the product. Up to a log increase in lymphocytes is collected in a PBSC collection compared to a bone marrow. Conversely, this increase in lymphocytes could aid in the patient's immune reconstitution and also impart a graft-versus-leukemia effect.

Peripheral blood progenitor cells are obtained for transplant by a procedure called **apheresis** or "leukapheresis." For 4 or 5 days before apheresis, normal donors are given G-CSF that increases the amount of stem cells released into the bloodstream. Typically, in the autologous setting, the patient is "mobilized," with G-CSF given for 7 to 10 days after myelosuppressive chemotherapy. Disease status and prior treatment influence the ability to mobilize autologous PBSCs. The levels of hematopoietic stem cells rise up to fiftyfold in the recovery phase after myelosuppressive chemotherapy and administration of G-CSF.

In apheresis the blood is removed through a central venous catheter or vein in the arm. The blood goes through a continuous-flow apheresis machine where mononuclear cells (presumably including the desired stem cells) are separated by centrifugation from the red blood cell (RBC) and plasma fractions, which are returned to the donor during the procedure. The process usually takes one or two sessions of 3 to 5 hours per collection. The collected cells are then cryopreserved (i.e., frozen) in liquid nitrogen for later use or transplanted into the recipient.

Similarly, stem cells from a newborn's cord blood (considered adult cells because they are not from embryos) produce only blood cells. In general, adult stem cells are scarcer in the body and more difficult to culture than embryonic cells, yet large numbers are needed for therapy.

TRANSPLANTATION

The high-dose chemotherapy given before transplant leads to prolonged cytopenias, which account for much of the morbidity and mortality associated with the procedure. After the bone marrow or PBSCs are transplanted into the recipient via a central catheter, the cells migrate to the bone marrow, where they begin to produce new blood cells in a process known as **engraftment.** The primary measure of

**Pre-Transplant Checklist for
Allogeneic Donor**

Name:_____   Medical Record #:_____

Date of Collection:_____   Pre-Test:_____ Where:_____

Contact:_____   Phone:_____ Fax:_____

Protocol:_____

HLA Typing Performed by _____   Date of Repeat HLA at Hospital:_____

Name of Recipient:_____   Medical Record #:_____

Type of Collection (circle):   Marrow/PBSC   Syngeneic/Related/Unrelated

Test	Required (÷)	Date Ordered	Date Report Received	Eligibility Criteria	Meets Eligibility (÷)
History and Physical	÷				
Transfusion History	÷				
Vaccination History	÷				
Chest X-Ray	÷				
EKG	÷				
Laboratory Tests					
ABO group / Rh type	÷				
HLA typing	÷				
Confirmatory HLA	÷				
Toxoplasma antibody	÷				
CMV	÷				
HSV I and II	÷				
Infectious Disease Markers					
HIV consent obtained	÷	Date:			
Anti-HIV 1 / 2	÷			**negative**	
HIV-1-Ag	÷			**negative**	
Anti-HTLV	÷				
HBsAg	÷				
Anti-HBc	÷				
HCV	÷				
RPR	÷				
CBC with differential	÷				
Electrolytes	÷				
BUN	÷				
Creatinine	÷				

Originated: 11/99   Form 9929
Revised:

Figure 32-1   Pretransplant checklist for allogeneic donor.

**Pre-Transplant Checklist for
Allogeneic Donor**

Test	Required (÷)	Date Performed	Date Report Received	Eligibility Criteria	Meets Eligibility (÷)
Beta HCG - **females only**				**negative**	
Liver Function Tests					
SGOT	÷				
SGPT	÷				
LDH	÷				
Alkaline phosphatase.					
Total bilirubin	÷				
Chimerism - peripheral blood					
Urinalysis	÷				
PT	÷				
PTT	÷				
High-risk behavior yes no		Comments:			

Additional Testing:

ABO compatibility	Donor ABO/Rh _____ Recipient ABO/Rh _____ compatible _____ major incompatibility _____ minor incompatibility _____
CMV Compatible yes no	Donor _____ Recipient _____
OR Date _____	
Autologous blood stored yes no	No. of units _____

PBSC donors

Sent to blood bank for donor evaluation	Date: _____ Cleared by blood bank yes no If no, comments _____

Request for Hematopoietic Progenitor Cell Product Collection Form #9904 completed	Date:
Informed Consent obtained and donor given opportunity to ask questions.	Date:

The above results have been reviewed, and the donor meets all eligibility criteria for donation of PBSC/Bone Marrow. Any abnormal results have been discussed with the donor.

Attending Physician

_____   _____
Signature   Date

Originated: 11/99   Form 9929
Revised:

Figure 32-1, cont'd

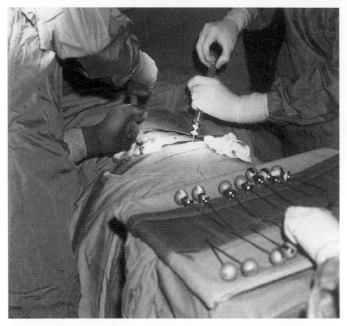

Figure 32-2   Bone marrow harvest from posterior iliac crest. *(Courtesy Bone Marrow Transplant Unit, Massachusetts General Hospital, Boston.)*

hematopoietic recovery, or engraftment, is when the neutrophil count reaches at least $0.5 \times 10^9/L$ for 3 consecutive days and a platelet count of $20 \times 10^9/L$ is maintained without platelet transfusion. Engraftment usually occurs within 2 to 4 weeks after infusion of stem cells. The type of transplant, source, and dose of stem cells are factors influencing engraftment times. Complete recovery of immune function takes much longer, up to several months for autologous transplant recipients and 1 to 2 years for allogeneic transplant recipients. Recent data show that patients receiving allogeneic PBSCs are less likely to have infections after transplantation than bone marrow recipients.

Transplant-Related Complications

Complications after transplantation of bone marrow or PBSCs can range from infection, GVHD, rejection, and organ damage to infertility and death. Early complications usually occur within the first 100 days after transplantation. After an allogeneic transplant, rejection rates can range between 1% and 2% in HLA-matched recipients and 5% to 10% in the mismatched recipients. GVHD can be attributed to many factors, including HLA mismatch between donor and recipient, conditioning regimen, viral exposure of donor and recipient, and the dose of T cells infused into the patient.

Acute GVHD affects at least 40% to 60% of allogeneic hematopoietic stem cell transplant patients after conditioning with myeloablative regimens and is a the major cause of early morbidity and nonrelapse mortality in these patients. Acute GVDH occurs within the first weeks after transplantation, is the result of complex interactions between the donor T cells, and involves the recognition of major histocompatibility complex (MHC) antigens on the recipient's organs (liver, gastrointestinal tract, skin, mucosal membranes).

Chronic GVHD occurs later and is defined as the presence or persistence of GVHD beyond 100 days since transplantation.

GVHD can be prevented or controlled by corticosteroids, calcineurin inhibitors (e.g., cyclosporin A, tacrolimus), and T-cell depletion of the graft.

Graft Manipulation and Storage

The processing of bone marrow and PBSCs varies from laboratory to laboratory, with different techniques to accomplish the same result. A bone marrow harvest results in the collection of a large volume of marrow that contains progenitor blood cells. Therefore, it is desirable to concentrate the marrow both in the autologous and allogeneic setting. The purpose is twofold: to reduce the volume and remove RBCs.

ABO incompatibility between donor and recipient is encountered in 23% to 30% of all hematopoietic cell transplants. A major incompatibility exists between donor and recipient when the recipient possesses antibodies against the RBC antigens of the donor, which would result in lysis of the transfused donor cells (e.g., group A donor and group O recipient).

Differences between donor and recipient's ABO or Rh blood groups have no effect on marrow engraftment, rejection, or GVHD. As long as the transplant recipient has antibodies against the RBCs of the donor, erythrocytes will be destroyed inside the marrow at an early stage. This could result in a state of "pure red cell aplasia" that can last for 4 to 6 weeks after the marrow infusion, although durations of up to 8 months have been reported.

To prevent acute hemolysis, the main objective of the laboratory is to remove as many RBCs as possible while preserving the hematopoietic progenitor cells to ensure timely engraftment. This is accomplished mainly by automated means, but manual methods are still used. Low-speed centrifugation sediments the cellular elements of the marrow so that the plasma and collection media can be removed and the WBC-rich buffy coat expressed into a separate container while the RBCs are retained in the original container. This manual method has an increased risk of contamination of the graft, depends on the technique of the technologist for good recovery of the cells, and is labor intensive.

Automated procedures involving apheresis equipment; such as the COBE Spectra and Fenwall CS-3000 Plus, use a closed, sterile system that rapidly recovers the desired mononuclear cells (Figure 32-3). The Fenwall CS-3000 Plus cell separator recovers mononuclear bone marrow cells in a 200-mL volume with greater than 95% reduction in contaminating RBCs and minimal granulocyte contamination.

Minor ABO mismatches are present in 15% to 20% of HLA-matched donor-recipient pairs. Patients who receive hematopoietic progenitor cells from a minor ABO-incompatible donor are at risk of developing immediate immune hemolysis caused by isohemagglutinins infused with the marrow or PBSCs or delayed hemolysis caused by isohemagglutinins produced by the donor lymphocytes (i.e., B cells). Immediate

The cryopreservation of the product is usually accomplished by the addition of 10% dimethyl sulfoxide (DMSO) and autologous plasma or 5% DMSO with 6% pentastarch, and 4% human albumin. DMSO and pentastarch are thought to keep the cells from "dehydrating" during the freezing process, which would cause them to lyse. The product is then frozen in a controlled-rate freezer, which reduces the temperature of the product by 1° to 3° C a minute, or by "dump" freezing in a −80° C freezer. After the product is frozen, it is kept in a liquid-nitrogen freezer, either vapor or liquid phase, until the time of transplant.

Cell Infusion

At transplant the product is thawed in a 37° C water bath in the laboratory or at the patient's bedside and is then infused without a filter through a central line. Toxicities and side effects have been associated with the infusion of cryopreserved products, mainly from the DMSO and volume overload. The most common symptoms are mild nausea, vomiting, and hypertension. Side effects of the infusion are rare and often mild. DMSO can cause patients to experience an immediate garlic-like taste. Sucking on hard candies during and after the infusion may help. Most patients undergoing allogeneic or syngeneic transplants do not experience this problem, because the cells most likely were not mixed with DMSO or cryopreserved.

TRANSPLANTS FROM UNRELATED DONORS

The National Marrow Donor Program (NMDP) is a nonprofit organization that facilitates unrelated marrow and blood stem cell transplants for patients who do not have matching donors in their families. This program has facilitated approximately 12,000 unrelated transplants. Through a network of national and international affiliates, the program aids in more than 130 transplants each month. Approximately 40% of the transplants facilitated by the NMDP involve a U.S. patient receiving stem cells from an international donor or an international patient receiving stem cells from a U.S. donor.

CURRENT DIRECTIONS

Research in techniques of gene transfer, gene expression, and hematopoietic stem cell manipulation remain under development and need to be improved before these techniques are able to change the course of diseases (e.g., cancer and AIDS). Recently, promising gene therapy work has been done in the field of bone marrow transplant and controlling GVHD in vivo. The use of donor T cells expressing the herpes simplex virus (HSV)–thymidine kinase gene ("suicide gene"), followed by ganciclovir treatment, could allow for specific modulation of the alloreactivity occurring after transplantation.

Donor and recipient matching is a significant factor in graft survival, but identification of minor HLA antigens and their significance in rejection might be of value in transplantation.

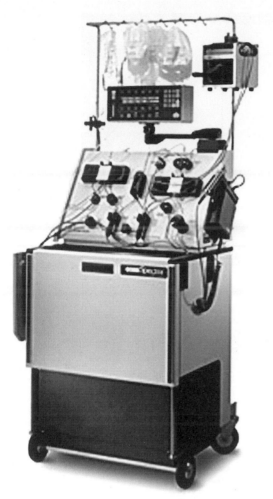

Figure 32-3 COBE Spectra Apheresis System. *(Courtesy Gambro BCT, Lakewood, Colo.)*

hemolysis can be avoided by simple removal of plasma from the graft before infusion. However, delayed hemolysis caused by antibody production from donor-derived B lymphocytes requires the ex vivo removal of lymphocytes or suppression of T-lymphocyte function by cyclosporine.

Removal of the plasma from the graft is used to minimize the risk of immediate hemolysis. This is accomplished by placing the marrow or PBSCs into standard blood transfer bags, centrifuging, and removing supernatant plasma. Normal saline or other media can be added to the product in a volume equivalent to about half the volume of the discarded plasma to dilute the remaining donor antibody and lower the hematocrit for easier infusion.

With the development of **monoclonal antibodies (MAbs),** there has been an increase in stem cell selection (e.g., CD34+ cells) and purging of grafts (e.g., CD19+/CD20+ B cells). These techniques have resulted in decreased tumor reinfusion into autologous recipients and decreases in the amount of T cells infused in allogeneic recipients. The Isolex 300i Magnetic Cell Selection system (Figure 32-4) has been shown to effect an approximate 4-log depletion of T cells, typically resulting in a residual T-cell content of 1×10^5/kg or less of recipient weight.

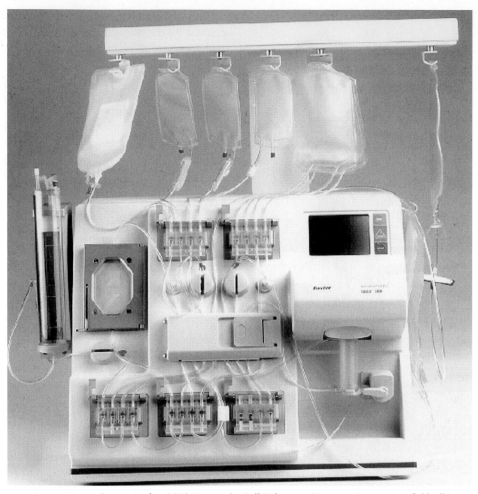

Figure 32-4 Baxter Isolex 300i Magnetic Cell Selector. *(Courtesy Baxter, Deerfield, Ill.)*

Donor leukocyte infusions are used for a *graft-versus-lymphoma* or *graft-versus-leukemia* (GVL) effect in the transplant setting. This treatment may kill any residual cancer cells but could simultaneously cause GVHD. Research is focusing on the ability to control the life-threatening GVHD while retaining the desired GVL effect from the T cells.

FUTURE DIRECTIONS

The following initiatives should be explored:
- Develop methods to deliver specific cell populations through positive or negative selection, activation, and possible expansion.
- Create and test new immunosuppressive drugs that are more effective in controlling rejection, less costly, and not as immunosuppressive as traditional agents.
- Focus new treatment programs on using highly specific MAbs directed at antigens present on lymphoma cells.
- Institute a nonmyeloablative approach to chemotherapy with bone marrow transplantation, because it is less

toxic to the patient and may result in **mixed chimerism.**

CASE STUDY

M.C. is an obese 46-year-old Caucasian woman with diabetes. She came to the emergency department with complaints of rectal bleeding and a feeling of significant fatigue.

History and Physical Examination

Medical History
The patient has a long-standing history of infected foot ulcerations that are not secondary to vascular insufficiency or diabetes. She received a prolonged course of chloramphenicol for the foot infections in Brazil. After treatment, she was found to be pancytopenic and required transfusions of packed RBCs and platelets on a regular basis.

Her medical history also includes a history of a positive PPD test, for which she received antituberculosis therapy for 4 months. She sustained facial fractures in a car accident several years ago.

Medications

The patient takes rifampin (300 mg PO daily), INH (300 mg PO daily), pyridoxine (50 mg PO daily), cyclosporine (Sandimmune), insulin morning and evening, and metformin (Glucophage).

Social History

Mrs. M.C. is a citizen of Brazil. Her husband died several years ago. She has three children, one living in the United States and two living in Brazil.

Allergies

She has no known allergies.

Family History

The patient's father died of heart disease at age 63; her mother died of cancer at age 48. The patient has nine siblings, six in Brazil and three in the United States. One sister, age 42, lives in United States and is HLA matched.

Physical Examination

The patient weighs 233 lb; her blood pressure is 120/70 mm Hg; and her pulse is 66 beats/min and regular.

Her temperature is 37.1° C. She has ecchymoses and petechiae of the skin with mild bruising on her left shoulder. She has multiple scars on her feet and legs. There are no other abnormal physical findings.

Laboratory Data

	Patient Result	Reference Range
White blood cell (WBC) count	2.1 × 10⁹/L	4.5-11 × 10⁹/L
Hematocrit (Hct)	20.4%	36%-46%
Hemoglobin (Hgb, Hb)	6.9 g/dL	12-16 g/dL
Red blood cell (RBC) count	1.83 × 10¹²/L	4-5.20 × 10¹²/L
Platelet count*	49 × 10⁹/L	150-350 × 10⁹/L
Mean corpuscular volume (MCV)	112 fL	80-100 fL
Red cell distribution width (RDW)	20.2%	11.5%-14.5%
Reticulocyte count	1.5%	0.5%-1.9%

Leukocyte Differential

Segmented neutrophils	27%	40%-70%
Lymphocytes	57%	22%-44%
Monocytes	13%	4%-11%
Eosinophils	0%	0%-8%
Basophils	0%	0%-3%

Variant lymphocytes: 3%
Anisocytosis: 2+
Hypochromia: 1+
Macrocytes: 3+

---

*Posttransfusion.

Blood Chemistry

Electrolytes: within normal limits.

Liver Function Tests

Alkaline phosphatase (ALP)	131 IU/L	30-100 IU/L
Alanine transaminase (ALT/SGPT)	167 IU/L	7-30 IU/L
Aspartate transaminase (AST/SGOT)	56 IU/L	9-25 IU/L
Lactic dehydrogenase (LDH)	266 IU/L	110-210 IU/L
Plasma glucose	123 mg/dL	70-110 mg/dL

Immunologic Studies

Hepatitis A antigen: positive.
Hepatitis B and hepatitis C screening tests: negative.

Follow-up Evaluation

A bone marrow biopsy was performed. Histologic study of the aspirate and clot revealed a hypocellular marrow with trilineage hematopoiesis and dyserythropoiesis. Cytogenetic studies were normal (karyotype: 46,XX). Flow cytometry revealed polyclonal (kappa+ and lambda+) CD19+ B cells and CD4+ and CD8+ T cells. The iron stain was normal.

HLA Typing

Patient: A11, 68	B18, 52	DR4, 15	DQ3, 6
Donor: A11, 28	B18, 52	DR4, 15	DQ3, 6

At 3 Months

The patient is feeling well. The pain and swelling in her right arm have resolved. She has had no fever, nausea, vomiting, diarrhea, rash, chest pain, shortness of breath, dysuria, hematuria, headache, or edema.

Medications

The patient was receiving fluconazole (Diflucan, 200 mg/day), ursodiol (Actigall, 300 mg/day), valganciclovir (Valcyte, 450 mg twice daily), cyclosporine (110 mg twice daily), sulfamethoxazole (Bactrim DS, 1 tablet PO Monday, Wednesday, and Friday), magnesium oxide (twice daily), norgestimate/ethinyl estradiol (Ortho Tri-Cyclen once daily).

Physical Examination

The patient now weighs 152.6 lb; her blood pressure is 139/93 mm Hg, temperature 35.9° C, and pulse 69 beats/min and regular. She has no skin rash.

Her eyes and mouth are without scleral icterus or mucositis, and the lungs are clear. Her heartbeat has a regular rate and rhythm. Her abdomen is soft and nontender without masses or organomegaly. Extremities are without edema. Her neurologic examination revealed no tremors.

Laboratory Data

Assay	Patient Result	Reference Range
Sodium (Na^+)	139 mEq/L	135-145 mEq/L
Potassium (K^+)	4.7 mEq/L	3.5-5 mmEq/L
Magnesium (Mg^{++})	1.6 mEq/L	1.4-2 mEq/L
Blood urea nitrogen (BUN)	28 mg/dL	8-25 mg/dL
Creatinine	1.8 mg/dL	0.6-1.5 mg/dL
Total bilirubin	0.2 mg/dL	0-1 mg/dL
Direct bilirubin	0.1 mg/dL	0-0.4 mg/dL
ALP	99 IU/L	30-100 IU/L
AST/SGOT	16 IU/L	9-25 IU/L
LDH	208 IU/L	100-210 IU/L
WBC count	3.7×10^9/L	4.5-11×10^9/L
Hct	39%	36%-46%
Platelet count	173,000	200-400×10^{12}/L

Impressions

1. Day +88 after HLA-matched donor stem cell transplantation for severe aplastic anemia: stable trilineage hematopoiesis. Mild leukopenia is probably a result of valganciclovir and/or sulfamethoxazole.
2. Right arm cellulitis: resolved.
3. Renal insufficiency secondary to focal glomerulosclerosis: persistent proteinuria (1.4 g/24 hr) and elevated BUN/creatinine (despite a low therapeutic cyclosporine level).

Treatment Plan

1. Check cyclosporine level today and adjust dose accordingly.
2. Refill norgestimate/ethinyl estradiol.
3. Continue sulfamethoxazole DS for *Pneumocystis carinii* (PCP) prophylaxis and valganciclovir for previous CMV infection.

Questions and Discussion

1. What is the etiology of this patient's aplastic anemia?

Extended treatment with high doses of chloramphenicol is notorious for causing aplastic anemia.

2. Did the patient have any other treatment options?

No. The patient had completed the normal course of treatment (e.g., cyclosporine and ATC) for aplastic anemia. It was unsuccessful. Because aplastic anemia is a life-threatening condition, the only remaining treatment option was a bone marrow transplant.

3. What are the risks involved in bone marrow transplant?

A patient faces the risk of bone marrow rejection and GVHD. In addition, because of the induced immunosuppression, patients are at risk of developing CMV infection, which is usually a reactivation of the disease. In addition, bacterial and particularly fungal infections are serious health threats.

4. What drug is highly effective in preventing rejection?

The drug that produced a significant breakthrough in transplantation survival is cyclosporine.

Diagnosis

Bone marrow transplantation, because of drug-induced aplastic anemia.

CHAPTER HIGHLIGHTS

- The goal of transplanting bone marrow or peripheral blood progenitor cells is to achieve a potential cure or to help patients recover from high-dose chemotherapy that has destroyed healthy stem cells or marrow cells.
- Bone marrow and peripheral blood progenitor cells are capable of reconstituting a patient's immune system because they contain the precursor to the cells that make up the blood. Some stem cells circulate in the bloodstream and are called peripheral blood stem cells (PBSCs).
- There are three major types of transplants: allogeneic, syngeneic, and autologous.
- Chemotherapy and radiation target rapidly dividing cells. These therapies are used to treat cancers because cancer cells divide more rapidly than healthy cells. Bone marrow cells also divide at a rapid rate and can be severely damaged or destroyed by high-dose treatments.
- Without healthy bone marrow, a patient cannot make the blood cells that are needed to fight off infections, carry oxygen, or prevent bleeding. Bone marrow and PBSC transplants can replace both the normal and abnormal cells that were destroyed during treatment.
- Factors that influence the eligibility for a bone marrow transplant include age, disease status, performance status for the recipient, organ function, infectious disease status, compatibility of the donor and recipient, and psychosocial status.
- The procedure for obtaining or "harvesting" bone marrow is the same for all types of transplants. The goal of the harvest procedure is to collect 10 to 15 mL of bone marrow per kilogram recipient weight.
- Complications that develop from transplantation of bone marrow or PBSCs range from infection, GVHD, rejection, and organ damage to infertility and death.

REVIEW QUESTIONS

1. The following diseases are treatable by stem cell transplantation:
   a. Acute lymphoblastic leukemia and acute myelogenous leukemia.
   b. Aplastic anemia and non-Hodgkin's lymphoma.
   c. Severe combined immunodeficiency disease and chronic myeloid leukemia.
   d. All the above.

2. Progenitor blood cells are:
   a. Pluripotent.
   b. Found only in bone marrow.
   c. Not useful in reconstituting a person's immune system.
   d. Determined by the exact number of CD34 and stem cells.

Questions 3-5. Match the following transplants:

3. _____ Allogeneic   a. Stem cells from identical twins.
4. _____ Autologous   b. Marrow from a related or unrelated donor.
5. _____ Syngeneic   c. Transplant of own cells.

6. Radiotherapy is most often used for:
   a. Myelodysplastic syndrome.
   b. Localized solid tumors.
   c. Hodgkin's disease.
   d. Both b and c.

7. Pretransplant evaluation includes:
   a. HLA tissue typing and hepatitis screening.
   b. ECG and CBC.
   c. Bone marrow biopsy and complete history of physical examination.
   d. All the above.

8. Bone marrow is usually aspirated from:
   a. Sternum.
   b. Anterior iliac crest.
   c. Posterior iliac crest.
   d. Vertebrae.

9. Peripheral blood stem cells (PBSCs) are obtained by:
   a. Phlebotomy.
   b. Apheresis.
   c. Leukapheresis.
   d. Both b and c.

10. Engraftment of bone marrow or PBSCs is:
    a. Cell production in the bone marrow.
    b. Matching the donor and patient.
    c. Measured by the number of lymphocytes in circulation.
    d. Antibody production.

11. Complications of bone marrow or PBSC transplantation include:
    a. Infection and graft-versus-host disease (GVHD).
    b. Acute rejection and organ damage.
    c. Chronic rejection and death.
    d. All the above.

12. Differences between donor and recipient's ABO or Rh blood groups have _____ effect on marrow engraftment.
    a. no
    b. some
    c. a major
    d. a total

13. Stem cell selection can be improved using the CD_____ cell surface marker.
    a. 4+
    b. 8+
    c. 34+
    d. 56+

14. Increased cell selection and purging of grafts using cell surface membrane markers has resulted in:
    a. Decreased risk of tumor reinfusion.
    b. Lesser GVHD.
    c. Transfusing fewer erythrocytes as contaminants.
    d. All the above.

15. Toxicity associated with infusion of cryopreserved products is mainly caused by:
    a. Dimethyl sulfoxide (DMSO).
    b. Pentastarch.
    c. Human albumin.
    d. Glycerol.

BIBLIOGRAPHY

Antin J et al: Peripheral blood stem cells for allogenic transplantation: a review, *Stem Cells* 19:108-117, 2001.

Barrett AJ: Mechanisms of graft-versus-leukemia reaction, *Stem Cells* 15:248-258, 1997.

Baynes RD et al: Bone marrow and peripheral blood hematopoietic stem cell transplantation: focus on autografting, *Clin Chem* 46(8B):1239-1251, 2000.

Bensinger W et al: Transplantation of bone marrow as compared with peripheral blood cells from HLA-identical relatives in patients with hematologic cancers, *N Engl J Med* 344:175-181, 2001.

Blaser B et al: Trans-presentation of donor-derived interleukin-15 is necessary for the rapid onset of acute graft-versus-host disease but not for graft-versus-tumor activity, *Blood* 108(7):2463-2469, 2006.

Blume KG et al: A review of autologous hematopoietic cell transplantation, *Biol Blood Marrow Transplant* 6:1-12, 2000.

Braziel RM et al: The Burkitt-like lymphomas: a Southwest Oncology group study delineating phenotypic, genotypic and clinical features, *Blood* 97:3713-3720, 2001.

Brecher ME, Lasky LC, Sacher RA, Issitt LA: *Hematopoietic progenitor cells: processing, standards and practice,* Bethesda, Md, 1995, American Association of Blood Banks.

Chabner BA, Longo DL, editors: *Cancer chemotherapy and biotherapy: principles and practice,* ed 3, Philadelphia, 2001, Lippincott–Williams & Wilkins.

Contassot E et al: Ganciclovir-sensitive acute graft-versus-host disease in mice receiving herpes simplex virus–thymidine kinase expressing donor T cells in a bone marrow transplantation setting, *Transplantation* 4:503-508, 2000.

Copelan EA: Hematopoietic stem cell transplantation, *N Engl J Med* 354(17):1813-1826, 2006.

Davies SM et al: Engraftment and survival after unrelated-donor bone marrow transplantation: a report from the National Marrow Donor Program, *Blood* 96:4096-4103, 2000.

Focosi D, Petrini M: More on donor-derived T-cell leukemia after bone marrow transplantation, *N Engl J Med* 355:2, 2006.

Franks LM, Teich NM: *Introduction to the cellular and molecular biology of cancer,* ed 3, New York, 1999, Oxford University Press.

Johnston LJ, Horning SJ: Autologous hematopoietic cell transplantation in Hodgkin's disease, *Biol Blood Marrow Transplant* 6:289-300, 2000.

Krause D et al: Isolation and flow cytometric analysis of T-cell-depleted CD34+ PBPCs, *Transfusion* 40:1475-1481, 2000.

Lasky LC, Warkentin PI: *Marrow and stem cell processing for transplantation,* Bethesda, Md, 1995, American Association of Blood Banks.

Laughlin MJ et al: Outcomes after transplantation of cord blood or bone marrow from unrelated donors in adults with leukemia, *N Engl J Med* 351(22):2265-2257, 2004.

Leisenrig WM et al: It's about time: a new prognostic tool for acute graft-versus-host disease, *Blood* 108:749-755, 2006.

Martin-Henao GA et al: Isolation of CD34+ progenitor cells from peripheral blood by use of an automated immunomagnetic selection system: factors affecting the results, *Transfusion* 40:35-43, 2000.

National Marrow Donor Program, 2001, www.nmdp.org.

Nikolic B et al: A novel application of cyclosporin A in nonmyeloablative pretransplant host conditioning for allogeneic BMT, *Blood* 96:1166-1172, 2000.

Penno K: Combining forces, *Adv Med Lab Prof* 17(10):18-20, 27, 2005.

Ross DW: *Introduction to oncogenes and molecular cancer medicine,* New York, 1998, Springer.

Sacher RA, AuBuchon JP: *Marrow transplantation: practical and technical aspects of stem cell reconstitution,* Bethesda, Md, 1992, American Association of Blood Banks.

Sacher RA, McCarthy LJ, Sibinga CS: *Processing of bone marrow for transplantation,* Arlington, Va, 1990, American Association of Blood Banks.

Sanz MA: Cord-blood transplantation in patients with leukemia: a real alternative for adults, *N Engl J Med* 351(22):2328-2338, 2004.

Serody JS et al: Comparison of granulocyte colony-stimulating factor (G-CSF)–mobilized peripheral blood progenitor cells and G-CSF–stimulated bone marrow as a source of stem cells in HLA-matched sibling transplantation, *Biol Blood Marrow Transplant* 6:434-440, 2000.

Socié G: Graft-versus-host disease: from the bench to the bedside? *N Engl J Med* 353(13):1396-1397, 2005.

Solano C et al: Chronic graft-versus-host disease after allogeneic peripheral blood progenitor cell or bone marrow transplantation from matched related donors: a case-control study. Spanish Group of Allo-PBT, *Bone Marrow Transplant* 12:1129-1135, 1998.

Spitzer TR: Nonmyeloablative allogeneic stem cell transplant strategies and the role of mixed chimerism, *Oncologist* 5:215-223, 2000.

Spitzer TR, McAfee SL: Bone marrow transplantation. In Ginns LC, Cosimi AB, Morris PJ, editors: *Transplantation,* Cambridge, 1999, Blackwell Science.

Spitzer TR et al: Intentional induction of mixed chimerism and achievement of antitumor response after nonmyeloablative conditioning therapy and HLA-matched donor bone marrow transplantation for refractory hematologic malignancies, *Biol Blood Marrow Transplant* 6:309-320, 2000.

Standards for hematopoietic progenitor cell services, ed 2, Bethesda, Md, 2000, American Association of Blood Banks.

Storek J et al: Immune reconstitution after allogeneic marrow transplantation compared with blood stem cell transplantation, *Blood* 97:3380-3389, 2001.

Sutherland R et al: The CD 34 antigen: structure, biology and potential clinical applications, *J Hematotherapy* 1:115-129, 1992.

Sykes M et al: Mixed lymphohaemopoietic chimerism and graft-versus-lymphoma effects after non-myeloablative therapy and HLA-mismatched bone marrow transplantation, *Lancet* 353:1755-1759, 1999.

Ullmann AJ et al: Posaconazole or fluconazole for prophylaxis in severe graft-versus-host disease, *N Engl J Med* 356(4):335-346, 2007.

Zambelli A et al: Clinical toxicity of cryopreserved circulating progenitor cells infusion, *Anticancer Res* 18:4705-4708, 1998.

Zhang C et al: Donor CD4+ T and B cells in transplants induce chronic graft-versus-host disease with autoimmune manifestations, *Blood* 107(7):2993-3000, 2006.

CHAPTER 33

Tumor Immunology

Benign Tumors
Malignant Tumors
Epidemiology
   Cancer in Adults
   Cancer in Children
   Risk Factors
Etiologic Factors in Human Cancer
   Environmental Factors
   Host Factors and Disease Associations
   Viruses
Stages of Carcinogenesis
Cancer-Predisposing Genes
Proto-oncogenes
   p53 Protein
Role of Oncogenes
   Mechanisms of Activation
   Viral Oncogenes
   Tumor-Suppressing Genes
Body Defenses against Cancer
   T Lymphocytes
   Natural Killer Cells
   Macrophages
   Antibodies

Tumor Markers
   Categories of Tumor Antigens
   Specific Tumor Markers
   Breast, Ovarian, and Cervical Cancer Markers
   Bladder Cancer
   Monocyte Chemotactic Protein
DNA Microarray Technology
Modalities for Treating Cancer
   Chemotherapeutic Agents
   Effects of Drug-Induced Immunosuppression
   Recent Advances
   What's New in Drug Therapy?
Prostate-Specific Antigen (PSA) Rapid Test in Seminal Fluid
Case Studies
Chapter Highlights
Review Questions
Bibliography

Learning Objectives

At the conclusion of this chapter, the reader should be able to:
- Compare the characteristics of benign and malignant tumors.
- Describe the epidemiology of cancer in adults and children.
- Explain the characteristics of the three major etiologic factors in human cancer.
- Compare the stages of carcinogenesis.
- Describe the aspects of cancer-related genes.

- Define and give examples of proto-oncogenes.
- Describe the role of oncogenes.
- Describe the characteristics of the major body defenses against cancer.
- Identify and discuss the characteristics of tumor markers.
- Compare various modalities for treating cancer.
- Analyze representative case studies.

Oncology is that branch of medicine devoted to the study and treatment of tumors. The term **tumor** is commonly used to describe a proliferation of cells that produces a mass rather than a reaction or inflammatory condition. Tumors are **neoplasms** and are described as **benign** or **malignant.** Most tumors are of epithelial origin (ectoderm, endoderm, or mesoderm); the remaining tumors are of connective tissue origin (Figure 33-1). The key distinction between benign and malignant tumors is the capacity of malignant tumors to invade normal tissue and to metastasize to other secondary sites.

BENIGN TUMORS

Benign tumors are often named by adding the suffix "oma" to the cell type (e.g., lipoma), but there are exceptions (e.g., lymphomas, melanomas, hepatomas). Benign tumors arising from glands are called *adenomas;* those from epithelial surfaces are named "polyps" or *papillomas.*

Benign tumors are characterized as:
- Usually being encapsulated.
- Growing slowly.
- Usually being nonspreading.

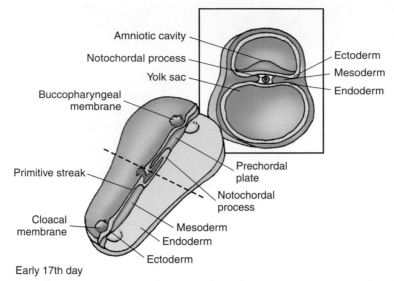

Figure 33-1 Embryonic primary germ layers. *(Redrawn from Larsen WJ: Human embryology, ed 3, Philadelphia, 2001, Churchill Livingstone.)*

- Having minimal mitotic activity.
- Resembling the parent tissue.

Other types of tumors include nonneoplastic lesions associated with an overgrowth of tissue that is normally present in the organ (e.g., hyperplastic tissue) and *choristomas,* normal tissue in a foreign location (e.g., pancreatic tissue in the stomach).

MALIGNANT TUMORS

A malignant neoplasm of epithelial origin is referred to as **carcinoma,** or cancer. Those arising from squamous epithelium (e.g., esophagus, lung) are called squamous cell carcinoma; those arising from glandular epithelium (e.g., stomach, colon, pancreas) are called adenocarcinomas, and those arising from transitional epithelium in the urinary system are called transitional cell carcinomas.

Other types of malignant tumors include amine precursor uptake and decarboxylational tumors. These are neuroendocrine tumors that commonly develop from neural crest and neural ectoderm, (e.g., small-cell carcinoma of lung). Sarcomas, malignant tumors of connective tissue origin (e.g., fibrosarcoma), and teratomas are derived from all three germ cell layers (e.g., teratoma of ovary or testis).

Malignant tumors are characterized by the following:
- Increase in the number of cells that accumulate.
- Usually, invasion of tissues.
- Dissemination by lymphatic spread or by seeding within a body cavity.
- Metastasis.
- Characteristic nuclear cellular features.
- Receptors for integrin molecules (e.g., fibronectin), which help malignant cells adhere to extracellular matrix; type IV collagenases, which dissolve basement membranes; and proteases.

- Secretion of transforming growth factor alpha (TGF-α) and beta (TGF-β) to promote angiogenesis and collagen deposition.
- Often, recurrence after attempts to eradicate the tumor by surgery, radiation, or chemotherapy.

Biologically distinct and relatively rare populations of "tumor-initiating" cells have been identified in cancers of the hematopoietic system, brain, and breast. Cells of this type have the capacity for self-renewal, the potential to develop into any cell in the overall tumor population, and the proliferative ability to drive continued expansion of the population of malignant cells. The properties of these tumor-initiating cells closely parallel the three features that define normal stem cells. Malignant cells with these functional properties have been termed *cancer stem cells* (Figure 33-2). Cancer stem cells can be the source of all the malignant cells in a primary tumor.

EPIDEMIOLOGY

Lung, colorectal, and breast cancer are the leading causes of cancer deaths in the United States. The types of cancer that are increasing in incidence are cancer of the lung, breast, prostate, pancreas, multiple myeloma, malignant melanoma, and Hodgkin's lymphoma. The types of cancer that are decreasing in incidence are cancer of the stomach, cervix, and endometrium.

Cancer in Adults

The lifetime probability of developing cancer is higher in men than in women. The three most common cancers in men are prostate, lung/bronchus, and colorectal, accounting for about 54% of all newly diagnosed cancers. The three most common cancers in women are breast, lung/bronchus, and colorectal, accounting for about 52% of estimated can-

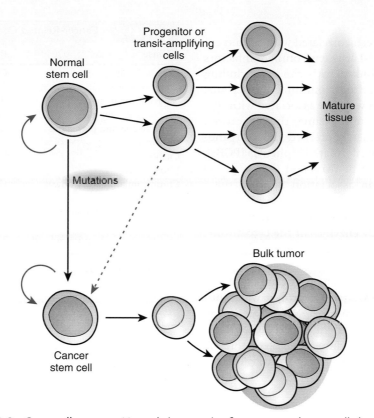

Figure 33-2 **Stem cell systems.** Normal tissues arise from a central stem cell that grows and differentiates to create progenitor and mature cell populations. Key properties of normal stem cells are the ability to self-renew (indicated by *curved arrow*), multilineage potential, and extensive proliferative capacity. Cancer stem cells arise by means of mutation in normal stem cells or progenitor cells and subsequently grow and differentiate to create primary tumors (*broken arrow* indicates that specific types of progenitors involved in the generation of cancer stem cells are unclear). As with normal stem cells, cancer stem cells can self-renew, give rise to heterogeneous populations of daughter cells, and proliferate extensively. *(Redrawn from Jordan CT, Guzman ML, Noble M: N Engl J Med 355(12):1255, 2006.)*

cer cases in women. Breast cancer alone is expected to account for 26% of all new cancer cases among women. Cancer accounts for more deaths than heart disease in persons under age 85 years.

Cancer in Children

Cancer is the second leading cause of death among children between 1 and 14 years old in the United States. Acute lymphoblastic leukemia continues to be the most common cause of pediatric cancer deaths, followed by tumors of the central and sympathetic nervous system, malignant lymphoma, soft tissue sarcomas, and renal tumors.

Risk Factors

Risk factors are important in specific cancers. Smoking is responsible for one third of cancers. Other risk factors include a high-fat, low-fiber diet, obesity, and a sedentary lifestyle. Certain types of cancer are more prevalent in specific populations. For example, African Americans have a 20% greater prevalence of cancer than Caucasians. The risk of breast cancer increases with age, and deaths are related to geography. Risk factors for breast cancer include family history, particularly breast cancer in a first-degree relative; first pregnancy after age 30 years; the presence of fibrocystic disease; probably the use of oral contraceptives or hormone replacement therapy; prior breast or chest wall radiation; prior breast cancer; and ethanol consumption.

Survivors of childhood and adolescent cancer are one of the higher-risk populations. The curative therapy (chemotherapy, radiation) administered for the cancer also affects growing and developing tissues. Such patients are at increased risk for early mortality caused by second cancers and cardiac or pulmonary disease. Two thirds of survivors have at least one chronic or late-occurring health problem.

ETIOLOGIC FACTORS IN HUMAN CANCER

Factors that cause the majority of neoplasms are unknown. Etiologic factors can be classified into environmental associations (e.g., chemical and radiation), host factors and disease associations, and viruses.

Environmental Factors

The incidence of cancer has been correlated with certain environmental factors. Table 33-1 lists environmental factors that have been definitively linked with cancer, including aerosol/industrial pollutants, drugs, and infectious agents. Radiation exposure is also known to be associated with specific types of cancer (e.g., acute leukemia, thyroid cancer, sarcomas, breast cancer). Women concerned about organochlorine substances (e.g., polychlorinated biphenyls [PCBs], dioxins, pesticides [DDT]) can be reassured that available evidence does not suggest an association between these chemicals and breast cancer.

Most chemical carcinogens are inactive in their native state and must be activated by enzymes in the cytochrome P-450 or other enzymes systems (e.g., bacterial enzymes or enzymes induced by alcohol).

In radiation carcinogenesis, ionizing particles (e.g., alpha and beta particles, gamma rays, x-rays) hydrolyze water into free radicals, which are mutagenic to DNA by activating proto-oncogenes. Ultraviolet (UV) light, especially UVB, induces the formation of thymidine dimers, which distort the DNA molecule, leading to skin cancers (e.g., basal cell carcinoma, malignant melanoma).

Table 33-1	Selected Environmental Factors Associated with Cancer
Factor	**Type of Cancer**
Aerosol/Industrial Pollutants	
Asbestos (silica)	Mesothelioma
Lead, copper, zinc, arsenic, cyclic aromatics, tobacco	Lung cancer
Vinyl chloride	Liver angiosarcoma
Benzene	Leukemia
Aniline dyes, coal	Skin and bladder carcinoma
Drugs	
Androgenic steroids	Hepatocellular carcinoma
Stilbestrol (prenatal)	Vaginal adenocarcinoma
Estrogen (postmenopausal)	Endometrial carcinoma
Hydantoins	Lymphoma
Chloramphenicol, alkylating agents	Leukemias, lymphomas
Infectious Agents	
Epstein-Barr virus	Burkitt's lymphoma, nasopharyngeal cancer? Hodgkin's disease
Human papillomavirus	Cervical cancer
Herpesvirus, type 2	Cervical cancer
Human immunodeficiency virus (HTLV-III)	Kaposi's sarcoma, non-Hodgkin's lymphoma, primary lymphoma of the brain, bladder cancer
HTLV-I	Non-Hodgkin's lymphoma
Hepatitis B	Hepatocellular carcinoma

Table 33-2	Cancer-Related Conditions
Disease	**Related Cancer**
Paget's disease	Osteogenic sarcoma
Cryptorchidism	Testicular cancer
Neurofibromatosis	Brain tumors, sarcoma
Esophageal webbing	Esophageal carcinoma
Achlorhydria and pernicious anemia	Gastric carcinoma
Cirrhosis	Hepatoma
Cholelithiasis	Gallbladder cancer
Chronic inflammatory bowel disease	Colon cancer
Migratory thrombophlebitis	Adenocarcinoma, especially pancreatic
Myasthenia gravis, pure red cell aplasia, T cell disorder	Thymoma
Nephrotic syndrome	Membranous carcinomas Lymphomas, especially Hodgkin's

Host Factors and Disease Associations

A variety of host factors have been linked to a higher-than-expected incidence of cancer. For example, the presence of certain genetic disorders (e.g., Down syndrome) is associated with an increased incidence of leukemia. The link between certain genetic abnormalities and leukemia is consistent with a germinal or somatic mutation in a stem cell line.

Familial clustering of germ cell tumors, malignant tumors arising in the testis, has been observed, particularly among siblings. Cryptorchidism and Klinefelter's syndrome are predisposing factors in the development of germ cell tumors arising from the testis and mediastinum, respectively.

The incidence of cancer is 10,000 times greater than expected in patients with immunodeficiency syndromes. The increased incidence of lymphomas in congenital, acquired, and drug-induced immunosuppression is consistent with the failure of normal immune mechanisms or antigen overstimulation with a loss of normal feedback control. Table 33-2 lists other cancer-related conditions.

Viruses

Viral causes of some cancers are known. Viruses associated with specific cancers are listed in Table 33-1. Nonpermissive cells that prevent an oncogenic RNA or DNA virus from completing its replication cycle often produce changes in the genome that result in activation of proto-oncogenes or inactivation of suppressor genes.

STAGES OF CARCINOGENESIS

Some precancerous conditions progress through a series of growth alterations before becoming cancerous. For example, cervical cancer progresses from squamous metaplasia to squamous dysplasia to carcinoma in situ and finally to invasive cancer. Endometrial cancer progresses from endometrial hyperplasia to atypical endometrial hyperplasia to carcinoma in situ and finally to invasive cancer.

Cancer (Box 33-1) results from a series of genetic alterations that can include:
- Activation of oncogenes that promote cell growth.
- Loss of tumor suppressor gene activity, which inhibits cell growth.

Mutation or overexpression of oncogenes produces proteins that can stimulate uncontrolled cell growth, whereas mutation or deletion of tumor suppressor genes results in the production of nonfunctional proteins that can no longer control cell proliferation. The mutant cell multiplies, and the succeeding generations of cells aggregate to form a malignant tumor.

Interleukin-24 (IL-24), initially named MOB-5, is a protein that is usually secreted by immune system cells in response to injury or infection. New research on colon cancer cells has demonstrated that IL-24 in conjunction with its receptors appears to give a cancer cell the ability to fuel its own growth. The secreted proteins are released from one cell to transmit a signal to grow, migrate, or survive to another cell. These proteins cannot act alone and must act through a receptor or receptors on the receiving cell.

CANCER-PREDISPOSING GENES

Cancer-predisposing genes may act in the following ways:
- Affect the rate at which exogenous precarcinogens are metabolized to actively carcinogenic forms that can damage the cellular genome directly.
- Affect a host's ability to repair resulting damage to DNA.
- Alter the immune ability of the body to recognize and eradicate incipient tumors.
- Affect the function of the apparatus responsible for the regulation of normal cell growth and associated proliferation of tissue.

Relatively few cancer-predisposing genes have been described. An absence of functional alleles at specific loci, however, allows the genesis of the malignant process (Table 33-3). For example, individuals with certain mutations in the gene BRCA2 are at a very high (up to 85%) risk for developing breast cancer and other cancers (e.g., ovarian) because a DNA repair path cannot properly repair ongoing wear and tear to the DNA.

Table 33-3	Examples of Tumors Associated with Homozygous Loss of Specific Chromosomal Loci	
Tumor Type		**Chromosomal Linkage**
Multiple endocrine neoplasia, type 2		1
Renal cell carcinoma		3
Lung carcinoma		3
Colon carcinoma, familial polyposis		5
Multiple endocrine neoplasia, type 2a		10
Wilms' tumor, hepatoblastoma, rhabdomyosarcoma		11
Retinoblastoma		13
Ductal breast carcinoma		13
Colon carcinoma		17
Acoustic neuroma, meningioma		22

A mutation in a gene thought to be responsible for colon cancer may initially cause it. This gene, APC, normally limits the expression of a protein, *survivin*. When APC is altered, survivin works overtime, and instead of dying, stem cells in the colon overpopulate, resulting in cancer. Survivin is overexpressed in colon cancer. Survivin prevents programmed cell death, or **apoptosis,** the process by which cells normally die. Rather than dying on schedule, cancer cells are instead growing out of control. The APC gene controls the amount of survivin by shutting down its production.

PROTO-ONCOGENES

Proto-oncogenes act as central regulators of the growth in normal cells that code for proteins involved in growth and repair processes in the body. Proteins, such as growth factors or transcription factors, are necessary for normal growth.

Genetic mutations in proto-oncogenes produce **oncogenes.** Oncogene activation causes overexpression of growth-promoting proteins, resulting in hypercellular proliferation and **tumorigenesis.** Tumor suppressor genes normally counteract proto-oncogenes by encoding proteins that prevent cellular differentiation. When mutations in tumor suppressor genes cause loss of function, the expressed tumor suppressor proteins are no longer able to suppress cellular growth.

For example, activation of proto-oncogenes (e.g., *ras*) that are involved in the growth process or inactivation of suppressor genes (e.g., p53), which keeps growth in check by binding and activating genes that put the brakes on cell division, is responsible for neoplastic transformation of a cell. Defects in the gene for p53 cause about half of all cancers.

p53 Protein

The **p53 gene** (tumor suppressor gene) is located on chromosome 17 and produces a protein that downregulates the cell cycle. A mutation of p53 is associated with an increased incidence of many types of cancer. The p53 tumor suppressor protein is dysfunctional in most human cancers. Even when p53 is not itself mutant, its regulators (e.g., p14^{ARF}, a p53-stabilizing protein) are often altered. The p53 protein is a key responder to various stresses, including DNA damage, hypoxia, and cell cycle aberrations. Specific molecular pathways that activate p53 depend on the nature of the stress and the cell type. Consequently, these determine the specific downstream effectors and cellular response: apoptosis, growth arrest, or senescence.

It is widely believed that the central role of p53 in tumor suppression is to mediate the response to DNA damage. If p53 is missing when damage occurs, cells do not undergo p53-mediated arrest or apoptosis. Cells that have sustained mutations in oncogenes or tumor suppressor genes because of the damage obtain a growth advantage that fuels the development of cancer.

Apparently, DNA damage itself is not the critical event that leads to cancer, as long as the oncogenic stress pathways that activate p53 are intact. For any given cancer type, p53 dysfunction generally correlates with poor treatment response and poor prognosis; therefore restoration of p53 function is a potential avenue for therapeutic development. Drugs in development enhance the function of kinases that activate p53 in response to DNA damage.

ROLE OF ONCOGENES

The genetic targets of carcinogens are oncogenes. Oncogenes have been associated with various tumor types (e.g., HER-2/*neu* with breast, kidney, and ovarian cancer). Oncogenes are considered altered versions of normal genes. Over a lifetime, a variety of mutations can convert a normal gene into a malignant oncogene.

Once an oncogene is activated by mutation, it promotes excessive or inappropriate cell proliferation. Oncogenes have been detected in about 15% to 20% of a variety of human tumors and appear to be responsible for specifying many of the malignant traits of these cells. More than 30 distinct oncogenes, some of which are associated with specific tumor types, have been identified (Table 33-4). Each gene has the ability to evoke many of the phenotypes characteristic of cancer cells.

Major classes of oncogene products involved in the normal growth process of cells include the following:
- Growth factors (e.g., *sis* oncogene)
- Epidermal growth factor receptors (EGFRs)
- Membrane-associated protein kinases (e.g., *src* oncogene)
- Membrane-related guanine triphosphate (GTP)–binding proteins (e.g., *ras* oncogene)
- Cytoplasmic protein kinases (e.g., *ras* oncogene)
- Transcription regulators located in the nucleus (e.g., *c-myc* oncogene)

In addition, tumor suppressor genes (*antioncogenes*) are guardians of unregulated cell growth (e.g., p53, Rb oncogenes).

Mechanisms of Activation

Point mutations, translocations (e.g., t8; 142 in Burkitt's lymphoma) and gene amplification (multiple copies of the gene with overexpression of products) are mechanisms of activation, as follows:
- Overexpression of the c-erbB-2 (HER-2/*neu*) oncogene is noted in up to 34% of patients with invasive ductal breast carcinoma and predicts poor survival.
- Activation of the *ras* proto-oncogene (point mutation) is associated with about 30% of all human cancers. About 25% of patients with acute myelogenous leukemia display this point mutation. *Ras* is mutated frequently in colon and pancreatic cancers; it appears that *ras* activation leads to unregulated expression of IL-24 and its receptors.
- Translocation of the *abl* proto-oncogene from chromosome 9 to chromosome 22 with formation of a large *bcr-abl* hybrid gene on chromosome 22 (Philadelphia chromosome) results in chronic myelogenous leukemia.
- Inactivation of suppressor genes (point mutations) leads to unrestricted cell division; inactivation of each of the RB1 suppressor genes on chromosome 13 is associated with malignant retinoblastoma in children; inactivation of the p53 suppressor gene on chromosome 17 accounts for one fourth to half of all malignancies involving the colon, breast, lung, and central nervous system.

Viral Oncogenes

Various RNA and DNA viruses have been associated with human malignancies (Box 33-2). Some viral agents have a clear causative role, such as the Epstein-Barr virus and certain papillomaviruses, which are the etiologic agents in Burkitt's lymphoma and cervical carcinoma, respectively.

Table 33-4	Examples of Oncogenes Formed by Somatic Mutation of Normal Genetic Loci
Oncogene	**Disorder**
ab1	Chronic myelogenous leukemia
myc	Burkitt's lymphoma
N-*myc*	Neuroblastoma
EGFR, HER-2	Mammary carcinoma
Ras type	Wide variety of tumors

EGFR, Epidermal growth factor receptor; *HER-2,* human EGFR-2.

Box 33-2	Oncogenic Viruses

Ribonucleic acid: leukemia, carcinoma viruses, mammary tumor viruses

Deoxyribonucleic acid: herpesviruses, adenoviruses, papillomaviruses

Viruses carry viral oncogenes into target cells, where they become firmly established. Clonal descendants then carry the viral genes, which maintain the malignant phenotype of the cell clones.

Tumor-Suppressing Genes

A very different class of cancer genes has recently been discovered. These tumor-suppressing genes in normal cells appear to regulate the proliferation of cell growth. When this type of gene is inactivated, a block to proliferation is removed, and cells begin a program of deregulated growth, or the genetically depleted cell itself may proliferate uncontrollably. Thus, tumor-suppressing genes are referred to as **antioncogenes.** In time their discovery will lead to the reformulation of ideas about how the growth of normal cells is regulated.

Much speculation surrounds the operation of tumor-suppressing genes in normal tissue. It is known that normal cells exert a negative growth influence on each other within a tissue. Normal cells also secrete factors that are negative regulators of their own growth and that of adjacent cells. Diffusible factors may also be released by normal cells to induce the end-stage differentiation of other cells in the immediate environment. Such factors include the following:

- Interferon beta (IFN-β)
- Transforming (tumor) growth factor (TGF)
- Tumor necrosis factor (TNF)

Normal gene products appear to prevent malignant transformation in some way. It is speculated that normal cells must have receptors that detect the presence of these growth-inhibiting and differentiation-inducing factors, which allow them to process the signals of negative growth and respond with appropriate modulation of growth. Genes may specify proteins necessary to detect and respond to the negative regulators of growth. If this process becomes dysfunctional as a result of inactivation or the absence of a critical component, such as the loss of chromosomal loci, a cell may continue to respond to mitogenic stimulation but lose its ability to respond to negative feedback to cease proliferation. Animal experiments suggest that humans carry a repertoire of genes, each of which is involved in the negative regulation of the growth of specific cell types. Somatic inactivation of these genes may be involved in the initiation of tumor cell growth or the transformation of benign tumors into malignant ones. Therefore the somatic inactivation of tumor-suppressing genes may be as important to carcinogenesis as the somatic activation of oncogenes.

BODY DEFENSES AGAINST CANCER

Although no single satisfactory explanation exists for the success of tumors in escaping the immune rejection process, it is believed that early clones of neoplastic cells are eliminated by the immune response. The growth of malignant tumors is primarily determined by the proliferative capacity of the tumor cells and by the ability of these cells to invade host tissues and metastasize to distant sites. It is believed that malignant tumors are able to evade or overcome the mechanisms of host defenses (Plate 9).

Tumor immunity has the following general features:

1. Tumors express antigens that are recognized as foreign by the immune system of the tumor-bearing host.
2. The normal immune response frequently fails to prevent the growth of tumors.
3. The immune system can be stimulated to kill tumor cells and rid the host of the tumor.

Host defense mechanisms against tumors are both *humoral* and *cellular*. Effector mechanisms include the following:

- T lymphocytes
- Natural killer cells
- Macrophages
- Antibodies

T Lymphocytes

Cytolytic T lymphocytes (CTLs) provide effective antitumor immunity in vivo. CTL-mediated rejection of transplanted tumors is the only established example of completely effective specific antitumor immunity in vivo. Mononuclear cells derived from the inflammatory infiltrate in human solid tumors, called *tumor-infiltrating lymphocytes,* also include CTLs with the capacity to lyse the tumor from which they were derived. CD4+ T cells may play a role in antitumor responses by providing cytokines for effective CTL development.

Natural Killer Cells

Natural killer (NK) cells can be activated by direct recognition of tumors or as a consequence of cytokines produced by tumor-specific T lymphocytes. These cells use the same lytic mechanisms as CTLs to kill cells, but they do not express T-cell antigen receptors, and they have a broad range of specificities. Research is also focused on the role of IL-2–activated NK cells in tumor killing. These cells, referred to as *lymphokine-activated killer cells,* are derived in vitro by culture of peripheral blood cells or tumor-infiltrating lymphocytes from tumor patients with high doses of IL-2.

The NK cells may play a role in immunosurveillance against developing tumors, especially those expressing viral antigens.

Macrophages

Activated macrophages produce the cytokine **tumor necrosis factor.** As the name implies, TNF can kill tumors but not normal cells. TNF kills tumors by direct toxic effects and indirectly by effects on tumor vasculature.

Antibodies

Antibodies are probably less important than T lymphocytes in mediating the effect of antitumor immune responses, but tumor-bearing hosts do produce antibodies against various tumor antigens. These serve as tumor markers.

Although malignant tumors may express protein antigens that are recognized as foreign by the tumor host, and despite the fact that immunosurveillance may limit the outgrowth of some tumors, the immune system often does not prevent the occurrence of cancer. The simplest explanation is that the rapid growth and spread of a tumor overwhelm the effector mechanisms of immune response.

TUMOR MARKERS

In tumor immunology, a fundamental tenet is that when a normal cell is transformed into a malignant cell, it develops unique antigens not normally present on the mature normal cell. Tumors frequently produce **tumor-specific antigens (TSAs)** to which the host may develop antibodies. Virus-induced cancers are the most antigenic; chemical-induced cancers are the least antigenic.

Tumor markers are substances present in or produced by tumors that can be used to detect the presence of cancer based on measurement in body fluids, cells, or tissue (Table 33-5). A tumor marker may be produced by the host in response to a tumor that can be used to differentiate a tumor from normal tissue or to determine the presence of a tumor. Nonneoplastic conditions can also exhibit tumor marker activity (Table 33-6). Some tumor markers are used to screen for cancer, but markers are more often used to monitor recurrence of cancer or to determine the degree of tumor burden in the patient. To be

of any practical use, the tumor marker must be able to reveal the presence of the tumor while it is still susceptible to destructive treatment by surgical or other means. Tumor markers can be measured quantitatively in tissues and body fluids using biochemical, immunochemical, or molecular tests (Table 33-7).

The search for tumor markers goes back more than 150 years. The earliest identified tumor marker was Bence Jones protein, a light-chain immunoglobulin, found in patients with multiple myeloma (see Chapter 27). Over the last decade, use of tumor markers in the United States has risen dramatically. Tumor markers play an especially important role in the diagnosis and monitoring of patients with prostate, breast, and bladder cancers.

Older, well-established markers include alkaline phosphatase and collagen-type markers in bone cancer, immunoglobulins in myeloma, catecholamines and their derivatives in neuroblastoma and pheochromocytoma, and serotonin metabolites in carcinoid. In addition, there are many breast tissue prognostic markers (e.g., hormone receptors, cathepsin-D, HER/*neu* oncogenes, plasminogen receptors and inhibitors). The list of tumor markers approved by the U.S. Food and Drug Administration (FDA) continues to grow (Table 33-8). Multiple-marker combinations are useful in the management of some cancers (Table 33-9), but the use of more than two markers is questionable.

Table 33-5	Common Biochemical Tumor Markers in Use	
Type of Molecule	**Tumor Marker**	**Type of Cancer Detected**
Enzyme	Prostate-specific antigen (PSA)	Prostate
Oncofetal proteins	Alpha-fetoprotein (AFP)	Hepatocellular/germ cell
	Carcinoembryonic antigen (CEA)	Colorectal
Hormones	Human chorionic gonadotropin (hCG)	Trophoblastic
	Calcitonin	Medullary thyroid
	Adrenocorticotropic hormone (ACTH)	Small cell lung
Mucins	CA 125, CA 19-9	Ovarian
	CA 27.29, CA 15-3	Breast
Immunoglobulins	Bence Jones protein	Multiple myeloma
Other proteins	Nuclear matrix protein 22 (NMP-22)	
	Bladder tumor–associated antigen (BTA)/complement factor H–related protein (CFHrp).	

Modified from Snyder J: *Adv Med Lab Prof* 16(22):44, 2004.

Table 33-6	Nonneoplastic Conditions with Elevated Serum/Plasma Concentrations of Tumor Markers	
Tumor Marker	**Concentration in Normal Serum**	**Nonneoplastic Conditions**
Carcinoembryonic antigen (CEA)	<2.5 ng/mL	Inflammatory bowel disease, pancreatitis, gastritis, smoker's chronic bronchitis, alcoholic liver disease, hepatitis
Alpha-fetoprotein (AFP)	<40 ng/mL	Pregnancy, regenerating liver tissue after viral hepatitis, chemically induced liver necrosis, partial hepatectomy, cystic fibrosis, ataxia-telangiectasia, premature infants, tyrosinemia
Beta subunit of human chorionic gonadotropin (β-hCG)	Negative	Pregnancy
Serum acid phosphatase	Negative	Pregnancy
Placental alkaline phosphatase	Negative	Pregnancy

Table 33-7	Tumor Markers in Neoplasms
Tumor Markers	**Clinical Value**
Carcinoembryonic antigen (CEA)	Monitors response to therapy of patients with various types of cancer
Alpha$_1$-fetoprotein	Diagnosis of germ cell and hepatic tumors
CA 125	Diagnosis of ovarian cancer
Beta subunit of chorionic gonadotropin (β-hCG)	Diagnosis of germ cell tumors
Prostate acid phosphatase	Diagnosis of prostate cancer

Categories of Tumor Antigens

Tumor cells manifest tumor antigens, as well as "self" HLA antigens. The four types of identified tumor antigens are as follows:

1. Tumor-specific antigens on chemically induced tumors
2. Tumor-associated antigens on virally induced tumors
3. Carcinofetal antigens
4. Spontaneous tumor antigens

Tumor-Specific Antigens

Chemically induced tumors are known to develop TSAs, which are uniquely associated with each tumor. These antigens are not found in normal cells. TSAs demonstrate little or no cross-reactivity between different tumors caused by the same carcinogen, perhaps because every tumor caused by chemical agents has unique surface characteristics.

Tumor-Associated Antigens

Tumor-associated antigens (TAAs) are cell surface molecules coded for by tumorigenic viruses. These antigens are not expressed on the virion but are synthesized by the host cell. In contrast to TSAs, TAAs are virus specific. Therefore, each specific virus induces the same antigens regardless of the tissue of origin or the animal species.

Carcinofetal Antigens

Well-differentiated tissue produces and secretes little or no fetal gene products. The abnormal behavior of malignant cells is believed to derepress genes normally expressed only during fetal life. Because the products of these fetally active

Table 33-8	Examples of Serum Markers				
Type of Cancer	**AFP**	**CEA**	**β-hCG**	**Neuronal Enolase**	**Other Hormones**
Adrenocortical	—	—	—	—	+
Breast	—	+	—	—	—
Choriocarcinoma	—	—	+	—	+
Colorectal	Rare	+	—	—	—
Esophageal	—	+	—	—	+
Gastric	Rare	+	—	—	—
Ovarian	—	Rare	—	—	+
Pancreatic	Rare	+	—	—	Rare
Parathyroid	—	—	—	+	+
Pheochromocytoma	—	—	—	+	+
Pulmonary (oat-cell)	—	—	+	+	+
Pulmonary (squamous)	—	+	+	—	+
Seminoma	—	—	—	—	—
Teratocarcinoma	+	—	+	—	—
Thyroid (colloid)	—	—	—	—	+
Thyroid (medullary)	—	—	—	+	+

Table 33-9	Applications of Tumor Markers
Markers	**Comments**
AFP and β-hCG	Valuable combination in therapy and follow-up in patients with germ cell tumors of the testes.
CEA, AFP, and LDH	Combination seems to help differentiate primary liver cancer from liver metastases related to another organ.
Ratio of free to total PSA	The ratio may distinguish benign prostatic hypertrophy (BPH) from prostate cancer.
CEA and numerous mucin-type markers	Combinations are being evaluated and compared for breast cancer applications (the markers are not necessarily useful as adjuncts to therapy, but may complement each other).
TAG-72, CEA, and CA 19-9	Evaluated for use in gastric cancer, but the combination offered no improvement in sensitivity over TAG-72 alone.
Serial assays of CA-125	Serial assays over a finite period of time may aid in initial diagnosis in ovarian cancer.

From Schwartz MK: New approaches to tumor marker testing. In *Tumor markers: challenges and solutions,* Washington DC, 1998, American Association for Clinical Chemistry.
AFP, Alpha-fetoprotein; *β-hCG,* beta subunit of chorionic gonadotropin; *CEA,* carcinoembryonic antigen; *LDH,* lactate dehydrogenase; *PSA,* prostate-specific antigen.

genes are recognized as self, they do not elicit either humoral responses or cell-mediated responses.

During malignant transformation, however, gene derepression is responsible for the production of increased concentrations of these gene products, which are known as *oncofetal proteins.* CEA is an example of a carcinofetal antigen.

Spontaneous Tumor Antigens

Tumors caused by no known mechanism are thought to produce antigens. Disagreement exists regarding whether these tumors are similar to those produced experimentally by chemical, viral, or physical agents. Although substantial evidence supports the contention that these tumors do not produce unique antigens, some evidence refutes this contention. The importance of these findings remains unclear.

Specific Tumor Markers

Specific tumor markers include the following:
- Alpha-fetoprotein (AFP)
- Beta subunit of human chorionic gonadotropin (β-hCG)
- CA 15-3
- CA 19-9
- CA 27.29
- CA 125
- Carcinoembryonic antigen (CEA)
- Prostate-specific antigen (PSA) and prostatic acid phosphatase
- Miscellaneous enzyme markers
- Miscellaneous hormone markers

Alpha-Fetoprotein

Alpha-fetoprotein is normally synthesized by the fetal liver and yolk sac. AFP is secreted in the serum in nanogram to milligram quantities in hepatocarcinoma, endodermal sinus tumors, nonseminomatous testicular cancer, teratocarcinoma of the testis or ovary, and malignant tumors of the mediastinum and sacrococcyx. In addition, a small percentage of patients with gastric and pancreatic cancer with liver metastasis may have elevated AFP levels. Both AFP and β-hCG should be quantitated initially in all patients with teratocarcinoma because one or both markers may be secreted in 85% of patients. The concentration of AFP may be elevated in nonneoplastic conditions such as hepatitis and cystic fibrosis.

Alpha-fetoprotein is a reliable marker for following a patient's response to chemotherapy and radiation therapy. Levels should be obtained every 2 to 4 weeks (metabolic half-life in vivo, 4 days).

Beta Subunit of Human Chorionic Gonadotropin

Beta-hCG, an ectopic protein, is a sensitive tumor marker with a metabolic half-life in vivo of 16 hours. A serum level of β-hCG greater than 1 ng/mL is strongly suggestive of pregnancy or a malignant tumor such as endodermal sinus tumor, teratocarcinoma, choriocarcinoma, molar pregnancy, testicular embryonal carcinoma, or oat cell carcinoma of the lung.

CA 15-3

CA 15-3 is a high-molecular-weight glycoprotein coded by the MUC-II gene and expressed on the ductal cell surface of most glandular epithelial cells. The main purpose of the assay is to monitor patients after mastectomy. Using a cutoff of 25 U/mL for CA 15-3, the detection rate is only 5% for stage I breast cancer. The sensitivity is much better in higher-stage disease, which makes it a good measure of tumor burden. CA 15-3 is positive in other conditions, including liver disease, some inflammatory conditions, and other carcinomas. A change in the CA 15-3 concentration is more predictive than the absolute concentration. Over time, tumor markers exhibit a steady state in the body, a balance between antigen production by the tumor and degradation and excretion. Changes in tumor burden are reflected by changes in the tumor marker concentration.

CA 19-9

CA 19-9 is a glycolipid, Lewis blood group carbohydrate. Elevated levels have been found in patients with pancreatic, hepatobiliary, colorectal, gastric, hepatocellular, pancreatic, and breast cancers. Its main use is as a marker for colorectal and pancreatic carcinoma. This marker has greater specificity for pancreatic cancers than CEA. CA 19-9 is also known as *gastrointestinal cancer–associated antigen.*

CA 27.29 (Breast Carcinoma–Associated Antigen)

Carcinoma of the breast often produces mucinous antigens that are high-molecular-weight glycoproteins with O-linked oligosaccharide chains. Monoclonal antibodies (MAbs) directed against breast carcinoma–associated antigen (CA 27.29) are available to quantitate the levels of this antigen in serum. The antibodies recognize epitopes of a breast cancer–associated antigen encoded by the human *MUC1* gene, which is also referred to as MAM6, milk mucin antigen, CA 27.29, and CA 15-3. This tumor marker may be useful in conjunction with other clinical methods for predicting early recurrence of breast cancer. It is not recommended as a breast cancer screening assay. Increased levels of CA 27.29 (>38 U/mL) may indicate recurrent disease in a woman with treated breast carcinoma and may indicate the need for additional testing or procedures. Some clinical investigators do not endorse the routine use of this new marker.

CA 125

CA 125, a mucinlike glycoprotein, is expressed on the surface of coelomic epithelium and human ovarian carcinoma cells. CA 125 is relatively more sensitive in low-stage ovarian cancer. It reacts against an MAb developed against a cell line from one patient's ovarian cystadenocarcinoma. It is elevated in carcinomas and benign disease of various organs (e.g., pelvic inflammatory disease, endometriosis), but it is most useful in ovarian and endometrial carcinomas.

Carcinoembryonic Antigen

The cell surface protein CEA is found predominantly on normal fetal endocrine tissues in the second trimester of gestation. If CEA is detected in mature individuals, it is of limited diagnostic value, but it is helpful in differentiating between benign and malignant pleural and ascites effusions. CEA was first described in 1965 as a tumor marker specifically elevated in patients with colon cancer; it was later found to be elevated in patients with breast, lung, liver, and pancreatic cancer. Plasma levels greater than 12 ng/mL are strongly correlated with malignancy. Elevated neoplastic states frequently associated with an increased CEA level are endodermally derived gastrointestinal neoplasms and neck and breast carcinomas. Also, 20% of smokers and 7% of former smokers have elevated CEA levels.

Carcinoembryonic antigen is used clinically to monitor tumor progress in patients who have diagnosed cancer with a high blood CEA level. If treatment leads to a decline to normal levels (<2.5 ng/mL), a rise in CEA may indicate a cancer recurrence to the clinician. A persistent elevation is indicative of residual disease or poor therapeutic response. In patients who have undergone colon cancer resection surgery, the rate of clearance of CEA levels usually return to normal within 1 month, but may take as long as 4 months. Blood specimens should be obtained 2 to 4 weeks apart to detect a trend.

Prostate-Specific Antigen and Prostatic Acid Phosphatase

Prostate cancer is a leading cause of cancer death in American men. There are two tumor markers for cancer of the prostate: PSA and prostatic acid phosphatase. PSA is a prostate tissue–specific marker, but not a prostate cancer–specific marker. PSA is a protease enzyme secreted almost exclusively by prostatic epithelial cells. Blood levels of PSA are increased when normal glandular structure is disrupted by benign or malignant tumor inflammation. Serum PSA is directly proportional to tumor volume, with a greater increase per unit volume of cancer compared with benign hyperplasia. Free PSA assists in distinguishing cancer of the prostate from benign prostatic hypertrophy (BPH). PSA levels appear useful for monitoring progression and response to treatment in patients with prostate cancer.

Other techniques that have been used in detection of prostate cancer include *PSA velocity* (incremental increase of PSA over time), PSA density (ratio of serum PSA to prostate volume), age-adjusted PSA (PSA increasing with age), biostatistically derived algorithms, free and total PSA, complexed PSA, and most recently, human kallikrein II, a molecule similar, but not identical, to PSA.

Prostatic acid phosphatase is another marker for prostate cancer. It is a serum enzyme exclusively diagnostic of prostatic carcinoma.

Isoforms of PSA represent the next generation of prostate cancer detection. An alternative marker is hK2. It is also elevated in the serum of men with prostate cancers. Another marker, early prostate cancer antigen-2 (EPCA-2) can specifically identify prostate cancer and distinguish aggressive from non-aggressive disease. These newer PSA-based screening assays will also be helpful in diagnosis and monitoring treatment. (See later PSA Rapid Test in Seminal Fluid.)

Miscellaneous Enzyme Markers

Lactic dehydrogenase (LDH) is the frequently measured enzyme of the glycolytic pathway. LDH is elevated in a wide variety of malignancies and other medical disorders. The level of LDH has been shown to correlate to tumor mass in solid tumors so it can be used to monitor progression of these tumors.

Neuron-specific enolase is an isoenzyme specific for all tumor cells derived from the neural crest. An enzyme increase has been detected in neuroblastoma, pheochromocytoma, oat cell carcinomas, medullary thyroid and C cell parathyroid carcinomas, and other neural crest–derived cancers. Serum levels are frequently elevated in disseminated disease.

Placental alkaline phosphatase (ALP) can be detected during pregnancy. ALA is also associated with the neoplastic conditions of seminoma and ovarian cancer.

Miscellaneous Hormone Markers

Elevated or inappropriate serum levels of hormones can function as tumor markers. Adrenocorticotropic hormone (ACTH), calcitonin, and catecholamines may be secreted by differentiated tumors of endocrine organs and squamous cell lung tumors. Oat cell carcinomas may produce β-hCG, antidiuretic hormone (ADH), serotonin, calcitonin, parathyroid hormone (PTH), and ACTH. These hormones can be used to follow a patient's response to therapy.

In addition, some breast cancers demonstrate progesterone and estradiol (estrogen) receptors, which are strongly correlated with a positive response to antihormone therapy. Patients with neuroblastoma and pheochromocytoma secrete catecholamine metabolites that can be detected in the urine. Neuroblastomas also release neuron-specific enolase and ferritin; these markers can be used for diagnosis and prognosis.

Breast, Ovarian, and Cervical Cancer Markers

For more than a decade, circulating breast cancer antigens have been used to monitor therapy and evaluate recurrence of the cancer. Estrogen and progesterone receptors are universally accepted as both prognostic markers and therapeutic choice indicators. A relatively new approach has been the use of the oncogene HER-2/*neu* as a prognostic indicator and a marker related to the choice of therapy. This has been particularly useful since the introduction of Herceptin as a chemotherapeutic agent that targets the HER-2/*neu* receptor. Breast cancer patients who express HER-2 in their cancers have a poor prognosis with shorter disease-free and overall survival than patients who do not express HER-2/*neu*. The evaluation of HER-2/*neu* has two clinical functions: (1) a predictive marker for response to Herceptin (trastuzamab) therapy and (2) a prognostic marker.

A new and more powerful predictor of the outcome of primary breast cancer in young women recently was reported. Microarray analysis of a previously established 70-gene profile demonstrated that a good-prognosis gene-expression signature was a strongly independent factor in predicting disease outcome.

Epidermal Growth Factor Receptor

Epidermal growth factor receptor (EGFR) and human epidermal growth factor receptor-2 (HER-2, HER-2/*neu*, or c-erB-2) are both transmembrane tyrosine kinase receptors expressed on normal epithelial cells but overexpressed in some cancer cells. A portion of both receptors is released from the cell surface and circulates in normal people and in abnormally high levels in cancer patients. The shed portions can be measured in serum or plasma using antibody-based immunoassays. These assays allow real-time assessment of the patient's HER-2/*neu* or EGFR status and repeat testing for patient monitoring and can be performed in a standardized and quantitative manner.

HER-2 and EGFR have been the targets of considerable pharmaceutical activity to develop therapies that will interfere with the oncogenic potential of these growth factor receptors. The therapies include small-molecule inhibitors that are designed to target and block the function of HER-2 protein overexpression. One drug, trastuzumab (Herceptin) is a humanized antibody that targets cells that overexpress the HER-2/*neu* and has been successfully used in combination with chemotherapy to increase the efficacy of the antibody-based treatment. An anti-ECFR antibody known as IMC-225 is directed against cells that overexpress the EGFR oncoprotein.

Molecular Diagnosis of Breast Cancer

The assessment of DNA content (aneuploid, diploid) and cell cycle analysis (G0G1, S, G2, M) can be of prognostic use in certain solid tumors (e.g., breast cancer). Cell cycle analysis can be performed on fresh or frozen tissue. In breast cancer, research indicates that low S-phase and diploid DNA content are associated with a relatively good prognosis; a high S-phase number of cells and aneuploid DNA content have a tendency to indicate a worse prognosis. The DNA content of a tumor is classified in order of worsening prognosis from diploid, near-diploid, tetraploid, aneuploid, hypertetraploid, and hypoploid. The ratio of tumor G0G1 DNA content to normal G0G1 DNA content is called the **DNA index.** Ploidy status and S-phase fraction should be combined with other indicators (e.g., hormone receptor status) to evaluate treatment options and prognosis.

Bladder Cancer

Bladder cancer tumor markers for the management of patients with bladder cancer have been actively investigated. Assays approved for clinical use include the following:
- Matritech nuclear matrix protein (NMP-22)
- Bard's BTA test

Almost all human tumors contain **telomerase,** a growth enzyme that promotes the malignant proliferation of cancer. Normal cells usually do not have the enzyme, but telomerase renews the DNA of tumor cells and permits indefinite replication.

Telomerase was first observed in ovarian cancer cells, and its presence was later established in virtually all cancers. It is not clear whether other vital cells need telomerase to function. For example, telomerase inhibition could adversely affect stem cells, which help produce blood cells and lymphocytes and may need the enzyme to function. Second, telomerase inhibition has not been proved or tested physiologically in the human system. Finally, a drug based on telomerase would have to reduce the ability of the cancer to spread. Screening for telomerase inhibitors and plans for future studies to discover and develop chemicals that block the action of telomerase may suggest a design of more effective anticancer drugs.

Monocyte Chemotactic Protein

Serum levels of a newer marker, monocyte chemotactic protein-1 (MCP-1) have been found to be helpful before and after vaccination with a HER-2/*neu* E75 peptide plus granulocyte-macrophage colony-stimulating factor vaccine. Levels of serum MCP-1 greater than 250 pg/mL correlated with favorable prognostic variables in breast cancer.

DNA MICROARRAY TECHNOLOGY

New developments in molecular genetics involve DNA microarray technology (see Chapter 14). Cancer can arise not only from mutations in oncogenes and tumor suppressor genes, but also from genes involved in cell cycle control, DNA repair, and apoptosis. Microarrays have the potential to uncover signature gene-expression patterns for specific cancers and ultimately assist in the staging of tumors, prognosis, and treatment. Microarrays may help disclose global gene expression pattern differences between healthy and diseased cells as more sensitive and specific diagnostic markers are developed, such as CD44+/CD24− gene-expression profile in breast cancer versus normal breast tissue. When differentially expressed genes were used to generate a 186-gene "invasiveness" gene signature (IGS), the IGS was strongly associated with metastasis-free survival and overall survival for four different types of tumors.

Proteomic technology uses two-dimensional polyacrylamide gel electrophoresis (2D-PAGE) and mass spectrometry. Although these techniques are not revolutionary, recent advances have improved their sensitivity. Expansion of computer-assisted bioinformatics has simplified the process of protein identification from mass spectra. Mass spectra are proving to be comparable to CA 125 in the detection of early-stage ovarian cancer.

In colorectal cancer, fecal DNA screening has been demonstrated to be useful. Oncogene mutations that characterize colorectal neoplasia are detectable in exfoliated epithelial cells in the stool. Neoplastic bleeding is intermittent, but epithelial shedding is continual, potentially making fecal DNA testing more sensitive.

MODALITIES FOR TREATING CANCER

Many different modes of therapy, including *angiogenesis inhibitors,* which keep tumors from building new blood vessels to supply themselves with food and oxygen, have demonstrated effectiveness in the treatment of cancer (Table 33-10).

Chemotherapeutic Agents

Drugs are used in cancer therapy for curing, palliation, and research to develop more effective therapy. The mechanisms of drug action are linked to the mitotic cell cycle, and thus antitumor drugs may be placed in the following three classes:

- Cell cycle active, phase specific
- Cell cycle active, phase nonspecific
- Non–cell cycle active

Cell Cycle Active, Phase Specific

Drugs in the cell cycle–active, phase-specific category act on the S, G2, or M phase of mitosis.

S-phase–active drugs are divided into antimetabolites, antifols, and synthetic enzyme inhibitors. Antimetabolites act through the incorporation of nucleotide analog into DNA, resulting in an abnormal nucleic acid (e.g., 5-fluorouracil, 6-mercaptopurine, 6-thioguanine, fludarabine). The antifols act as competitive inhibitors of the enzyme dihydrofolate reductase, which is necessary for the generation of CH3 groups required for thymidine synthesis (e.g., methotrexate). Synthetic enzyme inhibitors include DNA polymerase inhibitor (cytosine arabinoside) and nucleotide reductase inhibitor (hydroxyurea).

G2-phase–active drugs include bleomycin, which is thought to cause fragmentation of DNA, and etoposide (Eposin, Etopophos, Vepesid, VP-16), which is thought to cause double-stranded breaks in DNA by complexing with topoisomerase.

M-phase–active drugs include vinca alkaloids (e.g., vincristine, vinblastine), which are thought to inhibit mitotic spindle apparatus, and paclitaxel (Taxol), which stabilizes microtubules.

Cell Cycle Active, Phase Nonspecific

Drugs in the cell cycle–active, phase-nonspecific category are intercalating agents, alkylating agents, or 5-fluorouracil. Examples of intercalating agents are anthracyclines (Adriamycin, Daunomycin, Idarubicin, Mitoxantrone) and actinomycin D (dactinomycin [Cosmegan, Lyovac]). The alkylating agents in this category include cyclophosphamide and ifosfamide. These drugs act by distorting normal DNA through the insertion of flat, aromatic ring systems between the levels of base pairs into the DNA double helix.

Non–Cell Cycle Active

Drugs in the non–cell cycle–active category can be divided into five types: alkylating agents, L-asparaginase, corticosteroids, hormone antagonists, and miscellaneous. *Alkylating agents* (e.g., nitrogen mustard and mustard derivatives: mechlorethamine [Mustargen], cyclophosphamide [Cytoxan], chlorambucil [Leukeran], and melphalan [Alkeran]) act by interstrand cross-linking of DNA, thereby preventing normal DNA replication. This interference is not only cytotoxic, but also potentially mutagenic and carcinogenic. L-Asparaginase inhibits protein synthesis.

Glucocorticosteroids are the most frequently used steroids. Steroids control the damaging inflammatory immune response. The target cells are monocytes and T lymphocytes. Monocytes block interleukin-1 (IL-1) production, block TNF-γ, and reduce chemotaxis. The consequences are inhibition of T-cell activation, activation and recruitment of monocytes and neutrophils, and inhibition of the migration of cells to the site of inflammation. The steroids used in cancer oncology include glucocorticoids (prednisone), estrogens (diethylstilbestrol), androgens (testosterone proprionate), and progestational agents (medroxyprogesterone, megestrol acetate).

Table 33-10	Immunotherapy in Malignant Disease	
Approach	**Agent**	**Proposed Mechanism**
Active		
Specific	Modified or unmodified tumor cells, cell extract	Cellular and/or humoral response
Nonspecific systemic	Bacille Calmette-Guérin (BCG)	General immunocompetence
	Methanol-extracted residue of mycobacterial skeletal wall, *Corynebacterium parvum, Pseudomonas* vaccine	Increased mononuclear phagocyte system activity
	Levamisole, interferon	Restores immunocompetence
Local	BCG	Macrophage activation; killing of tumor with bystander effect
	Virus, hapten, dinitrochlorobenzene	
Passive		
Adoptive specific	Allogeneic organogenesis antibody	Removes soluble antigen or directly kills target cell
	Targeted monoclonal antibody	Conjugated with antitumor drug or radioisotope
	Lymphocytes, lymphocyte extract (i.e., immune RNA transfer factor)	Transfer of immunity
	Lymphokine-activated killer cells	Cytolysis of tumor cells

Table 33-11	Effects of Chemotherapy on the Immune Response			
	Antibody		Delayed Hypersensitivity	
	Primary Response	Secondary Response	Primary Response (Initial)	Secondary Response (Recall)
Corticosteroid	0	0	++	+
Methotrexate	++	+	+	0
6-Mercaptopurine	0	+	+	0
Azathioprine	0	+	+	0
6-Thioguanine	0	+	+	0
Cytosine arabinoside	+	++	0	0
Cyclophosphamide	++	0	+	0
L-asparaginase	+	0	0	0
Daunomycin	+	0	+	0

Hormone antagonists (e.g., tamoxifen) competitively bind to specific cytoplasmic receptors.

Cytokines

Cytokines constitute another group of cancer chemotherapy drugs (see Chapter 5). Interferon (IFN), interleukin-2 (IL-2), and colony-stimulating factors (CSFs) are being used to treat certain types of cancer in patients. Currently, IFNs are being used to treat patients with hairy cell leukemia, chromic myelogenous leukemia, and multiple myeloma. IL-2 is being used in the treatment of renal cell carcinoma and melanoma. CSFs decrease the duration of chemotherapy-induced neutropenia and may permit more dose-intensive therapy.

Interferon. The clinical development of recombinant IFN-α represents the most rapid development of any antineoplastic drug in the United States. IFN was first recognized as a naturally occurring antiviral substance in 1957 and identified for its antineoplastic properties. IFN-α appears to have activity in a wide range of malignancies.

Effects of Drug-Induced Immunosuppression

Drugs used to treat malignancies such as solid tumors or leukemia can have profoundly suppressive effects on the inflammatory response, delayed hypersensitivity, and specific antibody production (Table 33-11). Examples of the immune depression induced by drugs include depletion of T cells by corticosteroids, caused by the blocking of egress from the bone marrow into the circulation, and dysfunction of the antibody response caused by folate antagonists and purine analogs. For this reason, infection secondary to immune suppression is a major cause of death in cancer patients beginning therapy and those who are in clinical remission.

Recent Advances

Immunotherapy for tumors can take the form of active or passive therapy. *Active* host immune responses may be achieved by the following:
- Vaccination with killed tumor cells or with tumor antigens or peptides.

- Enhancement of cell-mediated immunity to tumors by expressing costimulators and cytokines and treating with cytokines that stimulate the proliferation and differentiation of T lymphocytes and NK cells.
- Nonspecific stimulation of the immune system by the local administration of inflammatory substances or by systemic treatment with agents that function as polyclonal activators of lymphocytes.
- For the first time in history of cancer treatment, gene therapy has apparently succeeded in shrinking and even eradicating large, metastatic tumors. Inserting genes into a patient's cells enables the body to fight a disease on its own without medication.

Passive immunotherapy consists of the following:
- Adoptive cellular therapy by transferring cultured immune cells with antitumor reactivity into a tumor-bearing host.
- Administration of tumor-specific MAbs for specific tumor immunotherapy.

What's New in Drug Therapy?

The list of drugs used for cancer therapy continues to grow. The website www.phrma.org lists 402 experimental drugs. The new therapeutic agents target various modes of action and applications (Table 33-12).

Table 33-12	Newer Therapeutic Agents	
Drug	Mode of Action	Application
Herceptin	Antigrowth; latches onto HER-2 receptor	Breast cancer
Rituximab	Monoclonal antibody, targeted cell membrane protein	Non-Hodgkin's lymphoma
Campath	Targeted cell destruction	Chronic lymphocytic leukemia
Gleevec	Antigrowth	Chronic myelogenous leukemia

Prostate-Specific Antigen (PSA) Rapid Test in Seminal Fluid

Principle

The principle of this test is the rapid, semiquantitative determination of PSA in seminal fluid by chromatographic immunoassay (CIA). Two monoclonal murine anti-PSA antibodies are active compounds. One of these antibodies is immobilized at the test region on the membrane. PSA at the sample will bind to the remobilized gold-labeled antibody and form a PSA-gold-antibody–labeled PSA-antibody complex. If a specimen contains PSA, the PSA-gold-antibody–labeled PSA-antibody complex will bind to the immobilized monoclonal antibody (MAb) of the test result region that recognizes another epitope on the PSA molecule, sandwich complex). The binding produces an additional third colored line on the fiber pad.

Specimen Collection and Preparation

Use Standard Precautions when handling seminal fluid specimens and performing the assay.
1. Seminal fluid should be diluted at least 1:500 before use because of its extremely high PSA concentration.
2. Use distilled water or standard buffer solutions at a neutral pH range (e.g., tris-buffered saline).
3. Semen stains or swabs can be extracted with buffer by incubating them on a shaker for 2 hours at 4° C. The PSA-containing supernatant is removed, briefly centrifuged for 3 minutes at 13,000 g, and if necessary, diluted. It is used as the sample for the test. Particles of tissue do not interfere with the test result.

Note: High viscosity of a sample might interfere with the capillary flow of the procedure.

Reagents, Supplies, and Equipment

The SeraTec PSA SemiQuant test kit contains 40 individually sealed tests per box, plastic pipettes, and one user instruction leaflet. Do not open pouch until ready to perform the assay.

A timer is required but not provided with the kit.

The test is stable up to the date of expiration printed on the sealed pouch. Tests can be stored at room temperature or refrigerated (4°-30° C). The test must remain unopened in the sealed pouch until use. Discard test if the pouch has been damaged or improperly stored.

Quality Control

The upstream control region and the region of the internal standard (between the control and test region) contain immobilized polyclonal goat antimouse antibodies. Through the capillary effect of the membrane, the reaction mixture of gold-antibody–labeled PSA-antibody complex will bind to the antimouse antibody at the control region and the region of the internal standard, thus developing two red lines (one at the control region; one at the region of the internal standard).

These two lines are independent of the existence of PSA in the sample and indicate only the correct performance of the test. The amount of antibody at the internal standard is adjusted to a color intensity of the line, which is equal to the color intensity of the test line at the PSA concentration of 4 ng/mL.

If the sample contains high amounts of PSA, it is possible that the color intensity of the test specimen can be weak.

Procedure

1. The test sample as well as the test device should be warmed up to room temperature before testing.
2. Remove the test device from the protective pouch, and label the device for specimen identification.
3. Add 5 drops (~200 μL) in the sample well. Retain the remaining specimen if additional testing (additional dilution) is necessary.
4. Observe the test reaction after 10 minutes of incubation at room temperature. No remaining fluid should be observed at this point.
5. An estimate of the amount of PSA can be made by comparison with the internal standard at exactly 10 minutes.

Reporting Results

Positive: Three colored lines in the result window.
Negative: Two colored lines in the result window; indicates no PSA in the probe, or PSA concentration below detection limit.

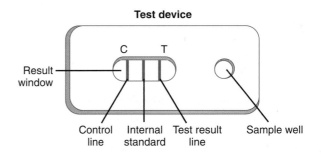

Test device

Test Device

Test result (T) reflects PSA concentration of the sample, visible in PSA-positive sample only.
- It may be helpful to compare the color the test line to the color of the 4-ng/mL internal standard.

Internal standard color intensity correlates with a concentration of approximately 4 ng/mL PSA.

Control line (C) control is for possible procedural errors and for the integrity of test components.
- If the internal standard line and/or the control line (C) is/are absent, the test result is invalid. Repeat the test with a new cassette.

Note: The upstream control region and the region of the internal standard (between the control and test region) contain immobilized polyclonal goat antimouse antibodies. A glass-fiber pad downstream of the membrane is used for sample loading and transmission to a second fiber pad with the dried and bold-labeled second monoclonal murine anti-PSA antibody.

Clinical Applications

Prostate-specific antigen is a glycoprotein produced in the prostate and secreted into the seminal fluid. PSA is one of the major proteins in seminal fluid, with concentrations of 0.2 to 3.0 mg/mL. Its main function is to liquefy the seminal fluid. PSA is an interesting marker in forensic science for the detection of even small amounts of seminal fluid; it is found at very low concentrations in vaginal fluid. PSA is a more specific than the acid phosphatase test.

Limitations

This assay is limited to seminal fluid.

Reference

SeraTec PSA SemiQuant package insert, Goettingen, Germany, 2005.

CASE STUDY

L.L., a 59-year-old Caucasian man, visited his primary care provider because of his need to urinate frequently and urgently. Over the last several years, his urine output had been in small volumes with a decreasing flow rate.

On physical examination, the patient had an enlarged prostate with a smooth, uniform surface. A PSA assay was ordered.

PSA Assay	Patient Result	Reference Range
Current (ng/mL)	5.5	0-3.5
1 year ago (ng/mL)	2.3	0-3.5

Questions and Discussion

1. Is the change in the patient's PSA results in 1 year significant?

The reference range of PSA increases with age and is age dependent. This patient's results were within range 1 year ago but are now above the reference range. The current results suggest the presence of a prostatic tumor.

2. What is the clinical significance of the patient's results?

The annual increase of PSA is defined as the *PSA velocity*. A rise in the PSA value greater than 0.7 ng/mL per year or an increase of greater than 20% per year is indicative of cancer.[1]

Some scientists believe that PSA results between 2 and 10 ng/mL are too insensitive and nonspecific to distinguish between BPH and prostate cancer, does not diagnose prostate cancer, and cannot distinguish between indolent and aggressive prostate cancer.

A number of new assays have been introduced to aid in the interpretation of PSA results between 4 and 10 ng/mL in determining whether a biopsy of the prostate should be performed. Free PSA and complexed PSA are two such assays. Free-PSA/PSA ratio can be determined. Other suggested biomarkers are isoforms of PSA and (-2)pPSA. Genomic and proteonomic approaches include transcriptional profiling on microarrays.[2]

3. What is the expected follow-up regimen for a patient with this profile?

A biopsy of multiple sites of the prostate would be a common follow-up procedure. In this case, specimens were obtained from six sites. Three of these sites revealed prostatic adenocarcinoma. A bone scan also was performed. No metastasis to the bone was seen. The patient subsequently underwent a radical prostatectomy.

4. After a radical prostatectomy, what PSA values would be expected?

No prostate tissue should remain after a radical prostatectomy. Because no PSA is produced after a radical prostatectomy, the laboratory results of a PSA assay should be 0 ng/mL. If the patient's postoperative PSA is above 0.1 ng/mL, this is considered to be reliable evidence of the persistence of the malignant tumor.

Diagnosis

Prostatic adenocarcinoma.

References

1. Rittenhouse-Diakun K: Clinical immunology No CI-4 2000, Tech Sample, *Am Soc Clin Pathol*, 2000, pp 23-27.
2. O'Kane DJ: Biomarkers for prostate cancer, *Adv Med Lab Prof* 14(12)18-20, 2002.

CASE STUDY

M.S., a 65-year-old African-American woman, visited her primary care provider for an annual examination, including a routine pelvic examination. Although she had gained some weight since her last examination, she reported that her general health was good, but that she had been experiencing some gastrointestinal problems over the last 6 weeks.

A palpable mass was discovered during her pelvic examination. A CA 125 assay and a transvaginal ultrasound examination were ordered.

The patient's CA 125 was 425 U/mL (reference range, <35 U/mL). The presence of a mass in the right side of the abdomen and abdominal ascites were confirmed.

The patient had a total abdominal hysterectomy with bilateral salpingo-oophorectomy; 4 weeks after operation, she began a chemotherapy series. The patient was judged to be in remission for 6 months when recurrence of the tumor was noted with diagnostic imaging. Subsequent chemotherapy was ineffective, and the patient died 8 months later.

Questions and Discussion

1. Is CA 125 an effective diagnostic blood serum tumor marker?

CA 125 is considered to be the best serum marker for ovarian cancer. About 50% of women in the earliest localized stage (stage I) of the disease exhibit an elevated level of this cancer antigen. The majority of patients with advanced ovarian cancer demonstrate elevated levels of CA 125.

2. Is CA 125 a specific tumor marker for ovarian cancer?

CA 125 is a useful component in the initial preoperative diagnosis of ovarian cancer, but it is not specific for ovarian cancer. Elevated levels can be demonstrated in various malignancies:

- Breast
- Lung
- Colon
- Pancreas
- Liver

Elevated levels of CA 125 can be observed in benign gynecologic conditions:

- Uterine fibroids
- Ovarian cysts
- Endometriosis

3. What is the major clinical use of CA 125?

The major clinical application of CA 125 is in postoperative monitoring of patients with a confirmed diagnosis of ovarian cancer. Declining levels correlate well with a positive response to chemotherapy and accompanying reduction in tumor mass. A rise in the level of CA 125 is a reliable indicator of disease recurrence.

Diagnosis

Ovarian cancer.

CHAPTER HIGHLIGHTS

- Tumors are neoplasms described as benign or malignant. A benign neoplasm is a nonspreading tumor; a malignant neoplasm is a growth that infiltrates tissues, metastasizes, and often recurs after attempts to remove it surgically.
- A malignant neoplasm can be referred to as carcinoma or cancer.
- The incidence of cancer has been correlated with certain environmental factors (occupational exposure to known carcinogenic agents) and host susceptibility.
- Cancer often begins when a carcinogenic agent damages the DNA of a critical gene in a cell. The mutant cell multiplies, and the succeeding generations of cells aggregate to form a malignant tumor.
- Proto-oncogenes act as central regulators of the growth in normal cells and are antecedents of oncogenes.
- The genetic targets of carcinogens, oncogenes have been associated with various tumor types, largely from preexisting genes present in the normal human genome. Oncogenes are considered altered versions of normal genes that promote excessive or inappropriate cell proliferation.
- Various RNA and DNA viruses have been associated with human malignancies (Epstein-Barr virus, certain papillomaviruses).
- Viruses carry viral oncogenes into target cells, where they become firmly established. Clonal descendants then carry the viral genes, which maintain the malignant phenotype of the cell clones.
- A very different class of cancer genes was discovered recently. Tumor-suppressing genes (antioncogenes) in normal cells appear to regulate the proliferation of cell growth. When this type of gene is inactivated, a block to proliferation is removed and cells begin a program of deregulated growth, or the genetically depleted cell itself may proliferate uncontrollably.
- No single satisfactory explanation exists for the success of tumors in escaping the immune rejection process. It is believed that early clones of neoplastic cells are eliminated by the immune response.
- Cells rather than immunoglobulins are believed to dominate tumor immunity.
- Four types of identified tumor antigens are tumor-specific antigens on chemically induced tumors, tumor-associated antigens on virally induced tumors, carcinofetal antigens, and spontaneous tumor antigens.
- A tumor marker is a characteristic of a neoplastic cell that can be detected in plasma or serum. Markers may be useful in diagnosis and selection of different treatment approaches, monitoring therapies, or prognoses.
- Tumor markers include CEA, AFP, β-hCG, neuron-specific enolase, prostatic acid phosphatase, and placental alkaline phosphatase.
- Various modalities are used to treat cancer. In addition to the classic therapies, new therapies (e.g., monoclonal antibodies) are being used.

REVIEW QUESTIONS

1. Benign tumors are characterized as:
   a. Growing slowly.
   b. Resembling the parent tissue.
   c. Usually invading tissues (metastasizing).
   d. Both a and b.

Questions 2-5. Match the following.

2. _____ Benign tumor arising from glands.

3. _____ Benign tumor arising from epithelial surfaces.

4. _____ Malignant tumor of connective tissue.

5. _____ Malignant tumor of glandular epithelium (e.g., colon).
   a. Sarcoma
   b. Adenoma
   c. Adenocarcinoma
   d. Papillomas

6. Which of the following factors is *not* a risk factor in the development of cancer?
   a. Smoking
   b. Low-fat diet
   c. Obesity
   d. Sedentary lifestyle

7. Risk factors associated with breast cancer include:
   a. First-degree family history of breast cancer.
   b. Pregnancy after 30 years of age.
   c. Use of estrogen (oral contraceptives or hormone replacement).
   d. All the above.

Questions 8-10. Indicate true statements with the letter "A," and false statements with the letter "B."

8. _____ Antibodies dominate body defenses against cancer.

9. _____ Tumors express antigens that can be recognized as foreign by the immune system of the tumor-bearing host.

10. _____ The normal immune response frequently fails to prevent the growth of tumors.

11. The cells involved in the immune response to tumors are:
    a. T lymphocytes, B lymphocytes, and macrophages.
    b. Cytotoxic T lymphocytes, NK cells, and macrophages.
    c. Neutrophils, lymphocytes, and monocytes.
    d. CD8+ lymphocytes, monocytes, and basophils.

12. Which of the following is *not* an environmental factor associated with carcinogenesis?
    a. Ultraviolet light
    b. Organically grown herbs
    c. Benzene
    d. Asbestos

13. The risk factor associated with the development of basal cell carcinoma or malignant melanoma is:
    a. Infrared light.
    b. Sunless tanning lotions.
    c. Ultraviolet light.
    d. Strobe lights.

14. Patients with Down syndrome have a higher incidence of:
    a. Leukemia.
    b. Breast cancer.
    c. Prostate cancer.
    d. Teratomas.

15. Tumor cells typically carry _____ genetic change(s).
    a. one
    b. two
    c. three to six
    d. multiple

16. Cancer-predisposing genes may:
    a. Affect a host's ability to repair damage to DNA.
    b. Increase cell cohesiveness.
    c. Decrease cell motility.
    d. Enhance the host's immune ability to recognize and eradicate incipient tumors.

17. Oncogenes are:
    a. Genetic targets of carcinogens.
    b. Altered versions of normal genes.
    c. Detectable in 15% to 20% of a variety of human tumors.
    d. All the above.

Questions 18 and 19. Match the following definitions.

18. _____ Mutation or overexpression of oncogenes

19. _____ Mutation or overexpression of tumor suppressor genes
    a. Results in the production of nonfunctional proteins that can no longer control cell proliferation.
    b. Produces proteins that can stimulate uncontrolled cell growth.

20. Which of the following is used to determine the risk of developing cancer?
    a. p53 gene
    b. c-erbB-2 gene
    c. Squamous cell carcinoma antigen
    d. Epidermal growth factor receptor (EGFR)

21. A tumor marker assay is most useful:
    a. To screen patients for malignancies.
    b. To monitor a cancer patient for disease recurrence.
    c. To determine the degree of tumor burden.
    d. All the above.

Questions 22-24. Match the following.

22. _____ Tumor-specific antigens

23. _____ Tumor-associated antigens

24. _____ Carcinofetal antigens

    a. Cell surface molecules coded for by tumorogenic viruses.
    b. Gene products resulting from gene derepression.
    c. Antigens uniquely related to each tumor.
    d. Probably do not produce unique antigens.

25. Which of the following tumor markers is classified as a tumor suppressor gene?
    a. BRCA1
    b. Carcinoembryonic antigen (CEA)
    c. Human chorionic gonadotropin (hCG)
    d. Nuclear matrix protein

25. Carcinoembryonic antigen is:
    a. An oncofetal protein, elevated in some types of cancer, found on normal fetal endocrine tissue in the last trimester of gestation.
    b. An oncofetal protein, strongly correlated with various malignancies, found on normal fetal endocrine tissue in the second trimester of gestation.
    c. Used clinically to monitor tumor progress in some type of patients, persistently elevated even in residual disease or poor therapeutic response.
    d. An alpha-fetoprotein, elevated in 20% of smokers, a cell surface protein found on normal epithelial tissue.

26. Alpha-fetoprotein (AFP):
    a. Is synthesized by the fetal liver and yolk sac.
    b. Can be elevated in some nonneoplastic conditions.
    c. Is a very reliable marker for monitoring a patient's response to chemotherapy and radiation therapy.
    d. All the above.

27. β-hCG is *not:*
    a. Elevated in normal pregnancy.
    b. A sensitive tumor marker.
    c. Elevated in squamous cell carcinoma of the lung.
    d. Elevated in teratocarcinoma and choriocarcinoma.

28. Prostate-specific antigen is:
    a. Prostate tissue specific.
    b. Prostate cancer specific.
    c. Not useful for monitoring response to therapy among patients with prostate cancer.
    d. Not proportional to tumor volume directly in prostate malignancies.

Questions 29-33. Match the following tumor markers and applications.

29. _____ CEA

30. _____ AFP

31. _____ CA 125

32. _____ CA 19-9

33. _____ CA 27-29

    a. Frequently elevated in endometrially derived gastrointestinal neoplasms.
    b. Most useful in ovarian and endometrial carcinomas.
    c. Increased levels may indicate recurrent breast carcinoma.
    d. May be elevated in patients with gastrointestinal malignancies.
    e. Should be quantitated with β-hCG initially in all patients with teratocarcinoma.

34. Which tumor marker is used to monitor patients with breast cancer for recurrence of disease?
    a. CA 15-3
    b. Estrogen receptor (ER)
    c. Cathepsin-D
    d. CA 50

Questions 35-38. Match an example of a therapeutic intervention with the appropriate mode of action (an answer may be used more than once).

35. _____ 6-Mercaptopurine

36. _____ Corticosteroids

37. _____ Alkylating agents or 5-fluorouracil

38. _____ Vinca alkaloids

    a. Cell cycle active, phase specific
    b. Cell cycle active, phase nonspecific
    c. Non–cell cycle active
    d. Hormone antagonist

39. Tamoxifen acts as a _____ pharmaceutical agent.
    a. cell cycle–active, phase-specific
    b. non–cell cycle active
    c. estrogen receptor–blocking
    d. both b and c

40. Active host immunotherapy responses may be achieved by:
    a. Transferring immune cells into host.
    b. Vaccination with killed tumor cells.
    c. Administration of tumor-specific MAbs.
    d. Administration of IFN-α.

Questions 41-45. Match the environmental factors and associated cancers.

41. _____ Benzene   a. Endometrial cancer

42. _____ Estrogen   b. Hepatocellular carcinoma

43. _____ Epstein-Barr   c. Burkitt's lymphoma virus

44. _____ Hepatitis B   d. Leukemia

45. _____ Asbestos   e. Mesothelioma

BIBLIOGRAPHY

Brugarolas J: Renal-cell carcinoma: molecular pathways and therapies, *N Engl J Med* 356(2):185-187, 2007.

Calle EE et al: Organochlorines and breast cancer risk, *CA Cancer J Clin* 52:301-307, 2002.

Carney WP, Williams J: HER-2/neu and EGFR oncoprotein expression in breast, ovarian and cervical cancers, *Adv Med Lab Prof* 13(13):18-20, 2001.

Check W: BRCA: what we now know, *CAP Today* 20(9):1, 78, 80-85, 2006.

Cohen HT, McGovern FJ: Renal cell carcinoma, *N Engl J Med* 353(23):2477-2490, 2005.

Delgado JC et al: Standardization of carcinoembryonic antigen testing in the setting of clinical laboratory consolidation, *Lab Med* 32:2, 2001.

Diamandis EP: Oncopeptidomics: a useful approach for cancer diagnosis? *Clin Chem* 53(6):1004-1006, 2007.

Eyre HJ, editor: News briefs, *CA Cancer J Clin* 52(5):248-251, 2002.

Friend SH, Dryja TP, Weinberg RA: Oncogenes and tumor-suppressing genes, *N Engl J Med* 318(10):618-623, 1988.

Gander TR et al: Driving forces in cancer diagnostics, *Med Lab Observer* 35(1):10-16, 2003.

Herbst RS, Lippman SM: Molecular signatures of lung cancer, *N Engl J Med* 356(1):76-78, 2007.

Holloway TL: Protein sustains cancer cells, *Adv Med Lab Prof* 14(8):12, 2002.

Holloway TL: Clinical clips: Scientists find possible origin of colon cancer, *Adv Med Lab Prof* 14(1):9, 2002.

Howlett NG et al: *Science,* June 13, 2002 (10.1126/science. 1073834).

Jenal A et al: Cancer statistics, 2007, *CA Cancer J Clin* 57(1):43-66, 2007.

Jordan CT, Guzman ML, Noble M: Cancer stem cells, *N Engl J Med* 35(12):1253-1260, 2006.

Karp JE, Broder S: Oncology, *JAMA* 270(2):237-240, 1993.

Kiluk J, Carter WB: Markers of angiogenesis in breast cancer, *Med Lab Observer* 38(8):10, 12, 16, 2006.

Krontiris TG: Molecular medicine: oncogenes, *N Engl J Med* 333(5):303-306, 1995.

Leavelle DE: *Interpretive data for diagnostic laboratory tests,* Rochester, Minn, 1997, Mayo Medical Laboratories.

Liu R et al: The prognostic role of a gene signature from tumorigenic breast-cancer cells, *N Engl J Med* 356(3):217-226, 2007.

Loeb S, Catalona WJ: PSA isoforms: the next generation of prostate cancer detection, *Clin Lab News* 33(3):12-13, 2007.

Lopez MF et al: A novel, high-throughput workflow for discovery and identification of serum carrier protein-bound peptide biomarker candidates in ovarian cancer samples, *Clin Chem* 53(6):1067-1074, 2007.

MabThera (Rituximab) product monograph. Hertfordshire, UK, 2004.

Mehltretter S: Clinical cytogenetics, *Adv Med Lab Prof* 7(13):6-9, 20, 1995.

Oeffinger KC, Hudson MM: Long-term complications following childhood and adolescent cancer: foundations for providing risk-based health care for survivors, *CA Cancer J Clin* 54(4):237, 2004.

Pennisi E: Tumor suppressor's structure revealed, *Sci News* 146(3):36, 1994.

Plaut D: Unraveling the complexities of cancer, *Adv Med Lab Prof* 18:36-44, 2006.

Schwartz RS: Jumping genes and the immunoglobulin V gene system, *N Engl J Med* 333(1):42-44, 1995.

Snyder J: Genomic, proteomic developments in tumor markers, *Adv Med Lab Prof* 16(22):42-48, 2004.

Thorn SH, Negrin RS, Contqg CH: Synergistic antitumor effects of immune cell–viral biotherapy, *Science* 311:1780-1784, 2006.

Van deVijuer MJ et al: A gene-expression signature as a predictor of survival in breast cancer, *N Engl J Med* 347:1999-2009, 2002.

Van Dyke T: p53 and tumor suppression, *N Engl J Med* 356(1):79-81, 2007.

Weiss RL, editor: *Guide to molecular diagnostics clinical laboratory testing,* Salt Lake City, Utah, 2001, Associated Regional and University Pathologists.

Witt E, Ashworth A: D-Day for BRCA2, June 2002, www.sciencexpress.org.

Woeste S: Diagnosing prostate cancer, *Lab Med* 36(7):399, 2005.

Woolf SH: A smarter strategy? Reflections on fecal DNA screening for colorectal cancer, *N Engl J Med* 351(26):2755-2758, 2005.

Wu JT: *Circulating tumor markers of the new millennium,* Washington, DC, 2002, AACC Press.

APPENDIX A

Answers to Review Questions

CHAPTER 1: AN OVERVIEW OF IMMUNOLOGY

1. e	8. b	15. a	22. a
2. a	9. d	16. a	23. a
3. b	10. b	17. a	24. c
4. c	11. c	18. b	25. a
5. d	12. d	19. b	26. b
6. c	13. c	20. b	
7. a	14. b	21. b	

CHAPTER 2: ANTIGENS AND ANTIBODIES

1. b	14. d	27. d	40. b
2. a	15. c	28. b	41. a
3. d	16. b	29. d	42. d
4. d	17. a	30. b	43. c
5. d	18. c	31. d	44. a
6. c	19. b	32. b	45. b
7. a	20. c	33. c	46. d
8. d	21. a	34. a	47. c
9. b	22. d	35. a	48. d
10. e	23. d	36. e	49. b
11. b	24. b	37. c	50. d
12. e	25. c	38. b	
13. a	26. a	39. d	

CHAPTER 3: CELLS AND CELLULAR ACTIVITIES OF THE IMMUNE SYSTEM: GRANULOCYTES AND MONONUCLEAR CELLS

1. c	11. b	21. b	31. d
2. d	12. c	22. a	32. c
3. a	13. b	23. c	33. b
4. b	14. d	24. d	34. b
5. d	15. c	25. b	35. d
6. d	16. a	26. d	36. a
7. a	17. a	27. a	37. b
8. d	18. c	28. c	38. d
9. a	19. a	29. c	39. a
10. e	20. b	30. c	40. c

CHAPTER 4: CELLS AND CELLULAR ACTIVITIES OF THE IMMUNE SYSTEM: LYMPHOCYTES AND PLASMA CELLS

1. b	15. d	29. d	43. a
2. c	16. a	30. b	44. d
3. d	17. c	31. d	45. c
4. b	18. c	32. d	46. b
5. d	19. c	33. b	47. b
6. a	20. d	34. d	48. c
7. c	21. b	35. a	49. c
8. b	22. b	36. b	50. b
9. c	23. c	37. b	51. c
10. a	24. a	38. a	52. a
11. c	25. c	39. c	53. d
12. a	26. c	40. d	
13. d	27. d	41. c	
14. b	28. b	42. b	

CHAPTER 5: SOLUBLE MEDIATORS OF THE IMMUNE SYSTEM

1. d	20. c	39. d	58. d
2. d	21. d	40. d	59. c
3. a	22. a	41. a	60. a
4. a	23. d	42. c	61. a
5. b	24. b	43. b	62. b
6. a	25. a	44. c	63. a
7. c	26. c	45. a	64. b
8. d	27. d	46. b	65. c
9. b	28. b	47. d	66. a
10. c	29. a	48. a	67. d
11. a	30. d	49. d	68. d
12. b	31. c	50. c	69. d
13. a	32. c	51. b	70. d
14. c	33. d	52. d	71. b
15. a	34. b	53. a	72. a
16. a	35. a	54. b	73. c
17. a	36. b	55. c	
18. a	37. a	56. a	
19. b	38. c	57. b	

CHAPTER 6: SAFETY IN THE IMMUNOLOGY-SEROLOGY LABORATORY

1. d	5. c	9. a	13. d
2. d	6. b	10. d	14. d
3. d	7. a	11. b	
4. a	8. a	12. b	

CHAPTER 7: QUALITY ASSURANCE AND QUALITY CONTROL

1. b	6. b	11. a	16. a
2. a	7. b	12. b	17. c
3. c	8. c	13. a	18. a
4. a	9. a	14. c	19. d
5. a	10. b	15. c	20. b

CHAPTER 8: BASIC SEROLOGIC LABORATORY TECHNIQUES

1. c	5. c	9. d	13. b
2. d	6. a	10. c	14. d
3. c	7. a	11. a	
4. d	8. d	12. b	

CHAPTER 9: POINT-OF-CARE TESTING

1. a	5. a
2. a	6. a
3. a	7. a
4. a	

CHAPTER 10: AGGLUTINATION METHODS

1. d	9. c	17. d	25. d
2. c	10. a	18. b	26. c
3. d	11. c	19. a	27. a
4. b	12. b	20. d	28. b
5. c	13. a	21. c	29. a
6. c	14. c	22. d	30. c
7. b	15. e	23. a	
8. d	16. d	24. b	

CHAPTER 11: ELECTROPHORESIS TECHNIQUES

1. c	5. a	9. b	13. d
2. d	6. b	10. d	14. a
3. c	7. a	11. d	15. d
4. b	8. a	12. c	16. a

CHAPTER 12: LABELING TECHNIQUES IN IMMUNOASSAY

1. d	5. a	9. a	13. a
2. a	6. b	10. c	14. b
3. b	7. b	11. b	15. c
4. d	8. c	12. a	16. d

CHAPTER 13: AUTOMATED PROCEDURES

1. b	4. c	7. b	10. b
2. c	5. a	8. a	11. d
3. b	6. b	9. c	12. d

CHAPTER 14: MOLECULAR TECHNIQUES

1. a	4. d	7. a	10. b
2. d	5. a	8. c	11. b
3. c	6. b	9. a	12. b

CHAPTER 15: THE IMMUNE RESPONSE IN INFECTIOUS DISEASES

1. d	7. c	13. a	19. c
2. b	8. d	14. d	20. a
3. d	9. c	15. c	21. b
4. a	10. b	16. d	22. c
5. c	11. c	17. d	23. a
6. a	12. a	18. a	24. b

CHAPTER 16: A PRIMER ON VACCINES

1. b	5. a	9. c	13. b
2. b	6. a	10. d	14. a
3. d	7. b	11. b	15. c
4. d	8. a	12. e	

CHAPTER 17: STREPTOCOCCAL INFECTIONS

1. b	6. b	11. c	16. c
2. a	7. d	12. a	17. b
3. d	8. a	13. b	18. b
4. b	9. b	14. b	19. b
5. a	10. d	15. a	20. c

CHAPTER 18: SYPHILIS

1. b	7. a	13. d	19. c
2. d	8. b	14. b	20. d
3. a	9. b	15. b	21. d
4. c	10. a	16. b	
5. c	11. a	17. b	
6. e	12. b	18. c	

CHAPTER 19: VECTOR-BORNE DISEASES

1. d	9. b	17. c	25. b
2. d	10. b	18. d	26. c
3. b	11. c	19. a	27. c
4. c	12. d	20. d	28. a
5. b	13. d	21. c	29. d
6. b	14. a	22. a	30. a
7. a	15. b	23. c	31. a
8. b	16. d	24. b	32. d

CHAPTER 20: TOXOPLASMOSIS

1. c	4. b	7. b
2. d	5. b	8. c
3. d	6. a	9. a

CHAPTER 21: CYTOMEGALOVIRUS

1. d	7. a	13. c	19. a
2. d	8. c	14. a	20. a
3. b	9. b	15. c	21. b
4. d	10. a	16. c	22. a
5. b	11. d	17. b	23. d
6. c	12. b	18. d	24. b

CHAPTER 22: INFECTIOUS MONONUCLEOSIS

1. d	6. d	11. c	16. a
2. b	7. d	12. b	17. b
3. b	8. d	13. c	
4. c	9. a	14. c	
5. d	10. c	15. c	

CHAPTER 23: VIRAL HEPATITIS

1. b	15. a	29. b	43. a
2. a	16. e	30. a	44. d
3. c	17. c	31. b	45. c
4. d	18. b	32. d	46. d
5. d	19. d	33. c	47. b
6. a	20. b	34. b	48. a
7. c	21. d	35. a	49. b
8. b	22. c	36. c	50. c
9. a	23. a	37. a	51. a
10. d	24. b	38. a	52. d
11. b	25. d	39. a	53. c
12. c	26. b	40. a	
13. d	27. a	41. b	
14. b	28. b	42. b	

CHAPTER 24: RUBELLA INFECTION

1. c	5. b	9. d	13. d
2. a	6. c	10. a	
3. d	7. c	11. a	
4. a	8. d	12. b	

CHAPTER 25: ACQUIRED IMMUNODEFICIENCY SYNDROME

1. b	8. d	15. e	22. b
2. b	9. c	16. b	23. c
3. d	10. c	17. c	24. d
4. d	11. a	18. c	25. b
5. c	12. b	19. a	26. c
6. b	13. d	20. b	27. b
7. c	14. a	21. d	28. a

CHAPTER 26: HYPERSENSITIVITY REACTIONS

1. d	8. d	15. d	22. d
2. a	9. b	16. b	23. d
3. c	10. b	17. c	24. d
4. b	11. c	18. a	25. d
5. d	12. a	19. a	
6. d	13. b	20. d	
7. d	14. a	21. b	

CHAPTER 27: IMMUNOPROLIFERATIVE DISORDERS

1. c	6. d	11. a	16. d
2. d	7. d	12. d	17. b
3. d	8. c	13. a	18. b
4. d	9. d	14. b	
5. c	10. c	15. a	

CHAPTER 28: AUTOIMMUNE DISORDERS

1. c	12. d	23. b	34. c
2. d	13. b	24. c	35. c
3. a	14. c	25. d	36. b
4. b	15. e	26. a	37. b
5. b	16. d	27. a	38. b
6. e	17. b	28. d	39. b
7. c	18. a	29. b	40. b
8. d	19. a	30. c	41. b
9. e	20. b	31. c	
10. a	21. a	32. d	
11. c	22. d	33. c	

CHAPTER 29: SYSTEMIC LUPUS ERYTHEMATOSUS

1. c	6. d	11. d	16. c
2. b	7. d	12. b	17. a
3. d	8. d	13. d	18. c
4. a	9. a	14. b	
5. c	10. d	15. a	

CHAPTER 30: RHEUMATOID ARTHRITIS

1. c	5. b	9. c	13. a
2. a	6. a	10. b	14. b
3. c	7. b	11. d	15. d
4. b	8. a	12. b	16. c

CHAPTER 31: SOLID ORGAN TRANSPLANTATION

1. b	7. c	13. a	19. c
2. a	8. e	14. a	20. b
3. c	9. d	15. c	21. b
4. d	10. d	16. b	22. d
5. b	11. d	17. d	23. b
6. a	12. b	18. a	24. c

CHAPTER 32: BONE MARROW TRANSPLANTATION

1. d	5. c	9. d	13. c
2. a	6. b	10. a	14. a
3. b	7. d	11. d	15. a
4. a	8. c	12. a	

CHAPTER 33: TUMOR IMMUNOLOGY

1. d	13. c	25. b	37. b
2. b	14. a	26. d	38. a
3. d	15. d	27. c	39. d
4. a	16. a	28. a	40. b
5. c	17. b	29. a	41. d
6. b	18. a	30. e	42. a
7. d	19. b	31. b	43. c
8. b	20. a	32. d	44. b
9. a	21. d	33. c	45. e
10. a	22. c	34. a	
11. b	23. a	35. a	
12. b	24. b	36. c	

Acetylcholine Receptor (AChR) Antibodies: Three types of AChR antibodies exist: binding, blocking, and modulating.

Components	Reference Interval
AChR-binding antibody	Negative: 0.0-0.4 nmol/L Positive: ≥0.5 nmol/L
AChR-blocking antibody	Negative: 0-15% blocking Indeterminate: 16%-24% blocking Positive: ≥25% blocking
AChR-modulating antibody	Negative: 0-20% modulation Indeterminate: 21%-25% modulation Positive: ≥26% modulation

Approximately 10% to 15% of individuals with confirmed myasthenia gravis have no measurable binding, blocking, or modulating antibody.

Acetylcholine Receptor (AChR)–Binding Antibody: Binding antibody can activate complement and lead to loss of ACh receptors at neuromuscular junctions of skeletal muscle. Useful in the diagnosis of myasthenia gravis; 85% to 90% of patients with myasthenia gravis express AChR.

Negative in ocular myasthenia, Eaton-Lambert syndrome, and in generalized myasthenia gravis if treated or inactive.

Acetylcholine Receptor (AChR)–Blocking Antibody: Measures antibody to AChRs that block binding of ^{125}I-α-bungarotoxin. Blocking antibody may impair AChR binding to the receptor, leading to poor muscle contraction. Found in about one third of patients with myasthenia gravis.

Acetylcholine Receptor (AChR)–Modulating Antibody: Modulating antibody causes receptor endocytosis, resulting in loss of AChR expression, which correlates most closely with clinical severity of disease.

Adrenal Antibody: Measures antibody to adrenal cortex cells. High antibody titers are characteristic of autoimmune hypoadrenalism in about three fourths of cases but are not found in tuberculous Addison's disease.

Alpha-1-Antitrypsin: Measures the quantity of alpha-1-antitrypsin, an acute-phase inflammatory reactant, in the blood. A deficiency of this protein is found if the alleles Z and S are present; moderate reduction is exhibited by the MS, and MZ phenotypes are increased in chronic or recurrent anterior uveitis and rheumatoid arthritis. The MZ phenotype is also associated with hepatoma and chronic hepatitis in adults. The ZZ phenotype predisposes an individual to the development of severe, early-onset pulmonary emphysema and to liver disease in infancy and childhood.

Alpha-Fetoprotein (AFP): AFP is normally produced during fetal development by the liver and yolk sac, as well as in small amounts by the gastrointestinal (GI) tract. After birth, serum AFP levels in neonates drop rapidly, and by 6 months the blood levels are very low. In pregnant females, AFP levels begin to rise at 12 to 14 weeks and peak during the third trimester.

AFP is a valuable tumor marker. Principal tumors that secrete AFP are endodermal sinus tumor (yolk sac carcinoma), neuroblastoma, hepatoblastoma, and hepatocellular carcinoma. In patients with AFP-secreting tumors, serum levels of AFP often correlate with tumor size. Resection is usually associated with decreased AFP levels, and serum levels are useful in assessing response to treatment.

Increased AFP levels have been observed in patients with primary hepatocellular carcinoma, ataxia-telangiectasia, nonseminomatous testicular carcinomas, and ovarian carcinomas, as well as in other epithelial tumors, especially those of the GI tract. AFP is useful in the management of nonseminomatous testicular cancer patients when used with information from the clinical evaluation and other diagnostic procedures.

AFP is also increased in some benign (nonmalignant) hepatic diseases, such as acute viral hepatitis and chronic active hepatitis and cirrhosis. This result cannot be interpreted as absolute evidence of the presence or absence of malignant disease.

AFP Reference Interval

0-14 days	5000-105,000 ng/mL
15 days-30 days	300-60,000 ng/mL
1 month	100-10,000 ng/mL
2 months	40-1000 ng/mL
3 months	11-300 ng/mL
4 months	5-200 ng/mL
5 months	0-90 ng/mL
6 months and older	0-15 ng/mL
Adult males and nonpregnant females:	0-15 ng/mL

Note: Results obtained with different assay methods or kits cannot be used interchangeably.

Alpha-Fetoprotein (Cerebrospinal Fluid): Using the Roche Modular E170 AFP method, increased cerebrospinal fluid (CSF) AFP concentrations have been observed in ataxia-telangiectasia, hereditary tyrosinemia, primary hepatocellular carcinoma, teratocarcinoma, GI tract cancers with and without liver metastases, and benign hepatic conditions such as acute viral hepatitis, chronic active hepatitis, and cirrhosis. The result cannot be interpreted as absolute evidence of the presence or absence of malignant disease. The result is not interpretable as a tumor marker in pregnant females.

AFP is a valuable aid in the management of nonseminomatous testicular cancer patients, when used with information from the clinical evaluation and other diagnostic procedures. This test is approved by the U.S. Food and Drug Administration (FDA) but is not labeled for use with CSF. Results obtained with different assay methods or kits cannot be used interchangeably

ANA: See Antinuclear Antibody.

ANCA: See Antineutrophil Cytoplasmic Antibody.

Anticardiolipin Antibody: Measures antibody directed to cardiolipin. The presence of antibody in systemic lupus erythematosus (SLE) is associated with arterial and venous thromboses, and in patients with placental infarcts in early pregnancy with or without SLE. Elevation of anticardiolipin antibody may be predictive of the risk of thrombosis or recurrent spontaneous abortions of early pregnancy.

Anticentromere Antibody: Measures anticentromere (antikinetocore) to chromosomal centromeres. Most patients with *c*alcinosis, *R*aynaud's phenomena, *e*sophageal dysfunction, *s*clerodactyly, *t*elangiectasia (CREST) syndrome demonstrate these antibodies. These antibodies are seen in about one third of patients with Raynaud's disease and approximately 10% of patients with systemic sclerosis.

Anti–DNase B Antibody: High levels of neutralizing antibody to deoxyribonuclease B (DNase B) are typically found in patients after group A streptococcal infection. Because it persists longer than other streptococcal antibodies (2-3 months), DNase B antibody is the preferred test in patients with chorea suspected to be caused by rheumatic fever. Because it is not influenced by the site of infection, DNase B antibody is more reliable than the streptolysin O antibody test in providing evidence for streptococcal infection in patients with postimpetigo glomerulonephritis. Elevated titers strongly suggest recent or current infection with group A streptococci. Fourfold increases in titer between acute and convalescent samples taken approximately 2 weeks apart are confirmatory.

Anti-dsDNA Antibody: Measures antibody to double-stranded deoxyribonucleic acid (dsDNA). Increased amounts (>25% by membrane assay) and decreased quantities of the C4 complement component confirm the diagnosis of systemic lupus erythematosus (SLE). These tests are useful in monitoring the activity and exacerbations of SLE. The absence of anti-DNA is demonstrated in about one fourth of SLE patients; therefore a negative test does not rule out SLE.

Antigliadin Antibodies (IgA and IgG): Gliadin antibodies are immunoglobulin G (IgG) and IgA antibodies against a group of proteins found in the gluten of wheat and rye grains. The enzyme-linked immunosorbent assay (ELISA) for gliadin antibodies is a reliable screening test for the evaluation of asymptomatic celiac disease in prepubertal children with short stature. Celiac disease results from an intolerance to dietary gluten, resulting in small intestinal villous atrophy with subsequent malabsorption and malnutrition. In celiac disease, IgG antibodies are more sensitive than IgA antibodies, but IgA antibodies are more specific than IgG antibodies. The level of IgA antibodies decreases with a gluten-free diet. IgA and IgG antibodies rise significantly during gluten challenge, sometimes several months before clinical relapse.

Anti–Glomerular Basement Membrane Antibody: Measures the amount of antibody to glomerular basement membrane (anti-GBM). High titers are suggestive of Goodpasture's syndrome (anti-GBM antibody disease) or anti-GBM nephritis. The test is useful for monitoring anti-GBM nephritis. Negative results, however, do not rule out Goodpasture's syndrome.

Anti–Intrinsic Factor (Intrinsic Factor Antibody): Measures antibodies to intrinsic factor (IF). The presence of IF-blocking antibodies is diagnostic of pernicious anemia and occurs in about 60% of patients.

Anti–Islet Cell Antibody: Measures antibodies to the islet cells of the pancreas. This test is useful as an early marker of beta pancreatic cell destruction.

Anti-Jo-1 Antibody: Anti-Jo-1 antibody is found in patients with pure polymyositis, pure dermatomyositis, or myositis associated with another rheumatic disease or with interstitial lung disease.

Anti–Liver-Kidney Microsomal (LKM) Antibody: Measures antibodies to components of renal and hepatic microsomes. The presence of a high titer is diagnostic of hepatic illness and suggests aggressive disease.

Antimitochondrial (M2) Antibody: Measures antibodies to cellular ultrastructures, the mitochondria. A high titer strongly suggests primary biliary cirrhosis (PBC); the absence of mitochondrial antibodies is strong evidence against PBC. Other forms of liver disease frequently exhibit low mitochondrial antibody titers.

Antimyelin Antibody: Measures antibody to components of the myelin sheath of nerves of myelin basic protein. Antibodies to myelin are associated with multiple sclerosis (MS) or other neurologic diseases. Myelin antibodies are not detectable in the cerebrospinal fluid of MS patients.

Antimyocardial Antibody: Measures antibody to components of the myocardium. The presence of myocardial antibodies is diagnostic of Dressler's syndrome (cardiac injury) or rheumatic fever.

Anti–Native DNA: See Anti-dsDNA Antibody.

Antineutrophil Antibody: Circulating antibodies to neutrophils can mediate neutropenia in a number of different disorders (e.g., SLE, Felty's syndrome, drug-induced neutropenia). Isoimmune destruction of neutrophils also occurs in febrile transfusion reactions and in isoimmune neonatal neutropenia. Antineutrophil antibodies may include anti-HLA antibodies.

Antineutrophil Cytoplasmic Antibody: Antineutrophil cytoplasmic antibodies (ANCAs) are autoantibodies specific for neutrophil lysosomal enzymes, particularly for proteinase 3 and myeloperoxidase. ANCA antibodies have been subdivided into c-ANCA (cytoplasmic) and p-ANCA (perinuclear). The p-ANCA pattern mimics antinuclear antibodies (ANAs). This perinuclear pattern reverts to c-ANCA, however, on formalin-fixed neutrophils. In about 80% of cases, c-ANCA has specificity for proteinase 3 and p-ANCA for myeloperoxidase.

Antinuclear Antibody: Measures antibody to nuclear antigens. Antinuclear antibodies (ANAs) are found in 99% of patients with untreated systemic lupus erythematosus (SLE).

Anti–Nuclear Ribonucleoprotein Antibody: Measures an antinuclear antibody (ANA), nuclear ribonucleoprotein (anti-nRNP). A high titer of this antibody is characteristic of mixed connective tissue disease (MCTD) or undifferentiated connective tissue disease. In MCTD, anti-nRNP is found in the absence of various other ANAs. Low titers of anti-nRNP are seen in about one third of SLE patients and are typically found in association with other ANAs (e.g., anti-DNA, anti-Sm).

Anti–Parietal Cell Antibody: Measures antibody to parietal cells (large cells on margin of peptic glands of stomach). The majority (80%) of patients with pernicious anemia have parietal cell antibodies. In the presence of these antibodies, gastric biopsy almost always demonstrates gastritis. Low antibody titers to parietal cells are often found with no clinical evidence of pernicious anemia or atrophic gastritis and are sometimes seen in elderly patients.

Antiphospholipid Antibody: See Anticardiolipin Antibody.

Antiplatelet Antibody: Measures immunologically attached IgG on platelets. The presence of platelet antibodies, measured indirectly, is associated with immune thrombocytopenia and systemic lupus erythematosus (SLE).

Antireticulin Antibody: Measures antibody to reticulin, an albuminoid or scleroprotein substance present in the connective framework of reticular tissue. The majority (80%) of patients with childhood gluten-sensitive enteropathy demonstrate reticulin antibodies. These antibodies can also be found in dermatitis herpetiformis and adult gluten-sensitive enteropathy and in about one fifth of patients with chronic heroin addiction.

Anti–Rheumatoid Arthritis Nuclear Antigen (Anti-RANA) Antibody: Measures antibody to a component of the Epstein-Barr virus. Antibody is found in the majority of patients with rheumatoid arthritis and in about 15% of SLE patients. Anti-RANA is not useful in diagnosis or differential diagnosis of arthritis. Also called *rheumatoid arthritis precipitin* (RAP).

Antiribosome Antibody: Measures the presence of antibodies to cellular organelles, the ribosomes. Ribosomal antibodies are found in about 10% of SLE patients.

Antiscleroderma (Anti–Scl-70) Antibody: Measures an antibody to a basic nonhistone nuclear protein. The presence of anti-Scl is diagnostic of systemic sclerosis; however, it is demonstrable in only about one fifth of patients with systemic sclerosis.

Antiskin (Dermal-Epidermal) Antibody: Measures antibody to the basement membrane area of the skin. Anti-

bodies are present in more than 80% of patients with bullous pemphigoid, but the absence of antibodies does not rule out the disorder.

Anti-Smith (Anti-Sm) Antibody: Measures Sm (Smith) antibody to acidic nuclear protein. Sm antibody is demonstrated by about one third of patients with systemic lupus erythematosus (SLE). Presence of the antibody confirms the diagnosis of SLE, but the absence of antibody does not exclude the diagnosis.

Anti–Smooth Muscle Antibody: Measures antibody to components of smooth muscle. A high and persistent titer suggests the autoimmune form of chronic active hepatitis. Anti-smooth muscle antibodies are also seen in viral disorders such as infectious mononucleosis.

Antisperm Antibody: Evaluates the presence of reproductive cell, or sperm, antibodies. Half of vasectomized men and 40% of men and women with fertility problems demonstrate the antibody.

Anti–SS-A (SS-A Precipitin, Anti-Ro) Antibody: Detects the presence of antibody to acidic nucleoprotein of human spleen extract. SS-A precipitins are demonstrable in more than 70% of patients with Sjögren's syndrome–sicca complex and are often found in a subset of these patients at risk for vasculitis. The antibody is also found in one third of patients with SLE or Sjögren's syndrome–rheumatoid arthritis, or the annular variety of subacute cutaneous lupus erythematosus (LE). In neonatal LE, autoantibodies to SS-A, discoid skin lesions, and congenital heart blocks are common.

Anti–SS-B (SS-B Precipitin, Anti-La) Antibody: Detects antibody to acidic nucleoprotein thymus. Anti–SS-B is demonstrated by most patients with Sjögren's syndrome–SLE. Half to three fourths of patients with Sjögren's syndrome–sicca complex have the antibody; it is frequently found in a subset of these patients at risk for vasculitis.

Antistriational Antibody: Measures antibody to components of striated muscle. Antibodies to striated muscle may be detected in patients with myasthenia gravis or thymoma or those receiving penicillamine treatment. Absence of the antibody in patients with myasthenia gravis generally rules out the presence of thymoma.

Antithyroglobulin and Anti–Thyroid Microsome Antibody: Evaluates the presence of antibody to the thyroid components: thyroglobulin, an iodine-containing protein secreted by the thyroid gland and stored within its colloid substance; and thyroid microsomes, particles derived from the endoplasmic reticulum. The presence of microsome antibodies is considered predictive of an elevated thyroid-stimulating hormone (TSH) level. A positive thyroid antibody test and an elevated TSH titer are associated with a risk of hypothyroidism. Absence of both antibodies is strong evidence against autoimmune thyroiditis.

Beta-Glucuronidase: Measures the enzyme activity of the enzyme beta-glucuronidase in cerebrospinal fluid. Increased levels of enzyme activity are associated with bacterial or fungal meningitis; extremely elevated enzyme levels are encountered in untreated leptomeningeal (pia or arachnoid) metastases. Treated cases of leptomeningeal carcinoma may demonstrate decreased enzyme levels. Normal enzyme levels are usually seen in primary brain tumors and parenchymal metastases.

Beta–Human Chorionic Gonadotropin (β-hCG): Human chorionic gonadotropin (hCG) is found in normal concentration during pregnancy. It can also be a valuable aid in the management of cancer patients with trophoblastic tumors, nonseminomatous testicular tumors, and seminomas when used with information from the clinical evaluation and other diagnostic procedures. Increased serum hCG concentrations have also been observed in melanoma; carcinomas of the breast, gastrointestinal tract, lung, and ovaries; and in benign conditions, including cirrhosis, duodenal ulcer, and inflammatory bowel disease.

Beta-2-Microglobulin: Measures the quantity of β_2-microglobulin in either serum or cerebrospinal fluid (CSF). Elevated levels of this protein are associated with central nervous system (CNS) involvement in patients with leukemia or lymphoma. Determination of β_2-microglobulin levels in both serum and CSF are of value in the early diagnosis of CNS involvement and in monitoring intrathecal (within the spinal canal) therapy.

C1 Esterase Inhibitor (C1 Inhibitor): Measures the activity and/or concentration of C1 inhibitor in serum. A deficiency of this protein is characteristic of hereditary angioedema. Some patients demonstrate catalytically inactive protein.

C1q: Evaluates the complement component C1q in serum. Decreased levels can be demonstrated in patients with hypocomplementemic urticarial vasculitis, severe combined immunodeficiency, or X-linked hypogammaglobulinemia.

C1q Binding: Measures the binding of immune complexes containing IgG1, IgG2, IgG3, and/or IgM to the complement component C1q. High values of C1q binding are associated with circulating immune complexes that interact with the classic pathway of complement activation. This test can be useful as a prognostic tool at diagnosis and during remission of acute myelogenous leukemia.

C2: Measures the second component of complement. An extremely low level of C2 component is suggestive of a lupuslike disease that may be caused by a genetic deficiency associated with HLA-A25, B18, or DR2. Approximately half the individuals with decreased levels of C2 have autoimmune disease; the other half are apparently normal but have an increased susceptibility to bacterial infection.

C3: Measures the third component of complement. Extremely decreased levels are seen in patients with poststreptococcal glomerulonephritis or inherited (C3) complement deficiency. This component is also decreased in cases of severe liver disease and in patients with systemic lupus erythematosus who have renal disease.

C3b Inhibitor (C3b Inactivator): Measures the C3b component of complement. This component causes low complement C3 levels, the absence of C3PA in serum, and high C3b levels. A deficiency of C3b inhibitor is associated with an increased predisposition to infection.

C3PA (C3 Proactivator, Properdin Factor B): Evaluates the level of the factor B component, which is consumed by activation of the alternate complement pathway. Assessment of C3PA indicates whether a decreased level of C3 is caused by the classic or alternate pathways of complement activation. A decreased level of complement components C3 and C4 demonstrates activation of the classic pathway. Decreased levels of C3 and C3PA with a normal level of C4 indicate complement activation via the alternate pathway.

Activation of the classic pathway (sometimes with accompanying alternate pathway activation) is associated with disorders such as immune complex diseases, various forms of vasculitis, and acute glomerulonephritis.

Activation of the alternate pathway is associated with many disorders, including chronic hypocomplementemic glomerulonephritis, diffuse intravascular coagulation, septicemia, subacute bacterial endocarditis, paroxysmal nocturnal hemoglobinuria, and sickle cell anemia.

In systemic lupus erythematosus, both the classic and the alternate pathway are activated.

C4a: Measures the level of component C4 of the classic complement activation pathway. A decreased C4 level with elevated anti-DNA and ANA titers confirms the diagnosis of systemic lupus erythematosus (SLE) in a patient. In SLE patients the periodic assessment of C4 can be useful in monitoring the progress of the disorder. Patients with extremely low C4 and CH50 levels in the presence of normal levels of the C3 component may be demonstrating the effects of a genetic deficiency of C1 inhibitor or C4.

C4 Allotypes: Evaluate the antigenically distinct forms of C4A and C4B, alleles located on the sixth chromosome in the major histocompatibility complex. Identification of C4 allotypes in conjunction with specific HLA antigens is a marker for disease susceptibility.

C5b (C5b-9): Measures the concentration of the C5 complement component. A genetic deficiency of the C5 component is associated with increased susceptibility to bacterial infection and is expressed as an autoimmune disorder (e.g., SLE). In the case of dysfunction of C5 (Leiner's disease), the patient is predisposed to infections of the skin and bowel, and the disease is characterized by eczema. In such a patient the level of C5 is normal, but the C5 component fails to promote phagocytosis.

C6: Measures the level of the C6 complement component. A decreased quantity of C6 predisposes an individual to significant *Neisseria* infections.

C7: Measures the quantity of the C7 complement component. A decreased level of this component is associated with severe bacterial infections caused by *Neisseria* species, Raynaud's phenomenon, sclerodactyly, and telangiectasia.

C8: Measures the level of the C8 complement component. A decreased quantity of this component is associated with systemic lupus erythematosus. A deficiency of C8 makes patients highly susceptible to *Neisseria* infections.

CA 125: CA 125 assay is useful in monitoring the response to therapy for patients with epithelial ovarian cancer. Serial testing for patient CA 125 values should be used in conjunction with other clinical methods for monitoring ovarian cancer. Elevations may be observed in patients with nonmalignant disease. A CA 125 assay result should not be interpreted as absolute evidence of the presence or absence of malignant disease.

CA 15-3: CA 15-3 is used to aid in the management of stage II and III breast cancer patients. Serial testing for patient CA 15-3 assay values should be used in conjunction with other clinical methods for monitoring breast cancer. Patients with confirmed breast carcinoma frequently have CA 15-3 assay values in the same range as healthy individuals, and elevations may be observed in patients with nonmalignant disease. This assay should not be interpreted as absolute evidence of the presence or absence of malignant disease.

CA 19-9: CA 19-9 is useful in monitoring pancreatic, hepatobiliary, gastric, hepatocellular, and colorectal cancer. The CA 19-9 assay value should not be interpreted as absolute evidence of the presence or absence of malignant disease.

CA 27.29: The CA 27.29 assay is intended for use as an aid in monitoring patients previously treated for stage II or III breast cancer. Serial testing in patients who are clinically free of disease should be used in conjunction with other clinical methods used for the early detection of cancer recurrence. The test is also intended as an aid in the management of breast cancer patients with metastatic disease by monitoring the progression or regression of disease in response to treatment. Patients with confirmed breast carcinoma frequently have CA 27.29 levels within the reference interval. Elevated levels of CA 27.29 can be observed in patients with nonmalignant diseases. This assay cannot be interpreted as absolute evidence of the presence or absence of malignant disease and should always be used in conjunction with other diagnostic procedures, including information from the patient's clinical evaluation.

Carcinoembryonic Antigen (CEA): Detects the presence of CEA in cerebrospinal fluid (CSF). An increased level of CEA in CSF is very suggestive of primary or secondary intradural malignancy. The level of CEA may decline with effective therapy.

Cardiolipin Antibody: See Anticardiolipin Antibody.

Ceruloplasmin: Detects the level of the protein ceruloplasmin in blood. Although increased or decreased levels of this protein are associated with a variety of clinical conditions, a severely decreased or complete absence of ceruloplasmin can be demonstrated in most homozygous patients with Wilson's disease. The absence or gross deficiency of ceruloplasmin in heterozygous carriers of the gene responsible for Wilson's disease is rare.

Cold Agglutinins: Evaluate the ability of antibodies to agglutinate group O erythrocytes at 4° C. The presence of an elevated titer of cold-reacting antibodies can cause acrocyanosis or hemolysis. These antibodies can be demonstrated in patients with primary (chronic) or secondary cold-agglutinin syndromes caused by bacterial or viral disease (e.g., *Mycoplasma pneumoniae,* Epstein-Barr virus) or neoplasms (e.g., lymphoma, histiocytic lymphoma).

Complement-Activation Products: Measure the protein fragments of C3 and C4 to reflect in vivo or in vitro activation. In vivo activation of complement (e.g., immune complex diseases), or in vitro activation (e.g., complement degradation), causes proteolytic digestion of these components and altered electrophoretic mobility. Assessment of these components is not considered to be of reliable diagnostic value.

Complement Components (C1r, C1s, C2, C3, C4, C5, C6, C7, C8): Assess various components of complement. These components are often elevated in certain inflammatory conditions, acute illnesses such as myocardial infarction, trauma, and some infectious diseases, such as typhoid fever. Homozygous component deficiencies predispose an individual to autoimmune diseases such as systemic lupus erythematosus, chronic glomerulonephritis, infections, arthritis, and vasculitis. Determination of complement levels in synovial (joint) fluid is of value. Increased levels may be demonstrated in Reiter's syndrome; decreased levels (relative to plasma concentrations) may be observed in rheumatoid arthritis.

C-Reactive Protein: Assesses one of the acute-phase inflammatory proteins, C-reactive protein (CRP). CRP is increased in inflammatory conditions.

Cryofibrinogen: Evaluates cold-precipitable fibrinogen and similar plasma proteins. The presence of cryofibrinogen suggests primary or secondary disorders. Secondary disorders include acute and chronic inflammation, lymphoproliferative and connective tissue disorders, necrosis, and tumors.

Cryoglobulins: Detect the presence of cold-precipitable immunoglobulins in serum. The major types of cryoglobulins and associated conditions include the following:

- Monoclonal IgM, IgG, or IgA without known antibody specificity, or monoclonal Bence Jones protein, associated with disorders such as Raynaud's phenomenon, myeloma, and macroglobulinemia.
- Monoclonal IgM, IgG, or IgA antibodies directed against polyclonal IgG associated with disorders such as Sjögren's syndrome, lymphoproliferative disorders, purpura, vasculitis, and macroglobulinemia.
- Mixed (usually IgM and IgG) polyclonal immunoglobulins associated with disorders such as Sjögren's syndrome, systemic lupus erythematosus, vasculitis, and purpura.

Diphtheria Antibodies: Measure the quantity of antibody present after the administration of diphtheria toxoid. The absence of antibody after immunization confirms a patient's inability to form new antibody (i.e., abnormal humoral immunity).

Ferritin: Evaluates the concentration of the storage form of iron, ferritin, in serum. In conjunction with abnormalities of erythrocyte tests (e.g., mean corpuscular volume, mean corpuscular hemoglobin), this assay is useful in establishing the diagnosis of iron deficiency anemia.

Histone Antibody: Histone antibodies are the predominant autoantibody in patients with systemic or drug-induced lupus erythematosus (SLE). Histone autoantibodies have been detected in 20% to 55% of patients with systemic SLE and 80 to 95% of patients with drug-induced SLE. Patients with idiopathic SLE have a variety of other autoantibodies in addition to histone autoantibodies. Histone antibodies of the IgG class have been shown to be SLE specific, whereas IgM antibodies are found in normal healthy people, as well as in some other non-SLE conditions. Histone antibodies occur in less than 20% of other types of connective tissue disorders.

HLA-B27: Assesses one of the human leukocyte antigens (HLAs) on the surface of lymphocytes. Detection of HLA-B27 is useful in establishing the diagnosis of ankylosing spondylitis (AS). The majority of white patients with AS are antigen positive, and about half of black patients with AS are antigen positive.

HLA-DR: Assesses one of the human leukocyte antigens (HLAs) on the surface of lymphocytes. Detection of HLA-DR is useful in predicting a person's susceptibility to disease and in estimating adverse reactions to certain drugs (e.g., hydralazine).

Identification of combinations of HLA alleles at various loci, such as HLA-A, B, C, and DR antigens, together with the inheritance of allotypes of C4 and allelic forms of C2 and properdin factor B (referred to as supratypes), is becoming a useful tool in diagnosing immunoregulatory abnormalities, as well as different types of clinical disease and susceptibility to infection.

HLA-DR3: Evaluates one of the human leukocyte antigens (HLAs) on the surface of lymphocytes. Detection of HLA-DR3 and an elevated titer of thyroid-stimulating hormone are prognostic for forms of Graves' disease that will not respond or will relapse with antithyroid medication.

Immunoglobulins: Measure the total immunoglobulin concentration in the serum. Increased concentration is representative of hyperglobulinemia. A major decrease in concentration, immunodeficiency, causes recurrent infections, atypical arthritis, or persistent diarrhea.

Immunoglobulin A (IgA): Quantitates the concentration of IgA. Normal concentrations rule out agammaglobulinemias in childhood and selective IgA deficiency. Selective deficiencies of IgA are the most common type of immunodeficiency.

Immunoglobulin D (IgD): Quantitates the concentration of IgD). It is found in very low concentrations in serum, and its functional role is not well characterized.

Immunoglobulin E (IgE): Measures IgE. Greatly increased values can be found in patients with immunodeficient states, especially cell-mediated immunodeficiency and atopic eczema; systemic fungal infections such as allergic bronchopulmonary aspergillosis; and invasive parasitic infections.

Immunoglobulin G (IgG): Quantitates the concentration of IgG. It is the major antibacterial, antifungal, and antiviral antibody. A severe deficiency is manifested by repeated infections.

Immunoglobulin G (IgG) Index: Compares the relative ratio of IgG to albumin in serum and cerebrospinal fluid. If the IgG index is increased (<0.7) and the IgG synthesis rate is increased in a specimen without oligoclonal immunoglobulins, plasma contamination may be present because of a leaky blood-brain barrier or a traumatic spinal tap.

Immunoglobulin G (IgG) Rheumatoid Factors: Measure the quantity of IgG antibodies reacting with human IgG. The role of IgG rheumatoid factor is considered of major pathogenic importance in rheumatoid arthritis.

Immunoglobulin G (IgG) Subclasses: Quantitate the subclasses IgG1, IgG2, IgG3, and IgG4 in serum. Increased levels of IgG4 can be demonstrated by patients with allergies who have normal IgE levels. A deficiency of IgG4 can be associated with severe recurrent sinopulmonary infections, symptomatic IgA deficiency, and common variable immunodeficiency (with pneumonia, bronchiectasis). In addition, elevated IgG4 is found in some highly allergic patients with normal IgE concentrations.

Immunoglobulin G (IgG) Synthesis Rate: Measures the rate of IgG synthesis in cerebrospinal fluid. Elevated rates are associated with demyelinating disease. Conditions associated with increased rates include multiple sclerosis, bacterial meningitis, subacute sclerosing panencephalitis, lupus-related central nervous system involvement, presenile dementia (Alzheimer's disease), IgG-synthesizing neoplasms, syphilis, cryptococcosis, chronic relapsing polyneuropathy, and acute cerebrovascular disease. If the immunoglobulin synthesis rate and IgG index are elevated, contamination of the specimen with plasma protein should be suspected.

IgM Antibodies (Antigen Specific): Provide identification of antigen-specific IgM antibodies in the presence of antigen-specific IgG and rheumatoid factor. The separation of IgM and IgG antibodies is important in the serodiagnosis of congenital infections.

IgM Rheumatoid Factor: Measure IgM antibodies to human IgG fixed to latex particles. Elevated levels of rheumatoid factor (RF) are associated with rheumatoid arthritis, but such elevations may also be seen in other disorders. Increased RF levels in combination with high levels of C-reactive protein are predictive of aggressive rheumatoid disease. In the case of a negative RF assay, a patient may be diagnosed through clinical signs and symptoms as having seronegative rheumatoid disease. See also *Rheumatoid Factor*.

Intrinsic Factor–Blocking Antibody: See Anti–Intrinsic Factor.

Islet Cell Antibody: See Anti–Islet Cell Antibody.

Jo-1 Antibody: Detects precipitins to an acidic nuclear protein from calf thymus. Approximately one third of patients with uncomplicated polymyositis and some patients with dermatomyositis demonstrate Jo-1 antibody.

Ku Antibody: Detects precipitins to an acidic nuclear protein from calf thymus. About half of patients with overlapping signs and symptoms of scleroderma and polymyositis demonstrate Ku precipitins.

Lyme Disease Testing: Current Centers for Disease Control and Prevention (CDC) recommendations for the serologic diagnosis of Lyme disease are to screen with a polyvalent enzyme-linked immunosorbent assay (ELISA) and confirm equivocal and positive results with Western blot (WB). Both IgM and IgG WBs should be performed on samples less than 4 weeks after appearance of erythema migrans. Only IgG WB should be performed on samples more than 4 weeks after the disease onset. IgM WB in the chronic stage is not recommended and does not aid in the diagnosis of neuroborreliosis or chronic Lyme disease. Submit requests for appropriate WB testing within 10 days.

Lymphocyte Mitogen Stimulation: Measures the rate of DNA synthesis by isolated lymphocytes. Decreased proliferation and DNA synthesis are diagnostic of a defect in cellular immunity. Cellular immunity is frequently defective in immunodeficiency disorders, infectious diseases, carcinoma, and occasionally in autoimmune disorders.

Lymphocyte Subset Panel: Differentiates and measures (using monoclonal antibodies to identify cell surface markers) the quantities of T cells and B cells in the circulating blood; useful in distinguishing T- and B-cell leukemias and lymphomas. Determination of T-cell subsets (helper/inducer, suppressor/cytotoxic) is helpful in monitoring treatment in patients with immunodeficiencies (e.g., HIV infection) or transplant recipients.

Myelin Basic Protein: Measures the concentration of myelin basic protein in cerebrospinal fluid. Elevated values indicate extensive and active demyelination of the central nervous system (CNS). Disorders in which the level of myelin basic protein can be increased include multiple sclerosis, subacute sclerosing panencephalitis, transverse myelitis, and optic neuritis. Increased values can also be observed in conditions producing damage to nervous tissue but in which demyelination is not the primary process (e.g., radiation or chemotherapy of neoplasms in or near CNS).

Oligoclonal Banding/Multiple Sclerosis: Evaluate the presence of abnormal bands of immunoglobulins in cerebrospinal fluid (CSF). Abnormal bands of monoclonal immunoglobulins are associated with disorders such as multiple sclerosis (MS), subacute sclerosing panencephalitis, paraprotein disorders, and infections.

Oligoclonal bands are present in the CSF of approximately 90% of MS patients. A patient is considered positive for CSF oligoclonal bands if there are two or more bands in the CSF Ig region that are not present in the serum. To confirm local production of oligoclonal IgG in CSF, a matched serum sample is required. Oligoclonal bands present in CSF, but not in serum, indicate CNS production.

Oligoclonal bands and elevated levels of CSF IgG may be present in other disease states, including meningoencephalitis, neurosyphilis, Guillain-Barré syndrome, and meningeal carcinomatosis. Up to 10% of patients with clinically supported MS are negative for oligoclonal bands.

Platelet-Associated IgG (PAIgG): Detects IgG found on the surface of platelets after thorough washing. Elevated levels of PAIgG with inversely proportional platelet counts are found in patients with immune thrombocytopenic purpura. Increased values can also be found in patients with systemic lupus erythematosus (SLE).

Platelet Antibody: Evaluates the quantity of platelets with immunologically attached IgG by the use of fluorescein-tagged antihuman immunoglobulin specific for the Fc portion of IgG. Antibodies can be demonstrated by this indirect test in less than half of patients with immune thrombocytopenia and the majority (82%) of SLE patients.

PM-1 Antibody: Detects antibodies to an acidic nuclear protein from calf thymus. These precipitins are found in the majority (87%) of patients with polymyositis scleroderma. More than half the patients with polymyositis demonstrate the antibody, but it is detected in less than one fifth of patients with dermatomyositis.

Prostate-Specific Antigen (PSA): Laboratory method approved as an aid in the detection of prostate cancer when used in conjunction with a digital rectal examination in men age 50 and older. Serial measurement of PSA can be of value in the prognosis and management of patients with prostate cancer. Elevated PSA concentrations can only suggest the presence of prostate cancer until biopsy is performed. PSA concentrations can also be elevated in benign prostatic hyperplasia or inflammatory conditions of the prostate. PSA is generally not elevated in healthy men or men with nonprostatic carcinoma.

Raji Cell Assay: Measures the binding of immune complexes to complement receptors on a lymphoblastoid cell line, Raji cells.

Rheumatoid Factor (RF): RF may be found in patients with a variety of autoimmune diseases, as well as in up to 10% of apparently healthy individuals. RF assays may be positive in some patients with syphilis, viral infections, chronic liver diseases, sarcoidosis, leprosy, neoplasms, and a variety of other chronic inflammatory conditions. High concentrations of RF are found in patients with rheumatoid arthritis (RA) and Sjögren's syndrome. Juvenile-onset RA is seldom associated with a positive test for RF. The RF test should be used with caution in the diagnosis of RA because of its low predictive value for this disease. The percentage of positive RF assays in the normal population increases with age.

Streptolysin O Antibody (ASO): In the past the antistreptolysin O antibody (ASO) test was routinely used to provide serologic evidence of previous group A streptococcal infection in patients suspected of having complications (e.g., acute glomerulonephritis, acute rheumatic fever). Use of the ASO for diagnosis of an acute group A streptococcal infection is rarely indicated at present unless the patient has received antibiotics that would render a culture negative.

An ASO performed on serum obtained during the presentation of a nonsuppurative complication that shows a titer two dilutions above the upper limit of normal is evidence for an antecedent streptococcal infection. It is recommended, however, to use a second test (e.g., anti–DNase B) to confirm antecedent infections. Elevated serum ASO titers are found in about 85% of individuals with rheumatic fever. When both ASO and anti–DNase B are used, the result is more than 95%.

Tetanus Antibody: Measures antibody to tetanus toxoid. If a patient has a history of immunization and antibodies are not demonstrable, abnormal humoral immunity is suspected.

Thyroid Peroxidase (TPO) Antibody: The thyroid microsomal antigen has been shown to be the enzyme thyroid peroxidase (TPO).

The measurement of low levels of TPO antibodies in serum can be useful in the assessment of a number of thyroid disorders. More than 90% of patients with autoimmune thyroiditis (Hashimoto's thyroiditis) have thyroglobulin or TPO antibodies. Although not diagnostic, detection of TPO antibodies can aid in predicting the progression of chronic thyroiditis and in further substantiating thyroid disease in patients with nonthyroidal illness.

Antibodies to TPO have also been found in most patients with idiopathic hypothyroidism (85%) and Graves' disease (50%) and less frequently in patients with other thyroid disorders. Low titers may also be found in 5% to 10% of normal individuals.

BIBLIOGRAPHY

ARUP's guide to clinical laboratory testing, Salt Lake City, April 2008, ARUP Laboratories, http://www.arup.com.

Specialty Laboratories Test Menu, Santa Monica, Calif, October 2002, http://www.specialtylabs.com.

A The nucleotide adenine.

abruptio placentae The premature separation of a normally situated placenta.

accuracy Degree of conformity of a measurement to a true value.

acquired Incurred because of external factors; not inherited.

acquired immunity See *adaptive immunity*.

acquired immunodeficiency A defect in the normal immune response caused by external factors or an existing disease or condition. Also called secondary immunodeficiency.

acquired immunodeficiency syndrome (AIDS) An immune disorder affecting T4 lymphocytes caused by the human immunodeficiency virus (HIV). Previously called "human T-lymphotropic retrovirus" (HTLV) or "lymphadenopathy-associated virus" (LAV).

activated partial thromboplastin time (aPTT) A coagulation procedure to detect factors that are active in the external mechanism (stage I) of blood coagulation.

active immunity The form of immunity produced by the body in response to stimulation by a disease-causing organism (naturally acquired active immunity) or by a vaccine (artificially acquired active immunity).

acute Referring to a condition of sudden and short duration.

acute glomerulonephritis A sudden inflammation of the small, convoluted mass of capillaries of the kidney, primarily the capsule.

acute-phase proteins A group of glycoproteins associated with nonspecific inflammation of body tissues. Also called acute-phase reactants.

adaptive immunity The augmentation of body defense mechanisms in response to a specific stimulus, which can cause the elimination of microorganisms and recovery from disease. This response frequently leaves the host with specific memory (acquired resistance), which enables the body to respond effectively if reinfection with the same microorganism occurs. Adaptive immunity is organized around T and B lymphocytes.

adenocarcinoma A malignant new growth derived from glandular tissue or from recognizable glandular structures.

adenoma A tumor derived from glandular tissue.

adenopathy Swelling or enlargement of the lymph nodes.

adjuvant Refers to a substance that enhances the effect of an antigen when the substance is given along with the antigen.

adrenal medulla The inner core of the small endocrine gland that rests on top of each kidney.

afferent lymphatic duct The vessel that carries transparent liquid and antigens into the lymph node.

affinity Propensity; the bond between a single antigenic determinant and an individual combining site.

agammaglobulinemia (common variable immunodeficiency) The absence of plasma gamma globulin, caused by a congenital or acquired condition.

agglutination Process of particulate antigens aggregating (clumping) to form a larger complex in the presence of a specific antibody.

agglutinin Previous term for *antibody*.

agglutinogen Earlier term for *antigen*.

aggregation See *agglutination*.

aliquot A representative portion of a larger sample or specimen.

allele An alternate form of one or more genes that occur at the same locus on homologous chromosomes.

allergen A substance that causes an allergic response when it enters the body.

allergic rhinitis Inflammation of the mucous membrane of the nose caused by a hypersensitivity reaction to environmental substances such as pollen or mold.

allergy (atopy) An abnormal or altered and often harmful response of the immune system to foreign substances, or antigens.

allergy march Progression of allergic disease.

alloantibodies Immunoglobulins (antibodies) produced in response to exposure of foreign antigens of the same species.

allogenic (allogeneic) Genetically different individuals of the same species.

allograft A graft of tissue from a genetically different member of the same species (e.g., human kidney).

alloimmunization A recipient who is immunocompetent can mount an immune response to the donor antigens when exposed to foreign red blood cells resulting in a variety of clinical consequences depending on the type of blood cells and specific antigens involved. The antigens most commonly involved are classified in the following categories: (1) HLAs, class I shared by platelets and leukocytes and class II present on some leukocytes; (2) granulocyte-specific antigens; (3) platelet-specific antigens (human platelet antigen [HPA]); and (4) RBC-specific antigens.

allotype The protein of an allele that may be detectable as an antigen by another member of the same species.

alopecia Loss of hair; baldness.

alpha-1 antitrypsin An acute-phase protein.

alternate pathway See *complement*.

alveolar Referring to an alveolus or alveoli; the thin-walled chambers of the lungs are referred to as *pulmonary alveoli*.

amniocentesis The process of removing fluid from the amniotic sac for study (e.g., biochemical analysis).

amplicon A DNA fragment produced by amplification of a specific DNA sequence.

amplification A process to produce multiple copies of a specific DNA sequence.

amyloidosis A condition of intercellular deposition of an abnormal protein with a waxy, translucent appearance in various tissues.

anaerobic metabolism The major, non-oxygen–associated, energy-yielding pathway connected with the breakdown of glucose (glycolysis) in body cells. Also referred to as the *Embden-Meyerhof glycolytic pathway* or *TCA cycle*.

anamnestic antibody response An antibody "memory" response. This secondary type of response occurs on subsequent exposure to a previously encountered and recognized foreign antigen and is characterized by the rapid production of IgG antibodies.

anaphylactic reaction A severe allergic reaction that can develop in IgA-deficient patients who have developed anti-IgA antibodies.

anaphylactic shock A severe allergic reaction.

anaphylactoid reaction A severe reaction to soluble constituents in donor plasma that produces edema.

anaphylatoxins   The complement components, C3a and C5a, which stimulate release by mast cells of their vasoactive amines.

anaphylaxis   An immediate (type I) hypersensitivity reaction characterized by local reactions such as urticaria (hives) and angioedema (redness and swelling) or by systemic reactions in the respiratory tract, cardiovascular system, gastrointestinal tract, and skin.

angioedema   Redness and swelling.

anicteric   Without icterus, or lacking a yellow discoloration of the skin and sclera.

anion   A negatively charged particle in solution.

anneal   The bonding or hybridization of two complementary nucleic acid strands to one another.

anomalies   Marked deviations from normal.

anorexia nervosa   An eating disorder prevalent in adolescent females.

antenatal   Before birth.

antibodies (antibody)   Specific glycoproteins (immunoglobulins) produced in response to an antigenic challenge. Antibodies can be found in blood plasma and body fluids (e.g., tears, saliva, milk). These serum globulins have a wide range of specificities for different antigens and can bind to and neutralize bacterial toxins or bind to the surfaces of bacteria, viruses, or parasites.

antibody affinity   See *affinity*.

antibody-dependent cell-mediated cytotoxicity reaction (ADCC)   A cellular activity exhibited by both K cells and phagocytic and nonphagocytic myelogenous-type leukocytes. The target cell in ADCC is coated with a low concentration of IgG antibody.

antibody-mediated immunity   See *humoral immunity*.

antibody titer   See *titer*.

anticore window   The period of time during which antigen cannot be detected in the circulating blood, such as in hepatitis B testing.

antigen (immunogen)   A foreign substance that can stimulate the production of antibodies (immune response).

antigenic determinant   See *epitope*.

antigen presentation   The activity associated with the conveying of an altered antigenic molecule to T and B cells by macrophages. This process is necessary for most adaptive responses.

antigen-presenting cell (APC)   Functionally defined cell capable of taking up antigens and presenting them to lymphocytes in a recognizable form.

antigenicity   Ability of an antigen to stimulate an immune response.

anti–human globulin reagent   An enhancement medium to promote agglutination.

antineutrophil antibody   An autoantibody divided into either antineutrophil cytoplasmic antibody (c-ANCA) or antibody producing a perinuclear staining of ethanol-fixed neutrophils (p-ANCA).

antioncogene   Tumor-suppressing genes that guard against unregulated cell growth.

antistreptolysin O antibody (ASO)   An antibody produced against streptolysin O, a hemolysin produced by streptococci, particularly group A.

antitoxins   Antibodies that interlock with and inactivate toxins produced by certain bacteria.

apheresis   The process of removing a specific component of the blood, such as platelets or plasma, and returning the remaining components (red blood cells) to the donor.

aplastic anemia   A deficiency of blood cells (e.g., erythrocytes) caused by the lack of cell production (hematopoiesis) in the bone marrow. This form of anemia may result from exposure to toxic chemicals or drugs such as chloramphenicol.

apoptosis   Programmed or normal cell death.

arteriosclerosis, artherosclerotic   Loss of elasticity (hardening) in the walls of blood vessels (e.g., arteries).

arthralgia   Pain in a joint.

arthritis   Inflammation of a joint.

arthropathy   Joint disease.

Arthus reaction   A type III hypersensitivity reaction.

aseptic technique   Handling of materials or specimens without the introduction of extraneous microorganisms.

asthma   Respiratory condition characterized by recurrent attacks of dyspnea (difficult or painful breathing) and wheezing caused by spasmodic constriction of the bronchi (larger air passages to or within the lungs).

astrocyte   A nerve cell characterized by fibrous or protoplasmic processes. Collectively these cells are called *macroglia* or *astroglia*.

asymptomatic   Exhibiting no symptoms of a disease or disorder.

ataxia   Irregularity of muscular action or faulty muscular coordination.

atopic eczema   Inflammation of the epidermis (skin) characterized by redness, itching, and weeping, which is caused by a hypersensitivity reaction.

atopy   Immediate hypersensitivity reaction caused by IgE antibody.

atrophy   Wasting or lack of growth of tissues or organs.

autoantibody (autoagglutinins)   An immunoglobulin produced against a "self" antigen.

autoimmune disorder   A disorder that results from the immune system attacking the body's own tissue because of failure to recognize self.

autoimmune hemolytic anemia   Destruction of erythrocytes by antibodies to self antigens.

autoimmunity   Condition in which the body's own antigenic structures stimulate an immune response and react with self antigens in a manner similar to the destruction of foreign antigens. This process may cause autoimmune disease.

autologous   A synonym for *self* or part of the same individual.

autonomic nervous system   The branch of the nervous system that functions without conscious control.

autosomal dominant gene   A genetic trait that expresses itself, if present, and is carried on one of the 1 through 22 pairs of (autosomal) chromosomes.

autosomal recessive gene   A genetic trait carried on one of the 1 through 22 pairs of chromosomes that is expressed only if present in a homozygous state.

avascular necrosis   Death of nonvascular cells or tissues.

avidity   Strength with which a multivalent antibody binds to a multivalent antigen.

B cell   See *B lymphocyte*.

B-cell growth factor-2   See *interleukin-5*.

B-cell–stimulating factor-1   See *interleukin-4*.

B-cell–stimulating factor-2   See *interleukin-6*.

B lymphocyte Lymphocyte subset type that secretes antibody, the humoral element of adaptive immunity. Also called B cell.

bacteremia Infection of the blood caused by bacterial microorganisms.

bare lymphocyte syndrome Infrequent cause of severe combined immunodeficiency (SCID).

base pair A nucleotide (adenine, guanine, cytosine, thymidine, or uracil) and its complementary base on the opposite strand.

BCG (bacille Calmette-Guerin) Tuberculosis vaccine that is also used to stimulate the immune system in patients with certain types of cancer.

Bence Jones (BJ) protein The abnormal protein frequently found in the urine of patients with multiple myeloma. It precipitates at 50° C, disappears at 100° C, and reappears on cooling to room temperature.

benign Nonmalignant or noncancerous.

bilirubin A breakdown product of erythrocyte catabolism. If increased levels of this substance accumulate in the circulation, it will be deposited in lipid-rich tissues such as the brain and will be manifested by the skin and sclera as jaundice/icterus.

biological response modifiers Substances that boost, direct, or restore normal immune defenses.

biometrics Refers in biological studies to the collection, synthesis, analysis, and management of quantitative data on biological communities. Also known as "biological statistics."

blast transformation The conversion of a B lymphocyte into a plasma cell.

blotting Transfer or fixation of nucleic acids onto a solid matrix (e.g., nitrocellulose) so that the nucleic acids may be hybridized with a probe.

bond Physiochemical forces that hold atoms together to form molecules.

bone marrow The spongy material inside bones that contains hematopoietic (blood-forming) tissues.

Bruton's disorder See *X-linked agammaglobulinemia.*

Burkitt's lymphoma An undifferentiated malignant neoplastic disorder of the lymphoid tissues.

bursa of Fabricius An outgrowth of the cloaca in birds that becomes the site of formation of lymphocytes with B-cell characteristics.

C The nucleotide cytosine.

C1 complex Interlocking enzyme system consisting of C1q, C1r, and C1s.

C3 The most abundant and important component of complement; produces a small (C3a) and a large peptide (C3b) when activated.

C5 The complement component split by C3b into C5a and C5b.

C6789 The lytic complement sequence that is activated by C5b and terminates in lysing the cell membrane, called the *membrane-attack complex* (MAC).

carcinoma An alternate term for malignant neoplasm of epithelial origin (cancer).

carrier molecule A molecule that, when coupled to a hapten, makes the hapten capable of stimulating an immune response. Also, a person with one normal gene and one corresponding gene for a recessive genetic disease, who usually does not have symptoms of the disease.

carrier state Asymptomatic condition of harboring an infectious organism. The term may also refer to a heterozygous individual or the carrier of a recessive gene.

catarrhal symptoms Term previously used to describe the manifestations of inflammation of the mucous membranes, particularly of the head or throat, with an accompanying discharge.

catecholamines Biologically active amines, including epinephrine and norepinephrine, that have a marked effect on the nervous and cardiovascular systems, metabolic rate and temperature, and smooth muscle.

cation A positively charged particle in solution.

CD4 The protein receptor on the surface of a target cell to which the gp 120 protein of the HIV viral envelope binds.

CD markers (cell surface markers) Molecules on the surface of lymphocytes that identify them to other immune system cells.

cDNA Complementary DNA, produced from mRNA using reverse transcriptase.

cell adhesion molecule (CAM) Proteins located on the cell surface involved with the binding with other cells or with the extracellular matrix in the process called *cell adhesion.*

cell-mediated immunity The type of immunity dependent on the link between T cells and macrophages.

cellulitis Inflammation within solid tissues, usually loose tissues beneath the skin, that is manifested by redness, pain, swelling (edema), and interference with function.

central tolerance Develops in the thymus during fetal development and eliminates cells that react with self antigens.

centromere The constricted portion of a chromosome.

cerebrospinal fluid (CSF) The fluid formed by the choroid plexus in the ventricles of the brain and found within the subarachnoid space, the central canal of the spinal cord, and the four ventricles of the brain.

cerebrovascular accident (CVA) Stroke.

ceruloplasmin Often measured as copper in the blood.

C_H Constant region of the immunoglobulin heavy-chain gene locus.

chancre A lesion that begins as a papule and erodes into a red ulcer. It is the primary wound of syphilis that occurs at the site of entry of the spirochete.

Chédiak-Higashi syndrome A rare inherited autosomal recessive trait characterized by the presence of large granules and inclusion bodies in the cytoplasm of leukocytes.

chemiluminescence Luminescence in which the light emission is caused by the products of a specific chemical reaction.

chemotactic factor See *interleukin-8.*

chemotaxis Release of substances that attract phagocytic cells as the result of traumatic or microbial damage.

chimeras Organisms whose bodies contain different cell populations of the same or different species, as in the exchange of tissue between fraternal twins before birth so that each recognizes tissue antigens of the other and accepts them, or as the result of transplantation of donor cells such as bone marrow.

cholestasis Blockage or suppression of the flow of bile.

choreoathetosis A condition characterized by rapid, jerky, involuntary movements or slow, irregular, twisting, snakelike movements seen mostly in the upper extremities (e.g., hands, fingers).

chorioretinitis Inflammation of the choroid (middle layer) and the retina (innermost layer) of the eye.

chromosomes   Strands of DNA that carry all the genes, with 23 pairs of chromosomes in each human cell.

chronic   Referring to a condition that persists for a long time.

chronic glomerulonephritis   An inflammation of long duration of the small, convoluted mass of capillaries of the kidney, primarily the capsule.

circulating immune complex   Antigen-antibody in the blood flow.

class switching   Change in isotype of antibody produced after a B lymphocyte has encountered an antigen.

clonal selection   Activation and proliferation of a lymphocyte when an individual lymphocyte encounters an antigen that binds to its unique antigen receptor site.

clone   Cells descended from the same single cell (daughter cells), all having identical phenotypes and growth characteristics as the original precursor cell.

cluster of differentiation (CD)   A surface marker that identifies a particular cell line or stage of cellular differentiation with a defined structure. Can be identified with a group or cluster of monoclonal antibodies (Mabs).

coagglutination (CoA)   A variation of latex agglutination. Visible agglutination of the coated particles indicate an antigen-antibody reaction.

coalesce   A fusion of components.

coefficient of variation   A statistical quality control calculation of variation from the average (mean).

collagen   A protein found in skin, tendons, bone, and cartilage.

collagen disease   Diseases of the skin, tendons, bone, and cartilage, such as systemic lupus erythematosus and rheumatoid arthritis.

collecting tubule   A small duct that receives urine from several renal tubules.

colony-stimulating factors (CSFs)   Molecular substances that stimulate hematopoietic progenitor cells to form colonies.

combining site   The portion of the Fab molecule that possesses specificity.

common immunocyte   Any cell of the lymphoid series that can react with an antigen to produce an antibody or participate in cell-mediated reactions.

common thymocyte   Lymphocytes arising in the thymus that precede mature (OKT 10, OKT6 surface antigen) thymocytes in development.

complement   A group of soluble blood proteins (enzymes) consisting of C1-C9. It is present in the blood and can produce inflammatory effects and lysis of cells when activated.

complement cascade   The sequential activation of plasma proteins that cause lysis of a cell.

complement fixation   This traditional procedure detects the presence of a specific antigen-antibody reaction by causing the in vitro activation of complement. If complement is not fixed, lysis of the preantibody-coated reagent erythrocytes occurs.

complement receptor   A part of the mediated innate immune system. Complement receptors are responsible for detecting pathogens by mechanisms not mediated by antibodies. Complement activity can be triggered by specific antigens. Therefore, complement (a group of proteins in the serum that help achieve phagocytosis and lysis of antigens) is also part of the humoral immune system.

complete antibody   Earlier term used for an IgM antibody.

confidence limits   Statistical standard deviations from a mean. Interval estimates are often desirable because the estimate of the mean varies from sample to sample.

congenital rubella syndrome   See *rubella syndrome.*

conjugate   Paired or joined. A laboratory substrate prepared by joining two substances, such as fluorescein to an immunoglobulin molecule.

conjugate vaccine   A vaccine in which easily recognizable proteins are linked to the outer coat of the disease-causing organism to stimulate an immune response.

constant region   The part of an antibody's structure that is alike in all antibodies of the same class.

control specimen   A specimen such as serum with known assay values that is tested concurrently with unknown patient specimens.

convalescence (convalescent) period   The time of recovery from conditions such as illness, injury, or surgery.

Coombs' test   Traditional term for the anti–human globulin (AHG) test that can be performed as both direct and indirect AHG.

cooperativity   Interaction of specific cellular elements (lymphocytes), cell products (immunoglobulins and cytokines), and nonlymphoid elements.

cortical-hypothalamic-pituitary axis   Interrelated associations among the outer layer of the brain, the structure located at the base of the cerebrum, and a small endocrine gland.

corticosteroid   Any of the hormones produced by the outer layer of the gland located on top of each kidney.

cosmopolitan   Referring to a wide distribution.

counterimmunoelectrophoresis (CIE)   A procedure in which oppositely charged antigen and antibody are propelled toward each other by an electrical field. Allows detection of concentrations of antigens and antibodies 10 times smaller than the lowest concentrations measurable by immunodiffusion or double diffusion.

cranial nerve neuritis   Inflammation of any of the nerves that are attached to the brain and pass through the openings of the skull.

C-reactive protein (C-RP)   A nonspecific, acute-phase reactant glycoprotein.

cross-reactivity   A condition in which some of the determinants of an antigen are shared by similar antigenic determinants on the surface of apparently unrelated molecules and a proportion of these antigens interact with the other kind of antigen.

cryoglobulin   An abnormal protein characterized as precipitating or forming a gel at $0°$ C and redissolving at warm temperatures.

cryptogenic cirrhosis   A condition of the liver with an obscure or doubtful cause.

cutaneous   Referring to the skin (epidermis).

cutaneous T-cell lymphoma   Malignant neoplasm with epidermal manifestations that involves the T subset of lymphocytes.

cytokines   Polypeptide products of activated cells (lymphocytes or macrophages) that control a variety of cellular responses and thereby regulate the immune system.

cytolysis   Rupture of a cell membrane with release of the cellular cytoplasm.

cytomegalovirus   A herpes-family virus that can cause congenital infections in the newborn and a clinical syndrome resembling infectious mononucleosis.

cytopenia   Severe decrease in hematologic cells.

cytotoxic T cell   Subset type of lymphocyte that can kill other cells infected by viruses, fungi, and some types of bacteria or cells transformed by malignancy.

cytotoxicity   A condition in which macrophages can kill some targets (possibly tumor cells) without phagocytizing them.

Dane particle   The intact, double-shelled hepatitis B virus.

Davidsohn differential test   The classic laboratory reference test for the diagnosis of infectious mononucleosis.

delta agent   An RNA virus that causes hepatitis but requires the coexistence of hepatitis B infection.

delayed hypersensitivity   An exaggerated immune response caused by chemicals released by sensitized T cells. Usually peaks at 24-48 hours after reexposure to the antigen. Type IV hypersensitivity reaction.

dementia   An irreversible condition of organic loss of mental function.

denaturation   The process of heating and separating two DNA strands.

denatured DNA   Double-stranded helix separates into two single strands. Hydrogen bonds break from heat, pH, nonphysiologic concentration of salts, organic solvents (e.g., alcohol), or detergents.

dendritic cells   The weakly phagocytic Langerhans cell of the epidermis and similar, nonphagocytic cells in the lymphoid follicles of the spleen and lymph nodes. These cells may be the main agent of T-cell stimulation, but their precise region has not yet been determined.

deoxyribonucleic acid (DNA)   The nucleic acid that forms the main structure of the genes.

dermatitis   An inflammation of the skin.

dermatomyositis   An inflammatory condition included in the collage disorders in which the skin, subcutaneous tissues, and muscles are involved. Necrosis of the muscles is characteristic.

D$_H$ Diversity region of the immunoglobulin heavy-chain gene locus.

diagnosis   Determination of the nature of a disorder or disease.

diapedesis   Ameboid movement of cells such as monocytes and polymorphonuclear neutrophils to a site of inflammation in phagocytosis.

DiGeorge syndrome   An immunodeficiency disease resulting from failure of the parathyroid and thymus glands to develop before birth.

dilution   Reducing the concentration of a chemical constituent in a solution.

direct agglutination   A general term in which macroscopic clumping can be observed because particulate reagents are used as an indicator of the presence of an antigen-antibody reaction.

direct antiglobulin test (DAT)   A test performed to detect the coating of erythrocytes with antibodies.

direct fluorescent antibody (DFA) test   A microscopic technique conjugating antibody to detect an antigen-antibody reaction.

discoid lupus   Term used to differentiate the benign dermatitis of cutaneous lupus from the cutaneous involvement of systemic lupus erythematosus (SLE).

disease   A pathologic condition characterized by a specific and unique set of signs and symptoms.

disorder   An abnormality of body function.

distal tubules   Ducts in the kidney located farthest from the center of the structure.

DNA (deoxyribonucleic acid)   A molecule, found in a cell's nucleus, that carries the cell's genetic information (genome).

DNA amplification   Ultrasensitive polymerase chain reaction (PCR) technique for the detection of HIV that amplifies minute amounts of viral nucleic acid in the DNA of lymphocytes.

DNA "dot-blot" hybridization   The rapid molecular biology technique used to detect the presence of a specific DNA in a specimen.

domain   Basic unit of an antibody structure. Variations between the domains of different antibody molecules are responsible for differences in antigen binding and in biologic function.

dot blot   Technique used to determine whether a particular nucleotide sequence is present in a patient's specimen.

downstream   Toward the 3′ end of a nucleic acid molecule.

dsDNA   Double-stranded DNA.

D^u   An outdated term now referred to as *weak D*, a phenotype of the Rh blood group system.

D^u Rosette test   An older procedure that uses D-positive indicator erythrocytes to form identifiable rosettes around individual D-positive fetal cells that may be in the maternal circulation.

dysplastic   Faulty or abnormal development of body tissue.

dyspnea   Difficulty in breathing.

dysproteinemia   An abnormality of the protein content of the blood.

early antigen (EA)   A "new" antigen expressed by B lymphocytes infected with Epstein-Barr virus in infectious mononucleosis. EA consists of early antigen-diffuse (EA-D), which is found in both the nucleus and cytoplasm of B cells, and early antigen-restricted (EA-R), which is usually found as a mass only in the cytoplasm.

early thymocyte   Immature T cell in the thymus that precedes the common thymocyte in maturational development.

ectopic pregnancy   The gestation of a fertilized egg outside of the uterus, most often in the fallopian tube.

eczema   An inflammatory condition of the skin (epidermis) characterized by redness, weeping, and itching.

edema (edematous)   Accumulation of fluid in the tissues that produces swelling.

EDTA   Ethylenediaminetetraacetic acid, disodium salt; a common in vitro anticoagulant.

effector cells   Active cells of the immune system that are responsible for destroying or controlling foreign antigens.

efferent lymphatic duct   The tubule through which semitransparent fluid (lymph) and possibly antigens exit the lymph node.

efficacy   Ability of a vaccine to produce the desired clinical effect at the optimal dosage and schedule.

EIA   See *enzyme immunoassay*.

electromagnetic spectrum   Form of radiation, including visible light, ranging from long to short wavelengths.

electrophoresis   A method of separating macromolecules such as proteins on the basis of net electrical charge and size (molecular weight). See also *serum electrophoresis*.

ELISA   See *enzyme-linked immunosorbent assay*.

eluate   The product of purposely manipulating a red cell suspension to break an antigen-antibody complex, with the subsequent release of the antibody into the surrounding medium.

elution   Removal of antibodies attached to antigen receptors on the red blood cell membrane.

embryogenesis   The growth and development of a living organism. In humans, this period is from the second to approximately the eighth week of gestation.

encephalopathy   Any degenerative disease of the brain.

endemic   Present at all times, such as the continual existence of a specific microorganism in a population of individuals or in a geographic location.

endocarditis   An inflammation of the inner lining of the heart (endocardium).

endothelial cell   The type of epithelial cell that lines body cavities such as the serous cavities, heart, and blood and lymphatic vessels.

endotoxemia   A condition of having bacterial cell wall heat-stable toxins in the circulation. These toxins are pyrogenic and increase capillary permeability.

end-stage renal disease   An irreversible, pathologic condition of the kidneys.

enterocolitis   An inflammation of the small intestine and colon.

env **gene**   A gene of a retrovirus such as HIV that encodes for a polyprotein that contains numerous glycosylation sites.

enzyme immunoassay (EIA)   A general term for quantitative testing of both antigens and antibodies. The method uses color-changed products of enzyme-substrate interaction or inhibition to measure the antigen-antibody reactions. Also called ELISA.

enzyme-linked immunosorbent assay (ELISA)   A quantitative method of laboratory analysis. Either antigen or antibody can be measured using enzyme-labeled antibody or antigen bound to a solid support. *Direct* ELISA measures antigen using competition for antibody-binding sites between enzyme-labeled antigen and patient antigen. *Indirect* ELISA measures antibody concentrations using bound antigen to interact with specimen antibodies.

epidemiology (epidemiologic)   The study of infectious disease or conditions in many individuals in the same geographic location at the same time.

epilepsy   A transient disturbance of nervous system function caused by abnormal electrical activity in the brain.

episomal DNA   An accessory, extrachromosomal-replicating genetic element.

epithelial cell   Cell of a type of body tissue that forms the covering of external and internal surfaces or composes a body structure, such as glandular epithelium.

epitope   A single antigenic determinant. It is functionally the portion of an antigen that combines with an antibody *paratope,* the part of the antibody molecule that makes contact with the antigenic determinant.

Epstein-Barr virus   A human DNA herpesvirus found in association with leukocytes and B lymphocytes. It is the causative agent of infectious mononucleosis in Western countries and Burkitt's lymphoma in Africa.

equivalence   The relative concentration of antibody and antigen that produces the maximal binding of antibody to antigen.

erysipelas   A febrile disease caused by group A streptococci. The disease is manifested by inflammation and redness of the skin and subcutaneous tissues and by fever, vomiting, or headache.

erythema   Redness of the skin caused by inflammation, infection, or injury.

erythematous   Characterized by erythema (redness).

erythrocyte   The scientific term for a red blood cell (RBC).

erythropoiesis   The process of producing red blood cells (RBCs).

estrogen   The term for the female sex hormones, including estradiol, estriol, and estrone.

etiology   A synonym for the study of or the cause(s) of disease.

exchange transfusion   The replacement of an infant's coated erythrocytes with donor blood until total blood volume transfer is accomplished.

extramedullary hematopoiesis   Production of erythrocytes outside the bone marrow, which can produce enlargement of the liver and spleen.

extravascular destruction   The destruction of an erythrocyte through phagocytosis and digestion by macrophages of the mononuclear phagocyte system.

extravascular hemolysis   The phagocytizing and catabolizing of erythrocytes by the mononuclear phagocyte system.

Fab fragments   Two of the three fragments formed if a typical monomeric IgG is digested with a proteolytic enzyme such as papain. These fragments retain the ability to bind antigens (specific receptors on cells) and are called *antigen-binding fragments.*

factor H   Major controlling event of the alternate complement pathway.

Fc portion   The third fragment formed in addition to the two Fab fragments if a typical monomeric IgG is digested with a proteolytic enzyme such as papain. This fragment is relatively homogeneous and sometimes crystallizable.

Fc receptor   The portion of an antibody responsible for binding to antibody receptors on cells and the C1q component of complement.

Fd fragment   The fragment consisting of a light chain and half of a heavy chain if the interchain disulfide bonds in the Fab fragment are disrupted.

febrile agglutinin   Antibodies demonstrated in microbial diseases that are manifested by a high fever.

febrile disease   A pathologic process in which an extremely high fever is a characteristic manifestation.

femur   Bone of the leg that extends from the pelvic girdle to the knee (the thigh bone).

fibrin   A meshy protein clot formed by the action of thrombin on fibrinogen.

fibroblast   An immature fiber-producing cell of connective tissue capable of differentiating into a cartilage-forming cell (chondroblast), a collagen-forming cell (collagenoblast), or a bone-forming cell (osteoblast).

fimbriae   Fringed or fingerlike structures.

FISH   See *fluorescent in situ hybridization.*

flocculation   Clumping together of particles to form visible masses.

flow cytometry   Computerized equipment is used for the separation, classification, and quantitation of particles (e.g., blood cells or antibodies). The technique is based on the passing of a monocellular stream of particles through a beam of laser light. The particles are categorized by size and then analyzed. Monoclonal antibodies can be used for the determination of specific subsets of cells. Also called flow cell cytometry.

flurochrome dye A stain for specific component or other markers.

fluorescent antibody A dye-antibody combination that emits light of another longer wavelength.

fluorescent antibody (FA) assay General term describing procedures that use the visual detection of fluorescent dyes coupled (conjugated) to antibodies that react with the antigen when present using fluorescent microscopy.

fluorescent in situ hybridization (FISH) A laboratory technique for demonstrating the presence of HIV-1 in lymphocytes in primary lymph nodes and in peripheral blood from HIV-infected patients.

Forssman antibody A heterophil type of immunoglobulin that is stimulated by one antigen and reacts with an entirely unrelated surface antigen present on cells from different mammalian species. It can be absorbed from human serum by guinea pig kidney cells.

Franklin's disease A dysproteinemia that is synonymous with *gamma heavy-chain disease*. This abnormality is characterized by the presence of monoclonal protein composed of the heavy-chain portion of the immunoglobulin molecule.

fulminant To occur suddenly with great intensity, such as lightninglike flashes of pain.

G The nucleotide guanine.

gag **gene** A gene of a retrovirus such as HIV that encodes for the major core structural protein.

gamma heavy-chain disease See *Franklin's disease*.

GALT See *gut-associated lymphoid tissue*.

gammopathy A disorder manifested by abnormality of gamma globulins.

gastroenteritis An inflammation of the lining of the stomach and intestine.

Gaussian curve A frequency distribution curve represented by deviations from the mean (average) of a test sample.

gene A unit of genetic material that codes for hereditary traits.

gene cloning A method for producing quantities of a specific DNA sequence.

gene expression profiling Measures the activity of thousands of genes at once, creating a global picture of cellular function. These profiles can distinguish between cells that are actively dividing, for example, or show how the cells react to a particular treatment. **Microarray** technology measures the relative activity of previously identified target genes.

genitalia The female and male reproductive organs and associated external structures such as the penis.

genome The complete DNA composition (hereditary factors).

genomics Study of an organism's entire **genome.**

gestation The period of development and growth of the unborn in viviparous animals (e.g., humans), from fertilization of the ovum to birth.

giant cell; epithelioid cell Macrophage-derived cells typically found at sites of chronic inflammation. A giant multinucleated cell is formed by the coalescing of cells into a solid mass, or granuloma.

giardiasis A parasitic infection associated with the unicellular *Giardia* species.

glial cell Also known as *neuroglial cell*. It is the non-nervous or supportive tissue of the brain and spinal cord known to produce minute amounts of CD4 or an alternate receptor molecule, which allows it to be infected with HIV virus.

glomerulonephritis See *acute glomerulonephritis* or *chronic glomerulonephritis*.

glomerulus (glomeruli) The small structure(s) in the malpighian body of the kidney composed of a cluster of capillary blood vessels in a cluster and enveloped in a thin wall.

glycolipids A molecule consisting of a carbohydrate plus a lipid.

glycoprotein A molecule consisting of a carbohydrate plus a protein.

goodness of fit The complementary matching of antigenic determinants and the antigen-binding sites of corresponding antibodies that influences the strength of bonding between antigens and antibodies.

grading Strength of agglutination rated from negative (0) to 4+.

grafting The transfer of cells or organs from one individual to another or from one site to another in the same individual.

graft-versus-host disease An intense and frequently fatal immunologic reaction of engrafted cells against the host caused by the infusion of immunocompetent lymphocytes into individuals with impaired immunity.

grand mal seizures A major epileptic attack with or without loss of consciousness.

granulocyte A type of leukocytic white blood cell.

granuloma A macrophage-derived lesion containing sequestered noxious agents such as foreign bodies, some types of bacteria, and others that cannot be eliminated.

granulomatous lesion A wound composed of granuloma.

Guillain-Barré syndrome A relatively rare disease of the nerves. Also called acute idiopathic polyneuritis.

gummas A granuloma that may result from delayed hypersensitivity. It is the soft tumor of the tissues characteristic of the tertiary stage of syphilis.

gut-associated lymphoid tissue (GALT) The GALT and bone marrow may play a role in the differentiation of stem cells into B lymphocytes; functions as the bursal equivalent in humans.

haplotype A single chromosome's set of genetic determinants.

hapten(s) Very small molecule(s) that can bind to a larger carrier molecule and behave as an antigen.

helper/inducer T-cell subset A major phenotypic lymphocyte subset of T lymphocytes. Also referred to as T4 subset, helper T cells.

hemagglutination A laboratory technique for the detection of antibodies that involves the agglutination of red blood cells.

hemagglutination inhibition technique (HAI) A laboratory technique for detecting antibodies that involves the blocking of agglutination of red blood cells.

hematopoiesis (hematopoietic tissues) Blood-producing structures of the body such as the liver, spleen, and bone marrow.

hematopoietic cells Blood-producing cells.

hemodynamic shock A physiologic condition (e.g., decreased blood pressure) resulting from the rapid loss of 15% to 20% or more of blood volume.

hemoflagellate A protozoan parasite found in the blood and body tissues.

hemolysin A substance such as streptolysin O and streptolysin S produced by most group A strains of streptococci that disrupts the membrane integrity of red blood cells, causing the release of hemoglobin.

hemolysis   Rupturing of the cell membrane (e.g., erythrocyte), with subsequent release of cytoplasmic contents (hemoglobin).

hemolytic anemia   A severe decrease in circulating erythrocytes and associated findings caused by the rupturing of circulating erythrocytes.

hemolytic disease of the newborn   An immunologic incompatibility between mother and fetus that can produce severe or fatal consequences in the unborn or newborn because of destruction of erythrocytes and the accumulation of breakdown products. Previously referred to as *erythroblastosis fetalis*.

hemolyzed   Referring to ruptured erythrocytes.

hemoptysis   Coughing and spitting up of blood as the result of bleeding from any part of the respiratory system.

hemostatic   Stoppage of bleeding.

hepatitis   Inflammation of the liver caused by a virus or other agents such as drugs.

hepatomegaly   Excessive enlargement of the liver.

hepatosplenomegaly   An enlarged liver and spleen.

herpesvirus   Any of a large group of DNA viruses such as herpes simplex and varicella.

heterogeneous   Different; a mixed or dissimilar population such as different types of cells or different ethnic groups mixed together.

heterosexual disease   A pathologic condition transmitted between individuals of the opposite gender.

heterozygous   Genetic state of having two dissimilar genes for the same trait.

hinge region   The area of an antibody molecule between the Fc and Fab regions that allows the two regions to operate independently.

histamine   An amine produced by the catabolism of histidine, which causes dilation of blood vessels.

histiocyte   A large phagocytic interstitial cell of the mononuclear phagocyte system, a macrophage.

histocompatibility (HLA) antigen   Cell surface protein antigen found on blood and body cells (e.g., leukocytes, platelets) that readily provokes an immune response if transferred into a genetically different (allogenic) individual of the same species.

histone   A simple protein found in combination with acidic substances such as nucleic acids.

Hodgkin's lymphoma, Hodgkin's disease   A major form of malignant lymphoma.

homogeneous   Uniform; the same. All of the individual cells or organisms are the same.

homozygous   In genetics, when the genes for a trait on homologous (paired) chromosomes are the same.

human B-cell lymphotropic virus (HBLV)   A herpesvirus that can interact with HIV in a way that may increase the severity of HIV infection.

human gonadotropic hormone (hCG)   A glucoprotein hormone secreted by the trophoblast of a developing embryo in early pregnancy.

human herpesvirus 6 (HHV-6)   A herpesvirus that can interact with HIV in a way that may increase the severity of HIV infection.

human immunodeficiency virus (HIV)   Causative agent of acquired immunodeficiency syndrome (AIDS), also called human immunodeficiency virus type 1 (HIV-1). Formerly referred to as "human T-lymphotropic virus (retrovirus) type III" (HTLV-III) and "lymphadenopathy-associated virus" (LAV).

human leukocyte antigens (HLA)   Antigens on the surface of cells that identify the cells as belonging to the specific body, rather than being foreign substances.

human T-lymphotropic virus type III (HTLV-III)   See *human immunodeficiency virus*.

humoral   Any fluid or semifluid in the body.

humoral immunity   A form of body defense against foreign substances represented by antibodies and other soluble, extracellular factors in the blood and lymphatic fluid.

hutchinsonian triad   The characteristic manifestation of congenital syphilis. The three major features are notched teeth, interstitial keratitis, and nerve deafness.

hyaluronidase   An enzyme that breaks down hyaluronic acid found in connective tissue. Also called spreading factor.

hybridization   Interaction between two single-stranded nucleic acid molecules to form a double-stranded molecule.

hybridoma   Cell lines created in vitro by fusion of two different cell types. A hybridoma is usually formed from a lymphocyte or plasma cells, one of which is a tumor cell.

hydrophilic   Water loving.

hydrophobic   Water hating.

hypercalcemia   A marked increase in ionized calcium in the circulating blood.

hypergammaglobulinemia   An increased gamma globulin fraction of plasma protein.

hyperkeratosis   A condition of increased growth of the upper layer of the skin (epidermis) or overgrowth of the cornea.

hypersensitivity   An unpleasant or damaging condition of the body tissues caused by antigenic stimulation. Hypersensitivity reactions include allergies such as hay fever.

hypervariable region   A part of an antibody molecule that enables the antibody to single out one antigen to attack.

hyperviscosity   An increase in the thickness (viscosity) of substances such as blood plasma.

hyperviscosity syndrome   A collection of symptoms resulting from increased resistance (viscosity) of the flow of blood in the circulation.

hypervolemia   An increase of total blood volume.

hypocomplementemia   A decrease or deficiency of complement in the blood circulation.

hypogammaglobulinemia   A decrease in the gamma globulin fraction of plasma protein.

hypoplastic   Defective or incomplete development of a tissue or organ.

hypothalamus   The portion of the brain beneath the thalamus at the base of the cerebrum that forms the floor and part of the walls of the third ventricle.

icterus (icteric)   Synonym for jaundice, or the yellow appearance of the skin and mucous membranes caused by accumulation of bilirubin (a product of red cell breakdown).

idiopathic   A disorder or disease without an identifiable external cause, or self-originated.

idiotope   An epitope in the variable region of an antibody.

idiotype   The antigenic characteristic of the antibody-variable region.

IgA   The second most abundant immunoglobulin in serum; the predominant form in tears, saliva and colostrum.

IgD   An immunoglobulin found in B-cell membranes; thought to play a role in B-cell response to antigens.

IgE   The immunoglobulin responsible for allergic reactions.

IgG   The most abundant immunoglobulin in serum; responsible for protection against viruses and bacteria.

IgM   The largest immunoglobulin molecule and the first antibody produced in response to an antigen.

iliac nodes   Small, rounded structure located in the lower three fifths of the small intestines from the jejunum to the ileocecal valve or in the inguinal region.

immature B cell   The receptor cell that is finally programmed for insertion of specific IgM molecules into the plasma membrane.

immediate hypersensitivity   A subset of the body's antibody-mediated mechanisms.

immune complex   The noncovalent combination of an antigen with its specific antibody. An immune complex can be small and soluble or large and precipitating, depending on the nature and proportion of the antigen and antibody.

immune deficiency (immunodeficiency) disease   A condition in which a defect exists in the ability to detect antigens and/or to produce antibodies against foreign antigens.

immune response   The reaction of the immune system to foreign antigens in the body.

immune status   The ability of a host (an individual) to recognize and respond to foreign (nonself) substances (e.g., antigens).

immune system   The structures (e.g., bone marrow, thymus, lymph nodes), cells (e.g., macrophages, lymphocytes), and soluble constituents of the circulating blood (e.g., complement) that allow the host to recognize and respond to foreign (nonself) substances such as antigens.

immunity   The process of being protected against foreign antigens.

immunization   A process of exposing the body to specific antigens to stimulate immunity.

immunoassay   A laboratory procedure for analyzing immunoglobulins.

immunoblot   See *Western blot*.

immunocompetent   The ability to mount an immune response; a host able to recognize a foreign antigen and build specific antigen-directed antibodies. The term specifically refers to lymphocytes that acquire thymus-dependent characteristics, which allow them to function in an immune response.

immunodeficiency   A dysfunction in body defense mechanisms that cause a failure in detection of foreign antigens and production of antibodies against these foreign (nonself) substances.

immunodiffusion   A laboratory method for the quantitative study of antibodies (e.g., radial immunodiffusion [RID]) or qualitative identity of antigens (e.g., Ouchterlony technique). Also called double diffusion. This classic technique is used to detect the presence of antibodies and determine their specificity by visualization of "lines of identity" (precipitin lines).

immunoelectrophoresis (IEP)   Two-step procedure involving the electrical separation of proteins, followed by the linear diffusion (immunofixation) of antibodies into the electrophoretic gel from a trough that extends through the length of the gel adjacent to the electrophoretic path. The reactions produce precipitin arcs at positions of equivalence.

immunofixation   Specific antibodies are used to produce sensitive and specific qualitative visual identification of paraproteins by electrophoretic position.

immunofluorescent assay (IFA)   A laboratory method that uses a fluorescent substance in immunologic studies. For example, particular antigens can be identified microscopically in tissues or cells by the binding of a fluorescent (light-emitting) antibody conjugate.

immunogen   A large organic molecule that is either protein or large polysaccharide and rarely, if ever, lipid.

immunogenic   See *antigen*.

Immunoglobulin (immune globulin, Ig)   Proteins produced by the immune system (i.e., antibodies). A synonym for antibody. The term has replaced the term gamma globulin because not all antibodies have gamma electrophoretic mobility. Immunoglobulins are divided into five classes: IgM, IgG, IgD, IgA, and IgE; IgG is the most abundant.

immunologic dysfunction   See *immune deficiency disease*.

immunology   The study of molecules, cells, organs, and systems responsible for recognition and disposal of nonself materials and how they work, or can be manipulated. All aspects of body defenses, such as antigens and antibodies, allergy, and hypersensitivity are included.

immunoprophylaxis   Prevention of an immune response.

immunosorbent agglutination assay (ISAGA)   An assay for detection of IgM antibodies against *Toxoplasma gondii*.

immunosuppression   Prevention of the recognition of antigen and/or production of antibody by repressing the normal adaptive immune response with drugs, chemicals, or other means. This process is frequently necessary before and after bone marrow or solid organ transplantation, or to alter a severe hypersensitivity reaction.

immunosuppressive agent   Drug, chemical, or other mechanism that prevents the immune system from recognizing and responding to nonself.

immunotherapy   Desensitization.

impetigo   A skin infection caused by streptococci that begins as a papule.

in vitro   A term used to designate outside the body (i.e., in test tube).

in vivo   A term used to designate as occurring in the living organism.

inactivated toxins   Toxins produced by bacteria and viruses that have been killed and are no longer capable of causing disease.

inactivated vaccine (killed vaccine)   A vaccine made from a whole microorganism (bacteria or virus) whose biologic ability to grow or reproduce is ended.

incomplete antibody   Formerly used term that refers to IgG-type antibodies.

indirect fluorescent antibody (IFA)   Procedure used to detect homogeneous antigen plus antigen with antiimmunoglobulins using fluorescent microscopy.

indirect hemagglutination technique   Laboratory method that uses erythrocytes passively coated with substances such as extracts of bacterial cells, rickettsiae, pathogenic fungi, protozoa, purified polysaccharides, or proteins to detect antibody. Also called passive hemagglutination technique.

infarction   An area of tissue, such as heart muscle, that undergoes necrosis (tissue breakdown) because of the lack of oxygen from the circulating blood. A condition of oxygen deprivation may be caused by a narrowing of blood vessels (stenosis) or a blockage of the blood circulation in the vessel (occlusion).

infection   A pathogenic condition caused by microorganisms (i.e., viruses or bacteria) that produce injurious effects.

infectious material   Body fluids or excretory products, or non-human substances contaminated with body fluids that contain disease-causing microorganisms.

infectious mononucleosis   A benign lymphoproliferative disorder.

inflammation   Tissue reaction to injury caused by physical or chemical agents, including microorganisms. Symptoms include redness, tenderness, pain, and swelling.

inflammatory response   See *inflammation*.

inguinal adenopathy   Enlarged lymph nodes in the region of the groin.

innate immunity (innate immune system)   Natural or inborn resistance to infection after microorganisms have penetrated the first line of resistance.

interferon alpha (IFN-α)   A protein that may be an immunosuppressive agent important in controlling the immune response in a negative manner. Originally called "leukocyte interferon."

interferon beta (IFN-β)   Originally called "fibroblast interferon" or "B-cell stimulatory factor-2" and now reclassified as *interleukin-6* (IL-6).

interleukin-1 (IL-1)   A cytokine whose most prominent biologic activity is activation of resting T cells. Originally called "lymphocyte-activating factor."

interleukin-2 (IL-2)   A cytokine best known for its ability to initiate proliferation or clonal expansion of activated T cells. IL-2 also dramatically enhances the cytolytic activity of a population of natural (lymphokine-activated) killer cells against certain tumor cells. Originally called "T-cell growth factor."

interleukin-3 (IL-3)   A cytokine that principally promotes the growth of early hematopoietic cell lines. Originally called "multicolony-stimulating factor" (mCSF).

interleukin-4 (IL-4)   A growth factor for the early activation of resting B cells that influences production of certain immunoglobulin synthesis. Originally called "B-cell–stimulating factor-1."

interleukin-5 (IL-5)   IL-5 shares many activities with IL-4, but it is not active on early lymphoid cells. Originally called "T-cell replacing factor" or "B-cell growth factor-2."

interleukin-6 (IL-6)   A cytokine that induces secretion of immunoglobulin and is a major factor in induction of the acute-phase reaction. Originally called "interferon beta-2" or "B-cell–stimulating factor-2."

interleukin-7 (IL-7)   A cytokine that stimulates early B-cell progenitor cells. Originally called "lymphopoietin-1."

interleukin-8 (IL-8)   An inflammatory cytokine that is chemotactic for both neutrophils and T cells. Originally called "monocyte-derived neutrophil chemotactic factor."

interleukin-9 (IL-9)   A cytokine that is a potent lymphocyte growth factor.

interleukin-10 (IL-10)   A cytokine that inhibits cytokine synthesis in various cells.

interleukin-11 (IL-11)   A regulator of hematopoiesis-stroma that stimulates the production of megakaryocyte and myeloid

progenitors; increases the number of immunoglobulin-secreting B lymphocytes.

interleukin-12 (IL-12)   Enhances the activity of cytotoxic effector T cells; acts as a growth factor for natural (lymphokine-activated) killer cells and for activated T cells of both the CD4+ and CD8+ subsets.

interleukin-13 (IL-13)   IL-13 possesses many biologic effects similar to IL-4. The major action of IL-13 on macrophages is to inhibit their activation and to antagonize interferon gamma (IFN-γ).

interleukin-14 (IL-14)   IL-14 acts as a B-cell growth factor (BCGF).

interleukin-15 (IL-15)   IL-15 is biologically similar to IL-2. Endogenous IL-15 is a key condition for IFN-γ synthesis.

interleukin-16 (IL-16)   IL-16 acts as a T-cell chemoattractant and participates in the regulation of many cytokines (IL-1, IL-4, IL-6, IL-10, IL-12, IFN-γ). Histamine and serotonin increase the production of IL-17. Mimics many of the proinflammatory actions of tumor necrosis factor (TNF) alpha and beta.

interleukin-18 (IL-18)   IL-18 acts as a synergist with IL-12 in some of their effects, especially in the induction of IFN-γ gamma production and inhibition of angiogenesis. It stimulates the production of IFN-γ by natural killer cells and T cells and synergizes with IL-12 in this response.

interleukin-19 (IL-19)   Biologic function of IL-19 is similar to that of IL-10. Regulates the functions of macrophages, suppresses the activities of T-helper cells (Th1 and Th2).

interleukin-20 (IL-20)   IL-20 plays an important role in skin inflammations.

interleukin-21 (IL-21)   IL-21 regulates hematopoiesis and immune response, influences the development of lymphocytes. Similar to IL-2 and IL-15 in antitumor defense system.

interleukin-22 (IL-22)   IL-22 is similar to IL-10 but does not prohibit the production of proinflammatory cytokines through monocytes.

interleukin-23 (IL-23)   Recently discovered cytokine that shares some in vivo functions with IL-12, including the activation of STAT-4 (signal transducer and activator of transcription factor 4).

interleukin-25 (IL-25)   A novel, secreted, bone marrow stroma–derived growth factor. Also called *SF-20*.

interstitial pneumonitis   An inflammation situated between or in the interspaces of the lung tissue.

intraperitoneal fetal transfusion (IPT)   Administration of blood to a fetus (unborn infant) via the abdominal cavity.

intrarenal obstruction   Blockage within the kidney.

intratubular precipitation   Formation of a solid mass from soluble substances within the tubules of the kidney.

intrauterine   Within the uterus.

intravascular coagulation   Formation of a clot within a vessel (i.e., blood vessels of the circulatory system).

intravascular destruction   An alternate pathway for erythrocyte breakdown, which normally accounts for less than 10% of red cell destruction.

intravascular hemolysis   An alternate pathway of red cell destruction in which the cells are lysed in the vessels of the circulatory system.

intravenous   Administration of drugs or fluids directly into the veins.

intravenous urography   Radiologic study of any part of the urinary tract by the administration through a vein of an opaque medium, which is rapidly excreted in the urine.

intrinsic coagulation mechanism   Initial stage of blood coagulation that can be activated by antigen-antibody complexes.

intrinsic factor (IF)   A substance secreted by the parietal cells of the mucosa in the fundus region of the stomach.

isoelectric focusing   Separation of molecules on the basis of their charge. Each molecule migrates to the point in the pH gradient where it has no net charge.

isoimmune   Possessing antibodies to antigens of the same system.

isotype   A term that refers to genetic variation within a family of proteins or peptides so that every member of the species will have each isotype of the family represented in its genome (e.g., immunoglobulin classes).

isotypic varion   The heavy-chain constant region structure associated with the different classes and subclasses. Isotopic variants are present in all healthy members of a species.

jaundice   A yellowish appearance of the skin, sclerae, and body excretions. See also *icterus*.

Kahler's disease   An alternate term for multiple myeloma.

Kaposi's sarcoma   A rare, malignant, metastasizing disorder chiefly involving the skin. An increased incidence of this malignancy has been observed in patients with AIDS.

keratinization   Development of or conversion into keratin, an extremely tough scleroprotein found in structures such as hair and nails.

kernicterus   Deposition of increased bilirubin, a red cell breakdown product, in lipid-rich nervous tissue such as the brain, which can produce mental retardation or death in the newborn. This condition can occur when circulating plasma bilirubin levels reach 20 mg/dL in a full-term infant and at lower levels in a premature infant.

killer T cells   Subset of lymphocytes that can kill cancer cells and cells infected with viruses, fungi, or certain bacteria. Also referred to as cytotoxic T cells and cytotoxic lymphocytes (CTLs).

kinetochore   A term for the centromere, the constricted area of the chromosome that demarcates the upper and lower arms of the structure.

kinetoplast   An accessory structure/body found in many protozoa. Also called micronucleus.

kinin   A small, biologically active peptide.

kinin system   A series of serum peptides sequentially activated to cause vasodilation and increased vascular permeability.

Kleihauer-Betke test   A testing method based on the differences in solubility between adult and fetal hemoglobin. The test is performed on a maternal blood specimen for the detection of fetal-maternal hemorrhage.

Kupffer cell   A phagocytic type of cell that lines the minute blood vessel (sinusoids) of the liver.

lag period   The period of time between a stimulus (i.e., antigenic stimulation) and a reaction (i.e., immunoglobulin response).

Langerhans cell   A macrophage found in the skin.

large granular lymphocyte (LGL)   Can be used synonymously with natural killer (NK) cell. About 75% of LGLs function as NK cells and appear to account fully for the NK activity in mixed-cell populations.

LASER   Light amplification by stimulated emission of radiation.

latent   Hidden or inactive.

latent infection   Persistent infections characterized by periods of reactivation of the signs and symptoms of the disease.

latex agglutination   A technique similar to hemagglutination except smaller, antigen-coated latex particles are substituted for erythrocytes for the detection of antibodies. Antibodies can be absorbed into the latex particles by binding to the Fc region of antibodies, leaving the Fab region free to interact with antigens present in the patient specimen.

lattice formation   The establishment of cross-links between sensitized particles such as erythrocytes.

leukocyte   White blood cell (WBC); functions in antigen recognition and antibody formation.

leukocytosis   A marked increase in the total circulating white blood cell concentration.

leukopenia   A marked decrease in the total circulating white blood cell concentration.

leukotriene   Recently identified class of compounds that mediate the inflammatory functions of leukocytes. These substances are a collection of metabolites of arachidonic acid, with powerful pharmacologic effects.

ligand   A linking or binding molecule.

light-chain disease (LCD)   A dysproteinemia of the monoclonal gammopathy type. In LCD only kappa or lambda monoclonal light chains, or Bence Jones proteins, are produced.

lipopolysaccharide (LPS)   The major component of some gram-negative bacterial cell walls, which protects them from phagocytosis but activates C3 directly. LPS can also act as a B-cell mitogen.

liposome   A particle of fatlike substance held in suspension in tissues.

liposome-enhanced testing   A variation of latex testing.

live, attenuated vaccine   A vaccine whose biologic activity has not been inactivated, but whose ability to cause disease has been weakened.

localized   Confined to a specific area.

localized inflammatory response   A tissue reaction confined to a specific area. This response is caused by physical or chemical agents, including microorganisms. The manifestations of the response include redness, tenderness, pain, and swelling.

LOCI   Luminescent oxygen-channeling immunoassay.

long terminal redundancy (LTR)   A structure that exists at each end of the proviral genome and plays an important role in the control of viral gene expression and the integration of the provirus into the DNA of the host.

lymphadenopathy   Disease of the lymph nodes.

lymph node   Any of the accumulations of lymphoid tissue organized as definite lymphoid organs along the course of lymphatic vessels.

lymphoblast   The most immature stage of the lymphocyte type of leukocyte.

lymphocyte   A small white blood cell found in lymph nodes and the circulating blood. Two major populations of lymphocytes are recognized: T and B cells.

lymphocyte recirculation   Process that enables lymphocytes to come in contact with processed foreign antigens and to disseminate antigen-sensitized memory cells throughout the lymphoid system.

lymphocyte-activating factor   See *interleukin-1*.

lymphocytopenia   A severe decrease in the total number of lymphocytes in the peripheral blood.

lymphocytosis   A significant increase in the total number of lymphocytes in the peripheral blood.

lymphokine   Soluble protein mediator released by sensitized lymphocytes on contact with an antigen. See *soluble mediator*.

lymphokine-activated killer (LAK) cells   A population of natural killer (NK) cells with enhanced cytolytic activity resulting from the addition of IL-2.

lymphoma   Solid, malignant tumor of the lymph nodes and associated tissues or bone marrow.

lymphopoietin-1   See *interleukin-7*.

lymphoproliferative disorder   A group of diseases characterized by the proliferation of lymphoid tissues and/or lymphocytes.

lymphosarcoma   Malignant neoplastic disorders of the lymphoid tissues, excluding Hodgkin's disease.

lyse   To break apart or dissolve.

lysis   Irreversible leakage of cell contents that occurs after membrane damage.

lysozyme (muramidase)   An enzyme secreted by macrophages that attacks the cell walls of some bacteria.

M protein   See *monoclonal protein*.

macroglobulin   A high-molecular-weight protein of the globulin type.

macrophage   A large, mononuclear phagocytic cell of the tissues that exists as either a wandering type or a fixed type that lines the capillaries and sinuses of organs such as the bone marrow, spleen, and lymph nodes. This cell phagocytizes, processes, presents antigens to T cells, and is also responsible for removing damaged tissue, cells, bacteria, and other substances from the host.

macrophage migration inhibitory factor (MIF)   A lymphocyte product that is chemotactic for monocytes. Other similar factors stimulate monocyte and macrophage functions.

macular lesion   A discolored, unraised spot on the skin.

maculopapular   A lesion with both macular and papular characteristics.

major histocompatibility complex (MHC)   A genetic region in humans and other mammals responsible for signaling between lymphocytes and antigen-bearing cells. It is also the major determinant of transplant compatability (or rejection).

malaise   A general feeling of tiredness or discomfort.

malignant (malignancy)   Cancerous.

manifestation   The development of the signs and symptoms of a disease or disorder.

mannose-binding lectin   A pattern-recognition molecule of the innate immune system.

mannose-binding lectin pathway   A complement activation pathway.

mast cell   A large tissue cell with basophilic granules containing vasoactive amines and heparin. When the cell is damaged, the granules release these inflammatory mediators, which increase vascular permeability and allow complement and phagocytic cells to enter damaged tissues from the circulating blood.

mature B cell   Concerned with synthesis of circulating antibodies.

mean   Statistical (arithmetic) average.

median   Half the numbers in a series of numbers are above the mean; half the numbers in the series are below the mean.

mediastinum   The tissues and organs such as the heart, trachea, esophagus, and lymph nodes that separate the sternum in the front (ventral side) from the vertebral column in the back (dorsal side) of the body.

megakaryocytic thrombocytopenic purpura   A severe deficiency of the cells (thrombocytes/platelets) related to blood clotting that causes large, purple discolorations of the skin.

melanocyte   A cell that produces melanin (the dark pigment normally found in structures such as the hair, eyes, and skin). It can also occur abnormally in certain tumors, melanomas.

membrane attack complex (MAC)   A unit created by action of the complement components (C7-9) that punctures the wall of a cell and allows cytoplasm and organelles to flow out.

memory   The immunologic response to an antigenic stimulus that usually leaves the immune system changed.

memory cells   Long-lived T or B lymphocytes that have been stimulated by a specific antigen and recall prior antigen exposure.

meningoencephalitis   An inflammation of the brain and its membranous covering (the meninges).

meningovascular   A term that refers to the blood vessels of the covering of the brain and spinal cord (meninges).

mesothelium   A type of epithelium, originally derived from the mesoderm lining the primitive embryonic body cavity, that becomes the serous membrane of body surfaces, such as the peritoneum (the membrane viscera and lining of the abdominal cavity, except the kidneys), the pleura (the membrane covering the lungs), the walls of the thoracic cavity (the chest and diaphragm), and pericardium (the sac enclosing the heart).

metastasis   Spreading of malignant cells from the primary site of malignancy.

meniscus   The upside down, half moon shape of aqueous liquids in a glass vessel such as a pipette or flask.

MHC   A condition in which a group of white blood cells is activated only if an antigen and specific type of MHC molecule are present.

microencephaly   Abnormally small brain.

microglia   The phagocytic cells of the brain, thought to be derived from incoming blood monocytes.

microplate   A compact plate of rigid or flexible plastic with multiple wells.

microspheres   Tiny, microscopic spheres that can carry vaccines or drugs and can pass easily through the body's tissues.

mitogen   A substance that stimulates cell division (mitosis).

mobility   The ability of specific and nonspecific cells of the immune system to circulate.

mode   The most frequent number in a group of numbers.

molecule   The smallest unit of a specific chemical substance that can exist alone.

monoclonal antibody (MAb)   Purified immunoglobulins produced by cells cloned from a single fusion-type hybridoma cell. Monoclonal antibodies are directed against antigens derived from a single cell line.

monoclonal gammopathy   A dysproteinemia in which a single type of immunoglobulin is increased. This immunoglobulin is secreted by a single clone of plasma cells.

monoclonal protein (M protein, paraprotein)   A protein characterized by a narrow peak or a localized band on electrophoresis, by a thickened bowed arc on immunoelectrophoresis, and by a localized band on immunofixation.

pleuritis An inflammation of the serous membrane lining, the pleura.

pluripotent See *multipotential stem cells.*

PMN See *polymorphonuclear leukocyte.*

Pneumocystis carinii A protozoan that causes interstitial plasma cell pneumonia. This microorganism is frequently observed as an opportunistic pathogen in patients with AIDS.

point-of-care A term used to designate laboratory testing at or near the patient.

pol **gene** A gene of a retrovirus (e.g., HIV) that encodes for reverse transcriptase, endonuclease, and proteases activities.

polyarthritis Inflammation of several joints.

polyclonal gammopathy A dysproteinemia in which the products of a number of different cell types are demonstrated.

polyendocrinopathies A disease condition that involves several endocrine glands.

polymerase chain reaction (PCR) This molecular biology technique uses amplification of low levels of specific DNA sequences in a sample to reach the threshold of detection. The reaction products are hybridized to a radiolabeled DNA segment complementary to a short sequence of the amplified DNA. After electrophoresis, the radiolabeled product of specific size is detected by autoradiography.

polymorphonuclear leukocyte (PMN) A short-lived scavenger blood cell whose granules contain powerful bactericidal enzymes. Also called *polymorphonuclear neutrophil leukocyte.*

polymyositis Inflammation of several muscles at the same time. This condition is manifested by a number of signs and symptoms, including pain, edema, deformity, and sleep disturbance.

polyneuropathy A disease involving several nerves.

polyserositis A condition of general inflammation of serous membrane with effusion (escape of fluid). The inflammation is progressive and especially prevalent in the upper abdominal cavity.

posterior cervical In the back (dorsal surface) and associated with the vertebral bone of the neck.

postnatal After birth.

postoccipital lobe The back portion (lobe) of the cerebral hemisphere that is shaped like a three-sided pyramid.

postpartum After birth.

post-zone Excess of antigen resulting in no lattice formation in an agglutination reaction.

potency The strength of a substance.

pre-B cell An early, rapidly dividing mature B-cell precursor.

Precipitate (precipitation) Formation of a solid mass from previously soluble components. An alternate definition is to occur suddenly or unexpectedly.

precision Also called reproducibility or repeatability; the degree to which further measurements or analysis produces the same or very similar results.

predictive value An expression of the probability that a given test result correlates with the presence or absence of disease. A positive predictive value is the ratio of patients with the disease who test positive to the entire population of individuals with a positive test result; a negative predictive value is the ratio of patients without the disease who test negative to the entire population of individuals with a negative test.

prenatal Before birth.

prime To give an initial sensitization to antigen.

primary antibody response An immunologic (IgM antibody) response that occurs after a foreign antigen challenge.

primary biliary cirrhosis Cirrhosis (interstitial inflammation of an organ) of the liver caused by chronic retention of bile. The causative agent (etiology) is unknown in the primary form of the disorder.

primary immunodeficiency Dysfunction in an immune organ such as the thymus.

primary immunoglobulin deficiency A genetically determined disorder associated with certain diseases.

primary lymphoid tissue or organ The bone marrow and thymus gland are classified as primary or central lymphoid tissues.

primitive stem cell The early form of uncommitted, multipotential blood cells that replicate themselves and generate more differentiated daughter cells.

procainamide A drug that functions as a cardiac depressant, used in the treatment of cardiac arrhythmias.

prodromal period (prodrome, prodromal) Earliest or initial sign or symptom of a developing disease or disorder. For example, the prodromal period of an infectious disease manifested by rash would be the time between the earliest symptoms and the appearance of the rash or fever.

proficiency testing A comparison of in-house laboratory assay results with results from external laboratories. A valuable continuous improvement (quality assurance) tool.

progenitor cells Precursor (immature) blood cells.

prognosis A forecast of the probable outcome of a condition, disorder, or disease.

progressive systemic sclerosis (PSS) A disorder of loss of tissue elasticity throughout the body that advances in severity over time.

properdin A normal protein of human plasma/serum.

prophylaxis A synonym for prevention.

prostaglandin Pharmacologically active derivative of arachidonic acid. Prostaglandins are naturally occurring, unsaturated fatty acids that stimulate and suppress the effects of many inflammatory processes and stimulate the contraction of uterine and other smooth muscle tissues. Different prostaglandins are capable of modulating cell mobility and immune responses.

prostration A condition of extreme exhaustion (lack of strength or energy).

proteins Large molecules, composed of amino acids, that are a major constituent of cells.

proteinuria Protein (albumin) in the urine.

proteolysis The breaking apart of a protein molecule.

proteolytic enzyme A substance able to break apart a protein molecule.

proteomics Large-scale study of proteins, particularly their structures and functions.

prothrombin time (PT) A blood coagulation test that assesses the process of clotting beginning with the formation of factor X.

protocol The steps usually followed in a situation such as laboratory testing or patient treatment.

proximal humerus The end portion of the upper bone of the arm nearest the center of the body (shoulder).

prozone phenomenon A possible cause of false-negative antigen-antibody reactions caused by an excessive amount of antibody.

pseudoagglutination   False clumping of cells or particles.

psychoneuroimmunology   The relationship between the mind and the body that combines research in basic science with psychologic and psychosocial factors.

psychosocial factors   Related to both psychologic and social factors.

PT   See *prothrombin time.*

purpura   An extensive area of red or dark-purple discoloration of the skin.

pyelonephritis   An inflammation of the kidney and pelvis region of the kidney (funnel-shaped expansion of upper end of ureter into which renal calices open).

pyoderma   Any purulent (pus-producing) skin disease.

pyogenic   Producing pus.

pyrogenic   Inducing fever.

pyroglobulin   An abnormal (IgM) globulin that precipitates on heating to 50° or 60° C but does not redissolve on cooling or intensified heating as do typical Bence Jones pyroglobulins.

quality assurance (QA)   Planned or systematic actions necessary to provide confidence that a laboratory assay result will satisfy the given requirements for quality.

quality control   A process used to ensure a certain level of quality in laboratory testing, including control of preanalytical, analytical, and postanalytical factors. The basic goal of quality control is to ensure that the results meet specific requirements and are dependable and satisfactory.

radial immunodiffusion (RID)   A quantitative variation of immunodiffusion. The diameter of the precipitin ring formed from evenly distributed antigen (or antibody) and its counterpart from the test sample diffuses into agar gel from a single well, resulting in a circular ring of precipitin around the sample well. The diameter of the precipitin ring is proportional to the concentration of specific antibody (or antigen) present in the test specimen. A comparison to known standards allows for quantitation of the test specimen.

radioallergosorbent test (RAST)   This procedure detects the presence of IgE (and IgG) antibodies to allergens.

radioimmunoassay (RIA)   An older and less frequently used laboratory technique involving the use of radioactive substances to evaluate immunoglobulins. Traditional RIA is done with specific antibodies in liquid solution. Solid-phase RIA uses antibody bound to solid support (e.g., tubes, glass beads).

Raynaud's phenomenon (Raynaud's disease)   A condition of episodic constriction of small arteries of the extremities (usually fingers or toes) induced by cold temperatures or emotional stress that would not affect an unafflicted person. The signs and symptoms of the condition include two forms: a pale appearance and numb feeling followed by redness and tingling or a swollen, red, and painful condition. Heat relieves the condition if the stimulus was cold induced.

reagin   An antibody-like protein that binds to a test antigen such as cardiolipid-lecithin–coated cholesterol particles in the Venereal Disease Research Laboratories (VDRL) serologic method of testing for syphilis: rapid plasma reagin (RPR) test. Also, former term for IgE with a specificity for allergens.

reagin antibodies   Nontreponemal antibodies produced by a patient infected with *Treponema pallidum* against components of their own or other mammalian cells.

reanneal   To reassemble or recombine two nucleic acid strands.

recessive   The term used to describe a gene that is not expressed unless it is in the homozygous form.

receptor   A cell surface molecule that binds specifically to particular proteins or peptides in the fluid phase.

recirculation   In reference to lymphocytes, mostly T cells, which pass from the circulating blood through the lymphatic system back to the circulating blood.

recombinant DNA technology   The technique in which genetic material from one organism is inserted into a foreign cell or another organism in order to mass-produce the protein encoded by the inserted genes. Also called recombinant genetic engineering.

recombinant vector vaccine   A vaccine that combines a *vector,* a harmless bacterium or virus used to transport an antigen into the body to stimulate protective immunity, and an antigen or immunogen from an organism other than the vector.

reference range   This term was previously referred to as normal values; typical laboratory results for specific groups of patients such as gender- or age-related average values.

refractory anemia   A form of anemia (decreased erythrocytes in the circulation) resistant to ordinary treatment.

regimen   A schedule of treatment.

regional adenopathy   Swelling or enlargement of the lymph nodes in a certain area or areas of the body.

relative lymphocytosis   An increase of lymphocytes in the circulating blood in relationship to the total number of leukocytes in the circulation.

reliability   Dependability of results.

renal impairment   Dysfunction of the kidneys.

renal insufficiency   Inadequate functioning of the kidneys.

replicability   The ability of specific and nonspecific cells of the immune system to produce daughter cells.

reproducibility   The ability to obtained similar results when the same specimen is repeatedly tested.

restriction endonuclease   Bacterial enzyme that recognizes short sequences of DNA and cleaves the DNA near this restriction site; each enzyme is named after the bacteria from which it has been isolated.

reticuloendothelial system   See *mononuclear phagocyte system.*

retinal hemorrhage   Extreme bleeding from the inner layer (retina) into the fluid-filled interior of the eye.

retinitis   An inflammation of the inner layer (retina) of the eye.

retroauricular   Behind the protruding portion of the external ear that surrounds the opening (auricle).

retrovirus   A type of virus that carries a single, positive-stranded RNA and uses a special enzyme, reverse transcriptase, to convert viral RNA into DNA.

reverse passive hemagglutination   A laboratory method that uses erythrocytes as an indicator cell to observe the absence of agglutination in the presence of antibodies.

reverse transcriptase (RT)   An enzyme found in the single, positive-stranded RNA core of a retrovirus. This enzyme converts (copies) RNA to DNA.

Reye's syndrome   An acute and frequently fatal childhood disease that may follow a variety of common viral infections within several hours or days. The signs and symptoms of disease include persistent vomiting followed by delirium caused by edema of the brain, hypoglycemia, dysfunction of the liver, convulsions, and coma.

RFLPs (restriction fragment length polymorphisms) A variation in the DNA sequence of a genome that can be detected by a laboratory technique known as gel electrophoresis. Analysis of RFLP variation is an important tool in genome mapping, localization of genetic disease genes, and determination of risk for a disease.

Rh factor This blood group antigen, named for the rhesus monkey, was originally identified because an antibody agglutinated the erythrocytes of all rhesus monkeys and 85% of humans. The antibody was later discovered to be the Landsteiner-Wiener antibody, which is dissimilar from the Rh antibody.

rheumatic disease A collection of rheumatoid disorders.

rheumatic fever A disease caused by the toxins produced by group A beta streptococci.

rhinorrhea Watery discharge from the nose.

RIA See *radioimmunoassay*.

rouleaux (rouleaux formation) Pseudoagglutination or the false clumping of erythrocytes when the cells are suspended in their own serum. This phenomenon is caused by an abnormal protein in the serum, plasma expanders (e.g., dextran), or Wharton's jelly from cord blood samples. Rouleaux formation appears as rolls resembling stacks of coins on microscopic examination.

RPR (rapid plasma reagin) test A veneral disease (syphilis) serologic test.

rubella The viral cause of measles.

rubella syndrome A number of congenital anomalies such as mental retardation and cardiovascular defects caused by the rubella virus.

sarcoma Malignant tumors of connective tissue origins.

scarlet fever An acute infectious disease caused by group A streptococcus. The rash and other signs and symptoms are caused by the erythema-producing toxin produced by the streptococci.

sclerodactyly A chronic disorder characterized by progressive fibrosis of the fingers and toes.

scleroderma A progressive fibrosis beginning with the skin.

sebum The oily secretion of the sebaceous glands whose ducts open into the hair follicles.

secondary immunoglobulin deficiency An acquired disorder associated with certain diseases.

secondary immune response The second and subsequent response by the immune system to the same antigen encountered; the secondary response is shorter, faster, and wider than the primary response.

secondary lymphoid tissue, secondary lymphoid organs The secondary tissues include the lymph nodes, spleen, and Peyer's patches in the intestine.

secretory component A protein in secretory IgA and IgM thought to protect against enzyme damage.

self-limiting Confined; able to resolve over time.

senescence The process of growing old.

sensitivity The frequency of positive results obtained in the testing of a population of individuals who are truly positive for antibody.

sensitization Physical attachment of antibody molecules to antigens on the erythrocyte membrane.

sepsis Microbial infection throughout the systemic circulation.

septic arthritis An inflammation of the joints caused by the presence of pathogenic microorganisms.

septicemia The presence of pathogenic microorganisms in the blood.

sequelae A disease condition occurring after or as a consequence of another condition or event.

serial dilution The stepwise dilution of a substance in solution.

seroconversion The development of a demonstrable antibody response to a disease or vaccine.

seroepidemiologic Pertaining to the evidence of antibodies to a disease in a defined population.

seronegative The lack of evidence of an antibody to a disease.

serositis An inflammation of the membrane consisting of mesothelium, a thin layer of connective tissue, having lines enclosing the body cavities.

serum Straw-colored fluid present after blood clots.

serum electrophoresis A technique for separating ionic molecules, principally proteins, into five fractions on a medium such as paper or cellulose acetate. The separation is based on the rate of migration depending on size and ionic charge of these individual components in an electrical field. The components can be visualized by staining and quantitated using a densitometer.

serum sickness A hypersensitivity reaction occurring after a single, large injection of serum from an animal of another species.

severe combined immunodeficiency disease (SCID) A life-threatening condition that results when a child is born without any major immune defenses.

sex-linked trait A genetic trait associated with the X chromosome.

sialic acid Found on red blood cell membranes; produces a negative surrounding charge.

sickle cell anemia An inherited form of anemia caused by a genetically defective hemoglobin.

silent carrier A carrier of a disease who manifests no clinically obvious symptoms or signs.

single-strand conformational polymorphism A technique used to detect subtle differences in nucleotide sequences; typically used to compare sequences from two or more individuals to determine whether or not they are identical or if a mutation has occurred.

sinusitis An inflammation of the cavity in a bone, such as in the paranasal sinuses.

sinusoid A specialized capillary found in locations such as the bone marrow, spleen, and liver through which blood passes to reach the veins, allowing the lining macrophages to remove damaged or antibody-coated cells.

SIRS (systemic inflammatory response syndrome) An inflammation that overwhelms the whole body.

Sjögren's syndrome An autoimmune disorder manifested by enlargement of the parotid glands, chronic polyarthritis, and dryness of the conjunctiva, throat, and mouth.

SLE See *systemic lupus erythematosus*.

solid-phase assay A laboratory method in which one of the reactants is bound to surface.

soluble Ability to be dissolved in or as if in a liquid and especially water.

soluble mediator A substance secreted by monocytes, lymphocytes, or neutrophils that provides the mechanism of cell-to-cell communication. Important lymphokines include IL-2, chemotactic factors, and IL-1. Also called lymphokine.

somnolence   A condition of prolonged drowsiness or a state resembling a trance.

sor **gene**   A gene of a retrovirus such as HIV. The product of the small, open-reading frame is a protein that induces antibody production in the natural course of infection.

Southern blot   A molecular biology laboratory technique used in DNA analysis. DNA from a patient specimen is denatured and treated with enzymes to produce DNA fragments; then the single-stranded DNA fragments are separated by electrophoresis. These fragments are further treated, and radiolabeling is introduced. The resulting DNA with the radiolabel, if present, is then detected by autoradiography. Applications include studying the HIV sequence in peripheral blood cells and tissues such as lymph nodes, liver, and kidney.

specificity   1. Ability of a particular antibody to combine with one antigen instead of another. 2. The proportion of negative test results obtained in the population of individuals who actually lack the antibody in question.

spirochete   A type of bacteria with a twisted or spiral appearance when viewed microscopically.

spleen   A large, glandlike organ located in the upper-left quadrant of abdomen under the ribs. The spleen is the body's largest reservoir of mononuclear phagocytic cells.

splenomegaly   Greatly enlarged spleen.

SQUID (superconducting quantum interference device)   Very sensitive magnetometers used to measure extremely small magnetic fields, based on superconducting loops containing Josephson junctions.

Standard Precautions (previously Uniform Precautions)   Specific regulations and practices, such as wearing gloves, that conform to current state and federal requirements. These precautions assume that *all* specimens (e.g., blood) have the potential for transmitting disease. Also called Universal Blood and Body Fluid Precautions (CDC).

stasis   Cessation of bleeding.

steric hindrance   Mutual blocking of dissimilar antibodies with the same binding constant, directed against antigenic determinants located in close proximity on a cell's surface.

streptokinase   An enzyme that dissolves clots by converting plasminogen to plasmin.

subclinical infection   An early or mild form of a disease without visible signs.

substrate   A substance on which another substance such as an enzyme acts.

supernatant   Fluid above the solid portion (e.g., cells in a centrifuged or sedimented specimen).

suppressor/cytotoxic   A major phenotypic lymphocyte subset of T lymphocytes. Also referred to as T8 cells.

supraglottic larynx   The area above the true vocal cords.

surface immunoglobulin (sIg)   Immunoglobulin, at first cytoplasmic and later surface bound, is the key feature of B cells, through which they recognize specific antigens.

surrogate testing   Procedures performed in place of specific tests for an infectious agent such as non-A, non-B hepatitis.

susceptibility   Having little resistance, such as resistance to infectious disease.

symptom   An indication of a disorder or disease, or a variation in normal body function.

symptomatic   A deviation from usual function or appearance.

syncytia   Giant, multinucleated groups or masses of cells.

syndrome   A collection of symptoms that occur together.

synergistic   The action of two or more agents that frequently produces a much greater effect than the expected sum of the individual agents.

systematic errors   Errors in testing that occur on a repeated and regular basis.

systemic   Throughout the body.

systemic circulation   Blood circulation throughout the body.

systemic lupus erythematosus (SLE)   An autoimmune disorder expressed as a group of multisymptom disorders that can affect practically every organ of the body.

systemic sclerosis   Loss of tissue elasticity of vessels such as blood vessels throughout the whole body.

T cell   See *T lymphocyte.*

T lymphocyte   The cells responsible for the cellular immune response and involved in the regulation of antibody reactions. Also called T cell.

tabes dorsalis   A slowly progressive degeneration of the nervous system caused by syphilis. In untreated patients this condition may appear from 5 to 20 years after the initial infection with *Treponema pallidum.*

tachycardia   An abnormally fast heart rate.

tart cell   When a blood preparation is microscopically examined for the presence of cells associated with systemic lupus erythematosus (SLE), tart cells may be seen. Tart cells usually represent monocytes that have phagocytized another whole cell or nucleus, often a lymphocyte. These cell formations can be mistaken for the classic LE cell connected with SLE.

TdT   See *terminal deoxynucleotidyl transferase.*

telangiectasia   A vascular lesion formed by the dilation of a group of capillaries and occasionally of terminal arteries.

teratomas   Malignant tumors derived from three germ layers.

terminal deoxynucleotidyl transferase (TdT)   An intracellular DNA polymerase found mainly in cortical, and therefore young, thymocytes. These cells are lost from the thymus after corticosteroid treatment.

thrombocytopenia   A severe deficiency of circulating blood platelets (thrombocytes).

thrombophlebitis   An inflammation of a vein that develops before the formation of a thrombus (clot).

thrombosis   A condition of formation of a blood clot or thrombus.

thrombus   A clot.

thymoma   A tumor derived from the epithelial or lymphoid elements of the thymus.

thymosin   A humoral factor secreted by the thymus that promotes the growth of peripheral lymphoid tissue. Also called thymic hormone.

thymus   A primary or central lymphoid tissue responsible for processes of lymphocytes into the T type of cell. This ductless, glandlike structure is located beneath the sternum (breastbone).

titer   The concentration or strength of an antibody expressed as the highest dilution of the serum that produces agglutination (e.g., 1:4, 1:8).

tolerance   Lack of immune response to self antigens initiated in fetal development.

toxic shock syndrome   A serious and potentially fatal disorder caused by toxins produced by *Staphylococcus aureus.*

Toxoplasma gondii   A protozoal microorganism that can be transmitted from an infected mother to an unborn infant. The disease can result in encephalomyelitis.

trans   A prefix meaning across, over, or through.

transaminase (ALT/SGPT)   A surrogate test for non-A, non-B hepatitis.

transforming growth factors   Cytokines identified as products of virally transformed cells. These molecules can induce phenotypic transformation in nonneoplastic cells.

transplacental hemorrhage   The entrance of fetal blood cells into the maternal circulation.

treponemes   Spirochetes of the genus *Treponema.*

tubular cell injury   Damage to cells of the renal tubules.

tumor   Proliferation of cells that produce a mass rather than a reaction or inflammatory condition.

tumor necrosis factor (TNF)   A cytokine that can destroy tumor cells.

tumor-specific antigen (TSA)   A tumor marker. An antigen that is only associated with a specific type of tissue.

ubiquitous   Existing everywhere.

ulcerative lesion   An open sore.

unilateral blindness   The lack of vision in one eye.

Universal Blood and Body Fluid Precautions   See *Standard Precautions.*

urticaria   Hives.

vaccination   A method of stimulating the adaptive immune response and generating memory and acquired resistance without contracting disease. A form of artificial active-acquired immunity.

vaccine   A suspension of killed or attenuated (inactivated) infectious agents administered to establish resistance to the disease.

variable region   The antigen-binding portion of an immunoglobulin molecule.

variable lymphocyte   A type of white blood cell that lacks the characteristics of a normal lymphocyte.

varicella   A virus that causes chickenpox.

varicosity   A condition of having distended veins.

vasculitis   An inflammation of a vessel such as a blood vessel.

vasoamine   Vasoactive amines (e.g., histamine, 5-hydroxytryptamine), produced by mast cells, basophils, and platelets and causing increased capillary permeability.

vector   A bacterium or virus that does not cause disease in humans and is used in genetically engineered vaccines.

venereal route   A sexually transmitted mode of infection.

viral capsid antigen (VCA)   A "new" antigen expressed by B lymphocytes infected with Epstein-Barr virus in infectious mononucleosis.

viremia   A systemic (blood) infection caused by a virus.

virion   A complete virus particle.

virulence   The degree of pathogenicity or ability to cause disease of a microorganism.

Waldenström's primary macroglobulinemia   A neoplastic proliferation of the lymphocyte–plasma cell system. Also called Waldenström's macroglobulinemia.

Wasserman test   The first diagnostic serologic test for syphilis; no longer in use.

Western blot (WB)   A molecular biology diagnostic technique similar to the Northern blot and Southern blot procedures. WB is used to detect antibodies to specific epitopes of electrophoretically separated subspecies of antigens. WB is often used to confirm the specificity of antibodies detected by an ELISA screening procedure.

Wiscott-Aldrich syndrome   A genetic disorder passed to males through the X chromosome that results in decreased production of specific antibodies and abnormal cellular immunity.

X-linked agammaglobulinemia   An inherited form, transmitted to males through the X chromosome, in which B cells fail to mature and to secrete immunoglobulins.

xenograft   A transplant (graft) between different species such as pigs to humans.

zeta potential   An electron cloud surrounding a red blood cell in solution (i.e., plasma).

zone of equivalence   Area in which optimum precipitation occurs because the number of multivalent sites of antigen and antibody are approximately equal.

zoonosis   Any infectious disease that is able to be transmitted (by a vector) from other animals, both wild and domestic, to humans or from humans to animals (the latter is sometimes called reverse zoonosis).

Index

A

ABO blood grouping procedure
  principle of, 23, 142-143
  quality control for, 23
  reagents, supplies and equipment for, 23
  results, reporting and interpretation of, 23
  sources of error, 23
  specimen collection and procedure, 23
  steps for, 23
  technical sources for, 24
Absolute lymphocyte count, 65, 65b
Absolute neutrophil count, 65
Accelerated rejection, 438
Acetaminophen, 404
Acetylcholine receptor (AChR)-binding antibody, 368-369
Acetylcholine receptor (AChR)-blocking antibody, 369
Acquired immunity
  components of, 4b
  passive versus active, 4, 5t
Acquired immunodeficiency syndrome (AIDS)
  blood donor, screening of, 318
  cell-mediated immunity and, 65
  classification system of, 311
  end stage of, 314
  epidemiology of, 311-313
  etiology of, 308-311
  evolution of, 315f
  genes and antigens, encoding of, 309t
  incidence of, 311
  infections from, 314, 314b
  infectious patterns of, 311
  progression of, 314-316
  signs and symptoms of, 313-316
  vaccine development, importance of, 198
  vaccine development for, 321b
  viral characteristics
    structure of, 308-309
  See also Human immunodeficiency virus (HIV)
Acquired rubella, 299
  manifestations of, 301-302
  signs and symptoms of, 300
Acquired toxoplasmosis, 248-249
Acridine orange (AO) stain, 239
Acrodermatitis chronica atrophicans (ACA), 229
Active immunity, 4
Acute glomerulonephritis, 396
Acute hepatitis, 283-284

Acute hepatitis C, 290
Acute inflammatory response, 38-39, 39f
Acute lymphoblastic leukemia, 448
Acute myelogenous leukemia (AML), 203
  multiple myeloma and, 353
Acute myeloid leukemia, 448
Acute phase, 128
Acute-phase protein
  C-reactive protein (CRP), 93
  examples of, 92t
  measurement of, 92b
  overview of, 92
  synthesis and catabolism of, 93
Acute-phase reactant, 92
Acute rejection, 438-439
Acute renal failure (ARF), 352
Acute rheumatic fever, 206
Adaptive immune system, 78
Adaptive immunity
  antigens and, 4-6
  comparative features of, 86t
  cytokines for, 85t
  innate immunity and, 6
ADCC reaction, 63
Addison's disease
  antigens implicated in, 368t
  cause of, 375
Adenoma, 461
Adherence, 34
Adrenal gland, 375
Advisory Committee on Immunization Practices (ACIP), 109
Afferent lymphatic duct, 55
Affinity, 19, 19f
Affymetrix GeneChip probe array, 184f
Agglutination
  antibody type and, 139
  antigen-antibody ratio and, 139
  influence of antibody types on, 21
  mechanisms of, 138-140
  methods for enhancing, 140
  patterns of, 136f
  principles of, 135
  process of, 21
  reactions
    false-positive/false-negative, 142t
    grading, 140-142, 140t
    reading, 141t
    using microplate, 142
  for rheumatoid factor (RF), 415
  in vitro inhibition, 136
Alkaline phosphatase (ALP), 471
Alkaloid, 450
Alkylating agent, 473, 450
Allele, nomenclature of, 426-427
Allele-specific oligonucleotide (ASO), 183
Allergen, 330

Allergy
  definition of, 330
  laboratory evaluation of, 334-335
  treatment for, 335
Alloantibody, production of, 16
Alloepitope, 428
Allogeneic transplant, 450
Allograft, 5
  definition of, 432t
  of heart valve, 433
  of skin, 433
Allotype determinant, 16, 17t
Alpha$_1$-antitrypsin, 95
Alpha-defensins 1, 2, and 3, 316
Alpha-fetoprotein, 470
Alternate pathway, 79, 82
Alternative activation pathway, 79
Alzheimer's disease, 380
Aminopterin, 21-22
Amplicon, 180
Amplification
  analysis of, 182-186
  conventional analysis of, 182
  DNA sequencing, 182
  technique for, 181-182
Amyotrophic lateral sclerosis (ALS), 380
Anamnestic response, 17
Anaphylactic reaction, 5t
Anaphylatoxin, 71
Anaphylaxis, 5
  mediators of, 333t
  stages of, 331
Anaphylotoxin, 331
Anaplasmosis, 238
Angioedema, 332
Anion, 147
Anthrax vaccine, 202
Antiadrenal antibody, 369
Antibody
  affinity of, 19, 19f
  agglutination and, 21, 139
  avidity of, 19, 19f
  cancer and, 467
  characteristics of, 10
  deficiency of, 65t, 68
  detection
    for cytomegalovirus, 193
    enzyme immunoassays for, 160-161
    fluorescent microsphere-based immunoassay for, 175f
    for HIV/AIDS, 318
    for Lyme disease, 235-237
  to DNA, 400-401
  function of, 10, 17-18
  to HBeAg and HBsAg, 283
  histones, 401
  to HIV-1, 317

Page number followed by t indicates table; b, box; f, figure.

513

Antibody—cont'd
  to nonhistone proteins, 401-402, 402t
  to nucleolar antigens, 402
  primary response, phases of, 17, 18f
  production of, 69
  response in Epstein-Barr virus, 268f
  secondary response, 17, 18f
  structure of, 12-16
  synthesis of, 17-18
  variants of, 16f
  viral infections and, 192-193
Antibody-dependent, cell-mediated cytotoxic
    (ADCC) activity, 62
  graft rejection and, 439
Antibody-forming cell blockade, 437
Antibody-mediated immunity, 4
Antibody testing, 128
Antibody titer
  concentration, determination of, 128
  definition of, 128
Anti-bone marrow antibody, 384
Anticardiolipin antibody, 369
Anticentriole antibody, 369
Anticentromere antibody, 369
Anticoagulant, 404
Antideoxyribonucleoprotein (anti-DNP),
    398
Anti-DNA antibody, 369
Anti-DNase (ADN-B), 209
Anti-EA-D, 269
Anti-EA-R, 269
Antigen
  adaptive immunity and, 4-6
  antibody test for, 373t
  autoimmune endocrine disease, 368t
  cell surface molecules as, 55
  characteristics of, 8-9
  chemical nature of, 9
  complexity of, 10
  degradability of, 9
  detection, enzyme immunoassays for,
    159-160
  Epstein-Barr nuclear, 269
  foreignness of, 9
  for HIV-1, 317, 318-319
  molecular weight of, 9
  physical nature of, 9-10
  processing and presentation to T cell, 59
  protein as, 9
  reaction to, 65
  structural stability of, 10
  T lymphocyte, recognition by, 59-62
  types of, 330
  viral capsid, 268
Antigen-antibody interaction, 18
Antigen-antibody ratio, 139
Antigen-antibody reaction
  detection of, 21
  molecular basis of, 20-21
  nephelometry and, 171f
  temperature and incubation period, 140
Antigen-binding fragment, 13f
Antigenic determinants, 8
  agglutination and, 139-140
  allotype class of, 16
  categories of, 16, 16f

Antigenic determinants—cont'd
  idiotype class of, 16-17
  isotype class of, 16
Antigen-nonspecific immunosuppression,
    440-441
Antigen-presenting cell, 5
Antigen-specific immunosuppression, 441
Anti-glomerular basement membrane
    antibody, 369
Anti-HBc, 283
Anti-HBs, 283
Antihuman globulin (AHG), 138
Antiimmunoglobins, 165
Anti-intrinsic factor antibody, 369
Anti-islet cell antibody, 369
Anti-liver kidney microsomal (anti-LKM)
    antibody, 369
Antilymphocyte globulin, 442-443
Antimalarial drug
  for rheumatoid arthritis, 418
  for SLE, 404
Antimetabolite, 450
Antimitochondrial antibody, 369
Antimyelin antibody, 369
Antimyocardial antibody, 369
Antineutrophil antibody, 369
Antinuclear antibody (ANA), 369, 392
Antinuclear antibody (ANA)
  autoimmune enzyme immunoassay
    screening test for, 408
  characteristics of, 400
  classification of, 400-401
  indirect immunofluorescent tests for,
    402-403
  patterns and disorders of, 403t
Antinuclear antibody visible method test,
    405-407
Anti-nuclear ribonucleoprotein (anti-nRNP)
    antibody, 369-370
Antinucleoprotein, rapid slide test for,
    407-408
Anti-oncogene, 467
Anti-parietal cell antibody, 369
Anti-perinuclear factor (APF), 416
Antiplatelet antibody, 369
Antireticulin antibody, 369
Anti-rheumatoid arthritis nuclear antigen
    (anti-RANA); RA precipitin), 369
Antiribosome antibody, 369
Anti-RNA polymerase II antibody, 383-384
Anti-Scl-70 antibody, 370
Anti-Scl antibody, 370
Antisepsis, 106b
Antiskin (dermal-epidermal) antibody, 370
Antiskin (interepithelial) antibody, 370
Antiskin antibody, 385-386
Anti-Sm antibody, 370
Anti-smooth muscle antibody, 370
Antisperm antibody, 370, 375
Anti-SS-A (SS-A precipitin; anti Ro)
    antibody, 370
Anti-SS-B (SS-B precipitin, anti-La)
    antibody, 370
Antistreptolysin) (ASO), 209
Antistriational antibody, 370
Antithymocyte globulin, 442-443

Antithyroglobulin antibody, 370
Antithyroid antibody test, 373t
Antithyroid microsome antibody, 370
Apheresis, 451
Arthralgia, 233
Arthritis
  Lyme disease and, 233
  in systemic lupus erythematosus, 397
  treatment for, 417-419
Arthrus reaction, 339
Aspergillosis, 191-192
Ataxia-telangiectasia, 70
Atopy, 330
Atrophic gastritis, 376-377
Autoagglutinin, 338
Autoantibody, 365
  detection of, 368-370
  myositis-specific, 385b
Autoantigen, 9, 331, 365
Autograft, 432t
Autoimmune disorder, 39, 340
  characteristics of, 365
  examples of, 340t, 365t, 366b
  immunopathogenic mechanisms of,
    367-368
  spectrum of, 365-367
Autoimmune disorder, 2
  examples of, 366f
  of skin, 385b
Autoimmune enzyme immunoassay ANA
    screening test, 161-163, 386, 408
Autoimmune gastritis, 376-377
Autoimmune hematologic disorder,
    378-380
Autoimmune hemolytic anemia, 338
Autoimmune hemolytic disease, 378-380
Autoimmune liver disease, 377
Autoimmune pancreatitis, 374-375
Autoimmunity
  definition of, 365
  factors influencing, 367
Autologous transplant, 450
Automated immunoassay
  analyzers for, 177t
  benefits of, 178b
  examples of, 177t
  trends in, 177-178
Automated testing, 170
Automatic dispenser/syringe, 125
Automatic pipette
  piston-type, steps in using, 124f
  sampling/sampling-diluting type of,
    123-125
Avascular necrosis, 397
Avidity, 19, 19f
Avidity test, 251-252
Azathioprine, 418
  as antirejection therapy, 441

B

Babesia, 239, 239f
Babesiosis, 239-240
Bacteria, 35
Bacterial agglutination, 138
Bacterial disease, 190
Bacterial sepsis, 380

Basophil, 33
BBLMonoSlide Test, 270
B-cell marker, 63
Bejel, 215
Bence Jones (BJ) protein, 149
    in multiple myeloma, 352, 354-355
    screening procedure for, 361-362
Benign tumor, 461-462
Beta chemokine, 310
Beta-hCG, 470
Biodefense, vaccination for, 198
Biohazard
    bags for, 108-109
    blood, disposal of, 107
    containers for, 108-109
    symbol for, 108f
Biologically activated molecule, 38
Biomarker, for rejection, 444-445
Biometrics, 117
Bladder cancer, 472
Blastomyces dermatitidis, 192
Blastomycosis, North American, 192
Bleach
    for decontamination, 107
    preparation of, 106t
Blood
    decontamination of spills, 107-108
    infectious disease transmission, 104
    as lymphoid organ, 52
    specimen preparation, 120-121
Blood cell, 31-32
Blood donor, screening of, 318
Blood group antigen, 9
Blood transfusion
    donor screening for, 318
    hemolytic reaction
        delayed, 337
        immediate, 336-337
    reactions, types of, 337b
Blotting, 183-184
B lymphocyte
    activation of, 63
    cell surface markers, types of, 63-64
    characteristics of, 65
    deficiency disorders of, 68
    electron photomicrograph of, 54f
    innate immunity and, 49
Body defense, 2-6
Body fluid
    decontamination of spills, 107-108
    infection, as defense against, 2, 3f
Bonding
    electrostatic force, 20
    goodness of fit, 20, 20f
    hydrogen, 20
    hydrophobic, 20
    types of, 20
    Van der Waals force, 20
Bone marrow, 52
    candidates for, evaluating, 451
    cell harvesting, 451
    indications for, 450
    myeloma cells in, 355f
Bone matrix autograft, 434
Booster vaccination, 4
Borrelia burgdorferi, 229, 231f

Branched DNA m(b-DNA), 182
Breast cancer
    marker for, 471-472
    molecular diagnosis of, 472
Breast carcinoma-associated antigen, 470
Brewster windows, 172-173
Bronchus-associated lymphoid tissue
    (BALT), 52
Bruton's X-linked agammaglobulinemia,
    68
Bull's eye rash, 234-235
Bullous disease, 385-386

C

C1 complex, 81
C1 esterase inhibitor (C1 inhibitor), 84
C1q, 84
C1q binding, 84
C1r, 84
C1s, 84
C2, 84
C3, 84
    pathways leading to, 79, 80f
C3 anaphylatoxin, 81
C3b inhibitor (C3b inactivator), 84
C3PA (C3 proactivator, Properdin Factor B),
    84-85
C4, 84-85
C4 allotype, 85
C5, 84-85
C6, 84-85
C7, 84-85
C8, 84-85
Ca 125, 470
CA 15-3, 470
CA 19-9, 470
CA 27.29, 470
Cancer
    in adult, 462-463
    body defenses against, 467-468
    chemotherapy and, 448-449
    in children, 463
    environmental factors associated with,
        464, 464t
    epidemiology of, 462-463
    etiologic factors in, 463-464
    human papillomavirus causing, 203
    immunodeficiency syndromes and, 464
    organ transplantation causing, 443
    predisposing genes, 465
    process of, 465b
    progenitor cell transplant, treating with,
        448-449
    radiotherapy for, 469-470
    related conditions, 464-465, 464t
    risk factors for, 463
    therapeutic agents for, 474t
    treatment for, 473-474
    vaccine development for, 203
    viral causes of, 464
Candida albicans, 190-192
Capillary electrophoresis (CE)
    microchip CE, comparing to, 156t
    separation techniques for, 155b
    types of, 155
Capillary isoelectric focusing (IEF), 155

Capillary zone electrophoresis (CZE), 155
Capture, 34
Capture EIA, 160-161
Carbohydrate, 9
Carcinoembryonic antigen, 471
Carcinofetal antigen, 469-470
Carcinogenesis, 464-465
Cardiovascular disorders, 370-371
Carditis, 207, 370-371
Card pregnancy test, 131-133, 132f
Catalase-positive bacteria, 41
Category A agent, 203
Cation, 147
CD25, 58
CD4, 310
CD4+, 310
    AIDS and, 314, 316
    differentiation of, 57f
    function of, 58f
    HIV and, 313
CD8+, 316
Celiac disease, 378
Cell adhesion molecule (CAM), 34, 62
Cell cycle-active, phase-specific drug, 473
Cell cytometry. *See* Flow-cell cytometry,
    173-174
Cell-mediated immunity, 4t, 5-6
    deficiency of, 65
    delayed hypersensitivity and, 5-6
    graft rejection and, 440
Cell sorting
    flow cytometry and, 174
    lasers and schematic for, 174f
Cell surface marker, 63
Cell surface receptor, 40
Cellular immunity, activation of, 437-438
Cellular replication, 192-193
Cellulitis, 208
Center for Biologics Evaluation and
    Research (CBER), 198
Centers for Disease Control and Prevention
    (CDC), 103-104
    inflammatory bowel disease, prevalence
        of, 377
    Lyme disease, definition of, 232-233
    PEP guidelines, 110
    Standard Precautions, 104-105
    vaccine approval, 198
Central tolerance, 368
Centrifugation, 120
Cephalosporin, 379
Cerebrospinal fluid, 236-237
Ceruloplasmin, 95
Cerumen. *See* Earwax
Cervical cancer marker, 471-472
Chédiak-Higashi syndrome, 41
Chemical carcinogen, 464
Chemiluminescence, 163-164
Chemiluminescent enzyme immunoassay,
    334
Chemokine
    as hematopoietic stimulator, 91
    target cells and biologic activities of, 90t
Chemokine coreceptor, 310
Chemotaxis, 33-34
Chemotherapeutic agent, 473-474

Chemotherapy
  as cancer treatment, 448-449
  types of drugs, 450
Chemotherapy agent, 450b
Chicken pox, 193-194
Children
  allergic disease in, 333
  cancer in, 463
  carditis in, 207
  leukemia in, 448
  rheumatic fever in, 207-208
  See also Juvenile rheumatoid arthritis
      (JRA)
  hepatitis B and, 285
Chinese, smallpox crust powder, 1
Cholestatic hepatitis, 277
Chronic active hepatitis, 377
Chronic glomerulonephritis, 396
Chronic granulomatous disease (CGD), 35,
    41
Chronic hepatitis, 284
Chronic hepatitis C, 290
Chronic liver disease, 280f
Chronic lymphocytic leukemia, 448
Chronic mucocutaneous candidiasis, 68
Chronic myeloid leukemia, 448
Chronic rejection, 439
Chyle, 121
Cirrhosis, idiopathic biliary, 377
C-kit ligand, 91
Classic pathway, 79
  activation of, 85
  components of, 81
  composition of, 81
Clinical and Laboratory Standards Institute
    (CLSI), 103-104, 120
Clinical Laboratory Improvement
    Amendments of 1988 (CLIA '88), 113
Clonal abortion
  of B-cell, 436
  of T-cell, 436
Clonal exhaustion, 436
Clonal expansion, 49-50, 52-55
Clonal selection, 6, 17, 55-56
Clot retraction, 120
Clumping, 140-142
Coagglutination, 135-136
Cobalamin-binding protein, 377t
Cobalamin transport, 376-377
COBE spectra apheresis system, 455f
Coccidioides immitis, 192
Coccidiomycosis, 192
Coefficient of variation (CV), 115
Cold autoimmune hemolytic anemia, 338,
    379
Colinearity, 172
Collagen vascular disorders, 371-372
College of American Pathologists (CAP),
    103-104
  standards for quality control, 113
Colloid antigen, 373
Colony-stimulating factor (CSF), 86, 91
Colorectal screening, 472-473
Colorimetric immunologic probe detection,
    164

Combining site, 18
Commission on Office Laboratory
    Accreditation (COLA), 113
Common variable immunodeficiency
    (CVID), 69
Competitive EIA, 160
Competitive immunoassay
  chemiluminescence and, 163
  format for, 163f
Complement
  activation, 79, 84-85
    effects of, 79-81
    enzyme activation, 79
    intravascular thrombosis, 83
  assessment of, 84-85
  breakdown products, detection of, 95
  components, 65
    function of, 82-84
  deficiency of, 83t, 85
  inactivation of, 121
  levels
    alteration of, 82-84
    decrease in, 83-84
    elevation of, 83
Complementary-determining region (CDR),
    12
Complement cascade, 79
Complement deficiency, 70, 70t
Complement fixation (CF), 17-18, 191
Complement-mediated cytotoxicity,
    429-430
Complement pathways
  activation
    initiators of, 79t
    types of, 80f
Complement protein, 3-4
  function of, 82-84
Complement receptor, 34, 79
Complement receptor 1 (CR1), 79
Complement receptor 3 (CR3)
  deficiency of, 41
  pathways leading to, 79, 80f
Complement system
  activities of, 79, 79t
  function of, 82
  overview of, 78-81
  proteolytic, amplification of, 81
  recognition unit of, 81
Complete blood cell (CBC) count, 65
Concentration
  calculation of, 126
  of dilution, 126
Congenital CMV, 190-192
Congenital infection, 193
Congenital rubella
  history of, 302f
  manifestations of, 302
  signs and symptoms of, 300-301
Congenital syphilis, 218, 218f
Congenital toxoplasmosis, 248b, 249
Constant (C) region, 12
Control specimen, 116
Convalescent phase, 128
Conventional CE, 155
Cooperation, in immune system, 1-2

Cornea transplant, 433
Corticosteroid
  for immunosuppressive therapy, 441-442
  for rheumatoid arthritis, 417
  for SLE, 404
Cowpox, 1
C-reactive protein (CRP), 92-93
  levels
    after cholecystectomy, 94f
    in disease states, 93
C-reactive protein rapid latex agglutination
    test, 95-97
Crohn's disease (CD), 377
Cross-reactivity, 18-19
Cryoglobulin, 172
Cryopreservation, 455
Cryptococcosis, 192
Cryptococcus neoformans, 192
Cryptosporidiosis, 314
Cutaneous lupus, 392
Cyclic citrullinated peptide (CCP) antibody,
    415
Cyclophosphamide, 418
Cyclosporine, 418
  for immunosuppressive therapy, 442
Cytokine, 5, 457
  activities of, 86
  assessment of, 91
  examples of, 85t
  host defense, role in, 86
  intracellular signaling pathways, initiation
      of, 86
  origin and immunoregulatory activities
      of, 87t
  overview of, 85-86
  production, defects in, 92t
  target cells and biologic activities of, 90t
Cytokine-release syndrome, 443
Cytolysis, 79
Cytolytic T lymphocyte (CTL), 467
Cytomegalovirus (CMV), 193, 196
  epidemiology of, 190
  etiology of, 189-190
  immunologic manifestations of, 192
  laboratory evaluation of, 191t, 192-194
  latent versus congenital infection, 190
  passive latex agglutination and, 193
  signs and symptoms of
    acquired infection, 191-192
    congenital infection, 192
  transmission of, 190
  vaccine development for, 202
Cytopenia, 451-454
Cytotoxic drug, 418, 441
Cytotoxic reaction, 5t
Cytotoxic T lymphocyte, 59
  tumor cell, effect on, 60f
Cytotoxicity, complement-mediated,
    429-430

D

Dacliximab (Zenapax), 443
Dane particle, 280
Darkfield microscopy, 219
Decline phase, 17

Decontamination. *See* Biohazard; Waste
Deer tick, 231f
Degranulation, 38
    of neutrophil, 35
Delayed hypersensitivity
    cell-mediated immunity and, 5
    testing for, 342
Deoxyribonucleic acid (DNA)
    antibodies to, 400-401
    polymerase chain reaction and, 180
    RNA converted to, 309
    synthesis and mitosis of, 65
    viruses involving, 193
Dermal-epidermal antibody, 385-386
Dermatomyositis, 385
Desensitization, 336f
Desert fever, 192
Diabetes, type 1, 368t
Diabetes mellitus, organ transplantation
        causing, 443-444
Diagnostic testing
    categories of, 131
    quality control standards for, 131
Diapedesis, 33-34, 38
Diarthrodial joint, 414
Differential agglutination test, 251
DiGeorge's syndrome, 66-68
Digestion, 35
Diluter-dispenser, 125
Dilution
    concentration
        calculation of, 126
        as expression of, 126
    five-tube twofold, 127f
    of specimen, 125
    See also Serial dilution; single dilution
Dilution factor, 125
    use of, 126
Diplococcus pneumoniae, 34-35
Direct antiglobulin test (DAT), 339, 379t
Direct bacterial agglutination, 138
Direct fluorescent antibody test, 165-166
Direct immunofluorescent assay (DFA)
    principle of, 164
    technique for, 164, 164f
Discoid lupus, 392, 396
Disease
    example of effects of, 148f
    prevalence and incidence of, 116
    prevention of, 109-111
    screening tests for, 109
    vaccine-preventable, 109
    See also Infectious disease; Vector-borne
        disease
Disease-modifying antirheumatic drug
        (DMARD), 417-418
Distribution curve, 117f
DNA chip (microarray), 184
DNA index, 472
DNA maturation, 180
DNA microarray technology, 472-473
DNA sequencing, 182
Domain, 12
Donor, 8-9
Dot blot, 183

Drug
    cell cycle-active, phase-specific, 473
    chemotherapeutic agents, 473-474
    immunosuppressive, 418
    non-cell cycle active, 473-474
Drug-induced hemolysis, 379-380
Drug-induced immunosuppression, 474
Drug-induced lupus, 392
Drug-induced positive antiglobulin test, 379t
Duncan's disease (X-linked
        lymphoproliferative disease), 69
Dust phagocyte, 37
Dye, fluorescent, 173
Dyspnea, 71-72

E

Early antigen, 269
Early antigen-diffuse (EA-D), 269
Early antigen-restricted (EA-R), 269
Earwax (cerumen), 2
Eczema, immunodeficiency with, 70
Efferent lymphatic duct, 55
Ehrlichia species, 237, 238f
Ehrlichiosis, 237-238
Eight-color immunofluorescence, 174-176
Elastase, 35
Electrical field
    application of, 148f
    in electrophoresis, 147
Electromagnetic spectrum, 173f
Electrophoresis, 147
    disease, effect of, 148f
    monoclonal immunoglobulin detection,
        356
    multiple myeloma and, 356-357
Electrophoretogram, 149
Electrostatic force, 20
Electrostatic potential, 139, 139f
Elution, 138-139
Endocrine gland disorder, 372-374
Endogenous pathway, 59
Endometriosis, 375
Endosome, 59
Endotoxin, 38
End-stage renal disease (ESRD), 352
Engraftment, 451-454
Engulfment, 34-35, 34f
Env gene, 309
Environmental Protection Agency (EPA),
        107
Environmental substance, 330
Enzyme activation, 79
Enzyme immunoassay (EIA), 110
    for antibody detection, 160-161
    for antigen detection, 159-160
    examples of, 158-161
    for hepatitis C detection, 289
    for HIV/AIDS
        false-positive/false-negative, 318t
        p24 antigen, 318
    uses for, 158-161
Enzyme-linked immunosorbent assay
        (ELISA), 22, 184
    for IgG antibody detection, 251
    for Lyme disease, 235

Eosinophil, 33
Eosinophilia-myalgia syndrome, 372
Eosinophilic cationic protein, 335
Epidermal growth factor receptor, 472
Epitope, 8
Epstein-Barr nuclear antigen (EBNA), 269
Epstein-Barr virus (EBV), 69, 193, 266
    antibody response, 268f
    characteristic diagnostic profile of, 269t
    lymphocytes in, 267f
    MonoSlide test for, 269-271
    serology of, 268
    signs and symptoms of, 267
Equilibrium constant, 138-139
Equipment
    decontamination of, 107
    preventive maintenance of, 114
Equivalence point, 147-148
Error
    causes of, 114b
    postanalytical, 115b
    preanalytical, 115b
    quality control and, 115
    sources of, 149
    types of, 114
Erysipelas, 208
Erythema chronicum migrans (ECM), 231,
        233f
Erythrocyte. *See* Red blood cell
Erythrocyte rosette formation (E technique),
        65
Erythrocyte sedimentation rate (ESR)
    indications of, 65
    inflammation, as sign of, 92
Erythrogenic toxin, 207
E technique (erythrocyte rosette formation),
        65
Exocrine gland disorder, 375-376
Exocytosis, 35
Exogenous pathway, 59
Extracellular matrix (ECM) components, 40
Extravasation, 33-34
Exudate, 32

F

Fab fragment, 13-14
Facial barrier, 105-106
False negative, 115-116
False-negative error, 114
False positive, 115-116
False-positive error, 114
Familial Mediterranean fever, 85
Fc fragment, 13-14
Fc receptor, 34
Felty's syndrome, 416
Field's test, 239
Fimbriae, 206
First aid, procedures for, 111
First-set rejection, 437-438
Five-tube twofold, 127f
Flea, 230t
Flocculation test, 138
Flow-cell cytometry, 172-177, 173f
    cell sorting, 174
    dot plots, 176f

Flow-cell cytometry—cont'd
principle of, 173-174
six-color, 176
Flow cytometry, 430
FlowMetrix system, 175-176
Fluid, body, 3f
infection, as defense against, 2
Fluorchrome, 173
Fluorescein isothiocyanate (FITC), 164
Fluorescein isothiocyanate (FITC), 173
Fluorescence-activated cell sorter (FACS), 165
Fluorescence in situ hybridization, 174
Fluorescence in situ hybridization (FISH), 168
Fluorescence polarization immunoassay, 167
Fluorescent antibody (FA), 164, 192
Fluorescent dye, 173
Fluorescent microsphere-based immunoassay, 175f
Fluorescent polarization immunoassay, 178
Fluorescent Treponemal antibody absorption test (FTA-ABS test), 223-226
control pattern examples, 224t
new conjugate titration, 223t
Fluorescent treponemal antibody adsorption (FTA-ABS) test, 219
Food allergy, rapid testing for, 342-343
Food and Drug Administration, 322
Free light chain (FLC), 355
assays for, 356t
production of, 355-356
serum immunoassay, benefits of, 355b
Functional deletion
of B-cell, 437
of T-cell, 436
Fungal disease, 190-192
testing methods for, 191t
Fungi, 190-191
Fusion inhibitor, 322

G

Gag gene, 309
Gallbladder, radiographs of, 94f
Gastritis, 376-377
Gastrointestinal disorder, 376-378
Gaucher's disease, 42
Gaussian curve, 116-117
Gaussian distribution, 116-117
Gel electrophoresis, 155, 180
two-dimensional polyacrylamide, 472
Gene
cancer-predisposing, 465
tumor-suppressing, 467
GeneChip, 185
eukaryotic target labeling for, 185f
gene expression on, 186f
Gene expression, 309
Genome, 6
German measles, 299
Germline-encoded receptor, 6
Glomerulonephritis, 208-209, 340
Gloves
for decontamination, 107
selection and use of, 105
Glucocorticoid, 417

Glucocorticosteroid, 473
Gluten, 378
Glycolipid, 8-9
Glycoprotein, 8-9
of HIV importance, 309
Goodpasture's syndrome, 338-339
gp120, 309, 310
gp160, 309
gp41, 309
Grading, agglutination reactions, 140-142, 140t
Graduated pipette, 121f, 122
Graft
manipulation and storage of, 454-455
people living with functioning, 432f
rejection of, 437-439, 438f
tissue antigen, importance of, 425
Graft-versus-host disease (GVHD)
cause of, 434-437
diagnostic evaluation of, 435
etiology and epidemiology of, 434
manifestations of, 435
prevention of, 435-436
requirements for, 434t
risk of, 451
signs and symptoms of, 435
transplantation and, 454
Gram-negative bacterial sepsis, 91
Granulocyte, 436
Granulocyte colony-stimulating factor (G-CSF), 450
Granulocyte-macrophage colony stimulating factor (GN-CSF), 450
Granuloma, 41
Graves' disease, 368t
Group A streptococcal antigen, 211-212
Group B streptococcal disease, 210-211
Guillain-Barré syndrome (GBS), 380-381
Gut-associated lymphoid tissue (GALT), 52

H

Hand
antisepsis of, 106b
hygiene of, 106
Handwashing
efficacy of, 106
guidelines for, 106b
importance of, 106
Haptens, 9
Hard-bodied tick, 229
Hashimoto's disease, 366
antigens implicated in, 368t
overview of, 372
thyroid gland in, 372f
HAT medium, 21-22
Hay fever, vaccine development for, 202
Heart transplant, 433
Heart valve replacement, 433
Heavy (H) chain, 12
Heavy-chain disease (HCD), 361
Heidelberger curve, 171
Helper T lymphocyte
differentiation of, 57f
function, alteration of, 64
subsets and role of, 57-59

Hemagglutination, 138-142
Hemagglutination inhibition (HAI), 302
Hematopoiesis, 31
Hematopoietic cell, 31-32
Hematopoietic stimulator, 91
Hemolysis, 79
Hemolysis, drug-induced, 379-380
Hemolytic disease of the newborn (HDN), 337-338
Hepadnavirus, 280
Hepatitis, chronic active, 377
Hepatitis B virus (HBV)
acute infection of, 283-284
carrier state, 284-285
chronic infection of, 284
prevention and treatment of, 285
Hepatitis A antigen (HA Ag), 276
Hepatitis A virus (HAV)
clinical sequelae of, 278f
diagnostic evaluation of, 278
electron micrograph of, 277f
etiology and epidemiology of, 276-278
immunologic manifestations of, 278
prevention and treatment of, 278
signs and symptoms of, 277-278
vaccine for, 278
Hepatitis B core antibody, 282-283
Hepatitis B core antigen (HBcAg), 280
Hepatitis B-related (HB-e) antigen, 282, 283
Hepatitis B surface antigen (HBsAg), 109, 278-280, 282
antibodies, development of, 283
carrier state, 284
test results, indications of, 283
Hepatitis B viral DNA, 283
Hepatitis B virus (HBV), 104
asymptomatic infection, 281
bleach and, 107
chronic liver disease, progression of, 280f
electron micrograph of, 277f
epidemiology of, 280
etiology of, 278-280
exposure to, 110
laboratory assays for, 281-283
panel interpretation for, 281t
prevention and treatment of, 285
serologic and clinical patterns observed, 282f
signs and symptoms of, 280-281
transmission of, 104
Hepatitis C virus (HCV), 287-291
acute and chronic, differentiating, 290
exposure to, 110
from needlestick injury, 287f
prevention of, 291
from transfusion, 288f
transmission of, 107
treatment for, 290-291
Hepatitis D virus (HDV), 285-287
Hepatitis E virus (HEV), 291-292
Hepatitis G virus (HGV), 292
Hepatitis virus
acute and chronic, differentiating, 283-285
electron micrograph of, 277f

Hepatitis virus—cont'd
  fluorescent microsphere-based
      immunoassay, 175f
  forms of, 276t
  incidence of, 276
  signs and symptoms of, 276
  transfusion-transmitted virus, 292-293
  types of, 275
  vaccine for, 279b
Hereditary angioedema, 85
Hereditary ataxia-telangiectasia, 70
Herpes simplex virus (HSV), 193
  congenital and neonatal, 193
  laboratory diagnosis of, 193
Herpesvirus, 193, 266
Heterogeneous, 148
Heterogenous immunoassay, 158
Heterograft, 432t
Heterophil antibody, 268
HG-U133A array, 186
Hidden-antigen theory, 368
Highly active antiretroviral therapy
      (HAART), 314
Hinge molecular component, 13-14
Histamine, 33-34
Histocompatibility antigen, 9
Histocompatibility testing, 429
Histone, 401
Histone-reactive antinuclear antibody
      (HR-ANA), 370
Histoplasmosis, 191
HLA-B27 antigen, 176-177, 428
Hodgkin's lymphoma, 448-449
Homogeneous, 148
Homogeneous immunoassay, 158
Homograft, 432t
Hormone antagonist, 474
Hospital Infection Control Practices
      Advisory Committee (HICPAC), 109
Human chorionic gonadotropin (hCG), 131,
      136
  beta subunit of, 470
Human ehrlichiosis, 237-238
Human Genome GeneChip, 185, 185f
Human Genome Project, 155
Human gonadotropin hormone (hCG), 120
Human herpesvirus-6, 194
Human IgG1, enzymatic cleavage of, 13f
Human immunodeficiency virus (HIV), 64
  asymptomatic, assessment of, 317t
  bleach and, 107
  blood donor, screening of, 318
  classification system of, 312b
  diagnostic evaluation of, 317-318
  drug resistance in, 322
  etiology of, 308
  life cycle of, 309-310, 309b
  mechanism for entering cell, 310f
  polymerase chain reaction and, 319
  postexposure prophylaxis, 322-323
  prevention of, 320-321
  proteins of, 309, 309t
  rapid antibody test, 323-325
  replication of, 309-311
  screening for antibodies to, 110

Human immunodeficiency virus (HIV)—
      cont'd
  Standard Precautions for, 104
  subtypes of, 308
  testing methods for, 318-320
  transmission of, 104, 107, 110-111,
      311-313
  treatment for, 321-323
  vaccine development
    expectations for, 202
    goal of, 201
    for immunity, 199-202
    problems in, 201-202
  vaccine development for, 320-321, 321b
  See also Acquired immunodeficiency
      syndrome (AIDS)
Human immunodeficiency virus Type 1
  AIDS development from, 316
  antibodies and antigens for, 317
  immunologic manifestations of, 316
  progression of, 314-316
  signs and symptoms of, 313
Human immunodeficiency virus Type 2, 311
Human intracisternal A-type particle (HIAP),
      416
Human leukocyte antigen (HLA), 9, 426
  applications of, 428
  disease and, 428b, 429t
  for kidney transplant, 430f
  molecules, classes of, 427
  naming system, 426t
  nomenclature of, 426-427
  role of, 427-428
  typing of, 429
Human monocytic ehrlichiosis (HME), 238
Human papillomavirus, 203
Human T-cell leukemia, 64
Human T-lymphotropic retrovirus (HTLV),
      308
Humoral, 3-4
Humoral-mediated immunity, 4-5, 4t
  graft rejection and, 440
Humoral system, 65
Hyaluronidase, 207
Hybridization, 182-184
Hybridoma, 21
Hydralazine, 392
Hydrogen bond, 20
Hydrophobic bond, 20
Hyperacute rejection, 438
Hypercholesterolemia, organ
      transplantation causing, 444
Hypergammaglobulinemia, 349, 377
Hyperimmunoglobulinemia E syndrome, 70
Hyper-M, 69
Hypersensitivity, 330
Hypersensitivity reaction
  in children, 333
  classification of, 5t, 331t
  delayed, 5
  immediate, 5
  laboratory evaluation of, 334-335
    chemiluminescent enzyme
      immunoassay, 334
    eosinophilic cationic protein, 335

Hypersensitivity reaction—cont'd
    first- and second-generation testing,
      334
    ImmunoCAP, 334, 334f, 335t
    protein microarray, 334
    third-generation method, 334-335
  triggers of, 330
  type 1
    anaphylactic reaction, 331
    anaphylactoid reaction, 331
    atopic reaction, 331-332
    etiology of, 330
    generalized reaction, 332-333
    immunologic activity, 331-332
    localized reaction, 332
    signs and symptoms of, 332-334
    testing for, 333-334
    treatment for, 335
  type II, 336-337
    affecting cell function, 339
    antibody-dependent, cell-mediated
      cytotoxicity, 338-339
    antibody-dependent reactions, 335-336
    hemolytic reaction, delayed, 337
    hemolytic reaction, immediate,
      336-337
    against solid tissue, 339
    testing for, 339
    transfusion reaction, 336-337
  type III
    cause of, 339-341
    manifestations of, 340
    testing for, 340-341
  type IV, 341
  types of, 330
Hypertension, organ transplantation
      causing, 444
Hypocomplementemia
  cause of, 83-84
  diseases association with, 83b
Hypoparathyroidism, idiopathic
  antigens implicated in, 375
  occurrence of, 375
Hyposensitization, 336f
Hypoxanthine, 21-22

I
Icteric serum, 121
Idiopathic adrenal atrophy, 375
Idiopathic biliary cirrhosis, 377
Idiopathic hypoparathyroidism
  antigens implicated in, 368t
  occurrence of, 368t
Idiopathic thrombocytopenia purpura, 380
Idiotype determinant, 16-17, 17t
IgE-dependent hypersensitivity, 5
Immediate hypersensitivity, 5
Immune complex, 19-20
Immune complexing, 379
Immune complex reaction, 5t
Immune-mediated disease, 71
Immune response, 85-91
Immune response gene-associated antigen,
      437
Immune senescence, 50-52

Immune system
aging, effects of, 64
cellular elements of, 2
chemotherapy, effects of, 474t
composition and characteristics of, 1
deficiency/dysfunction of, 2
HIV effect on, 316
Immunity
adaptive/acquired, 4-6
cell-mediated, 4t, 5-6
defects in, 64-65
desirable consequences of, 2
humoral-mediated, 4-5, 4t
natural, 3-4
Immunization
for disease prevention, 109
safer, 1
smallpox crust powder as, 1
Immunoassay
formats for, 158
for Group A streptococcal antigen,
211-212, 211f
labels, types of, 158
types of, 159t
Immuno blot calibration, 236f
ImmunoCAP, 334, 334f, 335t
Immunocompetence, 50
Immunocompetent host, 4
Immunodeficiency disorder
categories of, 66
cause of, 66
Immunodeficiency syndrome, 64-65, 65t
distribution of, 67f
with elevated IgM (Hyper M), 69
Immunodiffusion, 147-148, 192
Immunoelectrophoresis (IEP), 147-151
antigen-antiserum combinations, 149f
application of, 149
configuration of, 148f
immunofixation electrophoresis,
comparing to, 154f, 155t
immunoglobulin profile on, 150f
uses for, 357
Immunofixation electrophoresis
immunoelectrophoresis, comparing to,
154f, 155t
multiple myeloma and, 357
procedure for, 151-155
Immunofluorescence, 164-165
eight-color, 174-176
Immunofluorescence assay, 320
Immunogen. See Antigen
Immunoglobulin (Ig), 10
as bifunctional, 12
cellular immunodeficiency with, 67
comparing properties of, 18t
concentration of, 11f
configuration of, 12f
elevation of, 149
profile on immunoelectrophoresis, 150f
role in diagnostic tests, 21t
subclass deficiencies, 69
variants of, 16-17, 17t
Immunoglobulin (Ig) class
characteristics of, 10t
types of, 10-12

Immunoglobulin (Ig) family, 40
Immunoglobulin (Ig) molecule
domain of, 12
globular regions of, 13-14
Immunoglobulin A (IgA)
characteristics of, 11-12
molecule of, 15f
structure of, 14
toxoplasmosis and, 251
Immunoglobulin A (IgA) monomer, 12
Immunoglobulin D (IgD)
characteristics of, 12
molecule of, 15f
structure of, 14
Immunoglobulin deposit, 384f
Immunoglobulin E (IgE)
allergies and, 330
characteristics of, 12
molecule of, 16f
structure of, 16
test for
comparison of, 334t
ImmunoCAP, 335t
toxoplasmosis and, 251
Immunoglobulin G (IgG)
agglutination and, 139
anti-EA-D of, 269
anti-EA-R of, 269
avidity test for, 251-252
characteristics of, 11
differential agglutination test for, 251
ELISA-based test for, 251
IFA test for, 251
lateral blot rapid test, 252
polymerase chain reaction for, 252
Sabin-Feldman Dye Test for, 251
structure of, 13f
TORCH testing presence of, 195, 195t
toxoplasmosis and, 250, 251-252
Immunoglobulin M (IgM)
agglutination and, 139
characteristics of, 10-11
rubella, immunity to, 300
structure of, 14, 14f
TORCH testing presence of, 195, 195t
toxoplasmosis and, 250-251
Immunohematologic disease, 378t
Immunohistochemical staining, 320
Immunologic assay
IFA technique, examples performed by,
165b
indirect hemagglutination, 138b
latex particle agglutination, 136b
nephelometry, 171b
Immunologic organ, 49, 50f
Immunologic thrombocytopenic purpura
(ITP), 380
Immunologic tolerance, 436-437
Immunology
definition of, 1-2
function of, 2
history of, 1
milestones in, 2t
Immunomodulating drug, 404
Immunoprecipitation band, appearance of,
148-149

Immunoprophylaxis, 110
Immunosuppression
drug-induced, 474
graft rejection and, 439-440
protocols for, 443, 443b
treatment for, 440t
Immunosuppressive drug, 418
Immunotherapy
in malignant disease, 473t
for tumors, 474
Impetigo, 208, 208f
Inactivation, 121
Incubation, 140
Indirect anti-human globulin (AHG) assay,
339
Indirect fluorescent antibody (IFA), 165,
165b
for IgG antibody detection, 251
Indirect hemagglutination, 138b
Indirect immunofluorescence
principle of, 403
for SLE, 402-403
technique for, 403-404
Indirect immunofluorescent assay, 165
Infant
hereditary ataxia telangiectasia in, 70
transient hypogammaglobulinemia in, 69
Infection
active immunity and, 4
control of
protective techniques for, 105
safe work practice to, 105
defense, first line of, 2-3
defense against, natural body, 3f
Infectious agent, 330
Infectious disease
antibody significance with, 195
characteristics of, 189-190
development of, 190
examples of, 340t
immunoglobulin M (IgM) and, 195
multiple myeloma and, 352-353
organ transplantation causing, 443
prevention of transmission, 104-105
Infectious hepatitis. See Hepatitis A virus
Infectious mononucleosis
diagnostic evaluation of, 267, 267t
epidemiology of, 266-267
Epstein-Barr virus antibody response, 268f
etiology of, 266
immunologic manifestations of, 268-269
signs and symptoms of, 267
Infectious waste
disposal of, 108-109
See also Biohazard; Waste
Inflammation
characteristics of, 39
effects of, 38-39
eosinophils role in, 33
erythrocyte sedimentation rate (ESR) and,
92
lymphocyte-activating factor (IL-1) effect
on, 38
tissue damage and, 4
Inflammatory bowel disease (IBD), 377-378
Inflammatory myopathy, 385

Inflammatory polyneuropathy, 380-381
Influenza vaccine, efficacy of, 203
Inhibition immunofluorescent assay,
    164-165
Innate immune system, 6, 78
Innate immunity
    adaptive component of, 49
    adaptive immunity and, 6
    comparative features of, 86t
    cytokines for, 85t
Institute for Quality Laboratory Medicine,
    115
Insulin-dependent diabetes mellitus, 374
Integrase inhibitor, 322
Integrin family, 40
Intercalating agent, 473
Interferon (IFN)
    development of, 474
    overview of, 86-90
    types, origin and activities of, 87t
    viral infections and, 192-193
Interferon alpha-2a/b, 290
Interferon-gamma, 79
Interleukin (IL), 5, 86t
    function of, 86
    types, origin and activities of, 87t
Interleukin-1 (IL-1), 33-34
Interleukin-6 (IL-6), 350-351
Interphase FISH, 168
Intracellular signaling pathways, 86
Intrinsic factor (IF), 376-377
Invagination, 34-35
In vitro agglutination inhibition, 136
In vivo skin testing, 333-334
Isoelectric focusing (IEF), 155
Isoimmune thrombocytopenia, 380
Isolated error, 114
Isotachophoresis, 155
Isotachophoresis (ITP), 155
Isotype
    immune response and, 63-64
    signals of switching, 64
Isotype determinant, 16, 17t
Isotypic variant, 16
Ixodes scapularis
    babesiosis, as cause of, 239-240
    Lyme disease, as cause of, 229-231
Ixodid tick, 229-231

J

Jo-1 antibody, 370
Joint
    anatomy and physiology of, 414
    inflammation of, 418f
Juvenile rheumatoid arthritis (JRA), 416-417,
    416t

K

Kaposi's sarcoma, 314, 315f
Keratinization, 2
Keratoconjunctivitis, 375
Kidney transplantation
    history of, 433
    HLA typing for, 430f
K-type lymphocyte, 62-63
Ku antibody, 370

L

Labeling
    emerging technologies for, 166-168
    magnetic techniques for, 167, 167f
Laboratory
    automated testing in, 170
    decontamination in, 107-108
    hazards in, 107
    infectious waste, disposal of, 108-109
    policies for, 114
    procedure manual for, 114
    quality control for, 115
    test requisitioning, 114
Laboratory coat/gown, 106, 107
Lactate dehydrogenase (LDH), 471
Lag phase, 17
Lane soluble substance-B (SS-B), 398
Large granular lymphocyte (LGL), 62
Laser, 174f
Laser flow cytometry, 173f
Laser technology, 172-173
Latent CMV, 190
Latent syphilis, 217
Late-onset lupus, 397
Lateral blot rapid test, 252
Late syphilis, 217
Latex agglutination, 135-136, 136f
    immunologic assays performed by, 136b
    liposome-enhanced, 137f
    slide tests, 138
Latex sensitivity, 341-342
Lattice formation, 140
Lattice hypothesis, 139
LE cell, 398, 399f
Leukapheresis, 451
Leukemia
    bone marrow transplant for, 448
    in children, 448
    vaccine development for, 203
Leukocyte adhesion cascade, 34
Leukocyte adhesion deficiency (LAD), 42
Leukocyte integrin, 42-43
Leukopenia, 318, 354
Lice, 230t
Ligase chain reaction nucleic acid
    amplification, 182
Light (L) chain, 12
Light-chain disease (LCD), 349-350, 361
Line immunoassay (LIA), 320
Linkage disequilibrium, 427
Liposome-enhanced latex agglutination,
    137f
Liposome-enhanced testing, 135-136
Liquid-phase hybridization, 183
Listeria monocytogene, 166-167
Liver disease, 377
    hepatitis D as, 285-286
Liver transplant, 433-434
Live virus vaccine, 203-204
Log phase, 17
Long acting thyroid stimulator (LATS), 373
Long-acting thyroid stimulator protector
    (LATS-P), 373
Long terminal redundancy (LTR), 309
Luminescent oxygen-channeling
    immunoassay (LOCI), 166-167

Luminex Total System, 174-175
Lung transplant, 434
Lupus
    forms of, 392-394
    late-onset, 397
Lupus erythematosus, 396
Lyme disease, 229-237
    antibiotics for, 237
    antibody detection in, 235
    arthritis and, 233
    cardiac manifestations of, 233-234
    cases of
        by location, 232f
        per year, 232f
    cutaneous manifestations of, 233
    diagnosis of, 234-237, 235t
    enzyme-linked immunosorbent assay
        (ELISHA) for, 235
    epidemiology of, 231-232
    immunologic manifestations of, 234
    neurologic manifestations of, 239f
    polymerase chain reaction and, 236
    pregnancy and, 234
    prevalence and incidence of, 231
    PreVue *B. burgdorferi* antibody detection
        assay for, 235-236
    signs and symptoms of, 232-234
    treatment and prevention of, 237
    Western blot analysis, 236
Lymphadenopathy, 397
Lymphadenopathy-associated virus, 308
Lymph node, 52
    structure of, 54f
    view of, 53f
Lymphoblast, 49
Lymphocyte
    absolute count of, 65
    alterations in subsets of, 64
    characteristics of, 55t
    circulation of, 52-55
    cooperation and, 1-2
    development, sites of, 49-52
    electron photomicrograph of, 50f
    lymphoid organs, percentage in, 52t
    membrane marker development, 56f
    plasma cells and, 49-55
    radiation, effects of, 436
    specificity and memory, 1-2
    terminal differentiation of, 57
    testing of, 65
    virgin/naive, 64
Lymphocyte-activating factor (IL-1), 38
Lymphocyte recirculation, 52-55
Lymphocytopenia, 318
Lymphoid thyroiditis. *See* Hashimoto's
    disease
Lymphokine-activated killer cell, 467
Lymphoma, 448-449

M

Macroglobulinemia. *See* Waldenström's
    primary macroglobulinemia (WM)
Macrophage, 427, 467
    activation of, 37
    characteristics of, 35-37
    in culture, 36f

Macrophage—cont'd
electron micrograph of, 36f
as fixed/wandering cells, 37
function of, 37
phagocytosis and, 37, 38
Magnetic labeling technology, 167, 167f
Major histocompatibility complex (MHC), 5,
9, 35
class I and II, comparison of, 427t
genetic organization of, 426f
immune recognition, role in, 426
regions of, 427
role of, 427-428
Malignant tumor, 462
Mannose-binding lectin pathway, 79, 82
Manual pipette
pipetting with, 123b
technique for, 123
Margination, 34
Marker
categorization of, 55
development for lymphocyte membrane,
56f
Maternal rubella, 301t
Matrix metalloproteinase (MMP), 381
Mean, 116-117
Measles, 299
Median, 117
Membrane attack complex (MAC), 81
Membranoproliferative glomerulonephritis,
384
Memory, 1-2
Memory cell, 64
Meniscus, 123, 123f
Metaphase FISH, 168
Metastasis, 40
Methotrexate, 418
Methyldopa, 379-380
Mi-1 antibody, 370
Microarray (DNA chip), 184
Microbial disease, 2-6
Microchip CE
advantages and application of, 155
capillary electrophoresis, comparing to,
156t
Microhemagglutination for *Treponema
pallidum* (MHA-TP) test, 219
Microorganism, 4
Micropipetter, 123-125
Microplate, 142
Mite, 230t
Mixed-field agglutination, 143
Mode, 117
Molecular biology, 180-182
Molecular genetic testing, 180
Molecular weight, 9
Monoclonal antibody (MAb), 21-23
as antirejection therapy, 443
benefits of, 455
production of, 21-22, 22f
testing of, 55
uses of, 22-23
Monoclonal gammopathy
cause of, 349
characteristics of, 349-350

Monoclonal gammopathy—cont'd
diagnosis of, 149
disease progression in, 351f
for multiple bands, 361
multiple myeloma and, 356b
Monoclonal gammopathy of undetermined
significance (MGUS)
characteristics of, 360-361
diagnostic criteria for, 360t
Monoclonal paraproteinemia, 380
Monoclonal protein, 149
Monocyte, phagocytosis and, 37
Monocyte chemotactic protein, 472
Monocyte-macrophage
disorders of, 42
host defense and inflammation, 38
Mononuclear phagocyte
function of, 37, 38b
terminal stage of development, 37
Mononuclear phagocyte system, 5, 35-37,
37f
MonoSlide test, 269-271
Monospecific antisera, 151
Monovalent antisera, 151
Morula, 238
Mosquito, types and disease caused by,
230t
M protein, 149, 206
Multiple myeloma
bone marrow aspirate, view of, 355f
characteristics of, 350-358
diagnostic criteria for, 360t
diagnostic evaluation of, 354-357
disease progression in, 351t
epidemiology of, 351
etiology and pathophysiology of, 350
immunologic manifestations of, 353-354
immunologic testing for, 356-357, 357t
lesions, view of, 353f
monoclonal gammopathies, 356b
prognosis for, 357
signs and symptoms of, 352-353
treatment for, 357-358
Multiple sclerosis (MS), 381-383
immunologic manifestations of, 382b
Multiplex polymerase chain reaction, 181
Myalgia, 233
Myasthenia gravis
abnormalities associated with, 381b
overview of, 381
Mycobacterium tuberculosis, 35, 64
Mycophenolate mofetil, 442
Mycotic infection, 190-192
Myeloablation, 448
Myeloperoxidase deficiency, 41-42
Myocardium, inflammation of, 397
Myositis-specific autoantibody, 385, 385b

N

Naive lymphocyte, 64
National Marrow Donor Program (NMDP),
455
Natural immunity
characteristics of, 3-4
components of, 3b

Natural killer (NK) cell, 62-63
cancer and, 467
endometriosis and, 375
profile of, 62t
Natural Treg cell, 58
Necrotizing fasciitis, 206
Negative predictive value, 116
Negative selection, 52-55
Neisseria gonorrhoeae, 165
Neonatal HSV infection, 193
Neonatal SLE syndrome, 398
Neonatal varicella infection, 194
Neoplasm, 461
Neoplastic disease, 340t
Nephelometry, 170-172
advantages and disadvantages of, 172
immunologic assays performed by,
171b
measuring methods for, 172
optical system, 172
physical basis of, 171
principle of, 170-171, 171f
Neuromuscular disorder, 380-383
Neuropathy, 383-384, 383t
Neurosyphilis, 218
Neutropenia, 41
Neutrophil
abnormal function of, 41
absolute count of, 65
congenital abnormalities of, 41-42, 41b
degranulation of, 35
disorders of, 40-42
infection, role in, 39f
phagocytosis and, 32
Newborn
DiGeorge's syndrome, 66
hemolytic disease of, 337-338
Nezelof syndrome, 67
Nicotinamide-adenine dinucleotide
phosphate (NADPH), 35
Niemann-Pick disease, 42
Non-cell cycle active drug, 473-474
Noncompetitive EIA, 160
Noncovalent bond, 20
Nonhistone protein, 401-402, 402t
Non-Hodgkin's lymphoma, 448-449
Noninfectious neutrophil-mediated
inflammatory disease, 40-41, 40b
Non-instrument-based testing, 131
Nonnucleoside analog reverse-transcriptase
inhibitor (NNRTI), 321
Nonself
immunology and, 1
substances of, 2
Nonspecific activation, 63
Nonsteroidal antiinflammatory drug
(NSAID)
for rheumatoid arthritis, 417
for SLE, 404
Nontreponemal method, 219
Nonwaived assay, 113
North American blastomycosis, 192
Northern blot, 183
Nucleated cell (NC), 449t
Nucleic acid, 9

Nucleic acid sequence-based amplification, 182
Nucleolar antigen, 402
Nucleoside analog reverse-transcriptase inhibitor (NRTI), 321
Null allele, 426-427

O

Oat cell carcinoma, 471
Occlusive bandage, 105-106
Occupational Safety and Health Administration (OSHA), 103-104
  Bloodborne Pathogens Standard/ Occupational Exposure Standard, 104
  handwashing, 106
  infectious waste, definition of, 108
  personal protective equipment (PPE), 105
Oligoclonal band
  detection of, 382
  significance of, 382
Oligoclonal cerebrospinal fluid gamma globulins, conditions associated with, 383b
Oligonucleotide, 180
Oncofetal protein, 470
Oncogene
  examples of, 466
  genetic mutations causing, 465
  role of, 465-466
Oncogenic virus, 466-467, 466b
Oncology, 461
Opsonin, 34
Opsonization, 34, 79
Optical immunoassay, 211-212, 211f
Optical system, 172
Organ-nonspecific disease, 366, 367t
Organ-specific disease, 365-366, 367t
Organ transplantation
  complications from, 443-444
  facts about, 430-432
  history of, 425
  See also Transplantation
OSOM card pregnancy test, 131, 132f
Osteoporosis, organ transplantation causing, 443
Ostwald pipette, 121f
Otitis media, 71-72
Outer surface protein A (OspA), 237
Outer surface protein B (OspB), 237
Ovarian cancer marker, 471-472
Ovarian failure, premature, 375

P

p24, 309, 318-319
p25, 309
p39 antigen, 237
p53 protein, 465-466
Pain, multiple myeloma and, 352
Pancreas, 434
  autoimmune pancreatitis, 374-375
  insulin-dependent diabetes mellitus, 374
Papilloma, 461
Paraprotein, 149

Parasitic disease, 190
Parathyroid gland, 375
Parkinson's disease, 380
Paroxysmal cold hemoglobinuria, 379
Particle agglutination, 136f
Particle charge, 139
Passive immunity, 4
Pasteur, Louis, 1
Pasteur pipette, 142
Pathogen, 2
Pathogen-associated molecular pattern (PAMP), 6
Patient
  identification of, 114
  testing outcomes for, 117
Pattern-recognition receptor, 6
Peginterferon alpha, 290
Penicillin, 379
Peptide, 35
Perforin, 316
Peripheral blood progenitor cell, 451
Peripheral blood stem cell (PBSC), 449
Peripheral tolerance, 368
Pernicious anemia, 376-377
  characteristics of, 380
  hematologic and chemical findings in, 380t
Personal protective equipment (PPE)
  for decontamination, 107
  facial barrier and occlusive bandage, 105-106
  gloves, selection and use of, 105
  laboratory coat/gown, 106
  OSHA requirements for, 105
Personnel, competency of, 113
Peyer's patches, 52
pH, 140
Phagocyte
  cancer cells, activity against, 38
  function of, 38b
  myeloperoxidase deficiency, 41-42
Phagocytic cell, 3-4
  cell-mediated immunity and, 5
  deficiency of, 65t
Phagocytic engulfment, screening test for, 44-45
Phagocytosis
  bacteria and, 35
  facilitation of, 4
  inappropriate activation of, 40-41
  macrophages and, 38
  monocyte-macrophage and, 37
  neutrophil role in, 32
  parasitic disease and, 190
  process of, 33-35, 33f
Phagolysosome, 35
Phagosome, 34
Pharyngeal punch syndrome, 66
Phosphate-buffered saline (PBS), 223
Photon, 172
Pinta, 215
Pipette
  inspection of, 122-123
  pipetting with, 123b
  TD (to deliver), 122

Pipette—cont'd
  types of, 121f
  uses for, 121-123
Pipetting
  automatic dispensers/syringes, 125
  technique for, 122f, 123-125
  using automatic pipette, 123-125
  using diluter-dispensers, 125
  using manual pipette, 120
  using micropipettors, 123-125
Piston, of pipette, 123-124
Pituitary gland, 375
Placental transfer, 17-18
Plaques, 381
Plasmablast, 349
Plasma cell, 64
Plasmodium falciparum, 380
Plateau phase, 17
Platelet
  disorders of, 380
  radiation, effects of, 436
Plunger, of pipette, 123-124
Pluripotent, 449
PM-1 antibody, 370
Pneumocystis jiroveci (carinii), 314f
Point-of-care testing (POCT)
  categories of, 131
  definition of, 131
  pregnancy test as, 132f
  quality control standards for, 131
Pol gene, 309
Polio, 203
Polyclonal gammopathy, 149, 349, 350
Polyethylene glycol (PEG), 21-22
Polyglandular syndrome, 375
Polymerase chain reaction (PCR), 110, 181f
  applications of, 180
  cycles of, 180
  for hepatitis C detection, 289
  for HIV/AIDS, 319
  for IgG antibody detection, 252
  Lyme disease and, 236
  modification in technique, 181
  mulitplex, 181
  process of, 180-181
  real-time, 181
  reverse-transcriptase, 181
Polymorphonuclear neutrophilic (PMN) leukocyte, 31
Polymyositis, 385
Polyp, 461
Polysaccharide, 8-9
Polyvalent antiserum, 151
Positive predictive value, 116
Positive selection, 52-55
Postanalytical error, 115b
Postexposure prophylaxis (PEP), 109-111
Poststreptococcal glomerulonephritis, 206
Posttransfusion purpura, 380
Posttransplantation lymphoproliferative disorder (PTLD), 266
Postzone phenomenon, 139
Preanalytical error, examples of, 115b
Precipitation, 135
  zone of equivalence, 139

Precipitin band
abnormal curvature of, 151
appearance of
abnormal, 149-151
normal, 148-149
position of, 149-151
shortening, thinning and doubling of, 151
thickening and elongation of, 151
Predictive value (PV), 116
Pregnancy, Lyme disease and, 234
Pregnancy testing, 132f
protocols for, 137-138
urine for, 121
See also Card pregnancy test; Human gonadotropin chorionic hormone; OSOM pregnancy test
PreVue B. burgdorferi antibody detection assay, 235-236
Primary immunodeficiency disorder, 67b
Primary idiopathic myocarditis, 371
Primary immunodeficiency disorder, 66-70
complement deficiency as, 70, 70t
Primary lymphoid organ, 49
Primary lymphoid tissue, 49-52, 51f
Primary syphilis, 216, 217f
Primer annealing, 180
Probe, 168
Procainamide-induced disease, 392-393
Procedure manual, compliance of, 120
Procedure protocol, written, 114b
Proficiency testing (PT), 116
Progenitor cell, 49
peripheral blood, 451
as pluripotent, 449
Progenitor cell transplant, 448-449
Progressive systemic sclerosis, 371-372
Properdin deficiency, 85
Prostaglandins, 417
Prostate cancer, 471
Prostate-specific antigen (PSA), 471
rapid test in seminal fluid, 475-476
Prostatic acid phosphatase, 471
Protease inhibitor, 322
Protein
acute-phase, 92-93
antibodies to nonhistone, 401-402
as antigen, 9
of HIV importance, 309, 309t
Protein microarray, 334
Proto-oncogenesis, 465-466
Provirus, 309
Prozone phenomenon, 139, 149
Prozoning, 149
PSA density, 471
PSA velocity, 471
P-selectin, 34
Pseudoagglutination, 140-142
Pseudopodia, 34
Pulmonary alveolar macrophage, 37
Purified protein derivative (PPD), 65, 109
Pyogenic infection, 84
Pyrimidine analog, 441f
Pyrogenic exotoxin, 210

Q
Quality assurance (QA), 113
for OSOM card pregnancy test, 132
Quality control (QC), 113
activities for, 115
definitions for, 115
in laboratory, 114
monitoring of, 116
for OSOM card pregnancy test, 132
validating new procedures, 117
Quality Laboratory Medicine, Institute for, 115
QuantiFERON-TB Gold (QFT), 109
Quantum dots (Q dots), 166

R
Radiation carcinogenesis, 464
Radioimmunoassay (RIA), 158
Radiotherapy, 450
RANTES, 316
Rapid HIV antibody test, 323-325
Rapid latex agglutination, 419-421
Rapid plasma reagin card test (RPR test), 215, 219
Rapid testing
for antinucleoprotein, 407-408
for food allergy, 342-343
for HIV/AIDS, 320
prostate-specific antigen (PSA), 475-476
Raynaud's phenomenon, 396
Reaction, types of, 330
Reactive oxygen species (ROS), 35
Real-time polymerase chain reaction, 181
Recipient, 8-9
Recombinant fusion protein, 417
Red blood cell (RBC)
as immunogenic, 8-9
radiation, effects of, 436
Red wolf, 396
Reference range, 116-117
Regulatory T (Treg) cell, 57-59
types of, 58f
Rejection
accelerated, 438
acute, 438-439
biomarkers for, 444-445
chronic, 439
first-set and second-set, 437-438
of graft, 437-439
hyperacute, 438
mechanisms of, 439-444
Renal disease
anti-glomerular basement membrane antibody, 384-385
categories of, 384b
circulating immune complexes and, 384
multiple myeloma and, 352
in Waldenström's primary macroglobulinemia (WM), 358
Renal disorder, 384-385
Reproducibility, 115
Reproductive disorders, 375
Resistance testing, 318
Respiratory burst, 35

Restriction fragment length polymorphism (RFLP) analysis, 182, 183
Reticuloendothelial system. See Mononuclear phagocyte system
Retrovirus
replication of, 310-311
reverse-transcriptase and, 309
Reverse dot blot, 183
Reverse grouping, 24, 142-143
Reverse transcriptase, 309
Reverse-transcriptase polymerase chain reaction, 181
Rheumatic autoantibody, staining patterns of, 403
Rheumatic disease, 413
Rheumatic fever, 206
Rheumatic heart disease, 371
Rheumatoid arthritis (RA)
anti-perinuclear factor, antibodies to, 416
characteristics of, 413f
classification of, 413b
cyclic citrullinated peptide antibodies and, 415-416
cytokines, role of, 415f
diagnostic evaluation of, 414-416
diagnostic procedures for, 419
drugs for, 418t
etiology and epidemiology of, 412-413
extraarticular manifestations of, 413b
immunologic manifestations of, 414
signs and symptoms of, 413-414
Rheumatoid factor (RF), 414-415
Rheumatoid joint, inflammation of, 418f
Rhinitis, 330
Ribavirin, 290-291
Ribonucleic acid (RNA)
deoxyribonucleic acid, converting to, 309
viruses involving, 193
Ribonucleoprotein (RNP), 396
Rocky Mountain spotted fever, 237
Rosette
formation of, 65
in Giemsa-stained cytocentrifuged preparation, 66f
Rouleaux formation, 140-142
R protein, 377
Rubella, 109, 196
acquired versus congenital, 300
congenital malformations of, 301f
diagnostic evaluation of, 302-303
epidemiology of, 299-300
etiology of, 299
immune status serodiagnosis, 302t
immunologic manifestations of, 301-302
maternal, manifestations of, 301t
passive latex agglutination test for, 303-305
signs and symptoms of, 300-301
view of
in man, 300f
rash in child, 300f

S
Sabin-Feldman Dye Test, 251
Saline replacement, 140-142

Sandwich immunoassay
  chemiluminescence and, 163
  format for, 163f
Sanger method, 182
San Joaquin fever, 192
Scarlet fever, 208
Scavenger cell, 35
Schmidt's syndrome, 375
Scleroderma, 371-372
Screening tests, 109
Sebum infection, 2
Secondary immunodeficiency, 66, 71b
Secondary lymphoid tissue, 51f, 52
Secondary syphilis, 217, 217f
Second-set rejection, 437-438
Secretion, importance of, 2
Secretory IgA, 11
  molecule of, 15f
Selectin family, 40
Selective IgA deficiency, 69
Self antigen, 330
Seminal fluid, rapid PSA test in
Sendai virus, 21
Sensitivity, 115-116
Sensitization, in agglutination, 138-140
Sepsis, 39
  multiple myeloma and, 352-353
Septic shock, 91
Sequestered antigen theory, 368
Serial dilution
  calculation of, 126-127
  example of preparation of, 126t
  exercise for, 127-128
Serologic pipette, 121f, 122
Serologic testing
  importance of, 120
  microtechniques for, 142
Serositis, 397
Serum
  electrophoretic pattern of, 10f
  hepatitis C RNA titers in, 289-290
Serum electrophoresis, 147
Serum FLC immunoassay, benefits of, 355b
Serum marker, 469t
Serum protein electrophoresis procedure
  monoclonal immunoglobulin detection,
    356
  patterns in multiple myeloma, 356-357,
    357f
  principle of, 24
  quality control for, 24
  reagents, supplies and equipment for,
    24-25
  results and reference values for, 26
  specimen collection and procedure, 24
  steps for, 25-26
  storage and stability of, 24
Serum sickness, 340
Sheath, 173
Sheehan's syndrome, 375
Shingles, 193-194
  vaccine for, 199
Short-incubation hepatitis. See Hepatitis A
  virus

Signal amplification technology, 167
Single dilution, 126
Single nucleotide polymorphism (SNP),
  316
Sirolimus, 442
Six-color flow cytometry, 176
Sjögren's syndrome
  diagnosis of, 376t
  overview of, 375-376
Skeletal abnormality, 352
Skeletal muscle disorder, 385
Skin
  allografts of, 433
  autoimmune disorders of, 385b
  disorders of, 385-386
  keratinization of, 2
  transplantation rejection, 437b
Skin-associated lymphoid tissue, 52
Smallpox
  bioterrorism and, 203-204
  as Category A agent, 203
  vaccine for, 203-204
Smith (Sm) antigen, 398
Smoldering multiple myeloma, 350
Sodium hypochlorite solution, 107
Solid-organ transplantation. See Organ
    transplantation
Solid-phase enzyme immunosorbent assay
  for panel-reactive antibody (PRA)
      determination, 430
  principle of, 160f
Somatic cell hybridization, 21
Southern blot, 183
Specific activation, 63
Specific granule deficiency, 42
Specificity, 1-2, 115-116
Specimen
  blood, preparation of, 120-121
  dilution of, 125
  handling of, 121
  procurement and labeling of, 114
  transportation of, 107
  types of, 121
Spirochete bacterium
  Lyme disease, as cause of, 229
  transmission of, 231
Spleen, 52
Sporadic error, 114
Sporothrix schenckii, 192
Sporotrichosis, 192
SQUID technology, 166
Standard deviation (SD), 115, 117
Staphylococcus aureus, 41, 65
  Cowan strain of, 65
Stem cell factor (c-kit ligand), 91
Stem cell system, 463f
Stem cell transplantation
  disease treated with, 449t
  uses for, 448
Steric hindrance, 139-140
Still's disease, 417
Strand displacement amplification (SDA),
  181
Streptococcal disease, Group B, 210-211

Streptococcal infection
  characteristics of, 206
  epidemiology of, 207-208
  etiology of, 206
  extracellular products, 206-207
Streptococcal pharyngitis, 208
Streptococcal toxic shock syndrome (STSS),
  210
Streptococcosis, 208
Streptococcus pyogenes, 206, 207f
  complications of, 208-209
  diagnosis of, 209
  epidemiology of, 207-208
  immunologic manifestations of, 209
  signs and symptoms of, 208-209
Streptokinase, 207
Streptolysin O (SLO), 206
Streptolysin S (SLS), 206-207
Superantigen, 210
Supernatant, 140
Suppressor T lymphocyte, 59
  function, alteration of, 64
Surface immunoglobulin (sIg), 40
  B cells and, 63
Syngeneic transplant, 450
Syngraft, 432t
Syphilis
  congenital, 218, 218f
  diagnosis of, 219, 219t
  epidemiology of, 215
  etiology of, 215
  immunologic manifestations of, 218
  incidence of, 216
  latent, 217
  late/tertiary, 217
  primary, 216, 217f
  secondary, 217, 217f
  serologic tests, sensitivity of, 215, 220t
  signs and symptoms of, 216
  transmission of, 215-216
Systematic errors, elimination of, 114
Systemic lupus erythematosus (SLE)
  humoral aspects of Robert (ro) soluble
      substance-A (SS-A), 398
Systemic inflammatory response syndrome
    (SIRS), 39
Systemic lupus erythematosus (SLE), 340,
  392
  ACR classification of, 393t
  autoantibodies of, 398
  cellular aspects of, 398
  diagnostic evaluation of, 399-404
  drugs producing clinical/serologic
      features of, 393b
  epidemiology of, 394
  etiology of, 394
  facial rash from, 396f
  immunoglobulin deposit, view of, 384f
  immunologic assays for, 401t
  immunologic manifestations of, 397-399
  infections from, 396
  manifestations of, 395
  severity of, 392
  signs and symptoms of, 394-397, 395f

Systemic lupus erythematosus (SLE)—cont'd
  symptoms by case percentage, 395t
  treatment for, 404-405
Systemic sclerosis, 371-372, 383-384

T

T. gondii serologic profile (TSP), 250
Tacrolimus, 442
Target cell, 310
T-cell
  graft rejection, role in, 439-440
  tumor, response against, 61f
T-cell activation, 59
  defects in, 70
  profile of, 61t
T-cell dependent reaction, 5t
T-cell receptor (TCR), 40, 55
  peptide-MHC, recognition of, 61f
T-cell suppression, 436
Technical error, 114b
Temperature, antigen-antibody reaction, 140
Tertiary syphilis, 217
The Joint Commission (TJC), 103-104
  standards for quality control, 113
T-helper cell. *See* Helper T cell
Therapeutic agents, newer for cancer, 474t
Thoracic duct, 52
Three-day measles, 299
Thrombocytopenia, 380
Thrombocytopenia, immunodeficiency with, 70
Thrombosis, 83
Thucydides, 1
Thymidine, 21-22
Thymocyte, 50
Thymosin, 50
Thymus, 49-50, 51f
Thyroglobulin, 373
Thyroid disease, 372
Thyroid gland, 372f
Thyroid membrane receptor, 373
Thyroid microsome, 373
Thyronine, 373
Tick
  deer, 231f
  Lyme disease and, 229
  types and disease caused by, 230t
Tick-borne rickettsiae, 237
Time-resolved fluoroimmunoassay, 167
T-independent antigen, triggering of, 62
Tip, of pipette, 123-124
Tissue, damage to, 4
Titan Gel ImmunofiFix, 151
Titer
  concentration, determination of, 128
  definition of, 128
T lymphocyte
  aging, changes with, 64
  antigen recognition by, 59-62
  cancer and, 467
  cell-mediated immunity and, 5
  deficiency of, 50-52, 65t
  disorders of, 66-68
  electron photomicrograph of, 54f
  enumeration of, 72-73

T lymphocyte—cont'd
  innate immunity and, 49
  overview of, 55-62
  subsets of, 56-59
Tolerance, 368
  B-cell, 436-437
  immunologic, 436-437
  T-cell, 436
TORCH syndrome, 195
TORCH testing, 195-196, 195t
Toxoplasma gondii
  life cycle of, 248f
  toxoplasmosis, as cause of, 247
Toxoplasmic meningoencephalitis, 249f
Toxoplasmosis, 195-196
  acquired versus congenital, 248-249
  antibodies detected, 250-251
  cell culture for, 252
  diagnostic evaluation of, 250-252, 250t
  etiology and epidemiology of, 247
  histologic diagnosis of, 252
  manifestations of, 249-250
  prevention of, 248b
  signs and symptoms of, 248-249
Tracheobronchial aspirate, 314f
Transcobalamin II (TCII), 377
Transcription mediate amplification (TMA), 181
Transforming growth factor, 91
Transfusion reaction, 336-337
Transfusion-transmitted virus (TTV), 292-293
Transient hypogammaglobulinemia, 69
Transitional cell carcinoma, 462
Transplacental hemorrhage (TPH), 338
Transplantation
  cell infusion and, 455
  checklist for, 452f
  complications from, 443-444, 454
  direction of
    current, 455-456
    future, 456
  graft-versus-host disease and, 454
  high-dose chemotherapy and, 451-454
  immunogenicity of tissues, 437b
  problems in, 426-430
  recipient and donor, evaluation of, 428-430
  rejection from, 438f, 437
  scarcity of organs for, 432b
  survival rate, 5-year, 449t
  terminology for, 432, 432t
  types of, 432-434, 450
  from unrelated donor, 455
  waiting time for, 431
  See also Organ transplantation; progenitor cell transplant; stem cell transplantation
T-Regulatory lymphocyte. *See* Regulatory T (Treg) cell
Treponemal method, 219
Treponema pallidum
  diseases from, 216t
  etiology of, 215
  view of, 216f
Triiodothyronine, 373

Trimeric complex, 59
True negative, 115-116
True positive, 115-116
T-suppressor cell. *See* Suppressor T lymphocyte
Tuberculin (TB) Skin Test, 109
Tubulointerstitial nephritis, 385
Tumor
  benign versus malignant, 461
  immunotherapy for, 474
Tumor antigen
  categories of, 469-470
  spontaneous, 470
Tumor-associated antigen (TAA), 469
Tumor cell
  CD8+ T cell responses against, 61f
  cytotoxic T lymphocyte effect on, 60f
  metastasis of, 40
Tumor-infiltrating lymphocyte, 467
Tumor marker
  application of, 469t
  biochemical, 468t
  cancer and, 468-472
  in neoplasm, 469t
  serum/plasma concentration, 468t
Tumor necrosis factor (TNF)
  cancer and, 467
  role of, 90-91
  target cells and biologic activities of, 90t
Tumor necrosis factor-alpha (TNF-α)
  activities of, 91
  inflammation and, 38
Tumor necrosis factor-beta (TNF-β), 91
Tumorogenesis, 465
Tumor-specific antigen (TSA), 468, 469
Turbid serum, 121
Two-dimensional polyacrylamide gel electrophoresis (2D-PAGE), 472
Type III polyglandular syndrome, 375
Type II polyglandular syndrome, 375
Type I polyglandular syndrome, 375
Tyramide signal amplification (TSA), 167

U

Ulcerative colitis (UC), 377
Upper respiratory infection, 208
Urine, for pregnancy testing, 121
Urticaria, 332

V

Vaccination
  concept of, 198
  host response to, 199
  purpose of, 4
Vaccine
  administration of, 204
  AIDS and, 198
  for anthrax, 202
  in biodefense, 198
  for cancer, 203
  characteristics of, 199
  concerns about, 199
  development for HIV/AIDS
    expectations for, 202
    goal of, 201